Exercise for Pregnant Women with Pregestational
    Diabetes, 628
Exercise Tips for Pregnant Women, 141
Fluoride Supplementation, 430
Formula-Feeding, 427
Home Management of Preterm Labor, 716
Learning About Preeclampsia Condition, 566
Outcome Criteria, 516
Postterm Gestation, 719
Resumption of Sexual Intercourse, 483
Sponge Bathing, 384
Suggestions for Decreasing Sibling Rivalry, 482
Tub Bathing, 385

CULTURAL CONSIDERATIONS

Birth Practices in Different Cultures, 267
Cultural and Religious Aspects of Death, 821
Some Cultural Aspects of Women's Health Problems, 861
Some Cultural Beliefs about Breastfeeding, 412
Some Cultural Beliefs about Newborns, 378
Some Cultural Beliefs about Pain, 238

CLINICAL APPLICATION OF RESEARCH

Accuracy of Leopold's Maneuvers in Screening for
    Malpresentation, 693
Cesarean Birth Rate and Nurses' Care during Labor, 705
Effect of Fiber-Enriched Diets on Glucose Level in
    Pregnancy, 634
Effects of Maternal Position on Fundal Height
    Measurement, 149
Expectations and Experiences of Pain in Labor, 241
Factors Associated with Hypoglycemia, 333
Grandmother Social Support, Adolescent Mothering, and
    Infant Attachment, 742
Grieving after Termination of Pregnancy for Fetal
    Anomaly, 832
Health-Promoting and Health-Damaging Behaviors of
    Women, 852
Incontinence following Rupture of the Anal Sphincter
    during Birth, 443
Insufficient Milk Supply Syndrome, 422
Maternal-Fetal Attachment: Influence of
    Mother-Daughter and Husband-Wife Relationships,
    113
Maternity Blues and Postpartum Depression, 480
Measurement of Newborn Head
    Circumference, 366
Midline Episiotomy and the Risk of Third-Degree and
    Fourth-Degree Lacerations, 303
Nausea and Fatigue during Early Pregnancy, 106
Nipple-Feeding for Preterm Infants with
    Bronchopulmonary Dysplasia, 783
Pain Assessment in Premature Infants, 759
Pelvic Inflammatory Disease in HIV-Infected Women,
    863
Physical and Emotional Abuse in Pregnancy, 677
Physical Health and Psychologic Well-Being in Elderly
    Women, 843

Self-Described Lea
Sleeping Prone and
    Syndrome, 381
Social Networks ai
Thermoregulation Immediately after Birth, 376
Tympanic Thermometry for Taking Basal Body
    Temperatures, 43

LEGAL TIP

Abortion, 877
Cardiac and Metabolic Emergencies, 641
Care of Adolescents, 728
Definition of Live Birth, 826
Early Discharge, 483
Female Sterilization, 500
Fetal Monitoring Standards, 261
Infant Identification, 364
Informed Consent, 484
Informed Consent for Anesthetic, 240
Negligence during Neonatal Emergencies—Use of
    Malfunctioning Equipment, 753
Negligence during Neonatal Emergencies—Use of
    Warming Equipment, 763
Patient Abandonment, 468
Performance of Limited Ultrasound
    Examinations, 543
Prenatal Standards of Care, 136
Rubella Vaccination, 473
Standard of Care, 8
Standard of Care—Labor and Birth at Risk, 697
Standard of Care—Meconium Aspiration, 787
Standard of Care for the Preeclamptic Patient at Home,
    565
Standard of Care for Seizures and Bleeding Emergencies,
    591
Standards of Care for Labor, 279
Urine Drug Testing, 671

ETHICAL CONSIDERATIONS

Application of Genetic Technology, 85
Assisted Reproductive Therapies (ARTs), 875
Confidentiality, 596
Drug Screening, 675
Enforced Contraception, 494
Fetal Rights, 537
Forced Cesarean Birth, 702
HIV Screening, 135
Pregnant Women with Medical Complications, 629
Resuscitation of Extremely Premature Infants, 777

MATERNITY
Nursing

MATERNITY
Nursing

IRENE M. BOBAK, RN, PhD, FAAN
Professor Emerita, San Francisco State University
San Francisco, California

DEITRA LEONARD LOWDERMILK, RNC, PhD
Clinical Professor, School of Nursing
University of North Carolina—Chapel Hill
Chapel Hill, North Carolina

MARGARET DUNCAN JENSEN, RN, MS
Professor Emerita, San Jose State University
San Jose, California

ASSOCIATE EDITOR
SHANNON E. PERRY, RN, PhD, FAAN
Professor—School of Nursing, San Francisco State University
San Francisco, California

FOURTH EDITION

with 700 illustrations
with 42 color plates

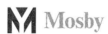 Mosby

St. Louis Baltimore Berlin Boston Carlsbad Chicago London Madrid
Naples New York Philadelphia Sydney Tokyo Toronto

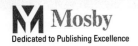

Mosby
Dedicated to Publishing Excellence

Publisher: Nancy L. Coon
Editor: Michael S. Ledbetter
Senior Developmental Editor: Teri Merchant
Associate Developmental Editor: Cecily Barolak
Project Managers: Karen Edwards and Linda McKinley

Production Editor: Aimee E. Noyes
Design Coordinator: Elizabeth Fett
Manufacturing Manager: Kathy Grone
Original art: Jack Reuter
Unit Opening Photographs: Cardine E. Brown

Great care has been used in compiling and checking the information in this book to ensure its accuracy. However, because of changing technology, recent discoveries, and research and individualization of prescriptions according to patient needs, the uses, effects, and dosages of drugs may vary from those given here. Neither the publisher nor the authors shall be responsible for such variations or other inaccuracies. We urge that before you administer any drug you check the manufacturer's dosage recommendations as given in the package insert provided with each product.

FOURTH EDITION

Copyright © 1995 by Mosby–Year Book, Inc.

Previous editions copyrighted 1983, 1987, 1991

Printed in the United States of America
Composition by The Clarinda Company
Printing/binding by Von Hoffmann Press, Inc.

Mosby–Year Book, Inc.
11830 Westline Industrial Drive
St. Louis, Missouri 63146

Library of Congress Cataloging in Publication Data
Maternity nursing/ [edited by] Irene M. Bobak, Deitra Leonard Lowdermilk, Maragaret Duncan Jensen; associate editor, Shannon E. Perry.—4th ed.
    p. cm.
    Rev. ed. of: Essentials of maternity nursing/Irene M. Bobak, Margeret Duncan Jensen. 3rd ed. c1991.
    Includes bibliographical references and index.
    ISBN 0-8016-7883-8
    1. Maternity nursing. 2. Pediatric nursing. I. Bobak, Irene M. Essentials of maternity nursing. II. Lowdermilk, Deitra Leonard. III. Jensen, Margaret Duncan, 1921-
    [DNLM: 1. Maternal-Child Nursing. 2. Ostetrical Nursing. WY
157 M4236 1994]
RG951. B66 1994
610.73'678—dc20
DNLM/DLC
for Library of Congress
                                              94-35006
                                              CIP

95 96 97 98 99 / 9 8 7 6 5 4 3 2 1

Contributors

KATHRYN RHODES ALDEN, RN, MSN
Clinical Assistant Professor
University of North Carolina—Chapel Hill
School of Nursing
Chapel Hill, North Carolina

JEAN A. BACHMAN, RN, DSN
Assistant Professor
University of Missouri—St. Louis
St. Louis, Missouri

IRENE M. BOBAK, RN, MS, PhD, FAAN
Professor Emerita
San Francisco State University
San Francisco, California

LINDA J. BOYNE, MS, RD/LD
Assistant Professor
Division of Medical Dietetics and Department of
   Pediatrics
The Ohio State University
Columbus, Ohio

KITTY CASHION, RNC, MSN
Clinical Nurse Specialist
Department of Obstetrics and Gynecology—
Division of Maternal-Fetal Medicine
University of Tennessee-Memphis College of Medicine
Memphis, Tennessee

CAROL FOWLER DUNHAM, RN, MSN
Clinical Assistant Professor
University of North Carolina—Chapel Hill
School of Nursing
Chapel Hill, North Carolina

CYNTHIA GARRETT, RNC, MSN
Women's Health Clinical Nurse Specialist
University of North Carolina Hospitals
Chapel Hill, North Carolina

PHYLLIS A. JOHNSON, RN, PhD
Associate Professor
Georgia State University School of Nursing
Atlanta, Georgia

CAROL LEE A. JOHNSTON, RN, MEd, MSN
Clinical Assistant Professor
University of North Carolina-Chapel Hill
Chapel Hill, North Carolina

PHYLLIS M. KLEIN, RN, BSN, MSN
Consultant
Maternal-Infant Nursing
Fairfax, Virginia

BARBARA J. LIMANDRI, RN, DNS
School of Nursing
Oregon Health Sciences University
Portland, Oregon

DEITRA LEONARD LOWDERMILK, RNC, PhD
Clinical Associate Professor
School of Nursing
University of North Carolina—Chapel Hill
Chapel Hill, North Carolina

SUSAN MATTSON, RNC, CTN, PhD
Associate Professor
College of Nursing
Arizona State University
Temple, Arizona

LILA PARAM, RNC, BSN
Neonatal Outreach Educator
Perinatal Outreach Services
The Medical Center at the University of California
San Francisco, California

SHANNON E. PERRY, RN, PhD, FAAN
Professor
School of Nursing
San Francisco State University
San Francisco, California

JUDITH H. POOLE, RNC, MN, FACCE
Perinatal Outreach Education Coordinator
Department of Obstetrics/Gynecology
Carolinas Medical Center
Charlotte, North Carolina

EDNA B. QUINN, RN, PhD, CNM
Professor of Nursing
Salisbury State University
Salisbury, Maryland

KATHLEEN RICE SIMPSON, RNC, MSN
Perinatal Clinical Nurse Specialist
St. John's Mercy Medical Center;
Lecturer
University of Missouri—St. Louis
St. Louis, Missouri

SARA RICH WHEELER, RN, MSN, Certified Grief Counselor
Principal
Grief, Ltd;
Associate Professor
Lakeview College of Nursing
Dansville, Illinois

RHEA P. WILLIAMS, RN, PhD
Assoiciate Professor—Nursing
California State University
Los Angeles, California

Clinical Consultants

BERNADINE ADAMS, BSN, MN
Associate Professor
School of Nursing
Northeast Louisiana University
Monroe, Louisiana

JOEA BIERCHEN, MSN, EdD
Professor of Nursing
St. Petersburg Junior College
St. Petersburg, Florida

CONSTANCE BOBIK, RN, BSN, MSN
Assistant Professor—Nursing
Brevard Community College
Cocoa, Florida

KAREN R. BOOTH, RN, MEd, MSN
Professor
Department of Nursing
Owens College
Toledo, Ohio

CHARLOTTE BREITHAUPT, RN, BSN, MN
Lecturer
Baylor University School of Nursing
Dallas, Texas

PENNY S. CASS, RN, PhD
Dean and Professor
College of Nursing
University of Wisconsin—Oshkosh
Oshkosh, Wisconsin

DOROTHY S. CROWDER, RN, BS, MS, CCE
Associate Professor—Maternal/Child Health Nursing
Virginia Commonwealth University
Medical College of Virginia School of Nursing
Richmond, Virginia

ALICE DAY, RN, BS, MS
Assistant Professor
South Georgia College
Douglas, Georgia

BONNIE K. GENSCH, RN
Coordinator, Resolve Through Sharing
Lutheran Hospital—La Crosse
La Crosse, Wisconsin

PHYLLIS M. KLEIN, RN, BSN, MSN
Consultant
Maternal-Infant Nursing
Fiarfax, Virginia

SUSAN K. KRUG-WISPE, MS, RD
Nutritionist
Department of Pediatrics
University of Cincinnati, Ohio
Cincinnati, Ohio

RANA LIMBO, RN, MS, MSN
Outpatient Therapist
Lutheran Hospital Recovery Centers;
Consultant
Grief, Ltd.
La Crosse, Wisconsin

EDWARD LOWDERMILK, BS, RPH
Lowdermilk Consultants
Chapel Hill, North Carolina

CAROL METCALF, RN, MPH
Department of Nursing
Truckee Meadows Community College
Reno, Nevada

LINDA MOORE, RN, MSN
Instructor
California State University, Fresno
Fresno, California

ROCHELLA S. NZE, RNC, MN
Perinatal Clinical Nurse Specialist
Greater Balimore Medical Center
Baltimore, Maryland

MARY L. OVERFIELD, RN, MN, IBCLC
Partner
Lactation Cosultants of North Carolina
Raleigh, North Carolina

ALICE SILLS
Central Piedmont Community College
Charlotte, North Carolina

KATHLEEN RICE SIMPSON, RNC, MSN
Perinatal Clinical Nurse Specialist
St. John's Mercy Medical Center;
Lecturer
School of Nursing
University of Missouri—St. Louis
St. Louis, Missouri

LUISE SPEAKMAN, RN, MA
Chair, Nursing Department
Cape Cod Community College
West Barnstable, Massachusetts

RACHEL SPECTOR, RN, PhD, CTN
Associate Professor
Boston College
Chestnut Hill, Massachusetts

RANDA FERGUSON SPERLING, RN, MSN
Faculty, Practical Nursing Program
Indiana Vocational Technical College
Evansville, Indiana

BETH M. WAGNER, RN, MSN
Staff Development Instructor for Obstetrics and Pediatrics
Pocono Medical Center
East Stroudsburg, Pennsylvania

SARAH E. WHITAKER, RN, MSN, DSNc
Lecturer
University of Texas—El Paso;
Perinatal Staff Nurse
R.E. Thomason Hospital
El Paso, Texas

Preface

Maternity and women's health nursing offers a unique combination of challenge and opportunity. Nurses are challenged to assimilate knowledge and to develop technical and critical thinking skills necessary to apply that knowledge to practice. Each woman presents a new challenge as her individual needs must be identified and met. The opportunities, however, are sufficiently extraordinary to make this one of the most fulfilling specialties of nursing practice.

The goal of nursing education is to prepare today's student to meet tomorrow's challenges. This preparation must extend beyond mastery of facts and skills. Nurses must be able to combine competence with caring. They must address both physiologic and psychosocial needs. Above all, they must look beyond the condition and see the woman as an individual with distinctive needs.

Maternity Nursing was developed to provide students with the knowledge they need to become competent nurses and the sensitivity they need to become caring nurses. This fourth edition has been revised and refined in response to comments and suggestions from both students and educators. It includes the most accurate, current, and clinically relevant information available; it presents that information in a clearly written, visually appealing, and logical format.

APPROACH

Professional nursing practice continues to evolve and adapt to society's changing health priorities. Today's consumers of maternity nursing care vary in age, ethnicity, culture, language, social status, and marital status. They seek care with physicians, nurse midwives, and other health care providers in a variety of health care setting, as well as in the home.

Nursing education must reflect these changes as well as the changing needs of nursing students. Today's nursing students are challenged to learn more than ever before and often in less time than their predecessors. Students are diverse. They may be new high school graduates, college students, or older adults with families. They

may be male or female. They may have college degrees in other fields and are interested in changing careers. They may be students for whom English is a second language and may need extra help or extra time to comprehend the required readings, take tests, and prepare written assignments.

This fourth edition of *Maternity Nursing* was designed to meet the unique needs of both maternity patients and students in all types of nursing programs in the 1990s. This edition presents content that is most relevant to current maternity care in a clear and easily readable manner while retaining the comprehensiveness of previous editions.

Care management has been used as an organizing framework for discussion in the nursing care chapters to ensure a logical and consistent presentation of material. This approach incorporates the nursing process and collaborative care to demonstrate how nursing care is combined with care by other health care providers to give the most comprehensive care to women and infants. Assessment, nursing diagnoses, expected outcomes, collaborative care, and evaluation of care are highlighted throughout the chapters for emphasis. Boxed case histories with assessment data and nursing plans of care reinforce the problem-solving approach to patient care. In chapters that focus on complications of childbearing, medical care is often the priority for patient care. Therefore in these discussions, the specific condition and medical therapy are presented first, followed by the nursing care management.

Health care today emphasizes *wellness*. This focus is an integral part of our philosophy that pregnancy and childbirth are part of the natural developmental process. Therefore we present the entire normal childbearing cycle before discussing potential complications. Likewise, the developmental changes a woman experiences throughout her life are considered to be natural and normal. In women's health care the goal is promotion of wellness for the woman through knowledge of her body and its normal functioning throughout her lifespan while developing an awareness of conditions that require professional intervention. We believe that students need to thoroughly understand and recognize the normal processes before they can identify complications and comprehend their implications for care. A new chapter on women's health promotion and screening has been added to emphasize the wellness focus of this aspect of nursing.

Teaching for self-care has become an essential component of nursing care. A new chapter on home care after childbirth discusses the nurse's role in teaching self-care and in providing follow-up care after today's shorter hospital stays. The chapter on women's health promotion and screening emphasizes teaching for self-care to promote wellness and to encourage preventive care. Special boxed elements highlight teaching approaches and home care throughout the text.

In order to implement *preventive care*, perinatal and women's health nurses must be able to recognize signs and symptoms of emergent problems. Throughout the discussions of assessment and care, we alert the nurse to signs of potential problems and provide references to pertinent content in the complications unit. Boxes throughout the text highlight warning signs and emergency situations.

Today's perinatal and women's health nurses will encounter women from diverse ethnic backgrounds. *Cultural* implications are integrated throughout the text to emphasize the wide range of ethnic diversity and its impact on maternity and women's health care. The revised family chapter focuses on specific customs related to childbearing and women's health. This chapter also stresses the importance of assessing both the nurse's and the patient's cultural beliefs. Boxes throughout the text highlight cultural aspects of care.

To truly meet the specific needs of each woman, the nurse must include family members and significant other in the plan of care. *Family dynamics* are rarely more prominent than in pregnancy and childbirth. The nurse is often the family's primary advocate. Three separate chapters on the family, including grandparents and siblings, in addition to integrated considerations throughout the text, demonstrate the importance of the entire family.

Nursing research has become an integral part of nursing education and practice. Examples of nursing research have been incorporated throughout the text to demonstrate how nursing research has affected the practice of perinatal and women's health nursing. In addition, boxed research highlights throughout the text demonstrate the *clinical* application of selected research studies.

FEATURES

The fourth edition's new design features larger, bolder print and a more spacious presentation. Students will find that the logical, easy-to-follow headings and attractive *two-color design* highlights important content and increases visual appeal. A new *full-color insert* features photographs of childbirth and newborn assessment. Hundreds of photographs and drawings illustrate important concepts and techniques to further enhance comprehension.

Each chapter begins with *learning objectives* to focus students' attention on the important content to be mastered. A list of *key terms* alerts students to new vocabulary; these terms are then boldfaced and defined within the chapter. *Related topics* are identified at the beginning of each chapter, and references are provided to help students locate information that needs to be reviewed or information about topics not yet covered. These references may be especially beneficial for students who need to prepare for clinical assignments regarding patients with complications that have not been discussed in class.

A new organizing framework, *care management*, is used consistently to discuss nursing care and collaborative care. The *nursing process* is incorporated into this framework. The five steps of the nursing process are similar to the five steps in care management. *Case histories* and nursing *plans of care* are included to help students apply the nursing process in the clinical setting. The plans of care include assessment data, use only NANDA-approved nursing diagnosis, include expected outcomes for patient care, provide rationales for interventions, and include evaluation of care. *Care path, procedure,* and *protocol* boxes are included to provide students with examples of various approaches to implement care.

Special boxed elements are highlighted and visually identifiable. *Teaching approaches* supplement the narrative and emphasize the importance of teaching for self-care. *Emergency* boxes alert the students to the signs and symptoms of various emergency situations and provide immediate nursing interventions. *Clinical application of research* boxes include a brief summary of the study and a discussion of the application to practice that stresses the relevance of current research to clinical practice.

Although childbearing is a normal process, complications may occur. During assessment the nurse must always be alert for *signs of potential complications;* therefore, we have included these signs in the assessment sections in the units that cover uncomplicated pregnancy and childbirth. Other new features include *cultural considerations* boxes that describes beliefs and practices about pregnancy, as well as childbearing and newborn care in relation to selected cultures; *legal tip* and *ethical considerations* boxes developed to provide students with relevant information to deal with these important areas in the context of perinatal and women's health nursing; and *home care* boxes that provide information to help students transfer learning from the hospital setting to the home.

At the end of each chapter, *key points* summarize important content. *Critical thinking exercises* guide the students in applying their knowledge and in increasing their ability to think critically. Current relevant references and bibliographies provide a basis for additional study and research in related topics.

ORGANIZATION

The fourth edition of *Maternity Nursing* comprises eight units organized to enhance understanding and learning and to facilitate easy retrieval of information.

Unit I, *Introduction to Maternity Nursing,* begins with an overview of contemporary perinatal and women's health nursing practice. It then addresses the family as a unit of care, incorporating cultural aspects of family-centered maternity care. The unit concludes with a review of the reproductive system.

Unit II, *Pregnancy,* describes nursing care of the woman and her family from conception through preparation for childbirth. A separate chapter on maternal and fetal nutrition emphasizes the important aspects of care, highlights the cultural variations on diet, and stresses the importance of early recognition and management of nutritional problems.

Unit III, *Childbirth,* focuses on collaborative care among physicians, nurse midwives, nurses, women, and their families during the process of labor and birth. Separate chapters deal with the nurse's role in the management of discomfort and fetal assessment. These chapters familiarize the students with current childbirth practices and focus on interventions to support and educate the woman and her family.

Unit IV, *The Newborn,* addresses the immediate assessment and care of the newborn. Information on the nutritional needs of the newborn and nursing care associated with breastfeeding and formula-feeding are highlighted in a separate chapter.

Unit V, *Postpartum Period,* deals with a time of significant change for the entire family. The mother requires both physical and emotional support as she adjusts to her new role. A separate chapter discusses family dynamics in response to the birth of a child. A new chapter on home care discusses the nurse's role in providing follow-up care after today's shorter hospital stays.

Unit VI, *Complications of Childbearing,* discusses the conditions that place the mother, fetus, newborn, and family at risk. Care management focuses on achieving the best possible outcome, as well as supporting the woman and family when expectations are not met. Separate chapters discuss high risk assessment and adolescent sexuality, pregnancy, and parenthood.

Unit VII, *Complications of the Newborn,* has been reorganized to address the trend of caring for the moderately compromised newborn in the normal newborn nursery. The unit presents general care of the newborn at risk, then describes the most common developmental and acquired conditions. A separate chapter on loss and grief discusses care management of the family experiencing a fetal, neonatal, or maternal loss.

Unit VIII, *Women's Health,* is a new unit that discusses health promotion and screening and then presents the common reproductive concerns.

The text concludes with a revised and expanded glossary of important terms, updated appendices that provide valuable resource information, and a detailed, cross-referenced index.

TEACHING AND LEARNING PACKAGE

A number of ancillaries to this textbook have been developed to assist instructors and students in the teaching and learning process. These include an *Instructor's Resource Manual* and *Test Bank, a Student Learning Guide,* a computerized test bank, a set of overhead transparency acetates, and a *Quick Reference for Maternity Nursing.*

The *Instructor's Resource Manual and Test Bank* is keyed chapter by chapter to the text to help coordinate course objectives to chapter content. Each chapter includes an outline of content with course guidelines, suggested learning activities, and student worksheets. These worksheets can be copied and used as a handout to reinforce learning and evaluate comprehension. The worksheets are also reproduced in the *Student Learning Guide,* which can be puchased separately or packaged with the text. The test bank includes more than 500 questions that parallel the new NCLEX format. The answer key provides page references and coding of questions according to the NCLEX test plan categories of nursing process and patient needs, as well as level of difficulty. In addition, a proposed class schedule and reading assignment for 5-to 7-week courses, as well as 12- to 14-week courses has been included to help educators use the text in the most essential way or in a more comprehensive manner.

CompuTest, a *computerized test bank,* is also available and aids instructors using computers in test construction. All questions on the disks are printed in the *Instructor's Resource Manual.*

The *overhead transparency* set of 50 two-color illustrations provides an additional resource for instructors. These illustrations were selected for their instructional value in lectures and classroom discussions.

The newly revised *Quick Reference for Maternity Nursing* is a valuable resource for students in the clinical setting. Thispocket-size reference features assessment guides, nursing interventions for various complications and emergency situations, and guidelines for medications commonly used in the perinatal and gynecologic settings. This handy resource is complimentary with each copy of the text.

Acknowledgments

I wish to thank everyone whose comments and suggestions prompted this collaboratove effort and reviewers who provided valuable criticism of the manuscript.

I offer thanks for shared expertise and photographs to the staffs of Lactation Consultants of North Carolina, University of North Carolina Hospitals, University of North Carolina at Chapel Hill School of Nursing Design Center, and Brett Thomas Photography, Woodstock, Illinois.

I would like to thank the following photographers: Marjorie Pyle, RNC, Lifecircle, Costa Mesa, California; Caroline E. Brown, RNC, MS, Hershey, Pennsylvania; and Kim Molloy, San Jose, California.

This edition contains artwork by George Wassilchenko, Broken Arrow, Oklahoma, whose precise, detailed anatomic drawings have made a substantial contribution to the study of complex theory. Many of the illustrations new to this edition have been drawn by Jack Reuter of St. Louis, Missouri.

Special words of gratitude are extended to Nancy Coon, Michael Ledbetter, Teri Merchant, Cecily Barolak, and Aimee Noyes of Mosby for their encouragement, inspiration, and assistance in preparation and production of this text. I thank Shannon Perry for her major role in this revision and appreciate the stimulation, support, and mutual respect generated by this collaboration. I thank Irene Bobak, without whose support, encouragement, and guidance I would not have undertaken co-authorship for this edition. I acknowledge the assistance and understanding of my husband Ed, without whose support my participation in this revision would not have been possible.

Deitra Leonard Lowdermilk

Contents in Brief

UNIT ONE **Introduction to Maternity Nursing,** 1

1 Contemporary Maternity Nursing, 3
Shannon E. Perry

2 The Family, A Unit of Care, 11
Rhea P. Williams

3 Anatomy and Physiology of Reproduction, 25
Cynthia Garrett

UNIT TWO **Pregnancy,** 56

4 Genetics, Conception, and Fetal Development, 59
Irene M. Bobak

5 Anatomy and Physiology of Pregnancy, 91
Phyllis M. Klein

6 Family Dynamics of Pregnancy, 109
Rhea P. Williams

7 Nursing Care during Pregnancy, 123
Phyllis M. Klein

8 Maternal and Fetal Nutrition, 172
Linda J. Boyne

UNIT THREE **Childbirth,** 202

9 Essential Factors and Processes of Labor, 205
Deitra Leonard Lowdermilk

10 Management of Discomfort, 221
Jean A. Bachman

11 Fetal Assessment, 246
Kathleen Rice Simpson

12 Nursing Care during Labor and Birth, 263
Deitra Leonard Lowdermilk

UNIT FOUR **The Newborn,** 318

13 The Newborn, 321
Shannon E. Perry

14 Nursing Care of the Newborn, 361
Shaonnon E. Perry

15 Newborn Nutrition and Feeding, 407
Shannon E. Perry

UNIT FIVE **Postpartum Period,** 436

16 Maternal Physiology during the Postpartum Period, 439
Kitty Cashion

17 Family Dynamics after Childbirth, 449
Rhea P. Williams

18 Nursing Care during the Postpartum Period, 463
Kitty Cashion
Carol Lee A. Johnston

19 Home Care, 506
Deitra Leonard Lowdermilk

UNIT SIX **Complications of Childbearing,** 530

20 Assessment for Risk Factors, 533
Susan Mattson

21 Hypertension, Hemorrhage, and Maternal Infections, 554
Judith H. Poole

22 Endocrine, Cardiovascular, and Medical-Surgical Problems during Pregnancy, 617
Kathryn Rhodes Alden
Carol Fowler Durham

23 Psychosocial Problems, 664
Barbara J. Limandri

24 Labor and Birth at Risk, 686
Deitra Leonard Lowdermilk

25 Adolescent Sexuality, Pregnancy, and Parenthood, 722
Phyllis A. Johnson

UNIT SEVEN **Complications of the Newborn,** 748

26 The Newborn at Risk, 751
Lila Param

27 Specific Problems of the Newborn at Risk, 767
Lila Param

28 Loss and Grief, 816
Sara Rich Wheeler

UNIT EIGHT **Women's Health,** 836

29 Health Promotion and Screening, 839
Edna B. Quinn

30 Common Reproductive Concerns, 857
Edna B. Quinn
Deitra Leanard Lowdermilk

Glossary, 896

Appendices

A Standards for the Nursing Care of Women and Newborns, 923
B NANDA-Approved Nursing Diagnoses, 929

C   Nursing Responsibilities in Implementing Intrapartum Fetal Heart Rate Monitoring, 931

D   Standard Laboratory Values, Pregnant, and Nonpregnant Women, 934

E   Human Fetotoxic Chemical Agents, 936

F   Standard Laboratory Values in the Neonatal Period, 939

G   Relationship of Drugs to Breast Milk and Effect on Infant, 941

H   Resources, 949

Contents

UNIT ONE

Introduction to Maternity Nursing, 1

1 Contemporary Maternity Nursing, 3

Trends in Fertility and Birthrate, 3
Number of Low-Birth-Weight Infants, 4
Infant Mortality in the United States, 5
Maternal Mortality Trends, 6
High-Risk Pregnancies Escalate, 6
Trend to High-Technology Care, 6
High Cost Trends and Issues, 7
Access Problems Continue, 7
Trends of Patient Involvement, Self-Care, and
    Focus on Health Care, 7
Changing Childbirth Practices, 7
Home Health Care Flourishes, 8
Legal Issues in the Delivery of Care, 8
Ethical Issues, 8
Research, 8
Future Trends, 8

2 The Family, A Unit of Care, 11

Defining the Family, 11
    Nuclear Family, 12
    Extended Family, 12
    Single-Parent Family, 12
    Blended Family, 13
    Homosexual Family, 13
    Family Unit, 13
Family Functions, 13
Family Dynamics, 15
Family Development, 15
    Implications for Maternity Nursing, 16
Key Factors in Family Health, 16
Cultural Factors, 16
    Cultural Context of the Family, 16

Childbearing Beliefs and Practices, 17
Family and Crisis, 18
    Maturational Crisis, 18
    Situational Crisis, 20
    Response to Crisis, 20

3 Anatomy and Physiology of Reproduction, 25

Female Reproductive System, 26
    External Structures, 26
    Internal Structures, 28
    Breasts, 38
    Menstrual Cycle, 39
Male Reproductive System, 44
    External Structures, 44
    Internal Structures, 47
Sexual Response, 48
    Physiologic Response to Sexual Stimulation, 48
    Nursing Implications, 50
Immunology, 50
    Body Defenses, 50
    Types of Immunity, 50
    Factors Associated with Immunologic
      Disease, 52
    Nursing Implications, 53

UNIT TWO

Pregnancy, 56

4 Genetics, Conception, and Fetal Development, 59

Genetics, 60
    Genes and Chromosomes, 60
    Cell Division, 60
    Gametogenesis, 61
    Chromosomal Abnormalities, 62
    Patterns of Genetic Transmission, 63

Conception, 65
Ovum, 66
Sperm, 66
Fertilization, 66
Implantation, 68
The Embryo and Fetus, 68
Embryonic Development, 75
Fetal Maturation, 79
Multifetal Pregnancy, 83
Genetic Counseling, 84
Nongenetic Factors Influencing
Development, 85
Preconception Care, 86

**5 Anatomy and Physiology
of Pregnancy,** 91

Gravidity and Parity, 92
Pregnancy Tests, 92
Adaptations to Pregnancy, 93
Signs of Pregnancy, 93
Reproductive System and Breasts, 94
Hypothalamus-Pituitary-Ovarian Axis, 94
Uterus, 94
Vagina and Vulva, 97
Breasts, 98
General Body Systems, 99
Cardiovascular System, 100
Respiratory System, 100
Renal System, 102
Integumentary System, 103
Musculoskeletal System, 104
Neurologic System, 104
Gastrointestinal System, 105
Endocrine System, 106

6 Family Dynamics of Pregnancy, 109

Maternal Adaptation, 110
Acceptance of Pregnancy, 110
Identification with Motherhood Role, 112
Mother-Daughter Relationship, 112
Partner Relationship, 112
Mother-Child Relationship, 113
Preparation for Childbirth, 114
Paternal Adaptation, 115
Acceptance of Pregnancy, 116
Identifcation with Fatherhood Role, 117
Partner Relationship, 117
Father-Child Relationship, 117
Anticipation of Labor, 118
Grandparent Adaptation, 118
Sibling Adaptation, 118

Parenthood After Age 35, 119
Multiparous Women, 119
Nulliparous Women, 120

7 Nursing Care during Pregnancy, 123

First Trimester, 124
Diagnosis of Pregnancy, 124
Estimated Date of Birth, 124
Second Trimester, 146
Third Trimester, 158

8 Maternal and Fetal Nutrition, 172

Weight Gain, 173
Weight Gain and Fetal Growth, 176
Pattern of Weight Gain, 176
Increased Nutrient Needs of Pregnancy, 178
Energy, 181
Protein, 182
Fluid, 182
Vitamins and Minerals, 182

UNIT THREE

Childbirth, 202

**9 Essential Factors and Processes
of Labor,** 205

Essential Factors in Labor, 206
Passenger, 206
Passageway, 209
Powers, 211
Position of the Mother, 215
Process of Labor, 215
Reproductive System Changes, 215
Stages of Labor, 216
Mechanism of Labor, 216
Adaptation to Labor, 218
Fetal Adaptation, 218
Maternal Adaptation, 218

10 Management of Discomfort, 221

Discomfort during Labor, 222
Neurologic Origins, 222
Expression of Pain, 222
Perception of Pain, 223
Nonpharmacologic Management
of Discomfort, 223
Childbirth Preparation Methods, 223
Relaxation and Breathing Techniques, 225
Pharmacologic Management of Discomfort, 228
Sedatives, 228
Analgesics and Anesthesia, 228

11 Fetal Assessment, 246

History, 246
Fetal Response to the Intrapartum Period, 247
  Baseline Fetal Heart Rate, 247
  Periodic Changes in FHR, 249
Monitoring Techniques, 254
  Periodic Auscultation: FHR, 254
  Electronic Fetal Monitoring (EFM), 255
Other Methods to Evaluate Fetal Well-Being, 257
  Fetal Blood Sampling, 257
  Fetal Stimulation, 257
EFM Pattern "Recognition, 259
  Reassuring and Nonreassuring FHR
    Patterns, 259
  Reassuring FHR Patterns, 259
  Nonreassuring FHR Patterns, 259
    Guidelines and Standards of Nursing Care
    Related to EFM, 261
  Nursing Liability, 261

12 Nursing Care during Labor
and Birth, 263

First Stage of Labor, 264
Second Stage of Labor, 291
Third Stage of Labor, 299
  Signs of Potential Problems, 301
  Nursing Considerations, 301
Interruption in Skin Integrity Related to
    Childhood, 302
  Episiotomy, 302
  Lacerations, 304
Fourth Stage of Labor, 304

UNIT FOUR

The Newborn, 318

13 The Newborn, 321

Biologic Characteristics, 321
  Cardiovascular System, 321
  Hematopoietic System, 323
  Respiratory System, 323
  Renal System, 324
  Gastrointestinal System, 325
  Hepatic System, 326
  Immune System, 328
  Integumentary System, 328
  Reproductive System, 330
  Skeletal System, 331
  Neuromuscular System, 331

Thermogenic System, 333
Behavioral Characteristics, 334
  Sleep-Wake Cycles, 335
  Other Factors Influencing Neonatal
    Behavior, 335
  Sensory Behaviors, 336
  Response to Environmental Stimuli, 338
Physical Assessment, 339

14 Nursing Care of the Newborn, 361

Therapeutic Interventions, 393
Anticipatory Guidance in Infant Care, 400

15 Newborn Nutrition and Feeding, 407

Infant Development and Nutritional Needs, 407
  Readiness for Feeding, 408
  Nutrient Needs, 408
Lactation, 410
  Breast Development, 410
  Lactation Process, 410
  Maternal Breastfeeding Reflexes, 412
  Cultural Aspects of Lactation, 412

UNIT FIVE

Postpartum Period, 436

16 Maternal Physiology during the
Postpartum Period, 439

Reproductive System and Associated
    Structures, 440
  Uterus, 440
  Cervix, 442
  Vagina and Perineum, 442
  Pelvic Muscular Support, 442
Endocrine System, 442
  Placental Hormones, 442
  Pituitary Hormones and Ovarian Function, 443
Abdomen, 443
Urinary System, 443
Gastrointestinal System, 444
  Mitility, 444
  Appetite, 444
  Bowel Evacuation, 444
Breasts, 444
  Nonbreastfeeding Mothers, 444
  Breastfeeding Mothers, 445
Cardiovascular System, 445
  Blood Volume, 445
  Cardiac Output, 445
  Vital Signs, 445

Blood Components, 445
Varicosities, 445
Neurologic System, 446
Musculoskeletal System, 446
Integumentary System, 447
Immune System, 447

17 Family Dynamics after Childbirth, 449

Parenting Process, 450
Cognitive-Motor Skills, 450
Cognitive-Affective Skills, 450
Parental Acquaintance, Bonding,
and Attachment, 450
Communication Between Parent
and Child, 451
Early Contact, 453
Extended Contact, 453
Parental Role after Childbirth, 453
Parental Tasks and Responsibilities, 454
Maternal Adjustment, 455
Paternal Adjustment, 456
Infant-Parent Adjustment, 457
Factors Influencing Parental Responses, 458
Sibling Adaptation, 459
Grandparent Adaptation, 460

**18 Nursing Care during the Postpartum
Period, 463**

Discharge from Hospital, 482
Sexual Activity, 483
Prescribed Medications, 483
Routine Mother and Baby Checkups, 483

19 Home Care, 506

The Health Care Environment that Supports
Early Discharge, 506
Potential Advantages of Short-Stay Maternity
Care, 507
Potential Disadvantages of Short-Stay Maternity
Care, 507
The Future of Early Postpartum Discharge, 508
Nursing Care and Early Postpartum Discharge:
Bridging Hospital and Home, 508
Care Path, 509
Postpartum Follow-Up Services, 509
Early Discharge Preparatory Instruction, 512
Instructions for the First Hours or Days at
Home, 513
The Trip Home, 514
Dealing with Activities of Daily Life, 514
Dealing with Visitors, 515
Postpartum Care, 515
Home Visits, 515

Telephone Follow-Up, 521
Warm Lines/Help Lines, 524
Support Groups, 527

UNIT SIX

Complications of Childbearing, 530

20 Assessment for Risk Factors, 533

Scope of the Problem, 533
Maternal Health Problems, 534
Fetal and Neonatal Health Problems, 534
High-Risk Factors, 535
Diagnostic Techniques, 537
Biophysical Assessment, 537
Biochemical Assessment, 544
Electronic Monitoring, 548

**21 Hypertension, Hemorrhage, and
Maternal Infections, 554**

Hypertension in Pregnancy, 555
Significance and Incidence, 555
Morbidity and Mortality, 555
Classification, 555
Etiology of Preeclampsia, 556
Pathophysiology of Preeclampsia, 556
Maternal Hemorrhagic Disorders, 572
Early Pregnancy Bleeding, 572
Late Pregnancy Bleeding, 581
Cord Insertion and Placental Variations, 585
Postpartum Hemorrhage, 586
Hemorrhagic Shock, 588
Care Management—Hemorrhagic Shock, 588
Clotting Disorders in Pregnancy, 591
Maternal Infections, 593
Sexually Transmitted Disease, 593
TORCH Infections, 597
Human Papillomavirus, 601
Genital Tract Infections, 602
Postpartum Infections, 603
General Infections, 605
Infection Control, 608

**22 Endocrine, Cardiovascular, and
Medical-Surgical Problems during
Pregnancy, 617**

Diabetes Mellitus, 618
Pathogenesis, 618
Classification, 620

Metabolic Changes during and after Pregnancy, 620
Pregestational Diabetes, 621
Preconceptional Counseling, 621
Maternal Risks and Complications, 621
Fetal/Neonatal Risks and Complications, 623
Gestational Diabetes Mellitus (GDM), 630
Hyperemesis Gravidarum, 636
Thyroid Disorders, 638
Hyperthyroidism, 638
Hypothyroidism, 639
Specific Cardiovascular Conditions, 647
Peripartum Heart Failure, 647
Rheumatic Heart Disease, 647
Infective Endocarditis, 648
Mitral Valve Prolapse, 648
Marfan's Syndrome, 648
Cerebrovascular Accidents, 649
Anemia, 649
Iron Deficiency Anemia, 649
Folic Acid Deficiency Anemia, 649
Sickle Cell Hemoglobinopathy, 650
Thalassemia, 650
Pulmonary Disorders, 650
Bronchial Asthma, 650
Adult Respiratory Distress Syndrome, 652
Cystic Fibrosis, 653
Gastrointestinal Disorders, 653
Cholelithiasis and Cholecystitis, 653
Inflammatory Bowel Disease, 653
Integumentary Disorders, 653
Neurologic Disorders, 654
Epilepsy, 654
Multiple Sclerosis, 654
Bell's Palsy, 654
Autoimmune Disorders, 654
Rheumatoid Arthritis, 655
Systemic Lupus Erythematosus, 655
Myasthenia Gravis, 655
Abdominal Surgery during Pregnancy, 656
Appendicitis, 656
Gynecologic Problems, 657
Truama during Pregnancy, 658

23 Psychosocial Problems, 664
Emotional Complications, 664
Mood Disorders, 665
Schizophrenia, 666
Psychoactive Substance Use, 668
Alcohol, 669
Cocaine, 669

Heroin, 672
Methamphetamine, 672
Phencyclidine (PCP), 672
Smoking, 673
Violence Against Women, 677
Dynamics of Abuse, 677
Care Management, 679
Poverty, 679
Factors Related to Poverty, 680
Migrant Families, 681
Preventive Health Care, 681
Reproductive Experience, 682

24 Labor and Birth at Risk, 686
Dystocia, 687
Dysfunctional Labor, 687
Alterations in Pelvic Structure, 687
Fetal Causes, 689
Position of the Mother, 692
Psychologic Response, 693
Abnormal Labor Patterns, 693
Preterm Labor and Birth, 711
Etiologic Factors, 711
Postterm Labor and Birth, 718
Nursing Considerations, 719

25 Adolescent Sexuality, Pregnancy, and Parenthood, 722
Adolescent Development, Sexuality, and Pregnancy, 722
Adolescence and Development, 723
Adolescent Sexuality, 724
Sexual Behavior, 725
Contraception, 725
Abortion, 726
Sex Education, 726
Sexually Transmitted Diseases and Human Immunodeficiency Virus, 727
Adolescent Pregnancy, 727
Developmental Tasks of Pregnancy, 727
Cultural Influences, 728
Family Reactions to Adolescent Pregnancy, 728
Adolescent Fathers, 728
Adolescent Parenthood, 729
Developmental Tasks of Parenthood, 729
The Extended Family, 729
Risks and Consequences of Pregnancy, 729
Physiologic Maternal Risk, 729
Physiologic Neonatal Risk, 730
Socioeconomic Risks, 730
The Pregnant Early Adolescent, 730

UNIT SEVEN

Complications of the Newborn, 748

26 The Newborn at Risk, 751

Transition to Extrauterine Life, 752
   Normal Transition, 752
   Dysfunctional Transition, 752

27 Specific Problems of the Newborn at Risk
767

Transient Tachypnea of the Newborn, 768
Sepsis Neonatorum, 768
Other Infections in the Newborn Population, 769
   Torch Infections, 769
   Chlamydia Infection, 773
   Human Immunodeficiency Virus-Acquired
      Immunodeficiency Syndrome, 774
   Candidiasis, 774
   Gonorrhea, 775
Gestational Age and Birthweight, 775
   Infant Mortality and Morbidity, 777
   The Premature of Preterm Infant, 777
Postterm and Postmature Infants, 785
Small-For-Gestational-Age Intrauterine Growth
     Retarded, Dysmature Infants, 787
Infants of Diabetic Mothers, 788
Hyperbilirubinemia, 793
   Rh Incompatibility, 793
   ABO Incompatibility, 793
   Kernicterus, 793
Congenital Anomalies, 793
   Prenatal Diagnosis, 794
   Perinatal Diagnosis, 794
   Postnatal Diagnosis, 794
   Genetic Diagnosis, 797
   Common Surgical Emergencies, 799
   Common Malformations, 801
   Parental Support, 805
Infant of the Substance Abusing Mother, 806
Discharge to Home for the Compromised
     Newborn, 813

28 Loss and Grief, 816

Grief Responses, 817
Tasks of Mourners, 818
Caring, 819
Other Losses, 832
   Perinatal Diagnosis with a Negative
     Outcome, 832

Adolescent Grief, 833
   Maternal Death, 833
   Complicated Bereavement, 833

UNIT EIGHT

Women's Health, 836

29 Health Promotion and Screening, 839

Well-Woman Health Care, 839
   Reasons for Entering the Health Care
     System, 840
   The Interview and History, 840
   Cultural Considerations, 843
   The Older Woman, 843
   The Woman with a Disbility, 844
   Abused Women, 844
   Schedule for Screening, 844
   Physical Examination, 844
   Laboratory and Diagnostic Procedures, 845
Anticipatory Guidance for Prevention and Health
     Promotion, 849
   Nutrition, 849
   Exercise, 851
   Stress Management, 851
   Substance Use, 853
   Sexuality Issues, 854

30 Common Reproductive Concerns, 857

Common Menstrual Disorders, 858
   Hypogonadotropic Amenorrhea, 858
   Dysmenorrhea, 858
   Premenstrual Syndrome, 859
   Endometriois, 859
Infections, 861
   Pelvic Inflammatory Disease, 861
Impaired Fertility, 864
   Special Considerations, 864
   Factors Associated with Infertility, 865
   Investigation of Female Infertility, 865
   Investigation of Male Infertility, 871
Reproductive Alternatives, 875
   Assisted Reproductive Therapies, 875
   Therapeutic Insemination, 875
   Tubal Reconstruction, 875
Therapeutic and Elective Abortion, 876
Normal Climacterium and Postclimacterium, 880
   Symptoms of Climacterium, 880
   Symptoms of Postclimacteric Period, 881

Sequelae of Childbirth Trauma, 884
    Alterations in Pelvic Support, 884
    Urinary Incontinence, 888
    Injuries to Pelvic Joints, 888
    Uterine Displacement, 888
    Genitial Fistulas, 890
Breast Cancer, 891

Glossary, 896

Appendices

A   Standards for the Nursing Care of Women and Newborns, 923

B   NANDA-Approved Nursing Diagnoses, 929

C   Nursing Responsibilities in Implementing Intrapartum Fetal Heart Rate Monitoring, 931

D   Standard Laboratory Values, Pregnant, and Nonpregnant Women, 934

E   Human Fetatoxic Chemical Agents, 936

F   Standard Laboratory Values in the Neonatal Period, 939

G   Relationship of Drugs to Breast Milk and Effect on Infant, 941

H   Resources, 949

Index, 955

UNIT One

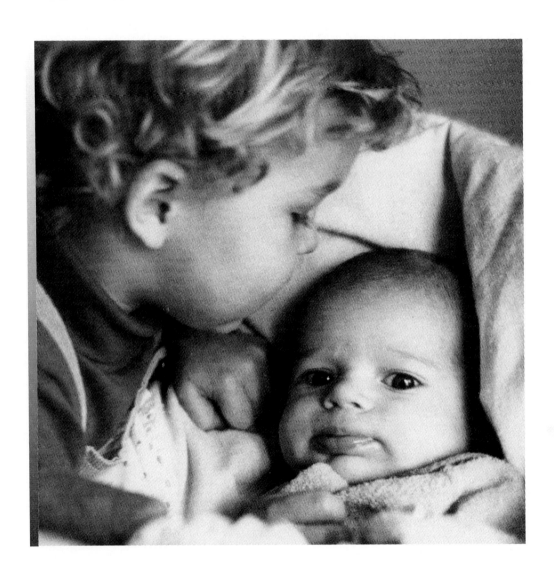

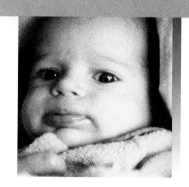

Introduction to Maternity Nursing

1 Contemporary Maternity Nursing

2 The Family, A Unit of Care

3 Anatomy and Physiology of Reproduction

1 Contemporary Maternity Nursing

SHANNON E. PERRY

LEARNING OBJECTIVES

Define the key terms listed.
Compare selected biostatistical data among races.
State contemporary issues in maternity nursing.
Describe social concerns in maternity care.

KEY TERMS

access to prenatal care
birthrate
family-centered care
fertility rate
infant mortality rate
low-birth-weight (LBW)
managed care
maternal mortality rate
self-care
standards of care

RELATED TOPICS

Childbirth education *(Chap. 7)* · Discharge teaching *(Chap. 18)* · Family-centered care *(Chap. 6)* · High-risk pregnancy *(Chap. 20)* · Prematurity *(Chap. 26)* · Prenatal care *(Chap. 7)*

Maternity nursing focuses on the care of child-bearing women and their families through all stages of pregnancy and childbirth, as well as the first 4 weeks after birth. Throughout the prenatal period, nurses, nurse-practitioners, and nurse-midwives provide care for women in clinics and doctors' offices, and teach classes to help families prepare for childbirth. They also care for the childbearing family during labor and birth in hospitals, in birthing centers, and, less frequently, in the home. Nurses with special training may provide intensive care for high-risk neonates in special care units and for high-risk mothers in antepartal units or at home. A large proportion of maternity nurses spend time teaching about pregnancy, the process of labor, birth and recovery, and parenting skills. Investment in health promotion during childbearing has the potential to make a significant difference not only in the health of individual women and their infants, but in society, as well.

The strength of a society rests on the health of its mothers and infants. In the United States serious problems related to the health and health care of mothers and infants exist (Box 1-1). Access to prepregnancy and pregnancy-related care for all women and the lack of reproductive health services for adolescents are both major concerns (Davidson, Gibbs, Chapin, 1991). This chapter discusses trends related to the health and health care of childbearing women.

TRENDS IN FERTILITY AND BIRTHRATE

Fertility trends and birthrates reflect women's needs for health care. The most recent statistics available are from 1991 (see Box 1-2 for an explanation of biostatistical terminology). The **fertility rate,** the number of births to women of childbearing age (15 to 44), was 68.3 live births per 1000 women in 1993. **Birthrate,** the number of live births per 1000 population in one year, is deter-

BOX 1-1

Facts about Maternal-Child Health Care in the United States

In 1991, the U.S. ranked twenty-second worldwide in infant mortality.

In 1988, the U.S. ranked twenty-second worldwide in under-five mortality rate (the annual number of deaths of children less than five years of age per 1,000 live births).

In 1991, the U.S. infant mortality rate for blacks (17.6) was more than twice that for whites (7.3)—a ratio that has remained unchanged for at least four decades.

In 1986, the U.S. infant mortality rate for blacks placed twenty-eighth worldwide; that for whites ranked eighteenth.

Between 1983 and 1985, nonwhite maternal mortality rose 10 percent nationally. Nonwhite women suffer a maternal death rate nearly four times that of white women.

42.7 percent of black children are poor; 37.1 percent of Hispanic children are poor; 19.8 percent of all children are poor.

Poor children are twice as likely as nonpoor children to be born at low birthweight. Low-birthweight infants are 20 times more likely to die during the first year of life than normal-birthweight infants.

In 1988, the U.S. ranked twenty-ninth worldwide in low-birthweight births.

The immunization status of the youngest American children is eroding: In 1985, a smaller percentage of two-year-olds was fully immunized against seven major childhood diseases than in 1980.

The number of cases of measles, rubella, and whooping cough in children has risen dramatically since 1983.

At least one-third of the homeless population are families with children.

The U.S. is the only industrialized nation except South Africa that does not ensure basic, minimal maternity and pediatric services for all women and children.

Based on data from Inglis AD: U.S. maternal and child health services, Part I: right or privilege? *Neonat Netw* 9(8):35; 1991, Wegman ME: Annual summary of vital statistics, 1992, *Pediatrics* 92:743, 1993. Used with permission.

TABLE 1-1 Birthrate According to Age—1989

AGE	RATE (/1000 WOMEN)
15 to 17	36.5
18 to 19	86.4
20 to 24	115.4
25 to 29	116.6
30 to 34	76.2
35 to 39	29.7
40 to 44	5.2

BOX 1-2

Maternal-Infant Biostatistical Terminology

Abortus—An embryo/fetus that is removed or expelled from the uterus at 20 weeks' gestation or less, or weighing 500 g or less, or measuring 25 cm or less.

Birthrate—Number of live births in one year per 1000 population.

Fertility rate—Number of births per 1000 women between the ages of 15 and 44 (inclusive), calculated on a yearly basis.

Infant mortality rate—Number of deaths of infants under one year of age per 1000 live births.

Maternal mortality rate—Number of maternal deaths from births and complications of pregnancy, childbirth, and puerperium (the first 42 days after termination of the pregnancy) per 100,000 live births.

Neonatal mortality rate—Number of deaths of infants under 28 days of age per 1000 live births.

Perinatal mortality rate—Number of stillbirths and the number of neonatal deaths per 1000 live births.

Stillbirth—An infant who, at birth, demonstrates *no* signs of life such as breathing, heartbeat, or voluntary muscle movements.

mined by age of the woman at the time of birth (Table 1-1). The overall birthrate in 1993 was 15.7 live births per 1000 population (National Center for Health Statistics, 1994). The greatest increases occurred in teenage and older mothers. In 1989 the birthrate for teens ages 15 to 17 was the highest in 15 years; 13% of all births were to teens (National Center for Health Statistics, 1991). This increase in the birthrate for teens directly relates to the increasing number of sexually experienced teenagers; currently, 51% of 17-year-old girls are sexually experienced). The high birthrates for the 20 to 24 and 25 to 29 year-old groups reflect the peak childbearing years. The number of women ages 30 to 34 who were giving birth increased, and the birthrate for this group was the highest since 1967. Women ages 35 to 44 who postponed marriage and childbearing had higher birthrates too. For women ages 40 to 44, the birthrate increased 8% over the previous year.

Birthrates vary according to age and racial groups. For example, a large proportion of Hispanic births are to teenage mothers. In Table 1-2, note that those groups with low rates of teen births tend to have high rates of births to women over 30 years old.

NUMBER OF LOW-BIRTH-WEIGHT INFANTS

Babies born weighing less than 2500 grams (5 lbs, 8 oz) are classified as **low-birth-weight (LBW)** and their risks

CLINICAL APPLICATION OF RESEARCH

SOCIAL NETWORKS AND HELP-SEEKING OF PREGNANT TEENS

Pregnant teens are at risk for delaying entry into prenatal care and for having low-birth-weight babies. Social support is related to positive health practices in adults, but little is known about the social networks of teens.

For this study the researcher interviewed 31 single, low-income, pregnant teens using questions that assessed social support and a structured interview to bring out help-seeking behaviors. The researcher found that the length of pregnancy and social network size have a negative correlation to emotional, tangible, and prenatal support. The researcher found that families and friends provided greater support for younger teens than for older teens. Teen mothers most often relied upon their own mothers their babies' fathers for support. Emotional and financial assistance was the type of help most often needed by teenage mothers. In conclusion, the researcher's findings indicated a gap

between the needs of teenage mothers and their available resources, and that the differences in teens' sources of support have implications for nursing care. These findings support the conclusions of other researchers about the high-risk status of teens. Without assistance, teens may not receive prenatal care, which places them at greater risk.

In their encounters with pregnant teens, nurses can inquire about social support and involve the teen's mother and the baby's father in the prenatal care. Referrals to sources of financial support are also appropriate. Nurses can provide the best form of support for a young woman in her teens by assuming a major role in education about family planning.

Reference: May KM: Social networks and help-seeking experiences of pregnant teens, *JOGNN* 21(6):497, 1992.

TABLE 1-2   Birthrate According to Age and Race

BIRTHS/1000 POPULATION

RACE	Teens	AGE 30+ Years
Chinese	1	57
Japanese	3	59
Filipino and other Asian	6	38 to 46
White	11	31
Hawaiian	17	20 to 21
Native American	20	20 to 21
African-American	23	20 to 21

Note that the rates are in inverse order; the races that have low teen birthrates have high 30+ birthrates.

for morbidity and mortality increase. By reducing the number of LBW infants, the health of infants improves. In 1991, 7.1% of infants born were LBW, the highest level since 1978 (National Center for Health Statistics, 1994). The greatest risk for LBW outcome occurs among women giving birth in their teens. The proportions of LBW infants differ according to race, for example, 5.8% of white infants were LBW in 1993 compared to 13.2% of African-American infants. The steady increase in the number of preterm births, those births occurring before 38 weeks of gestation, accounts for the increase in LBW births. In 1989, 10.6% of births were preterm, with 8.8% of those preterm births occurring in whites and 18.9% in African-Americans.

Although lifesaving techniques after birth have been perfected and give LBW infants a better chance of survival, the number of LBW and preterm infants has not decreased. For decreases to occur, the risk factors asso

ciated with LBW and preterm birth must be reduced too (National Commission to Prevent Infant Mortality, 1990).

INFANT MORTALITY IN THE UNITED STATES

The **infant mortality rate** indicates the adequacy of prenatal care and the health of a nation. The United States attained its lowest rate of infant mortality ever with 8.5 deaths per 1000 live births in 1991. This rate remains higher than rates for 21 of the other industrialized countries (Wegman, 1993). Infant mortality continues to be higher for African-American babies than for white babies (17.6 vs. 7.3) (Fig. 1-1), an ever-widening gap since the mid-1970s (National Center for Health Statistics, 1994).

Some researchers attribute this high infant mortality rate to limited maternal education, young maternal age, unmarried status, poverty, and lack of prenatal care (Brecht, 1989). In a study of disadvantaged African-Americans in Washington, D.C., the city with the highest infant mortality rate in the country, researchers found that factors other than socioeconomic status and demographic characteristics contribute significantly to their higher infant mortality rate (Boone, 1982). These factors include lack of prenatal care, poor nutrition, smoking and alcohol use, and maternal conditions such as poor health or hypertension. Thus access to health care programs emphasizing nutrition education and support, health and parenting education, smoking cessation, drug and alcohol abuse treatment, pediatric care, immunizations, and accident prevention education may help reduce the gap between African-Americans and whites in

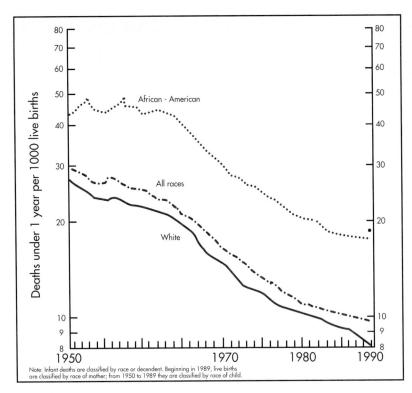

FIG. 1-1 Infant mortality rates by race: United States, 1950-1989.

infant mortality rate (Boone, 1982; National Commission to Prevent Infant Mortality, 1990). To effect changes in mortality rates, the focus must shift from high-technology medical interventions to improving access to preventive care.

MATERNAL MORTALITY TRENDS

In 1991 310 U.S. women died from complications of pregnancy, childbirth, and puerperium, for a **maternal mortality rate** of 7.6 deaths per 100,000 live births (National Center for Health Statistics, 1994). The record low was 6.6 in 1987. The mortality rate for African-American women in 1989 was 18.4, and 5.6 for white women. Thus African-American women were more than three times as likely to die from complications of pregnancy, childbearing, and puerperium than white women.

HIGH-RISK PREGNANCIES ESCALATE

High-risk pregnancies have increased, which means that a greater number of pregnant women are at risk for poor pregnancy outcomes. Escalating drug use (between 11% and 27% of pregnant women, depending on the geographic location) has contributed to higher incidences of prematurity, LBW, congenital defects, learning disabili-

ties, and withdrawal symptoms in infants (National Commission to Prevent Infant Mortality, 1990). Alcohol use during pregnancy has been associated with miscarriages (spontaneous abortions), mental retardation, LBW, and fetal alcohol syndrome. Syphilis, which contributes to congenital defects and infant deaths, increased 40% between 1980 and 1987. In addition, other sexually transmitted diseases during pregnancy (which can be associated with defects and diseases in the newborn) also increased, as did the incidence of acquired immunodeficiency syndrome (AIDS) in childbearing women and children. The rate of unmarried mothers giving birth increased 64% since 1980, and babies born to unmarried mothers are twice as likely to die as those born to married mothers. Teens also are twice as likely to have an LBW infant. This need not be the case. Adequate prenatal care focusing on health and reduction of risk factors can improve pregnancy outcomes (National Commission to Prevent Infant Mortality, 1990).

TREND TO HIGH-TECHNOLOGY CARE

Advances in scientific knowledge and the large number of high-risk pregnancies have contributed to a health care system that emphasizes high-technology care. In general, high-technology care has flourished while "health" care has become relatively neglected. These technologic advances have also contributed to higher health care costs (Queenan, 1991).

HIGH COST TRENDS AND ISSUES

The cost of health care is one of the fastest growing sectors of the U.S. economy. National health expenditures are 14.3% of the gross domestic product, or one seventh of the U.S. economy (Statistical Bulletin, 1994). A shift in demographics, an increased emphasis on high-cost technology, and liability costs of a litigious society created the cost crisis (Queenan, 1991). Most researchers agree that the costs of caring for the increased number of LBW infants in intensive care units have also contributed significantly to the overall health care costs, especially since 19% of all uninsured women gave birth to an LBW infant (National Commission to Prevent Infant Mortality, 1990).

Managed care, a method of guiding care for a patient during a hospital stay, is gaining popularity as a means of controlling care costs (Marr, Reid, 1992). Managed care focuses on meeting the patient's needs while promoting efficiency and cost-effectiveness (Hicks, Stallmeyer, Coleman, 1992). Throughout this text, the concept of care management will be applied to maternal and newborn nursing. Approaches, such as *protocols* and critical paths, will be utilized where applicable.

ACCESS PROBLEMS CONTINUE

Access to prenatal care continues to be an issue in the 1990s. Between 1980 and 1987, there was an increase in the number of women not receiving prenatal care (a 26% increase for African-Americans and a 17% increase for whites). In addition, many women with access to prenatal care entered the health care system late or came only sporadically. Thus one in three pregnant women received inadequate prenatal care (care beginning after the first 3 months and with fewer than 13 total visits). Although 79% of white mothers began prenatal care in the first trimester, only 61% of African-American women did so (National Commission to Prevent Infant Mortality, 1990).

Many women are unable to pay for health care. According to Miller and associates (1989), 35% of the women of childbearing age are without public or private health insurance. In addition, 25% of the women of childbearing age with some insurance do not have maternity coverage. Thus many women remain uninsured (Health Insurance Institute, 1989). In fact, women and children are disproportionately represented in the group with limited access to care as the result of their inability to pay (Health Insurance Institute, 1989: National Commission to Prevent Infant Mortality, 1990).

TRENDS OF PATIENT INVOLVEMENT, SELF-CARE, AND FOCUS ON HEALTH CARE

In the late 1960s patients began to demand information about medical technology and their medical care. A movement toward self-help and assuming responsibility for wellness also occurred. No longer do patients passively accept and comply with the advice of health care providers, rather, patients demand information and take active roles. **Self-care** has been appealing to both patients and the health care system because of its potential to reduce health care costs.

Maternity patients are usually well when they enter the health care system. As a result, their care focuses on enhancing health and wellness, a focus that is especially well-suited to self-care. Visits to health care providers present opportunities for them to address topics such as nutrition education, stress management, smoking cessation, alcohol and drug treatment, improvement of social supports, and parenting education.

CHANGING CHILDBIRTH PRACTICES

Maternity care has changed dramatically. Maternity nurses have played active roles in shaping the health care system so that it meets the needs of contemporary women (Boeke, 1991). Often times women can choose either a physician or a nurse-midwife as their primary care provider. In 1991 physicians attended 94.7% of all births and nurse-midwives attended 4.1%, an increase from the 3.4% reported in 1988; the remaining 1.2% of births were unattended (Wegman, 1993). Women can now choose to give birth in a hospital labor room (rather than a delivery room), a birthing room, a birthing center, or at home. The method of anesthesia and positions for labor and birth vary according to the mother's condition and choice. With **family-centered care,** fathers, grandparents, siblings, and friends may be present for labor and birth. Fathers may attend cesarean births. Newborn infants stay with their mothers and may breastfeed immediately after birth. Prebirth education classes are common and encourage the participation of a support person, teach breathing/relaxation techniques, and give general information about birth.

Nursing care is changing to single-room maternity care, which permits a woman to labor, give birth, and recover in the same room (Labor-Delivery-Recovery, LDR). In some settings, the entire hospital stay for a birth may occur in the same room (Labor-Delivery-Recovery-Postpartum, LDRP). Instead of having one nurse care for the mother and another care for the infant, some hospitals have one nurse caring for the mother and baby as a unit. In some hospitals, central nurseries have been eliminated so that the babies may "room-in" with their mothers.

In the past mothers stayed in the hospital 3 to 4 days after the birth. Now, with "early discharge," mothers may go home 6 to 48 hours after the birth. This creates a growing need for follow-up or home care (NAACOG, 1991; Stotland, 1990). Nurses may establish "warm lines" or incorporate follow-up telephone calls or home visits into their practice as they assist families needing information and reassurance.

HOME HEALTH CARE FLOURISHES

A shift in settings from acute care institutions to the home has been occurring. Even high-risk childbearing women are increasingly cared for in the home. New technology, previously available only in the hospital, is now found in the home. This has affected the organizational structure of care, the skills required in providing such care, and the costs to patients (deLissovoy, Feustle, 1991).

LEGAL ISSUES IN THE DELIVERY OF CARE

Nursing standards of practice in perinatal and women's health nursing have been described by several organizations, including the American Nurses Association (ANA) (which publishes standards for maternal-child health nursing) and the Association for Women's Health, Obstetric and Neonatal Nurses (AWHONN). These standards reflect current knowledge and represent levels of practice agreed on by health care providers and leaders in the specialty. Because nursing practice, society, and the health care system are dynamic rather than static, standards will continue to change over time. In addition to these more formalized standards, agencies often have their own policy and procedure books that outline standards to be followed in that setting. In determining legal negligence, the care given is compared to the **standards of care.** If the standard was not met and harm resulted, then negligence occurred. The number of legal suits in the perinatal area has typically been high. As a consequence, malpractice insurance costs have risen dramatically for physicians, nurse-midwives, and nurses (Lang, Marek, 1991; Pellegrino, Siegler, Singer, 1991; Rhodes, 1989).

 LEGAL TIP: **Standard of Care**
When you are uncertain about how to perform a procedure, consult the agency procedure book and follow the guidelines printed in the book. These guidelines are the standard of care for that agency.

ETHICAL ISSUES

Advances in the science of obstetrics and neonatology have contributed to ethical dilemmas. Intrauterine fetal surgery, artificial insemination, genetic engineering, surrogate childbearing, infertility surgery, fetal research, and treatment of very low-birth-weight (VLBW) newborns have resulted in questions about informed consent and allocation of resources. Regulations, guidelines, and ethics committees have become commonplace. Experts in ethics are increasingly consulted to examine theories for ethical decision making, to assist in applying abstract theories to concrete situations, and to educate the public about methods for making moral decisions. Nursing can play a constructive role in this area by providing rational, knowledgeable, and experienced voices (Pellegrino, Siegler, Singer, 1991; Styles, 1990).

RESEARCH

The incorporation of research findings into practice is essential to develop a science-based practice. Practicing nurses can identify problems and read research literature to identify studies that address their clinical concerns. They can develop protocols and procedures based on published research. Health care providers need to support researchers in their endeavors; for example, they may participate in research as data collectors.

FUTURE TRENDS

Maternity nurses specialize in providing care for women throughout the childbearing cycle. Recent trends indicate that a new approach to women's health during the childbearing cycle is critical to the improvement of the overall health and well-being of women and their infants. Increased access to preventive care must become the focus. Maternity nurses can play an important role in this process (Styles, 1990).

KEY POINTS

- There are serious deficits in the health and health care of women in the childbearing years.
- Fertility and birthrate trends reflect women's need for health care.
- Biostatistical data differ based on age and race.

- Knowledgeable patients no longer play passive roles in their health care; they wish to be participants in health care decision making.
- Major changes in childbirth practices have created a more family-centered approach to care.
- Nurses have played active roles in shaping the health care system, making it more responsive to women.

CRITICAL THINKING EXERCISES

1. Infant mortality differs by state. What is your state's infant mortality? What demographic characteristics of the state contribute to infant mortality? Describe the health care services available to women without insurance in your state. As a nurse, what can you do about mortality and the availability of health care services?

2. Interview two nurses working in different maternity settings. How do the childbirth practices differ in these settings? Interview two women in their last trimester of pregnancy. What childbirth practices do they prefer? Have they expressed those preferences to their health care providers? If their preferences differ from what is available in the maternity setting, what do you think will happen to their childbirth satisfaction?

References

Boeke A: Beyond reproduction: a paradigm shift in women's health, *JOGNN* 20(1):12, 1991.

Boone MS: A socio-medical study of infant mortality among disadvantaged blacks, *Hum Org* 41(3):227, 1982.

Brecht M: The tragedy of infant mortality, *Nurs Outlook* 37(1):18, 1989.

Davidson ED, Gibbs CE, Chapin J: The challenge of care for the poor and underserved in the United States. An American College of Obstetricians and Gynecologists' perspective on access to care for underserved women. *Am J Dis Child* 145(5):546, 1991.

deLissovoy G, Feustle JA: Advanced home health care, *Health Policy* 17:227, 1991.

Development in health care costs—an update, *Statistical Bulletin* 75:30, 1994.

Health Insurance Institute: *Source book of health insurance data*, New York, 1989, Health Insurance Institute.

Hicks L, Stallmeyer JM, Coleman JR: Nursing challenges in managed care, *Nurs Econ* 10(4):265, 1992.

Inglis AD: US maternal and child health services Part I: right or privilege? *Neonat Netw* 9(8):35, 1991.

Lang NM, Marek KD: The policy and politics of patient outcomes, *J Nurs Qual Assur* 5(2):7, 1991.

Marr JA, Reid B: Implementing managed care and case management: the neuroscience experience, *J Neurosci Nurs* 24(5):281, 1992.

Miller CL et al: Barriers to implementation of a prenatal care program for low income women, *Am J Public Health* 79(1):62, 1989.

NAACOG: NAACOG endorses health care reform plan, *NAACOG Newsletter* 18(9):1, 1991.

National Center for Health Statistics: Advance report of final natality statistics, 1989, *Monthly Vital Statistics Report* 40(8 Supp):1, Hyattsville, MD: Public Health Service, 1991.

National Center for Health Statistics: Births, marriages, divorces, deaths, 1993, *Monthly Vital Statistics Report* 42:19, Hyattsville, MD: Public Health Service, 1994.

National Commission to Prevent Infant Mortality: *Troubling trends: the health of America's next generation*, Washington, DC, 1990.

Pellegrino ED, Siegler M, Singer PA: Future directions in clinical ethics, *J Clin Ethics* 2(1):5, 1991.

Queenan JT: White House action on US health care, *Contemp OB/GYN* 36(6):8, 1991.

Rhodes AM: Minimizing the liability risk of genetic counseling, *MCN* 14:313, 1989.

Stotland NL: Social change and women's reproductive health care, *Soc Change Reproduc Health Care* 1(1):4, 1990.

Styles MM: Challenges for nursing in this new decade, *MCN* 15(6):347, 1990.

Wegman ME: Annual summary of vital statistics, 1992, *Pediatrics* 92:743, 1993.

Bibliography

Covington C, Collins JE: Back to the future of women's health and perinatal nursing in the 21st century, *JOGNN* 23(1):183, 1994.

Craft I, al-Shawaf T: Outcome and complications of assisted reproduction, *Curr Opin Obstet Gynecol* 3(5):668, 1991.

Dixon J: US health care. I: The access problem, *BMJ* 305(6857):817, 1992.

Himmelstein DU, Woolhandler S, Wolfe SM: The vanishing health care safety net: new data on uninsured Americans, *Int J Health Serv* 22(3):381, 1992.

Kermani EJ: Issues of child custody and our moral values in the era of new medical technology, *J Am Acad Child Adolesc Psychiatry* 31(3):533, 1992.

Krieger JW, Connell FA, LoGergo JP: Medicaid prenatal care: a comparison of use and outcomes in fee-for-service and managed care, *Am J Public Health* 82(2):185, 1992.

Lappe M: Ethical issues in manipulating the human germ line, *J Med Philos* 16(6):621, 1991.

Mason JO: Reducing infant mortality in the United States through "healthy start," *Public Health Rep* 106(5):479, 1991.

McGinnis JM, Richmond JB, Brandt EN et al: Health progress in the United States: results of the 1990 objectives for the nation, *JAMA* 268(18):2545, 1992.

Mendoza FS, Ventura SJ, Valdez RB et al: Selected measures of health status for Mexican-American, mainland Puerto Rican, and Cuban-American children, *JAMA* 265(2):227, 1991.

Rockefeller J: Health care reform: prospects and progress, *Acad Med* 67(3):141, 1992.

CHAPTER

2 The Family, A Unit of Care

RHEA P. WILLIAMS

RELATED TOPICS

Family dynamics of pregnancy *(Chap. 6)* • Family dynamics after childbirth *(Chap. 17)*

Every newborn comes into this world surrounded by a family, be it a single-parent family or a large extended family. Regardless of the family structure, the maternity nurse is in a unique position to influence the care and well-being of these childbearing families. Thus the nurse acknowledges the family unit as the focus of care.

The family is one of society's most important institutions. It represents a primary social group that influences and is influenced by other people and institutions. People recognize the family as the fundamental social unit because most people have more continuous contact with this social group than with any other. The family assumes major responsibility for the introduction and socialization of persons. It transmits the fundamental cultural background of a given family to its members. Despite modern stresses and strains, the family forms a social network that acts as a potent support system for its members.

To deliver safe, comprehensive, and holistic care within the context of the nursing process, nurses working with childbearing families need a clear understanding of the family as an institution in our society.

DEFINING THE FAMILY

Families are defined in many ways. Definitions of the family involve explaining family *structure, functions, composition,* and *affectional ties.* The people who occupy a housing unit make up a household. Although a majority of households consist of a family-type of living arrangement, many do not. The U.S. Bureau of the Census (1992) identified two major categories of households as family and nonfamily. A *family* or *family household* requires the presence of at least two people, the householder and one or more additional family members related to the householder through birth, adoption, or marriage. A *nonfamily household* is composed of a householder who either lives alone or with people who are not related to the householder.

Friedman (1992) offers a broad definition of family, emphasizing the importance of emotional involvement as a necessary characteristic. She says, the family is "two or more persons who are joined together by bonds of sharing and emotional closeness and who identify themselves as part of the family." This definition includes a variety of family forms such as the extended family living in two or more households, cohabiting couples, childless families, gay and lesbian families, and single-parent families.

Nuclear Family

The **nuclear family** consists of parents and their dependent children. The family lives apart from either the husband's or wife's family of origin, and is usually economically independent.

The nuclear family has long represented the "traditional" American family. In this family group, different sex parents are expected to play complementary roles of husband-wife and father-mother in giving emotional and physical support to each other and their children. Recent trends in contemporary society, however, have caused many variations in this often considered "ideal" family structure. The "idealized" two-parent, two-child nuclear family, where the father is the sole provider and the mother is the homemaker, is a myth of the past (Fig. 2-1). Libman (1988), states that today couples in an intact first marriage, with two children and the mother at home, represent only 8% of the nation's families.

Extended Family

The **extended family** includes the nuclear family and other blood-related persons. These people are called "kin" and include grandparents, aunts, uncles, and cousins (Fig. 2-2) (Friedman, 1992). The family is a central focus for all members who live together as a group. Through its kinship network, the extended family provides role models and support to all members.

Variations of the traditional nuclear and extended families have always existed. Until recently, most of these *alternative family forms* have been considered deviations from the norm. Today single parenthood, unintentional or planned, is becoming an acceptable option in the United States. Single parenthood can be a voluntary choice that does not result in rejection by family and society, or the loss of job. In addition, biologic and adoptive parenthood is becoming a socially acceptable option for women and men who do not choose to marry; les-

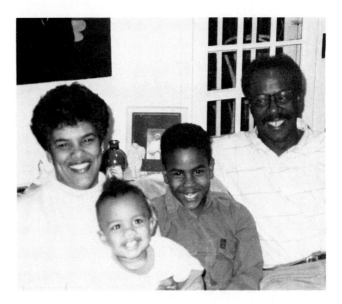

FIG. 2-1 Nuclear family.

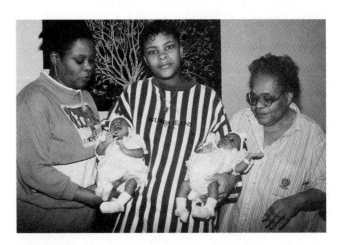

FIG. 2-2 An extended family. (Courtesy Caroline E. Brown, Hershey, PA.)

bian and gay parenthood is yet another alternative (Evans et al, 1989). The emergence of single parenthood as a planned choice reflects a belief that one has the "right" to choose to be a parent.

Single-Parent Family

The **single-parent family** is becoming an increasingly recognized structure in our society. The single-parent family may result from the loss of a spouse by death, divorce, separation, or desertion; from the out-of-wedlock birth of a child; or from the adoption of a child. The 1992 U.S. Bureau of the Census reveals that there were 10.7 million one-parent (female household, no husband present) family groups in 1990. Of all children 17 years old or younger, approximately 26% live in a family with a single parent, another relative, or a non-relative. Fewer than 4% live with fathers in a single-parent household (Evolving American Family, 1993).

The single-parent family tends to be vulnerable economically and socially. Unless buttressed by a concerned society, it may create an unstable and deprived environment for the growth potential of children (Norton, Glick, 1986).

For other adults, the single-parent family is a chosen life-style that provides a free and open system for development of parents and children. In these families decision making and communication are seen as joint commitments between parent and child, and the parent-child relationship is considered a major source of life fulfillment.

Blended Family

The **blended family,** also called a "reconstituted" or "combined family," includes stepparents and stepchildren. Separation, divorce, and remarriage are common in the United States, where approximately 50% of marriages end in divorce. Divorce and remarriage may occur at any time in the family life cycle and, therefore, will have different impacts on family function. Whatever the timing, effort is required to restabilize old family groups and to constitute and stabilize new family groups. This emotional work must be accomplished before family and individual development can proceed.

Homosexual Family

Homosexual families are being recognized increasingly in Western society. Children in such families may be the offspring of previous heterosexual unions, conceived by one member of a lesbian couple through artificial insemination, or adopted. Homosexual couples have the same biologic and psychologic needs as do heterosexual couples. They too seek quality care for themselves and for their children.

Family Unit

Although people find it difficult to define the family precisely, members of a family can readily describe its composition. Family members know who is kin and who is not, how the family has affected their lives, and in what family style they believe.

However the family is defined, the *family unit* is incomplete without an adult. From an adult's perspective, the family can be composed of people of any age or sex bound by a blood or love relationship. From the child's perspective, the family is a set of relationships between the child's dependent self and one or more protective adults.

Regardless of the form a family assumes or the society in which it is found, the family possesses enduring characteristics that have far-reaching personal and societal effects. According to Blehar (1979):

Despite disagreement about the state of the family and its definition, a consensus might be reached on three points: (1) the family is currently in a state of flux precipitated by economic and social pressures; (2) imperfect though it may be, it is difficult to imagine substituting an alternative that could perform all its functions as well; and (3) it is more desirable to bolster families than to attempt to supplant them with untried structures.

What then are the functions that families must perform, and how can nurses best support families facing economic and social pressures?

FAMILY FUNCTIONS

As the family progresses through its life cycle (see Table 2-1), from young adulthood to the commitment of two people to share a life and ending with the dissolution of the family through death or other separations, it carries out certain functions for the well-being of family members. The **family functions** extend over five basic areas: biologic, economic, educational, psychologic, and sociocultural (WHO, 1978). The interdependent functions depend on the physical and mental health of family members. Each family develops common *beliefs, values,* and *sentiments* that are used as criteria in the choice of alternative actions.

Biologic functions include reproduction, care and rearing of children, nutrition, maintenance of health, and recreation. The ability to carry out such functions implies certain prerequisites: healthy genetic inheritance, fertility management, care during the maternity cycle, good dietary behavior, intelligent use of health services, companionship, and nurturing of family members.

Economic functions include earning enough money to carry out the other functions, developing family budgets, and ensuring the financial security of family members. To accomplish these tasks the family must have the necessary skills, opportunities, and knowledge.

Educational functions include the teaching of skills, attitudes, and knowledge relating to the other functions. Family members must have access to resources and the necessary skills to use these resources to be able to do this.

The psychologic function of the family is expected to provide an environment that promotes the natural development of personality. Families should offer optimum psychologic protection, and promote the ability to form relationships with people outside the family circle. These tasks require stable emotional health, common bonds of affection as well as the abilities to be mutually supportive, to tolerate stress, and to cope with crises.

Sociocultural functions are associated with the socialization of children. These functions include the transfer of values relating to behavior, tradition, language, reli-

TABLE 2-1 Stages of the Family Life Cycle

FAMILY LIFE CYCLE STAGE	EMOTIONAL PROCESS OF TRANSITION: KEY PRINCIPLES	SECOND-ORDER CHANGES IN FAMILY STATUS REQUIRED TO PROCEED DEVELOPMENTALLY
Leaving home: single young adults	Accepting emotional and financial responsibility for self	Differentiation of self in relation to family of origin Development of intimate peer relationships Establishment of self re work and financial independence
The joining of families through marriage: the new couple	Commitment to new system	Formation of marital system Realignment of relationships with extended families and friends to include spouse
Families with young children	Accepting new members into the system	Adjusting marital system to make space for child(ren) Joining in child-rearing, financial, and household tasks Realignment of relationships with extended family to include parenting and grandparenting roles
Families with adolescents	Increasing flexibility of family boundaries to include children's independence and grandparents' frailties	Shifting of parent child relationships to permit adolescent to move in and out of system Refocus on midlife marital and career issues Beginning shift toward joint caring for older generation
Launching children and moving on	Accepting a multitude of exits from and entries into the family system	Renegotiation of marital system as a dyad Development of adult-to-adult relationships between grown children and their parents Realignment of relationships to include in-laws and grandchildren Dealing with disabilities and death of parents (grandparents)
Families in later life	Accepting the shifting of generational roles	Maintaining own and/or couple functioning and interests in face of physiologic decline; exploration of new familial and social role options Support for a more central role of middle generation Making room in the system for the wisdom and experience of the elderly, supporting the older generation without overfunctioning for them Dealing with loss of spouse, siblings, and other peers and preparation for own death; life review and integration

From Carter B, McGoldrick M: *The changing family life cycle: a framework for family therapy*, ed 2, New York, 1988, Gardner Press, Inc.

gion, and prevailing or previous social moral attitudes. As a result, family members become conditioned to a variety of behavioral norms set by their society, which are appropriate to all stages of adult life. To do this, the family must possess "accepted standards" and be sensitive to the varying social needs of children according to their ages. A family must also accept and exemplify society's behavioral norms and be willing to explain, defend, and promote these standards. Although certain functions are relegated to or emphasized more in one phase of the family's life cycle than another (e.g., the care and socialization of children are part of the childbearing and childrearing phase of the cycle), many of the functions are continuous for the family's survival and progress.

FAMILY DYNAMICS

Families work cooperatively to accomplish family functions. Through **family dynamics,** family members assume appropriate social roles. Social roles are learned in the family, and learned in pairs (e.g., mother-father, parent-child, and brother-sister). A social role does not exist by itself, but is designed to work with a role partner. Role pairing enables social interactions to take place in an orderly, predictable manner—the roles are said to be complementary. Some families maintain a traditional pairing of roles, whereas other families change behavior patterns to suit a change in family life-style. Rather than mother-father, brother-sister, the roles may be mother-daughter, mother-son. *Negotiation* brings these pair roles into a new alignment. Negotiation is essential to maintain family equilibrium.

Each family sets up *boundaries* between itself and society. People are extremely conscious of the difference between "family members" and "outsiders," people without kinship status. Some families isolate themselves from the outside community. Others have a wide community network to help in times of stress. Although boundaries exist for every family, family members set up *channels* through which they interact with society. These channels also ensure that the family receives its share of social resources.

Ideally the family uses its resources to provide a safe, intimate environment for the biopsychosocial development of the family members. The family provides for the *nurturing* of the newborn and the gradual *socialization* of the growing child. It serves as the source of first relationships with others. The earliest and closest relationships children form are with their parents, or parenting persons, and continue throughout a lifetime. For better or worse, parent-child relationships influence a person's self-worth and ability to form later relationships. The family influences the child's perceptions of the outside world. The family provides the growing child with an identity that possesses both a past and a sense of the future. Cultural values and rituals are passed from one generation to the next through the family (Friedman, 1992).

Through everyday interactions, the family develops and uses its own patterns of verbal and nonverbal *communication.* These patterns give insight into the emotional exchange within a family and act as reliable indicators of interpersonal functioning. Family members not only react to the communication or actions of other family members, but also interpret and define them.

Over time the family develops protocols for *problem solving,* particularly regarding important decisions such as having a baby, buying a house, or sending children to college. The criteria used in making decisions are based on *family values* and *attitudes* concerning the appropriateness of the behavior and the moral, social, political, and economic events of society. The *power* to make critical decisions is given to a family member through tradition or negotiation. This power is not always stated. Power reflects the family's concepts of male or female dominance and the cultural practices, social customs, and community norms. As a result, family members attain certain *statuses* or *hierarchies.* They play out these statuses by assuming various *roles.* Most families have a member who "takes charge" or "is supportive" or "can't be expected to do anything."

FAMILY DEVELOPMENT

Many academic disciplines study the family and have developed theories that provide differing perspectives for assessment. Knowledge of these theories provides nurses with guidelines to understand family functioning and dynamics. For example, it is useful for nurses to view the family from a developmental perspective.

The **developmental theory** used to study the family incorporates ideas from a number of theoretical and conceptual approaches such as the social systems approach, structural-functional approach, life cycle concepts of developmental needs and tasks, and concepts of interacting personalities. The central theme in the developmental theory notes "the changes in the process of internal development with the dimensions of time as central" (Bower, Jacobson, 1978). The family is a *small group, semiclosed* system engaging in interactive behavior within the larger cultural social system. The significant unit in this theory is the *person* rather than the role. The family process is one of *interaction* over the family's *life cycle.*

Family members pass through phases of growth, from dependence through active independence to interdependence. The family also demonstrates variations in structure and function over time. Together these constitute the *family life cycle.* Carter and McGoldrick (1988) outlined the stages and tasks of the family life cycle in Table 2-1.

Mercer (1989) summarizes the essence of the developmental approach in family nursing:

> Developmental concepts include movement to a higher level of functioning. This implies continuous, unidirectional progression. However, during transitional periods from one stage or phase to the next, disequilibrium occurs, during which time the individual may revert to an earlier level of developmental responses. Families face normative and unexpected transitions that also create a period of disorganization, during which the family functions at a lower level than usual. Resolution of the disequilibrium or crisis has potential to lead to a higher level of family functioning.

Implications for Maternity Nursing

The developmental perspective provides many useful insights into family functioning. Knowledge of problem types, identified during certain phases of the life cycle, can assist nurses in providing anticipatory guidance for families. For example, helping childbearing families prepare for the birth of a newborn may minimize the development of crisis situations.

The family as a group and the family as individuals are simultaneously engaged in developmental tasks (Duvall, 1977; Erikson, 1968). If the developmental task of the family is not in tune with the developmental task of the person, disharmony occurs. Many examples of such dissonance exists. The adolescent father grappling with the need to break from his own family ties while also expected to establish monetary and other support for his new family. A toddler learning socially acceptable behaviors, when introduced to a new sibling may revert to infantile behavior. Knowing the implications of these situations can be useful when helping a family develop appropriate coping mechanisms.

The developmental approach presents a constantly evolving concept of family that becomes more in tune with reality. The phases of the life cycle in the nuclear family are easier to plot than in an extended family, because the extended family may involve many generations. Sometimes it is difficult to document the life cycle of a family; it often changes or disintegrates before we can grasp its significance.

Developmental theory offers the maternity nurse one basis for understanding the family unit and a familiar approach for using the nursing process to promote family health among childbearing families.

KEY FACTORS IN FAMILY HEALTH

Certain factors have proved important in determining the quality of family health. For example, family dynamics (previously discussed on p. 15) encompasses the coordination of intrafamilial roles, the distribution of power within the family, and the decision making process. Family dynamics also affect the use of health services.

Family socioeconomic characteristics are important. Social class affects expectations, obligations, and rewards, all of which affect the use of health services. In addition, the family acts as the primary economic unit in which incomes may be pooled, expenditure decisions made jointly, and services rendered internally.

Friedman (1992) considers a family's social class as the prime molder of family lifestyle. Social class, she says, and cultural background:

> . . . Exert the greatest overall influence on family life, influencing our early socialization, the role expectations we hold, the values we stress, the types of behavior we consider acceptable or deviant, or the world experiences we have.

CULTURAL FACTORS
Cultural Context of the Family

The family process within its **cultural context** is a central concern in nursing. A culture's beliefs and practices regarding childbearing are embedded in its economic, religious, kinship, and political structures. All cultures have behavioral norms and expectations for each stage of the perinatal cycle. These norms and expectations relate to each culture's view of how people stay healthy and prevent illness. With multiculturalism and the expansion of international nursing, nurses need to focus on cultural variations in perceptions of life events and the use of health care systems. Patients have a right to expect that their health care needs, both physiologic and psychologic, will be met, and that their cultural beliefs will be respected.

Culture has many definitions. Helman (1990) views culture as a set of guidelines, which individuals inherit as members of a particular society, that tell people how to view the world and how to relate to other people, supernatural forces, and the natural environment. Cultural knowledge includes beliefs and values about each facet of life. These guidelines have been tested over time. They relate to food, language, religion, art, health and healing practices, kinship relationships, and all other systems of behavior.

Many subcultures may be found within each culture. *Subculture* refers to a group existing within a larger cultural system that retains its own characteristics. A subculture may be an ethnic group or a group organized in other ways. For example, in the varied culture of the United States, there are many ethnic subcultures (African-Americans, Asian-Americans, Mexican-Americans). Within the culture of health care providers, the subcultures of nursing and medicine exist.

Each subculture holds rich and complex traditions, including health practices that have proven effective over time. These traditions vary from group to group. In a multicultural society, many groups can influence these traditions and practices. As cultural groups come in contact with each other, acculturation and assimilation may occur.

Acculturation refers to changes that take place in one or both groups when people from different cultures come in contact with one another. People may retain some of their own culture while adopting some of the cultural practices of the dominant society. This familiarization among cultural groups results in much overt behavioral similarity. Individuals exchange and adopt mannerisms, styles, and practices of the other group. Dress, language patterns, food choices, and health practices especially show differences among cultural groups within a society. An example of acculturation would be the adoption of ethnic food practices in the United States.

Assimilation, on the other hand, occurs when a cultural group loses its identity and becomes a part of the dominant culture. According to Friedman (1992), "Assimilation denotes the more complete and one-way process of one culture being absorbed into the other." Assimilation is the process by which groups "melt" into the mainstream, thus accounting for the notion of a "melting pot," a phenomenon that has been said to occur in the United States. In contrast, Spector (1991) asserts that in the United States, the "melting pot," with its dream of a common culture "has proved to be a myth and faded; it is now time to identify and both accept and appreciate the differences among people."

Nurses must recognize that a wide range of cultural diversity exists within society. Assessment of the beliefs and practices of a group, and those within the group, is essential for the health care provider striving to provide culturally appropriate health care. Nurses must also be aware of factors that may prevent some health care providers from providing optimum care. Understanding the concepts of ethnocentrism and cultural relativism may be helpful to nurses caring for families in a multicultural society.

Ethnocentrism "is the view that one's culture's way of doing things is the right and natural way" (Galanti, 1991). Essentially, ethnocentrism supports the notion "my group is the best," whether an ethnic or social group. For example, socialization into the profession of nursing occurs within the framework of the Western health care system. This system emphasizes the biomedical model, which is based primarily on the white, middle-class value system in the United States. This biomedical model represents pregnancy and childbirth as phenomena with inherent risk, most appropriately managed through specific knowledge and technology. The nurse, when encountering behavior in women who are unfamiliar with this model, may become frustrated and impatient. The women's behavior may be labeled inappropriate and in conflict with "good" health practices. If the Western health care system provides the nurse's only standard for judgment, the behavior of the nurse is called *ethnocentric.*

Cultural relativism, the opposite of ethnocentrism, involves learning about and applying the standards of another person's culture to activities within that culture. To be culturally relativistic, the nurse recognizes that people from different cultural backgrounds actually see the same objects and situations differently. For the most part, viewpoints are culturally determined.

Cultural relativism does not require nurses to *accept* the beliefs and values of another culture, rather, nurses should recognize that other's behavior may be based on a system of logic different from their own. Cultural relativism affirms the uniqueness and value of every culture. Spector (1991) states that ". . . because health care providers learn from their culture the way and the how of being healthy or ill, it behooves them to treat each patient with deference to his own cultural background."

Childbearing Beliefs and Practices

Nurses working with childbearing families in the United States and Canada care for families from different cultures and ethnic groups. To provide a high level of care to all families, the nurse should be aware of the cultural beliefs and practices important to these families. Countless beliefs and practices stem from a religious or an ethnic origin and may or may not still be observed by families with differing cultural backgrounds.

Table 2-2 provides examples of *some* cultural beliefs and practices surrounding childbearing that may be important to Mexican-Americans, Asian-Americans, and African-Americans. Most of these cultural beliefs and customs reflect the traditional culture and are not universally practiced by all members of the cultural group in every part of the country. Variables, such as degree of acculturation, educational and income levels, and amount of contact with the older generations, influence the extent to which people practice these customs. Women from these cultural-ethnic groups may adhere to some, all, or none of the practices listed.

The nurse needs to become familiar with each woman as an individual, and validate the cultural beliefs, if any, that are meaningful to her. Equipped with this knowledge, the nurse supports and nurtures those beliefs that promote physical or emotional adaptation to pregnancy. However, if certain beliefs are identified that might be harmful, the nurse should carefully explore those beliefs with the patient, and use the beliefs in the reeducation and modification process.

TABLE 2-2 (Traditional*) Cultural Beliefs and Practices: Childbearing and Parenting

PREGNANCY	CHILDBIRTH	PARENTING
MEXICAN-AMERICAN (Galanti, 1991; Kay, 1978; Williams, 1989)		
Pregnancy desired soon after marriage	**Labor** Use of "partera" or lay midwife preferred in some places, may prefer presence of mother, rather than husband	**Newborn** Breastfeeding begun after the third day; colostrum may be considered "filthy" or "spoiled"
Expectant mother influenced strongly by mother or mother-in-law	After birth of baby, mother's legs brought together to prevent air from entering uterus	Olive oil or castor oil given to stimulate the passage of meconium
Cool air in motion considered dangerous during pregnancy	Loud behavior in labor	Male infant not circumcised
Unsatisfied food cravings thought to cause a birthmark		Female infant's ears pierced
Some pica observed in the eating of ashes or dirt (not common)	**Postpartum** Diet may be restricted after birth, for first 2 days only boiled milk and toasted tortillas permitted (special foods to restore warmth to the body)	Belly band used to prevent umbilical hernia
Milk avoided because it causes large babies and difficult births		Religious medal worn by mother during pregnancy; placed around infant's neck
Many predictions about the sex of the baby	Bed rest for 3 days after birth	Infant protected from the "evil eye"
May be unacceptable and frightening to have pelvic examination by male health care provider	Keep warm Mother's head and feet protected from cold air—bathing permitted after 14 days	Various remedies used to treat "Mal ojo" and fallen fontanel (depressed fontanel)
Use of herbs to treat common complaints of pregnancy	Mother often cared for by her own mother	
Drinking chamomile tea thought to assure effective labor	40-day restriction on sexual intercourse	

*There are variations in some beliefs and practices among Asian subcultures.
NOTE: Most of these cultural beliefs and customs reflect the traditional culture and are not universally practiced. These lists are not intended to stereotype patients, rather to serve as guidelines while discussing meaningful cultural beliefs with a patient and her family. Examples of other cultural beliefs and practices are found throughout this text.

FAMILY AND CRISIS

For the family system, stress can arise internally and externally. Although many families cope with stress, the situation may become acute and take on the characteristics of a crisis. Crisis may be defined as a disturbance of habit: a disruption in a family's or an individual's usual means of maintaining control over a situation. When faced with a crisis, the family or individual first uses customary values and behaviors to resolve the crisis. If these behaviors can not resolve the crisis adequately, new behavior patterns must be developed through crisis intervention. Crisis intervention strives to help patients learn new ways of dealing with conflicts or problems. Although patients may seek help for a specific problem, the strategies they learned may apply to future difficulties. Crises can center around maturational or situational events.

Both maturational and situational events accompany the childbearing experience. This experience represents a significant turning point in a family's life. Childbearing is often considered a time of crisis. Maternity nurses, who understand crisis theory, can readily assist families unable to cope with the stress of these events.

Maturational Crisis

Maturational crises develop as a result of normal growth and development. They characteristically evolve over time and involve *role* and *status* changes. They include events such as birth, infancy, childhood, adolescence, adulthood, and old age. Each phase of the family life cycle produces characteristic crises or events capable of creating stress that can affect the health of one or more family members.

The birth of a child represents one of the most important events in a family's life. Births and the subsequent child-care require parental, intellectual, and psychologic maturity. This may account for periods of crisis in a family.

TABLE 2-2   (Traditional) Cultural Beliefs and Practices: Childbearing and Parenting—cont'd

PREGNANCY	CHILDBIRTH	PARENTING

AFRICAN-AMERICAN
(Carrington, 1978; Galanti, 1991; Williams, 1989)

PREGNANCY	CHILDBIRTH	PARENTING

Acceptance of pregnancy depends on economic status
Pregnancy thought to be state of "wellness," which is often the reason for delay in seeking prenatal care, especially by lower income African-Americans
Old wives tales include having a picture taken during pregnancy will cause stillbirth; reaching up will cause the cord to strangle the baby
Craving for certain foods including chicken, greens, clay, starch, dirt
Pregnancy may be viewed by African-American men as a sign of their virility
Self-treatment for various discomforts of pregnancy including constipation, nausea, vomiting, headache, and heartburn
	Labor
	Use of "Granny midwife" in certain parts of the country
	Varied emotional responses: some cry out, some display stoic behavior to avoid calling attention to selves
	Patient may arrive at hospital in far-advanced labor
	Emotional support often provided by other women, especially own mother
	
	Postpartum
	Vaginal bleeding seen as sign of sickness; tub baths and shampooing of hair prohibited
	Sassafras tea thought to have healing power
	Eating liver thought to cause heavier vaginal bleeding because of its high "blood" content
		Newborn
		Feeding very important:
		  "Good" baby thought to eat well
		  Early introduction of solid foods
		  May breastfeed or bottle feed; breastfeeding may be considered embarrassing
		Parents fearful of spoiling baby
		Commonly call baby by nicknames
		May use excessive clothing to keep baby warm
		Belly band used to prevent umbilical hernia
		Abundant use of oil on baby's scalp and skin
		Strong feeling of family, community, and religion

ASIAN-AMERICAN
(Chung, 1977; Galanti, 1991; Williams, 1989)

PREGNANCY	CHILDBIRTH	PARENTING

Pregnancy considered time when mother "has happiness in her body"
Pregnancy seen as natural process
Strong preference for female health care provider
Belief in theory of hot and cold
May omit soy sauce in diet to prevent dark-skinned baby
Prefer soup made with ginseng root as general strength tonic
Milk is usually excluded from diet because it causes stomach distress
	Labor
	Mother attended by other women, especially her own mother
	Father does not actively participate
	Labor in silence
	
	Postpartum
	Must protect self from Yin (cold forces) for 30 days
	  Ambulation limited
	  Shower and bathing prohibited
	  Warm room
	  Chinese mother avoids fruits and vegetables
	Diet
	  Warm fluids
	  Some patients are vegetarians
	  Korean mother is served seaweed soup with rice
	  Chinese diet high in hot foods
		Concept of the family is important and valued
		Father is head of the household; wife plays a subordinate role
		The birth of a boy is preferred
		May delay naming child
		Some groups (e.g., Vietnamese) believe colostrum is dirty, therefore, they may delay breastfeeding until milk comes in

Nurses assist with the birth of children and can provide support as the adults undertake active parenting roles. They can provide parents with a knowledge of human psychosocial development, which will help parents see their children realistically and establish appropriate criteria for children's behavior. Nurses may use this unique relationship with a family to promote birth as a family-centered event. Ideally, the birth of a child can help the growth of all family members.

Situational Crisis

Situational crises include such events as preterm birth, mental or physical illness, loss of financial or social support, changed body image, experience of violence or serious illness, divorce, death, and grief. These crises involve a threat to an individual's self-worth or the loss of a valued object or position. Anxiety and depression are characteristic responses. If the situational crisis causes severe strain, it can result in health impairment.

Response to Crisis

In both maturational and situational crises, the family plays a critical role in reducing distress, successful adaptation, and healthy rehabilitation. Knowledge of how a family reacts to crisis helps the nurse understand the family's ability to withstand stress. The nurse can help the family use its problem-solving abilities to deal with the crisis.

Aguilera (1994) has devised a stratagem for assessing a family's or an individual's potential or actual response to a crisis. She maintains that three key areas or components act as balancing factors affecting equilibrium: (1) the patient's perception of the crisis event, (2) the patient's coping mechanisms, and (3) the patient's support system. The interplay among these three areas is critical for the outcome or resolution of a problem.

Perception of the Event

What one person considers a crisis may or may not be perceived as a crisis by someone else. Factors, such as *age* and *prior experience*, can alter perception. For example, an event viewed as a crisis by an adolescent may not be seen as a crisis by an adult. *Emotional states, anxiety,* or *hostility* may influence perception. The highly anxious, first-time mother may become disorganized by her infant's crying, whereas a mother of four may accept the crying as normal.

Nursing intervention, relative to a patient's perception of a crisis-provoking event, may be limited to helping the patient state "what the problem is." More nursing intervention is required if the event can have a negative effect on the patient, the infant, or the family. For example, in some cultures such as Southeast Asians (D'Avanzo, 1992), pregnancy is seen as such a natural event that does not require medical or nursing supervision. Since complications of pregnancy can arise, with detrimental effects for mother and child, the nurse should encourage the family to participate in ongoing health care.

Coping Mechanisms

Coping mechanisms can be defined as patterns of behavior that people or families develop for dealing with threats to their sense of well-being (Stuart, Sundeen, 1995). Coping mechanisms may be constructive or destructive. *Constructive coping mechanisms* lead to the resolution of a problem. *Destructive coping mechanisms* can distort reality, interfere with interpersonal relationships, and limit working ability.

Nurses use knowledge of human coping mechanisms to identify an individual's or a family's defense mechanism and evaluate the success of the mechanism in reducing problems. When necessary, attempts are made to substitute more beneficial behaviors, while supporting and reinforcing constructive coping. Coping mechanisms, whether constructive or destructive, appear to be essential for all individuals and groups in order to maintain emotional stability.

Support Systems

Support systems refer to the network from which people receive help in times of crisis. Caplan (1959), one of the crisis intervention developers, maintains that successful resolution of a crisis often depends on the patient's support system. Patients with a strong support system may only need minimal intervention to resolve a crisis and to recover. If the patient has a weak support system, disorganization may occur and the patient may not recover without considerable intervention from health care professionals.

A patient's support system may include family, friends, and significant others. Other people functioning as part of support systems are health care providers or "community caretakers" (Caplan, 1959). Community caretakers are people working in agencies that represent a community's organized health resources. With their knowledge and experience, these individuals can assist patients who are unable to handle crises on their own or with help from family and friends. Maternity nurses are in an ideal position to offer help throughout the maternity cycle. Their assistance may take the form of teaching or counseling, or involve helping patients learn the procedures for enlisting the aid of other community agencies. For example, nurses have developed *parent education programs* to provide women and men with skills for coping with the stress of labor. These programs also help parents learn about their infants' needs and about child-care activities. This way parents are better able to cope with the changing needs of a growing child and to understand the impact of a newborn on the family.

Key factors such as family dynamics, socioeconomic status, cultural patterns, and coping responses should all be considered as nurses formulate nursing care plans for the childbearing family.

Care Management

✦ ASSESSMENT

To plan for the care of a family or an individual family member, the nurse must remember that a family operates as a system. That means, no one family member has a problem; if a problem exists, the whole family has a problem. Solutions to problems can evolve best through family participation.

Data Collection Process

The *process* of an assessment in planning family care is often more difficult and complicated than assessing a patient's physical health. It requires adept communication skills and the ability to establish a trusting relationship with each family member simultaneously. Families often have varying degrees of openness and privacy. All groups resent interrogation by an outsider. The reasons for obtaining information must be explained to family members in a clear, nonthreatening, and culturally appropriate manner.

Generally, family members freely give information such as the address, marital status, and ages. To attain other information: (1) *observe* and note relationships, attitudes, and stress responses (who is doing what), (2) *listen* to conversation about community and family involvements or hopes and aspirations, and (3) *ask questions* in a culturally appropriate manner.

Stern (1980) developed a useful model for improving communication between patients from different ethnic and cultural backgrounds and their Western health care providers. This model identifies barriers in communication that exist on three levels: approach, custom, and language.

Approach includes numerous factors considered in interpersonal relationships. Americans approach most issues in health care by addressing the problem directly. With many cultures, such as Asians and Native Americans, engaging in small talk is vital before beginning a serious discussion. Some cultures equate commenting on flowers or pictures and having tea or a cold drink with showing respect. To begin talking to an expectant mother about the need for prenatal care before commenting on the other children, the pretty chair, or the weather, could set up an atmosphere of distrust. In some cultures such as Asian-Americans and Mexican-Americans, women prefer a caregiver of the same sex. Therefore an initial encounter with a female caregiver may be critical. Showing respect and patience is essential in building trust.

Custom includes practices and behaviors characteristic of a culture. Understanding that a cultural reason exists for all behaviors and making a sincere effort to know the

person's rationale for behavior are important steps in establishing trust. Patients themselves may be the best source in helping the nurse understand cultural logic and individual differences. An assessment of health beliefs and practices is essential to achieve a holistic approach to care. For patients, adherence to a particular cultural custom provides a sense of constancy with their cultural heritage.

Language is an important factor. Stern (1980) emphasizes the use of clear, jargon-free English. When the family does not speak English, a bilingual nurse is ideal for assessing the family. If a bilingual nurse is not available, use either a family member or a member of the same cultural group as an interpreter. When using an interpreter, address questions and responses to the patient and not to the interpreter.

Ways to elicit cultural explanations regarding childbearing are listed in Cultural Considerations.

A nurse cannot be expected to know everything about every culture and subculture, as well as the many lifestyles within each culture. To come to a better realization of why people believe as they do, people must first understand their own culture. Understanding patients' cultures, through interview, study, contact, and sincere interest, is invaluable, because understanding enables nurses to give culturally appropriate nursing care.

Analysis, Synthesis, Validation

Following the data-gathering phase, the nurse analyzes and synthesizes the findings and makes inferences about the data. By asking: What are the significant stressors influencing this family? Do the family's beliefs reflect cultural variations? Do these beliefs promote physical or emotional well-being, or might they be harmful to the family? Is this family's immediate support system adequate for coping with potential crises during childbearing? Does family communication respect all family mem-

 CULTURAL CONSIDERATIONS

QUESTIONS TO OBTAIN CULTURAL EXPLANATIONS ABOUT CHILDBEARING

1. What do you and your family think you should do to remain healthy during pregnancy?
2. What are the things you can do or not do to improve your health and the health of your baby?
3. Who do you want with you during your labor?
4. What things or actions are important to you and your family to do after the baby's birth?
5. What do you and your family expect from the nurse or nurses caring for you?
6. How will family members participate in your pregnancy, childbirth, and parenting?

bers in light of individual's developmental stage?

Since inferences are subjective and based not only on the nurse's competence level but also on individual values and beliefs, the nurse needs to validate the interpretation of the data with the patient. The development of nursing diagnoses follows validation of inferences.

✜ NURSING DIAGNOSES

Nursing diagnoses reflect the family's perception of its needs, as well as the nurse's perception. *It is important to determine the family's perception of its nursing care needs rather than the perception of any one family member.*

Examples of nursing diagnoses (Christensen, Kenney, 1995) commonly encountered with childbearing families include:

Altered parenting related to
- Impaired parent-infant attachment

Altered family processes related to
- Birth of a child with a defect

Anxiety related to
- Expectations of parenting experience

Knowledge deficit related to
- Infant care activities

Social isolation related to
- Lack of interaction with peers

Spiritual distress related to
- Conflict between ideal and personal religious practices associated with childbearing

The nurse should keep in mind that nursing diagnosis may vary with cultural groups. For example, when diagnosing "Impaired maternal attachment," the nurse must consider the family's cultural beliefs. Galanti (1991) describes the Vietnamese tradition of delaying naming the child, a tradition that Western health care providers often misinterpret as poor bonding. Traditionally, Vietnamese families decide on the baby's name in a family naming ceremony.

Once the nursing diagnoses are established, the nurse takes time to explore personal value judgments about the family that may affect and impede nursing interventions. It is also essential for nurses to validate the diagnoses, to make sure their perceptions are objective and accurate. In addition to direct validation with the family, a review of literature, an analysis of cultural norms, and discussion with other family members are also means of validation.

✜ EXPECTED OUTCOMES

The nurse sets expected outcomes related to each diagnosis. The nurse establishes these expected outcomes with the family. Family members evaluate the expected outcomes for realism and acceptance. They establish both short-term and long-term expected outcomes. The expected outcomes are assessed to determine priority. Certain health needs require immediate attention (e.g., unexplained vaginal bleeding). Other health needs require more time to resolve (e.g., grief over birth of a child with a defect).

Working with the available data, the nursing diagnoses, and the health goals, the nurse proceeds to organize a plan for implementing the most appropriate interventions. The nurse identifies the nursing role, that is, whether the role is to teach, provide direct care, or refer the patient to a more appropriate resource.

The nurse must be able to teach at various levels so that individual family members feel understood and supported. Different strategies may be necessary for each family member. As a direct care provider, the nurse promotes activities that will lead to the family's own self-care and independence.

✜ COLLABORATIVE CARE

Nurses put the preventive, curative, or rehabilitative actions into practice. Then they tailor these actions to meet the individual needs of the family and its members. Nurses may also use their knowledge and skills to guide family members who will participate in the implementation. The nurse may also refer the family to appropriate internal and community support systems, and determine the family's willingness to use these resources.

✜ EVALUATION

The nurse works with the family to evaluate expected outcomes using outcome criteria. These need to be stated precisely and behaviorally in order to measure the degree of realization. The criteria need to be realistic and flexible enough to permit modification as circumstances change.

Friedman (1992) suggests six questions to ask when evaluating the family nursing process.

1. Were family expectations set in relative and accurate terms?
2. Is there a consensus between the family and other health care team members on the evaluation?
3. What additional data need to be collected to evaluate progress?
4. Were the nursing diagnoses, goals, and approaches realistic and accurate?
5. If the family's behavior and perception indicate that the problem has not been satisfactorily resolved, what are the reasons?
6. Were there any unforeseen outcomes that need to be considered?

KEY POINTS

- The family forms a social network that acts as an important support system for its members.
- Ideally, the family provides a safe, intimate environment for the biopsychosocial development of children and its adult members.
- Family developmental theory provides nurses with a familiar guide to understand family function.
- A family's life cycle may be difficult to document.
- The reproductive beliefs and practices of a culture are embedded in its economic, religious, kinship, and political structures.

- The expression of parental roles and how children are viewed reflect cultural differences.
- North American culture is a pluralistic one in which varying family forms are recognized and accepted in differing degrees.
- In both maturational and situational crises the family plays a critical role in reducing distress, successful adaptation, and healthy rehabilitation.
- Balancing factors affecting equilibrium in a family include the patient's perception of the crisis event, coping mechanisms, and support system.

CRITICAL THINKING EXERCISES

1. Select a family whose cultural origins are different from your own. Interview an adult member of the family regarding cultural variations related to childbearing and child-rearing activities. Pay particular attention to cultural taboos. How can these cultural beliefs or traditions be incorporated into nursing care during pregnancy and birth.
2. Analyze a childbearing family using the major concepts identified in developmental theory.

References

Aguilera DC: *Crisis intervention: theory and methodology,* ed 7, St Louis, 1994, Mosby.

Blehar MC: Families and public policy. In Corfman E, editor: *Families today,* vol 2, National Institute of Mental Health, Division of Scientific and Public Information, Science Monograph No 1, Washington, DC, 1979, US Government Printing Office.

Bower F, Jacobson M: Family theories: frameworks for nursing practice. In Archer S and Fleshman R, editors: *Community health nursing: patterns and practice,* N Scituate, MA, 1978, Duxbury Press.

Caplan G: *Concepts of mental health and consultation,* Children's Bureau, US Department of Health, Education and Welfare, Washington, DC, 1959, US Government Printing Office.

Carrington BW: The Afro-American. In Clark AL, editor: *Culture/child-bearing/health professionals,* Philadelphia, 1978, FA Davis Co.

Carter B, McGoldrick M: *The changing family life cycle: a framework for family therapy,* ed 2, New York, 1988, Gardner Press, Inc.

Christensen P, Kenney S: *Nursing process: application of theories, frameworks, and models,* ed 4, St Louis, 1995, Mosby.

Chung HQ: Understanding the oriental maternity patient, *Nurs Clin North Am* 12:67, March 1977.

D'Avanzo CE: Bridging the cultural gap with Southeast Asians, *MCN* 17(4):204, 1992.

Duvall ER: *Marriage and family development,* ed 5, Philadelphia, 1977, JB Lippincott Co.

Erikson EH: *Identity: youth and crisis,* New York, 1968, WW Norton & Co, Inc.

Evans MI et al: *Fetal diagnosis and therapy: science, ethics, and the law,* Philadelphia, 1989, JB Lippincott Co.

Evolving American Family, *Statistical Bulletin* 74:2, 1993.

Friedman MM: *Family nursing theory and assessment,* New York, 1992, Appleton-Century-Crofts.

Galanti G: *Caring for patients from different cultures: case studies from American hospitals.* Philadelphia, 1991, University of Pennsylvania Press.

Helman CG: *Culture, health and illness,* London, 1990, Wright.

Kay MA: The Mexican-American. In Clark AL, editor: *Culture/ child-bearing/health professionals,* Philadelphia, 1978, FA Davis Co.

Libman J: The American ideal is kin through thick and thin, *Los Angeles Times,* November 20, 1988.

Mercer RT: Theoretical perspective on the family. In Gillis CL et al, editors: *Toward a science of family nursing,* Menlo Park, CA, 1989, Addison-Wesley Publishing Co, Inc.

Norton A, Glick P: One parent families: a social and economic profile, *Fam Relations* 35(1):9, 1986.

Spector RE: *Cultural diversity in health and illness,* New York, 1991, Appleton-Century-Crofts.

Stern PN et al: Culturally-induced stress during childbearing: the Filipino-American experience, *Issues Health Care Women* 2(3-4):67, 1980.

Stuart GW, Sundeen SJ: *Principles and practice of psychiatric nursing,* ed 5, St Louis, 1995, Mosby.

US Bureau of the Census: *1990 Census of population and housing: summary population and housing characteristics United States,* Washington, DC, 1992, US Department of Commerce, Economics and Statistics Administration, Bureau of the Census.

Williams RP: Issues in women's health care. In Johnson BS, editor: *Psychiatric mental health nursing: adaptation and growth,* Philadelphia, 1989, JB Lippincott Co.

World Health Organization: *Health and the family: studies in the demography of family life cycles and their health implication,* Geneva, 1978, The Organization.

Bibliography

Balcazar H, Cole G, Hartner J: Mexican-Americans' use of prenatal care and its relationship to maternal risk factors and pregnancy outcome, *Am J Prev Med* 8(1):1, 1992.

Burks JA: Factors in the utilization of prenatal services by low-income black women, *Nurse Pract* 17(4):34, 1992.

Geissler EM: *Pocket guide to cultural assessment*, St Louis, 1994, Mosby.

Lazarus ES, Philipson EH: A longitudinal study comparing the prenatal care of Puerto Rican and white women, *Birth* 17(1):6, 1990.

Mattson S, Lew L: Culturally sensitive prenatal care for Southeast Asians, *JOGNN*, 21(1):48, 1992.

Quimby CH, Women and the family of the future, *JOGNN* 23(1):113, 1994.

Scupholme A, Robertson EG, Kamons AS: Barriers to prenatal care in a multiethnic, urban sample, *J Nurse Midwifery* 36(2):111, 1991.

3 Anatomy and Physiology of Reproduction

CYNTHIA GARRETT

LEARNING OBJECTIVES

Define the key terms listed.
Identify the internal, external, and accessory structures of both the female and male reproductive systems.
Explain the functions of the structures of both the female and male reproductive systems.
Summarize the menstrual cycle in relation to hormonal response, ovarian response, and endometrial response.
Identify the four phases of the sexual response cycle.
Compare natural and acquired immunity in the immunocompetent patient.
Explain antibody-mediated and cell-mediated immunity.
Discuss the effects of age, lifestyle, environment, and nutrition on the immune system.

KEY TERMS

acquired (adaptive) immunity
active immunity
climacterium
endometrial cycle
fertilization
hypothalamic-pituitary cycle
immunocompetent
immunology
menarche
menopause
menstruation
natural immunity
ovarian cycle
ovulation
passive immunity
perineum
prostaglandins
pubarche
sexual response cycle
vaccination

RELATED TOPICS

AIDS *(Chap. 21)* • Basal body temperature *(Chap. 18)* • Dysmenorrhea *(Chap. 30)* • Essential factors of labor *(Chap. 9)* • Fertilization and implantation *(Chap. 4)* • Hemolytic disease of the newborn *(Chap. 27)* • Incompetent cervix *(Chap. 21)* • Infertility *(Chap. 30)* • Menopause *(Chap. 30)* • Multifetal pregnancy *(Chap. 4)* • Osteoporosis *(Chap. 30)* • Pap smear *(Chap. 29)* • Prostaglandins for induction of labor *(Chap. 24)* • Prostaglandins for therapeutic abortion *(Chap. 30)* • Rubella infection *(Chap. 21 and 27)* • Toxoplasmosis *(Chap. 21 and 27)*

The purposes of this chapter are to review sexual and reproductive anatomy and physiology, and to present a brief overview of the immune system. Nurses providing health care to women require a greater depth and breadth of knowledge of female and male anatomy and physiology than is usually taught in general courses. To plan, implement, and evaluate nursing care of the maternity patient and her family, knowledge of the anatomy and physiology of female and male structures involved in reproduction is essential.

Although the female and male reproductive systems look different, their structures are homologous (having the same embryonic origin). Each structure performs a vital role in continuing the human species, expressing human sexuality, and generating and maintaining secondary sexual characteristics. Through hormonal influences,

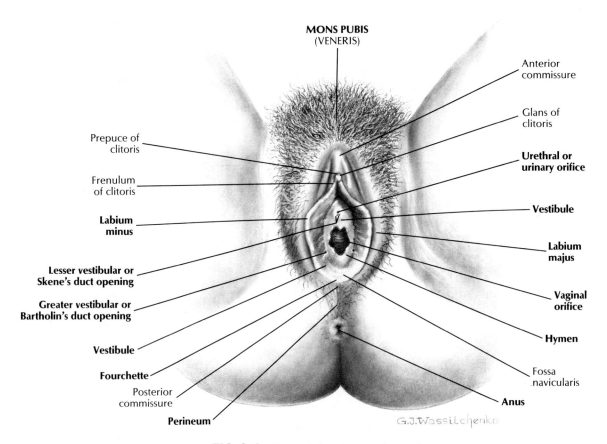

FIG. 3-1 External female genitals.

the genitals, pelvis, and breasts acquire the unique adaptations necessary to childbearing. Both female and male reproductive systems consist of the following four principal components:

1. External genitals
2. A pair of primary sex glands (gonads)
3. Ducts leading from the gonads to the body's exterior
4. Secondary (accessory) sex glands

FEMALE REPRODUCTIVE SYSTEM

The female reproductive system consists of internal organs, located in the pelvic cavity and supported by the pelvic floor, and external genitals, located in the perineum. The female's internal and external reproductive structures develop and mature in response to estrogens and progesterones, which start in fetal life and continuing through puberty and the childbearing years. The reproductive structures *atrophy* (decrease in size) with age or a drop in ovarian hormone production. An extensive and complex innervation and a generous blood supply support the functions of these structures. The appearance of the external genitals varies greatly from woman to woman; heredity, age, race, and number of children a woman has borne determine the size, shape, and color.

External Structures

The external structures or the *vulva* are presented in the following order (from anterior to posterior): Mons pubis (mons veneris), labia majora and minora, clitoris, prepuce of clitoris, vestibule, fourchette, and perineum. The external genitals are illustrated in Fig. 3-1.

Mons Pubis

The mons pubis, or mons veneris, is the rounded, soft fullness of subcutaneous fatty tissue and loose connective tissue over the symphysis pubis. It contains many sebaceous (oil) glands and develops coarse, dark, curly hair at **pubarche,** about 1 to 2 years before the onset of the menses. **Menarche** (the onset of menses) occurs, on the average, at 13 years of age. Characteristics of pubic hair vary from sparse and fine among Oriental women to thick, coarse, and curly among African-American women. The functions of the mons are to play a role in sensuality and to protect the symphysis pubis during coitus (sexual intercourse). As a woman ages, the amount of fatty tissue found in her body decreases, and her pubic hair thins.

Labia Majora

The labia majora are two rounded, lengthwise folds of skin-covered fat and connective tissue that merge with the mons. They extend from the mons downward around the labia minora, ending in the perineum in the midline. The labia majora protect the labia minora, urinary meatus, and vaginal introitus (opening to the vagina). In the woman who has never experienced vaginal childbirth, the labia majora lie close together in the midline, covering the underlying structures. Some labial separation and even gaping of the vaginal introitus follow childbirth and perineal or vaginal injury. Declining hormone production causes the labia majora to atrophy.

On their lateral surfaces the labial skin is thick, usually pigmented darker than the surrounding tissues, and covered with coarse hair (similar to that of the mons) that thins out toward the perineum. The medial (inner) surfaces of the labia majora are smooth, thick, and without hair. They contain an abundant supply of sebaceous glands and sweat glands and are highly vascular. The extreme sensitivity of the labia majora to touch, pain, and temperature is caused by the extensive network of nerves, which also function during sensual arousal.

Labia Minora

The labia minora, located between the labia majora, are narrow, lengthwise folds of hairless skin extending downward from beneath the clitoris and merging with the fourchette. Whereas the lateral and anterior aspects of the labia are usually pigmented, their medial surfaces are similar to vaginal mucosa: pink and moist. Their rich vascularity gives them a reddish color and permits marked turgescence (swelling) of the labia minora with emotional or physical stimulation. The glands in the labia minora also lubricate the vulva. A rich nerve supply makes them sensitive, enhancing their erotic function. The space between the labia minora is called the vestibule.

Clitoris

The clitoris is a short, cylindric, erectile organ fixed just beneath the arch of the pubis. The visible portion is about 6 × 6 mm or less in the unaroused state. The tip of the clitoral body is called the glans and is more sensitive than its shaft. When a woman is sexually aroused, the glans and shaft increase in size.

Sebaceous glands of the clitoris secrete smegma, a cheeselike fatty substance with a distinctive odor that serves as a pheromone (an organic compound that provides olfactory communication with other members of the same species to elicit a certain response, which in this case is erotic stimulation of the human male). The term *clitoris* comes from a Greek word meaning "key," because the clitoris was seen as the key to female sexuality. Its rich vascularity and innervation make the clitoris highly sensitive to temperature, touch, and pressure sensation. The main function of the clitoris is to stimulate and elevate levels of sexual tension.

Prepuce of Clitoris

Near the anterior junction, the right and left labia minora separate into medial and lateral portions. The lat-

eral portions unite above the clitoris to form its prepuce, a hoodlike covering; the medial portions unite below the clitoris to form its frenulum. Sometimes the prepuce covers the clitoris. As a result, this area looks like an opening that can be mistaken for the urethral meatus if the nurse does not identify vulvar structures carefully. Attempts to insert a catheter into this sensitive area can cause considerable discomfort.

Vestibule

The vestibule is an ovoid or boat-shaped area formed between the labia minora, clitoris, and fourchette. The vestibule contains the openings to the urethra, paraurethral (lesser vestibular or Skene's) glands, the vagina, and the paravaginal (greater vestibular, vulvovaginal, or Bartholin's) glands. The thin, almost mucosal surface of the vestibule is easily irritated by chemicals (feminine deodorant sprays, bubble bath salts), heat, discharges, and friction (tight jeans).

Although not a true part of the reproductive system, the *urinary* (urethral) *meatus* is considered here because of its closeness and relationship to the vulva. The meatus is a pink or reddened opening of varying shapes, often with slightly puckered margins. The meatus marks the terminal, or distal, part of the urethra. It is usually about 2.5 cm (1 inch) below the clitoris.

The *lesser vestibular glands* are short tubular structures situated posterolaterally just inside the urethral meatus, at about the 5 and 7 o'clock positions around the meatus. They produce a small amount of mucus, which functions as lubrication.

The *hymen* (see Fig. 3-1) is a partial, rarely complete, elastic but tough mucosa-covered fold around the *vaginal introitus*. In virginal females the hymen may be an impediment to vaginal examination, insertion of menstrual tampons, or coitus. The hymen may be elastic and allow distention, or it may be torn easily. Occasionally the hymen covers the orifice completely, resulting in an imperforate hymen that prevents passage of menstrual flow, instrumentation (e.g., with a speculum), or coitus. A hymenotomy may be necessary in some cases. After instrumentation, use of tampons, coitus, or vaginal birth residual tags of the torn hymen (hymenal caruncles or carunculae myrtiformes) may be seen.

One common myth is that the condition of the hymen tells whether a female is a virgin. Sexually active and even parous women may have intact hymens. For other women, the hymen may be torn during strenuous physical work or exercise, masturbation, or use of tampons. Some cultural groups cleanse the female infant so vigorously that the hymen is torn, leaving only hymenal tags. Therefore the "test for virginity"—evidence of bleeding following the first sexual intercourse—is unreliable.

The *greater vestibular glands* are two compound glands at the base of the labia majora, one on either side of the vaginal orifice. Several ducts, about 1.5 cm long, drain each gland. Each opens into the groove between

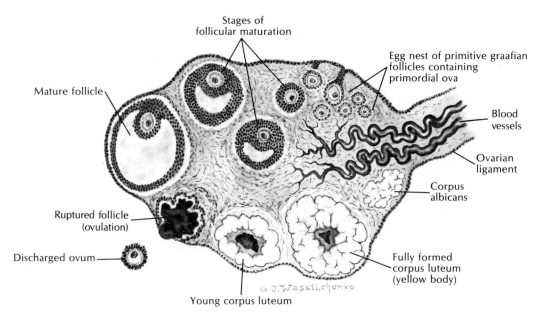

FIG. 3-2 Cross section of ovary.

the hymen and the labia minora. Usually the gland openings are not visible or noticeable. The glands secrete a small amount of clear, sticky mucus, especially during coitus. The alkaline pH of the mucus is supportive of sperm.

Fourchette

The fourchette is a thin, flat, transverse fold of tissue formed where the tapering labia majora and minora merge in the midline below the vaginal orifice. A small depression, the fossa navicularis, lies between the fourchette and the hymen.

Perineum

The **perineum** is the skin-covered muscular area between the vaginal introitus and the anus. The perineum forms the base of the perineal body (see Fig. 3-13, p. 36). The terms *vulva* and *perineum* occasionally, but inaccurately, are used interchangeably.

Internal Structures

The internal reproductive organs are discussed in the order that reflects the ovum's path. Supportive tissues are discussed along with the internal reproductive organs they support. Internal organs include the ovaries, uterine (fallopian) tubes, uterus, and vagina. A brief description of the bony pelvis follows.

Ovaries

One ovary is located on each side of the uterus, below and behind the uterine tubes. Two ligaments hold the ovaries in place, the mesovarian portions of the uterine *broad ligament,* which suspend them from the lateral pelvic side walls at about the level of the anterosuperior iliac

crest, and the *ovarian* ligaments (see Figs. 3-3 and 3-7), which anchor them to the uterus. The ovaries are moveable with palpation.

The ovaries are similar in origin (homologous) to the male testes. Each ovary resembles a large almond in size and shape (Fig. 3-2). At the time of ovulation, ovarian size may double temporarily. The oval-shaped ovaries are firm in consistency and slightly tender. The ovary's surface is smooth before menarche. After sexual maturity, scarring from repeated ruptures of follicles and ovulation roughens the nodular surface.

The two functions of the ovaries are **ovulation** and hormone production. At birth the normal female's ovaries contain countless primordial (primitive) ova. At intervals during the reproductive life (generally monthly) one or more ova mature and undergo ovulation. The ovary is also the major site of production of steroid sex hormones (estrogens, progesterone, and androgens) in amounts required for normal female growth, development, and function.

Fallopian Tubes (Uterine Tubes)

The paired uterine tubes are attached to the uterine fundus (Figs. 3-3, 3-4, and 3-7). The tubes extend laterally, enter the free ends of the broad ligament, and curl around each ovary.

The tubes are approximately 10 cm (4 inches) long and 0.6 cm (¼ inch) in diameter. Each tube has an outer coat of peritoneum, a middle, thin muscular coat, and an inner mucosa. The mucosal lining consists of columnar cells, some of which are ciliated and others of which are secretory. The mucosa is at its thinnest during menstruation. Each tube, along with its mucosa, is continuous with the mucosa of the uterus and of the vagina.

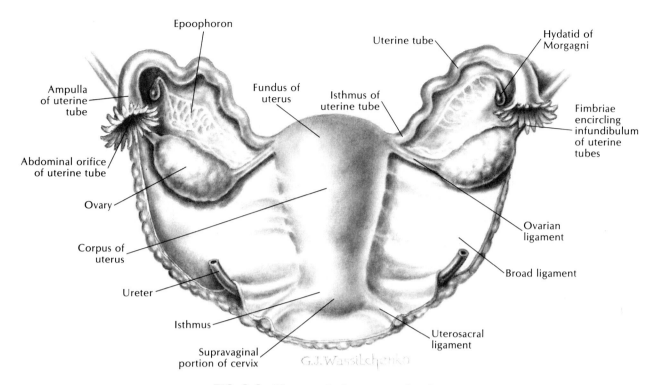

FIG. 3-3   Uterus and adnexa, posterior view.

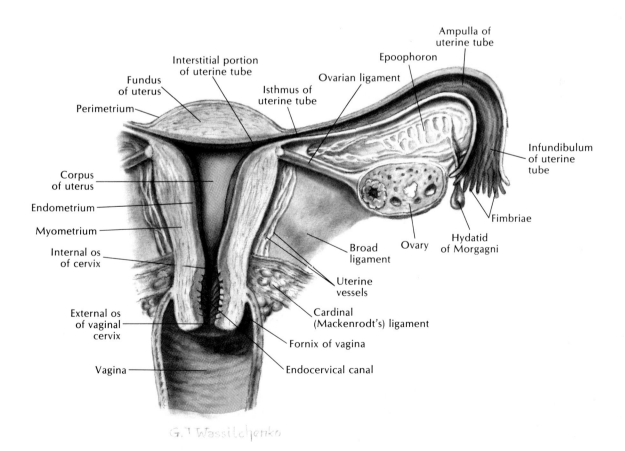

FIG. 3-4   Cross section of uterus, adnexa, and upper vagina.

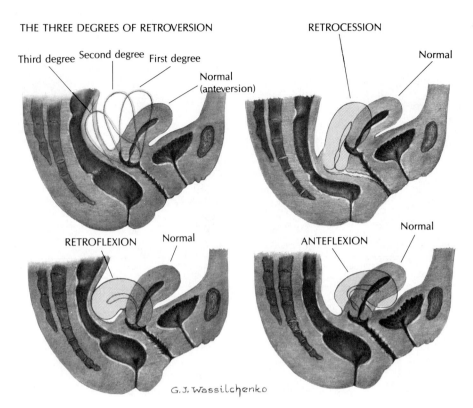

THE THREE DEGREES OF RETROVERSION

Third degree   Second degree   First degree

Normal (anteversion)

RETROCESSION

Normal

RETROFLEXION   Normal

ANTEFLEXION   Normal

Normal

G. J. Wassilchenko

FIG. 3-5 Uterine positions.

The structure of the uterine tube changes along its length. Four distinctive segments can be identified (Figs. 3-3 and 3-4): (1) the infundibulum, (2) the ampulla, (3) the isthmus, and (4) the interstitial. The *infundibulum* is the most distal portion. Its funnel, or trumpet-shaped opening, is encircled with fimbriae. The fimbriae become swollen, almost erectile, at ovulation. The *ampulla* makes up the distal and middle segment of the tube. The sperm and the ovum unite and **fertilization** occurs in the ampulla.

The *isthmus* is proximal to the ampulla. It is small and firm, much like the round ligament. The *interstitial* (or intramural) portion passes through the myometrium between the fundus and the body of the uterus, and has the smallest lumen (tunnel), measuring less than 1 mm in diameter. Before the fertilized ovum can pass through this lumen, it has to discard its crown of granulosa cells.

The uterine tubes provide a passageway for the ovum. The fingerlike projections (fimbriae) of the infundibulum pull the ovum into the tube with wavelike motions. The ovum is propelled along the tube, partially by the cilia but primarily by the peristaltic movements of the muscular coat, toward the uterine cavity. Estrogen and prostaglandins influence peristaltic motion. Peristaltic activity of the uterine tubes and the secretory function of their mucosal lining are greatest at the time of ovulation. The columnar cells secrete a nutrient to sustain the ovum while it is in the tube.

Uterus

Between birth and puberty the uterus descends gradually into the true pelvis from the lower abdomen. After puberty the uterus is usually located in the midline in the true pelvis posterior to the symphysis pubis and urinary bladder and anterior to the rectum.

For most women, with the urinary bladder empty, the uterus is anteverted (tipped forward) and slightly anteflexed (bent forward), with the corpus (body) lying over the top of the posterior wall of the bladder. The cervix is directed downward and backward toward the tip of the sacrum so that it is usually at approximately a right angle to the plane of the vagina. For other women the uterus may be in the midposition or tipped backward (retroverted). A uterus that is bent more than usual, so that the fundus (top) is closer to the cervix, is called anteflexed, or retroflexed (Fig. 3-5).

A full bladder pushes the uterus back toward the rectum. A full rectum moves the uterus forward against the bladder. Uterine position also changes depending on the woman's position (e.g., lying supine, prone, on her side, or standing), her age, and pregnancy. The free mobility permits the uterus to rise slightly during the sexual response cycle (p. 49) so that the cervix is placed in a position to increase the likelihood of fertilization.

Ligaments and muscles of the pelvic floor support the uterus, including the perineal body. A total of 10 ligaments stabilize the uterus within the pelvic cavity

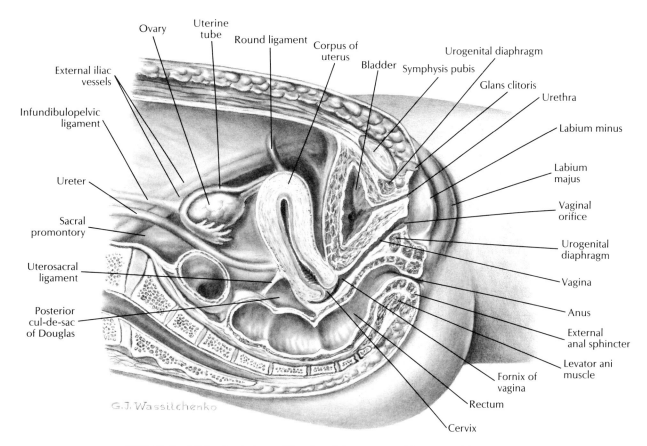

FIG. 3-6   Midsagittal view of female pelvic organs, with woman lying supine.

(see Figs. 3-1, 3-4, and 3-7): four paired ligaments—broad, round, uterosacral, and cardinal (transverse or Mackenrodt's); and two single ligaments—anterior (pubocervical) and posterior (rectovaginal). The posterior ligament forms the deep rectouterine pouch known as the *cul-de-sac of Douglas* (Figs. 3-6 and 3-13).

The uterus is a flattened, hollow, muscular, thick-walled organ that looks somewhat like an upside-down pear (Fig. 3-6). In the adult woman who has never been pregnant, the uterus weighs 60 g (2 oz). The uterus normally is symmetric in shape and nontender, smooth, and firm to the touch. The degree of firmness varies with several factors. For example, the uterus is spongier during the secretory phase of the menstrual cycle, softer during pregnancy, and firmer after menopause.

The uterus has three parts (see Figs. 3-3 and 3-4): the *fundus,* which is the upper, rounded prominence above the insertion of the uterine tubes; the *corpus,* or main portion, encircling the intrauterine cavity; and the *isthmus,* which is the slightly constricted portion that joins the corpus to the cervix and is known during pregnancy as the lower uterine segment.

Three functions of the uterus are cyclic menstruation with rejuvenation of the endometrium, pregnancy, and labor. These functions are essential to reproduction, but not necessary for a woman's physiologic survival.

Uterine Wall

The uterine wall comprises three layers: the endometrium, the myometrium, and a partial outer layer of parietal peritoneum (see Fig. 3-4).

The highly vascular *endometrium* is a lining of mucous membrane composed of three layers: a compact surface layer, a spongy middle layer of loose connective tissue, and a dense inner layer that attaches the endometrium to the myometrium. (The upper two layers are also referred to as the functional layer, and the inner layer as the basal layer.) During menstruation and following birth, the compact surface and middle spongy layers slough off. Just after menstrual flow ends, the endometrium is 0.5 mm thick; near the end of the endometrial cycle, just before menstruation begins again, it is about 5 mm (less than ¼ inch) thick.

Layers of smooth muscle fibers that extend in three directions (longitudinal, transverse, and oblique) make up the thick *myometrium* (Fig. 3-7). The smooth muscle fibers interlace with elastic and connective tissues and blood vessels throughout the uterine wall and blend with the dense inner layer of the endometrium. The myometrium is particularly thick in the fundus, thins out as it nears the isthmus, and is thinnest in the cervix.

Longitudinal fibers make up the *outer* myometrial layer, found mostly in the fundus, making this layer well-

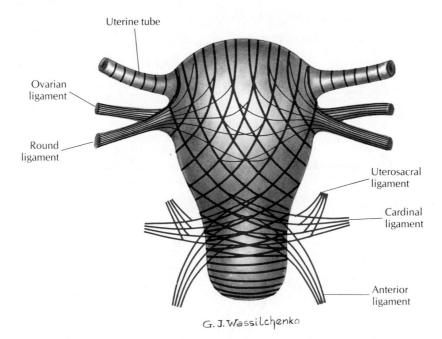

Uterine tube

Ovarian ligament

Round ligament

Uterosacral ligament

Cardinal ligament

Anterior ligament

G. J. Wassilchenko

FIG. 3-7 Schematic arrangement of directions of muscle fibers. Note that uterine muscle fibers are continuous with supportive ligaments of uterus.

suited for expelling the fetus during the birth process. In the thick *middle* myometrial layer, the interlaced muscle fibers form a figure-eight pattern encircling large blood vessels. Contraction of the middle layer produces a hemostatic action (Fig. 3-8). Only a few circular fibers of the *inner* myometrial layer are found in the fundus. Most of the circular fibers are concentrated in the cornua (the place where the uterine tubes join the uterine body) and around the internal os (opening). The sphincter action of this layer prevents the regurgitation of menstrual blood out of the uterine tubes during menstruation. This sphincter action around the internal cervical os helps retain the uterine contents during pregnancy. Injury to this sphincter can weaken the internal os and result in an incompetent internal cervical os.

Remember, the myometrium works as a whole. The structure of the myometrium, which gives strength and elasticity, presents an example of adaptation to function:

1. To thin out, pull up, and open the cervix and to push the fetus out of the uterus, the fundus must contract with the most force.
2. Contraction of interlacing smooth muscle fibers that surround the blood vessels controls blood loss after abortion and childbirth. Because of their ability to close off (ligate) blood vessels between them, the smooth muscle fibers of the uterus are referred to as the *living ligature* (Fig. 3-8).

The *parietal peritoneum,* a serous membrane, coats all of the uterine corpus except for the lower one fourth of the anterior surface, where the bladder is attached, and the cervix. Diagnostic tests and surgery involving the uterus can be performed without entering the abdominal cavity because parietal peritoneum does not completely cover the uterine corpus.

Cervix

The lowermost portion of the uterus is the cervix, or neck. The attachment site of the uterine cervix to the vaginal vault divides the cervix into the longer supravaginal (above the vagina) portion (see Fig. 3-3) and the shorter vaginal portion (see Fig. 3-4). The length of the cervix is about 2.5 to 3 cm, of which about 1 cm protrudes into the vagina in the nonpregnant woman.

The cervix is composed primarily of fibrous connective tissue with some muscle fibers and elastic tissue. The cervix of the nulliparous woman is a rounded, almost conical, rather firm, spindle-shaped body. The narrowed opening between the uterine cavity and the endocervical canal (canal inside the cervix that connects the uterine cavity with the vagina) is the *internal os.* The narrowed opening between the endocervix and the vagina is the *external os,* a small, circular opening in women who have not borne children. Childbirth changes the circular os to a small transverse opening dividing the cervix into an anterior and a posterior lip (Fig. 3-9).

When a woman is not ovulating or not pregnant, the tip of the cervix feels firm, much like the end of the nose, with a dimple in the center. This dimple marks the site of the external os.

The most significant characteristic of the cervix is its ability to stretch during vaginal childbirth. Several factors contribute to cervical elasticity: high connective tissue and elastic fiber content, numerous infoldings in the endocervical lining, and a 10% muscle fiber content.

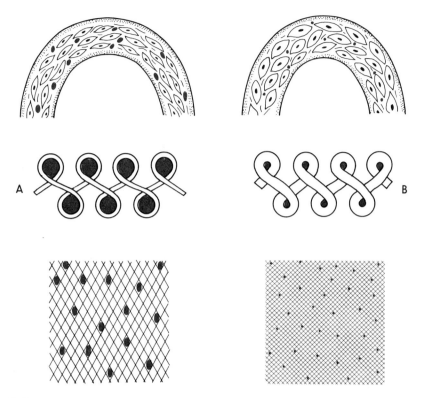

FIG. 3-8 The living ligature: interlacing smooth muscle fibers of the thick middle myometrium. **A,** Relaxed muscle fibers. **B,** Contracted muscle fibers ligating the blood vessels.

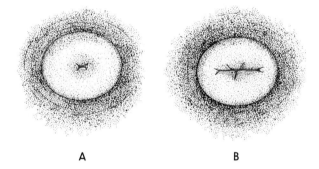

FIG. 3-9 External cervical os as seen through speculum. **A,** Nonparous cervix. **B,** Parous cervix.

Canals

Two cavities within the uterus are known as the uterine and cervical canals (see Fig. 3-4). The uterine canal in the nonpregnant state is compressed by thick muscular walls so that it is only a potential space, flat and triangular. The fundus forms the base of the triangle. The uterine tubes open into either end of the base. The apex of the triangle points downward and forms the internal os of the cervical canal.

The endocervical canal, with its many infoldings, has a surface layer of tall, columnar, mucus-producing cells. *Columnar epithelium* is beefy red, deeper, and rougher looking than the epithelial outer covering of the cervix. After menarche, *squamous epithelium* covers the outside

of the cervix (ectocervix). This external covering of flat cells gives a glistening pink color to the cervix. A deeper bluish-red color is seen when the woman is ovulating or pregnant. A reddened (hyperemic) cervix may indicate inflammation.

The two types of epithelium meet at the *squamocolumnar junction*. This junction line is usually just inside the external cervical os, but may be found on the ectocervix in some women. The squamocolumnar junction is the most common site of neoplastic cellular changes. Therefore cells for cytologic study, the Papanicolaou (Pap) smear, are scraped from this junction.

The columnar epithelial cells produce odorless and nonirritating mucus in response to ovarian endocrine hormones—estrogen and progesterone.

Blood Vessels

The abdominal aorta divides at about the level of the umbilicus and forms the two iliac arteries. Each iliac artery divides to form two arteries, the major one of which is the hypogastric artery. The uterine arteries branch off from the *hypogastric arteries.* The closeness of the uterus to the aorta ensures an ample blood supply to meet the needs of the growing uterus and conceptus.

In addition, the ovarian artery, a direct subdivision of the aorta, first supplies the ovary with the blood and then proceeds to join the uterine artery, thus adding to the blood supply (Fig. 3-10).

In the nonpregnant state, the uterine blood vessels are

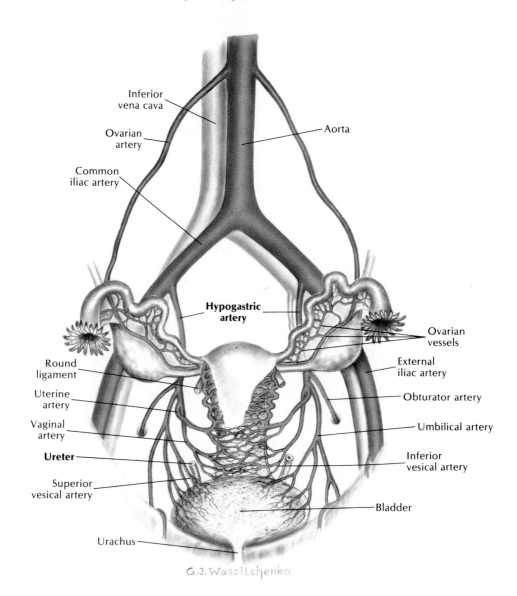

Inferior
vena cava

Ovarian
artery

Aorta

Common
iliac artery

**Hypogastric
artery**

Ovarian
vessels

Round
ligament

External
iliac artery

Uterine
artery

Obturator artery

Vaginal
artery

Umbilical artery

Ureter

Inferior
vesical artery

Superior
vesical artery

Bladder

Urachus

G.J. Wassilchenko

FIG. 3-10 Pelvic blood supply.

coiled and tortuous (twisted). With advancing pregnancy and an enlarging uterus, these blood vessels straighten. The uterine veins follow along the arteries and empty into the internal iliac veins.

Vagina

The vagina, a tubular structure located in front of the rectum and behind the bladder and urethra (see Fig. 3-6), extends from the introitus (the external opening in the vestibule between the labia minora of the vulva) to the cervix. When a woman is standing, the vagina slants backward and upward. It is supported mainly by its attachments to the pelvic floor musculature and fascia.

The vagina is a thin-walled, collapsible tube capable of great distention. Because of the way the cervix protrudes into the uppermost portion of the vagina, the length of the anterior wall of the vagina is only about 7.5 cm, while that of the posterior wall is about 9 cm. The recesses formed all around the protruding cervix are

called fornices: right, left, anterior, and posterior. The posterior fornix is deeper than the other three (see Figs. 3-4 and 3-13).

Glandular mucous membrane lines the smooth muscle walls. During the reproductive years this mucosa is arranged in transverse folds called *rugae*.

The vaginal mucosa responds promptly to estrogen and progesterone stimulation. The mucosa loses cells, especially during the menstrual cycle and pregnancy. Cells scraped from the vaginal mucosa can be used to estimate steroid sex hormone levels.

Vaginal fluid is derived from the lower or upper genital tract. The fluid should be slightly acidic. Interaction between vaginal lactobacilli and glycogen maintain acidity. If the pH rises above 5, the incidence of vaginal infection increases. The continuous flow of fluid from the vagina maintains relative cleanliness of the vagina. Therefore *vaginal douching in normal circumstances is neither necessary, nor recommended.*

A *Papanicolaou smear,* used throughout the world for

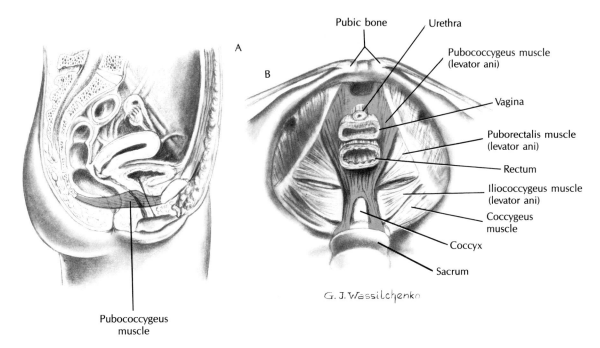

FIG. 3-11 Upper pelvic diaphragm. **A,** Pubococcygeus portion of levator ani muscles, mid-sagittal view. **B,** View from above.

cancer detection by cell examination (cytology), is a spread of vaginal mucus from the posterior vaginal fornix and a scraping from the squamocolumnar junction of the cervix fixed in ethyl ether and alcohol and then treated with trichrome nucleocytoplasmic stain.

The copious blood supply to the vagina is derived from the descending branches of the uterine artery, vaginal artery, and internal pudendal arteries (see Fig. 3-10).

The vagina is relatively insensitive. There is some innervation from the pudendal and hemorrhoidal nerves to the lowest one third of the vagina. Due to this minimal innervation and lack of special nerve endings, the vagina is the source of little sensation during sexual excitement and coitus, and causes less pain during the second stage of labor than if this tissue were well-supplied with nerve endings.

The *G-spot* is an area on the anterior vaginal wall beneath the urethra defined by Graefenberg as analogous to the male prostate gland. During sexual arousal, the G-spot may be stimulated to the point of orgasm with ejaculation into the urethra of fluid similar in nature to prostatic fluid (Herbst et al, 1992).

The vagina functions as the organ for coitus and as the birth canal.

Pelvic Floor and Perineum

The pelvic diaphragm, the urogenital diaphragm or triangle, and the muscles of the external genitals and anus compose the pelvic floor and perineum. The perineum is sometimes defined as including all the muscles, fascia, and ligaments of the upper (pelvic) and lower (urogenital) diaphragms. The perineal body adds strength to these structures.

The *upper pelvic diaphragm,* composed of muscles and their fascia and ligaments, extends across the lowest part of the pelvic cavity like a hammock (Fig. 3-11). The largest and most significant portion of the diaphragm is formed by the pair of broad, thin *levator ani muscles* that extend sheetlike between the ischial spines and coccyx, and the sacrum. The levator ani group of muscles is made of three muscle pairs: puborectalis, iliococcygeus, and pubococcygeus muscles. The pubococcygeus muscle is significant, because it plays a role in sexual sensory function, in bladder control, in controlling perineal relaxation during labor, and in expulsion of the fetus during birth.

The second paired muscles of the upper pelvic diaphragm are the closely joined *coccygeus muscles.* These muscles extend from the ischial spines to the coccyx and lower sacrum. The parts of the pelvic diaphragm provide a slinglike support to abdominal and pelvic viscera.

The strength and resilience of this sling are derived from the way in which the layered parts of this sling are interwoven and interlaced. *The layers are not fixed; that is, they slide over each other.* This unique arrangement strengthens the supportive capacity of the pelvic diaphragm, allows for dilation of the vagina during the birth process and for its closure after birth, and assists with constriction of the urethra, vagina, and anal canal, which pass through the diaphragm.

The *lower pelvic diaphragm* is located in the hollow of the pubic arch and consists of the transverse perineal muscles, which originate at the ischial tuberosities and insert into the perineal body. The strong muscle fibers provide support to the anal canal during defecation and to the lower vagina during birth. The deep transverse perineal muscles join to form a central seam, or raphe.

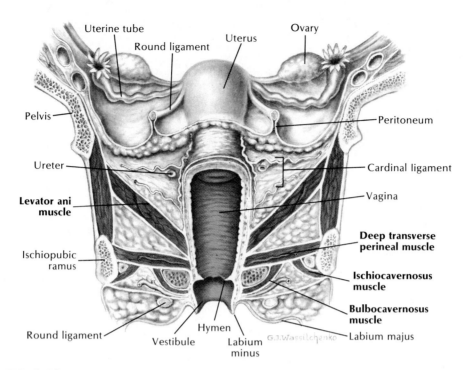

FIG. 3-12 Levator ani muscles of upper pelvic diaphragm and urogenital (lower pelvic) diaphragm, anterior view.

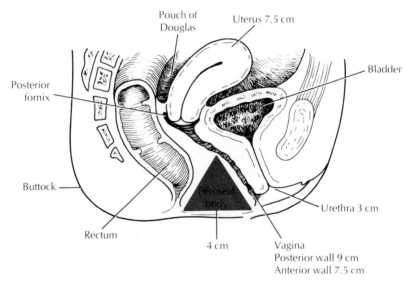

FIG. 3-13 Perineal body. Location and size relative to surrounding tissues, with woman sitting.

Some of their fibers encircle the urinary meatus and vaginal sphincters.

The *perineum* is located below the upper and lower pelvic diaphragms. Its muscles and fascia reinforce the strength of the pelvic diaphragm, and aid in constricting the urinary, vaginal, and anal openings. The *bulbocavernosus muscle* (Fig. 3-12) fibers originate in the perineal body and surround the vaginal opening as the muscle fibers pass forward to insert into the pubis.

The *ischiocavernosus muscles* originate in the tuberosi-ties of the ischium and continue at an angle to insert next to the bulbocavernosus muscles (see Fig. 3-12). These muscle fibers contract to cause erection of the clitoris.

Anal sphincter muscle fibers originate at the coccyx, separate to pass on either side of the anus, fuse, and then insert into the transverse perineal muscles.

The bulbocavernosus, transverse perineal, and anal sphincter muscle fibers can be strengthened through Kegel exercises (for a description of Kegel exercises, see Chapter 7).

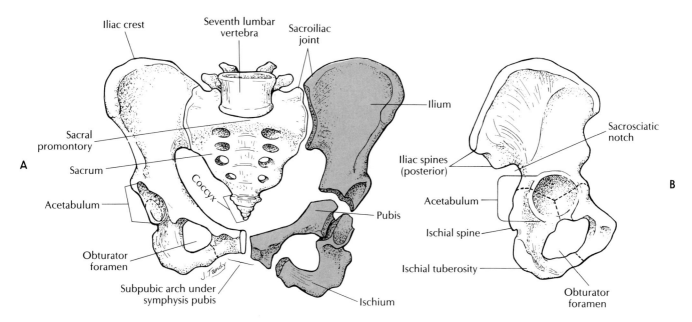

FIG. 3-14   Adult female pelvis. **A,** Anterior view. **B,** External view of innominate bone (fused).

The *perineal body,* the wedge-shaped mass between the vaginal and anal openings, serves as an anchor point for the muscles, fascia, and ligaments of the upper and lower pelvic diaphragms (Fig. 3-13). The skin-covered base of the body is known as the perineum. The perineal body is continuous with the septum between the rectum and vagina. This tissue is flattened and stretched as the fetus moves through the birth canal.

Bony Pelvis

The nurse needs to be thoroughly familiar with the bony pelvis to understand the female reproductive tract and perineum. The pelvis serves three primary purposes: (1) its bony cavity produces a protective cradle for pelvic structures, (2) its architecture is of special importance in accommodating a growing fetus throughout pregnancy and during the birth process, and (3) its strength provides stable anchorage for the attachment of supportive muscles, fascia, and ligaments.

In a study of the bony pelvis, the following structures and *landmarks* are especially important (Fig. 3-14): iliac crest and superior, anterior iliac spine; sacral promontory; sacrum; coccyx; symphysis pubis; subpubic arch; ischial spines; and ischial tuberosities.

The pelvis (Fig. 3-14, *A*) is made of four bones: (1) the right and (2) the left innominate bones, each of which comprises the right or left pubic bone, ilium, and ischium, which fuse after puberty; (3) the sacrum; and (4) the coccyx. The two *innominate bones* (hip bones) form the sides and front of the bony passage, and the *sacrum* and *coccyx* form the back.

Below the *ilium* is the *ischium,* a heavy bone terminating posteriorly in the rounded protuberances known as the *ischial tuberosities* (see Fig. 3-14, *B*). The tuberosities bear the body's weight in the sitting position. The *ischial spines,* the sharp projections from the posterior border of the ischium into the pelvic cavity, may be blunt or prominent.

The *pubis,* forming the front portion of the pelvic cavity, is located beneath the mons. In the midline the two pubic bones are joined by strong ligaments and a thick cartilage to form the joint called the symphysis pubis. In the female the angle formed by the subpubic arch optimally measures slightly more than 90 degrees.

Five fused vertebrae form the *sacrum.* The upper anterior portion of the body of the first sacral vertebra, the promontory, forms the posterior margin of the pelvic brim.

The *coccyx* (tailbone), composed of three to five fused vertebrae, articulates with the sacrum. The coccyx projects downward and forward from the lower border of the sacrum.

The pelvis is divided into two sections, the shallow upper basin, or false pelvis, and the deeper lower, or true pelvis (Fig. 3-15, *A*). The *false pelvis* lies above the linea terminalis (brim or inlet) and varies considerably in size in different women. The *true pelvis* consists of the brim, or inlet, and the area below.

Pelvic planes include those of the *inlet,* the *midpelvis,* and the *outlet.* The cavity of the (true) midpelvis resembles an irregularly curved canal (Fig. 3-15, *B*) with unequal anterior and posterior surfaces. The anterior surface is formed by the length of the symphysis. The posterior surface is formed by the length of the sacrum.

Age, sex, and race are responsible for the greatest variations in pelvic shape and size. There is considerable change in the pelvis during growth and development. Pelvic ossification is complete at about 20 years of age or slightly later. Smaller people have smaller, lighter bones than larger people.

Breasts

The breasts are paired mammary glands located between the second and sixth ribs (Fig. 3-16). About two thirds of the breast overlies the pectoralis major muscle, between the sternum and midaxillary line, with an exten-

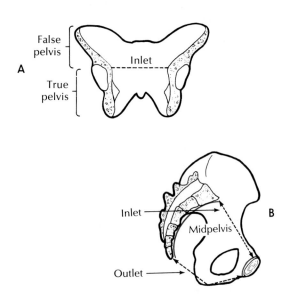

FIG. 3-15 Female pelvis. **A,** Cavity of false pelvis is shallow. **B,** Cavity of true pelvis is an irregularly curved canal *(arrows).*

sion to the axilla referred to as the tail of Spence. The lower one third of the breast overlies the serratus anterior muscle. The breasts are attached to the muscles by connective tissue or fascia.

The breasts of healthy mature women are approximately equal in size and shape, but are often not absolutely symmetric. The size and shape vary depending on the woman's age, heredity, and nutrition. However, the contour should be smooth with no retractions, dimpling, or masses.

True glandular tissue is called *parenchyma;* supporting tissues, the fat, and fibrous connective tissue are called *stroma.* The relative amount of stroma determines the size and consistency of the breast.

Estrogen stimulates growth of the breast by inducing fat deposition in the breasts, development of stromal tissue (i.e., increase in its amount and elasticity), and growth of the extensive ductile system. Estrogen also increases the vascularity of breast tissue.

Once ovulation begins in puberty, progesterone levels increase. The increase in progesterone causes maturation of mammary gland tissue, specifically the lobules and acinar structures. During adolescence, fat deposition and growth of fibrous tissue contribute to the increase in the gland's size. Full development of the breasts is not achieved until after the end of the first pregnancy or in the early period of lactation.

Each mammary gland is made of 15 to 20 lobes, which are divided into lobules. Lobules are clusters of acini. An acinus is a saclike terminal part of a compound gland emptying through a narrow lumen or duct. In dis-

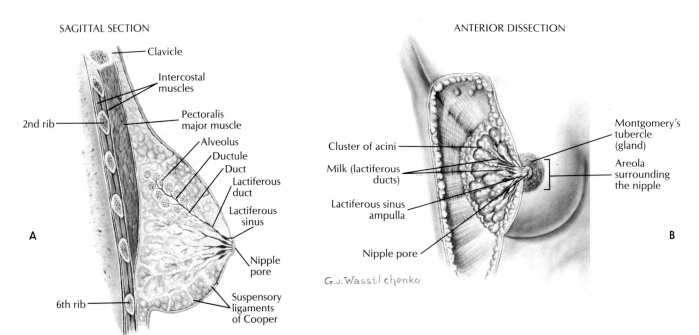

FIG. 3-16 Position and structure of mammary gland. **A,** Sagittal section. **B,** Anterior dissection. (**A,** From Seidel HM et al: *Mosby's guide to physical examination,* St Louis, 1987, Mosby.)

cussions of mammary glands, the correct anatomic term *(acinus)* is often used interchangeably with *alveolus.* The acini are lined with epithelial cells that secrete colostrum and milk. Just below the epithelium is the myoepithelium (*myo,* or muscle), which contracts to expel milk from the acini (Fig. 3-17).

The ducts from the clusters of acini that form the lobules merge to form larger ducts draining the lobes. Ducts from the lobes converge in a single nipple (mammary papilla) surrounded by an areola. Just as the ducts converge, they dilate to form common lactiferous sinuses, which are also called ampullae. The lactiferous sinuses serve as milk reservoirs. Many tiny lactiferous ducts drain the ampullae and exit in the nipple.

The glandular structures and ducts are surrounded by protective fatty tissue and are separated and supported by fibrous suspensory *Cooper's ligaments.* Cooper's ligaments provide support to the mammary glands while permitting their mobility on the chest wall.

The round nipple is usually slightly elevated above the breast. On each breast the nipple projects slightly upward and laterally. It contains 15 to 20 openings from lactiferous ducts. The nipple is surrounded by fibromuscular tissue and covered by wrinkled skin. Except during pregnancy and lactation, there is usually no discharge from the nipple.

The nipple and surrounding areola are usually more deeply pigmented than the skin of the breast. The rough appearance of the areola is caused by sebaceous glands, *Montgomery tubercles* (see Fig. 3-16), directly beneath the skin. These glands secrete a fatty substance, thought to lubricate the nipple. Smooth muscle fibers in the areola contract to stiffen the nipple to make it easier for the breastfeeding infant to grasp.

The vascular supply to the mammary gland is abundant. In the nonpregnant state the skin does not have an obvious vascular pattern. The normal skin is smooth without tightness or shininess.

The skin covering the breasts contains an extensive superficial lymphatic network that serves the entire chest wall and is continuous with the superficial lymphatics of the neck and abdomen. In the deeper portions of the breasts, the lymphatics form a rich network as well. The primary deep lymphatic pathway drains laterally toward the axillae.

Besides their function of lactation, breasts function as organs for sexual arousal in the mature adult.

The breasts change in size and nodularity in response to cyclic ovarian changes throughout reproductive life. Increasing levels of both estrogen and progesterone in the 3 to 4 days before menstruation increase vascularity of the breasts, induce growth of the ducts and acini, and promote water retention. The epithelial cells lining the ducts proliferate in number, the ducts dilate, and the lobules distend. The acini become enlarged and secretory, and lipid (fat) is deposited within their epithelial cell lin-

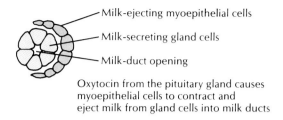

Oxytocin from the pituitary gland causes myoepithelial cells to contract and eject milk from gland cells into milk ducts

FIG. 3-17 Acinus in cross section.

ing. As a result, breast swelling, tenderness, and discomfort are common symptoms just before the onset of menstruation. After menstruation, cellular proliferation begins to regress, acini begin to decrease in size, and retained water is lost.

After breasts have undergone changes numerous times in response to the ovarian cycle, the proliferation and involution (regression) are not uniform throughout the breast. In time, after repeated hormonal stimulation, small persistent areas of nodulations may develop. This normal physiologic change must be remembered when breast tissue is examined. Nodules may develop just before and during menstruation, when the breast is most active. The physiologic alterations in breast size and activity reach their minimum level about 5 to 7 days after menstruation stops. Therefore breast self-examination is best carried out during this phase of the menstrual cycle (Fig. 3-18).

Menstrual Cycle

Knowledge of the menstrual cycle is important for nurses providing care to women across the life span. Nurses should be knowledgeable about menstrual myths, menarche, the endometrial cycle, the hypothalamic-pituitary cycle, the ovarian cycle, other cyclic changes, and the climacterium.

Menstrual Myths

Many myths have their origin in the mystery that surrounded the woman, her hidden reproductive organs, and her uniqueness in adding new members to society. As a consequence, a vast store of folklore, fancies, and superstitions evolved. Because of their recurring nature and similar sequence, menstrual cycles were thought to be under the control of the moon. Before the discovery of ovulation in humans, people thought that an egg was produced during menstruation only when fruitful intercourse had occurred. Not until the nineteenth century was knowledge available about the existence of the human egg, ovulation, and ovarian functioning.

As late as the second half of this century, the many behavioral changes falsely attributed to women during their menstrual cycles have been used to argue, for example, why electing a woman president of the United States would be unwise. Historical literature contains many references to dangers attributed to menstruating

The *proliferative phase* is a period of rapid growth lasting from about the fifth day to the time of ovulation, which would be, for example, day 10 of a 24-day cycle, day 14 of a 28-day cycle, or day 18 of a 32-day cycle. The endometrial surface is completely restored in approximately 4 days, or slightly before bleeding ceases. From this point on an eightfold to tenfold thickening occurs with a leveling off of growth at ovulation. The proliferative phase depends on estrogen stimulation derived from ovarian (graafian) follicles.

The *secretory phase* extends from the day of ovulation to about 3 days before the next menstrual period. After ovulation, larger amounts of progesterone are produced. An edematous, vascular, functional endometrium is now apparent.

At the end of the secretory phase the fully matured secretory endometrium reaches the thickness of heavy, soft velvet. It becomes luxuriant with blood and glandular secretions, a suitable protective and nutritive bed for a fertilized ovum, should one be available.

Implantation (nidation) of the fertilized ovum generally occurs about 7 to 10 days after ovulation. If fertilization and implantation do not occur, the corpus luteum (yellow body), which secretes estrogen and progesterone, regresses. With the rapid fall in progesterone and estrogen levels, the spiral arteries go into a spasm. During the *ischemic phase,* the blood supply to the functional endometrium is blocked and necrosis develops. The functional layer separates from the basal layer, and menstrual bleeding begins, marking day 1 of the next cycle.

Hypothalamic-Pituitary Cycle

Toward the end of the normal menstrual cycle, blood levels of estrogen and progesterone fall (Fig. 3-18). Low blood levels of these ovarian hormones stimulate the hypothalamus to secrete gonadotropin-releasing hormone (Gn-RH). Gn-RH, in turn, stimulates anterior pituitary secretion of follicle stimulating hormone (FSH). FSH stimulates development of ovarian graafian follicles and their production of estrogen. Estrogen levels begin to fall, and hypothalamic Gn-RH triggers the anterior pituitary release of lutenizing hormone (LH). A marked surge of LH and a smaller peak of estrogen (day 12; Fig. 3-19) precede the expulsion of the ovum from the graafian follicle by about 24 to 36 hours. LH peaks about the thirteenth or fourteenth day of a 28-day cycle. If fertilization and implantation of the ovum have not occurred by this time, regression of the corpus luteum follows. Therefore the levels of progesterone and estrogen decline, menstruation occurs, and the hypothalamus is once again stimulated to secrete Gn-RH. This process is called the **hypothalamic-pituitary cycle.**

Ovarian Cycle

The primitive graafian follicles contain immature oocytes (primordial ova) (see Fig. 3-2). Before ovulation, from 1 to 30 follicles begin to mature in each ovary under the influence of FSH and estrogen. The preovulatory surge of LH affects a selected follicle. Within the chosen follicle, the oocyte matures, ovulation occurs, and the empty follicle begins its transformation into the corpus luteum. This *follicular phase* (preovulatory phase) (Fig. 3-19) of the ovarian menstrual cycle varies in length from woman to woman. *Almost all variations in* **ovarian cycle** *length are the result of variations in the length of the follicular phase.* On rare occasions (i.e., 1 in 100 menstrual cycles), more than one follicle is selected, and more than one oocyte matures and undergoes ovulation.

After ovulation, estrogen levels drop. For 90% of women, only a small amount of *withdrawal bleeding* occurs so that it goes unnoticed. In 10% of women, there is sufficient bleeding for it to be visible, resulting in what is known as *midcycle bleeding.*

The *luteal phase* begins immediately after ovulation and ends with the start of menstruation. This postovulatory phase of the ovarian cycle usually requires *14 days* (range of 13 to 15 days). The corpus luteum reaches its peak of functional activity 8 days after ovulation, secreting both of the steroids estrogen and progesterone. Coincident with this time of peak luteal functioning, the fertilized egg is implanted in the endometrium. If no implantation occurs, the corpus luteum regresses, and steroid levels drop. Two weeks after ovulation, if fertilization and implantation do not occur, the functional layer of the uterine endometrium is shed through menstruation.

Other Cyclic Changes

When the hypothalamic-pituitary-ovarian axis functions properly, other tissues undergo predictable responses. Before ovulation the woman's basal body temperature (BBT) is lower, often below 98.6° F (37° C); after ovulation, with rising progesterone levels, her BBT rises (see Clinical Application of Research). Changes in the cervix and cervical mucus follow a generally predictable pattern (Figs. 3-20 and 3-21). Preovulatory and postovulatory mucus is viscous (sticky) so that sperm penetration is discouraged. At the time of ovulation, cervical mucus is thin and clear. It looks, feels, and stretches like egg white. This stretchable quality is termed *spinnbarkheit* (Fig. 3-20). Some women experience localized lower abdominal pain called *mittelschmerz* that coincides with ovulation.

These, and other cyclic changes, enhance fertility awareness and form the basis for the symptothermal method used for conception and contraception. The subjective and objective signs are biologic markers of the phases of the menstrual cycle (Table 3-1). Examination of women with impaired fertility includes a thorough documentation of the presence or absence of these biologic markers.

CLINICAL APPLICATION OF RESEARCH

TYMPANIC THERMOMETRY FOR TAKING BASAL BODY TEMPERATURES

Basal body temperature is commonly used in family planning to monitor ovulation for achieving and preventing pregnancy. First morning oral, rectal, and vaginal temperatures using glass/mercury or electronic thermometers are satisfactory for this purpose. Tympanic membrane (TM) thermometry has been shown to be accurate and to correlate with other methods. This study was undertaken to compare TM with oral and rectal digital and glass thermometry in detection of ovulation. Twelve regularly menstruating women between the ages of 18 and 42 participated. For one month the women recorded first morning temperatures daily at three sites (oral, rectal, and tympanic membrane) with three types of thermometers (oral digital, oral and rectal glass/mercury, and TM recording device). They recorded their temperatures from the right and left sublingual areas of the mouth simultaneously using digital and glass/mercury thermometers, from the rectum using a glass/mercury thermometer, and from the right ear with the TM recording device. The rectal temperature was the most ac-

curate, and the other recordings were compared to it. The researchers found that the day of ovulation detected with the TM was the same as that noted from rectal temperature graphs in 9 out of 10 instances; one women had a discrepancy of one day. The mercury thermometers for both the oral and rectal routes showed the same day of ovulation. There was a one day discrepancy between the oral digital and the rectal temperature recordings. A greater difference in temperature existed between the luteal phase and the proliferative phase for the TM temperatures than for the oral or rectal readings. Participants reported that they preferred the TM device over the other types of thermometry. Nurses may recommend use of TM thermometry for its rapidity of recording and simplicity of use. They should become familiar with such devices and be prepared to provide patient teaching for patients who use the device.

Reference: Wolf GC, Baker CA: Tympanic thermometry for recording basal body temperatures, *Fertil Steril* 60:922, 1993.

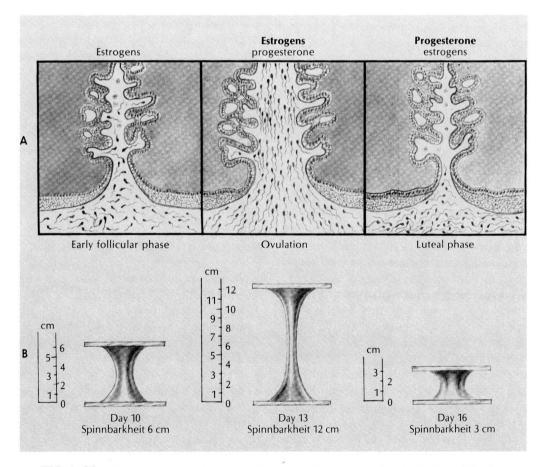

FIG. 3-20 Changes in cervical mucus and cervix during menstrual cycle. **A,** Early follicular. **B,** Ovulation. **C,** Luteal phase.

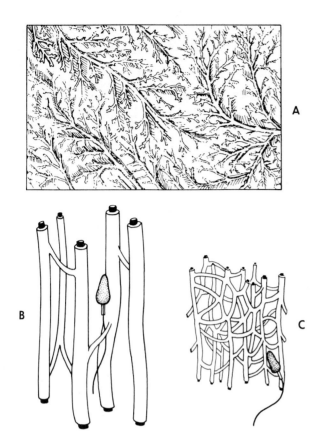

FIG. 3-21 Cervical mucus changes during menstrual cycle. **A,** Fern pattern. **B,** Mucus receptive to sperm passage. **C,** Mucus nonreceptive to sperm passage.

Prostaglandins

Prostaglandins (PGs) are oxygenated fatty acids now classified as hormones. The different kinds of PGs are distinguished by letters (PGE, PGF), numbers (PGE_2), and letters of the Greek alphabet ($PGF_{2\alpha}$).

PGs are produced in most organs of the body, but most notably by the prostate and the endometrium. Therefore semen and menstrual blood are potent prostaglandin sources. PGs are metabolized quickly by most tissues. They are biologically active in minute amounts in the cardiovascular, gastrointestinal, respiratory, urogenital, and nervous systems. They also exert a marked effect on metabolism, particularly on glycolysis. Prostaglandins play an important role in many physiologic, pathologic, and pharmacologic reactions. $PGF_{2\alpha}$, PGE_4, and PGE_2 are most commonly used in reproductive medicine.

Prostaglandins affect smooth muscle contractility and modulation of hormonal activity. Indirect evidence supports PGs' effects on: ovulation, fertility, changes in the cervix and cervical mucus that affect receptivity to sperm, tubal and uterine motility, sloughing of endometrium (menstruation), onset of abortion (spontaneous and induced), and onset of labor (term and preterm).

After exerting their biologic actions, newly synthe-sized PGs are rapidly metabolized by tissues in such organs as the lungs, kidneys, and liver.

PGs may play a key role in ovulation. If PG levels do not rise along with the surge of LH, the ovum remains trapped within the graafian follicle. After ovulation, PGs may influence production of estrogen and progesterone by the corpus luteum.

The introduction of PGs into the vagina or into the uterine cavity (from ejaculated semen) increases the motility of uterine musculature, which may assist the transport of sperm through the uterus and into the oviduct. High concentration of PGs in the semen (about 55 μg/ml) may be necessary for normal fertility in males.

PGs produced by the woman cause regression (return to an earlier state) of the corpus luteum, regression of the endometrium, and sloughing of the endometrium, which results in menstruation. PGs increase myometrial response to oxytocic stimulation, enhance uterine contractions, and cause cervical dilation. They may be one factor in the initiation or maintenance of labor, or both. They may also be involved in the following pathologic states: male infertility, dysmenorrhea, hypertensive states, preeclampsia-eclampsia, and anaphylactic shock.

Climacterium

The **climacterium** (perimenopause) is a transitional phase during which ovarian function and hormone production decline. This phase spans the years from the onset of premenopausal ovarian decline to the postmenopausal time when symptoms stop. **Menopause** (from the Latin *mensis,* month, and Greek *pausis,* to cease) refers only to the last menstrual period. Unlike menarche, however, menopause can be dated only with certainty 1 year after menstruation ceases. The average age at natural menopause is 51.4 years, with an age range of 35 to 60 years.

MALE REPRODUCTIVE SYSTEM

The male reproductive system consists of external genitals and internal organs located in the pelvic cavity. The male's reproductive system begins to develop in response to testosterone during early fetal life. Essentially, no testosterone is produced during childhood. Resumption of testosterone production at the onset of puberty stimulates growth and maturation of reproductive structures and secondary sex characteristics. The size and appearance of the external genitals vary with age, heredity, race, and culture.

External Structures

The structures that make up the external genitals are presented in the following order: mons pubis, penis, and scrotum.

At maturity, pubic hair is long, dense, coarse, and

TABLE 3-1   Signs and Symptoms of the Phases of the Menstrual Cycle

SIGN	PREOVULATION	OVULATION	AT LEAST 2 DAYS AFTER OVULATION UP TO MENSES
SUBJECTIVE SIGNS			
Physical Discomfort			
Breasts	Unreported	Unreported	Heaviness, fullness; enlarged, tender*
Abdomen	Dysmenorrhea: uterine cramping; nausea, vomiting, and diarrhea; dizziness	Intermenstrual pain (mittelschmerz) occurs 1.7 days after peak of cervical mucus and 2.5 days before increase in BBT	Premenstrual syndrome: backaches; feeling of increasing pelvic fullness
General	Increased weight; feeling of heaviness	Unreported	Headache†; acne
Affective Changes‡			
Moods	Some depression may persist from premenses	Sense of well-being	Premenstrual syndrome (PMS): increased irritability, passivity, depression
Libido	Unreported	Increased sexual desire	Unreported
Energy levels	Unreported	Unreported	Spurt of energy, followed by fatigue
OBJECTIVE SIGNS			
BBT	Individualized, often below 98.6° F (37° C)	Slight drop in BBT	Rise of about 0.4° to 0.8° F (0.2 to 0.4° C)
Respiration	Unreported	Unreported	Hyperventilation with decrease in alveolar P_{CO_2}
Heart rate	Unreported	Unreported	Increased slightly
Breasts	Time of least hormonal effect and smallest breast size	Increased nipple erectility; increased areolar pigmentation	Increased nodularity; enlarged
Cervix (see Figs. 3-20 and 3-21)	"Dry" (no mucus) progressing to viscous, opaque; no ferning	Abundant, thin, clear (egg-white) mucus with spinnbarkheit (4 cm, often up to 10 cm) that dries in a fern pattern (arborization); facilitates sperm transport	Cloudy, sticky, impenetrable to sperm; dries in granular pattern (no ferning)
Mucus pH	About 7.0	7.5	Unreported
Os	Gradual, progressive widening	Open, with mucus seen spilling out	Gradual closing of os
Color of exocervix	Pink	Hyperemic (red)	Gradual return to pink
Body	Firm to touch (like tip of nose)	Soft (like earlobe)	Gradual return to firm

*Sociocultural influences may affect symptoms reported by women. Breast tenderness is rarely reported by Japanese women.
†Headaches reported with greater frequency by Nigerian women.
‡NOTE: Literature usually attributes negative premenstrual symptoms to biology, while good moods and rational behavior are not. When men and women are compared in activity patterns, mood changes, and symptoms, similar variability has been found in *both* men and women even though the changes in women are given more attention by society.

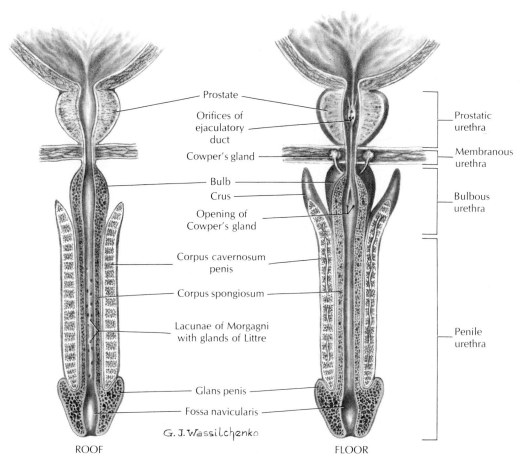

Prostate
Orifices of
ejaculatory
duct
Cowper's gland
Bulb
Crus
Opening of
Cowper's gland
Corpus cavernosum
penis
Corpus spongiosum
Lacunae of Morgagni
with glands of Littre
Glans penis
Fossa navicularis
G. J. Wassilchenko
Prostatic
urethra
Membranous
urethra
Bulbous
urethra
Penile
urethra
ROOF
FLOOR

FIG. 3-22 Anatomy of urethra and penis.

curly, forming a diamond-shaped pattern from the umbilicus to the anus. The area over the symphysis pubis is referred to as the *mons pubis.*

The *penis,* an organ of urination and copulation, consists of the shaft, or body, and the glans (Fig. 3-22). The shaft of this external male reproductive organ, which enters the vagina during coitus, is composed of three cylindric layers and erectile tissue, two lateral *corpora cavernosa* and a *corpus spongiosum,* which contains the urethra. These corpora terminate distally in the smooth, sensitive *glans penis,* which is the counterpart of the female glans clitoris.

Skin and fascia loosely envelop the penis to permit enlargement during erection. The glans is the enlarged end of the penis that contains many sensitive nerve endings and a urethral meatus at the tip (usually). The *prepuce* (foreskin), an extended fold of skin, covers the glans in uncircumcised males (Fig. 3-23). In the newborn the foreskin is generally not retractable and may not be retractable for 4 to 6 months or even as long as 13 years. It is easily retractable in the adolescent and the adult. With sexual arousal, neurocirculatory factors cause considerable increase in blood flow to the erectile tissue of the corpora, and enlargement and erection of the penis occur.

The *urethra* is a common passageway for both urine and semen (see Figs. 3-22 and 3-23).

The *scrotum,* a wrinkled pouch of skin, muscles, and fascia (see Fig. 3-23), is divided internally by a septum, and each compartment normally contains one *testis, epididymis,* and *vas deferens* (seminal duct). The left side of the scrotum hangs somewhat lower (about 1 cm) than the right side. The skin is abundantly supplied with sebaceous and sweat glands and is sparsely covered with hair. Contraction and relaxation of smooth muscles under the skin result in retraction of the testes to protect them from external trauma and cold. During hot external (environmental) or internal (fever) temperature the muscle relaxes, lowering the testes away from the body. Conversely, cold external temperature stimulates contraction of the muscle to bring the testes close to the body.

The purpose of this mobility is to maintain the testes within an optimum temperature range for the production and viability of sperm. Hot tubs, tight underwear (jockey shorts) and pants, and long-term sitting (such as in long-distance truck driving or cycling) present too hot an external environment or prevent testicular mobility so that spermatogenesis and sperm are jeopardized.

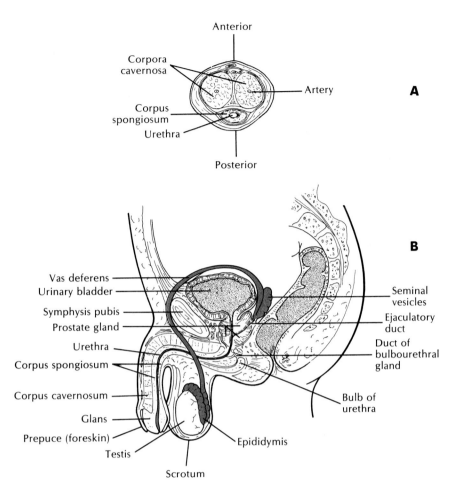

FIG. 3-23   Fascial planes of the male lower genitourinary tract. **A,** Transverse section of penis. **B,** Relationship of bladder, prostate, seminal vesicles, penis, urethra, and scrotal contents.

Internal Structures

Internal structures (see Figs. 3-22 and 3-23) include testes, ducts of the testes, and accessory reproductive tract glands.

Testes

The testes are two small ovoid glands located within the scrotal sac. Both are suspended by attachment to scrotal tissue and the spermatic cord. Originally located in the abdomen, the testes descend through the inguinal canal by the end of the seventh lunar month of fetal life. At term birth, one or both of the testes may still be within the inguinal canals with final descent into the scrotal sac occurring in the early postnatal period. The testes must be within the scrotum for spermatogenesis to occur.

The testes are similar in origin (homologous) to the ovaries in the female. Each testis is whitish, somewhat flattened from side to side, and measures about 4 or 5 cm in length. White fibrous tissue encases each testis and divides it into several lobules. Within each lobule are one to three long (about 75 cm), narrow, coiled *seminiferous* tubules and clusters of *interstitial cells* (Leydig's cells).

Spermatids attach to the germinal epithelium (Sertoli cells) within the seminiferous tubules, and develop into sperm. The interstitial cells are large connective and supportive tissue (stromal) cells responsible for the production of the androgen hormone testosterone.

The two principal functions of the testes are spermatogenesis and hormone production. Primitive sex cells (spermatogonia) are present in the seminiferous tubules of the male newborn. Spermatogenesis, the maturation process that results in sperm, begins during puberty and normally continues throughout a man's lifetime. The testes secrete the steroid sex hormone testosterone in the amounts required for normal male growth, development, and function.

Ducts (Canals) of the Testes

For sperm to exit the body, they must travel the full length of the duct system in succession: seminiferous tubules (mentioned earlier), epididymides (pl.), vasa deferentia (pl.), ejaculatory ducts, and the urethra. Each testis has one tightly coiled tube, about 6 m (20 ft) in length. This tube, the *epididymus* (see Fig. 3-23) lies along the top and side of each testis. The epididymides are storage sites for maturing sperm and produce a small part of the seminal fluid (semen). Seminiferous tubules are continuous with the epididymides, which in turn connect to the vasa deferentia.

Accessory Reproductive System Glands

Accessory reproductive glands secrete fluids that support the life and function of sperm. These glands include the paired *seminal vesicles,* located along the lower posterior surface of the bladder; the *prostate gland,* which surrounds the prostatic urethra; and the *bulbourethral* (or Cowper's) *glands,* located below the prostate, one at either side of the membranous urethra (see Figs. 3-22 and 3-23).

Semen

Semen is the fluid ejaculated at the time of orgasm. Semen contains sperm and secretions from the seminal vesicles, prostate gland, and bulbourethral glands. An average volume per ejaculate is 2.5 to 3.5 ml (range: 1 to 10 ml) after several days of continence (no ejaculations). The volume of semen and sperm count decrease rapidly with repeated ejaculations. Semen contains constituents that provide nourishment, support and enhance sperm motility, and buffer the acidic environment of the cervical and vaginal fluids.

Semen is white to opalescent with a specific gravity of 1.028. The pH is alkaline, ranging from 7.35 to 7.5. Sperm count averages 100 million/ml with fewer than 20% abnormal forms. About 60% of the total fluid is derived from the seminal vesicles, about 20% from the prostatic glands. Some fluid is secreted by the bulbourethral glands and probably by the urethral glands.

Less than 5% of the ejaculate consists of sperm and fluid from the testes and epididymides. A vasectomy affects only the production of this portion of the ejaculate, so there is no noticeable change in volume, even after sperm are no longer available for transport through the remaining canal system.

The seminal vesicles produce a high concentration of prostaglandin, however, their function in semen production is not fully understood (Ganong, 1987). Prostaglandins are discussed on p. 44.

SEXUAL RESPONSE

The hypothalamus and anterior pituitary gland in females and males regulate the production of FSH and LH. The target tissue for these hormones is the gonad: an ovary or testis. In the female the ovary produces ova and secretes estrogen and progesterone; in the male the testis produces sperm and secretes testosterone. A *feedback mechanism* between hormone secretion from the gonads, hypothalamus, and anterior pituitary aids in the control of the production of sex cells and steroid sex hormone secretion (Figs. 3-19 and 3-24).

Physiologic Response to Sexual Stimulation

Although the first outward appearance of maturing sexual development occurs at an earlier age in females, both females and males achieve physical maturity at about the age of 17. However, individuals' development rates vary greatly. Anatomic and reproductive differences notwithstanding, women and men are more alike than different in their physiologic response to sexual excite-

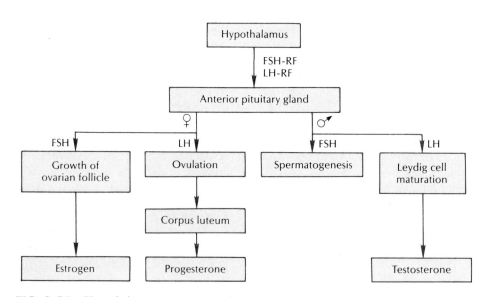

FIG. 3-24   Hypothalamic-pituitary-gonadal axis. Comparison of male and female releasing factors (RF).

ment and orgasm. For example, the glans clitoris and the glans penis are embryonic homologues. Not only is there little difference between female and male sexual response, but the physical response is essentially the same whether stimulated by coitus, fantasy, or mechanical or manual masturbation.

Physiologically, according to Masters and Johnson (1966), sexual response can be analyzed in terms of two processes: vasocongestion and myotonia.

Sexual stimulation results in vasocongestion reflex dilation of penile blood vessels (erection in the male) and circumvaginal blood vessels (lubrication in the female), causing engorgement and distention of the genitals. Venous congestion is localized primarily in the genitals, but also occurs to a lesser degree in the breasts and other parts of the body.

Arousal is characterized by *myotonia* (increased muscular tension), resulting in voluntary and involuntary rhythmic contractions. Examples of sexually stimulated myotonia are pelvic thrusting, facial grimacing, and spasms of the hands and feet (carpopedal spasms).

The **sexual response cycle** is arbitrarily divided into

TABLE 3-2 Four Phases of Sexual Response

REACTIONS COMMON TO BOTH SEXES	FEMALE REACTIONS	MALE REACTIONS
EXCITEMENT PHASE Heart rate and blood pressure increase. Nipples become erect. Myotonia begins.	Clitoris increases in diameter and swells. External genitals become congested and darken. Vaginal lubrication occurs; upper two thirds of vagina lengthen and extend. Cervix and uterus pull upward. Breast size increases.	Erection of the penis begins; penis increases in length and diameter. Scrotal skin becomes congested and thickens. Testes begin to increase in size and elevate toward the body.
PLATEAU PHASE Heart rate and blood pressure continue to increase. Respirations increase. Myotonia becomes pronounced; grimacing occurs.	Clitoral head retracts under the clitoral hood. Lower one third of vagina becomes engorged. Skin color changes occur—red flush may be observed across breasts, abdomen, or other surfaces.	Head of penis may enlarge slightly. Scrotum continues to grow tense and thicken. Testes continue to elevate and enlarge. Preorgasmic emission of 2 or 3 drops of fluid appears on the head of the penis.
ORGASMIC PHASE Heart rate, blood pressure, and respirations increase to maximum levels. Involuntary muscle spasms occur. External rectal sphincter contracts.	Strong rhythmic contractions are felt in the clitoris, vagina, and uterus. Sensations of warmth spread through the pelvic area.	Testes elevate to maximum level. Point of "inevitability" occurs just prior to ejaculation and is an awareness of fluid in the urethra. Rhythmic contractions occur in the penis. Ejaculation of semen occurs.
RESOLUTION PHASE Heart rate, blood pressure, and respirations return to normal. Nipple erection subsides. Myotonia subsides.	Engorgement in external genitalia and vagina resolves. Cervix and uterus descend to normal position. Breast size decreases. Skin flush disappears.	Fifty percent of erection is lost immediately with ejaculation; penis gradually returns to normal size. Testes and scrotum return to normal size. Refractory period (time needed for erection to occur again) varies according to age and general physical condition.

four phases: excitement phase, plateau phase, orgasmic phase, and resolution phase. The four phases occur progressively with no sharp dividing line between any two phases. Specific body changes take place in sequence. The time, intensity, and duration for cyclic completion also vary for individuals and situations. Table 3-2 compares male and female body changes during each of the four phases of the sexual response cycle.

Nursing Implications

Nurses are in a unique position to help adults with health maintenance and detection of problems concerning sexuality. The role of sex educator is an important one for nurses working with families during the childbearing and child-rearing years. Parents often need help teaching their children about sex because adults are commonly misinformed about many aspects of reproduction and how their bodies function. Parents, therefore, need accurate sex information to teach their children to be healthy, responsible sexual beings.

Besides helping with childhood and adult sexuality, nurses can help prepare patients for the sexual problems and changes occurring with age. Many nurses have not been aware of the importance of sex education for older people because of the myth that the elderly are no longer interested in sex.

Sexual dysfunction problems often begin after children are born. The mother, especially, may become so involved with child-rearing activities that her relationship with her husband suffers. At the same time, the husband may be actively involved in career establishment, thereby leaving little energy for home life. Nurses need to be aware of how the demands of parenting can adversely affect the marital relationship. Simple counseling provided during these early years may prevent serious marital problems later.

The older woman in particular, who has been able to move gracefully into old age and who continues to recognize herself as a sexual being, is probably better able to accept the sexuality of the young. As a result, she may accept the pregnancy of a daughter as a continuation of her own sexuality rather than as a threat or reminder of her lost youth.

A knowledgeable, nonjudgmental nurse who recognizes personal sexual biases can contribute greatly to the sexual health of young families. The nurse can recognize potential problems within the marriage and either intervene or refer the couple for further counseling.

IMMUNOLOGY

Immunology is the study of the molecules, cells, organs, and systems responsible for the recognition and disposal of foreign (nonself) material, and how the human body defends itself against this material. The human immune system is necessary for survival. Nonself substances can be as diverse as life-threatening infectious microorganisms or a lifesaving organ transplant. The desirable consequences of immunity include natural resistance, recovery, and acquired resistance to infectious diseases.

Body Defenses

The first barrier to infection is unbroken skin and mucosal membrane surfaces. These surfaces form a physical barrier against many microorganisms. Secretions, such as mucus or those produced in the process of eliminating liquid and solid wastes (e.g., the urinary and gastrointestinal processes), are also important as nonspecific mechanisms for removing potential pathogens from the body. The acidity and alkalinity of the fluids of the stomach and intestinal tract, and the acidity of the vagina, can destroy many potentially infectious microorganisms. These fluids can also have chemical properties that defend the body. For example, lysozyme is an enzyme found in tears and saliva that attacks the cell wall of susceptible bacteria.

The body has a wide variety of barrier-assisting defenses that initially protect the body against disease. Although these barriers vary between individuals, they do assist in the general resistance to infectious organisms. When barrier-assisting defenses break down, the potential for disease increases. For instance, when the new mother's skin integrity is impaired (e.g., through episiotomy or lacerations) or when she has drying or cracking of the nipples, she is at increased risk for infection. In older women, the pH and amount of vaginal fluid is altered, resulting in the increased risk of yeast infection (i.e., *Candida albicans*).

Types of Immunity
Natural Immunity

Natural (innate or inborn) resistance is one of two ways the body resists infection after microorganisms have penetrated the first line of resistance. The second form, acquired or adaptive resistance, specifically recognizes and selectively eliminates exogenous (or endogenous) agents.

Natural immunity is characterized as a nonspecific mechanism. If a microorganism penetrates the skin or mucosal membranes, cellular and humoral defense mechanisms become operational. The elements of natural resistance are phagocytic cells, complement, and the acute inflammatory reaction. Despite their relative lack of specificity, these components are essential, because they are largely responsible for natural immunity to many environmental microorganisms (Table 3-3).

Cellular Components	Humoral Components
Mast cells (tissue basophils)	Complement
Neutrophils	Lysozyme
Macrophages	Interferon

TABLE 3-3 Immune Functions of Specific Leukocytes

IMMUNE DIVISION	LEUKOCYTE	FUNCTION
Inflammation	Neutrophil	Nonspecific ingestion and phagocytosis of microorganisms and foreign protein
	Macrophage	Nonspecific recognition of foreign proteins and microorganisms; ingestion and phagocytosis
	Monocyte	Destruction of bacteria and cellular debris; matures into macrophage
	Eosinophil	Weak phagocytic action; releases vasoactive amines during allergic reactions
	Basophil	Releases histamine and heparin in areas of tissue damage
Antibody-mediated immunity	B lymphocyte	Becomes sensitized to foreign cells and proteins
	Plasma cell	Secretes immunoglobulins in response to the presence of a specific antigen
	Memory cell	Remains sensitized to a specific antigen and can secrete increased amounts of immunoglobulins specific to the antigen
Cell-mediated immunity	T lymphocyte helper cell	Enhances immune activity through secretion of various factors, cytokines, and lymphokines
	Cytotoxic T cell	Selectively attacks and destroys nonself cells, including virally infected cells, grafts, and transplanted organs
	Natural killer cell	Nonselectively attacks nonself cells, especially body cells that have undergone mutation and have become malignant; also attacks grafts and transplanted organs

From Ignatavicius DD, Bayne MV: *Medical-surgical nursing: a nursing process approach,* Philadelphia, 1991, WB Saunders.

Acquired Immunity

If a microorganism overwhelms the body's natural resistance, another form of defensive resistance, **acquired** or **adaptive immunity,** allows the body to recognize, remember, and respond to a specific stimulus—an antigen. Acquired immunity can eliminate microorganisms, and commonly leaves the host with antigen-specific immunologic memory. This condition of memory or recall, *acquired resistance,* allows the host to respond more effectively if reinfection with the same microorganism occurs. Acquired immunity, like natural immunity, is composed of cellular and humoral components.

Cellular Components	Humoral Components
T lymphocytes	Antibodies
B lymphocytes	Lymphokines
Plasma cells	

The major cellular component of this mechanism is the lymphocyte; the major humoral component is the antibody. Lymphocytes selectively respond to nonself materials—antigens—which leads to immune memory and a permanently altered pattern of response or adaptation to the environment. The two categories of the adaptive response are antibody-mediated and cell-mediated immunity (see Table 3-3). Antibody-mediated immunity is the primary defense against bacterial infection. Cell-mediated immunity is the primary defense against viral and fungal infections, intracellular organisms, tumor antigens, and graft rejections.

Antibody-Mediated Immunity

If specific antibodies have been formed to antigenic stimulation, they are available to protect the body against foreign substances. The recognition of foreign substances and subsequent production of antibodies to these substances is the specific meaning of immunity. Antibody-mediated immunity to infection occurs when the antibodies are formed by the host or received from another source. These two types of immunity (Table 3-4) are called *active* and *passive* immunity, respectively.

Active immunity can be acquired by natural exposure in response to an infection or natural series of infections, or acquired by injection of an antigen. This intentional injection of antigen, called **vaccination,** effectively stimulates antibody production and memory (acquired resistance) without suffering from the disease. The selected antigenic agent should produce the antibodies without the clinical signs and symptoms of the disease in an **immunocompetent** host (a person whose immune system is able to recognize a foreign antigen and build specific antigen-directed antibodies) and produce permanent antigenic memory. Booster vaccinations may be needed in some cases to expand the pool of memory cells.

Artificial **passive immunity** is achieved by infusion of serum or plasma containing high concentrations of antibody. This provides immediate antibody protection against microorganisms such as hepatitis A or antigens such as Rh-positive (fetal) red blood cells. The antibod-

TABLE 3-4 Types of Acquired Antibody-Mediated Immunity

TYPE	MODE OF ACQUISITION	ANTIBODY PRODUCED BY HOST	DURATION OF IMMUNE RESPONSE
ACTIVE			
Natural	Infection	Yes	Long*
Artificial	Vaccination	Yes	Long*
PASSIVE			
Natural	Transfer in vivo or through colostrum (maternal antibodies)	No	Short
Artificial	Infusion of serum/plasma (Rh$_o$IG)	No	Short

*In the immunocompetent host.

ies have been produced by another person or animal that has been actively immunized, not by the ultimate recipient. As long as the antibodies persist in the circulation, recipients will benefit from passive immunity. Passive immunity can also be acquired naturally by the fetus through the transfer of antibodies by the maternal circulation in utero. Maternal antibodies are also transferred to the newborn after parturition in the prelactation fluid, called *colostrum*. For the newborn to have lasting protection, active immunity must occur.

Cell-Mediated Immunity

Cell-mediated immunity consists of immune activities that differ from those of antibody-mediated immunity. Cell-mediated immunity is moderated by the link between T-lymphocytes and phagocytic cells (i.e., monocyte-macrophage cells) (see Table 3-3). Lymphocytes (T-cells) do not directly recognize the antigens of microorganisms or other living cells, such as an *allograft* (a graft of tissue from a genetically different member of the same species [e.g., a human kidney]) but do so when the antigen is present on the surface of an antigen-presenting cell—the macrophage. Lymphocytes are immunologically active through various types of direct cell-to-cell contact, and by the production of soluble factors, such as *lymphokines,* for specific immunologic functions. These include the recruitment of phagocytic cells to the site of inflammation. The term *delayed hypersensitivity* is often used synonymously with the term *cell-mediated immunity.* Delayed hypersensitivity, however, refers to the slow appearance of a secondary response in the skin. The term dates back to when antibody responses were detected by immediate hypersensitivity and reflected the subtle difference in the length of time that it took for a delayed response to occur (e.g., tuberculin skin test).

Under some conditions, the activities of cell-mediated immunity may not be beneficial. Suppression of the normal adaptive immune response *(immunosuppression)* by drugs or other means is necessary in conditions such as

organ transplantation, hypersensitivity, and autoimmune disorders.

Factors Associated with Immunologic Disease

Factors such as general health and the age of an individual are important considerations in the functioning of the immune system in defense against infectious disease. In the case of noninfectious diseases or disorders, however, additional factors may be important.

In the maternity and gynecologic setting, nurses must consider the development of the immune system in the fetus and newborn, environmental factors, nutritional status, and lifestyle considerations.

Immunity in the Newborn

Although nonspecific and specific body defenses are present in unborn and newborn infants, many of these defenses are not completely developed in this group. A healthy newborn does not sweat, has no tears, and is not born with "normal" skin or intestinal microbial flora. Young children are at greater risk for diseases, particularly infectious diseases. If the integrity of the skin is broken, the newborn becomes predisposed to tissue and blood invasion by foreign cells, such as bacteria. Infants who are preterm, small for gestational age, or postterm have different skin qualities that increase their susceptibility to invasive agents.

Full-term infants usually have passively acquired natural immunity because of the presence of maternal antibodies. These antibodies are transferred from mother to infant through the placental circulation and provide short-term resistance (3 months) to the specific antigens to which the mother produced antibodies. The preterm infant may be deficient in this type of immunity, especially if born before the thirty-sixth week of gestation. Another passively acquired antibody is present in colostrum and can be acquired in the newborn by breastfeeding.

Environment

Each person's environment significantly determines the challenges posed to the immune system. The environment—the quality of air, water, and food, as well as the ventilation, refrigeration, crowding, and cleanliness available in the setting—contribute to the risks that people in that environment encounter from microorganisms and substances. The environment greatly influences the acquisition and transmission of infectious diseases, such as tuberculosis and toxoplasmosis. Not everyone is exposed to the tubercle bacillus or to the parasite that causes toxoplasmosis, only people who live where tubercle bacillus is endemic (e.g., an urban, overcrowded area with poor ventilation) have a greater risk of exposure. The cat owner, whose pet harbors the toxoplasmosis parasite, is at increased risk of acquiring the disease, especially if the person has contact with the cat's feces (i.e., by emptying the litter pan). Toxoplasmosis can be transmitted from mother to fetus via placental transfer.

Nurses can exert some control to effect fewer challenges to the immune defense system, of patients staying in the hospital. People with infectious diseases should be carefully screened, and a meticulous medical aseptic technique should be used in the nursery. This does not suggest that normal newborns should have a sterile environment, but that there is no reason to overtax a relatively meager set of immune defense mechanisms. An overwhelming systemic infection, such as that caused by herpes virus in the neonate, can interfere with the healthy growth and development of the parent-child relationship, because of prolonged separation, and can also threaten the newborn's life. For this reason, the environment into which a fetus will be born must be assessed for risk potential in posing harm to the newborn.

Nutritional Status

Good nutrition promotes good health. Not only is nutrition important to growth and development, but a healthy diet also affects the aging process and the *triad of nutrition, immunity, and infection*. The consequences of diet on multiple aspects of the immune response have been documented in many disorders. Nutritional intake appears to influence every constituent of body defenses, including phagocytosis and humoral and cellular immunity. Deficient or excessive intake of some dietary components, such as vitamins and minerals, can negatively affect the immune response. Therefore a healthy diet is important for the immune system to function well.

Breast milk supports the body's immune defense system by favoring the growth of *Lactobacillus bifidus* in the infant's intestinal system. This microorganism converts lactose into lactic acid. Lactic acid diminishes the growth of pathogenic organisms in the intestinal tract. Breast milk also provides the necessary nutrients, such as proteins and essential minerals, that support the healthy functioning of the immune system.

Lifestyle

Certain infectious diseases are associated with the patterns of living that people establish for themselves. For instance, people with multiple sex partners are more likely to acquire sexually transmitted diseases, such as syphilis and gonorrhea. Many other aspects comprise the concept of *lifestyle* besides sexual preference patterns and sexual behavior. These factors include the numerous health behaviors people practice, such as patterns of rest, exercise, food and drug intake, relaxation, work performance, self-care, and use of health care professionals. Nurses need to carefully access the many details about their patients' lifestyles, because these factors affect susceptibility to invasion by harmful substances. For instance, a pattern of heavy *alcohol consumption* is associated with certain nutritional deficiencies (notably the B vitamin complex) that decrease the individual's immune responsiveness to vaccines and depress the cell-mediated and humoral lymphocytic activity (Whitney, Cataldo, 1983). Individuals who assume responsibility for their health, and who practice health maintenance and preventive strategies (such as acquiring artificial active immunity), are more likely to enjoy a competent immune defense system.

Nursing Implications

When a patient shows any degree of compromised immune responsiveness, the nurse must take steps to ensure protection from sources of infection in the hospital and the home environments. Scrupulous attention must be given to practicing medical asepsis by all caregivers who come in contact with the patient. This will help prevent superimposed iatrogenic nosocomial infections. In some cases reverse or protective isolation should be instituted to further protect the patient.

It is essential that nurses appreciate the complexity of the immune system and fully understand how to:

1. Support patients' healthy defense mechanisms.
2. Protect and care for patients with impaired immune responsiveness.
3. Avoid unintentional stimulation of potentially dangerous (allergic) defense mechanisms.

To devise an individualized plan, nurses should assess for factors that would place their patients at risk such as their age, overall health status, environment, and lifestyle. Patients require supportive therapy to maintain good fluid and nutritional status, and to maintain the integrity of this first-line defense mechanism. In some situations patients are further protected with passive immunity support with IgG antibody injections. Patients who have a poor prognosis (such as those with AIDS) and their families also need to have supportive psychosocial care and opportunities to discuss and design their futures. Specific care needs for patients with immunologic problems are discussed throughout the text (see Related Topics).

KEY POINTS

- The myometrium of the uterus is uniquely designed to expel the fetus and promote hemostasis after birth.
- Normal feedback regulation of the menstrual cycle depends on an intact hypothalamic-pituitary-gonadal mechanism.
- The female's reproductive tract structures and breasts respond predictably to changing levels of sex steroids across her life span.
- Prostaglandins play an important role in reproductive functions by their effect on smooth muscle contractility and modulation of hormones.

- Nurses need to be aware of their own feelings and values regarding sexuality before they can adequately and competently help patients meet their information needs or refer them for further counseling.
- The desirable consequences of immunity include natural resistance, recovery, and acquired resistance to infectious diseases.
- Vaccination is an effective method of stimulating antibody production and memory.
- Factors such as fetal/neonatal development, lifestyle, environment, and nutrition affect the functioning of the immune defense system.

CRITICAL THINKING EXERCISES

The local high school has asked your clinical group to teach some classes to high school seniors. The subjects to be covered are male and female anatomy and the immune system. One half of the group will teach each class.

1. The first group must outline the essential content on the anatomy and physiology of the male and female reproductive systems, as well as se-

lect appropriate teaching methods. Justify the content selection and teaching methods.

2. The second group must outline the essential content on the functioning of the immune system in relation to age, lifestyle, environment, and nutrition. Appropriate teaching methods should be identified. Justify the content selection and teaching methods.

References

Ganong WE: *Review of medical physiology,* ed 13, Norwalk, CT, 1987, Appleton & Lange.

Herbst AL et al: *Comprehensive gynecology,* ed 2, St Louis, 1992, Mosby.

Ignatavicius DD, Bayne MV: *Medical-surgical nursing: a nursing process approach,* Philadelphia, 1991, WB Saunders.

Masters WH, Johnson VE: *Human sexual response,* 1966, Little, Brown & Co.

Whitney EN, Cataldo CB: *Understanding normal and clinical nutrition,* New York, 1983, West Publishing.

Bibliography

Barkauskas VH et al: *Health and physical assessment,* St Louis, 1994, Mosby.

Groër M: Psychoneuroimmunology: an emerging discipline gives new theoretical support to nursing care of the "body-mind," *Am J Nurs* 91(8):33, 1991.

Long BC, Phipps WJ, Cassmeyer VL: *Medical-surgical nursing: a nursing process approach,* ed 3, St Louis, 1993, Mosby.

Masters WH, Johnson VE, Kolodny RC: *Masters and Johnson on sex and human loving,* 1988, Little, Brown, & Co.

Mudge-Grout C: *Immunologic disorders, Mosby's clinical nursing series,* vol 9, St Louis, 1992, Mosby.

RN Update: Measles outbreak: implications for nurses, *RN* 53(3):10, 1990.

Sarrel PM: Sexuality and menopause, *Obstet Gynecol* 75(4):26(suppl), 1990.

Scott JR et al: *Danforth's obstetrics and gynecology,* ed 6, Philadelphia, 1990, JB Lippincott.

Seidel HM et al: *Mosby's guide to physical examination,* ed 3, St Louis, 1995, Mosby.

Thibodeau GA, Patton K: *Anatomy and physiology,* ed 2, St Louis, 1993, Mosby.

Thompson JM et al: *Mosby's clinical nursing,* ed 3, St Louis, 1993, Mosby.

US Department of Health and Human Services: Universal precautions for prevention of transmission of HIV, hepatitis B virus, and other blood borne pathogens in health care settings, *MMWR* 37:377, 1988.

Wilkin TJ: Receptor autoimmunity in endocrine disorders, *N Engl J Med* 323(19):1318, 1990.

UNIT
Two

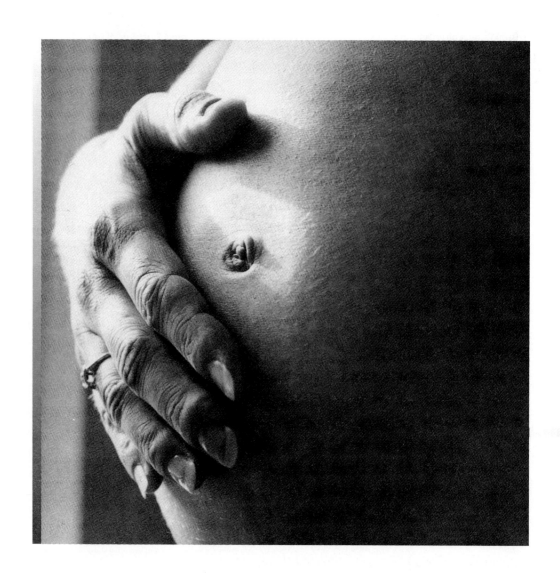

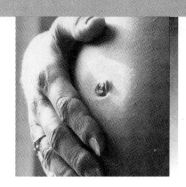

Pregnancy

4   **Genetics, Conception, and Fetal Development**

5   **Anatomy and Physiology of Pregnancy**

6   **Family Dynamics of Pregnancy**

7   **Nursing Care during Pregnancy**

8   **Maternal and Fetal Nutrition**

4 Genetics, Conception, and Fetal Development

IRENE M. BOBAK

LEARNING OBJECTIVES

Define the key terms listed.
Summarize the fertilization process.
Explain the basic principles of genetics.
Describe the development, structure, and functions of the placenta.
Describe the composition and functions of the amniotic fluid.
Identify common teratogens.
Identify the potential effects of teratogens during the vulnerable periods of embryonic and fetal development.
Describe the nurse's role in genetic and preconception counseling.

KEY TERMS

amniotic fluid
autosomes
blastocyst
cephalocaudal
    development
chorionic villi
chromosomes
conception
decidua basalis
dizygotic twins
dominant
Down syndrome
ductus arteriosus
embryo
fertilization
fetal membranes
fetus
foramen ovale
gametes
genes
human chorionic
    gonadotropin (hCG)
implantation

karyotype
lanugo
lecithin/
    sphingomyelin
    (L/S) ratio
meconium
monozygotic twins
morula
mutation
neural tube defect
placenta
preconception care
quickening
recessive
sex chromosomes
surfactants
teratogens
umbilical cord
vernix caseosa
viability
X-linked dominant
    inheritance disorders
X-linked recessive
    inheritance disorders
zygote

RELATED TOPICS

Abortion *(Chap. 30)* · Acoustic stimulation *(Chap. 20)* · Adolescent sexuality *(Chap. 25)* · Amniocentesis *(Chap. 20)* · Chorionic villi sampling *(Chap. 20)* · Contraception *(Chap. 18)* · Exercise tips *(Chap. 7)* · Hazards *(Chap. 29)* · Menstrual cycle *(Chap. 3)* · Nutrition *(Chap. 8)* · Pregnancy tests *(Chap. 5)* · Prenatal care *(Chap. 7)* · Rh sensitization *(Chap. 27)* · Risk factors *(Chap. 20, 29)* · Safer sex practices *(Chap. 18)* · Sexually transmitted diseases (Chap. 21 and 27)* · Violence *(Chap. 23)*

The maternity nurse is in the unique position of providing nursing care to the unborn. Pregnant women and their families have many questions about fetal development, such as "When is our baby due?" "How big is my baby now?" "My friend had a baby with blue eyes, but she and the father have brown eyes. Is that possible?" These questions commonly crop up in childbirth classes and private conversations with the woman or her partner. The wide media coverage of substances that affect the unborn can disturb parents. The knowledgeable nurse can advise parents based on understanding of conception and normal fetal development. This chapter is designed to help nurses answer these questions. It introduces the nurse's role in genetic counseling and preconception care, and gives a brief overview of the genetic basis of inheritance and normal embryonic and fetal development from conception to full-term gestation.

GENETICS

Human development is a complicated process. This process depends on the systematic unraveling of instructions found in the genetic material of the united egg and sperm. Although the progress from conception to birth of a normal, healthy baby occurs without incident in most cases, occasionally some anomaly in the genetic code of the embryo creates a birth defect or disease. Parents then wonder what went wrong, which parent might be "responsible," or, most significantly, what are the chances of the problem recurring with the next pregnancy. The science of genetics seeks to explain the underlying causes of disorders present at birth, as well as the patterns in which inherited disorders pass from generation to generation. A basic understanding of genetics will help the professional nurse assist new families in locating the right sources (often genetics counselors) to help them cope with the questions and fears surrounding birth defects.

Genes and Chromosomes

The hereditary material carried in the nucleus of each of the somatic (body) cells determines an individual's physical characteristics. This material, called deoxyribonucleic acid (DNA), forms threadlike strands known as **chromosomes.** Each chromosome is composed of many smaller segments of DNA referred to as **genes.** Genes, or combinations of genes, contain coded information that determine an individual's unique characteristics. The "code" is found in the specific linear order of the molecules that combine to form the strands of DNA.

All normal human somatic cells contain 46 chromosomes arranged as 23 pairs of homologous (matched) chromosomes; one chromosome of each pair is inherited from each parent. There are 22 pairs of **autosomes,** which control most traits in the body, and one pair of **sex chromosomes,** which primarily control sex determination. The large female chromosome is called the X; the tiny male chromosome is the Y. Generally, the presence of a Y chromosome causes an embryo to develop as a male; in the absence of a Y chromosome, the individual develops as a female. Thus in a normal female the homologous pair of sex chromosomes would be XX, and in a normal male the homologous pair would be XY.

Each person has two genes for every trait, because each gene occupies a specific chromosome location, and because chromosomes are inherited as homologous pairs. In other words, if an autosome has a gene for hair color, its partner will also have a gene for hair color, and they will be in the same location on the chromosome. Although both genes code for hair color, they may not code for the *same* hair color. Different genes coding for different variations of the same trait are called alleles. An individual having two copies of the same allele for a given trait is said to be homozygous for that trait; with two different alleles, the person is heterozygous for the trait.

Some genes are **dominant,** and their characteristics are expressed even if another allele is present on the other chromosome. Other genes are **recessive,** and their characteristics will be expressed only if they are carried by both homologous chromosomes. For example, the gene for brown eyes is dominant over the gene for blue eyes. Thus a person with one gene for brown eyes and one gene for blue eyes will have brown eyes. When an egg and a sperm unite, the combination of alleles becomes that individual's entire genetic makeup, or genotype, which includes all the genes that the person carries and that can be passed to offspring. The genotype determines an individual's physical appearance, or phenotype, but this determination is affected by the nature of the dominant or recessive allele. To continue the example, an individual with two brown eye alleles at the gene for eye color will have the same phenotype as someone with one allele for brown eyes and one for blue eyes; that is, both individuals will have brown eyes.

The pictorial analysis of the number, form, and size of an individual's chromosomes is known as a **karyotype.** A karyotype can be obtained from a blood sample that has been specially treated and stained to make the replicating chromosomes visible under a microscope. The photographed chromosomes are cut out and arranged in a specific numeric order according to their length and shape. Fig. 4-1 illustrates the chromosomes in a body cell. Karyotypes can be used to determine what sex a child will be, and whether any gross chromosomal abnormalities are present.

Cell Division

Cells are reproduced by two different methods: mitosis and meiosis. In mitosis, body cells replicate to yield two

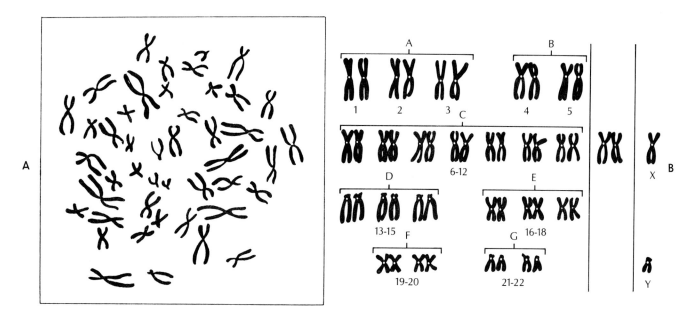

FIG. 4-1   Chromosomes during cell division. **A,** Example of photomicrograph. **B,** Chromosomes arranged in karyotype; female and male sex-determining chromosomes.

cells with the same genetic makeup as the parent cell. First the cell makes a copy of its DNA; then it divides, and each daughter cell receives one copy of the genetic material. The purpose of mitotic division is for growth and development or cell replacement.

Meiosis produces **gametes** (egg and sperm). Each homologous pair of chromosomes receives one gene from the mother and the other from the father, therefore, it is easy to understand that meiosis results in cells containing one of each of the 23 pairs of chromosomes. Because these germ cells contain 23 single chromosomes, half of the genetic material of a normal somatic cell, they are called haploid. This halving of the genetic material is accomplished by replicating the DNA once and then dividing twice. In mitosis, the DNA is replicated once and followed by a single cell division. When the female gamete (egg or ovum) and the male gamete (spermatozoan) unite to form the **zygote,** the diploid number of human chromosomes (46 or 23 pairs) is restored.

The process of DNA replication and cell division in meiosis allows different alleles for genes to be distributed at random by each parent, and then rearranged on the paired chromosomes. The chromosomes then separate and proceed to different gametes. Many combinations of genes are possible on each chromosome because parents have genotypes derived from four different grandparents. This random mixing of alleles accounts for the variation of traits seen in the offspring of the same parents.

Gametogenesis

When a male reaches puberty, his testes begin the process of spermatogenesis. The cells that undergo meiosis in the male are called spermatocytes. The primary spermatocyte, which undergoes the first meiotic division,

contains the diploid number of chromosomes. Remember, however, that the cell has already copied its DNA before division, so four alleles for each gene are actually present. The cell is still considered diploid because the copies are bound together—one allele plus its copy on each chromosome. During the first meiotic division, two haploid secondary spermatocytes are formed. Each secondary spermatocyte contains 22 autosomes and one sex chromosome; one contains the X chromosome (plus its copy), and the other has the Y chromosome (plus its copy). During the second meiotic division, the male produces two gametes with an X chromosome and two gametes with a Y chromosome, all of which will develop into viable sperm (Fig. 4-2, *A*).

Oogenesis, the process of egg (ovum) formation, begins in the female's fetal life. At birth, a woman's ovaries contain all of the cells that may undergo meiosis in her lifetime. The majority of the estimated 2 million primary oocytes (the cells that undergo the first meiotic division) degenerate spontaneously. Only 400 to 500 ova will mature during the approximately 35 years of a woman's reproductive life. The primary oocytes begin the first meiotic division (i.e., they replicate their DNA) during fetal life, but remain suspended at this stage until puberty (Fig. 4-2, *B*). Then, usually monthly, one primary oocyte matures and completes the first meiotic division, yielding two unequal cells, the secondary oocyte and a small polar body. Both contain 22 autosomes and one X sex chromosome. At ovulation, the second meiotic division begins, however, the ovum does not complete the second meiotic division unless fertilization occurs. At fertilization, a second polar body and the zygote (the united egg and sperm) are produced (Fig. 4-2, *C*). If fertilization does not occur, the ovum degenerates.

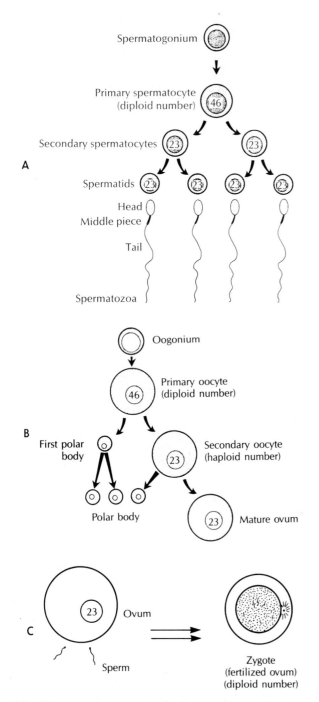

A

B

C

FIG. 4-2 **A,** Spermatogenesis. Gametogenesis of the male produces four mature gametes, the sperm. **B,** Oogenesis. Gametogenesis in the female produces one mature ovum and three polar bodies. Note the relative difference in overall size between the ovum and sperm. **C,** Fertilization results in the single-cell zygote and the restoration of the diploid number of chromosomes.

Chromosomal Abnormalities

Errors resulting in chromosomal abnormalities can occur in either mitosis or meiosis. Abnormalities of number or structure occur in either the autosomes or the sex chromosomes. Even small deviations in chromosomes without the presence of obvious structural malformations can cause problems in fetal development.

Autosomal Abnormalities

Autosomal abnormalities result from unequal distribution of the genetic material during gamete formation. Discussion regarding some of the causes and clinical effects of these genetic problems follows.

Abnormalities of Chromosome Number

Abnormalities of chromosome number, aneuploidy, are most often caused by nondisjunction. Nondisjunction occurs during meiosis when a pair of chromosomes fails to separate, and one resulting cell contains both chromosomes while the other contains none. The product of the union of a normal gamete with a gamete containing an extra chromosome is a trisomy. The resulting individual has 47 chromosomes in each cell.

The most common trisomal abnormality is **Down syndrome,** or trisomy 21. The affected individual has an extra chromosome 21. The clinical characteristics include a broad, small skull; flat facial profile; epicanthal folds with slanted palpebral fissures in the eyes; flat, low-set ears (Fig. 4-3, *A*); protruding tongue; short neck with fat pads at the nape; short, broad hands with a single transverse (simian) crease (Fig. 4-3, *B*); and hypotonic muscles with hypermobility of joints. Mental retardation is the major limitation, although there are also increased incidences of congenital heart disease, infectious diseases, and acute childhood leukemia in individuals with Down syndrome. The incidence of Down syndrome increases with maternal or paternal age (Carothers, 1987). Many affected embryos are spontaneously aborted, and some affected fetuses are stillborn.

The product of the union of a normal gamete (ovum or sperm) with a gamete that is missing a chromosome is known as a monosomy. This individual would have only 45 chromosomes in each cell. Missing an autosomal chromosome always results in the death of the embryo.

Nondisjunction can also occur during mitosis. If this occurs early in development, when cell lines are forming, then the individual has a mixture of cells, some with a normal number of chromosomes and others either missing a chromosome or containing an extra chromosome. This condition is known as mosaicism. Mosaicism in the autosomes is most commonly seen as another form of Down syndrome. Depending on when the nondisjunction occurs during development, different body tissues will have different numbers of chromosomes. The clinical characteristics of Down syndrome may be present mildly or with varying degrees of severity depending on the number and location of the abnormal cells. However, an individual with mosaic Down syndrome may have normal intelligence.

Abnormalities of Chromosome Structure

Abnormalities of chromosome structure involve chromosome breakage that results from one of two events: (1) translocation and (2) additions and/or deletions. Translocation occurs when genetic material is transferred from one chromosome to another different chromosome. Thus instead of two normal pairs of chromosomes, the individual contains one normal chromosome of each pair, plus a third chromosome that is a fusion of the other two. As long as the cell retains all genetic material, the individual is unaffected, but is a carrier of balanced translocation. Problems may arise for offspring, if this individual's genetic material divides unequally during meiosis.

Whenever a portion of a chromosome is deleted from one chromosome and added to another, the gamete produced may contain either extra copies of genes or too few copies. The clinical effects produced may be mild or severe depending upon the amount of genetic material involved. Two of the more commonly described conditions are the deletion of the short arm of chromosome 5 (*cri-du-chat syndrome*) and the deletion of the long arm of chromosome 18. Cri-du-chat syndrome, so named after the typical mewing cry of the affected infant, causes severe mental retardation with microcephaly and unusual facial appearance. Deletion of the long arm of chromosome 18 causes severe psychomotor retardation with multiple organ malformations.

Sex Chromosome Abnormalities

Several sex chromosome abnormalities have been identified that are caused by nondisjunction during gametogenesis in either parent. The most common deviation in females is *Turner's syndrome*, or monosomy X. The affected female is missing an X chromosome and exhibits juvenile external genitalia with undeveloped ovaries. She is usually short in stature with webbing of the neck. Intelligence may be impaired. Most affected embryos abort spontaneously.

The most common deviation in males is *Klinefelter's syndrome*, or trisomy of the sex chromosomes XXY. The affected male has an extra X chromosome and exhibits poorly developed secondary sexual characteristics and small testes. He is infertile, usually tall, and effeminate. Males mosaic for Klinefelter's syndrome may be fertile. Subnormal intelligence is usually present.

Patterns of Genetic Transmission

Heritable characteristics are those that can be passed on to offspring. The number of genes involved in the expression of a trait affects the patterns by which genetic material is transmitted to the next generation. Although many phenotypic characteristics result from two or more genes found on different chromosomes and acting together (referred to as multifactorial inheritance), others are controlled by a single gene (unifactorial inheritance).

Unlike chromosomal abnormalities, defects at the gene level cannot be determined by conventional laboratory methods, such as karyotyping. Instead, genetic counselors predict the probability of the presence of an abnormal gene from the known occurrence of the trait in the individual's family and the known patterns by which the trait is inherited.

Unifactorial Inheritance

If a single gene controls a particular trait, disease, or defect, its pattern of inheritance is referred to as unifactorial mendelian, or single-gene inheritance. Unifactorial or single-gene disorders follow the inheritance patterns of dominance, segregation, and independent assortment described by Mendel. These disorders include autosomal dominant, autosomal recessive, and X-linked recessive and dominant modes of inheritance.

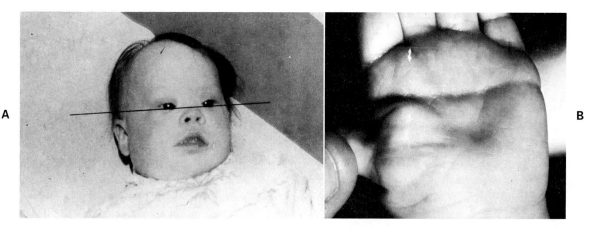

FIG. 4-3   Trisomy 21 (Down syndrome). **A,** Low-set ears. **B,** Simian crease.

Autosomal Dominant Inheritance

Autosomal dominant inheritance disorders are those in which the abnormal gene for the trait is expressed even when the other member of the pair is normal. A disorder may occur in a family for the first time if an abnormal gene appears as a result of a **mutation,** a spontaneous and permanent change in the normal gene structure. Usually, an affected individual comes from multiple generations having the disorder. An affected parent who is heterozygous for the trait has a 50% chance of passing the abnormal gene to each offspring. Males and females are equally affected.

Autosomal dominant disorders are not always expressed with the same severity of symptoms. The parent may have a minor abnormality that had not been diagnosed until the birth of a more severely affected child. There is no way to predict whether an offspring will have a minor or a severe abnormality.

Examples of common autosomal dominantly inherited disorders are Marfan's syndrome (disorder of connective tissue resulting in skeletal, ocular, and cardiovascular abnormalities) (Blackburn, Loper, 1992), achondroplasia (dwarfism), polydactyly (extra digits), Huntington's chorea, and polycystic kidney disease (PKD).

Autosomal Recessive Inheritance

Autosomal recessive inheritance disorders are those in which both genes of a pair must be abnormal for the disorder to be expressed. Heterozygous individuals have only one abnormal gene and are unaffected clinically because their normal gene overshadows the abnormal gene. They are known as carriers of the recessive trait. These recessive traits are inherited by generations of the same family, as a result an increased incidence of the disorder occurs in consanguinous matings (closely related parents). In order for the trait to be expressed, two carriers must each contribute the abnormal gene to the offspring (Fig. 4-4). There is a 25% chance of the trait occurring in each child. A clinically normal offspring may be a carrier of the gene. Males and females are equally affected.

Most recessive disorders tend to have severe clinical manifestations, and affected offspring do not often reproduce. If they do, all of their offspring will be carriers for the disorder.

Most inborn errors of metabolism, such as phenylketonuria (PKU), galactosemia, maple syrup urine disease, Tay-Sachs disease (Chapter 27), sickle cell anemia, and cystic fibrosis, are all autosomal recessive inherited disorders.

Inborn Errors of Metabolism

Disorders of protein, fat, or carbohydrate metabolism reflecting absent or defective enzymes generally follow a recessive pattern of inheritance (Nyhan, 1991). Enzymes, the actions of which are genetically determined, are essential for all the physical and chemical processes that sustain body systems. Defective enzyme action interrupts the normal series of chemical reactions from the affected point onward. The result may be an accumulation of a damaging product, such as phenylalanine, or the absence of a necessary product, such as thyroxin or melanin (see Appendix F for screening tests for inborn errors of metabolism).

Phenylketonuria (PKU) is an uncommon disorder caused by autosomal recessive genes. Genetic screening methods may identify heterozygous carriers and affected infants. A deficiency in the liver enzyme phenylalanine hydroxylase results in failure to metabolize the amino acid phenylalanine, allowing its metabolites to accumulate in the blood. The incidence of this disorder is 1 per every 10,000 to 20,000 births. The highest incidence is found in Caucasians (from northern Europe and the United States). It rarely occurs in Jewish, African, or Japanese populations.

Tay-Sachs disease, inherited as an autosomal recessive trait, results from a deficiency of hexosaminidase. It occurs primarily in Jewish families. Until 4 to 6 months of age, infants appear normal; in fact their facial features are considered very beautiful. Then the clinical symptoms appear: apathy and regression in motor and social development and decreased vision. Death occurs between 3

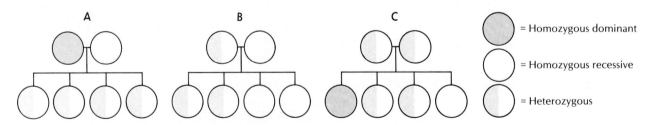

FIG. 4-4 Possible offspring in three types of matings. **A,** Homozygous-dominant parent and homozygous-recessive parent. Children all heterozygous, displaying dominant trait. **B,** Heterozygous parent and homozygous-recessive parent. Children 50% heterozygous display dominant trait; 50% homozygous display recessive trait. **C,** Both parents heterozygous. Children 25% homozygous-dominant trait; 25% homozygous-recessive; 50% heterozygous display dominant trait.

and 4 years of age. As yet there is no known treatment for Tay-Sachs disease. In subsequent pregnancies amniocentesis (for a discussion of amniocentesis, see Chapter 20) may be performed on women who have given birth to infants with this condition.

Cystic fibrosis (mucoviscidosis or fibrocystic disease of the pancreas) is inherited as an autosomal recessive trait, and is characterized by generalized involvement of exocrine glands. Clinical features are related to the altered viscosity of mucus-secreting glands throughout the body. This serious chronic disease occurs primarily in Caucasians, but can appear in those of mixed ancestry. Overall incidence is 1 per every 2000 births. It is thought that the carrier state is 1:20 to 25. Advances in diagnosis and treatment have improved the prognosis, so now many affected individuals live to adulthood. Some affected women have borne children, but men are generally sterile (MacMullen, Brucker, 1989). If the mother has cystic fibrosis and the father has no family history, offspring have a 50% chance of inheriting the gene for cystic fibrosis.

Meconium ileus occurs in about 10% of newborns with cystic fibrosis. In these newborns no meconium is passed during the first 24 to 48 hours, although an initial stool may be passed from the rectum. The abdomen becomes increasingly distended, and eventually the newborn requires a laparotomy for diagnosis and treatment of the condition.

X-Linked Recessive Inheritance

Abnormal genes for **X-linked recessive inheritance disorders** are carried on the X chromosome (Fig. 4-5). Females may be heterozygous or homozygous for traits carried on the X chromosome because they have two. Males are hemizygous because they have only one X chromosome carrying genes with no alleles on the Y chromosome. Therefore X-linked recessive disorders are most commonly manifested in the male with the abnormal gene on his single X chromosome. The male receives the defective gene from his carrier mother on her affected X chromosome. Female carriers (those heterozygous for the trait) have a 50% probability of transmitting the abnormal gene to each offspring. An affected male can only pass the abnormal gene to his daughters on the X chromosome. The daughters will be carriers of the trait if they receive a normal gene on the X chromosome from their mother. They can be affected only if they receive an abnormal gene on the X chromosome from their mother also.

Hemophilia, color blindness, and Duchenne's muscular dystrophy are all X-linked recessive disorders.

X-Linked Dominant Inheritance

X-linked dominant inheritance disorders occur both in males and heterozygous females. The effects are more severe in affected males because females also have a nor-

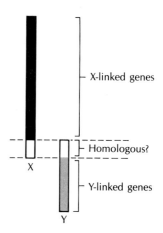

X and Y chromosomes.

FIG. 4-5 X and Y chromosomes.

mal gene. Affected males can only transmit the abnormal gene to their daughters on the X chromosome. Heterozygous females have a 50% chance of transmitting the abnormal gene to each offspring. An example of these extremely rare disorders is vitamin D-resistant rickets.

Fragile-X syndrome is a relatively new diagnosis. The "fragile site" on the X chromosome was identified in a central nervous system disorder affecting males and heterozygous carrier females. Affected individuals are mentally handicapped.

Multifactorial Inheritance

Most of the common congenital malformations result from multifactorial inheritance, a combination of genetic and environmental factors. Examples are cleft lip, cleft palate, congenital heart disease, neural tube defects, and pyloric stenosis. Each malformation may range from mild to severe, depending on the number of genes present for the defect or the amount of environmental influence. A **neural tube defect** may range from spina bifida, a bony defect in the lumbar region of the vertebrae with little or no neurologic impairment, to anencephaly, absence of brain development, which is always fatal. Some malformations occur more often in one sex or the other. For example, pyloric stenosis and cleft lip occur more often in males, and cleft palate is more common in females. Multifactorial disorders also tend to occur in families.

A discussion of environmental conditions and exposures that adversely affect development occurs in Chapter 20.

CONCEPTION

Conception, formally defined as the union of a single egg and sperm, marks the beginning of a pregnancy. This event does not occur in isolation, rather, a series of events surround it. These include gamete (egg and sperm) formation, ovulation (release of the egg), union of the ga-

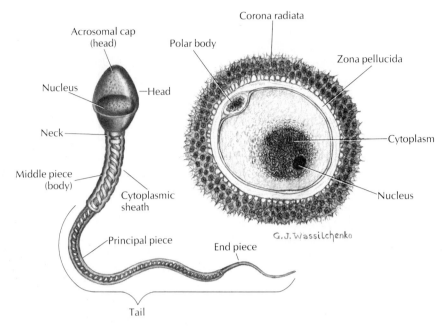

FIG. 4-6 Sperm and ovum.

metes, and implantation of the embryo in the uterus. Only after all of these events are successfully completed can the process of embryonic and fetal development begin.

Ovum

As previously discussed meiosis in the female produces an egg, or ovum. This process occurs in the ovaries, specifically in the ovarian follicles. Each month, one ovum matures with a host of surrounding supportive cells.

At the time of ovulation, the ovum bursts from the ruptured ovarian follicle. High estrogen levels increase the motility of the uterine tubes so that their cilia will be able to capture the ovum and propel it through the tube toward the uterine cavity. The ovum cannot move by itself.

Two protective layers of tissue surround the ovum (Fig. 4-6). The first is a thick, shapeless membrane, the zona pellucida. The outer ring, the corona radiata, is composed of elongated cells held together by hyaluronic acid.

Ova are considered fertile for about 24 hours after ovulation. If unfertilized by a sperm, the ovum degenerates and is reabsorbed.

Sperm

Ejaculation during sexual intercourse normally propels less than a teaspoon of semen, containing as many as 200 to 500 million sperm, into the vagina. The sperm swim with the flagellar movement of their tails. Some sperm can reach the site of fertilization within 5 minutes, but the average transit time is 4 to 6 hours. *Sperm remain viable* within the woman's reproductive system for 2 to 3 days. Most sperm are lost in the vagina, within the cer-

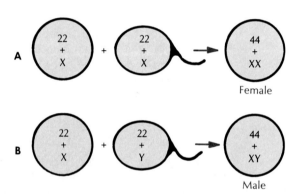

FIG. 4-7 Fertilization. **A,** Ovum fertilized by X-bearing sperm to form female zygote. **B,** Ovum fertilized by Y-bearing sperm to form male zygote.

vical mucus, in the endometrium, or they enter the tube that contains no ovum. As the sperm travel through the uterine tubes, enzymes produced there aid in capacitation of the sperm. *Capacitation* is a physiologic change that removes the protective coating from the heads of the sperm (the acrosomes). Then small perforations form in the acrosome, allowing enzymes (e.g., hyaluronidase) to escape. These enzymes are necessary for the sperm to penetrate the protective layers of the ovum before fertilization.

Fertilization

Fertilization takes place in the ampulla (outer third) of the uterine tube. When a sperm successfully penetrates the membrane surrounding the ovum, both sperm and ovum are enclosed within the membrane, and the membrane becomes impenetrable to other sperm. This is termed the zona reaction. The second meiotic division of the oocyte is completed, and the ovum nucleus be-

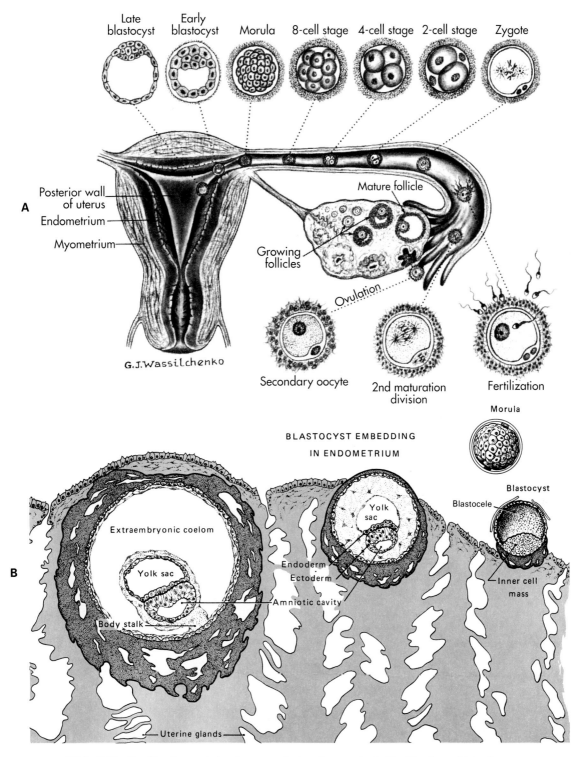

FIG. 4-8   Fertilization and development during first week. **A,** Fertilization within the outer third of the uterine tube approximately 12 to 24 hours following ovulation. **B,** After zona pellucida disappears, blastocyst begins to embed in endometrium. Germ layers begin to form. (**A,** From Thompson JM et al: *Mosby's clinical nursing,* ed 3, St Louis, 1993, Mosby. **B,** Adapted from Langley LL et al: *Dynamic human anatomy and physiology,* ed 5, New York, 1980, McGraw-Hill copyright Mosby.)

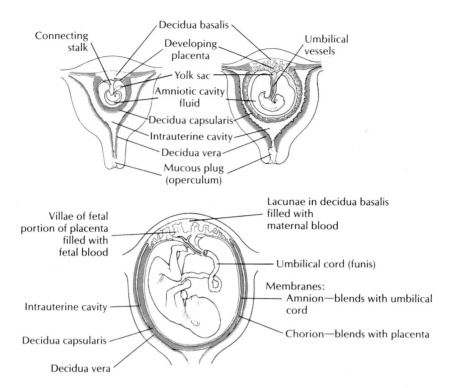

FIG. 4-9 Development of fetal membranes. Note gradual obliteration of intrauterine cavity as decidua capsularis and decidua vera meet. Also note thinning of uterine wall. Chorionic and amniotic membranes are in opposition to each other but may be peeled apart.

comes the female pronucleus. The head of the sperm enlarges to become the male pronucleus, and the tail degenerates. The nuclei fuse and the chromosomes combine, restoring the diploid number (46) (Fig. 4-7). Conception, the formation of the zygote (the first cell of the new individual), has been achieved.

Mitotic cellular replication, called cleavage, begins as the zygote travels the length of the uterine tube into the uterus. This voyage takes 3 to 4 days. Because the fertilized egg divides rapidly with no increase in size, successively smaller cells, blastomeres, form with each division. A 16-cell **morula,** a solid ball of cells, is produced within 3 days (Fig. 4-8). The morula is still surrounded by the protective zona pellucida. Further development occurs as the morula floats freely within the uterus. Fluid passes through the zona pellucida into the intercellular spaces between the blastomeres. A cavity forms within the cell mass as the spaces come together, forming a structure called the **blastocyst.** Formation of the blastocyst signals the first major differentiation of the embryo. The inner solid mass of cells develop into the embryo and the embryonic membrane called the *amnion.* The outer layer of cells surrounding the cavity is the trophoblast, from which develops the other embryonic membrane, the *chorion,* and the embryonic part of the placenta.

Implantation

The zona pellucida degenerates, and the trophoblast attaches itself to the uterine endometrium, usually in the anterior or posterior fundal region. Between 7 and 10 days after conception, the trophoblast secretes enzymes that enable it to burrow into the endometrium until the entire blastocyst is covered. This is known as **implantation.** Endometrial blood vessels erode, and some women experience slight implantation bleeding (very slight spotting or bleeding during the time of the first missed menstrual period). **Chorionic villi,** fingerlike projections, develop out of the trophoblast and extend into the blood-filled spaces of the endometrium. These villi are vascular processes that obtain oxygen and nutrients from the maternal bloodstream and dispose of carbon dioxide and waste products into the maternal blood.

After implantation, the endometrium is called the decidua. The portion directly under the blastocyst, where the chorionic villi tap the maternal blood vessels, is the **decidua basalis.** The portion covering the blastocyst is the decidua capsularis, and the portion lining the rest of the uterus is the decidua vera (Fig. 4-9).

THE EMBRYO AND FETUS

Pregnancy lasts approximately 10 lunar months, 9 calendar months, 40 weeks, or 280 days. *Length of pregnancy is computed from the first day of the last menstrual period (LMP)* until the day of birth* (see discussion of

Text continued on p. 75.

---

*The first day of the last menstrual period refers to the first day of menstrual flow.

TABLE 4-1   Milestones in Human Development Before Birth Since LMP

4 WEEKS	8 WEEKS
EXTERNAL APPEARANCE	
Body flexed, C-shaped; arm and leg buds present; head at right angles to body	Body fairly well formed; nose flat, eyes far apart; digits well formed; head elevating; tail almost disappeared; eyes, ears, nose, and mouth recognizable

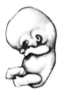

4 WEEKS	8 WEEKS
CROWN-TO-RUMP MEASUREMENT (CM), WEIGHT (G)	
0.4 to 0.5 cm; 0.4 g	2.5 to 3 cm; 2 g
GASTROINTESTINAL SYSTEM	
Stomach at midline and fusiform; conspicuous liver; esophagus short; intestine a short tube	Intestinal villi developing; small intestines coil within umbilical cord; palatal folds present; liver very large
MUSCULOSKELETAL SYSTEM	
All somites present	First indication of ossification—occiput, mandible, and humerus; fetus capable of some movement, definitive muscles of trunk, limbs, and head well represented
CIRCULATORY SYSTEM	
Heart develops, double chambers visible, begins to beat; aortic arch and major veins completed	Main blood vessels assume final plan; enucleated red cells predominate in blood
RESPIRATORY SYSTEM	
Primary lung buds appear	Pleural and pericardial cavities forming; branching bronchioles; nostrils closed by epithelial plugs
RENAL SYSTEM	
Rudimentary ureteral buds appear	Earliest secretory tubules differentiating; bladder-urethra separates from rectum
NERVOUS SYSTEM	
Well-marked midbrain flexure; no hindbrain or cervical flexures; neural groove closed	Cerebral cortex begins to acquire typical cells; differentiation of cerebral cortex, meninges, ventricular foramens, cerebrospinal fluid circulation; spinal cord extends entire length of spine
SENSORY ORGANS	
Eye and ear appearing as optic vessel and otocyst	Primordial choroid plexuses develop; ventricles large relative to cortex; development progressing; eyes converging rapidly; internal ear developing
GENITAL SYSTEM	
Genital ridge appears (fifth week)	Testes and ovaries distinguishable; external genitals sexless but begin to differentiate

Modified from Wong DL: *Whaley and Wong's nursing care of infants and children,* ed 5, St Louis, 1995, Mosby.

Continued.

TABLE 4-1 Milestones in Human Development Before Birth Since LMP—cont'd

12 WEEKS	16 WEEKS

EXTERNAL APPEARANCE

Nails appearing; resembles a human; head erect but disproportionately large; skin pink, delicate	Head still dominant; face looks human; eyes, ears, and nose approach typical appearance on gross examination; arm-leg ratio proportionate; scalp hair appears

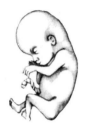 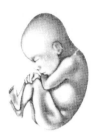

CROWN-TO-RUMP MEASUREMENT (CM), WEIGHT (G)

6 to 9 cm; 19 g	11.5 to 13.5 cm; 100 g

GASTROINTESTINAL SYSTEM

Bile secreted; palatal fusion complete; intestines have withdrawn from cord and assume characteristic positions	Meconium in bowel; some enzyme secretion; anus open

MUSCULOSKELETAL SYSTEM

Some bones well outlined, ossification spreading; upper cervical to lower sacral arches and bodies ossify; smooth muscle layers indicated in hollow viscera	Most bones distinctly indicated throughout body; joint cavities appear; muscular movements can be detected

CIRCULATORY SYSTEM

Blood forming in marrow	Heart muscle well developed; blood formation active in spleen

RESPIRATORY SYSTEM

Lungs acquire definite shape; vocal cords appear	Elastic fibers appear in lungs; terminal and respiratory bronchioles appear

RENAL SYSTEM

Kidney able to secrete urine; bladder expands as a sac	Kidney in position; attains typical shape and plan

NERVOUS SYSTEM

Brain structural configuration roughly complete; cord shows cervical and lumbar enlargements; fourth ventricle foramens developed; suckling present	Cerebral lobes delineated; cerebellum assumes some prominence

SENSORY ORGANS

Earliest taste buds indicated; characteristic organization of eye attained	General sense organs differentiated

GENITAL SYSTEM

Sex recognizable; internal and external sex organs specific	Testes in position for descent into scrotum; vagina open

TABLE 4-1 Milestones in Human Development Before Birth Since LMP—cont'd

20 WEEKS	24 WEEKS
EXTERNAL APPEARANCE	
Vernix caseosa appears; lanugo appears; legs lengthen considerably; sebaceous glands appear	Body lean but fairly well proportioned; skin red and wrinkled; vernix caseosa present; sweat glans forming

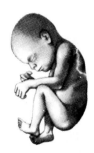

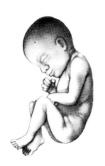

CROWN-TO-RUMP MEASUREMENT (CM), WEIGHT (G)

16 to 18.5 cm; 300 g	23 cm; 600 g

GASTROINTESTINAL SYSTEM

Enamel and dentine depositing; ascending colon recognizable

MUSCULOSKELETAL SYSTEM

Sternum ossifies; fetal movements strong enough for mother to feel

CIRCULATORY SYSTEM

Blood formation increases in bone marrow and decreases in liver

RESPIRATORY SYSTEM

Nostrils reopen; primitive respiratory like movements begin	Alveolar ducts and sacs present; lecithin begins to appear in amniotic fluid (weeks 26 to 27)

RENAL SYSTEM

NERVOUS SYSTEM

Brain grossly formed; cord myelination begins; spinal cord ends at level S-1	Cerebral cortex layered typically; neuronal proliferation in cerebral cortex ends

SENSORY ORGANS

Nose and ears ossify	Can hear

GENITAL SYSTEM

Testes at inguinal ring in descent to scrotum

Continued.

TABLE 4-1 Milestones in Human Development Before Birth Since LMP—cont'd

28 WEEKS	30-31 WEEKS
EXTERNAL APPEARANCE	
Lean body, less wrinkled and red; nails appear	Subcutaneous fat beginning to collect; more rounded appearance; skin pink and smooth; has assumed birth position

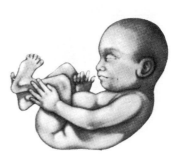

28 WEEKS	30-31 WEEKS
CROWN-TO-RUMP MEASUREMENT (CM), WEIGHT (G)	
27 cm; 1100 g	31 cm; 1800 to 2100 g
GASTROINTESTINAL SYSTEM	
MUSCULOSKELETAL SYSTEM	
Astragalus (talus, ankle bone) ossifies; weak, fleeting movements, minimum tone	Middle fourth phalanxes ossify; permanent teeth primordia seen; can turn head to side
CIRCULATORY SYSTEM	
RESPIRATORY SYSTEM	
Lecithin forming on alveolar surfaces	L/S ratio = 1.2:1
RENAL SYSTEM	
NERVOUS SYSTEM	
Appearance of cerebral fissures, convolutions fast appearing; indefinite sleep-wake cycle; cry weak or absent; weak suck reflex	
SENSORY ORGANS	
Eyelids reopen; retinal layers completed, light receptive; pupils capable of reacting to light	Sense of taste present; aware of sounds outside mother's body
GENITAL SYSTEM	
	Testes descending to scrotum

TABLE 4-1 Milestones in Human Development Before Birth Since LMP—cont'd

36 WEEKS	40 WEEKS
EXTERNAL APPEARANCE	
Skin pink, body rounded; general lanugo disappearing; body usually plump	Skin smooth and pink, scant vernix caseosa; moderate to profuse hair; lanugo on shoulders and upper body only; nasal and alar cartilage apparent
CROWN-TO-RUMP MEASUREMENT (CM), WEIGHT (G)	
35 cm; 2200 to 2900 g	40 cm; 3200+ g
GASTROINTESTINAL SYSTEM	
MUSCULOSKELETAL SYSTEM	
Distal femoral ossification centers present; sustained, definite movements, fair tone, can turn and elevate head	Active, sustained movement; good tone; may lift head
CIRCULATORY SYSTEM	
RESPIRATORY SYSTEM	
L/S ratio $\geq$ 2:1	Pulmonary branching only two thirds complete
RENAL SYSTEM	
Formation of new nephrons ceases	
NERVOUS SYSTEM	
End of spinal cord at level (L-3); definite sleep-wake cycle	Myelination of brain begins; patterned sleep-wake cycle with alert periods; cries when hungry or uncomfortable; strong suck reflex
SENSORY ORGANS	
GENITAL SYSTEM	
	Testes in scrotum; labia majora well developed

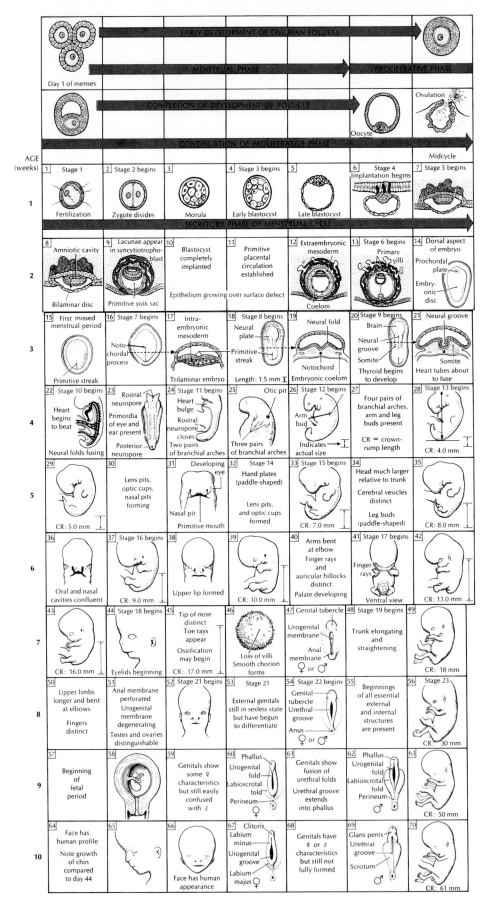

FIG. 4-10 Timetable of human prenatal development from LMP and weeks 1 to 10 following fertilization. Within large boxes are small boxes with numbers in upper left corner. These numbers refer to days since fertilization. (From Moore KL: *Before we are born: basic embryology and birth defects,* ed 3, Philadelphia, 1989, WB Saunders.)

Nägele's rule, and adjustment for longer and shorter cycles, p. 124). However, conception occurs approximately 2 weeks after the first day of the LMP. Thus the postconception age of the fetus is 2 weeks less for a total of 266 days or 38 weeks. Postconceptional age will be used to discuss fetal development.

Intrauterine development is divided into three stages: ovum, embryo, and fetus. Table 4-1 summarizes this development. The stage of the ovum lasts from conception until day 14. This period covers cellular replication, blastocyst formation, initial development of the embryonic membranes, and establishment of the primary germ layers.

Embryonic Development

The stage of the **embryo** lasts from day 15 until approximately 8 weeks after conception or until the embryo measures 3 cm (1.2 inches) from crown to rump. This stage is the most critical time in the development of the organ systems and the main external features. Developing areas with rapid cell division are the most vulnerable to malformation by environmental teratogens. At the end of the eighth week, all organ systems and external structures are present, and the embryo in unmistakably human (Fig. 4-10).

Placenta

Structure

During the third week after conception, the trophoblast cells of the chorionic villi continue to invade the decidua basalis. As the uterine capillaries are tapped, the endometrial spiral arteries (the spaces formed) fill with maternal blood. The chorionic villi grow into the spaces with two layers of cells: the outer syncytium and the inner cytotrophoblast. A third layer develops into anchoring septa, dividing the projecting decidua into separate areas called cotyledons. In each of the 15 to 20 cotyledons, the chorionic villi branch out with a complex system of fetal blood vessels forming. Each cotyledon is a functional unit. The whole structure is the **placenta.**

The maternal-placental-embryonic circulation is in place by day 17, when the embryonic heart starts beating. By the end of the third week, embryonic blood circulates between the embryo and the chorionic villi. In the intervillous spaces (between the villi), maternal blood supplies oxygen and nutrients to the embryonic capillaries in the villi (Fig. 4-11). Waste products and carbon dioxide diffuse into the maternal blood. The placenta functions as a means of metabolic exchange. Exchange is minimal at this time, because the two cell layers of the villous membrane are too thick. Permeability increases as the cytotrophoblast thins and disappears by the fifth month, leaving only the single layer of syncytium between the maternal blood and the fetal capillaries. The

syncytium is the functional layer of the placenta. By the eighth week, genetic testing may be done by obtaining a sample of chorionic villi by aspiration biopsy. The placenta's structure is complete by the twelfth week. The placenta continues to grow wider until 20 weeks, it covers about one half of the uterine surface. Then, the placenta continues to grow thicker. The branching villi continue to develop within the body of the placenta, increasing the functional surface area.

Functions

One of the early functions of the placenta is as an endocrine gland with the production of four hormones necessary to maintain the pregnancy and support the embryo-fetus. The hormones are produced in the syncytium.

The protein hormone, **human chorionic gonadotropin (hCG)** is detected in the maternal serum by 8 to 10 days after conception, shortly after implantation. This hormone is the basis for pregnancy tests. The hCG preserves the function of the ovarian *corpus luteum,* ensuring a continued supply of estrogen and progesterone needed to maintain the pregnancy. If the corpus luteum stops functioning before 11 weeks, when the placenta produces sufficient estrogen and progesterone, then spontaneous abortion occurs. The hCG reaches its maximum level at 50 to 70 days, then begins to decrease.

The other protein hormone produced by the placenta is *human placental lactogen (hPL).* This is a growth hormone-like substance that stimulates maternal metabolism, in order to supply needed nutrients for fetal growth. This hormone facilitates glucose transport across the placental membrane and stimulates breast development to prepare for lactation.

The placenta eventually produces more of the steroid hormone *progesterone* than the corpus luteum does during the first few months of pregnancy. Progesterone maintains the endometrium, decreases the contractility of the uterus, and stimulates development of breast alveoli and maternal metabolism.

By 7 weeks, the placenta produces most of the maternal *estrogens,* steroid hormones. The major estrogen secreted by the placenta is estriol, while the ovaries produce mostly estradiol. Measuring estriol levels is a clinical assay for placental functioning. Estrogen stimulates uterine growth and uteroplacental blood flow. It also causes a proliferation of the breast glandular tissue. Estrogen stimulates myometrial contractility. Placental estrogen production increases markedly toward the end of pregnancy. One theory for the cause of the onset of labor is the decrease in circulating levels of progesterone and the increased levels of estrogen.

The metabolic functions of the placenta may be summarized as respiration, nutrition, excretion, and storage. Oxygen *diffuses* from the maternal blood across the pla-

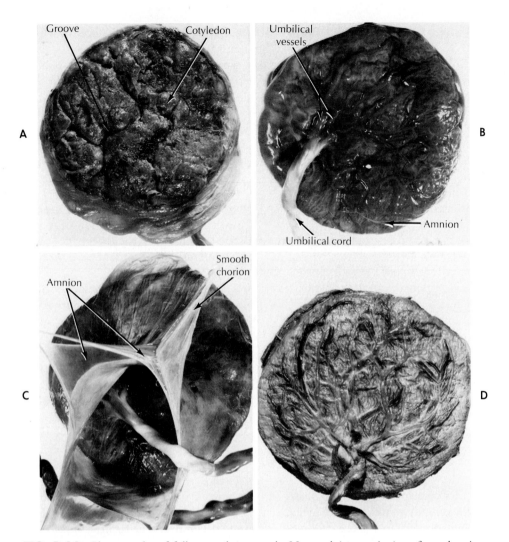

FIG. 4-11 Photographs of full-term placentas. **A,** Maternal (or uterine) surface, showing cotyledons and grooves. **B,** Fetal (or amniotic) surface, showing blood vessels running under amnion and converging to form umbilical vessels at attachment of umbilical cord. **C,** Amnion and smooth chorion are arranged to show that they are (1) fused and (2) continuous with margins of placenta. **D,** Placenta with a marginal attachment of the cord, often called a battledore placenta because of its resemblance to bat used in medieval game of battledore and shuttlecock. (From Moore KL: *Before we are born: basic embryology and birth defects,* ed 3, Philadelphia, 1989, WB Saunders.)

cental membrane into the fetal blood, and carbon dioxide diffuses in the opposite direction. In this way, the placenta functions as the fetal lungs.

Water, inorganic salts, carbohydrates, proteins, fats, and vitamins pass from the maternal blood supply across the placental membrane into the fetal blood supplying nutrition. Water and most electrolytes with a molecular weight less than 500 readily diffuse through the membrane. Hydrostatic and osmotic pressures aid the bulk flow of water and some solutions. *Facilitated and active transport* assist in the transfer of glucose, amino acids, calcium, iron, and substances with higher molecular weight. Amino acids and calcium are transported against the concentration gradient between the maternal blood

and fetal blood. The fetus requires a higher level of these nutrients, as well as glucose. The fetal concentration of glucose is lower than the glucose level in the maternal blood, because of its rapid metabolism by the fetus. This requires transport of larger amounts of glucose from the maternal blood than would be supplied by diffusion alone.

Pinocytosis is a mechanism used for transferring large molecules, such as albumin and gamma globulins, across the placental membrane. This mechanism conveys the maternal immunoglobulins that render early passive immunity to the fetus.

Metabolic waste products cross the placental membrane from the fetal blood into the maternal blood. The

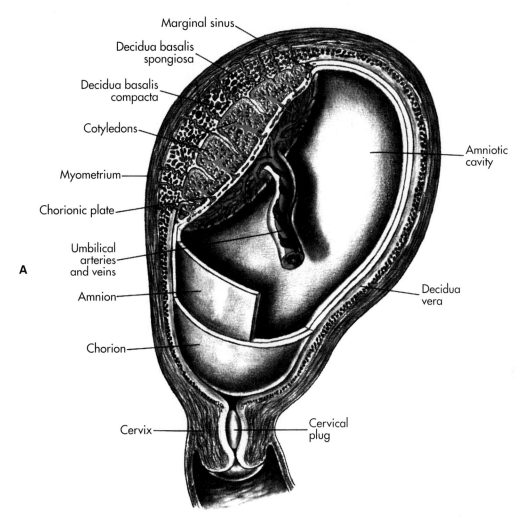

Marginal sinus
Decidua basalis spongiosa
Decidua basalis compacta
Cotyledons
Myometrium
Chorionic plate
Umbilical arteries and veins
Amnion
Chorion
Cervix

Amniotic cavity
Decidua vera
Cervical plug

A

FIG. 4-12   Placenta. **A,** Pregnant uterus showing placenta and membranes.   *Continued.*

maternal kidneys then excrete them.

Many viruses can cross the placental membrane and infect the fetus. Some bacteria and protozoa first infect the placenta and then infect the fetus.

Drugs can also cross the placental membrane and may harm the fetus. Caffeine, alcohol, nicotine, carbon monoxide and other toxic substances in cigarette smoke, and prescription and recreational drugs (such as cocaine and marijuana) readily cross the placenta. More examples of these drugs are listed in Appendix E.

Although there is no direct link between the fetal blood in the vessels of the chorionic villi and the maternal blood in the intervillous spaces, only one cell layer separates them. Breaks in the placental membrane occasionally occur. Fetal erythrocytes then leak into the maternal circulation, and the mother may develop antibodies to the fetal red blood cells. *This is often how the Rh-negative mother becomes sensitized to the erythrocytes of her Rh-positive fetus.*

Carbohydrates, proteins, calcium, and iron are stored in the placenta for ready access to meet fetal needs.

Even though the placenta and fetus are living tissue

transplants, the host mother does not destroy them (Cunningham et al, 1993). The placental hormones suppress the immunologic response, or the tissue evokes no response (Willson, Carrington, 1991).

Placental function depends on the maternal blood pressure supplying circulation. Maternal arterial blood, under pressure in the small uterine spiral arteries, spurts into the intervillous spaces (Fig. 4-12, *B*). As long as rich arterial blood continues to be supplied, pressure is exerted on the blood already in the intervillous spaces, pushing it toward drainage by the low-pressure uterine veins. At term gestation, 10% of the maternal cardiac output goes to the uterus. If there is interference with the circulation to the placenta, the placenta cannot supply the embryo-fetus. Vasoconstriction, such as that caused by hypertension and cocaine use, diminishes uterine blood flow. Decreased maternal blood pressure or cardiac output also diminishes uterine blood flow. For example, this occurs when the woman lies on her back with the pressure of the uterus compressing the vena cava, diminishing blood return to the right atrium (for discussion of supine hypotension, see p. 102). Excessive mater-

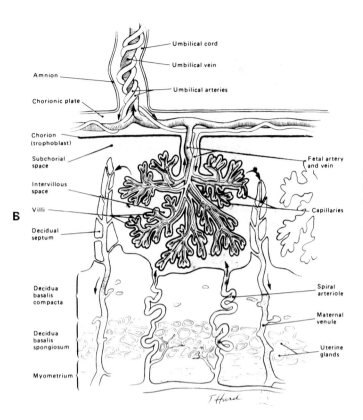

Umbilical cord
Umbilical vein
Amnion
Umbilical arteries
Chorionic plate
Chorion
(trophoblast)
Subchorial
space
Intervillous
space
Fetal artery
and vein
Villi
Capillaries
Decidual
septum
B
Decidua
basalis
compacta
Spiral
arteriole
Decidua
basalis
spongiosum
Maternal
venule
Myometrium
Uterine
glands

FIG. 4-12, cont'd. **B,** Cross section through placenta. Arrows indicate direction of blood flow. **(A,** From Thompson JM et al: *Mosby's clinical nursing,* ed 3, St Louis, 1993, Mosby. **B,** From Langley LL, Telford IR, Christensen JB: *Dynamic human anatomy and physiology,* ed 5, New York, 1980, McGraw-Hill; copyright Mosby.)

nal exercise that diverts blood to the muscles away from the uterus compromises placental circulation. Optimum circulation is achieved when the woman lies at rest on her side. It is also believed that Braxton Hicks contractions (see p. 96) enhance the movement of blood through the intervillous spaces, aiding placental circulation. However, prolonged contractions or too-short intervals between contractions during labor reduce blood flow to the placenta.

Membranes

At the time of implantation, two **fetal membranes,** which will surround the developing embryo, begin to form (Fig. 4-12, *A*). The chorion develops from the trophoblast and contains the chorionic villi on its surface. The villi burrowing into the decidua basalis increase in size and complexity as the vascular processes develop into the placenta. The chorion becomes the covering of the fetal side of the placenta. It contains the major umbilical blood vessels as they branch out over the surface of the placenta. As the embryo grows, the decidua capsularis becomes stretched. The chorionic villi on this side atrophy and degenerate, leaving a smooth chorionic membrane.

The inner cell membrane, the amnion, develops from the interior cells of the blastocyst. The cavity that develops between this inner cell mass and the outer layer of cells (trophoblast) is the amniotic cavity (Fig. 4-8, *B*). As it grows larger, the amnion forms on the side opposite to the developing blastocyst (Fig. 4-9). The developing embryo draws the amnion around itself, forming a fluid-filled sac. The amnion becomes the covering of the umbilical cord and covers the chorion on the fetal surface of the placenta. As the embryo grows larger, the amnion enlarges to accommodate both the embryo-fetus and its surrounding **amniotic fluid.** The amnion eventually comes in contact with the chorion surrounding the fetus.

Amniotic Fluid

Initially, the amniotic cavity derives its fluid by diffusion from the maternal blood. The amount of fluid increases weekly, so that at term there is normally between 800 and 1200 ml of transparent, slightly yellow liquid. The amniotic fluid volume changes constantly. The fetus swallows fluid, and fluid flows into and out of the fetal lungs. The fetus urinates into the fluid, greatly enhancing its volume. Having less than 300 ml of amniotic fluid *(oligohydramnios)* is associated with fetal renal abnormalities. Having greater than 2 L of amniotic fluid *(hydramnios)* is associated with gastrointestinal and other malformations.

There are many functions served by amniotic fluid for the embryo-fetus. It cushions the fetus from trauma by blunting and dispersing the forces. It allows freedom of movement for musculoskeletal development. It keeps the embryo from tangling with the membranes, which facilitates symmetric growth of the fetus. If the embryo does intersect with the membranes, extremity amputations or other deformities can occur from constricting amniotic bands (Reed, Claireaux, Bain, 1989). Amniotic fluid helps maintain a constant body temperature. It serves as a source of oral fluid and as a waste repository.

Amniotic fluid contains albumin, urea, uric acid, creatinine, lecithin, sphingomyelin, bilirubin, fructose, fat, leukocytes, proteins, epithelial cells, enzymes, and lanugo hair. Study of the amniotic fluid via amniocentesis yields much information about the fetus. Genetic studies (karyotyping) provide knowledge about the sex and normality of chromosome number and structure. Other studies determine the health or maturity of the fetus.

Yolk Sac

While the amniotic cavity and amnion are forming, another blastocyst cavity forms on the other side of the developing embryonic disk (Fig. 4-8, *B*). This cavity becomes surrounded by a membrane, forming the yolk sac. This aids in transferring maternal nutrients and oxygen, which have diffused through the chorion to the embryo.

Blood vessels form to aid transport. By the third week, blood cells and plasma are manufactured in the yolk sac. At the end of the third week, the primitive heart begins to beat to circulate the blood through the embryo, connecting stalk, chorion, and yolk sac.

Part of the yolk sac becomes incorporated into the embryo's body as the primitive digestive system during the folding in of the embryo in the fourth week. Primordial germ cells arise in the yolk sac and migrate into the embryo. The shrinking remains of the yolk sac degenerate (Fig. 4-9). By the fifth or sixth week, the remnant has separated from the embryo. In about 2% of adults the intra-abdominal part of the yolk stalk persists as a diverticulum of the ileum known as *Meckel's diverticulum* (Moore, 1989).

Primary Germ Layers

During the second week after conception, the embryonic disk differentiates into three primary germ layers: the ectoderm, mesoderm, and endoderm or entoderm (Fig. 4-8, *B*). From these three layers develop all tissues and organs of the embryo.

The *ectoderm*, the upper layer of the embryonic disk, gives rise to the epidermis, glands, nails and hair, the central and peripheral nervous systems, eye lens, tooth enamel, and the floor of the amniotic cavity.

The middle layer, the *mesoderm,* develops into the bones and teeth, muscles (skeletal, smooth, and cardiac), dermis, and connective tissue, the cardiovascular system and spleen, and the urogenital system.

The lower layer, the *endoderm,* gives rise to the epithelium lining the respiratory tract and digestive tract, including the oropharynx, the liver and pancreas, urethra, bladder, and female vagina. The endoderm forms the roof of the yolk sac.

Umbilical Cord

By day 14 after conception, the embryonic disk, amniotic sac, and yolk sac are attached to the chorionic villi by the connecting stalk. During the third week, the blood vessels develop to supply the embryo with maternal nutrients and oxygen. During the fifth week, after the embryo has curved inward on itself from both ends, bringing the connecting stalk to the ventral side of the embryo, the connecting stalk becomes compressed from both sides by the amnion forming the narrower **umbilical cord** (Fig. 4-9). Two arteries carry blood from the embryo to the chorionic villi, and one vein returns blood to the embryo. One percent of umbilical cords contain only two vessels, one artery and one vein. This occurrence is sometimes associated with congenital malformations.

The cord rapidly increases in length. At term, the cord ranges from 30 to 90 cm long (average 55 cm) and is 2 cm in diameter. It twists spirally on itself and loops around the embryo-fetus. A true knot is rare, but false

knots occur as folds or kinks in the cord. Connective tissue, called Wharton's jelly, prevents compression of the blood vessels to ensure continued nourishment of the embryo-fetus. Compression can occur if the cord lies between the fetal head and the pelvis or twists around the fetal body. When the cord is wrapped around the fetal neck, it is called a *nuchal cord.*

As the placenta develops from the chorionic villi, the umbilical cord is usually located centrally. A peripheral location is less common and known as a *battledore placenta* (Fig. 4-11). The blood vessels are arrayed out from the center to all parts of the placenta.

Fetal Maturation

The stage of the **fetus** lasts from 9 weeks until the pregnancy ends. Changes in the fetal period are not as dramatic, since refinement of structure and function are taking place. The fetus is less vulnerable to teratogens (see p. 85), except for those affecting central nervous system functioning.

Viability refers to the capability of the fetus to survive outside the uterus. In the past, the earliest age at which fetal survival could be expected was 28 weeks after conception. With modern technology and advancements in maternal and neonatal care, viability has now been possible at 20 weeks after conception (22 weeks since LMP; fetal weight $\geq$500 g). The limitations on survival outside the uterus are based on central nervous system functions and oxygenation capability of the lungs (Moore, 1989).

Fetal Circulatory System

The cardiovascular system is the first organ system to function in the developing human. Blood vessel and blood cell formation begin in the third week to supply the embryo with oxygen and nutrients from the mother. By the end of the third week, the tubular heart begins to beat and the primitive cardiovascular system links the embryo, connecting stalk, chorion, and yolk sac. During the fourth and fifth weeks, the heart develops into the four-chambered organ. By the end of the embryonic stage, the heart is developmentally complete.

The fetal lungs do not function for respiratory gas exchange, so a special circulatory pathway exists that bypasses the lungs.

Oxygen-rich blood from the placenta flows rapidly through the umbilical vein into the fetal abdomen (Fig. 16-1). When the umbilical vein reaches the liver, it divides into two branches. One circulates some oxygenated blood through the liver. Most of the blood passes through the ductus venosus into the inferior vena cava. There it mixes with the deoxygenated blood from the fetal legs and abdomen on its way to the right atrium. Most of this blood passes straight ahead through the right atrium and through the **foramen ovale,** an opening into the left atrium. There it mixes with the small amount of blood returning deoxygenated from the fetal lungs through the pulmonary veins. The blood flows into the left ventricle and is squeezed out into the aorta. Here, the arteries supplying the heart, head, neck, and arms receive the major part of the oxygen-rich blood. This pattern, supplying the highest levels of oxygen and nutrients to the head, neck, and arms, enhances the **cephalocaudal** (head-to-rump) **development** of the embryo-fetus.

Deoxygenated blood returning from the head and arms enters the right atrium through the superior vena cava. This blood is directed downward into the right ventricle, where it is squeezed into the pulmonary artery. A small amount of blood circulates through the resistant lung tissue, but the majority follows the path with less resistance through the **ductus arteriosus** into the aorta, distal to the point of exit of the arteries supplying the head and arms with oxygenated blood. The oxygen-poor blood flows through the abdominal aorta into the internal iliac arteries, where the umbilical arteries direct most of it back through the umbilical cord to the placenta. There, the blood gives up its wastes and carbon dioxide in exchange for nutrients and oxygen. The blood remaining in the iliac arteries flows through the fetal abdomen and legs, ultimately returning through the inferior vena cava to the heart.

There are three special characteristics that enable the fetus to obtain sufficient oxygen from the maternal blood:

1. Fetal hemoglobin carries 20% to 30% more oxygen than maternal hemoglobin.
2. The fetal hemoglobin concentration is about 50% greater than that of the mother.
3. The fetal heart rate (FHR) is 120 to 160 beats per minute, making the fetal cardiac output per unit of body weight higher than that of an adult.

Hematopoietic System

Beginning in the third week hematopoiesis, the formation of blood, occurs in the yolk sac (Fig. 4-9). Hematopoietic stem cells seed the fetal liver during the fifth week. During the sixth week, hematopoiesis begins in the fetal liver, and accounts for its relatively large size between the seventh and ninth weeks. Stem cells seed the fetal bone marrow, spleen and thymus, and lymph nodes between weeks 8 and 11.

The antigenic factors that determine blood type are present in the erythrocytes soon after the sixth week. For this reason, the Rh-negative woman is at risk for isoimmunization with any pregnancy that lasts longer than 6 weeks after fertilization.

Respiratory System

Fetal lung development begins between gestational weeks 5 and 17 with the formation of bronchi and terminal bronchi. Most commonly, fetal pulmonary maturity coincides with the establishment of surfactants during gestational week 35.

Pulmonary Surfactants

The detection of the presence of pulmonary **surfactants,** surface-active phospholipids, in amniotic fluid has been used to determine the degree of fetal lung maturity, or the ability of the lungs to function after birth. Lecithin is the most critical alveolar surfactant required for postnatal lung expansion. It increases in amount after the twenty-fourth week. Another pulmonary phospholipid, sphingomyelin, remains constant in amount. Thus the measure of **lecithin** (L) in relation to **sphingomyelin** (S), or the **L/S ratio** of 2:1, is used to determine fetal lung maturity. This occurs at approximately 35 weeks of gestation (Creasy, Resnik, 1994).

Certain maternal conditions alter fetal lung development. Those conditions that accelerate lung maturity generally cause decreased maternal placental blood flow. The resulting fetal hypoxia apparently stresses the fetus, increasing blood levels of corticosteroids that accelerate alveolar and surfactant development. Conditions such as maternal hypertension, placental dysfunction, infection, or corticosteroid use accelerate maturity. Conditions such as gestational diabetes and chronic glomerulonephritis can retard fetal lung maturity.

The recent approval of the use of intrabronchial synthetic surfactant in the treatment of respiratory distress syndrome in the newborn has greatly improved the chances of survival of preterm infants (Paynton, 1991).

Fetal respiratory movements have been seen on ultrasound as early as the eleventh week. These fetal respiratory movements may aid in development of the chest wall muscles and regulate lung fluid volume. The fetal lungs produce fluid that expands the air spaces in the lungs. The fluid drains into the amniotic fluid or is swallowed by the fetus. Before birth, secretion of lung fluid decreases. The normal birth process squeezes out approximately one third of the fluid. Infants of cesarean births do not benefit from this squeezing process; as a result, they have more respiratory difficulty at birth. The fluid remaining in the lungs at birth is usually reabsorbed into the infant's bloodstream within 2 hours of birth.

Renal System

The permanent kidneys form during the fifth week. Urine formation is present during the third month. Urine is excreted into the amniotic fluid and accounts for a major part of the amniotic fluid volume. *Oligohydramnios,* an abnormally small amount of amniotic fluid, is indicative of renal dysfunction. The placenta acts as the organ of excretion and maintains fetal water and electrolyte balance, so that an infant does not need functioning kidneys during fetal life. At birth, however, the kidneys are required immediately for excretory and acid-base regulatory functions.

A fetus with a renal malformation can be diagnosed in utero. Either corrective or palliative fetal surgery can successfully treat renal malformation, or plans can be made for treatment immediately after birth.

At term the fetus has fully developed kidneys. However, the glomerular filtration rate (GFR) is low, and the kidneys lack the ability to concentrate urine. This makes the newborn more susceptible to both overhydration and dehydration.

Most newborns void within 24 hours of birth. With the loss of the swallowed amniotic fluid and the metabolism of placenta-provided nutrients, voidings for the first days of life are scanty until fluid intake increases.

Neurologic System

The nervous system originates from the ectoderm at 18 days after fertilization. The open neural tube forms during the fourth week. It initially closes at what will be the junction of the brain and spinal cord, leaving both ends open. The embryo folds in on itself lengthwise at this time, forming a head fold in the neural tube at this junction. The cranial end of the neural tube closes, then the caudal end. During week 5, different growth rates cause more flexures in the neural tube, delineating three brain areas: the forebrain, midbrain, and hindbrain.

The forebrain develops into the eyes (cranial nerve II) and cerebral hemispheres. The development of all areas of the cerebral cortex continues throughout fetal life and into childhood. The olfactory system (cranial nerve I) and thalamus also develop from the forebrain. Cranial nerves III and IV (oculomotor and trochlear) form from the midbrain. The hindbrain forms the medulla, pons, cerebellum, and the remainder of the cranial nerves. Brain waves can be recorded on an electroencephalogram by week 8.

The spinal cord develops from the long end of the neural tube. Another ectodermal structure, the neural crest, develops into the peripheral nervous system. By the eighth week, nerve fibers traverse throughout the body. By week 11 or 12, the fetus makes respiratory movements, moves all extremities, and changes position in utero. The fetus can suck his or her thumb and swim in the amniotic fluid pool, turning somersaults and possibly tying a knot in the umbilical cord. When the movements are strong enough to be perceived by the mother as "the baby moving," **quickening** has occurred. For the nullipara, this sensation is usually noted after 16 weeks. For the multipara, the perception occurs earlier. At this time, the mother becomes aware of the sleeping and waking cycles of the fetus.

Sensory Awareness

Purposeful movements of the fetus have been demonstrated in response to a firm touch transmitted through the mother's abdomen. Invasive procedures to be done on a fetus now require anesthesia.

Fetuses have been shown to respond to sound by 24 weeks. Different types of music evoke different movements. The fetus can be soothed by the sound of the mother's voice. Acoustic stimulation can be used to evoke an FHR response (Bar-Hava, Barnhardt, 1994). The fetus does become accustomed to noises heard repeatedly.

The fetus is able to distinguish taste. By the fifth month, when the fetus is swallowing amniotic fluid, a sweetener added to the fluid causes the fetus to swallow twice as fast (Poole, 1986). The fetus also reacts to temperature changes. A cold solution placed into the amniotic fluid can cause fetal hiccups.

The fetus can see. Eyes have both rods and cones in the retina by the seventh month. A bright light shone on the mother's abdomen in late pregnancy causes abrupt fetal movements. During sleep time, rapid eye movements (REMs) have been observed similar to those occurring in children and adults while dreaming (Poole, 1986).

At term the fetal brain is approximately one fourth the size of an adult brain. Neurologic development continues. Stressors on the fetus and neonate, such as chronic poor nutrition or hypoxia, drugs, environmental toxins, trauma, or disease, cause damage to the central nervous system long after the vulnerable embryonic time for malformations in other organ systems. Neurologic insult can result in cerebral palsy, neuromuscular impairment, mental retardation, and learning disabilities.

Gastrointestinal System

During the fourth week, the embryo changes from almost straight to a "C" shape as both ends fold in toward the ventral surface. A portion of the yolk sac is incorporated into the body from head to tail as the primitive gut (digestive system).

The foregut produces the pharynx, part of the lower respiratory tract, the esophagus, the stomach, the first half of the duodenum, the liver, the pancreas, and the gallbladder. These structures evolve over the fifth and sixth weeks. The malformations that can occur in these areas are esophageal atresia, hypertrophic pyloric stenosis, duodenal stenosis or atresia, and biliary atresia.

The midgut becomes the distal half of the duodenum, the jejunum and ileum, the cecum and appendix, and the proximal half of the colon. The midgut loop projects into the umbilical cord between weeks 5 and 10. A malformation (omphalocele) results if the midgut fails to return to the abdominal cavity, and intestines protrude from the umbilicus. Meckel's diverticulum is the most common malformation of the midgut (see p. 79). It occurs when a remnant of the yolk stalk that has failed to degenerate attaches to the ileum, leaving a blind sac.

The hindgut develops into the distal half of the colon, the rectum and parts of the anal canal, the urinary bladder, and urethra. Anorectal malformations are the most common abnormalities of the digestive system.

The fetus swallows amniotic fluid beginning in the fifth month. Gastric emptying and intestinal peristalsis occur. The placenta takes care of fetal nutrition and elimination needs. As the fetus nears term, fetal waste products have accumulated in the intestines as dark green to black, tarry **meconium.** Normally, this substance is passed through the rectum within 48 hours of birth. Sometimes with a breech birth or fetal hypoxia, meconium is passed in utero in the amniotic fluid. The failure to pass meconium after birth could be indicative of atresia somewhere in the digestive tract, an imperforate anus, or a meconium ileus with a firm meconium plug blocking passage. This is seen in infants with cystic fibrosis.

The metabolic rate of the fetus is relatively low, but the infant has great growth and development needs. Beginning in week 9, the fetus synthesizes glycogen for storage in the liver. Between 26 to 30 weeks, the fetus begins to lay down stores of *brown fat* in preparation for extrauterine cold stress (see Chapter 13). Thermoregulation in the neonate requires increased metabolism and adequate oxygenation.

The gastrointestinal system is mature by 36 weeks. Digestive enzymes are present in sufficient quantity except pancreatic amylase and lipase. The neonate cannot digest starches or fats efficiently. Little saliva is produced.

Hepatic System

The liver and biliary tract develop from the foregut during the fourth week of gestation. Hematopoiesis begins during the sixth week, requiring that the liver be large. The embryonic liver is prominent and occupies most of the abdominal cavity. Bile, a constituent of meconium, begins to form in the twelfth week.

Glycogen is stored in the fetal liver beginning at week 9 or 10 and continuing for extrauterine needs. At term, glycogen stores are twice those of the adult. Glycogen is the major source of energy for the fetus and neonate who is stressed by in utero hypoxia or by extrauterine loss of the maternal glucose supply, by the work of breathing, or by cold stress.

The fetal liver stores iron. If the maternal intake is sufficient, enough iron can be stored to last for 5 months after birth.

During fetal life, the liver does not have to conjugate bilirubin for excretion, because the unconjugated bilirubin is cleared by the placenta. Therefore the fetal liver has less glucuronyl transferase enzyme needed for conjugation than is required after birth. This predisposes the neonate to hyperbilirubinemia.

Coagulation factors II, VII, IX, and X cannot be synthesized in the fetal liver because of the *lack of vitamin K synthesis* in the sterile fetal gut. This coagulation deficiency persists after birth for several days, and is the rationale for the prophylactic administration of vitamin K to the newborn.

Endocrine System

The thyroid gland develops with structures in the head and neck during the third and fourth weeks. The secretion of thyroxine begins during the eighth week. Maternal thyroxine does not readily cross the placenta. As a result, the fetus, who does not produce thyroid hormones, will be born with congenital hypothyroidism. If untreated, this can result in severe mental retardation. All neonates are screened for hypothyroidism with a blood test after birth (Appendix F).

The adrenal cortex is formed during the sixth week and produces hormones by the eighth or ninth week. As term approaches, the fetus produces *more cortisol.* This is believed to aid in *initiation of labor* by decreasing the maternal progesterone and stimulating production of prostaglandins.

The pancreas forms from the foregut during the fifth through eighth weeks. The islets of Langerhans develop during the twelfth week. Insulin is produced by the twentieth week. In infants of mothers with uncontrolled diabetes, maternal hyperglycemia produces fetal hyperglycemia, stimulating hyperinsulinemia and islet-cell hyperplasia. This results in an excessive sized fetus. The hyperinsulinemia also blocks lung maturation, placing the neonate at risk for respiratory distress and hypoglycemia when the maternal glucose source is lost at birth. Control of the maternal glucose level during pregnancy minimizes the problems for the infant.

Reproductive System

Until the seventh week, there is no sex differentiation in the embryo. Then the Y chromosome in the male dictates the formation of testes. By the end of the embryonic period, testosterone is being secreted and causes formation of the male genitalia. By week 28, the testes begin descending into the scrotum. After birth, low levels of testosterone continue to be secreted until the pubertal surge.

The lack of a Y chromosome in the female brings about the formation of ovaries and female external genitalia. Female and male external genitalia are indistinguishable until after the ninth week. By the sixteenth week, oogenesis has been established. At birth, the ovaries contain the female's lifetime supply of ova. The female lacks most female hormone production until puberty, however, the fetal endometrium responds to the maternal hormones. Withdrawal bleeding (pseudomenstruation) or vaginal discharge may occur at birth when these maternal hormones are lost. The high level of maternal estrogen also stimulates mammary engorgement and secretion of fluid (witch's milk).

Immunologic System

During the last trimester, albumin and globulin are present in the fetus. The only immunoglobulin that crosses the placenta is IgG, providing passive acquired immunity to specific bacterial toxins. The fetus produces IgM immunoglobulins by the end of the first trimester. These are produced in response to blood group antigens, gram-negative enteric organisms, and some viruses. IgA immunoglobulins are not produced by the fetus; however, colostrum, the precursor to breast milk, contains large amounts and can provide passive immunity to the neonate.

The normal neonate can fight infection, but not as effectively as an older child. The preterm infant is at much greater risk for infection.

Musculoskeletal System

Bones and muscles develop from the mesoderm by the fourth week of embryonic development. At that time the cardiac muscle is already beating. The mesoderm beside the neural tube forms the vertebral column and ribs. The parts of the vertebral column grow toward each other to enclose the developing spinal cord. Ossification or bone formation begins. If there is a defect in the bony fusion, spina bifida may occur. A large defect affecting several vertebrae may allow the membranes and spinal cord to pouch out from the back, producing neurologic deficits and skeletal deformity.

The flat bones of the skull develop during the embryonic period, and ossification continues throughout childhood. At birth connective tissue sutures exist where the bones of the skull meet. The areas where more than two bones meet, called *fontanels,* are especially prominent. The sutures and fontanels allow the bones of the skull to mold, or move during birth, enabling the head to pass through the birth canal. The larger fontanel remains open until the second year of life.

The bones of the shoulders, arms, hips, and legs appear in the sixth week as a continuous skeleton with no joints. Differentiation occurs, producing separate bones and joints. Ossification will continue through childhood to allow growth.

Beginning during the seventh week, muscles contract spontaneously. Arm and leg movements are visible on ultrasound, although the mother does not perceive them until the sixteenth to the twentieth week.

Integumentary System

The epidermis begins as a single layer of cells derived from the ectoderm at 4 weeks. By the seventh week, there are two layers of cells. The superficial layer cells are sloughed and become mixed with the sebaceous gland secretions to form the white, greasy **vernix caseosa,** the material that protects the skin of the fetus. The vernix is thick at 24 weeks, but becomes scant by term. The basal layer of the epidermis is the germinal layer, which replaces the lost cells. Until 17 weeks, the skin is very thin and wrinkled, with blood vessels visible underneath. The

skin thickens, and all layers are present at term. After 32 weeks, as subcutaneous fat is deposited under the dermis, the skin is less wrinkled and red in appearance.

By 16 weeks, the epidermal ridges are present on the palms of the hands, the fingers, the bottom of the feet and the toes. This makes the hand and footprints unique to that infant.

Hairs form from hair bulbs in the epidermis, which project into the dermis. Cells in the hair bulb keratinize to form the hair shaft. As the cells at the base of the hair shaft proliferate, the hair grows to the surface of the epithelium. The very fine hairs, called **lanugo,** appear first at 12 weeks on the eyebrows and upper lip. By 20 weeks, they cover the entire body. At this time, the eyelashes, eyebrows, and scalp hair are beginning to grow. By 28 weeks, the scalp hair is longer than the lanugo, which is thinning and may disappear by term gestation.

Fingernails and toenails develop from thickened epidermis at the tips of the digits beginning during the tenth week. They grow slowly. Fingernails usually reach the fingertips by 32 weeks, and toenails reach toetips by 36 weeks. Table 4-1 summarizes embryonic and fetal development.

Multifetal Pregnancy
Twins

The woman who produces two mature ova in one ovarian cycle has the potential for both to be fertilized by separate sperm. This results in two zygotes or **dizygotic twins.** (Fig. 4-13). There are always two amnions, two

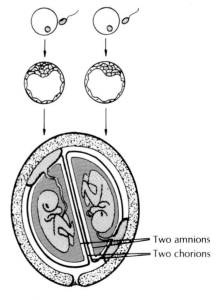

Two amnions
Two chorions

FIG. 4-13 Formation of dizygotic twins. There is fertilization of two ova, two implantations, two placentas, two chorions, and two amnions. (From Whaley LF: *Understanding inherited disorders,* St Louis, 1974, Mosby.)

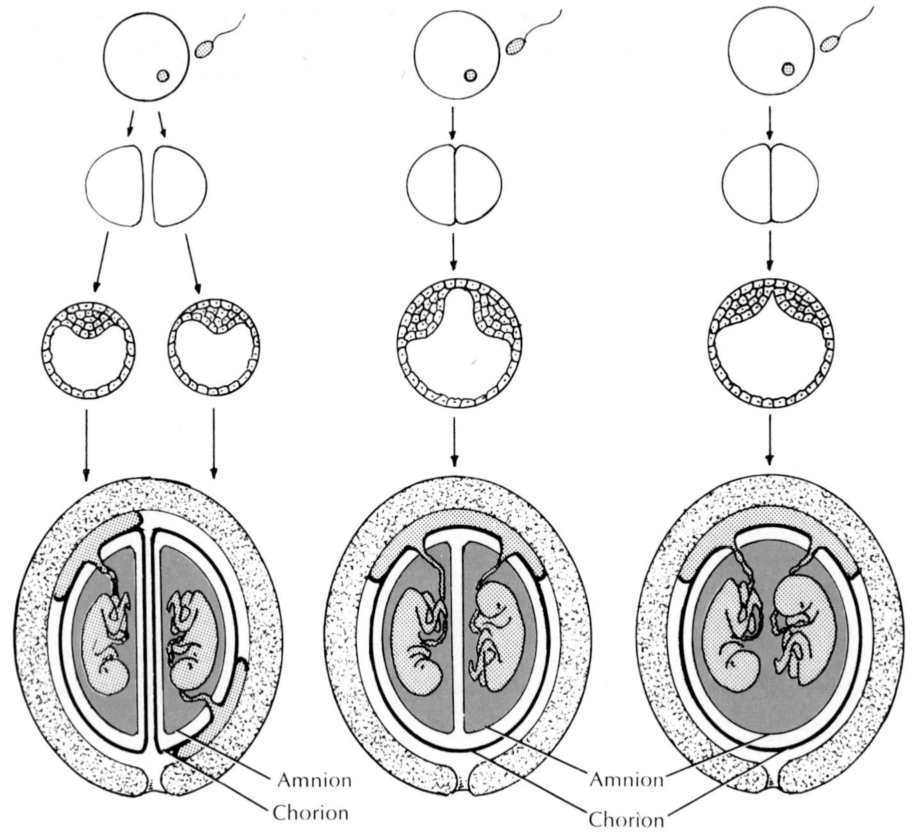

FIG. 4-14 Formation of monozygotic twins. **A,** One fertilization: blastomeres separate, resulting in two implantations, two placentas, and two sets of membranes. **B,** One blastomere with two inner cell masses, one fused placenta, one chorion, and separate amnions. **C,** Later separation of inner cell masses, with fused placenta and single amnion and chorion. (From Whaley LF: *Understanding inherited disorders,* St Louis, 1974, Mosby.)

chorions, and two placentas that may be fused together. These fraternal twins may be the same sex or different sexes and are genetically no more alike than siblings born at different times. Dizygotic twinning occurs in families, more often among African-American women than white women and least among Asian women. It increases in frequency with maternal age up to 35 years, with parity, and with the use of fertility drugs.

Identical twins develop from one fertilized ovum, which then divides (hence the term **monozygotic twins**) (Fig. 4-14). They are the same sex and have the same genotype. If division occurs soon after fertilization, then two embryos, two amnions, two chorions, and two placentas that may be fused will develop. Most often, division occurs between 4 and 8 days after fertilization, and there are two embryos, two amnions, one chorion, and one placenta. Rarely, division occurs after the eighth day after fertilization. In this case, there are two embryos within a common amnion and a common chorion with one placenta. This commonly causes circulation problems because the umbilical cords tangle together, and one or both fetuses may die. If division occurs very late, cleavage may not be complete, and conjoined or

"Siamese" twins could result.

Monozygotic twinning occurs in approximately 1 of 250 births (Cunningham et al, 1993). There is no association with race, heredity, maternal age, or parity. Fertility drugs do increase the incidence (Derom et al, 1987).

Other Multifetal Pregnancies

The occurrence of multifetal pregnancies with three or more fetuses has increased with the use of fertility drugs and in vitro fertilization. Triplets occur once in about 7600 pregnancies. They can occur from the division of one zygote into two, with one of the two dividing again, producing identical triplets. Triplets can also be produced from two zygotes, one dividing into a set of identical twins and the second zygote a single fraternal sibling, or from three zygotes. Quadruplets, quintuplets, sextuplets, and so on, likewise, have similar possible derivations.

Genetic Counseling

Rapid expansion in the identification, understanding, and diagnosis of genetic disease has been accompanied by effective medical or surgical therapies in a small number of cases. For the majority of genetic conditions, therapeutic or preventive measures are nonexistent or disappointingly limited. Consequently, the most useful means of reducing the incidence of these disorders is by preventing their transmission. With the accumulation of knowledge about genetic disease, the probability of recurrence in any given situation can be predicted with increased accuracy.

Patients Seeking Genetic Counseling

The reasons people seek genetic counseling vary. People may or may not be affected themselves. Those who seek counseling commonly fall into the following categories:

1. People who want to know if they have a genetic disorder or if they are carriers of a genetic disorder
2. People who are concerned about being at risk for producing a child with a specific genetic disorder
3. People who are planning parenthood and want to know the implications (prognosis and treatment) of a genetic disorder afflicting one or both partners
4. People seeking help in making a decision about prenatal diagnosis, selective abortion, artificial insemination by donor, or adoption
5. People seeking help for a child affected with a genetic disorder

For all pregnancies, it is standard practice to assess for heritable disorders in order to identify potential patients (Creasy, Resnik, 1994). The interviewer inquires about the health status of family members, abnormal reproductive outcomes, history of maternal disorder (e.g., diabetes, PKU, and cystic fibrosis), drug exposures, and illness (Fanaroff, Martin, 1992). Advanced maternal and paternal ages are noted.

Ethnic origin should be recorded, since some disorders appear more frequently in some groups (Creasy, Resnik, 1994). Examples include: Tay-Sachs disease in Jewish individuals of Ashkenazic or Sephardic descent, β-thalassemia in Italians and Greeks, sickle cell anemia in African-Americans, α-thalassemia in Southeast Asians and Filipinos, and tyrosinemia in French Canadians from the Lac St. Jean-Chicoutimi region of Quebec (Fanaroff, Martin, 1992).

Role of Nurse in Genetic Counseling

Nurses are assuming an increasingly important role in counseling people about genetically transmitted or genetically influenced conditions. Diagnosis and treatment of genetic disorders require medical skills; the complexities of determining risk factors for many diseases and for individual circumstances require a geneticist's expertise. Nurses, who are actively involved in counseling, require a minimum of a master's degree in genetics or in a related subject. Nurses without advanced preparation in genetics can still be productive members of a counseling service.

All nurses, especially those involved in the care of mothers and children, need to: (1) have an understand-

ETHICAL CONSIDERATIONS

APPLICATION OF GENETIC TECHNOLOGY

Prenatal diagnostic tests such as amniocentesis and chorionic villus biopsy, which reveal birth defects and fetal sex, raise the specter of *elective abortion* for sex selection. This rationale for elective abortion raises serious ethical questions for health care providers faced with these situations.

Another technology with ethical implications is the use of *fetal tissue transplantation* (Erlen, 1990; Gero, Giordano, 1990). Current research suggests that fetal neurologic, liver, and pancreatic tissues transplanted into adults with Parkinson's disease, metabolic disorders, or head and spinal cord injury could hold promise of recovery for those adults. The important ethical issue is to reduce any pressure for fetal tissues on a mother who is contemplating an elective abortion (Council on Scientific Affairs and Council on Ethical and Judicial Affairs, 1990). Elective abortion continues to be a controversial issue, with many ethical issues yet to be resolved.

ing of genetic theory and the nature of more common genetic disorders in order to recognize cues that may indicate a genetically related problem, (2) be able to help families obtain counseling services, (3) augment the counseling process (Stringer, Librizzi, Weiner, 1991), and (4) be aware of the legal and ethical issues involved (Barber, 1991) (see Ethical Considerations). Nurses assist with preparation of patients for procedures and counseling, as well as with diagnostic procedures and therapeutic programs. Nurses also interpret and reinforce counseling, maintain follow-up care, support the family's coping capacities, and assist them in problem solving. To provide supportive care for families involved in genetic counseling, nurses need an understanding of the process and some of the procedures that the family will experience.

Nurses are in the best position to sustain a close relationship and provide follow-up care (e.g., community health nurses who have already established a rapport with many families). Interviewing and counseling skills are an integral part of a nurse's professional practice.

Nongenetic Factors Influencing Development

Not all congenital disorders are inherited. Congenital simply means that the condition was present at birth. Some congenital malformations may be the result of **teratogens,** defined as environmental substances or exposures that cause adverse effects (Bernhardt, 1990). Although teratogens are not genetic material per se, they

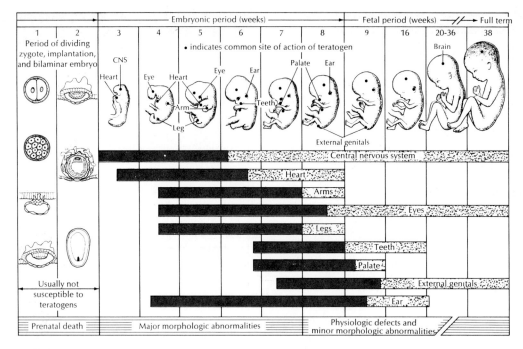

FIG. 4-15 Sensitive, or critical, periods in human development. Dark color denotes highly sensitive periods; light color indicates stages that are less sensitive to teratogens. (From Moore KL: *Before we are born: basic embryology and birth defects,* ed 3, Philadelphia, 1989, WB Saunders.)

frequently produce their ill effects by altering the normal expression of the embryonic genome in some fashion. Known human teratogens are drugs and chemicals (for embryonic fetal effects, see Appendix E) (Thomson, Cordero, 1989; Brown, Bellinger, Matthews, 1990), infections, exposure, and certain maternal conditions (see Box 4-1). A teratogen has the greatest effect on the organs and parts of an embryo during its periods of rapid differentiation. This occurs during the embryonic period, specifically from days 15 to 60. During the first 2 weeks of development, teratogens either have no effect on the embryo, or their effects are so severe that they cause spontaneous abortion (Moore, 1989). Brain growth and development continue during the fetal period, and teratogens can severely affect mental development throughout gestation (Fig. 4-15).

Besides the genetic makeup and the influence of teratogens, the adequacy of maternal nutrition also influences development. The embryo and fetus must obtain the nutrients they need from the mother's diet; they cannot tap the maternal reserves. Malnutrition during pregnancy produces low-birth-weight newborns, who are more susceptible to infection. Malnutrition also affects brain development during the latter half of gestation, resulting in learning disabilities in the child.

Preconception Care

A relatively new concept, **preconception care,** is as important to perinatal services as prenatal care. Preconception care is care designed for health maintenance. It stresses healthy behaviors that promote health of the woman and her potential fetus. Some women do not desire pregnancy. With the exception of sterilization, any form of contraception can fail and result in pregnancy. Fifty percent of all pregnancies in the United States are unplanned (Centers for Disease Control, 1992). Therefore preconception care should be available to all women with reproductive potential who are sexually active with a male partner.

The *rationale* for preconception care includes the following:
- Establish lifestyle behaviors to maintain optimum health
- Identify and treat risk factors (e.g., medical conditions, substance abuse) before conception
- Conceive a pregnancy without unnecessary risk factors
- Prepare people psychologically for pregnancy and the responsibilities that come with parenthood

Every woman of childbearing age should be viewed as a potential mother. Therefore, identifying and treating risk factors and anticipatory guidance with emphasis on healthy lifestyles may be the key to improving the health of the next generation (Commentary, 1990). The *components* of preconception care, such as health promotion, risk assessment, and interventions as needed, are outlined in Box 4-2.

The more the health care provider knows about a woman's state of health and lifestyle the better. For ex-

BOX 4-1

Human Teratogens

DRUGS AND CHEMICALS

Alcohol
Androgens
Anticoagulants (warfarin and dicumarol)
Antithyroid drugs (propylthiouracil, iodide, and methimazole)
Chemotherapeutic drugs (methotrexate and aminopterin)
Diethylstilbestrol (DES)
Lead
Lithium
Organic mercury
Phenytoin
Polychlorinated biphenyls (PCBs)
Isoretinoin*
Streptomycin
Tetracycline
Thalidomide
Trimethadione paramethadione
Valproic acid

INFECTIONS

Cytomegalovirus
Rubella
Syphilis
Toxoplasmosis
Varicella

EXPOSURES

Radiation

MATERNAL CONDITIONS

Diabetes mellitus
Phenylketonuria

From Reed, Claireaux, Bain, editors: *Diseases of the fetus and newborn: pathology, radiology, and genetics,* St Louis, 1989, Mosby.
*Trade name: Accutane, a synthetic derivative of vitamin A.

BOX 4-2

Components of Preconception Care

HEALTH PROMOTION: GENERAL TEACHING

Nutrition
  Healthy diet
  Optimum weight
Exercise and rest
Avoidance of substance abuse (tobacco, alcohol, "recreational" drugs)
Use of "safer sex" practices
Attending to family and social needs

RISK FACTOR ASSESSMENT

Medical history
  Immune status (e.g., *Rubella*)
  Illnesses (e.g., infections)
  Genetic disorders
  Current use of medication (prescription, nonprescription)
Reproductive history
  Contraceptive
  Obstetric
Psychosocial history
  Spouse/partner and family situation, including domestic violence
  Availability of family or other support systems
  Readiness for pregnancy (e.g., age, life goals, stress)
Financial resources
Environmental (home, workplace) conditions
  Safety hazards
  Toxic chemicals
  Radiation

INTERVENTIONS

Anticipatory guidance/teaching
Treatment of medical conditions and results
  Medications
  Cessation/reduction in substance abuse
  Immunizations (e.g., *Rubella*, tuberculosis, hepatitis)
Nutrition, diet and weight management
Referral for genetic counseling
Referral to and use of
  Family planning services
  Family and social needs management

ample, women with insulin-dependent diabetes mellitus, who maintain excellent control of blood sugar at the time of conception, could reduce the risk for congenital anomalies (malformations) in the fetus (Centers for Disease Control, 1992). Women who have an adequate periconception (before and after conception) folic acid intake (0.4 mg/d) decrease the possibility of neural tube defects (Werler, Shipiro, Mitchell, 1993).

Some of the areas to be explored are listed in Box 4-3.

Role of Nurse in Preconception Care

Thoughtful assessment always provides a basis for identifying potential risks, developing outcome criteria, planning for care, and intervening.

The *management* of preconception care is directed by findings from the interview, physical examination, and laboratory studies. If a couple is planning a pregnancy, the primary health care provider may assist them with timing of conception after having had time to implement

lifestyle recommendations for their health. These recommendations could include diet and weight management, physical conditioning (Ratts, 1993), and immunizations. If pregnancy is not desired, the risk of unintended pregnancy is discussed, and the same lifestyle behaviors are recommended. Recommendations can be reinforced with videotapes or audio tapes, illustrations, and printed teaching aids (Scherger, 1993).

Prevention should be the focus of self-care in any plan

BOX 4-3

Preconception Assessment

INTERVIEW

Lifestyle
  Nutrition
  Exercise, rest
  Substance use: alcohol, tobacco, other
  Occupation
  Psychosocial: stress, anxiety, depression; support from partner, family, friends; domestic violence
  Financial resources
Immunization status
  Rubella
  Hepatitis
Medications
  Over-the-counter, nonprescription (e.g., aspirin)
  Prescription
Medical conditions: review of systems
  Hypertension
  Seizure disorders
  Diabetes mellitus
  Renal disease
  Autoimmune disorders (e.g., lupus, rheumatoid arthritis)
Reproductive system
  Fertility problems; endometriosis
  Contraceptive history
  Obstetric history (e.g., prior pregnancies, miscarriages, child with a disorder)
  Abnormal Pap smear results
  Sexually transmitted diseases (STDs)
  Sexual practices
Family history, including father of baby
  Medical conditions
  Genetic conditions (e.g., sickle cell disease, Tay-Sachs disease, cystic fibrosis, bleeding disorders, phenylketonuria [PKU])
  Birth defects

PHYSICAL EXAMINATION:

General medical with emphasis on:
  Thyroid gland
  Breasts
  Pelvic structures

LABORATORY STUDIES

General: CBC, urinalysis, blood type and Rh, rubella immunity, STDs (e.g., syphilis, gonorrhea, *Chlamydia*), hepatitis B surface antigen, Pap smear, and cervical culture
Depending on risk:
  PPD
  HIV
  Toxicology screen
  Thalassemia

of care. Preventive measures are suggested throughout this text for infection, nutrition, substance abuse, and other health-related concerns. Eight percent to 10% of birth defects occur as a result of environmental factors, and may be amenable to nursing interventions (Pletsh, 1990). Cleanliness, ventilation, adherence to manufacturer's directions for use and disposal of materials, use of protective gear to shield against known and unknown hazards, and avoidance of exposure are examples of strategies to reduce risk.

In some instances safer materials can be substituted for potentially hazardous ones. For example, most household cleaning needs can be met with baking soda, table salt, distilled white vinegar, lemon juice, trisodium phosphate (TSP; which does not emit fumes), a plunger, and some common sense. These substances clean drains, wash windows, degrease, prevent mold and mildew, disinfect, and scour (Dadd, 1987).

Nurses must implement self-protective measures when working with radiation therapy (Lowdermilk, 1990). The patient's room should be identified with the radioactivity logo and posted with the radiology department's precautionary protocol for the type of therapy being administered, for example, wearing gloves while handling bodily fluids. The three principles for radiation safety are time, distance, and shielding. A film badge or thermoluminescent dosimeter (TLD) badge must be worn to monitor the nurse's minute-by-minute exposure.

Industrial nurses must be alert to conditions in the workplace that may affect reproductive health of workers and their partners. Stress reduction through relaxation and guided imagery, as well as moderate exercise and rest, are useful (see index for these content areas).

As private citizens, nurses must become involved in their professional and political organizations to promote and support legislation to control pollution of the environment. Nurses can teach about alternative ways to clean the home and care for yards and gardens to reduce exposure to potentially harmful substances.

Evaluation of short-term results is possible to some extent. The birth of a healthy baby with no apparent disorder or disease, the uncomplicated recovery of the new mother, continued fertility, and demonstration of a lifestyle that supports good reproductive health are some expected outcomes if preconception and pregnancy care were effective. Long-term effects may not be known for many years or generations.

KEY POINTS

- Genes are the basic units of heredity, and are responsible for all human characteristics. They comprise 23 pairs of chromosomes: 22 pairs of autosomes and one pair of sex chromosomes.
- Mitosis is the process by which body cells replicate for growth, development, and cell replacement of the organism.
- Meiosis is the process by which gametes are formed for reproduction of the organism.
- Chromosomal abnormalities of number and structure occur in both autosomes and sex chromosomes.
- Genetic disorders follow mendelian inheritance patterns of dominance, segregation, and independent assortment of normal genetic transmission.
- Multifactorial inheritance includes both genetic and environmental contributions.
- Human gestation is approximately 280 days after the last menstrual period or 266 days after conception.

- Fertilization occurs in the uterine tube within 24 hours of ovulation. The zygote undergoes mitotic divisions, creating a 16-cell morula.
- Implantation occurs between 7 and 10 days after fertilization.
- The ovum stage ends with the formation of the embryonic membranes, the amnion and chorion, and the formation of the three germ layers: the ectoderm, mesoderm, and endoderm.
- The embryo stage lasts from the third to the eighth week after fertilization. The organ systems and external features develop, and the embryo becomes unmistakably human.
- The stage of the fetus lasts from the ninth week until birth. Refinement of structure and function occur, and the fetus becomes capable of extrauterine survival.
- There are critical periods in human development during which the embryo-fetus is vulnerable to environmental teratogens.

CRITICAL THINKING EXERCISES

1. Your family, friends, and co-workers know that you are a nursing student. All of these people view you as a resource person in health matters. As part of your nursing experience, you are attending and participating in parent education classes.

   You may encounter the following questions. Choose one question to discuss. In lay terms (terminology understood by the general public), briefly determine what additional information you need from the questioner. Then formulate your response, keeping in mind genetics and stages of development from conception to term gestation:
   a. "When is our baby due?"
   b. "How big is my baby now?"
   c. "My friend had a baby with blue eyes, but both of the parents have brown eyes. Is that possible?"

   d. "My baby sometimes jerks every couple of minutes for a short period of time. My mother said the baby is hiccuping. Is that true?"
   e. "How does the baby breathe in there?"
   f. "Everyone smokes in the office where I work. Will it hurt the baby?"
   g. "Will having sex (late in pregnancy) put holes in the baby's head or in his heart?"

2. Make a list of the household chemicals used in your home. In a group, compile a master list. Select some examples from the list, identify their purpose, describe why they are hazardous to the reproductive health of women and men and to the developing embryo/fetus. List what alternatives can be substituted to accomplish the same purpose.

References

Barber HRK: Ethics, morals, and gene control, *The Female Patient* 16(10):13, Oct 1991.

Bar-Hava I, Barnhard Y: Fetal vibracoustic stimulation, *The Female Patient* 19(5): 63, 1994.

Bernhardt JH: Potential workplace hazards to reproductive health: information for primary prevention, *JOGNN* 19:53, 1990.

Blackburn ST, Lopez DL: *Maternal, fetal, and neonatal physiology: a clinical perspective,* Philadelphia, 1992, WB Saunders.

Brown MJ, Bellinger D, Matthews J: In utero lead exposure, *MCN* 15(2):94, March/April 1990.

Carothers GP: Down syndrome and maternal age: the effect of erroneous assignment of parental origin, *Am J Hum Genet* 40:147, 1987.

Centers for Disease Control: Recommendation for use of folic acid to reduce number of spina bifida cases and other neural tube defects, *MMWR* 41:RR-14, 1992.

Commentary: Preconception care: risk reduction and health promotion in preparation for pregnancy, *JAMA* 264(9): 1147, Sept 1990.

Council on Scientific Affairs and Council on Ethical and Judicial Affairs: Medical applications of fetal tissue transplantation, *JAMA* 263(4):565, 1990.

Creasy RK, Resnik JR, editors: *Maternal-fetal medicine: principles and practice,* ed 3, Philadelphia, 1994, WB Saunders.

Cunningham FG et al: *Williams obstetrics,* ed 19, Norwalk, CT, 1993, Appleton & Lange.

Dadd DL: Nontoxic cleaners for your home, *San Francisco Chronicle,* p C8, April 1, 1987.

Derom C et al: Increased monozygotic twinning rate after ovulation induction, *Lancet* 1:1237, 1987.

Erlen JA: Anencephalic infants as sources of organs: issues and implications for nurses, *JOGNN* 19(3):249, May/June 1990.

Fanaroff AA, Martin RJ, editors: *Neonatal-perinatal medicine: diseases of the fetus and infant,* ed 5, St Louis, 1992, Mosby.

Gero E, Giordano J: Ethical considerations in fetal tissue transplantation, *J Neurosci Nurs* 22(1):9, Feb 1990.

Lowdermilk D: Nursing care update: internal radiation therapy, *NAACOG's Clin Issu Perinat Womens Health Nurs:* 1:532, 1990.

MacMullen NJ, Brucker MC: Pregnancy made possible for women with cystic fibrosis, *MCN* 14(3):196, May/June 1989.

Moore KL: *Before we are born: basic embryology and birth defects,* ed 3, Philadelphia, 1989, WB Saunders.

Nyhan WL: Diagnosing inborn errors of metabolism antenatally, *Contemp OB/GYN* 36(11):62, Nov 1991.

Paynton A: Synthetic surfactant: giving premature infants a better chance for survival, *Nursing 91* 21(3):64, 1991.

Pletsh P: Birth defect prevention: nursing interventions, *JOGNN* 19:482, 1990.

Poole RM editor: *The incredible machine,* Washington, DC, 1986, National Geographic Society.

Ratts, VS: Women and exercise: effects on the reproductive system, *The Female Patient* 18(7):59, July 1993.

Reed GB, Claireaux AE, Bain AD, editors: *Diseases of the fetus and newborn: pathology, radiology and genetics,* St Louis, 1989, Mosby.

Scherger JE: Preconception care: a neglected element of prenatal services, *The Female Patient* 18(7):78, July 1993.

Stringer M, Librizzi R, Weiner S: Establishing a prenatal genetic diagnosis: the nurse's role, *MCN* 16(3):152, May/June 1991.

Thomson EJ, Cordero JF: The new teratogens: accutane and other vitamin-A analogs, *MCN* 14(4):244, July/Aug 1989.

Werler MM, Shipiro S, Mitchell AA: Periconceptional folic acid exposure and risk of occurrent neural tube defects, *JAMA,* 269:1257, 1993.

Willson JR, Carrington ER: *Obstetrics and gynecology,* ed 9, St Louis, 1991, Mosby.

Wong DL: *Whaley and Wong's nursing care of infants and children,* ed 4, St Louis, 1995, Mosby.

Bibliography

Arias F: *Practical guide to high-risk pregnancy and delivery,* ed 2, St Louis, 1992, Mosby.

England MA: *Color atlas of life before birth: normal fetal development,* St Louis, 1990, Mosby.

Gjerdingen DK, Fontaine P: Preconception health care: a critical task for family physicians, *J Am Board Fam Pract* 4:237, 1991.

Groër M: Psychoneuroimmunology: an emerging discipline gives new theoretical support to nursing care of the "body-mind", *Am J Nurs* 91(8):33, 1991.

Heins HC: Your health pregnancy: hazards at home and on the job, *Am Baby* 53:10, March 1991.

Jack BW, Culpepper L: Preconception care: risk reduction and health promotion in preparation for pregnancy, *JAMA,* 264:1147, 1990.

Kitzmiller JL, Gavin LA, Gin GD et al: Preconception care of diabetes: glycemic control prevents congenital anomalies, *JAMA* 265:731, 1991.

Patterson E, Freese M, Goldenberg R: Seeking safe passage: utilizing health care during pregnancy, *Image J Nurs Sch* 22(1):27, 1990.

Polin RA, Fox WW: *Fetal and neonatal physiology,* vols 1 and 2, Philadelphia, 1991, WB Saunders.

Seidel HM et al: *Mosby's guide to physical examination,* ed 3, St Louis, 1995, Mosby.

5 Anatomy and Physiology of Pregnancy

P H Y L L I S   M.   K L E I N

LEARNING OBJECTIVES

Define the key terms listed.
Describe various pregnancy tests.
Explain the expected maternal anatomic and physiologic adaptations to pregnancy.
Identify the maternal hormones produced during pregnancy and their target organs. Relate their major effects on pregnancy.
Describe gravidity and parity using the 5-digit system.
Differentiate among presumptive, probable, and positive signs of pregnancy.
Compare the abdomen, vulva, and cervix of the nullipara and multipara.

KEY TERMS

amenorrhea
ballottement
Braxton Hicks' sign
Chadwick's sign
chloasma
colostrum
diastasis recti abdominis
epulis
ferning
friability
funic souffle
Goodell's sign
gravidity
  gravida
    multigravida
    nulligravida
    primigravida
Hegar's sign
hirsutism
hyperplasia
hypertrophy
leukorrhea
lightening

linea nigra
McDonald's sign
mean arterial pressure (MAP)
Montgomery's tubercles
operculum
palmar erythema
parity
  multipara
  nullipara
  primipara
parturient
preterm
pyrosis
ptyalism
quickening
radioimmunoassay
signs of pregnancy
  positive
  presumptive
  probable
striae gravidarum
telangiectasias
term
uterine souffle
viability

RELATED TOPICS

Anemia *(Chap. 22)* • Cardiovascular disorders of pregnancy *(Chap. 22)* • Diabetes mellitus and pregnancy *(Chap. 22)* • Fetal heart rate assessment *(Chap. 11)* • Human chorionic gonadotropin *(Chap. 3)* • Iron supplementation in pregnancy *(Chap. 8)* • Pregnancy-induced hypertension *(Chap. 21)* • Respiratory disorders in pregnancy *(Chap. 22)* • Supine hypotensive syndrome *(Chap. 7)*

healthy pregnancy with a physically safe and emotionally satisfying outcome for both mother and infant is the expected outcome of maternity care. Consistent health supervision and surveillance are of utmost importance. Many maternal adaptations are unfamiliar to pregnant women and their families. The knowledgeable maternity nurse can help the pregnant woman recognize the relationship between her physical status and the plan for her care. Sharing information encourages the pregnant woman to participate in her own care, depending upon her interest, need to know, and readiness to learn.

GRAVIDITY AND PARITY

An understanding of the following terms used to describe the pregnant woman is essential to the study of maternity care:

gravida A woman who is pregnant.

parturient A woman in labor.

gravidity Pregnancy.

parity The number of *pregnancies* in which the fetus or fetuses have reached viability, not the number of fetuses born. Whether the fetus is born alive or is stillborn after viability is reached does not affect parity.

nulligravida A woman who has never been pregnant.

primigravida A woman who is pregnant for the first time.

multigravida A woman who has had two or more pregnancies.

nullipara A woman who has *not* completed a pregnancy with a fetus or fetuses who have reached the stage of fetal viability.

primipara A woman who has completed one pregnancy with a fetus or fetuses who have reached the stage of fetal viability.

multipara A woman who has completed two or more pregnancies to the stage of fetal viability.

viability Capacity to live outside the uterus; about 22 menstrual (20 gestational) weeks or greater than 500 g.

term Born between the beginning of the thirty-eighth week and the end of the forty-second week of gestation.

preterm Born after 20 weeks of gestation but before completion of 37 weeks of gestation.

Usually a 5-digit code is used to represent a woman's pregnancy history (GTPAL):

G, Gravida (number of pregnancies)
T, Term Pregnancies (number of term pregnancies)
P, Preterm pregnancies
A, Abortions (number of spontaneous and/or elective)
L, Living children (number of children alive now)

A woman who is pregnant for the first time and gives birth to twins at 35 weeks that survive, would be coded as: G-1, T-0, P-1, A-0, L-2. Further examples of pregnancy histories can be found in Table 5-1.

PREGNANCY TESTS

All tests that are in current use detect the presence of human chorionic gonadotropin (hCG). Early detection of pregnancy allows early initiation of care. Human chorionic gonadotropin can be measured by radioimmunoassay and detected in the blood as early as 6 days after conception, or about 20 days since the last menstrual period (LMP). Its presence in the urine in early pregnancy is the basis of the various laboratory tests for pregnancy, and it can sometimes be detected in the urine as early as 14 days after conception (Ganong, 1989). Less specific tests may not be accurate until 4 to 10 days after the missed menstrual period or 3 weeks after conception.

A first-voided morning urine specimen (urine that is at least a 6-hour concentrate) contains levels of hCG approximately the same as those in serum, whose levels increase exponentially between days 21 and 70 (counting from the first day of the LMP). Random urine samples usually have lower levels. The ability to recognize the beta subunit of hCG is the newest innovation in the evolution of endocrine tests for pregnancy. The wide variety of tests precludes discussion of each, however, several

TABLE 5-1 Gravidity and Parity Using Five-Digit System

CONDITION	FIVE-DIGIT SYSTEM				
	PREGNANCIES	TERM BIRTH	PRETERM BIRTH	ABORTIONS	LIVING CHILDREN
Judith is pregnant for the first time.	1	0	0	0	0
She carries the pregnancy to term, and the neonate survives.	1	1	0	0	1
She is pregnant again.	2	1	0	0	1
Her second pregnancy ends in abortion.	2	1	0	1	1
During her third pregnancy, she delivers preterm twins.	3	1	1	1	3

categories of tests are described here. The nurse should read the manufacturer's directions for the test to be used.

Latex agglutination inhibition (LAI) tests are easy to do and give results in 2 minutes. They are accurate from 4 to 10 days following missed menses. Examples of this type of test include the Gravindex slide, Pregnosticon slide, and UCG Beta slide.

Hemagglutination inhibition (HAI) tests are more sensitive than LAI tests, but require 1 to 2 hours to obtain results. However, Neocept, which gives accurate results at or before missed menses, all HAI tests are accurate about 4 days following missed menses. Also on the market is e.p.t. (early pregnancy test), an HAI in-home test available for consumer purchase (Doshi, 1986).

The *radioreceptor assay* is one of the newest categories of pregnancy tests. This 1-hour serum test requires fairly sophisticated equipment. Radioreceptor assays are usually accurate at time of missed menses (14 days after conception) (Brucker, MacMullen, 1985). Biocept G is an example of this type of test.

Radioimmunoassay pregnancy tests for the beta subunit of hCG use radioactively labeled markers, which require the testing to be done in a laboratory. Depending on the degree of sensitivity required, the test time ranges from 1 to 48 hours. Radioimmunoassays are the most sensitive pregnancy tests available today (Brucker, MacMullen, 1985). Pregnancy can be diagnosed 8 days after ovulation or 6 days before missed menses.

Enzyme immunoassays use complex monoclonal anti-hCG with enzymes.* A color change makes the results easy to read. This new test holds promise for the future. Confidot is an immunoenzymatic assay home pregnancy test. The manufacturers of Confidot claim that this self-administered test confirms pregnancy 10 days after fertilization, about 4 days before missed menses.

Enzyme-linked immunosorbent assay (ELISA) testing is the most popular testing procedure for pregnancy (Batzer, 1985; Scott et al, 1990). It uses a specific monoclonal antibody produced by hybrid cell-line technology (News, 1985). An enzyme, rather than a radioactive compound, identifies the antigen of the substance to be measured. The enzyme induces a simple color-change reaction. The endpoint of the test can be read with either the eye or a spectrometer.

ELISA testing has many advantages. The antigen enzyme conjugate and test reagents are stable, the equipment needs are simple, and there are no nuclear waste products. As an office or home procedure, ELISA requires minimum time and offers results in 5 minutes coupled with sensitivities from 25 to 50 mIU/ml of hCG in the specimen. ELISA technology is the basis for the new over-the-counter tests. Most pharmacies make these over-the-counter tests available for women to do in the

privacy of their own homes. The manufacturer provides directions for collection of specimen (serum, plasma, or urine), care of specimen, testing procedure, and reading of results.

Interpretation of the results of pregnancy tests requires some judgment. The type of pregnancy test and its degree of *sensitivity* (ability to detect low levels of a substance) and *specificity* (ability to discern the absence of a substance) are interpreted in conjunction with the woman's history, which includes the date of the last normal menstrual period (LNMP), usual cycle length, and results of previous pregnancy tests. It is important to know if the woman is a substance abuser. Interactions with other drugs can give false results. Improper collection of the specimen, hormone-producing tumors, and laboratory errors may be responsible for false reports (Doshi, 1986). Where there is any question, serial testing may be the answer (Batzer, 1985). Speed and convenience need to be weighed against sensitivity and specificity.

ADAPTATIONS TO PREGNANCY

This chapter provides the basis for preventive, curative, and rehabilitative maternity care. Maternal adaptations are attributed to the *hormones* of pregnancy and to *mechanical pressures* arising from the enlarging uterus and other tissues. These adaptations protect the woman's normal physiologic functioning, meet the metabolic demands pregnancy imposes on her body, and provide for fetal developmental and growth needs. Although pregnancy is a normal phenomenon, problems can occur. The nurse needs an adequate foundation in normal maternal physiology to accomplish the following:

1. Identify potential or actual deviation from normal adaptation to initiate remedial care.
2. Help the mother understand the anatomic and physiologic changes during pregnancy.
3. Allay the mother's (and family's) anxiety, which may result from lack of knowledge.
4. Teach the mother (and family) signs and symptoms that must be reported to the health care provider.

Along with the expected adjustments to pregnancy, some disease states also cause changes. Some examples are low hemoglobin levels, a high erythrocyte sedimentation rate, dyspnea at rest, and alterations in cardiac function and endocrine balance. These changes reflect the body's effort to protect the mother and the fetus. An understanding of these changes is necessary for anyone who participates in the care of the mother and the fetus.

Signs of Pregnancy

Some of the physiologic changes that occur during pregnancy are recognized as **signs of pregnancy.** The three

---

*Read package inserts for a description of "monoclonal anti-hCG with enzymes."

categories are **presumptive,** those changes felt by the woman (e.g., amenorrhea, fatigue, breast changes); **probable,** those changes observed by an examiner (e.g., Hegar's sign, ballottement, pregnancy tests); and **positive** (e.g., sonography, fetal heart tone). Box 5-1 summarizes these signs of pregnancy.

REPRODUCTIVE SYSTEM AND BREASTS
Hypothalamus-Pituitary-Ovarian Axis

During pregnancy elevated levels of estrogen and progesterone suppress secretion of follicle-stimulating hormone (FSH) and luteinizing hormone (LH). The maturation of a follicle and release of an ovum do not occur. Menstrual cycles cease (often a presumptive sign of pregnancy). Although the majority of women experience **amenorrhea** (absence of menses), at least 20% have some slight, painless spotting for unexplained reasons during early gestation. A great majority of these women continue to term and have normal infants.

After implantation the fertilized ovum and the chorionic villi produce hCG, which maintains the corpus luteum's production of estrogen and progesterone for the first 8 to 10 weeks of pregnancy until the placenta takes over their production (Scott et al, 1990).

Uterus

The phenomenal uterine growth in the first trimester occurs in response to the hormonal stimulus of high levels of estrogen and progesterone. Enlargement results from (1) increased vascularity and dilatation of blood vessels, (2) hyperplasia (production of new muscle fibers and fibroelastic tissue) and hypertrophy (enlargement of preexisting muscle fibers and fibroelastic tissue), and (3) development of the decidua (Fig. 5-1). By 7 weeks the

uterus is the size of a large hen's egg; by 10 weeks it has grown to the size of an orange (twice its nonpregnant size); by 12 weeks the uterus is the size of a grapefruit. Table 5-2 compares uterine measurements for the nonpregnant and pregnant uterus at 40 weeks of gestation. After the third month uterine enlargement is primarily the result of mechanical pressure from the growing fetus (Seidel et al, 1995).

As the uterus increases in size, it also changes in weight, shape, and position. The muscular walls strengthen and become more elastic. At conception the uterus is shaped like an upside-down pear. During the second trimester it is spheric or globular. Later, as the fetus lengthens, the uterus becomes larger and more

---

BOX 5-1

Signs of Pregnancy

PRESUMPTIVE (changes felt by the woman)
amenorrhea
fatigue
breast soreness
breast enlargement
morning sickness
quickening

PROBABLE (changes observed by the examiner)
Hegar's sign
ballottement
pregnancy tests
Goodell's sign

POSITIVE
sonography
fetal heart tone
visualization and palpation of fetal movement by
  examiner

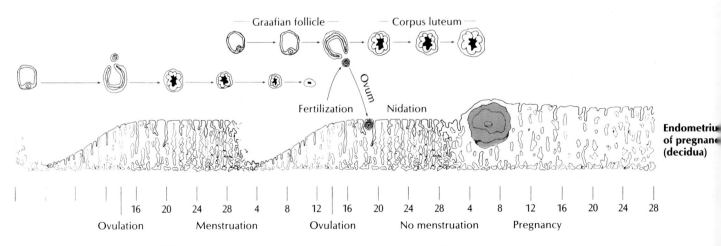

FIG. 5-1 Changes in endometrium and corpus luteum if pregnancy occurs (in days).

ovoid, and rises out of the pelvis into the abdominal cavity. In the nonpregnant woman the uterine cavity holds about 10 ml of fluid; during pregnancy, its capacity increases to 5 to 10 L or more (Cunningham et al, 1993).

In most normal pregnant women, a reasonably accurate correlation of *uterine enlargement* and the duration of amenorrhea is possible from the sixth week to term. Variation in the positions of the fundus or the fetus, variations in the amount of amniotic fluid present, or the presence of more than one fetus reduces the accuracy of the estimation of the pregnancy's duration.

The pregnancy may "show" after the fourteenth week, although this depends to some degree on the woman's height and weight. *Abdominal enlargement* may be less apparent in the primigravida with good abdominal muscle tone (Fig. 5-2). Posture also influences the type and degree of abdominal enlargement seen.

During the early weeks of pregnancy an increase in uterine blood flow and lymph causes pelvic congestion and edema. As a result, the uterus, cervix, and isthmus soften perceptibly and progressively, and the cervix takes on a bluish color (**Chadwick's sign,** a probable sign of pregnancy).

At about the seventh to eighth week the following patterns of uterine softening are noted: isthmic softening and compressibility (**Hegar's sign;** Fig. 5-3), cervical softening (**Goodell's sign),** and easy flexion of the fundus on the cervix (**McDonald's sign).** These are probable signs of pregnancy. After the eighth week general enlargement and softening of the uterine corpus and cervix are likely to occur.

Some believe that the nonsteroid ovarian hormone, *relaxin,* may act synergistically with progesterone (Cunningham et al, 1993; Scott et al, 1990). Relaxation not only occurs in the uterus, but throughout various parts of the body, such as on the joints and walls of blood vessels.

As the uterus grows, it is elevated out of the pelvic areas and may be palpated above the symphysis pubis sometime between the twelfth and fourteenth weeks of pregnancy (Fig. 5-4). The softness of the isthmus results in exaggerated uterine anteflexion during the first 3

months of pregnancy. The fundus pressing on the urinary bladder, along with edema of the bladder wall, causes the woman to experience *urinary frequency.* The uterus rises gradually to the level of the umbilicus at about 20 gestational weeks, and nearly reaches the xiphoid process at term. Between weeks 38 and 40, fun-

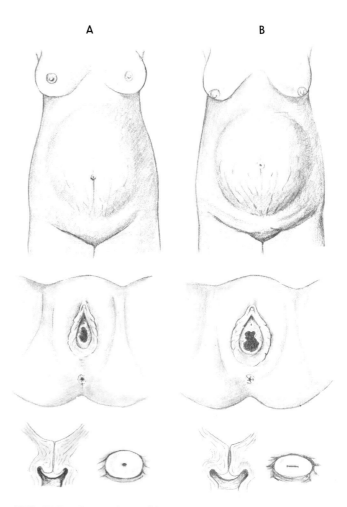

FIG. 5-2 Comparison of breasts, abdomen, vulva, and cervix in nullipara, **A,** and multipara, **B,** at the same stage of pregnancy and parturition.

TABLE 5-2 Comparison of Measurements for Nonpregnant and Pregnant Uterus at 40 Weeks*

MEASUREMENT	NONPREGNANT	PREGNANT (40 WEEKS)
Length	6.5 cm (2½ in)	32 cm (12½ in)
Width	4 cm (1½ in)	24 cm (9½ in)
Depth	2.5 cm (1 in)	22 cm (8½ in)
Weight	60 to 70 g (2½ oz)	1100 to 1200 g (2½ lb)
Volume	≤10 ml	5000 ml

*Note that references vary as to the exact values, but all references agree on the magnitude of the growth the uterus undergoes during pregnancy.

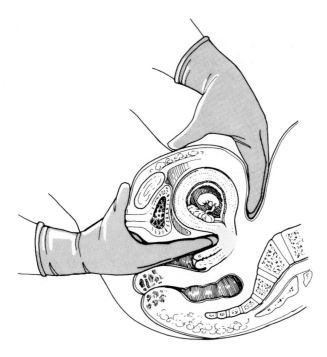

FIG. 5-3 Hegar's sign. Bimanual examination for assessing softening of isthmus while the cervix is still firm.

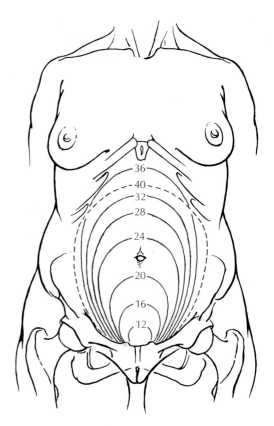

FIG. 5-4 Height of fundus by weeks of normal gestation with a single fetus. Dotted line indicates height after lightening. (Adapted from Malasanos L et al: *Health assessment*, ed 4, St Louis, 1990, Mosby.)

dal height drops as the fetus begins to engage in the pelvis **(lightening).**

Generally, the uterus rotates to the right as it elevates, probably because of the presence of the rectosigmoid colon on the left side. The extensive **hypertrophy** (enlargement) of the round ligaments keeps the uterus in line. Eventually, the growing uterus touches the anterior abdominal wall and displaces the intestines to either side of the abdomen. When a pregnant woman stands, the major part of her uterus rests against the anterior abdominal wall, contributing to her altered center of gravity.

Soon after the fourth month of pregnancy, uterine contractions can be felt through the abdominal wall. These contractions are referred to as the **Braxton Hicks' sign,** a probable sign of pregnancy. Braxton Hicks' contractions are a continuation of the irregular, painless contractions that occur intermittently throughout each menstrual cycle. The contractions are felt as uterine firmness through the abdominal wall, or are evident because they raise and push the uterus forward. Contractions facilitate uterine blood flow and thereby promote oxygen delivery to the uterus. Ordinarily, Braxton Hicks' contractions are not painful, but some women do complain that they are annoying. After the twenty-eighth week, contractions become much more definite, especially in slender women. Generally, these contractions cease with walking or exercise. Women rarely perceive them as painful. During the last few weeks of pregnancy, these contractions may become strong enough to be confused with the contractions of beginning labor.

Blood flow increases rapidly as the uterus increases in size. Although uterine blood flow increases twenty-fold, the size of the conceptus grows more rapidly. Consequently, more oxygen is extracted from the uterine blood during the latter part of pregnancy (Ganong, 1989). In a normal term pregnancy, one sixth of the total maternal blood volume is within the uterine vascular system. The rate of blood flow through the uterus averages 500 ml/min, and oxygen consumption of the gravid uterus averages 25 ml/min. Maternal arterial pressure, contractions of the uterus, and maternal position influence blood flow. Estrogens also play a role in uterine blood flow.

Using an ultrasound device or a fetal stethoscope, the health care provider or nurse may hear (1) the **uterine souffle** or bruit, a rushing sound of maternal blood going to the placenta that is synchronous with the maternal pulse, (2) the **funic souffle,** which is synchronous with the fetal heart rate and caused by fetal blood coursing through the umbilical cord, and (3) the *fetal heart rate (FHR)*. These sounds are all positive signs of pregnancy.

Passive movement of the unengaged fetus is called **ballottement.** Usually, ballottement can be identified between the sixteenth and eighteenth week. Ballotte-

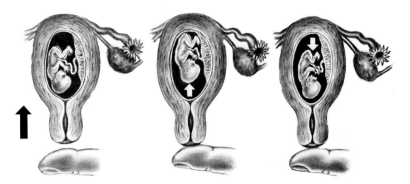

FIG. 5-5 Internal ballottement (18 weeks).

ment is a technique of palpating a floating structure by bouncing it gently and feeling it rebound. The examiner's finger within the vagina taps gently upward; the fetus rises. Then the fetus sinks, and a gentle tap is felt on the finger (Fig. 5-5). Internal ballottement of a fetus within a uterus is a probable objective sign of pregnancy.

The first recognition of fetal movements, or "feeling life," by the multiparous woman may occur as early as the fourteenth to sixteenth week. The nulliparous woman may not notice these sensations until the eighteenth week or later. **Quickening,** a presumptive sign of pregnancy, is commonly described as a flutter, and is difficult to distinguish from peristalsis. Noting the week in which quickening occurs provides a tentative clue in dating the duration of gestation.

A softening of the cervical tip may be observed about the beginning of the sixth week in a normal, unscarred cervix. This probable sign of pregnancy, Goodell's sign, is brought about by increased vascularity, slight hypertrophy, and **hyperplasia** of the muscle and its collagen-rich connective tissue, which becomes loose, edematous, highly elastic, and increased in volume. The glands near the external os proliferate beneath the stratified squamous epithelium, giving the cervix the velvety consistency characteristic of pregnancy. The changes in the cervix and in the vagina help prepare the birth canal for the fetus's passage through each of them (Fig. 5-6). **Friability** increases, that is, the cervix bleeds easily when scraped or touched. Increased friability is the cause of the few drops of blood seen after coitus with deep penetration or vaginal examination. These few drops are usually within normal limits.

The cervix of the nullipara is rounded. Lacerations of the cervix almost always occur during the birth process. With or without lacerations, following childbirth the cervix becomes more oval in the horizontal plane, and the external os appears as a transverse slit (see Fig. 5-2).

Vagina and Vulva

Pregnancy hormones prepare the vagina for distention during labor by producing a thickened vaginal mucosa, loosened connective tissue, hypertrophied smooth

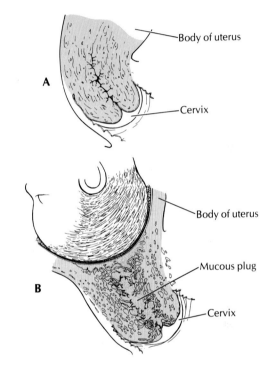

FIG. 5-6 **A,** Cervix in nonpregnant woman. **B,** Changes in cervix during pregnancy.

muscle, and an increase in the length of the vaginal vault. Increased vascularity results in a violet-bluish color to the vaginal mucosa and cervix. The deepened color, termed Chadwick's sign, a probable sign of pregnancy, may be evident as early as the sixth week, but is easily noted at the eighth week of pregnancy. Desquamation (or exfoliation) of the vaginal, glycogen-rich cells occurs under estrogen stimulation. The cells that are shed contribute to the thick, whitish vaginal discharge, leukorrhea.

During pregnancy the pH of vaginal secretions becomes less acidic. The pH changes from 4 to 6.5. *The rise in pH makes the pregnant woman more vulnerable to vaginal infections,* especially yeast infections. A diet of large quantities of sugars can make the vaginal environment even more suitable for a yeast infection.

The increased vascularity of the vagina and other pel-

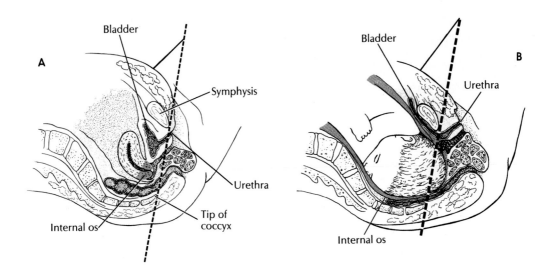

FIG. 5-7 **A,** Pelvic floor in nonpregnant woman. **B,** Pelvic floor at end of pregnancy. Note marked projection (growth of tissue) below line joining tip of coccyx and inferior margin of symphysis. Note elongation of bladder and urethra as a result of compression. Fat deposits are increased.

vic viscera results in a marked increase in sensitivity. The *increased sensitivity may lead to a high degree of sexual interest and arousal,* especially during the second trimester of pregnancy. The increased congestion, plus the relaxed walls of the blood vessels and the heavy uterus, may result in edema and varicosities of the vulva. The edema and varicosities usually resolve during the postpartum period.

External structures of the *vulva* are enlarged during pregnancy because of an increase in vasculature, hypertrophy of the perineal body, and deposition of fat (Fig. 5-7). The labia majora of the nullipara approximate and obscure the vaginal introitus; those of the parous woman separate and gape after childbirth and perineal or vaginal injury. Torn residual tags of the hymen remain after the use of tampons, coitus, and vaginal birth. Fig. 5-2 compares the nullipara and the multipara in relation to several characteristics: pregnant abdomen, vulva, and cervix.

Leukorrhea is a white or slightly gray mucoid discharge with a faint musty odor. Increased estrogen and progesterone stimulation of the cervix produces copious mucoid fluid. The fluid is whitish because of the presence of many exfoliated vaginal epithelial cells caused by normal pregnancy hyperplasia. This vaginal discharge is never pruritic or blood stained. **Ferning** (see Fig. 3-21) does *not* occur in the dried cervical mucous smear because of the progesterone effect. The mucus fills the endocervical canal, resulting in the formation of the mucous plug (**operculum;** Fig. 5-6). The operculum acts as a barrier against bacterial invasion during pregnancy.

Breasts

Fullness, heightened sensitivity, tingling, and heaviness of the breasts begin as early as the sixth week of gestation.

These breast changes are presumptive signs of pregnancy. Breast sensitivity varies from mild tingling to sharp pain. Nipples and areolae become more pigmented, a secondary pinkish areola develops, and nipples become more erectile. Hypertrophy of the sebaceous (oil) glands embedded in the primary areola, called **Montgomery's tubercles** (see Fig. 3-16), may be seen around the nipples. These sebaceous glands may have a protective role in that they keep the nipples lubricated. Suppleness of the nipples is jeopardized if the protective oils are washed off with soap.

The richer blood supply dilates the vessels beneath the skin. Once barely noticeable, the blood vessels now become visible, often appearing in an intertwining blue network beneath the surface of the skin. Venous congestion in the breasts is more obvious in primigravidas. Striae may appear at the outer aspects of the breasts (see p. 103).

During the second and third trimesters growth of the mammary glands accounts for the progressive increase in breast size. The high levels of luteal and placental hormones in pregnancy promote proliferation of the lactiferous ducts and lobule-alveolar tissue, so that the palpation of the breasts reveals a generalized, coarse nodularity. The increase in glandular tissue displaces connective tissue, and as a result, the tissue becomes softer and looser. Overstretching of the fibrous suspensory Cooper's ligaments (see Fig. 3-16) supporting the breasts may be prevented with a well-fitted maternity brassiere.

Although development of the mammary glands is functionally complete by midpregnancy, lactation is inhibited until a drop in estrogen level occurs after birth of the fetus and placenta. A thin, clear, viscous precolostrum secretion, however, may be expressed from the

nipples by the end of the sixth week (Seidel et al, 1995).*
This secretion thickens as term approaches and is then
known as colostrum. **Colostrum,** the creamy, white to
yellowish premilk fluid, may be expressed from the
nipples during the third trimester. See discussion of pituitary prolactin p. 107.

GENERAL BODY SYSTEMS
Cardiovascular System

Maternal adjustments to pregnancy involve extensive
changes in the cardiovascular system, both anatomic and
physiologic. Cardiovascular adaptations protect the
woman's normal physiologic functioning, meet the
metabolic demands pregnancy imposes on her body, and
provide for fetal developmental and growth needs.

Slight cardiac hypertrophy (enlargement) or dilatation
is probably secondary to increased blood volume and cardiac output. As the diaphragm is displaced upward, the
heart is elevated upward and rotated forward to the left
(Fig. 5-8). The apical impulse, point of maximum impulse (PMI), is shifted upward and laterally about 1 to
1.5 cm (½ in). The degree of shift depends on the duration of pregnancy and on the size and position of the
uterus.

Auscultatory changes accompany changes in heart size
and position. Increases in blood volume and cardiac output also contribute to auscultatory changes common in
pregnancy. There is more audible splitting of S_1 and S_2.
S_3 may be readily heard after 20 weeks of gestation. Additionally, grade II systolic ejection murmurs may be
heard over the pulmonic area.

Between 14 and 20 weeks, the *pulse* increases slowly,
up to 10 to 15 beats per minute, which then persists to
term. Palpitations may occur.

Blood Pressure

Arterial blood pressure (brachial artery) varies with age.
Additional factors must be considered. These factors include maternal position, maternal anxiety, and size of
cuff. Maternal position affects readings, because it can
cause the uterus to impede venous return, thus decreasing the carciac output (CO) and lowering the blood pressure. Brachial blood pressure is highest when the woman
is sitting, lowest when she is lying in the left lateral recumbent position, and intermediate when she is supine.
Therefore the same maternal position and the same arm
are used at each visit. The position and arm used are
noted along with the reading. During the first half of
pregnancy, there is a decrease in both systolic and diastolic pressure of 5 to 10 mm Hg. The decrease in blood

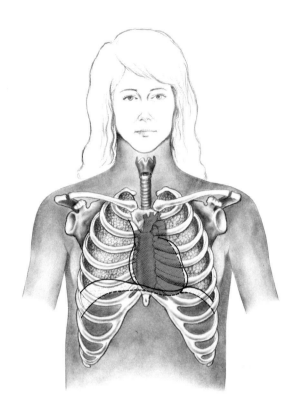

FIG. 5-8   Changes in position of heart, lungs, and thoracic
cage in pregnancy. *Broken line,* nonpregnant. *Solid line,* change
that occurs in pregnancy.

pressure is probably the result of peripheral vasodilatation from hormonal changes during pregnancy. During
the third trimester maternal blood pressure should return
to the values obtained during the first trimester.

The **mean arterial pressure (MAP)** increases the diagnostic value of the findings. The MAP is estimated by
adding one third of the *pulse pressure* to the diastolic
pressure. Pulse pressure is the difference between the systolic and diastolic values.

Example
Blood pressure: 106/70 at 22 weeks
Pulse pressure (106 − 70): 36 ÷ 3 = 12
MAP: (diastolic) 70 + 12 = 82

MAP readings of 82 at 22 weeks are within the normal
range for the length of gestation.

Some degree of compression of the vena cava occurs
in all women who lie on their back during the second
half of pregnancy. Some women experience a fall of ≥30
mm Hg systolic. After 4 to 5 minutes a reflex bradycardia is seen, cardiac output is reduced by half, and the
woman feels faint.

Edema of the lower extremities and varicosities results
from obstruction of the iliac veins and inferior vena cava
by the uterus, as well as causes increased *venous pressure.*

---
*References differ as to the gestational week during which precolos-
trum can be expressed. Some references cite week 16 as the earliest
time that fluid may be expressed from the breasts.

Blood Volume and Composition

The degree of blood volume expansion varies considerably (Cunningham et al, 1993). Blood volume increases by approximately 1500 ml* (normal value: 8.5% to 9% of body weight). The increase is made up of 1000 ml *plasma* plus 450 ml *red blood cells* (RBCs). The increase in volume starts about the tenth to twelfth week, peaks at about 30% to 50% above the nonpregnant levels at 20 to 26 weeks, and levels off after the thirtieth week. The increased volume is a protective mechanism. It is essential for (1) the hypertrophied vascular system of the enlarged uterus, (2) adequate hydration of fetal and maternal tissues when the woman assumes an erect or supine position, and (3) fluid reserve for blood loss during the birth and puerperium. Peripheral vasodilatation maintains a normal blood pressure despite the increased blood volume in pregnancy.

During pregnancy there is an accelerated production of RBCs (normal 4 to 5.5 million/mm^3). The percentage of increase depends on the amount of iron available. The RBC mass increases by 30% to 33% by term if an iron supplement is taken. If no supplement is taken, the RBC increases by only 17% in some women.

Despite an increase in RBC production, there is an apparent decrease in normal *hemoglobin* values (12 to 16 g/dl blood) and *hematocrit* values (37% to 47%). This condition is referred to as *physiologic anemia*. The decrease is more noticeable during the second trimester, when rapid expansion of blood volume takes place. If the hemoglobin value drops to 10 g/dl or less, or if the hematocrit drops to 35% or less, the woman is anemic.

The total *white cell count* increases during the second trimester and peaks during the third trimester. This increase is primarily in the granulocytes. The lymphocyte count stays about the same throughout pregnancy. See Appendix D for laboratory values during pregnancy.

Cardiac Output

Cardiac output increases from 30% to 50% by the thirty-second week of pregnancy; it declines to about a 20% increase at 40 weeks. The elevated cardiac output is largely a result of increased stroke volume, and in response to increased tissue demands for oxygen (normal value is 5 to 5.5 L/min) (Fig. 5-9). Cardiac output in late pregnancy is appreciably higher when the woman is in the lateral recumbent position than when she is supine. In the supine position, the large heavy uterus often impedes venous return to the heart. Cardiac output increases with any exertion such as labor and birth.

Circulation and Coagulation Times

The circulation time decreases slightly by week 32. It almost returns to normal near term.

There is a greater *tendency to coagulation* during pregnancy, because of increases in various clotting factors (factors VII, VIII, IX, X, and fibrinogen). Fibrinolytic activity (the splitting up or the dissolving of a clot) is depressed during pregnancy and the postpartum period, which makes the woman more vulnerable to thrombosis.

Respiratory System

Structural and ventilatory adaptations occur during pregnancy to provide for both maternal and fetal needs. Maternal oxygen requirements increase in response to the acceleration in metabolic rate and the need to add to the tissue mass in the uterus and breasts. The conceptus requires oxygen and a way to eliminate carbon dioxide.

Elevated levels of estrogen cause the ligaments of the rib cage to relax, permitting increased chest expansion (see Fig. 5-8). In preparation for the enlarging uterus, the length of the lungs decreases. The transverse diameter of the thoracic cage increases by about 2 cm (¾ in), and the circumference increases by 5 to 7 cm (2 to 2¾ in) (Cunningham et al, 1993). The costal angle of approximately 68 degrees before pregnancy increases to about 103 degrees in the third trimester. The lower rib cage appears to flare out. After birth, the chest may not return to its prepregnant state (Seidel et al, 1995).

The level of the diaphragm is displaced by as much as 4 cm (1½ in) during pregnancy. With advancing pregnancy, as the enlarging uterus moves up in the abdominal cavity, thoracic breathing replaces abdominal breathing, and descent of the diaphragm with inspiration becomes less possible.

Increased vascularization in response to elevated levels of estrogen also occurs in the upper respiratory tract. As the capillaries become engorged, edema and hyperemia develop within the nose, pharynx, larynx, trachea, and bronchi. This congestion within the tissues of the respiratory tract gives rise to several conditions commonly seen during pregnancy. These conditions include nasal and sinus stuffiness, epistaxis (nosebleed), changes in the voice, and marked inflammatory response to even a mild upper respiratory infection.

Increased vascularity also swells tympanic membranes and eustachian tubes, giving rise to symptoms of impaired hearing, earaches, or a sense of fullness in the ears.

Pulmonary Function

The pregnant woman breathes deeper (increases *tidal volume*, the volume of gas moved into or out of the respiratory tract with each breath) but increases her respiratory rate only slightly (about two breaths per minute). The increase in respiratory tidal volume, associated with the normal respiratory rate, results in an increase in respiratory minute volume by approximately 26%. The increase in the respiratory minute volume is the *hyperventilation of pregnancy*, which is responsible for a decreased

---

*Expansion of blood volume: primigravidas, 1250 ml; multigravidas, 1500 ml; twin pregnancies, 2000 ml.

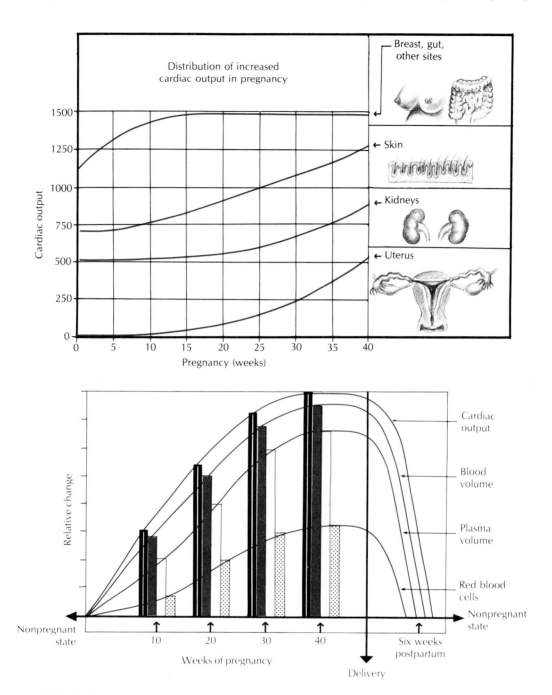

FIG. 5-9 Distribution of increased cardiac output in pregnancy and 6 weeks postpartum.

concentration of carbon dioxide in alveoli. The increased levels of progesterone apparently causes the hyperventilation of pregnancy, since hyperventilation has been mimicked in males given progesterone (Scott et al, 1990).

During pregnancy, changes in the respiratory center result in a lowered threshold for carbon dioxide. Progesterone and estrogen are presumed to be responsible for the increased sensitivity of the respiratory center to carbon dioxide. In addition, pregnant women experience increased awareness of the need to breathe; some may complain of dyspnea at rest.

Although pulmonary function is not impaired by pregnancy, diseases of the respiratory tract may be more serious during gestation (Cunningham et al, 1993). One important factor may be the increased oxygen requirements.

Basal Metabolism Rate

The basal metabolism rate (BMR) usually rises by the fourth month of gestation. It is increased by 15% to 20% by term. The BMR returns to nonpregnant levels by 5 to 6 days postpartum. The elevation in BMR reflects increased oxygen demands of the uterine-placental-fetal unit, as well as oxygen consumption from increased maternal cardiac work. Peripheral vasodilatation and acceleration of sweat gland activity assist in dissipating the excess heat resulting from the increased metabolism during pregnancy. Pregnant women may experience heat intolerance, which annoys some women. Many women in early pregnancy describe *lassitude* and *fatigability* after only slight exertion. These feelings may persist, along with a greater need for sleep. Lassitude and fatigability may be caused in part by the increased metabolic activity (see thyroid gland discussion later in this chapter).

Acid-base Balance

By about the tenth week of pregnancy there is a decrease of about 5 mm Hg in Pco_2. Progesterone may be responsible for increasing the sensitivity of the respiratory center receptors so that tidal volume increases, Pco_2 falls, the base excess (HCO_3, or bicarbonate) falls, and pH rises (becomes more basic). These alterations in acid-base balance indicate that *pregnancy is a state of respiratory alkalosis* compensated by mild metabolic acidosis.

Renal System

The kidneys are vital excretory organs. Their purpose is to maintain the body's internal environment in the relatively constant homeostatic state that is necessary for the efficient functioning of the body at the cellular level. The kidneys are responsible for maintenance of electrolyte and acid-base balance, regulation of extracellular fluid volume, excretion of waste products, and the conservation of essential nutrients.

Anatomic Changes

Changes in renal structure result from hormonal activity (estrogen and progesterone), pressure from an enlarging uterus, and an increase in blood volume. As early as the tenth week of pregnancy, the renal pelvis and the ureters dilate. Dilatation of the ureters is more pronounced above the pelvic brim, in part because they are compressed between the uterus and the pelvic brim. Dilatation above the pelvic brim is more marked on the right side. In most women, the ureters below the pelvic brim are of normal size. The smooth muscle walls of the ureters undergo hyperplasia, hypertrophy, and relaxed muscle tone. The ureters elongate, become tortuous, and form single or double curves. In the latter part of pregnancy the right renal pelvis and ureter dilate more than the left as a result of the displacement of the heavy uterus to the right by the rectosigmoid colon.

These changes cause the pelvis and ureters to hold a larger volume of urine and also slows the urine flow rate. Urinary stasis or stagnation has several consequences:

1. There is a lag between the time urine is formed and when it reaches the bladder. Therefore, clearance test results may reflect substances contained in glomerular filtrate several hours before.

2. Stagnated urine is an excellent medium for the growth of microorganisms. In addition, the urine of pregnant women contains greater amounts of nutrients, including glucose. Therefore, during pregnancy, women are more susceptible to urinary tract infection.

Bladder irritability, nocturia, and *urinary frequency* and *urgency* (without dysuria) are commonly reported in early pregnancy. Near term, bladder symptoms may return.

Urinary frequency results from an increased bladder sensitivity and later from a compression of the bladder (see Fig. 5-7). In the second trimester, the bladder is pulled up and out of the true pelvis into the abdomen. The urethra lengthens to 7.5 cm (3 in) as the bladder is displaced upward. The pelvic congestion of pregnancy is reflected in hyperemia of the bladder and urethra. This increased vascularity causes the bladder mucosa to be traumatized and bleed easily. There may be a decrease in bladder tone, which permits distention of the bladder to approximately 1500 ml. At the same time, the enlarging uterus compresses the bladder, resulting in the urge to void even if the bladder contains only a small amount of urine.

Renal Function Changes

In normal pregnancy, renal function is altered considerably. Glomerular filtration rate (GFR) and renal plasma flow (RPF) increase early in pregnancy (Cunningham et al, 1993). The woman's kidneys must manage the increased metabolic and circulatory demands of the maternal body and also excretion of fetal waste products. Changes in renal function are caused by pregnancy hormones, an increase in blood volume, the woman's posture, physical activity, and nutritional intake.

Renal function is most efficient when the woman lies in the lateral recumbent position and least efficient when the woman assumes a supine position. When the pregnant woman is lying supine, the heavy uterus compresses the vena cava and the aorta, and cardiac output decreases. The result is a drop in maternal blood pressure and fetal heart rate (vena cava or *hypotensive syndrome*) and a drop in the volume of blood to the kidneys. When cardiac output drops, blood flow to the brain and heart continues at the expense of other organs, including the kidneys and uterus.

Fluid and Electrolyte Balance

Selective renal tubular reabsorption maintains sodium and water balance regardless of changes in dietary intake and losses through sweat, vomitus, or diarrhea. Normally, from 500 to 900 mEq of *sodium* is retained during pregnancy to meet fetal needs. The need for increased maternal intravascular and extracellular fluid volume requires additional sodium to expand fluid volume and to maintain an isotonic state. To prevent excessive sodium depletion, the maternal kidneys undergo a significant adaptation by increasing tubular reabsorption. As efficient as the renal system is, it can be overstressed by excessive dietary sodium intake or restriction, or by use of diuretics. *Severe hypovolemia and reduced placental perfusion are two consequences.*

The capacity of the kidneys to excrete water during the early weeks of pregnancy is more efficient than later in pregnancy. Occasionally in early pregnancy, the extent of water loss may cause some women to feel thirsty. The pooling of fluid in the legs in the latter part of pregnancy decreases renal blood flow and GFR. The diuretic response to the water load is triggered when the woman lies down, preferably on her side, and the pooled fluid reenters general circulation. This pooling of blood in the lower legs is sometimes referred to as *physiologic edema,* which requires no treatment.

Normally, the kidney reabsorbs almost all of the glucose and other nutrients from the plasma filtrate. In pregnant women, tubular reabsorption of glucose is impaired so that *glucosuria* does occur at varying times and to varying degrees. Normal values are 0 to 20 mg/dl. That is, during any one day, the urine is sometimes positive and sometimes negative. When it is positive, the amount of glucose varies from 1+ to 4+.

In nonpregnant women, blood glucose levels must be at 160 to 180 mg/dl before glucose is "spilled" into the urine (not reabsorbed). During pregnancy, glucosuria occurs when maternal glucose levels are lower than 160 mg/dl. Why glucose, as well as other nutrients such as amino acids, is wasted during pregnancy is not understood, nor has the exact mechanism been discovered. Although glucosuria may be found in normal pregnancies (indeed 1+ levels may be seen with increased anxiety states), the possibility of diabetes mellitus must be kept in mind.

Albumin and globulin are proteins that are not normal constituents of urine at any time. Small (trace) amounts of protein may occasionally be found in concentrated urine or in first-voided urine following sleep. However, a measurable amount (over 150 mg in 24 hours) of protein in the urine is a significant sign of renal disease at any time.

Integumentary System

Alterations in hormonal balance and mechanical stretching are responsible for several changes in the integumentary system during pregnancy. General changes include increases in skin thickness and subdermal fat, hyperpigmentation, hair and nail growth, accelerated sweat and sebaceous gland activity, and increased circulation and vasomotor activity. There is greater fragility of cutaneous elastic tissues, resulting in striae gravidarum, or stretch marks. Cutaneous allergic responses are enhanced.

Pigmentation is caused by the anterior pituitary hormone melanotropin, which increases during pregnancy. Facial melasma, also called **chloasma** or *mask of pregnancy,* is a blotchy, brownish hyperpigmentation of the skin over the malar prominences and the forehead, especially in dark-complexioned pregnant women. Chloasma appears in 50% to 70% of pregnant women, beginning after the sixteenth week and increasing gradually to birth. The sun intensifies this pigmentation in susceptible women. Chloasma caused by normal pregnancy usually fades after birth. Darkening of the nipples, areolae, axillae, and vulva occurs at about the same time, and they fade after birth.

The **linea nigra** is a pigmented line extending from the symphysis pubis to the top of the fundus in the midline. This line is known as the linea alba before hormone-induced pigmentation. In primigravidas the extension of the linea nigra, beginning in the third month, keeps pace with the rising height of the fundus; in multigravidas the entire line often appears earlier than the third month. Not all pregnant women develop the linea nigra.

Striae gravidarum, or stretch marks (seen over lower abdomen in Fig. 5-2), which appear in 50% to 90% of women during the second half of pregnancy, may be caused by action of adrenocorticosteroids. Striae reflect separation within the underlying connective (collagen) tissue of the skin. These slightly depressed streaks tend to occur over areas of maximum stretch (i.e., abdomen, thighs, and breasts). The stretching sometimes causes a sensation similar to itching. Tendency to the development of striae may be familial. After birth they usually fade, although they never disappear completely. In the multipara, in addition to the reddish striae of the present pregnancy, glistening silvery lines representing the cicatrices (scars) of previous striae are commonly seen. Striae may be evident on the breasts as a result of stretching as they increase in size.

Angiomas or **telangiectasias** are commonly referred to as *vascular spiders.* They are tiny, stellate or branched, slightly raised and pulsating end-arterioles. The spiders, a result of elevated levels of circulating estrogen, are usually found on the neck, thorax, face, and arms. They are also described as focal networks of dilated arterioles radiating about a central core. The spiders are bluish in color and do not blanch with pressure. Vascular spiders appear during the second to the fifth month of pregnancy in 65% of white women and 10% of African-American women. The spiders usually disappear after birth.

Pinkish red, diffuse mottling or well-defined blotches are seen over the palmar surfaces of the hands in about 60% of white women and 35% of African-American women during pregnancy (Cunningham et al, 1993). These pigmentation changes and **palmar erythema** may also be seen in some women taking oral hormonal contraceptives.

Epulis (gingival granuloma gravidarum) is a red, raised nodule on the gums that bleeds easily. This lesion

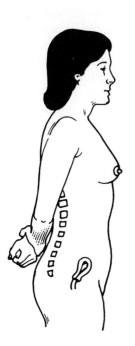 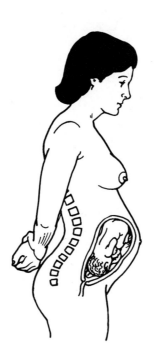 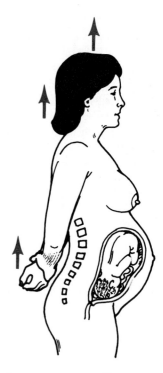

FIG. 5-10 Postural changes during pregnancy. **A,** Nonpregnant. **B,** Incorrect posture. **C,** Correct posture.

may develop around the third month, and usually continues to enlarge as pregnancy progresses. Treatment by excision is initiated only if it becomes excessive in size, causes pain, or bleeds excessively.

Nail growth accelerates during pregnancy. *Oily skin* and *acne vulgaris* may occur during pregnancy. For other women, the skin clears and looks radiant. **Hirsutism** is commonly reported. An increase in fine hair growth may occur. The fine hair tends to disappear after pregnancy. Growth of coarse or bristly hair does not usually disappear after pregnancy. Some women comment that their hair is thickest and most abundant during pregnancy.

Musculoskeletal System

The gradually changing body and increasing weight of the pregnant woman cause marked alterations in posture (Fig. 5-10) and walking. The great abdominal distention that gives the pelvis a forward tilt, decreased abdominal muscle tone, and increased weight bearing in late pregnancy require a realignment of the spinal curvatures. The woman's center of gravity shifts forward. An increase in the normal lumbosacral curve develops, and a compensatory curvature in the cervicodorsal region (exaggerated anterior flexion of the head) is required to maintain balance. Large breasts and a stoop-shouldered stance will further accentuate the lumbar and dorsal curves. Locomotion is more difficult, and the waddling gait of the pregnant woman, called "the proud walk of pregnancy" by Shakespeare, is well known. The ligamentous and muscular structures of the mid and lower spine may be

severely stressed. These and related changes often cause musculoskeletal discomfort.

The young, well-muscled woman may tolerate these changes without complaint. However, older women, those with a back disorder, or women with a faulty sense of balance may have a considerable amount of back pain during and just after pregnancy.

Slight relaxation and increased mobility of the pelvic joints are normal during pregnancy. This is secondary to exaggerated elasticity and softening of connective and collagen tissue, and to the result of increased circulating steroid sex hormones. These adaptations permit enlargement of pelvic dimensions. The degree of relaxation varies, but considerable separation of the symphysis pubis and the instability of the sacroiliac joints may cause pain and difficulty in walking. Obesity and multifetal pregnancy tend to increase the pelvic disability.

The muscles of the abdominal wall stretch and ultimately lose some tone. During the third trimester, the rectus abdominis muscles may separate (Fig. 5-11), allowing abdominal contents to protrude at the midline. The umbilicus flattens or protrudes. After birth, the muscles gradually regain tone, however, separation of the muscles (**diastasis recti abdominis**) may persist.

Neurologic System

Little is known regarding specific alterations in function of the neurologic system during pregnancy, aside from hypothalamic-pituitary neurohormonal changes. Specific physiologic alterations resulting from pregnancy may

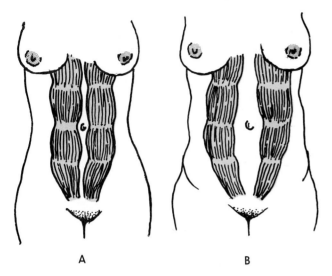

FIG. 5-11 Possible change in rectus abdominis muscles during pregnancy. **A,** Normal position in nonpregnant woman. **B,** Diastasis recti in pregnant woman.

cause the following neurologic or neuromuscular symptomatology:

1. Compression of pelvic nerves or vascular stasis caused by enlargement of the uterus may result in sensory changes in the legs.
2. Dorsolumbar lordosis may cause pain because of traction on the nerves or compression of the nerve roots.
3. Edema involving the peripheral nerves may result in *carpal tunnel syndrome* during the last trimester. The edema compresses the median nerve beneath the carpal ligament of the wrist. The syndrome is characterized by paresthesia (abnormal sensation such as burning or tingling because of a disorder of the sensory nervous system) and pain in the hand, radiating to the elbow. The dominant hand is usually affected the most.
4. Acroesthesia (numbness and tingling of the hands) is caused by the stoop-shouldered stance (see Fig. 5-10, *B*) assumed by some women during pregnancy. The condition is associated with traction on segments of the brachial plexus.
5. Tension headache is common when anxiety or uncertainty complicates gestation. Headaches may also be attributed to vision problems such as refractive errors, sinusitis, or migraine.
6. "Lightheadedness," faintness, and even syncope (fainting) are common during early pregnancy. Vasomotor instability, postural hypotension, or hypoglycemia may be responsible.
7. Hypocalcemia may cause neuromuscular problems such as muscle cramps or tetany.

Gastrointestinal System

The functioning of the gastrointestinal tract during pregnancy presents a curiously interesting picture. The appetite increases. Intestinal secretion is reduced. Liver function is altered, and absorption of nutrients is enhanced. The colon is displaced laterally upward and posteriorly. Peristaltic activity (motility) decreases. As a result bowel sounds are diminished, and constipation, nausea, and vomiting are common. Blood flow to the pelvis increases as does venous pressure, contributing to hemorrhoid formation in later pregnancy.

Mouth

The gums are hyperemic, spongy, and swollen. They tend to bleed easily because the rising levels of estrogen cause selective increased vascularity and connective tissue proliferation (a nonspecific gingivitis). There is no increase in secretion of saliva. Women do complain of **ptyalism** (excessive salivation). This perceived increase is thought to be caused by the decrease in unconscious swallowing by the woman when nauseated. Epulis and bleeding gums are discussed under Integumentary System.

Teeth

The pregnant woman requires about 1.2 g of calcium and approximately the same amount of phosphorus every day during her pregnancy. This is an increase of about 0.4 g of each of these elements over nonpregnant needs. A well-balanced diet satisfies these requirements. Serious dietary deficiency, however, may deplete the mother's osseous stores of these elements, but it does not draw on calcium in her teeth. Demineralization of teeth does not occur during pregnancy. Hence, the old adage "for every child a tooth" is untrue. Poor dental hygiene during pregnancy, or anytime, and gingivitis may contribute to dental caries, which could result in the loss of a tooth.

Appetite

Appetite changes during pregnancy. The first trimester often sees a decrease in appetite because of nausea and/or vomiting. These symptoms occur in approximately half of all pregnancies, and are the result of changes in the GI tract and higher systemic levels of hCG (see Clinical Application of Research). By the second trimester, nausea and vomiting occur less frequently and the appetite increases. This increase in appetite is attributed to the growth needs of the fetus.

Esophagus, Stomach, and Intestine

Herniation of the upper portion of the stomach (*hiatal hernia*) occurs after the seventh or eighth month of pregnancy in about 15% to 20% of pregnant women. This condition results from upward displacement of the stomach, which causes a widening of the hiatus of the diaphragm. This occurs more often in multiparas and older or obese women.

Increased estrogen production causes decreased secretion of hydrochloric acid. Therefore peptic ulcer forma-

CLINICAL APPLICATION OF RESEARCH

NAUSEA AND FATIGUE DURING EARLY PREGNANCY

Nausea and vomiting are common problems during early pregnancy. Many women with nausea also report fatigue. Van Lier and associates studied 51 women, who were less than 16 weeks pregnant, and who were being cared for in one of two nurse-midwifery practices, to determine whether nausea and fatigue were related. The participants completed the Pearson-Byars fatigue feeling checklist, a nausea scale, and a demographic data form. The majority of women reported nausea (88%). Fatigue that ranged from mildly to extremely distressing was also reported by 88% of the women, but not by the same women. The researchers found that women with nausea were no more likely to report fatigue than women without nausea. However, women with severe nausea reported greater fatigue. From the study it remains unclear whether fatigue and nausea influence each other. The researchers suggest that treatment of nausea in pregnancy needs to expand beyond dietary recommendations. Such treatment needs to include control of fatigue by encouraging pregnant women to incorporate rest periods into their daily routine and to ask for assistance from family or friends. Nurses working with pregnant women who complain of nausea should attempt to relieve these uncomfortable symptoms of pregnancy by questioning them about their fatigue levels and by recommending adequate rest and assistance from a support network.

Reference: Van Lier D et al: Nausea and fatigue during early pregnancy, *Birth* 20(4):193, 1993.

tion or flare-up of existing peptic ulcers is uncommon during pregnancy.

Increased progesterone production causes decreased tone and motility of smooth muscles, so that there is esophageal regurgitation, increased emptying time of the stomach, and reverse peristalsis. As a result, women may experience "acid indigestion" or *heart-burn* (**pyrosis**).

In response to increased needs during pregnancy, iron is absorbed more readily in the small intestine. In general, if the individual is deficient in iron, iron absorption increases.

Increased progesterone (causing loss of muscle tone and decreased peristalsis) results in an increase in water absorption from the colon. *Constipation* may result. In addition, constipation is secondary to hypoperistalsis (sluggishness of the bowel), unusual food choice, lack of fluids, abdominal distention by the pregnant uterus, and displacement of intestines with some compression. *Hemorrhoids* (varicose veins of the rectum and anus) may be everted or may bleed during straining at stool. Bowel habits and a characteristic type of stool are established early in life. Variations will be noted with concern and may be perceived as a disease process. A mild ileus (sluggishness, lack of movement) following birth, as well as postbirth fluid loss and perineal discomfort, contribute to continuing constipation.

Gallbladder and Liver

The gallbladder is quite often distended because of its decreased muscle tone during pregnancy. Increased emptying time and thickening of bile are typical. These features, together with slight hypercholesterolemia from increased progesterone levels, may account for the common development of *gallstones* during pregnancy.

Hepatic function is difficult to appraise during gestation, however, only minor changes in liver function develop during pregnancy. Occasionally, intrahepatic cholestasis (retention and accumulation of bile in the liver, caused by factors within the liver) in response to placental steroids, occurs late in pregnancy and may result in *pruritus gravidarum* (severe itching) with or without jaundice. Oatmeal baths and lotions help ease the itching. These distressing symptoms subside promptly after birth.

Abdominal Discomfort

Intraabdominal alterations that can cause discomfort include pelvic heaviness or pressure, round ligament tension, flatulence, distention and bowel cramping, and uterine contractions. In addition to displacement of intestines, pressure from the expanding uterus increases venous pressure in the pelvic organs. Although most abdominal discomfort is a consequence of normal maternal alterations, the health care provider is constantly alert to the possibility of disorders such as bowel obstruction or an inflammatory process.

Appendicitis may be difficult to diagnose. The *appendix* is displaced upward and laterally, high and to the right, away from McBurney's point.

Endocrine System

Profound endocrine changes occur that are essential for pregnancy maintenance, normal fetal growth, and postpartum recovery.

Thyroid Gland

During pregnancy there is moderate enlargement of the thyroid gland caused by hyperplasia of the glandular tissue and increased vascularity (Cunningham et al, 1993;

Scott et al, 1990). Oxygen consumption and BMR increase secondary to the metabolic activity of the products of conception. For a discussion of changes in thyroid hormone production see Cunningham et al (1993) and Scott et al (1990).

Parathyroid Gland

Pregnancy induces a slight secondary hyperparathyroidism, a reflection of increased requirements for calcium and vitamin D. When the needs for growth of the fetal skeleton are greatest (during the last half of pregnancy), plasma parathormone levels are elevated, that is, the peak level occurs between 15 and 35 weeks of gestation.

Pancreas

The fetus requires significant amounts of glucose for growth and development. To meet its need for fuel, the fetus not only depletes the store of maternal glucose, but also decreases the mother's ability to synthesize glucose by siphoning off her amino acids. Maternal blood glucose levels fall. Maternal insulin does *not* cross the placenta to the fetus. As a result, in early pregnancy, the pancreas decreases its production of insulin.

As pregnancy continues, the placenta grows and produces progressively larger amounts of hormones (i.e., human placental lactogen [hPL], estrogen, and progesterone). Cortisol production by the adrenals also increases. Estrogen, progesterone, hPL, and cortisol collectively decrease the mother's ability to utilize insulin. Cortisol simultaneously stimulates increased production of insulin and increases the mother's peripheral resistance to insulin (i.e., the tissues cannot use the insulin). Insulinase is an enzyme produced by the placenta to deactivate maternal insulin. Decreasing the mother's ability to use her own insulin is a protective mechanism that ensures an ample supply of glucose for the needs of the fetoplacental unit.

As a result, the pregnant woman's body demands more insulin. The normal beta cells of the islets of Langerhans in the pancreas can meet the demand for insulin, which continues to increase steadily until term.

Pituitary Prolactin

In pregnancy, serum prolactin begins to rise in the first trimester and increases progressively to term. It is generally believed that although all the hormonal elements (estrogen, progesterone, thyroid, insulin, and free cortisol) necessary for breast growth and milk production are present in elevated concentrations during pregnancy, the high levels of estrogen inhibit active alveolar secretion by blocking the binding of prolactin to breast tissue, thus inhibiting the milk-producing effect of prolactin on the target epithelium (Scott et al, 1990).

Endocrine System and Maternal Nutrition

Progesterone causes the deposit of fat in subcutaneous tissues over the abdomen, back, and upper thighs. The fat serves as an energy reserve for both pregnancy and lactation. Several other hormones affect nutrition. *Aldosterone* conserves sodium. *Thyroxin* regulates metabolism. *Parathyroid hormone* controls calcium and magnesium metabolism. *Human placental lactogen (hPL)* acts as a growth hormone. *Human chorionic gonadotropin (hCG)* induces nausea and vomiting in some women during early pregnancy.

KEY POINTS

- The biochemical, physiologic, and anatomic adaptations that occur during pregnancy are profound, and return almost completely to the nonpregnant state following birth and lactation.
- Maternal adaptations are attributed to the hormones of pregnancy and to mechanical pressures arising from the enlarging uterus and other tissues.
- The understanding of these adaptations to pregnancy remains a major goal. Without such knowledge, it is difficult, if not impossible, to understand the disease processes—pregnancy-induced or coincidental—that can threaten women during pregnancy and the postpartum.
- The ability to recognize the beta subunit of hCG through monoclonal antibody technology has revolutionized endocrine tests for pregnancy.
- Signs of pregnancy often mimic other conditions and, therefore, are considered to be either presumptive, probable, or positive signs of pregnancy.

- Adaptations to pregnancy protect the woman's normal physiologic functioning, meet the metabolic demands pregnancy imposes, and provide for fetal developmental and growth needs.
- The rise in pH of the pregnant woman's vaginal secretions makes her more vulnerable to vaginal infections.
- Increased vascularity and sensitivity of the vagina and other pelvic viscera may lead to a high degree of sexual interest and arousal.
- Some adaptations to pregnancy result in discomforts such as fatigue, urinary frequency, nausea, and breast sensitivity.
- Balance and coordination are affected by changes in joints and the woman's center of gravity as pregnancy progresses.

CRITICAL THINKING EXERCISES

1. Interview three pregnant women (and partner, if present) at different stages of their pregnancy:
   a. How does each pregnant woman feel about changes in her body related to anatomic and physiologic adaptations?
   b. Which changes do they find pleasant?
   c. Which changes do they find uncomfortable or troublesome?
   d. What is their level of understanding of these adaptations?
   e. What complaints or questions were asked by them related to anatomic or physiologic changes?

Analyze your findings. Use your findings to develop a protocol for assessment for the different stages of this pregnancy:
   ▪ Formulate interview questions.
   ▪ Describe the physical examination.
   ▪ List appropriate laboratory or diagnostic tests.
   ▪ Justify your decisions.

2. Explore your own emotions and attitudes regarding the changes a woman's body undergoes during pregnancy.

3. Obtain one over-the-counter pregnancy test. Read the instructions. Are they easy to follow? How would you teach women to use that pregnancy test?

References

Batzer FR: Guidelines for choosing a pregnancy test, *Contemp OB/GYN* 26:37, Oct 1985 (special issue).

Blackburn ST, Loper DL: *Maternal, fetal, and neonatal physiology: a clinical perspective*, Philadelphia, 1992, WB Saunders.

Brucker MC, MacMullen NJ: What's new in pregnancy tests? *JOGN Nurs* 14:353, Sept-Oct 1985.

Cunningham FG et al: *Williams obstetrics*, ed 19, Norwalk, CT, 1993, Appleton & Lange.

Doshi ML: Accuracy of consumer performed in-home tests for early pregnancy detection, *Am J Public Health* 76:512, 1986.

Ganong WF: *Review of medical physiology*, ed 13, Norwalk, CT, 1989, Appleton & Lange.

News: Monoclonals: new frontiers in reproductive medicine in Technology 1986, *Contemp OB/GYN* 26:75, Oct 1985.

Scott JR et al: *Danforth's obstetrics and gynecology*, ed 6, Philadelphia, 1990, JB Lippincott.

Seidel HM et al: *Mosby's guide to physical examination*, ed 3, St Louis, 1995, Mosby.

Bibliography

Austin DA, Davis PA: Valvular disease in pregnancy, *J Perinat Neonat Nurs* 5(2):13, Sept 1991.

Barkauskas VH et al: *Health and physical assessment*, St Louis, 1994, Mosby.

Chez RA: Advising pregnant women about nutrition, *Contemp OB/GYN* 36(1):80, Jan 1991.

Elkayam U, Gleicher N: *Changes in cardiac findings during normal pregnancy*. In Elkayam U, Gleicher N, editors: *Cardiac problems in pregnancy*, ed 2, New York, 1990, Alan R. Liss.

Groer M: Psychoneuroimmunology, *AJN* 91(8):33, Aug 1991.

Hart JL: Low back pain, radiculopathies, and pregnancy, *Pain Management* 3:103, March/April 1990.

Institute of Medicine, National Academy of Sciences, Food and Nutrition Board: *Nutrition during pregnancy. Part I: Weight gain. Part II: Nutrient supplements.* Washington, DC, 1990, National Academy Press.

Terhaar M, Schakenbach L: Care of the pregnant patient with a pacemaker, *J Perinat Neonat Nurs* 5(2):1, Sept 1991.

Willson JR, Carrington ER: *Obstetrics and gynecology*, ed 9, St Louis, 1991, Mosby.

6 Family Dynamics of Pregnancy

R H E A   P.   W I L L I A M S

LEARNING OBJECTIVES

Define the key terms listed.

Examine maternal adaptation to pregnancy in regard to acceptance, identification with motherhood role, family relationships, and anticipation of labor.

Examine paternal adaptation to pregnancy in regard to acceptance, identification with fatherhood role, family relationships, and anticipation of labor.

Discuss sibling adaptation to pregnancy.

Discuss grandparent adaptation to pregnancy.

Discuss pregnancy after age 35.

KEY TERMS

announcement phase
attachment
body boundaries
couvade
emotional lability
expressive style
fantasy child
focusing phase
instrumental style
maturational crisis
mitleiden
moratorium phase
observer style
rite of passage

RELATED TOPICS

Adolescent pregnancy *(Chap. 25)* • Cultural beliefs *(Chap. 2)* • Family dynamics after childbirth *(Chap. 17)* • Prebirth education *(Chap. 7)*

Pregnancy involves all family members. Because "conception is the beginning, not only of a growing fetus but also of the family in a new form with an additional member and with changed relationships," each family member must adapt to the pregnancy and interpret its meaning in light of his or her own needs (Grossman, Eichler, Winckoff, 1980).

This process of family adaptation to pregnancy takes place within a cultural environment that is influenced by societal trends. There have been dramatic changes in the fabric of Western society in recent years, and the nurse must be prepared to support single-parent families, reconstituted families, and dual-career families, as well as traditional families in the childbirth experience. Because much of the research on family dynamics in pregnancy and childbirth preparation in the United States and Canada has been done with white, middle-class families, findings may not apply to culturally diverse families, or families who do not fit the traditional American model. The terms *spouse, husband,* and *wife* are used consistently in the literature. The nurse may have to adapt these terms to apply to corresponding roles in many families. The reality of today's family may differ significantly from the image of the ideal family described by research in traditional terms.

To give a more accurate picture of today's American family, research must be expanded to include subjects from culturally diverse families and nontraditional family forms. Table 2-2 provides examples of some traditional cultural beliefs surrounding pregnancy that may be important to some African-American, Asian-American, and Mexican-American families.

American culture has also been influenced by the changing role of women. In most families women participate actively in the economic, social, and political life of their communities. This has resulted in a corresponding role change for many men—the role of father now includes more direct participation in childbirth preparation, the birth process, and in caring for the child. More research is needed to assess the impact of this involvement on the family, but it has been reported that increasingly a father's involvement fosters positive attitudes and behaviors toward the mother and child (Jones, 1986; Westney, Cole, Munford, 1988). Another trend related to the changing role of women is the tendency to postpone childbearing (see discussion p. 119).

MATERNAL ADAPTATION

Women, from teenagers to women in their 40s, use the 9 months of pregnancy to adapt to the maternal role. This is a complex social and cognitive process that is not intuitive but learned (Rubin, 1967a; Affonso and Sheptak, 1989). In becoming a mother, the teenager must shift from being mothered to mothering. The adult, in contrast, must move from "well-established routines to the unpredictable context created by an infant" (Mercer, 1981). The nullipara, or the woman without child, becomes the woman with child; and the multipara, the woman with child, becomes the woman with children (Lederman, 1984).

Subjective experience of time and space changes during pregnancy as plans and commitments become regulated by the expected date of birth (EDB) (Rubin, 1984). Early in pregnancy nothing seems to be happening, and there may be a resistance to giving up the full days of social demands and activities for a "burdensome, empty time." A lot of time is spent sleeping. With quickening in the second trimester there is a reduction of time and space, both geographic and social, as the woman turns her attention inward to her pregnancy and to relationships with her mother and other women who have been or are pregnant. With the third trimester there is a slower pace and a sense that time is running out as the woman's activities are curtailed (Rubin, 1984).

Pregnancy is a **maturational crisis** that can be stressful but rewarding as the woman prepares for a new level of caring and responsibility. Her self-concept must change in readiness for parenthood as she prepares for her new role. Gradually, she moves from being self-contained and independent to being committed to a life-long concern for another human being. This growth requires mastering certain developmental tasks: accepting the pregnancy, identifying the role of mother, reordering the relationships between mother and daughter and between herself and her partner, establishing a relationship with the unborn child, and preparing for the birth

experience (Rubin, 1967a; Lederman, 1984; Stainton, 1985). Studies indicate that the partner's emotional support is an important factor in the successful accomplishment of these developmental tasks (Entwistle, Doering, 1981; Mercer, 1981). Unwed adolescent fathers may also provide significant support to young mothers who must master the developmental tasks of pregnancy superimposed on those of adolescence (Westney, Cole, Munford, 1988).

Acceptance of Pregnancy

The first step in adapting to the maternal role is acceptance of the idea of pregnancy and assimilation of the pregnant state into the woman's way of life (Lederman, 1984). The degree of acceptance is reflected in the woman's readiness for pregnancy and her emotional responses.

Readiness for Pregnancy

The availability of birth control means that pregnancy for many women is a joint commitment between responsible partners. Planning a pregnancy, however, does not necessarily ensure acceptance of the pregnancy (Entwistle, Doering, 1981). Other women view pregnancy as a natural outcome of the marital relationship that may or may not be desired, depending on circumstances. For some women, including many adolescents, pregnancy can result from sexual experimentation using no contraception.

Women prepared to accept a pregnancy are prompted by early symptoms to seek medical validation of the pregnancy. Some women who have strong feelings of "not me," "not now," and "not sure," may postpone seeking supervision and care (Rubin, 1970). Some women may postpone medical validation, however, because of limited access to care, modesty, and cultural reasons. For others, pregnancy is viewed as a natural occurrence, and there is no perceived need for early medical validation.

Once pregnancy is confirmed, a woman's emotional response may range from great delight to shock, disbelief, and despair. The reaction of many women is the "someday but not now" response:

> There is a real pleasure in finding oneself functionally capable of becoming pregnant. There is pleasure in learning that others are pleased with the promise of having, and being given, a child. But these feelings exist independently of the question of time. Personally and privately she is not ready, not now (Rubin, 1970).

Other women may simply accept the pregnancy as nature's intent. Many women are dismayed initially at finding themselves pregnant. However, eventual acceptance of pregnancy parallels the growing acceptance of the reality of a child. Nonacceptance of the pregnancy should not be equated with rejection of the child. A woman may dislike being pregnant but feel love for the child to be born.

Emotional Responses

Women who are happy and pleased about their pregnancies often view it as biologic fulfillment and part of their life plan. They have high self-esteem and tend to be confident about outcomes for themselves, their babies, and other family members. Even though a general state of well-being predominates, an **emotional lability** expressed as rapid mood changes is commonly encountered in pregnant women.

These rapid mood changes and increased sensitivity to others are disconcerting to the mother-to-be and those around her. Increased irritability, explosions of tears and anger, and feelings of great joy and cheerfulness alternate, apparently with little or no provocation. According to one father-to-be:

> ▪ I sometimes think she is crazy—we're going somewhere she wants to go, out to dinner or a concert. She goes upstairs happy as a lark and in 2 minutes is down again in a regular temper, won't go, and shouts at me. I really feel bewildered by it all.

Profound hormonal changes that are part of the maternal response to pregnancy may be responsible for mood changes, much as they are before menstruation or during menopause. Other reasons such as sexual concerns or fear of pain during the birth have also been postulated to explain this seemingly erratic behavior.

As pregnancy progresses, the woman becomes more open about her feelings toward herself and others. She is willing to talk about matters previously not discussed or discussed only within the family and seems to believe that her thoughts and symptoms will be of interest to the listener whom she deems protective. This openness, coupled with a readiness for learning, enhances opportunites for working with pregnant women and increases the likelihood of supportive care being therapeutically effective.

When the child is wanted, the discomforts associated with pregnancy tend to be considered as irritations, and measures taken to relieve them are usually successful. Pleasure derived from thinking about the unborn child and a feeling of closeness to the child helps the mother adjust to these discomforts.

In some instances the woman who commonly complains about physical discomforts may be asking for help with conflicts regarding the mothering role and its responsibilities. Further assessment of coping measures and tolerance is indicated (Lederman, 1984).

Response to Changes in Body Image

The physiologic changes of pregnancy result in rapid and profound changes in body contour. During the first trimester body shape changes little, but by the second trimester obvious bulging of the abdomen, thickening of the waist, and enlargement of the breasts proclaim the state of pregnancy. The woman develops a feeling of an overall increase in the size of her body and of occupying more space. This feeling intensifies as pregnancy advances (Jessner, 1970). There is a gradual loss of definite **body boundaries** that serve to separate the self from the nonself and provide a feeling of safety. Fawcett and York (1978) describe this feeling as an awareness of the "perceived zone of separation between self and nonself."

The woman's attitude about her body is thought to be influenced by her values and personality traits. This attitude often changes as pregnancy progresses. A positive body attitude is usually expressed during the first trimester. As the pregnancy advances, however, the feelings become more negative. For most women the feeling of liking or not liking their bodies in the pregnant state is temporary and does not cause permanent changes in their perception of themselves.

Ambivalence during Pregnancy

Ambivalence is defined as simultaneous conflicting feelings, such as love and hate toward a person, thing, or state of being. Ambivalence is a normal response experienced by persons preparing for a new role. Most women have some ambivalent feelings during pregnancy.

Even women who are pleased to be pregnant may experience feelings of hostility toward the pregnancy or unborn child from time to time. Such things as a partner's chance remark about the attractiveness of a nonpregnant woman or hearing about a colleague's promotion when the decision to have a child means relinquishing a job can give rise to ambivalent feelings. Body sensations, feelings of dependence, and realization of the responsibilities associated with child care can trigger such feelings.

Intense feelings of ambivalence that persist through the third trimester may indicate unresolved conflict with the motherhood role (Lederman, 1984). Upon the birth of a healthy child, memories of these ambivalent feelings are usually dismissed. If a child with a defect is born, a woman may look back at the times of not wanting the child and feel intensely guilty. Without proper education and support, she may believe that her ambivalence caused the defect in her child.

Rite of Passage

Pregnancy functions as a **rite of passage,** indicative of reaching maturity in a society that has no other obvious rituals. In many states the pregnant woman is legally an adult regardless of her age and may give personal consent for any type of care for herself or for her newborn. She is entitled to financial and other aid from a government source if needed and, if unwed, is considered to be the sole legal guardian of her child. As such she has the right to care for the child herself, place the child in a foster home, or give the child up for adoption.

Identification with Motherhood Role

The process of identifying with the motherhood role begins early in each woman's life, with the memories she has of being mothered as a child. Her social group's perception of what constitutes the feminine role can also make her lean more toward motherhood or a career, toward being married or single, or toward being independent rather than interdependent. Stepping-stone roles, such as playing with dolls, baby-sitting, and taking care of siblings, may increase her understanding of what being a mother entails.

Many women have always wanted a baby, liked children, and looked forward to motherhood. They are highly motivated to become parents, which affects acceptance of pregnancy and eventual prenatal and parental adaptation (Grossman, Eichler, Winckoff, 1980; Lederman, 1984). Other women apparently have not considered in any detail what motherhood means to them. During pregnancy conflicts such as not wanting the pregnancy and child-related or career-related decisions need to be resolved.

Mother-Daughter Relationship

The woman's relationship with her mother has been shown to be significant in adaptation to pregnancy and motherhood (Rubin, 1967a, b; Mercer, Hackley, Bostrom, 1982). Lederman (1984) noted the importance of four components in the pregnant woman's relationship with her mother: the mother's availability (past and present), her reactions to the daughter's pregnancy, respect for her daughter's autonomy, and the willingness to reminisce.

The availability of the mother to a daughter during childhood often means the mother will also be available and supportive during pregnancy. "With the common bond of motherhood and mutual availability, subjects often described a closeness that appeared to facilitate the development and adaptation of both individuals" (Lederman, 1984).

The mother's reaction to the daughter's pregnancy signifies her acceptance of the grandchild and of her daughter. If the mother is supportive, the daughter has an opportunity to discuss pregnancy and labor and her feelings of joy or ambivalence with a knowledgeable and accepting woman. Rubin (1975) noted that, if the pregnant woman's mother is not pleased with the pregnancy, the daughter begins to have doubts about her self-worth and the eventual acceptance of her child by others.

Mothers who respect their daughters' autonomy prompt feelings of self-confidence in their daughters. Grandparents who have helped their children become independent are seen as being willing to help rather than interfere or dominate.

Reminiscing about the pregnant woman's early childhood and sharing the grandmother-to-be's account of her childbirth experience help the daughter anticipate and prepare for labor and birth. Hearing about themselves as young children makes pregnant women feel loved and wanted. They draw closer to their parents and begin to feel that, despite the errors they might make in their own mothering experiences, they will continue to be loved by their children.

Partner Relationship

The most important person to the pregnant woman is usually the father of her child (Richardson, 1983). There is increasing evidence that the woman who is nurtured by her male partner during pregnancy has fewer emotional and physical symptoms, fewer labor and childbirth complications, and an easier postpartum adjustment (Grossman, Eichler, Winckoff, 1980; May, 1982a). Women have expressed two major needs within this relationship during pregnancy (Richardson, 1983). The first is to receive signs that she is loved and valued. The second need is to secure her partner's acceptance of the child and assimilate the infant into the family. Rubin (1975) states that the pregnant woman must "ensure the necessary social and physical accommodation within the family and within the household for a new member."

The marital or committed relationship is not static but evolves over time. The addition of a child changes forever the nature of the bond between partners. Lederman (1984) reported that wives and husbands grew closer during pregnancy. In this study pregnancy had a maturing effect on the wife-husband relationship as they assumed new roles and discovered new aspects of one another. Additional research is necessary to determine if these findings are also true for nonmarried partners.

Sexual Relationship

Sexual expression during pregnancy is highly individual. Some couples express satisfaction with their sexual relations, whereas others express concern. These varied feelings are affected by physical, emotional, and interactional factors, including myths about sex during pregnancy, sexual dysfunction problems, and physical changes in the woman.

As pregnancy progresses, changes in body shape, body image, and levels of discomfort influence both partners' desire for sexual expression. During the first trimester the woman's sexual desire often decreases, especially if she experiences nausea, fatigue, and sleepiness. As she progresses into the second trimester, her combined sense of well-being and increased pelvic congestion may profoundly increase her desire for sexual release. In the third trimester increased somatic complaints and physical bulkiness may account for decreased pleasure and decreased interest in sex (Rynerson, Lowdermilk, 1993).

Partners need to feel free to discuss their sexual re

CLINICAL APPLICATION OF RESEARCH

MATERNAL-FETAL ATTACHMENT: INFLUENCE OF MOTHER-DAUGHTER AND HUSBAND-WIFE RELATIONSHIPS

Attachment theorists postulate a link between early attachment relationships and subsequent attachments. The purpose of this study was to study relationships among a pregnant woman's original attachment with her mother, her present attachment with her husband, and her developing attachment with her fetus. The sample included 115 pregnant women who were attending prenatal classes. The women were "caucasian, reared by their own mothers, married and living with their husbands, 18 years or older, expecting their first liveborn infant, 28 weeks or more gestation without preexisting medical condition or illness, and fluent in English" (p. 39). Data were collected using "Relationship with Mother" and "Relationship with Husband" subscales of Lederman's Prenatal Self-Evaluation Questionnaire and the Cranley Maternal-Fetal Attachment Scale. The author found that mother-daughter and husband-wife attachments were re-

lated, but that these attachments were not related to maternal-fetal attachment. Rather maternal-fetal attachment was related to weeks gestation. These findings support the theory that early mother-child relationships are associated with adult relationships. Since attachment increases with increasing gestational age, nurses working with pregnant women should be alert for patients' comments indicating that a maternal-fetal relationship is not developing as pregnancy advances. These women may need additional support or counseling. Whether these findings apply to women of other ethnic/racial groups is unknown. These relationships need to be investigated further.

Reference: Zachariah R: Maternal-fetal attachment: influence of mother-daughter and husband-wife relationships, *Res Nurs Health* 17:37, 1994.

---

sponses during pregnancy. Sensitivity to each other and a willingness to share concerns can strengthen their sexual relationship. Communication between the couple is important. Partners who do not understand the seemingly rapid physiologic and emotional changes of pregnancy can become confused by the other's behavior. By talking to each other about the changes they are experiencing, couples are able to define problems and offer the needed support. Nurses can facilitate communication between partners by talking to pregnant couples about possible changes in feelings and behaviors a couple may experience as pregnancy progresses (Rynerson, Lowdermilk, 1993).

Concerns about the Fetus

Parental concern for the health of the child seems to vary during the course of pregnancy (Gaffney, 1988a). The first concern appears in the first trimester and relates to the possibility of losing the pregnancy. Many women delay telling others about the pregnancy until this time passes. As the child becomes more of a reality, with movement and an audible heartbeat, parental anxiety focuses on possible defects in the child. Parents may talk openly about these anxieties and press for confirmation that the child will be all right. In the later stages of pregnancy fear about the death of the child is less identifiable; this possibility is evidently remote for parents.

Mother-Child Relationship

Emotional **attachment** to the child begins during the prenatal period as women use fantasizing and daydreaming to prepare themselves for motherhood (Rubin, 1975;

Gaffney, 1988a). They think of themselves as mothers and imagine maternal qualities they would like to possess. Expectant parents desire to be warm, loving, and close to their child. They try to anticipate changes in their lives the child will bring and wonder how they will react to noise, disorder, less freedom, and caregiving activities. They question their ability to share their love for other children with the unborn child. Rubin (1967a,b) found that women "try on" and test the motherhood role by taking their own mothers or substitute mothers as role models who serve as confidantes, support persons, or sources of information and experience.

The mother-child relationship progresses through pregnancy as a developmental process (Rubin, 1975). Three phases in the developmental pattern become apparent.

In Phase 1

The woman accepts the biologic fact of pregnancy. She needs to be able to state, "I am pregnant" and incorporate the idea of a child into her body and self-image.

Early in pregnancy the mother's thoughts center around herself and the immediate reality of the pregnancy itself. The child is viewed as part of oneself, and most women think of their fetus as unreal during the early period of pregnancy (Lumley, 1980, 1982).

In Phase 2

The woman accepts the growing fetus as distinct from the self and as a person to nurture. She can now say, "I am going to have a baby."

During the second trimester, usually by the fifth

month, there is a growing awareness of the child as a separate being. This differentiation of the child from the woman's self permits the beginning of the mother-child relationship that involves not only *caring* but also *responsibility*. Women who plan pregnancy are pleased with their pregnancy and develop attachment to the child earlier than other women (Koniak-Griffin, 1988).

With acceptance of the reality of the child (hearing the heartbeat and feeling the child move) and an overall feeling of well-being, the woman enters a quiet period and becomes more introspective. A **fantasy child,** or dream child becomes precious to the woman. As she seems to withdraw and to concentrate her interest on the unborn child, her partner sometimes feels left out, and other children in the family become more demanding in their efforts to redirect the mother's attention to themselves.

In Phase 3

The woman prepares realistically for the birth and parenting of the child. She expresses the thought "I am going to be a mother" and defines the nature and characteristics of the child.

Although the mother alone experiences the child within, both parents and siblings believe the unborn child responds in a very individualized, personal manner. Family members may interact a great deal with the unborn child by talking to the fetus and stroking the mother's abdomen, especially when the fetus shifts position (Fig. 6-1).

Gaffney (1988b) has summarized selected studies that fail to show consistent significant relationships among factors believed to affect maternal-fetal attachment. More research relating psychologic variables to prenatal attachment and maternal-fetal interaction with maternal-infant interaction is needed. These studies may yield results that help nurses better understand the factors that promote early attachment and reduce the risk of negative long-term sequelae such as child neglect and abuse.

Preparation for Childbirth

Many women, especially nulliparas, prepare actively for birth. They read books, view films, attend parenting classes, and talk to other women (mothers, sister, friends, strangers). They will seek the best caregiver possible for advice, monitoring, and caring (Patterson, Freese, Goldenberg, 1990). The multipara has her own history of labor and birth, which influences her approach to preparation for this childbirth experience.

Anxiety can arise from concern about a safe passage for herself and her child during the birth process (Rubin, 1975). This may not be expressed overtly, but cues are given as the nurse listens to plans women make for care of the new baby and other children in case "anything should happen." These feelings persist despite statistical evidence about the safe outcome of pregnancy for

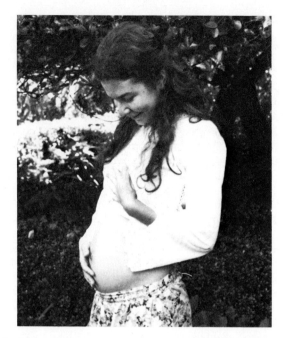

FIG. 6-1 Mother talks to her baby: "How are you doing in there?"

the mother. Many women fear the pain of birth or mutilation because they do not understand anatomy and the birth process. Education by the nurse can alleviate many of these fears. Women also express concern over what behaviors are appropriate during the birth process and how the persons who will be caring for them will accept them and their actions. The best preparation for labor has been found to be "a healthy sense of the realistic—an awareness of work, pain, and risk balanced by a sense of excitement and expectation of the final reward" (Lederman, 1984).

Readiness for Childbirth

Toward the end of the third trimester breathing is difficult and movements of the fetus become vigorous enough to disturb the mother's sleep. Backaches, frequency and urgency of urination, constipation, and varicose veins can become troublesome. The bulkiness and awkwardness of her body interfere with the woman's ability to care for other children, perform routine work-related duties, and assume a comfortable position for sleep and rest.

By this time most women become impatient for labor to begin, whether the birth is anticipated with joy, dread, or a mixture of both. A strong desire to see the end of pregnancy, to be over and done with it, makes women at this stage ready to move on to childbirth.

Second-Time Mothers

Mothers expecting their second child have different concerns in pregnancy (Merilo, 1988). They may have unresolved feelings about their first labor. They may be so focused on their first child that they are less excited and think less about the second baby than they did about the first. They are concerned about the first child's reaction to separation at the sibling's birth and aware that a change in their relationship with the first child will occur after the new baby is born. These concerns may lead to a sense of loss and sadness. Friends and family, assured of the mother's ability to care for an infant, may offer less attention and help.

The nurse needs to recognize that there are dependency needs with every pregnancy. Nurses can help second-time mothers meet their dependency needs by encouraging them to take time out to focus on the second child and their own needs. These expectant mothers need to set realistic expectations for themselves, arranging for household help and child care and reducing outside commitments. Prenatal classes in which second-time mothers are able to share concerns and experiences can help these women recognize that their needs are legitimate and will promote a positive adaptation to the many demands of their new role (Merilo, 1988).

PATERNAL ADAPTATION

There is little scientific evidence to validate the impressions of health care providers on paternal adaptation to pregnancy. Indeed, it has only been within the past two decades that researchers have addressed the importance of the father in parenthood (Henderson, Brouse, 1991). It is generally thought, however, that expectant fathers, like expectant mothers, have been preparing for parenthood throughout their lives. Subconsciously or consciously men think about having a wife and children. During courtship and early marriage discussion of future plans may even include the number, spacing, and names of their children-to-be.

The father's beliefs and feelings about the ideal mother and father and his cultural expectation of appropriate behavior during pregnancy will affect his response to his partner's need for him.

One man may engage in nurturing behavior. Another may feel lonely and alienated as the woman becomes physically and emotionally engrossed in the unborn child. He may seek comfort and understanding outside the home or become interested in a new hobby or involved with his work. Some men view pregnancy as proof of their masculinity and their dominant role. To others, pregnancy has no meaning in terms of responsibility to either mother or child. However, for most men pregnancy can be a time of preparation for the parental role with intense learning.

How fathers adjust to the parental role is the subject of increasing contemporary research (Fawcett, 1986a; Strickland, 1987). In older societies the man is expected to subject himself to various behaviors and taboos associated with pregnancy and giving birth (May, 1982a; Schodt, 1989). These practices are known as **couvade** (French, "to hatch"). By enacting the *couvade*, the man's responses are channeled into acceptable modes of expression, and this new status is recognized and endorsed. His behavior acknowledges his psychosocial and biologic relationship to the mother and child. In Western societies participation of fathers in childbirth is now commonplace.

The man's emotional responses to becoming a father, his concerns, and informational needs change during the course of pregnancy. Phases of the developmental pattern become apparent. May (1982c) described three phases characterizing the three developmental tasks experienced by the expectant father: the announcement phase, the moratorium phase, and the focusing phase.

The early period, the **announcement phase,** may last from a few hours to a few weeks. The developmental task is to accept the biologic fact of pregnancy. The man needs to be able to state, "She is pregnant and I am the father." Men react to the confirmation of pregnancy with joy or dismay depending on whether the pregnancy is desired or unplanned or unwanted. Realization of the reality of the pregnant state seems to come more slowly for the father who does not experience the early symptoms of pregnancy and sees little physical change in his partner in the first trimester of pregnancy. On seeing a sonograph of his son at 12 weeks, one man remarked, "Until I saw his picture, it was all unreal. I knew intellectually my wife was pregnant, but it didn't mean anything to me. It was amazing—in a few minutes I became a father."

The second phase, the **moratorium phase,** is the period of adjusting to the reality of pregnancy. The developmental task is to accept the pregnancy and to be able to state, "We are going to have a baby, and we are changing." Men appear to put conscious thought of the pregnancy aside for a time. They become more introspective and engage in many discussions about their philosophy of life, religion, childbearing, and child-rearing practices and their relationships with family members and friends. Depending on the man's readiness for the pregnancy, this phase may be relatively short or persist until the last trimester.

The third phase, the **focusing phase,** begins in the last trimester and is characterized by the father's active involvement in both the pregnancy and his relationship with his child. The developmental task is to negotiate with his partner the role he is to play in labor and to prepare for parenthood. He needs to be able to state, "I know my role during the birth process, and I am going to be a parent." In this phase the man concentrates on his own experience of pregnancy, and in doing so he feels more in tune with his partner. He begins to redefine himself as a father and the world around him in terms of his future fatherhood.

Acceptance of Pregnancy
Readiness for Pregnancy

May (1982c) found that fathers' readiness for pregnancy was reflected in three areas: (1) a sense of relative financial security, (2) stability in the couple relationship, and (3) a sense of closure to the childless period in their relationship.

Many men express concern for the family's *economic security*. Today most young married women as well as men are employed outside the home. Although pregnant women and mothers with young children may continue their employment, many childbearing and child-rearing women have a phase of unemployment. Financial adjustments must be made to accommodate decreased income and increased expenses of an additional family member.

Those couples who have a *stable relationship* before pregnancy tend to draw closer as a result of their coming parental roles (Lederman, 1984).

Their partners' pregnancies bring *to closure the childless period* in men's lives. Many men view having children and being a father as an integral part of their life plan. Couples who plan for pregnancy are more accepting of pregnancy (Lederman, 1984). If pregnancy is unplanned or unwanted, some men find the alterations in life plans and lifestyles difficult to accept and do not necessarily become reconciled to the pregnancy (May, 1982c).

Emotional Responses

Men display varied emotional responses (styles of involvement) to their partners' first-time pregnancy. In studies conducted by May (1980, 1982a) three characteristic styles (observer, expressive, and instrumental) were noted. Her description provides useful information to nurses working with pregnant families.

Observer style was defined as a detached approach to involvement in the pregnancy. The fathers in this category fell into two major groupings, those who wanted the pregnancy and those who did not. Those who were happy about the pregnancy were supportive of their partners and wanted to be good fathers. However, because of cultural values or shyness, they needed to distance themselves from such activities as prenatal classes, decisions about breastfeeding, and choosing professional care. If by nature unemotional and matter-of-fact, some men appeared to need an emotional buffer zone and the pregnancy did not change them.

The other group who were not happy about the pregnancy reported feelings of ambivalence about pregnancy and the role of father. These men needed time to adjust to the idea of pregnancy and fatherhood and responded to the feelings of ambivalence by becoming involved in careers and resisting their partners' attempts to involve them in preparations for the coming child. "Men established an emotional distance from the pregnancy in relation to the amount of ambivalence they experienced.

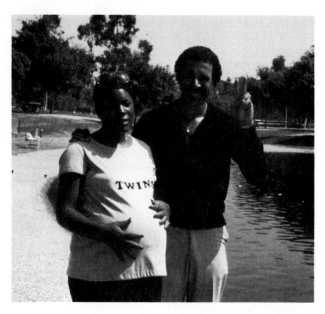

FIG. 6-2 Mother and father walk together. Women respond positively to their partner's interest and concern. (Courtesy Marjorie Pyle, RNC, *Lifecircle*, Costa Mesa, CA.)

Women often sensed this distance and attempted to involve their partners more closely. Often the man responded by withdrawing more" (May, 1982c).

Expressive style was observed as a strong emotional response to pregnancy and a desire to be a full partner in the project (Fig. 6-2). These husbands showed awareness of their wives' needs for support and were conscious of the times when they were not able to give their wives the support needed. They experienced the same emotional lability and ambivalence that characterizes pregnant women. They were excited and pleased about the baby, but also worried about their ability to be good fathers. These fathers may experience the discomforts usually associated with women in pregnancy, such as nausea, lassitude, and various aches and pains. **Mitleiden** (suffering along), or psychosomatic symptoms of expectant fathers, has long been recognized as a phenomenon of expectant fatherhood.

The **instrumental style** was adopted by men who emphasized tasks to be accomplished and saw themselves as "caretakers or managers of the pregnancy" (May, 1980). They asked questions, became interested in the role of labor coach, and planned for photographs during pregnancy, birth, and the neonatal period. They felt responsible for the outcome of pregnancy and were protective and supportive of their wives.

The three styles of involvement emphasize the different ways some men experience pregnancy. Each needs to feel free to define his role in pregnancy just as the woman does. Not all men are able or willing to attend childbirth classes or act as labor coaches because of cultural conditioning or a different supportive style. More research is needed to determine if similar styles of involvement occur in partners of multiparous women.

Identification with Fatherhood Role

Every father brings to pregnancy attitudes that affect the manner in which he adjusts to pregnancy and the parental role (Cronenwett and Kunst-Wilson, 1981; Kunst-Wilson and Cronenwett, 1981; Lederman, 1984).

The father's memories of fathering by his own father, the experiences he has had with child care, and the perceptions of the male and father role within his culture and social group will guide his selection of the tasks and responsibilities he will assume. Some men are highly motivated to nurture and love a child. They may be excited and pleased about the anticipated role of father. Men who have reasonable self-esteem and control of financial resources and working conditions seem more able to incorporate fatherhood into their life plans. Similar to expectant mothers, expectant fathers need support as they prepare for this new role. Jordon's (1990) study with expectant fathers highlights this need. Men in the study reported being recognized as helpers or breadwinners but said they felt excluded from the pregnancy experience. They believed they had no role models to help them become new fathers.

Four types of support necessary for preparing for fatherhood, as outlined by House (1981), provide useful guides for nurses working with expectant fathers.

1. *Emotional support.* The man's primary source of support is his partner. This support has to be modified to permit nurturing of the baby and the additional nurturing his partner needs. Therefore the father needs to seek support from family and friends.
2. *Instrumental support.* The father needs to know that he can depend on family or friends for help if necessary.
3. *Informational support.* The father needs to know who is available (e.g., professionals or relatives) to provide tips on how to solve immediate problems.
4. *Appraisal support.* The father needs to find others to provide criteria against which he can measure his performance.

Partner Relationship

The partner's role in pregnancy can be one of nurturance, responding to the pregnant woman's feelings of vulnerability in both her biologic state and in her relationship with her own mother. The man's support indicates to his mate his involvement in the pregnancy and his preparation for attachment to their child (Lederman, 1984; Diamond, 1986).

In psychoanalytic literature some aspects of the father's behavior indicate rivalry. Direct rivalry with the

fetus may be evident, especially during sexual activity. Husbands may protest that fetal movements prevent sexual gratification.

The woman's increased introspection may cause her partner to experience a sense of uneasiness as she becomes preoccupied with thoughts of the child and of her mother, with her growing dependence on her health care provider, and with her reevaluation of their relationship. He may sense that his partner's support—his key support—is being withdrawn (Jordan, 1990).

Father-Child Relationship

The father-child attachment can be as strong as the mother-child relationship, and fathers can be as competent as mothers in nurturing their infants (Jones, 1981; Cronenwett, 1982). Paternal behavior toward children does not differ significantly from maternal behavior, with the exception of play with the infants (Field, 1978).

Men prepare for fatherhood in many of the same ways as women do for motherhood—reading, fantasizing, and daydreaming about the baby. They may adjust previous commitments to include new responsibilities to enable them to spend time with their new families.

Daydreaming is a form of role playing or anticipatory psychologic preparation for the infant most common in the last weeks before birth. Rarely do men confide their daydreams unless they are reassured that daydreams are normal and fairly common. Questions such as the following help the nurse and the parent in identifying concerns and allow for reality testing:

1. What do you expect the child to look and act like?
2. What do you think being a father will be like?
3. Have you thought about the baby's crying? Changing diapers? Burping the baby? Being awakened at night? Sharing your partner with the baby?

The father may not wish to share his answers with the nurse at the moment, but may need time to think them through or discuss them with his partner.

If an expectant father can imagine only an older child and has difficulty visualizing or talking about the infant, this area needs to be explored. The nurse can give information about the unborn child's ability to respond to light, sound, and touch and encourage the father to feel and talk to the fetus. Plans for seeing, holding, and examining his newly born child can be made.

Some fathers become involved by picking the child's name and anticipating the child's sex. As early as the first month, the name of the child may be selected. Family tradition, religious mandate, and continuation of one's own name or names of relatives and friends are sometimes important in the selection process.

At the time of birth, most parents can accept the sex of their infant, but occasionally disappointment is evident and voiced. The parents may experience a grief reaction and a sense of loss at birth as they release the fantasized child and begin to accept the real child.

Anticipation of Labor

The days and weeks immediately preceding the expected day of birth are characterized by anticipation and anxiety. Boredom and restlessness are common as the couple focuses on the birth process.

The father's major concerns are getting the mother to a medical facility in time for the birth and not appearing ignorant. Many fathers want to be able to recognize labor and to determine when it is appropriate to leave for the hospital or call the health care provider. They may fantasize several situations and plan what they will do or rehearse the routes to the hospital, timing each route at different times of the day. Suitcase, car, and essential telephone numbers are readied.

Many fathers have questions about the labor suite's furniture, nursing staff, location, and availability of health care provider and anesthesiologist. Others want to know what is expected of them when their partners are in labor. The father may have fears of mutilation and death for his partner and child.

With the exception of parent education classes, a father has few opportunities to learn how to be an involved and active partner in this rite of passage into parenthood. Tensions and apprehensions of the unprepared, unsupportive father are readily transmitted and may increase the mother's fears. His own self-doubts and fear of inadequacy may be realized if he is not supported. Self-confidence comes from achieving realistic goals and earning the approval of others.

GRANDPARENT ADAPTATION

The definition of *grand* is extensive and includes descriptions such as impressive or imposing; stately, majestic, dignified; highest, or very high, in rank or official dignity; of great importance or distinction; first rate, very good, splendid; princely, regal, royal, and exalted. A grandparent is an ancestor, one generation more remote—a founder or originator of a family. Grandparents are a vital link between generations (Horn, Manion, 1985). Much research is needed to explain grandparent adaptation to their child's pregnancy and its effect on the pregnancy.

Expectant grandparenthood can be a maturational crisis for the parent of an expectant parent. The pregnancy is undeniable evidence that one is now old enough to have a child who is soon to bear a grandchild. Many think of a grandparent as old, white haired, and becoming feeble of mind and body. Being old carries a stigma for some in predominantly youth-oriented societies. Some people face grandparenthood when still in their 30s and 40s. Occasionally a mother-to-be announcing her pregnancy to her mother may be greeted by, "How *dare* you do that to me! *I* am not ready to be a grandmother!" Both daughter and mother may be startled and hurt by the outburst. Some grandparents-to-be not only are non-

supportive but also use subtle means to decrease the self-esteem of the young parents-to-be. Mothers may talk about their terrible pregnancies; fathers may discuss the endless cost of rearing children, and mothers-in-law may describe the neglect of their son as the concern of others is directed toward the pregnant daughter-in-law.

However, most grandparents are delighted with the prospect of a new baby in the family. It reawakens their feelings of their own youth, the excitement of giving birth, and their delight in the behavior of the parents-to-be when they were infants. They set up a memory store of first smiles, first words, and first steps, which can be used later for claiming the newborn as a member of the family. Satisfaction comes with the realization that continuity between past and present is guaranteed.

The grandparent is the historian who transmits the history of the family and provides continuity with the present, a resource person who shares knowledge based on experience, a role model, and a support person. The grandparent's presence can strengthen family systems by widening the circle of support and nurturance (Barranti, 1985). Other sources of information cannot replace the unique contribution that grandparents make.

Recent research indicates the importance of the grandparent-grandchild relationship. Grandparents act as a potential resource for families. Their support can strengthen family systems by widening the circle of support and nurturance (Barranti, 1985). The parent acts as negotiator in establishing the grandparent-grandchild relationship (Greene, Polivka, 1985). Many women report that their pregnancies bridged the final gap between them and their own mothers. The estrangement that began in adolescence disappeared as the now-pregnant daughter experienced joys, concerns, and anxieties similar to those her mother had felt before her.

To be truly *family-oriented*, maternity care must include the grandparent in implementing the nursing process with childbearing families. Grandparents' classes represent one method of facilitating the adjustment to the grandparenting role, of incorporating the grandparents into the family system, and of encouraging communication between the generations (Maloni, McIndoe, Rubenstein, 1987).

Grandparents' anxieties and concerns and their relationships with expectant parents and grandchildren should be discussed during courses for expectant parents as well. The expectant parents may use this opportunity to begin to resolve conflicts and perceived differences with their parents, a task that can enhance their ability to relate to their own children.

SIBLING ADAPTATION

Sharing the spotlight with a new brother or sister may be the first major crisis for a child. The older child often experiences a sense of loss or feels jealous on being "re-

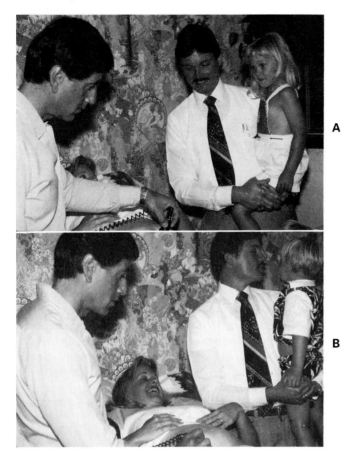

FIG. 6-3   Father and siblings accompany mother on prenatal visit. **A,** Daughter's attention is focused on nurse listening to baby's heart. **B,** Son is reluctant to watch as fetal heart rate is assessed. (Courtesy Marjorie Pyle, RNC, *Lifecircle*, Costa Mesa, CA).

By the third or fourth year of age children like to be told the story of their own beginning and accept its being compared to the present pregnancy. They like to listen to heartbeats and feel the baby moving in utero (Fig. 6-3). Sometimes they worry about how the baby is being fed and what it wears.

School-age children take a more clinical interest in their mother's pregnancy. They may want to know in more detail, "How did the baby get in there?" and "How will it get out?" Children in this age group notice pregnant women in stores, churches, and schools and sometimes seem shy if they need to approach a pregnant woman directly. On the whole they look forward to the new baby, see themselves as "mothers" or "fathers," and enjoy buying baby supplies and readying a place for the baby. Because they still think in concrete terms and base judgments on the here and now, they respond positively to their mother's current good health.

Early and middle adolescents preoccupied with the establishment of their own sexual identity may have difficulty accepting the overwhelming evidence of the sexual activity of their parents. They reason that if they are too young for such activity, certainly their parents are too old. They seem to take on a critical parental role and may ask, "What will people think?" or "How can you let yourself get so fat?" Many pregnant women with teenage children will confess that their teenagers are the most difficult factor in their current pregnancy.

Late adolescents do not appear to be unduly disturbed. They think that they soon will be gone from home. Parents usually report they are comforting and act more as other adults than as children.

PARENTHOOD AFTER AGE 35

Two groups of older parents have emerged in the population of women having a child late in their childbearing years. One group consists of women who have many children or who have a child during the menopausal period. The other group of older parents includes relative newcomers to maternity care. These are women who have deliberately delayed childbearing until their 30s or early 40s.

Multiparous Women

Multiparous women may be those who have never used contraceptives because of personal choice or lack of knowledge concerning contraceptives, or they may be women who have used contraception successfully during the childbearing years. As menopause approaches, women in the latter group may cease to menstruate regularly, stop using contraception, and consequently become pregnant. The older multiparous woman often experiences displacement, feeling that pregnancy alienates her from her peer group and that her age interferes with close associations with young mothers (Hogan, 1979).

placed" by the new baby. Some of the factors that influence the child's response are age, the parents' attitudes, the role of the father, the length of separation from the mother, the hospital's visitation policy, and how the child has been prepared for the change (Spero, 1993; Fortier et al, 1991).

The mother with other children must devote much time and energy to reorganizing her relationships with existing children. She needs to prepare siblings for the birth of the child and to begin the process of role transition in the family by including the children in the pregnancy and being sympathetic to older children's protests against losing their places in the family hierarchy. No child willingly gives up a familiar position.

Siblings' responses to pregnancy vary with age and dependency needs. The 1-year-old seems to be largely unaware of the process, but the 2-year-old notices the change in mother's appearance and may comment, "Mommy's fat." The 2-year-old child's need for sameness in the environment makes the child aware of any changes. Toddlers may exhibit more clinging behavior and may revert to dependent behaviors in toilet training or eating.

Other parents welcome the unexpected infant as evidence of continuing maternal and paternal roles.

Including the family in preparation for the birth is important. The other children in the family may be teenagers. Women often welcome the professional person's support and suggestions concerning how to best involve them. Because older siblings often assume aspects of the parental role, the child develops in a multiparent household.

Nulliparous Women

The number of first-time pregnancies in women between the ages of 35 and 40 years has increased by 40%. Births in this age-group have increased by 37% since 1985. It is no longer uncommon to see women in their late 30s or even in their early 40s pregnant for the first time. Reasons include advanced education, career priorities, and better contraceptive measures.

These women choose parenthood as opposed to the alternative, a child-free lifestyle. They often are successfully established in a career and a lifestyle with a partner that includes time for self-attention, establishment of a home with accumulated possessions, and freedom to travel. When questioned as to why they chose pregnancy late in life, many reply, "because time is running out." Sheehy (1977) points out that age 35 brings a biologic

boundary into view. Deutch (1945) refers to the late desire for a child as a biologic "closing of the gates."

The dilemma of choice includes recognition that being a parent will have both positive and negative consequences (Chervenak, Kardon, 1991). Couples need to discuss the consequences of childbearing and child rearing before committing themselves to a lifelong venture. Partners in this group seem to share the preparation for parenthood, the planning for a family-centered birth, and the desire to be loving and competent parents. Robinson et al (1987) determined that older women were less troubled by pregnancy and remained better adjusted as they entered the last trimester of pregnancy. However, the reality of child care may prove difficult for these parents. The mother who is accustomed to the stimulation of and contact with other adults may find the isolation with her infant difficult to accept. Anger and resentment toward the father (or infant) can result, even with preparation for these aspects of parenting.

During pregnancy, both mother and father explore the possibilities and responsibilities of changing identities and new roles. They must prepare a safe and nurturing environment during pregnancy and after birth. They must also integrate the child into an established family system and negotiate new roles (parent roles, sibling roles, grandparent roles) for family members.

KEY POINTS

- Pregnancy involves all family members, who react to pregnancy and interpret its meaning in light of their own needs and the needs of the others affected.
- The process of family adaptation to pregnancy takes place within a cultural environment.
- Pregnancy presents several developmental tasks to the mother- and father-to-be as they prepare for new levels of caring and responsibility.
- Since pregnancy is a developmental crisis, it is a time of emotional upheaval for both the man and the woman, necessitating adequate communication between them.

- The parent-child, sibling-child, and grandparent-child relationships start during the pregnancy.
- Maternal and familial adaptations to pregnancy generate needs that the nurse can anticipate and meet by providing support, and teaching/counseling/advocacy.
- The psychosocial aspects of care are paramount and may well affect the whole course of pregnancy, childbirth, and the adjustment of the new family.

CRITICAL THINKING EXERCISE

1. You are participating in a health screening fair. Melanie B. approaches you and asks, "What can you tell me about pregnancy for a woman past 35?" What assumptions would you make? What further information do you need before responding? Discuss at least four phases experienced during pregnancy by women between ages 35 and 40.

2. Jennifer P., pregnant with her second child, confides in you, "I don't know how my 18-month-old will take to a new sister or brother. To make matters worse, the grandparents are trying to outdo each other in telling us what to do!" What assumptions would you make? What further information do you need before responding? Briefly discuss at least two interventions you might consider, and justify your choices.

3. Develop a table or chart outlining characteristics of adaptation to pregnancy—maternal, paternal, sibling, and grandparental. Interview prospective parents and other family members, comparing and contrasting their adjustments with expected adaptation.

4. Check libraries and bookstores for popularized accounts of pregnancy and childbirth processes (the how-to approach). Choose one book to critique for the class in terms of its accuracy compared with the discussion of the possible effect such books might have on the pregnant woman.

References

Affonso DD, Sheptak S: Maternal cognitive themes during pregnancy, *Matern Child Nurs J* 18(2):147, 1989.

Barranti C: The grandparent/grandchild relationship: family resource in an era of voluntary bonds, *Fam Relat* 34:3, July 1985.

Chervenak JL, Kardon NB: Advanced maternal age; the actual risks, *Female Patient* 16:17, 1991.

Cronenwett LR, Kunst-Wilson W: Stress, social support, and the transition to fatherhood, *Nurs Res* 30:196, 1981.

Diamond MJ: Becoming a father: a psychoanalytic perspective on the forgotten parent, *Psychoanal Rev* 73(4):445, 1986.

Entwistle DR, Doering SG: *The first birth: a family turning point,* Baltimore, 1981, Johns Hopkins University Press.

Fawcett J: Body image and the pregnant couple, *MCN* 3:227, 1978.

Fawcett J, York R: Spouses' physical and psychological symptoms during pregnancy and the postpartum, *Nurs Res* 35(4):144, 1986.

Field T: The three Rs of infant-adult interactions: rhythms, repertoires, and responsivity, *J Pediatr Psychol* 3:131, 1978.

Fortier JC et al: Adjustment to a newborn: sibling preparation makes a difference, *J Obstet Gynecol Neonatal Nurs* 20(1):73, 1991.

Gaffney KF: New directions in maternal attachment, research, *J Pediatr Health Care* 2:181, 1988a.

Gaffney KF: Prenatal maternal attachment, *Image J Nurs Sch* 20(2):106, 1988b.

Greene R, Polivka J: The meaning of grandparent day cards: an analysis of the intergenerational network, *Fam Relat* 34:2, 1985.

Grossman FK, Eichler LS, Winckoff SA: *Pregnancy, birth, parenthood,* San Francisco, 1980, Jossey-Bass.

Henderson AD, Brouse AJ: The experiences of new fathers during the first 3 weeks of life, *J Adv Nurs* 16(3):293, 1991.

Hogan LR: Pregnant again—at 41, *Matern Child Nurs J* 4:174, 1979.

Horn M, Manion J: Creative grandparenting: bonding the generations, *J Obstet Gynecol Neonatal Nurs* 14:233, 1985.

House JS: *Work, stress and social support,* Reading, MA, 1981, Addison-Wesley.

Jessner L et al: The development of parental attitudes during pregnancy. In Anthony EJ, Benedek T, editors: *Parenthood,* Edinburgh, 1970, Churchill Livingston.

Jones C: Father to infant attachment: effects of early contact and characteristics of the infant, *Res Nurs Health* 4:193, 1981.

Jones LC: A meta-analytic study of the effects of childbirth education on the parent-infant relationship, *Health Care for Women International* 7:357, 1986.

Jordan P: Laboring for relevance: expectant and new fatherhood, *Nurs Res* 39:1, 1990.

Koniak-Griffin D: The relationship between social support, self-esteem, and maternal-fetal attachment in adolescents, *Res Nurs Health* 11:269, 1988.

Kunst-Wilson W, Cronenwett L: Nursing care for the emerging family: promoting paternal behavior, *Res Nurs Health* 4:201, 1981.

Lederman RP: *Psychosocial adaptation in pregnancy: assessment of seven dimensions of maternal development,* Englewood Cliffs, NJ, 1984, Prentice-Hall.

Lumley J: Attitudes to the fetus among primigravidas, *Aust Pediatr J* 18:106, 1982.

Lumley J: The development of maternal-fetal bonding in first pregnancy. In Zichella LJ, editor: *Emotions and reproduction,* New York, 1980, Academic Press.

Maloni JA, McIndoe JE, Rubenstein G: Expectant grandparents class, *J Obstet Gynecol Neonatal Nurs* 16:26, 1987.

May KA: A typology of detachment and involvement styles adopted during pregnancy by first-time expectant fathers, *West J Nurs Res* 2:445, 1980.

May KA: The father as observer, *MCN* 7:319, 1982a.

May KA: Father participation in birth: fact and fiction, *J Calif Perinat Assoc* 2:41, 1982b.

May KA: Three phases of father involvement in pregnancy, *Nurs Res* 31:337, 1982c.

Mercer RT: A theoretical framework for studying factors that impact on the maternal role, *Nurs Res* 30:2, 1981.

The prenatal period is a preparatory one, both physically, in terms of fetal growth and maternal adaptations, and psychologically, in terms of anticipation of parenthood. Becoming a parent represents one of the maturational crises of our lives and as such can represent a time of growth in responsibility and concern for others. It is a time of intense learning for the parents and for those close to them, as well as a time for development of family unity.

Regular prenatal visits, ideally beginning soon after the first missed menstrual period, offer opportunities to ensure the health of the expectant mother and her infant. Prenatal health supervision permits diagnosis and treatment of maternal disorders that may have preexisted or may develop during the pregnancy. It is designed to follow the growth and development of the fetus and to identify abnormalities that may interfere with the course of normal labor. The woman and her family can seek support for stress and learn parenting skills.

FIRST TRIMESTER

The initial visit of the woman to either the health care provider's office or an obstetric clinic is important in setting the tone for her care. The woman needs to feel welcomed and important. The initial visit may include diagnosing the pregnancy and establishing the data base, depending on the duration of gestation. If pregnancy is too early and cannot be verified, her next appointment is scheduled in 2 weeks.

Pregnancy spans 9 calendar months, 10 lunar months, or approximately 40 weeks. Pregnancy is divided into three 3-month periods or trimesters. The first trimester covers weeks 1 through 13; the second, weeks 14 through 26; the third, weeks 27 through term gestation (38 to 40 weeks).

Once pregnancy is diagnosed, prenatal care is instituted. Nursing care follows the nursing process: assessment, analysis and formulation of nursing diagnoses, planning, implementation, and evaluation.

Diagnosis of Pregnancy

The clinical diagnosis of pregnancy before the second missed period may be difficult in at least 25% to 30% of women. Physical variability, lack of relaxation, obesity, or tumors, for example, may confound even the experienced obstetrician or midwife. Accuracy is most important, however, because emotional, social, medical, or legal consequences of an inaccurate diagnosis, either positive or negative, can be extremely serious. A correct date for the **last (normal) menstrual period (LMP),** the date of intercourse, or the basal body temperature (BBT) record may be of great value in the accurate diagnosis of pregnancy. Reexamination in 2 to 4 weeks may be required for verifying the diagnosis.

Great variability is possible in the subjective and objective symptoms of pregnancy. The diagnosis of pregnancy is classified as follows: presumptive, probable, and positive. Many of the signs and symptoms of pregnancy are clinically useful in the diagnosis of pregnancy.

The *presumptive signs and symptoms* of pregnancy can be caused by conditions other than gestation. Therefore these signs alone are not reliable for diagnosis. For example, amenorrhea may be caused by an endocrine disorder; lassitude and fatigue may signify anemia or infection; and nausea or vomiting may be caused by a gastrointestinal upset or allergy.

Presumptive findings include subjective symptoms and objective signs. Subjective symptoms may include amenorrhea, nausea and vomiting **(morning sickness),** *breast fullness* and sensitivity, *urinary frequency,* lassitude or fatigue, weight gain, and mood swings. Quickening may be noted between weeks 16 and 20. Objective signs include a variety of demonstrable anatomic and physiologic changes, elevation of BBT, skin changes such as striae gravidarum and deeper pigmentation (chloasma, linea nigra), breast changes, abdominal enlargement, and changes in the uterus and vagina.

Probable signs of pregnancy are observed by an examiner. When combined with presumptive signs and symptoms, they strongly suggest pregnancy. Objective signs include uterine enlargement, Braxton Hicks contractions and souffle, ballottement, and positive pregnancy test results.

The positive signs of pregnancy are demonstration of a fetal heart distinct from that of the mother, appreciation of fetal movement by someone other than the mother, and visualization of the fetus with a technique such as ultrasound (Scott et al, 1990).

Estimated Date of Birth

Following the diagnosis of pregnancy the woman's first question usually concerns when she will give birth. This date has traditionally been termed the estimated date of confinement (EDC). To promote a more positive perception of both pregnancy and birth, however, the term **estimated date of birth** (EDB) is usually used. Because the precise date of conception generally must remain conjectural, many formulas or rules of thumb have been suggested for calculating the EDB. None of these rules of thumb are infallible, but Nägele's rule is reasonably accurate and is the method usually used.

Nägele's Rule. Nägele's rule is as follows: add 7 days to the first day of the LMP, subtract 3 months, and add 1 year. For example, if the first day of the LMP was July 10, 1994, the EDB is April 17, 1995. In simple terms, add 7 days to the LMP and count forward 9 months.

Nägele's rule assumes that the woman has a 28-day cycle and that the pregnancy occurred on the fourteenth day. An adjustment is in order if the cycle is longer or shorter than 28 days. With the use of Nägele's rule, only about 4% to 10% of pregnant women give birth spontaneously on the EDB. Most women give birth during the period extending from 7 days before to 7 days after the EDB.

Care Management

✤ ASSESSMENT

The process of assessment continues throughout the prenatal period. It begins when a woman makes contact with health professionals because she suspects she is pregnant. Assessment techniques include the interview, physical examination, and laboratory tests. Any deviations from the normal findings may indicate a complication; further tests and assessments must be done.

A checklist of care needs spanning pregnancy is a valuable tool. It provides the team of care providers with a communication tool to prevent gaps and identify areas of repeated concern for patients. When shared with patients, the checklist items validate their universality among pregnant women and their families. Knowledge that items are common to many offers some reassurance. Reading the checklist also reminds patients of otherwise forgotten data (Box 7-1).

BOX 7-1

First-Trimester Checklist

Diagnosis and expected date of birth	Nutrition
	Sexuality
Schedule and events of visits	Cultural variation
Counseling for self-care:	Warning signs of potential complications
Birth plan	Resources
Adaptations/discomforts	Education
	Dental evaluation
Breast changes	Medical service
Urinary frequency	Social service
Nausea and vomiting	Emergency room
Nasal stuffiness and epistaxis	Diagnostic tests Specify
Gingivitis and epulis	Other
Leukorrhea	
Fatigue	
Psychosocial responses and family dynamics	
Exercise and rest	
Relaxation	

Interview

The initial assessment interview establishes the therapeutic relationship between the nurse and the pregnant woman. It is planned, purposeful communication that focuses on specific content. Two sources are usually used in collecting data: the patient's subjective interpretation of health status and the nurse's objective observations. During the interview the nurse observes the patient's affect, posture, body language, skin color, and other physical and emotional signs. These observations become important data in the assessment.

The initial evaluation includes a comprehensive health history emphasizing the current pregnancy, previous pregnancies, the family, a psychosocial history, a cultural history, a physical assessment, diagnostic testing, and an overall risk assessment (NAACOG, 1991). A prenatal history form (Box 7-2, pp. 126-127) is the best method to document the history on the initial visit and record follow-up visits.

Often the woman is accompanied by a family member or members. The nurse builds a relationship with these persons as part of the social context of the patient. They also are helpful in recalling and validating information related to the woman's health problem. With the woman's permission, those accompanying her can be included in the initial prenatal interview. Wright and Leahey (1984) offer excellent guidance to the nurse in developing skills for interviewing families and assessing the interaction between family members. Observations and information about the patient's family are part of the interview. For example, if the patient is accompanied by small children, the nurse can inquire about her plans for child care during the forthcoming labor and birth.

Reason for Seeking Care

The patient's description of the purpose for the request for care is quoted verbatim in the record. For example, "I think I am pregnant," or "My legs get so swollen I can hardly walk." This statement does not constitute a diagnosis because the woman's condition needs to be confirmed by the nurse or primary care provider before any care is instituted. Recording the chief purpose of a visit in the patient's own words alerts other personnel to the priority of need as seen by the patient.

Current Pregnancy

It is usually the presumptive signs of pregnancy that bring a woman for care. A review of symptoms she is experiencing, and how she is coping with them, helps establish a data base to develop a plan of care. A calculation of EDB may be done at this time.

Obstetric/Gynecologic History

Data are gathered on age of menarche and menstrual history, any infertility, any gynecologic anomalies (e.g., fibroids), history of any sexually transmitted diseases

FAIRFAX HOSPITAL

PRENATAL RECORD

Name		Religion	Date

Address		Telephone

Occupation	Business Address	Business Telephone

Husband's Name	Business Address	Business Telephone

Husband's Occupation	Referred by

Age	Gravida	Para	Term	Premature	Abortions	Living

LMP	PMP	Quickening	EDD

Significant History

Significant Findings

Date													
Wt. ( )													
B.P.													
Edema													
Ht. of Fundus													
Position													
F.H.													
Urine Sug/Pro													
Gestation													
Movement													
Initials													
RTC													

Blood Group	Rh	STS	Hgb. HCT.	Pap	HBsAg

Rubella	Glucola	Alpha Feto Protein	GC	HIV

Ppd	Chest X-Ray	Vitamin Supplement	Breast Bottle	Anesthesia Preference	Pediatrician

PROBLEM LIST

_____

_____

_____

_____

_____

_____

_____

_____

_____

_____

_____

☐ Family Planning Information

FAIRFAX HOSPITAL
PRENATAL RECORD Continuation

Name:

PRESENT PREGNANCY

Nausea:	Vomiting:	Other Symptoms of Pregnancy:	
Bleeding:	Cramping:	Pain:	Edema:
Pregnancy Test	Date		

PREVIOUS PREGNANCIES

No.	Date Delivered	Feed-ing	Sex	Wt.	Wks. Preg.	Condition Birth	Condition Now	Duration of Labor	Type of Delivery	Remarks
1										
2										
3										
4										
5										
6										

PAST HISTORY

Menstruation Onset	Frequency	Duration	Flow	Pain
Usual Childhood Illnesses	Rheumatic Fever		Heart Disease	Pulmonary Disease
Convulsions	Venereal Disease		Allergies	Blood Transfusion
Injuries	Operations		Urinary Disease	
Alcohol	Smoking		Drugs	Medication

FAMILY HISTORY

Mother	Father	Siblings:	Other
Diabetes:		Twins:	

PHYSICAL EXAMINATION

General:	Ht.:	B.P. /	Eyes:	Fundi:
Ears:	Mouth:	Teeth:	Throat:	Thyroid:
Chest:	Breasts:	Nipples:	Heart:	Lungs:
Abdomen:	Extremities:			

Ext. Genitalia:	Perineum:
Vagina:	Cervix:
Uterus:	
Adnexa:	

B.I.: c.m.	D.C.: c.m.	Arch:	
Sacrum		Spines:	
Post. Sagittal:	S.S. Ligaments:	Coccyx:	

_____ ,M.D.

SIGNATURE

Form 923
R87

(STDs), sexual history, all pregnancies, including the present pregnancy, and their outcomes.

Medical History

The interviewer records information such as the woman's menstrual history, sexual activity, and previous pregnancies and their outcomes. The conduct of the *present pregnancy* is predicated on the reports of previous pregnancies.

The medical history describes medical or surgical conditions that may affect the course of pregnancy or that may be affected by the pregnancy. For example, the pregnant woman who has diabetes or epilepsy requires special care. Because most patients are anxious during the initial interview, reference to cues such as a Medic-Alert bracelet helps the patient explain allergies, chronic diseases, or medications being used (e.g., cortisone, insulin, anticonvulsants). If the woman is using any medication, she is asked to list them and describe their use.

Previous surgeries are described. Uterine surgery or extensive repair of the pelvic floor may necessitate cesarean birth; appendectomy rules out appendicitis as cause of right lower quadrant pain; spinal surgery may contraindicate spinal or epidural anesthesia. Any *injury* involving the pelvis is noted particularly.

Often women who have adapted well to chronic or handicapping conditions forget to mention them because they are so integrated into their lifestyle. Special shoes or a limp may indicate a pelvic structural defect, which is an important consideration in pregnancy. The nurse who observes these special characteristics and can inquire about them sensitively obtains individualized data that will provide the basis for a comprehensive nursing care plan. Observations are vital components of the interview process because they prompt the nurse and the pregnant woman to focus on the specific needs of the woman and her family.

Nutritional History

This is an important component of the prenatal history. The nutritional status of a pregnant woman has a direct effect on the growth and development of the fetus, and motivation to learn about good nutrition is high in the woman. A dietary assessment can reveal special diet practices, food allergies, eating behaviors, and other factors related to nutritional status.

Drug Use

Past and present drug use needs to be assessed. The woman needs to be questioned as to the use of both legal (over-the-counter, tobacco, prescription, caffeine, alcohol) and illegal (marijuana, cocaine) drug use. Many substances cross the placenta and may adversely affect the developing fetus. Periodic urine toxicology screens are often recommended during pregnancy for women who have a history of illegal drug use.

Family History

The family history provides information about the patient's immediate family, including parents, siblings, and children. This helps identify familial or genetic disorders and conditions that could affect the health status of the woman or fetus.

Social History

Situational factors such as the woman's and partner's occupation, education, marital status, ethnic and cultural backgrounds, and socioeconomic status are determined in the social history.

Perception of this pregnancy is explored. Is this pregnancy wanted or not, planned or not? Is the woman (couple) pleased, displeased, accepting, or nonaccepting? Is the pregnancy "hers" or "theirs"? What problems arise because of the pregnancy: financial, career, and living accommodations? The *family support* system is determined. What primary support is available to the mother? Are there changes needed to promote adequate support for the mother? What are the existing relationships between mother, father, siblings, and inlaws? What preparations are being made for the care of the woman and dependent family members during labor and for the care of the infant after birth? Is community support needed, for example, financial, educational? What are the woman's (couple's) ideas about childbearing, expectations of infant's behavior, and outlook on life and the female role? Questions that need to be asked include: What will it be like to have a baby in the home? How is your life going to change by having a baby? What plans does having a baby interrupt? During interviews throughout the pregnancy the nurse remains alert for potential parenting disorders such as depression, lack of family support, and inadequate living conditions. What is the woman's (couple's) attitude toward health care, particularly during childbearing? What is expected of the primary caregiver, and how is the relationship between the woman (couple) and nurse viewed?

Coping mechanisms and patterns of interacting are identified. Early in the pregnancy the nurse determines the woman's (couple's) knowledge of pregnancy, maternal changes, fetal growth, care of self, and care of the newborn, including feeding. It is important to ask about attitudes toward unmedicated or medicated childbirth and about parental knowledge of availability of parenting skills classes. Before planning for nursing care, the nurse needs information about the woman's (couple's) decision-making abilities and living habits (e.g., exercise, sleep, diet, diversional interests, personal hygiene, clothing).

Attitudes concerning the range of *acceptable sexual behavior* during pregnancy are explored. Questions such as the following could be asked: What has your family (partner, friends) told you about sex during pregnancy? What are your feelings about sex during pregnancy? *Sexual self-*

concept is given more emphasis by employing questions such as: How do you feel about the changes in your appearance? How does your partner feel about your body now? Do maternity clothes make pregnant women attractive?

Birth Plan

The woman's preparation for the childbirth experience is assessed. Is she planning to attend parent education classes (with or without her partner) during the first trimester? Is the couple considering a birth plan? Attendance at parent education classes and the development of a birth plan may vary with the woman's culture, usual means of coping (classes and reading material or other), and feelings about the role of the health caregivers. Some women may come with a form of birth plan; for example, after the birth of an ill infant, the woman anticipating a second birth may prefer to give birth at a tertiary care center with a neonatal intensive care unit. A highly dependent woman may allow the health care team to make decisions about birth plans, assuming that its decisions would be the wisest. A more independent, assertive woman may seek health care that is within her philosophy of care and her beliefs and knowledge; she wants her wishes honored during pregnancy, labor and birth, and the postpartum period. The birth plan is discussed later in this chapter.

Woman with a Disability

Women with serious and handicapping physical or emotional disorders—the deaf, the blind, the depressed, the physically disabled, the mentally retarded, the brain injured—must all be respected and the assessment approach adapted to their needs. Women who are emotionally restricted may not be able to give an effective history, but they must be respected, and the history should be obtained from *them* to the extent possible. Their points of view and their attitudes matter. Still, when necessary, the family, other health professionals involved in care, and the patient's record must be queried to get the complete story. Each woman must be fully respected and fully involved to the limit of emotion, cognitive capacity, or physical handicap.

Physical Examination

The initial physical examination provides the baseline for assessing subsequent changes. The examiner should determine the patient's needs for basic information regarding the structure of the genital organs and provide this information, along with a demonstration of the equipment that may be used and an explanation of the procedure itself. The interaction requires an unhurried, sensitive, and gentle approach with a matter-of-fact attitude.

It is important that the examiner ensure the cleanliness of the facilities, equipment, supplies, and hands. All equipment necessary for the procedure should be in

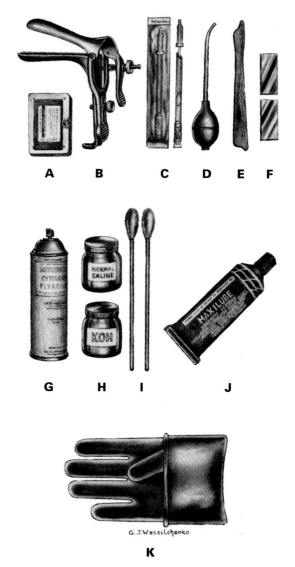

FIG. 7-1   Equipment used for pelvic examination. **A,** Thayer-Martin medium for isolation of *Neisseria gonorrhoeae.* **B,** Vaginal speculum. **C,** Culturette, modified Stuart's bacterial transport medium with self-contained sterile swab. **D,** Vaginal pipette with a rubber bulb. **E,** Wooden spatula for Pap test and cytology specimens. **F,** Slides for cytology specimens (Pap test) or for wet mounts for diagnosing cause of vaginitis. **G,** Spray can of fixative for slide specimens. When dry, slides are packaged for transport to laboratory. **H,** Normal saline and 10% potassium hydroxide (KOH) for wet mounts of vaginal fluids. **I,** Cotton pledget stick for drying cervix. **J,** Sterile lubricant. **K,** Glove for vaginal (sterile) and rectal (clean) exams.

place to avoid interrupting the examination (Fig. 7-1).

The woman is ensured privacy for the examination without unexpected intrusions. She is given a cover gown and drape for modesty. The environment is comfortably warm and pleasant.

The physical examination begins with assessment of vital signs, height and weight, and blood pressure. Because the bladder must be empty before pelvic examination, the urine specimen is obtained before the examination.

Each examiner has developed a routine for proceeding with the physical examination; most choose the head-to-toe progression. Heart and breath sounds are evaluated, and extremities are examined. Distribution, amount, and quality of body hair is of particular importance because the findings reflect nutritional status, endocrine function, and general emphasis on hygiene. The thyroid gland is assessed carefully. The typical basic examination is usually completed without much difficulty for the healthy woman.

The examiner needs to remain alert to the woman's clues that give direction to the remainder of the assessment and that indicate imminent untoward response such as supine hypotension.

Thyroid Gland

The thyroid gland is the largest endocrine gland in the body and the only one accessible to direct physical examination. Assessment of thyroid function or possible dysfunction includes more than observation and palpation of the area where the thyroid gland is located. Metabolic rates and rhythms, including menstrual regularity in the woman of childbearing age, are governed by the thyroid gland. The effects of thyroid activity are widespread. Therefore observations of behavior, appearance, skin, eyes, hair, and cardiovascular status are important. Several findings require further attention (e.g., enlargement, coarse and gritty consistency, nodules).

Breasts

The gynecologic examination includes an evaluation of the breasts primarily to establish a data base of normal findings. However, the practitioner needs to be alert to the possibility of carcinoma at all times. Early detection of potential malignancies has been and continues to be the single most important factor in the successful treatment of this disease. Since professional assessment is done only periodically, each woman is advised to do a breast self-examination (BSE) on a monthly basis at the time when the breast is least affected by menstrual changes, 4 to 10 days after the last menstrual period (see Chapter 29). Due to changes in the breast tissue during pregnancy and lactation, BSE is not as reliable during pregnancy.

Abdomen

The examination of the abdomen is done carefully and systematically. The skin is assessed for general condition, color, rashes, lesions, scars, striae, dilated veins, turgor, texture, and hair distribution. Contour, symmetry, and presence of hernias are noted. Bowel sounds are auscultated. The height of the fundus is noted if the first examination is done late in the pregnancy.

Pelvic Examination

The pelvic examination may be deferred to the next prenatal visit if the woman is anxious, tense, or refuses to have one at this visit. The vagina enlarges, and supporting structures are more relaxed as pregnancy advances. When the examination is performed, the tone of the pelvic musculature and need for and knowledge of **Kegel's exercises** (p. 137) are assessed. During the pelvic examination the nurse remains alert for symptoms of supine hypotension (see Emergency Box, p. 131).

Many women are intimidated by the gynecologic portion of the physical examination. The nurse in this instance can take an advocacy approach that supports a partnership relationship between the patient and the care provider.

The woman is assisted into the **lithotomy position** (Fig. 7-2, *A*) for the pelvic examination. When she is in the lithotomy position, the woman's hips and knees are flexed with the buttocks at the edge of the table and her feet supported by heel or knee stirrups. Some women prefer to keep their shoes or socks on, especially if the stirrups are not padded.

Many women express feelings of vulnerability and strangeness when in the lithotomy position. During the procedure the nurse assists the woman with relaxation techniques; the primary caregiver's and nurse's behavior toward her at this point adds to her ability to relax. One method of helping the woman relax is to have her place her hands on her chest at about the level of the diaphragm, breathe deeply and slowly (in through her nose and out through an O-shaped mouth), concentrate on the rhythm of breathing, and relax all body muscles with each exhalation (Barkauskas et al, 1994). This breathing technique is particularly helpful for the adolescent or the woman whose introitus may be especially tight, or for whom the experience may be new and may provoke tension.

Some women relax when they are encouraged to become involved with the examination by using a mirror to see the area being examined. This type of participation helps with health teaching as well. Distraction is another technique that can be used effectively, for example, placement of interesting pictures or mobiles on the ceiling over the head of the table.

The nurse is reminded that the woman *must not squeeze her eyes closed or clench her fists;* tightening these muscles also tightens the perineal muscles.

Many women find it distressing to attempt to converse in the lithotomy position. Most patients appreciate an explanation of the procedure as it unfolds as well as coaching for the type of sensations they may expect. But in general women prefer not to have to respond to questions until they are again upright and at eye level with the examiner. Questioning during the procedure, especially if they cannot see their questioner's eyes, may make women tense.

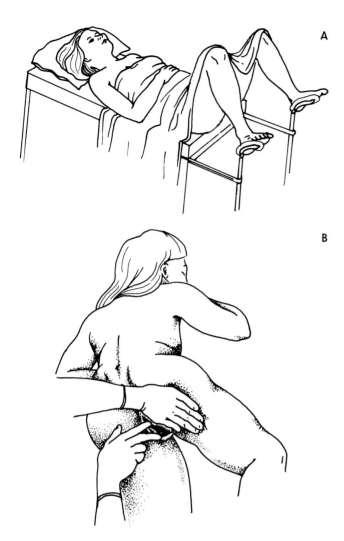

FIG. 7-2 A, Lithotomy position. **B,** Left lateral position, alternate position for examination of genitals.

E M E R G E N C Y

SUPINE HYPOTENSION

SIGNS/SYMPTOMS
Pallor
Dizziness, faintness, breathlessness
Tachycardia
Nausea
Clammy (damp, cool) skin; sweating

INTERVENTIONS
Position woman on her side until her signs/symptoms subside and vital signs stabilize within normal limits (WNL).

perineum are visualized. After childbirth or other trauma there may be healed scars.

External Palpation

The examiner proceeds with the examination using palpation* and inspection. The examiner wears sterile gloves (without lubricant) for this portion of the assessment. The labia are spread apart to expose the structures in the vestibule: urinary meatus, Skene's glands, vaginal orifice, and Bartholin's glands. To assess Skene's glands, the examiner inserts one finger into the vagina and milks the area of the urethra. Any exudate from the *urethra* or *Skene's glands* is collected for culture. Masses and erythema of either structure are assessed further. Ordinarily, the openings to Skene's glands are not visible; prominent openings may be seen if the glands are infected (e.g., with gonorrhea). During the examination, the examiner keeps in mind the findings from the review of systems, such as history of burning on urination.

The *vaginal orifice* is examined. Carunculae myrtiformes (hymenal tags) are normal findings. With one finger still in the vagina, the examiner repositions the index finger near the posterior part of the orifice. With the thumb outside the posterior part of the labia majora, the examiner compresses the area of *Bartholin's glands* located at the 8 o'clock and 4 o'clock positions and looks for swelling, discharge, and pain.

The *support* of the anterior and posterior *vaginal wall* is assessed. The examiner spreads the labia with the index and middle finger and asks the woman to strain down. Any bulge from the anterior wall (urethrocele or cystocele) or posterior wall (rectocele) is noted and compared with the history, such as difficulty to start the stream of urine or constipation.

Supine Hypotension

When a woman is lying in the lithotomy position (see Fig. 7-2, *A*), the weight of abdominal contents may compress the vena cava and aorta, resulting in a drop in blood pressure **(supine hypotension)**. Pallor, breathlessness, and clammy skin are other objective signs. Nursing actions include positioning the woman on her side until her signs and symptoms subside. If the woman is unable to tolerate the lithotomy position, the lateral position may be used for genital examination (Fig. 7-2, *B*).

External Inspection

The examiner sits at the foot of the table for the inspection of the external genitals and for the speculum examination. To facilitate open communication and to help the woman relax, the woman's head is raised on a pillow and the drape is arranged so that eye-to-eye contact can be maintained. In good lighting, external genitals are inspected for sexual maturity, and the clitoris, labia, and

---

*As a sign of caring and to assist the woman to feel more at ease, the woman should receive a verbal cue and a cue through touch on a nonemotionally charged body part (e.g., knee) before experiencing touch on her genitals. The back of the hand, lightly touching the inner aspect of the thigh, often works well.

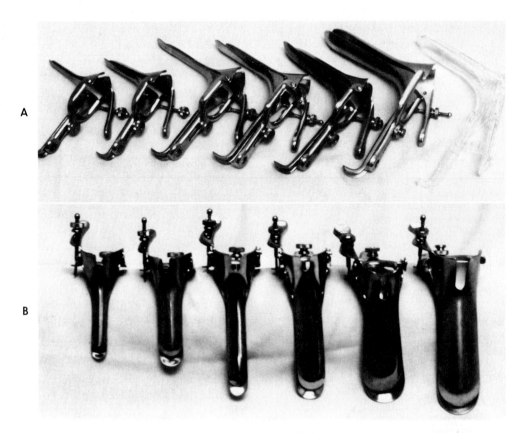

FIG. 7-3 Vaginal specula. **A** *(left to right),* Short-billed pediatric, pediatric, small Pederson, Pederson, small Graves, large Graves, plastic Graves. **B** *(left to right),* Short-billed pediatric, pediatric, small Pederson, Pederson, small Graves, large Graves. (From Seidel H et al: *Mosby's guide to physical examinations,* ed 3, St Louis, 1995, Mosby.)

The *perineum* (area between the vagina and anus) is assessed for scars from old lacerations or episiotomies, for thinning, fistulas, masses, lesions, and inflammation. The *anus* is assessed for hemorrhoids, hemorrhoidal tags, and integrity of the anal sphincter. Occasionally, following traumatic birth with lacerations that extended into the anal sphincter, the muscle may not have been correctly repaired; for example, the examiner will see a dimple over two ends of separated muscle, and the wink reflex is incomplete. If the anal sphincter was not repaired correctly, the woman may have given a history of incontinence. The anal area is also assessed for lesions, masses, abscesses, tumors. If there is a history of sexually transmitted disease, the examiner may want to collect a specimen from the anal canal for culture at this time.

Throughout the genital examination, the examiner notes the odor of the perineal area. Odor may indicate infection and poor hygienic practices.

Internal Examination

When the woman made the appointment for her examination, she was asked to refrain from douching or using vaginal medications for the previous 24 hours. (*Note:* Douching is *not* recommended at any time.) These ac-

tions cloud diagnosis based on secretions, cells, and odor. In addition, douching removes vaginal secretions, making insertion of the vaginal speculum more difficult. Some women have a hard time complying with this request; they cannot go to the primary caregiver feeling unclean in the genital region.

Vaginal specula consist of two blades and a handle. Specula come in a variety of types and styles (Fig. 7-3). Vaginal specula are used to view the vaginal vault and cervix. The pelvic examination is detailed in Procedure 7-1.

The speculum blades are opened to reveal the cervix and are locked into the open position. The cervix is inspected: position and appearance of os, position of cervix, color, lesions, bleeding, and discharge. Cervical findings not within normal limits (for example, ulcerations, masses, inflammation, excessive protrusion into the vaginal vault), anomalies (for example, cock's comb [protrusion over cervix that looks like a rooster's comb], hooded, or collared cervix [seen in DES daughters]), and polyps are noted.

Collection of specimens for cytologic examination is an important part of the gynecologic examination. *Infection* can be diagnosed through examination of speci-

PROCEDURES 7-1

ASSISTING WITH PELVIC EXAMINATION

Wash hands.

Ask woman to empty her bladder before the examination (obtain clean-catch urine specimen as needed).

Assist with relaxation techniques. Have the woman place her hands on her chest at about the level of the diaphragm, breathe deeply and slowly (in through her nose and out through an O-shaped mouth), concentrate on the rhythm of breathing, and relax all body muscles with each exhalation (Barkauskas et al., 1994).

Encourage the woman to become involved with the examination if she shows interest. For example, a mirror can be placed so that she can see the area being examined.

Remind the woman *not* to squeeze her eyes closed, clench her fists, or squeeze the nurse's hand.

Assess for and treat signs of problems such as supine hypotension (see Emergency Box, p. 131).

Warm the speculum in warm water if a prewarmed one is not available.

Instruct the woman to bear down when the speculum is being inserted.

Apply gloves and assist the examiner with collection of specimens for cytologic examination, such as Pap test. After handling specimens, remove gloves and wash hands.

Assist the woman at completion of the examination to a sitting position and then a standing position.

Lubricate the examiner's fingers with water or water-soluble lubricant before bimanual examination.

Provide tissues to wipe lubricant from perineum.

Provide privacy for the woman while she is dressing.

---

mens collected during the pelvic examination. These infections include gonorrhea, *Chlamydia trachomatis,* beta-streptococcus, *Trichomonas vaginalis,* and herpes simplex types 1 and 2. Once the diagnoses have been made, treatment can be instituted. *Carcinogenic conditions,* potential or actual, can be determined by examination of cells from the cervix collected during the pelvic examination using a **Papanicolaou (Pap) test.**

After the specimens are obtained, the vagina around the cervix is viewed by rotating the speculum. The speculum blades are unlocked and partially closed. As the speculum is withdrawn, it is rotated and the vaginal walls are inspected for color, lesions, rugae, fistulas, and bulging.

Incontinence of urine during straining is not a normal finding and is noted. A variety of factors can cause incontinence, including pubococcygeal muscles that are weak from lack of exercise (Kegel's) or trauma from childbirth (see Kegel's exercises, p. 137).

Bimanual Palpation

The examiner stands for this part of the examination. A small amount of lubricant is dropped* onto the fingers of the gloved hand for the internal examination. To avoid tissue trauma and contamination, the thumb is abducted and the ring and little fingers are flexed into the palm (Fig. 7-4).

The vagina is palpated for distensibility, lesions, and tenderness. The cervix is examined for position, shape, consistency, motility, and lesions. The fornix around the cervix is palpated.

The other hand is placed on the abdomen halfway be-

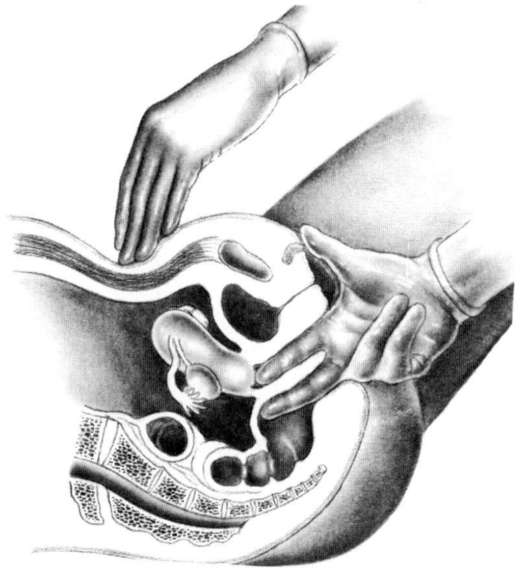

FIG. 7-4 Rectovaginal palpation. (From Seidel H et al: *Mosby's guide to physical examinations,* ed 3, St Louis, 1995, Mosby.)

tween the umbilicus and symphysis pubis and exerts pressure downward toward the pelvic hand. Upward pressure from the pelvic hand traps reproductive structures for assessment by palpation. The uterus is assessed for position (see Fig. 3-5), size, shape, consistency, regularity, motility, masses, and tenderness.

Moving the abdominal hand to the right lower quadrant and the fingers of the pelvic hand in the right lateral fornix, the examiner assesses the adnexa for position, size, tenderness, and masses. The examination is repeated on her left side. Pelvic measurements are assessed.

Just before the intravaginal fingers are withdrawn, the woman is asked to tighten her vagina around the fingers

---

*If the contaminated glove touches the tube, the tube is discarded.

as much as she can. If the muscle response is weak, the woman is assessed for her knowledge about Kegel's exercises (see Kegel's exercises, p. 137).

Rectovaginal Palpation

To prevent contamination of the rectum from organisms in the vagina (e.g., gonorrhea) it is best to change gloves, add fresh lubricant, and then reinsert the index finger into the vagina and the middle finger into the rectum (see Fig. 7-4). Insertion is facilitated if the woman strains down. The maneuvers of the abdominovaginal examination are repeated. The rectovaginal examination permits assessment of the rectovaginal septum, the posterior surface of the uterus, and the region behind the cervix.

After the pelvic examination, the woman is assisted into a sitting position, given tissues or wipes to cleanse herself, and privacy to dress. The woman often returns to the examiner's office for a discussion of findings, prescriptions for therapy, and counseling.

Laboratory Tests

The data obtained from laboratory examination of specimens add important information concerning the symptoms of pregnancy and health status. Both nursing and medical diagnoses stem from such information.

Specimens are collected at the initial visit so that results of their examination will be ready for the next scheduled visit (Table 7-1). A clean-catch urine specimen is tested. Tine or purified protein derivative of tuberculin (PPD) tests are administered for exposure to tuberculosis. During the pelvic examination cervical and vaginal smears for cytology and for infection are obtained. Blood may be drawn to test for a variety of conditions: tests for syphilis; HIV test for AIDS antibodies; complete blood count (CBC) with hematocrit, hemoglobin, and differential values; blood type and Rh factor; antibody screen (rubella, toxoplasmosis, and anti-Rh); sickle cell anemia; level of folacin when indicated. Urine is tested for glucose, protein, and acetone; culture and sensitivity tests are ordered as necessary.

TABLE 7-1 Laboratory Tests in Prenatal Period

LABORATORY TEST	PURPOSE
Hemoglobin/hematocrit/WBC, differential	Detects anemia/detects infection
Hemoglobin electrophoresis	Identifies women with hemoglobinopathies (e.g., sickle cell anemia, thalassemia)
Blood type, Rh, and irregular antibody	Identifies those fetuses at risk for developing erythroblastosis fetalis or hyperbilirubinemia in neonatal period
Rubella titer	Determines immunity to rubella
Tuberculin skin testing; chest film after 20 weeks' gestation in women with reactive tuberculin tests	Screens high-risk population for exposure to tuberculosis
Urinalysis, including microscopic examination of urinary sediment; pH, specific gravity, color, glucose, albumin, protein, RBC, WBC, casts, acetone; hCG	Identifies women with unsuspected diabetes mellitus, renal disease, hypertensive disease of pregnancy; infection; pregnancy
Urine culture	Identifies women with asymptomatic bacteriuria
Renal function tests: BUN, creatinine, electrolytes, creatinine clearance, total protein excretion	Evaluates level of possible renal compromise in women with a history of diabetes, hypertension, or renal disease
Pap test	Screens for cervical intraepithelial neoplasia and herpes simplex type 2
Vaginal or rectal smear for *Neisseria gonorrhoeae*, *Chlamydia*, HPV	Screens high-risk population for asymptomatic infection
VDRL/FTA-ABS	Identifies women with untreated syphilis
HIV* antibody, hepatitis B surface antigen, toxoplasmosis	Screens for infection
1-hour glucose tolerance	Screens for gestational diabetes; done at initial visit for women with risk factors; done at 28 weeks for all pregnant women
3-hour glucose tolerance	Screens for diabetes in women with elevated glucose level after 1-hour test; must have elevated fasting or two elevated readings for diagnosis
Cardiac evaluation: ECG, chest x-ray film, and echocardiogram	Evaluates cardiac function in women with a history of hypertension or cardiac disease

BUN, Blood urea nitrogen; *ECG*, electrocardiogram; *FTA-ABS*, fluorescent treponemal antibody absorption test; *hCG*, human chorionic gonadotropin; *HPV*, human papillomavirus.
*With patient permission.

Fetal Development

A summary of the development of the fetus is presented in Box 7-3.

Early in pregnancy (at about 12 weeks), before the uterus is an abdominal organ, the fetal heart tones (FHTs) can be heard with an ultrasound fetoscope or an ultrasound stethoscope (see Fig. 7-8). The instrument is placed in the midline just anterior to the symphysis pubis. Firm pressure is needed as the scope is used. The woman and her family can be offered the opportunity to listen to the FHTs.

Risks to the fetus are mainly from insult to the developing organs from toxins. Spontaneous abortion from unknown etiology occurs in approximately one in six pregnancies (The Boston Women's Health Book Collective, 1992).

✤ NURSING DIAGNOSES

Each woman and family have a unique set of responses to pregnancy. To attend to these responses, the nurse begins by formulating appropriate nursing diagnoses from the following list that arise from analysis of assessment findings during the first trimester:

Anxiety related to
- Concern about herself
- Physical changes with pregnancy
- Her (or others') feelings about the pregnancy
- Early discomforts of pregnancy

Altered family processes related to
- Family's response to diagnosis of pregnancy

Knowledge deficit related to
- Own role in health and pregnancy management

Altered nutrition: less than body requirements related to
- Morning sickness

BOX 7-3

Fetal Development at 13 Weeks

Differentiation of tissues complete as period of organogenesis ends
Human appearance
Sex distinguishable
Skeleton ossifying
Tooth buds forming
Respiratory activity evident
Insulin secreted (since eighth week)
Kidneys secreting
Intestine returns to abdomen
Head is one third of total length
Length: 9 cm (3½ in)
Weight: 15 g (½ oz)
Fetus less susceptible to malformation from teratogenic agents

---

Altered sexuality patterns related to
- Discomforts of early pregnancy
- Fear of injury to the fetus

✤ EXPECTED OUTCOMES

Planning care for patients during the first trimester is based on the biopsychosocial assessment of the woman and her family. For each woman a plan is developed that relates specifically to her clinical and nursing problems. The information in this chapter is general; that is, not all women experience all problems discussed or require all facets of the care described. The nurse selects those aspects of care relevant to the woman and her family based on the following expected outcomes related to physiologic and psychosocial care:

1. The woman will demonstrate pertinent knowledge of the adaptation of the maternal body to a developing fetus as a basis for understanding the rationale and necessity for modalities of care.
2. The woman will use knowledge of nutritional needs, sexual needs, activities of daily living, discomforts of pregnancy, and self-care.
3. The woman will recognize symptoms that indicate deviations from normal progress and will report them.
4. The woman and her family will actively participate in her care during the first trimester of pregnancy.

✤ COLLABORATIVE CARE

Although other health care providers are involved in giving prenatal care to women, the nurse-patient relation-

---

ETHICAL CONSIDERATIONS

HIV SCREENING

Pregnant women are ethically obligated to seek reasonable care during pregnancy and to avoid causing harm to the fetus. Maternity nurses should be advocates for the fetus, but not at the expense of the pregnant woman.

Mandatory HIV screening involves ethical issues related to privacy invasion, discrimination, social stigma, and reproductive risks to the pregnant woman. Incidence of perinatal transmission from an HIV-positive mother to her fetus ranges from 25% to 35%. Methods of preventing maternal-fetal transmission and fetal treatment currently are not available. Until there is a change in technology that alters the diagnosis or treatment of the fetus, testing of the pregnant woman should be voluntary. Health care providers have an obligation to make sure the pregnant woman is well informed about HIV symptoms and testing.

ship is critical in setting the tone for further interactions. The techniques of listening with an attentive expression, touching, and using eye contact have their place, as does recognition of the woman's feelings and her right to express them. The intervention may occur in various formal or informal settings. For certain persons, involvement in goal-directed health groups is neither feasible nor acceptable. Encounters in hallways or clinic examining rooms, home visits, or telephone conversations may provide the only opportunities for contact and can be used effectively. Sometimes women seek information about a particular problem repeatedly, not so much for the advice given, but to direct the nurse's attention toward themselves. The nurse can help these women by asking for a patient-generated solution and a report of its effectiveness.

In supporting a patient one must remember that both the nurse and the patient are contributing to the relationship. The nurse has to accept the patient's responses as a factor in trying to be of help. An example of one nurse-patient relationship follows:

▪ Mrs. _____ had been very forthright in saying that this pregnancy was unplanned but had countered this statement with comments such as "All things happen for the best," "We always wanted the boys to have a family to turn to," and "Children bring their own love."

Over time, as our relationship developed to one of *mutual* trust, she complained increasingly of her fear of pain, her hating to wear maternity clothes, and her having to give up helping the family. Finally I ventured to say, "Sometimes when a pregnancy is unplanned, women resent it very much and are angry about it." Her relief was evident. She said, "Oh, you don't know how angry I've been."

As a result the whole tenor of support being offered changed, and the plan was adjusted to meet her real needs.

LEGAL TIP:

Prenatal Standards of Care
Providing a standard of care for pregnancy includes:
Assessing for risks, need for referrals, maternal and fetal well-being
Administering medications
Providing support
Maintaining accurate patient records

The nurse also needs to accept the fact that the woman must be a willing partner in a purely voluntary relationship. As such, the relationship can be refused or terminated at any time by the pregnant woman or her family.

Supportive care involves developing, augmenting, or changing the mechanisms used by women and families in coping with stress. An effort is made to promote active participation by the individuals in the process of solving their own problems. Patients are helped to gather pertinent information, explore alternative actions, make decisions as to choice of action, and assume responsibility for the outcomes. These outcomes may be any or all of the following: living with a problem as it is; mitigating effects of a problem so that it can be accepted more readily; or eliminating the problem through effecting change.

Expectations of success in the area of emotional supportive care must be flexible. It is not within the province of any outsider to ensure another person a rewarding, satisfying experience. The mother and persons significant to her are crucial elements in this process. Many of their problems are beyond the scope or capabilities of any professional worker. However, this should not deter nurses from encouraging women to use the decision-making process as a means of coping with problems.

At other times a successful outcome can be readily documented. A woman who early in her pregnancy had predicted a severe depressive state in the postbirth period was elated when such a state did not materialize. She remarked to the nurse who had provided support during the pregnancy and birth, "You're the best nerve medicine I've ever had!"

Education for Self-Care

Health maintenance is an important aspect of prenatal care. Patient participation in the care ensures prompt reporting of untoward responses to pregnancy. Patient assumption of responsibility of health maintenance is prompted by understanding of maternal adaptations to the growth of the unborn child and a readiness to learn. Nurses in their role of teacher provide patients with the information necessary for compliance with health care measures.

The expectant mother needs information about many subjects. During the initial health assessment, the woman may have indicated a need to learn self-care activities such as prevention of urinary tract infection and Kegel's exercises.

Prevention of Urinary Tract Infection

Urinary tract infections may be asymptomatic. Whether symptomatic or not, urinary tract infections present a risk to both mother and fetus. Prevention of these infections is essential. The woman's understanding and use of general hygiene measures are assessed. Before developing a plan of care, the nurse needs to elicit feelings or ideas concerning cultural, ethnic, religious, or other factors affecting health practices.

The woman may need to learn that every woman should always wipe from front to back after urinating or moving her bowels and use a clean piece of toilet paper for each wipe. Wiping from back to front may carry bacteria from the rectal area to the urethral opening and increase risk of infection. Soft, absorbent toilet tissue, preferably white and unscented, should be used because harsh, scented, or printed toilet paper may cause irritation. Women need to change panty shields or sanitary napkins often. Bacteria can multiply on soiled napkins. Women need to wear underpants and pantyhose with a cotton crotch. They should avoid wearing tight-fitting slacks or jeans or panty shields for long periods. A buildup of heat and moisture in the genital area may contribute to the growth of bacteria.

Some women do not have an adequate fluid and food intake. After eliciting her food preferences, the nurse should advise the woman to drink 2 to 3 quarts (8 to 12 glasses) of liquid a day. Eight to 10 ounces of cranberry juice may be included because cranberry juice is more acidic than other fluids and can lower the pH of the urinary tract, making it less hospitable to developing bacteria. Yogurt and acidophilus milk may also help prevent urinary tract and vaginal infections.

The nurse should review with the woman healthy urination practices. Women should urinate frequently. They need to maintain fluid intake to ensure urination and not limit fluids to reduce frequency of urination. They should not ignore signals that indicate the need to urinate. Holding urine increases the time bacteria are in the bladder and allows them to multiply. Women should plan ahead when entering situations where urination must be delayed (e.g., a long car ride). They should always urinate before going to bed at night. Bacteria can be introduced during intercourse. Therefore women are advised to urinate before and after intercourse, then drink a large glass of water to promote additional urination.

The nurse can be reasonably assured that teaching was effective if the woman does not develop a urinary tract infection.

Kegel's Exercises

Kegel's exercises (exercises for the pelvic floor) strengthen the muscles around the reproductive organs and improve muscle tone.

Many women are not aware of the muscles of the pelvic floor (see Figs. 3-11 and 3-12) until it is pointed out that these are the muscles used when urinating and during sexual intercourse and are therefore consciously controlled. Since pelvic floor muscles encircle the outlet through which the baby must pass, it is important that they be exercised, because an exercised muscle can stretch and contract readily at the time of birth.

To help pelvic floor muscles return to normal functioning, Kegel's exercises should be started immediately after birth (see Teaching Approaches box). Kegel's exercises strengthen these muscles and improve muscle tone. If practiced regularly, the exercises help prevent prolapsed uterus and stress incontinence later in life.

The nurse can be reasonably assured that teaching was effective if the woman reports increased muscle tone to control urine flow and during sexual intercourse.

Additional Teaching

Other subjects about which patients need information include diet, exercise, sleep, bowel habits, smoking, alcohol ingestion, medication usage, and sexual relations. It is impossible to impart at one visit all of the information the woman and her family may need at the time her pregnancy is diagnosed. She can be given printed information* at this time, either in the form of notes that are prepared by the health care provider or as a listing of the books pertaining to pregnancy that have been written for lay persons. If the latter, the health care provider should have read the books carefully to be certain they supply the kind of information desired.

Nutritional intake is an important factor in the maintenance of maternal health during pregnancy and in the provision of adequate nutrients for embryonic/fetal development. Assessing nutritional status and providing nutritional information or referral to a dietitian are part of the nurse's responsibilities in prenatal care.

 TEACHING APPROACHES

KEGEL'S EXERCISES

THE EXERCISE

The muscles that stop the flow of urine are the pubococcygeal muscles. Doing Kegel's exercises during urination helps the woman know whether she is doing them correctly. If she can stop the stream of urine, her tone is good.

After a woman has located the correct muscles, Kegel's exercises can be done in the following ways:

1. *Slow:* Tighten the muscle, hold it for the count of three, and relax it.
2. *Quick:* Tighten the muscle, and relax it as rapidly as possible.
3. *Push out, pull in:* Pull up the entire pelvic floor as though trying to suck up water into the vagina. Then bear down as if trying to push the imaginary water out. This uses abdominal muscles also.

PRACTICE

This exercise needs to be practiced several times a day to be effective. It must be done every day for the rest of the woman's life.

This exercise can be done 10 times in a row at least 3 times or more a day. Although some people recommend doing this exercise as many as 100 times in a row, this only fatigues the pelvic floor muscles.

A good time to practice is during trips to the bathroom, but additional practice at other times is even more beneficial.

---

*The nurse must determine, in a sensitive manner, that the woman can read the material given to her. Some women do not use reading as a means of coping, so that other means may be more appropriate (e.g., videotapes or audio cassettes).

SIGNS OF POTENTIAL COMPLICATIONS

FIRST TRIMESTER

SIGNS/SYMPTOMS	POSSIBLE CAUSES
Severe vomiting	Hyperemesis gravidarum
Chills, fever	Infection
Burning on urination	Infection
Diarrhea	Infection
Abdominal cramping; vaginal bleeding	Spontaneous abortion, miscarriage

Formal classes in childbirth and parenthood education have proved successful for some women and families. "Early bird" classes provide fundamental information to meet the needs of most expectant parents during the first trimester (p. 164). Allowing the expectant mother or family the opportunity to ask questions and express any anxieties or fears she or they may have is also important.

Schedule for Care

During the initial visit, women appreciate knowing the schedule for return prenatal visits. Most women can expect to return every 4 weeks until the twenty-eighth week of pregnancy, every 2 weeks until the thirty-sixth week of pregnancy, and then every week from week 37 until delivery. More frequent visits may be needed to accommodate the woman's individual needs. The initial prenatal visit is usually lengthy. Women can be reassured by knowing what to expect on subsequent visits

Signs of Potential Complications

One of the first responsibilities of persons involved in the care of the pregnant woman is to alert her to signs and symptoms that indicate a potential complication of pregnancy. The woman needs to know how to report such warning signs (see Potential Complications above). When one is stressed by a disturbing symptom, it is difficult to remember specifics. Therefore the pregnant woman and her family are reassured if they receive a printed form listing the signs and symptoms that warrant an investigation and the phone numbers to call in an emergency.

Discomforts of Pregnancy

Women pregnant for the first time are confronted with symptoms that would be considered abnormal in the nonpregnant state. Much of prenatal care requested by such women relates to explanations of the causes of the discomforts and what measures can be taken to relieve them. The discomforts are fairly specific to each trimester of pregnancy. Information about the physiology, prevention, and treatment of discomforts experienced during the first trimester is given in Table 7-2.

Nurses can anticipate these symptoms and provide anticipatory guidance for women. Women who have a knowledge of the physical basis for the discomforts of pregnancy are less apt to become overly anxious concerning their health. An understanding of the rationale for treatment promotes their participation in their own care. Nurses need to use terminology the woman (or couple) can understand.

Employment

Continued assessment during the prenatal period is necessary to determine if working is causing undue fatigue or stress. It may be possible for the woman to change the type of work being done with a recommendation from her health care provider. Some women may lose interest in work as they become more introverted during the second trimester of pregnancy. This response may be difficult to accept for the woman who has always been competent and independent before pregnancy.

Activities that depend on a good sense of balance should be discouraged, especially during the last half of pregnancy. Commonly, excessive fatigue is the deciding factor in the termination of employment. Women in sedentary jobs need to walk around at intervals and should neither sit nor stand in one position for long periods. Activity is necessary to counter the usual sluggish, dependent circulation that potentiates development of varices and thrombophlebitis. The pregnant woman's chair should provide adequate back support. A footstool can prevent pressure on veins, relieve strain on varices, and minimize swelling of feet. Work breaks are best spent resting in the lateral side-lying position. It is recommended that employers have an area where women can lie down. Standards for maternity care and employment of mothers in industry have been recommended by the United States Children's Bureau to safeguard expectant mothers' interests.

The nurse can encourage each woman to consider the effects of working postnatally on herself and her newborn. Flexible scheduling of working hours, if possible, can allow for breastfeeding. Also, women who plan to

TABLE 7-2   Discomforts Related to Maternal Adaptation During the First Trimester

DISCOMFORT	PHYSIOLOGY	EDUCATION FOR SELF-CARE
Breast changes, new sensations: pain, tingling	Hypertrophy of mammary glandular tissue and increased vascularization, pigmentation, and size and prominence of nipples and areolae caused by hormone stimulation	Supportive maternity brassiere with pads to absorb discharge may be worn at night; wash with warm water and keep dry; see Maternal physiology and sexual counseling
Urgency and frequency of urination	Vascular engorgement and altered bladder function caused by hormones; bladder capacity reduced by enlarging uterus and fetal presenting part	Kegel's exercises; limit fluid intake before bedtime; reassurance; wear perineal pad; refer to primary health care provider for pain or burning sensation
Languor and malaise; fatigue (early pregnancy, usually)	Unexplained; may be caused by increasing levels of estrogen, progesterone, and hCG or to elevated BBT; psychologic response to pregnancy and its required physical/psychologic adaptations	Reassurance; rest as needed; well-balanced diet to prevent anemia
Nausea and vomiting, morning sickness—occurs in 50% to 75% of pregnant women; starts between first and second missed periods and lasts until about fourth missed period; may occur any time during day; if mother does not have symptoms, expectant father may; may be accompanied by bad taste in mouth	Cause unknown; may result from hormonal changes, possibly hCG; may be partly emotional, reflecting pride in, ambivalence about, or rejection of pregnant state	Avoid empty or overloaded stomach; maintain good posture—give stomach ample room; stop or decrease smoking; eat dry carbohydrate on awakening; remain in bed until feeling subsides, or alternate dry carbohydrate 1 hour with fluids such as hot tea, milk, or clear coffee the next hour until feeling subsides; eat five to six small meals per day; avoid fried, odorous, spicy, greasy, or gas-forming foods; consult primary care provider if intractable vomiting occurs; reassurance
Ptyalism (excessive saliva) may occur starting 2 to 3 weeks after first missed period	Possibly caused by elevated estrogen levels; may be related to reluctance to swallow because of nausea	Astringent mouth wash; chewing gum; support
Psychosocial dynamics, mood swings, mixed feelings	Hormonal and metabolic adaptations; plus feelings about female role, sexuality, timing of pregnancy, and resultant changes in one's life and lifestyle	Treatment same as prevention; both partners need reassurance and support; support significant other who can reassure woman about her attractiveness, etc.; improved communication with her partner, family, and others; refer to social worker, if needed, or supportive services (financial assistance, food stamps)

return to work after giving birth may appreciate information about daycare centers.

Travel

If traveling for long distances, periods of activity and rest should be scheduled. While sitting, the woman can practice deep breathing, foot circling, and alternating contracting and relaxing different muscle groups. Fatigue should be avoided.

Although travel in itself is not a cause of either abortion or preterm labor, certain precautions are recommended. A woman who does not wear automobile restraints risks injury to herself and her fetus. Maternal death as a result of injury is the most common cause of fetal death (Crosby, 1983). The next most common cause is placental separation. Body contours change in reaction to the force of a collision. The uterus as a muscular organ can adapt its shape to that of the body. The

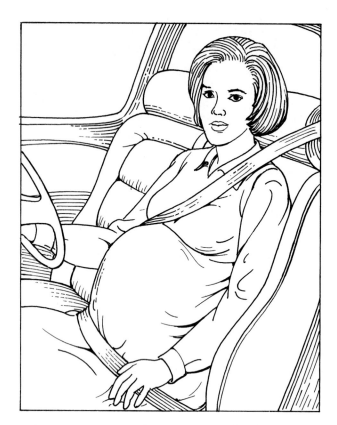

FIG. 7-5 Proper use of seat restraint and head rest.

TEACHING APPROACHES

SAFETY DURING PREGNANCY

Maternal adaptations to pregnancy involve relaxation of joints, alteration to center of gravity, faintness, and discomforts. Problems with coordination and balance are common. Therefore the woman should follow these guidelines:

- Use good body mechanics.
- Use safety features on tools/vehicles; safety seat belts, shoulder harnesses, and head rests, goggles, helmets, as specified.
- Avoid activities requiring coordination, balance, and concentration.
- Take rest periods; reschedule daily activities to meet rest and relaxation needs.

Embryonic and fetal development is vulnerable to environmental teratogens. Many potentially dangerous chemicals are present in the home, yard, and workplace: cleaning agents, paints, sprays, herbicides, and pesticides. The soil and water supply may be unsafe. Therefore the woman should follow these guidelines:

- Read all labels for ingredients and proper use of product.
- Ensure adequate ventilation with clean air.
- Dispose of wastes appropriately.
- Wear gloves when handling chemicals.
- Change job assignments or workplace as necessary.
- Avoid high altitudes (not in pressurized aircraft), which could jeopardize oxygen intake.

placenta lacks the resiliency to change, and placental separation can occur. A combination lap belt and shoulder harness is the most effective automobile restraint (Fig. 7-5) (Hammond, 1990). Both shoulder and lap belts should be used. The lap belt should be worn low across the hip bones and as snug as is comfortable. The shoulder belt should be worn above the pregnant uterus and below the neck to avoid chafing. The pregnant woman should sit upright. The headrest should be used to avoid a whiplash injury.

In high-altitude regions, lowered oxygen levels may cause fetal hypoxia, especially if the pregnant woman is anemic (Barry, Bia, 1989). Women who travel extensively expose themselves to the risk of serious accident and may find themselves far removed from good maternity care. In addition, fatigue or tension, as well as altered regular personal habits and diet during arduous travel, may be detrimental.

If long-distance travel is necessary, the trip should be made by air. U.S. flight regulations do not permit pregnant women aboard during the last month without a statement from the health care provider. Most foreign airlines have a cutoff of 35 weeks' gestation. Air travel itself carries little risk. Magnetometers used at airport security checkpoints are not harmful to the fetus. Sitting in a cramped seat of an airliner for prolonged periods may increase the risk of superficial and deep thrombophlebitis. A 15-minute walk around the aircraft for every hour of travel is recommended to minimize this risk.

Many women experience a sense of uneasiness when traveling by any vehicle. They describe feelings of fear for the safety of their unborn baby (Teaching Approaches).

Physical Activity

Many women exercise regularly and strenuously in the nonpregnant state. They are concerned about loss of physical fitness during an enforced period of decreased activity during pregnancy (Culpepper, 1990; Mittelmark, 1991). Women who have led sedentary lifestyles need to begin with physical activity of very low intensity and advance activity levels gradually (Fishbein and Phillips, 1990). A number of researchers have recommended moderate exercise during pregnancy (Culpepper, 1990; Mittelmark, 1991) (see Home Care box). However, activities continued to the point of exhaustion or fatigue compromise uterine perfusion and fetoplacental oxygenation. If the woman is accustomed to jogging, she may continue; however, she should not reach the point of fatigue. Heat stress may also endanger the fetus. Furthermore, as gestation advances, the woman's center of gravity changes, her bony pelvic support loosens, her coordination usually decreases, and she notices a sensation of awkwardness. Connective tissue laxity increases the risk

HOME CARE

EXERCISE TIPS FOR PREGNANT WOMEN

Consult your health care provider when you know or suspect you are pregnant. Discuss your medical and obstetric history, your current regimen, and the exercises you would like to continue throughout pregnancy.

Seek help in determining an exercise routine that is well within your limit of tolerance, especially if you have not been exercising regularly.

Consider decreasing weight-bearing exercises (jogging, running) and concentrate on non–weight-bearing activities such as swimming, cycling, or stretching. If you are a runner, starting in your seventh month you may wish to walk instead.

Avoid risky activities such as surfing, mountain climbing, skydiving, and racquetball. Activities requiring precise balance and coordination may be dangerous. Avoid activities that require holding your breath and bearing down (Valsalva's maneuver). Jerky, bouncy motions also should be avoided.

Exercise regularly at least three times a week, as long as you are healthy, to improve muscle tone and increase or maintain your stamina. Sporadic exercises may put undue strain on your muscles.

Limit activity to shorter intervals. Exercise for 10 to 15 minutes, rest for 2 to 3 minutes, then exercise for another 10 to 15 minutes.

Decrease your exercise level as your pregnancy progresses. The normal alterations of advancing pregnancy, such as decreased cardiac reserve and increased respiratory effort, may produce physiologic stress if you exercise strenuously for a long time.

Take your pulse every 10 to 15 minutes while you are exercising. If it is more than 140 beats/min, slow down until it returns to a maximum of 90. You should be able to converse easily while exercising. If you cannot, you need to slow down.

Avoid becoming overheated for extended periods. It is best not to exercise for more than 35 minutes, especially in hot, humid weather. As your body temperature rises, the heat is transmitted to your fetus. Prolonged or repeated fetal temperature elevation may result in birth defects, especially during the first 3 months. Your temperature should not exceed 100.4° F (38° C).

Avoid hot tubs and saunas.

Warm-up and stretching exercises prepare your joints for more strenuous exercise and lessen the likelihood of strain or injury to your joints. No exercise should be performed flat on your back after the fourth month of gestation.

A cool-down period of mild activity involving your legs after an exercise period will help bring your respiration, heart, and metabolic rates back to normal and avoid pooling of blood in the exercised muscles.

Rest for 10 minutes after exercising, lying on your left side. As the uterus grows, it puts pressure on a major vein on the right side of your abdomen, which carries blood to your heart. Lying on your left side removes the pressure and promotes return circulation from your extremities and muscles to your heart, increasing blood flow to your placenta and fetus. Care should be taken to rise gradually from the floor to avoid feeling dizzy or fainting (orthostatic hypotension).

Drink two or three 8-ounce glasses of water after you exercise, to replace the body fluids you lost through perspiration. While exercising, drink water whenever you feel the need.

Increase your caloric intake to replace the calories burned during exercise and to provide the extra energy needs of pregnancy. Choose high-protein foods such as fish, cheese, eggs, and meat.

Take your time. This is not the time to be competitive or train for activities requiring long endurance.

Wear a supportive bra. Your increased breast weight may cause changes in posture and put pressure on the ulnar nerve.

Wear supportive shoes. As your uterus grows, your center of gravity shifts and you compensate by arching your back. These natural changes may make you feel off balance and more likely to fall.

Stop exercising immediately and consult your health care provider if you experience shortness of breath, dizziness, numbness, tingling, pain of any kind, more than four uterine contractions per hour, decreased fetal activity, or vaginal bleeding.

Modified from Paglone A, Worthington S: Cautions and advice on exercise during pregnancy. *Contemp OB/GYN* 25:160, 1985 (special issue); Fishbein EG, Phillips M: How safe is exercise during pregnancy? *JOGNN* 19:45, 1990, ACOG: *Home exercise program: exercise during pregnancy and the postnatal period,* Washington, DC, ACOG, 1985.

of joint injury; therefore stretches should not be taken to the point of maximum resistance. Deep flexion or extension of joints must be avoided. Any activity such as jumping, jarring motions, or rapid changes in direction are contraindicated because of joint instability (Fishbein, Phillips, 1990). Awkwardness may cause the woman to lose balance and fall, injuring herself.

Exercises such as those depicted in Fig. 7-6 are taught either at prenatal classes or by the nurse in the clinic or the health care provider's office. The exercises promote comfort and help prepare the woman for labor. Other topics for discussion and demonstration are posture and the correct method used to lift and move objects safely to counteract the awkwardness and prevent the discomfort often experienced starting in the second trimester of pregnancy.

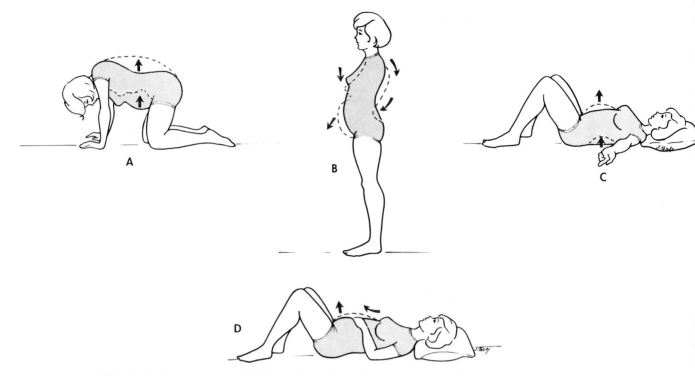

FIG. 7-6 Exercises. **A** to **C,** Pelvic rocking relieves low backache (excellent for relief of menstrual cramps as well). **D,** Abdominal breathing aids relaxation and lifts abdominal wall off uterus.

Dental Health

Dental care during pregnancy is especially important. Nausea during pregnancy may lead to poor oral hygiene, and dental caries may develop. No physiologic alteration during gestation can cause dental caries. Calcium and phosphorus in the teeth are fixed in enamel. Therefore the old adage "for every child a tooth" need not be true.

There is no scientific evidence that filling teeth or even dental extraction with the use of local or nitrous oxide–oxygen anesthesia causes abortion or preterm labor. Antibacterial therapy should be considered for sepsis, however, especially in pregnant women who have had rheumatic heart disease or nephritis. Extensive dental surgery is postponed until after birth for the woman's comfort, if possible.

Medications

Although much has been learned in recent years about fetal drug toxicity (Appendix E,) the possible teratogenicity of many drugs, both prescription and over the counter (OTC), is still unknown. This is especially true for new medications and combinations of drugs. Moreover, certain subclinical errors or deficiencies in intermediate metabolism in the fetus may convert an otherwise harmless drug into a hazardous one. The greatest danger of causing developmental defects in the fetus from drugs exists from fertilization through the first trimester. Self-treatment must be discouraged. All drugs, including aspirin, should be limited, and a careful record of therapeutic agents used should be kept (Dicke, 1989).

Immunization

There has been some concern over the safety of various immunization techniques during pregnancy (Barry, Bia, 1989; Cunningham et al, 1993). Immunization with live or attenuated live viruses is contraindicated during pregnancy because of potential teratogenicity. Vaccines with killed viruses may be used. Live virus vaccines include measles (rubeola and rubella) (Burgess, 1990) and mumps. Some women may need immunization against influenza. For immediate protection following exposure, inactivated polio vaccine (IPV) may be used. Immunization against cholera, typhoid, and poliomyelitis may be needed if the woman must travel to areas where these diseases are endemic. Tetanus toxoid or varicella immune globulin may be given when necessary.

Alcohol, Cigarette Smoke, and Other Substances

No safe level of alcohol consumption has yet been established. Although occasional alcoholic beverages *may* not be harmful to the mother or her developing embryo or fetus, complete abstinence is strongly advised. Maternal alcoholism is associated with high rates of spontaneous abortion; the risk for spontaneous abortion is dose related (three or more drinks per day) in the first trimester (Cook et al, 1990).

Cigarette smoking or continued exposure to a smoke-filled environment (even if the mother does not smoke) is associated with fetal growth retardation and an increase in perinatal and infant morbidity and mortality. Smoking also increases the frequency of preterm labor, premature rupture of membranes (PROM), abruptio placentae, placenta previa, and fetal death (McDonald, Armstrong, Sloan, 1992). Laboratory studies indicate a lowered Po_2 level in both mother and fetus during exposure to cigarette smoke. Smoking may result in a lessened supply of milk during lactation, and harmful substances may be transferred to the infant in the milk.

If the woman is a smoker, the nurse needs to discuss the options she has regarding methods designed to help her quit. If she is resistant to the idea of quitting, the nurse can try to offer ways in which she can cut down (Ershoff et al, 1989).

Most studies of human pregnancy report no association between caffeine consumption and birth defects or low birth weight (Leviton, 1988; Cunningham et al, 1993). Other effects are unknown. Therefore, pregnant women are advised to limit caffeine intake.

Any mind-altering substance has a deleterious effect on the fetus and should not be used. Marijuana, heroin, and cocaine (Peters, Theorell, 1991) are well-known examples of such substances.

Birth Plan

The birth plan is a natural evolution of the contemporary wellness-oriented lifestyle. It is a tool by which parents can explore their childbirth options and choose those which are most important to them. Many parents have already indicated some of their preferences by the type of health care provider and birth setting (hospital and the options it offers or free-standing birth center) they have chosen. Some pregnant women enlist the services of the health care provider only after an interview and a tour of the birth facility. Others do not give conscious thought to the conduct of their pregnancy, labor and birth, recovery, and early parenthood. These women may need help with decision making. After the confirmation of pregnancy, couples tend to focus on the reality of their situation and their emotional responses. However, it is acceptable for the nurse to initiate a discussion of a birth plan during the first and second prenatal visit. Some maternity clinics have printed material describing available options and answers to frequently asked questions. In addition, tours of the birth setting are offered by almost all facilities that provide perinatal services.

Patients' expectations must be reasonable for the resources available in the community. The nurse can provide couples with pertinent information for informed decision making, alerting them to various options and the advantages and consequences of each. The nurse assesses patients' readiness to learn. Some health care providers supply birth plan lists. A discussion of the printed list serves as a means of starting couples to think about, discuss, and identify what is personally important.

Topics for discussion and decision making may include any or all of the following:

- *Partner's participation.* Attend prenatal visits? Parent education classes? Present during labor? During birth? During cesarean birth?
- *Birth setting.* Hospital delivery room or birthing room (if available)? Birthing center?
- *Labor management.* Would you like to walk around during labor? Use a rocking chair? Use a shower? Jacuzzi (available in many new labor, delivery, recovery, and postpartum [LDRP] rooms)? Perineal preparation or enema (if they are still done routinely at that particular setting)? Consider an electronic fetal monitor? Consider stimulation of labor? Consider medication—what kind? Be interested in having music or dimmed lighting? Older children or other people present?
- *Birth.* Have you considered the various positions for birth—side lying, on hands and knees, kneeling or squatting? Or using a birthing bed? Or delivery table? Will you be photographing or filming any of the labor or birth? Who would you like to be present—partner, older siblings, other family member(s), or friend(s)? What are your feelings about forceps, episiotomies? Will your partner choose to cut the umbilical cord?

Other relevant topics might best be presented during the second trimester.

The birth plan also can serve as a tool for open communication between the pregnant woman and her partner and between them and health care providers. Early introduction to the idea of a birth plan allows the couple time to think about events or situations that could make their childbearing experience meaningful and those they would prefer to avoid. The nurse-patient interaction concerning the birth plan needs to occur in an accepting atmosphere in which women can see themselves as unique and yet normal.

Sexual Counseling during Pregnancy

Sexual counseling includes countering misinformation, providing reassurance of normalcy, and suggesting alternative behaviors. The uniqueness of each couple is considered within a biopsychosocial framework.

Counseling couples concerning sexual adjustment during pregnancy demands self-assessment by the nurse as well as a knowledge of the physical, social, and emotional responses to sex during pregnancy (Rynerson, Lowdermilk, 1993). Not all maternity nurses are comfortable dealing with the sexual concerns of their patients. Nurses who are aware of their personal strengths and limitations in dealing with sexual content are in a better position to make referrals when necessary.

A significant number of patients merely need *permission* to be sexual during pregnancy. Many other clients need *information* about the physiologic changes that occur during pregnancy and to have myths associated with sex during pregnancy debunked. Giving permission and providing information are within the purview of the maternity nurse and should be an integral component of providing health care (Teaching Approaches).

A few couples must be referred for either *sex therapy* or *family therapy*. Couples with sexual dysfunction problems of long standing that are intensified by pregnancy are referred for sex therapy. When a sexual problem is a symptom of a more serious interactional problem, the couple would benefit from family therapy.

Couples are relieved to learn that their fears and concerns do not make them "weird" or "crazy." It is important for the counselor to view sexuality in its broadest sense. Kissing, hugging, massaging, petting, and increased gentleness and sensitivity are valid forms of sexual expression and signs of affection. Each of these behaviors is pleasurable in itself and is not always a preliminary behavior leading to intercourse. When a couple cannot have, or chooses not to have, penile-vaginal intercourse, the need for closeness and intimacy can be expressed in many other ways.

To date research has not proved conclusively that coitus and orgasm are contraindicated at any time during pregnancy for the obstetrically and medically healthy woman (Enkin, 1989; Scott et al, 1990; Cunningham et al, 1993). However, a history of more than one spontaneous abortion or a threatened abortion in the first trimester, impending miscarriage in the second trimester, or premature rupture of membranes, bleeding, or abdominal pain during the third trimester may warrant precaution against coitus and orgasm (Rynerson, Lowdermilk, 1993).

Solitary and mutual masturbation and oral-genital intercourse may be used by couples as alternatives to penile-vaginal intercourse. Men who enjoy cunnilingus (oral stimulation of female genitalia) may feel turned off by the normal increase in amount and odor of vaginal discharges during pregnancy. Couples who practice cunnilingus should be cautioned concerning the blowing of air into the vagina, particularly during the last few weeks of pregnancy. There have been cases reported of maternal death and near-fatal cases from air emboli caused by forceful blowing of air into the vagina (Bernhardt et al, 1988). If the cervix is slightly open (as it may be near term), there is the possibility that air will be forced between the membranes and the uterine wall. Some air may enter the maternal placental lakes, thus gaining entrance into the maternal vascular bed.

Pictures of possible variations of *coital position* are often helpful. The female-superior, side-by-side, and rear-entry positions are possible alternative positions to the

TEACHING APPROACHES

SEXUALITY IN FIRST TRIMESTER OF PREGNANCY

- Be aware that maternal physiologic changes, such as breast enlargement, nausea, fatigue, abdominal changes, perineal enlargement, leukorrhea, pelvic vasocongestion, and orgasmic responses, may affect sexuality and sexual expression.
- Discuss responses to pregnancy with your partner.
- Keep in mind that cultural prescriptions (dos) and proscriptions (don'ts) may affect your responses.
- Although your libido may be depressed during the first trimester, it increases during the second and third trimesters.
- Discuss and explore with your partner:
  —Alternative behaviors (e.g., mutual masturbation, foot massage, cuddling)
  —Alternative positions (e.g., female superior, side-lying) for sexual intercourse
- Intercourse is safe as long as it is not uncomfortable. There is no correlation between intercourse and spontaneous abortion, but observe the following precautions:
  —Abstain from intercourse if you experience uterine cramping or vaginal bleeding; report event to your caregiver as soon as possible.
  —Abstain from intercourse (or any activity that results in orgasm) if you have a history of cervical incompetence, until it is corrected.
- Continue to use "safer sex" behaviors. Women at high risk for acquiring or transmitting sexually transmitted diseases are encouraged to use condoms during sexual intercourse throughout pregnancy.

male-superior position. The woman astride (superior position) allows her to control the angle and depth of penile penetration as well as to protect her breasts and abdomen. The side-by-side position is the one of choice, especially during the third trimester, since it requires reduced energy and pressure on the pregnant abdomen. (For other positions the reader is referred to Rynerson, Lowdermilk, 1993).

Multiparous women have reported severe *breast tenderness* in the first trimester. A coital position that avoids direct pressure on the woman's breasts and decreased breast fondling during love play can be recommended. The woman should also be reassured that this condition is normal and temporary. *Lactating mothers* lose milk in uncontrolled spurts in response to sexual stimulation. The couple that is forewarned can be prepared for this eventuality.

The National Family Planning and Reproductive Health Association, Washington, DC, suggests that for some women, *use of the condom should be continued* throughout the pregnancy. The objective is prophylaxis against the acquisition and transmission of sexually transmitted diseases (e.g., herpes simplex virus [HSV], gonorrhea, acquired immunodeficiency syndrome [AIDS]) (Goldsmith, 1989).

Cultural Variation in Prenatal Care

Prenatal care as we know it is a phenomenon of Western medicine. The Western biomedical model of care encourages women to seek prenatal care as early as possible in their pregnancy. Visits are usually routine and follow a systematic sequence, with the initial visit followed by monthly and then weekly visits. Monitoring weight and blood pressure, testing blood and urine, teaching specific information about diet, rest, and activity, and preparing for childbirth are common components of prenatal care.

This model not only is unfamiliar but commonly seems strange to many groups (Lee, 1989; Kulig, 1990; Green, 1990). Many **cultural variations** in prenatal care exist. Even when the prenatal care described is familiar, some practices may conflict with a subcultural group's beliefs and practices. Because of these and other factors, such as lack of money, lack of transportation, and poor communication on the part of health care providers, many groups do not participate in the prenatal care system (Lazarus, Philipson, 1990; Leatherman, Blackburn, Davidhizar, 1990; Scupholme, Robertson, Kamons, 1991). Their behavior may be misinterpreted by nurses as uncaring, lazy, or ignorant.

A concern for *modesty* is also a deterrent for prenatal care for many persons. Exposing one's body parts, especially to a man, can be a major violation of modesty. Thus many women prefer a female health care provider over a male health care provider. Most women value and appreciate efforts to maintain modesty.

Although pregnancy is considered normal by many, certain practices are expected of women of all cultures to ensure a good outcome. *Prescriptions* tell women what to do, and *proscriptions* establish *taboos*. The purposes of these practices are to prevent maternal illness from a pregnancy-induced imbalanced state and protect the vulnerable fetus. Prescriptions and proscriptions are related to emotional response, clothing, activity and rest, sexual activity, and dietary practices.

Emotional Response

Virtually all cultures emphasize the importance of a socially harmonious and agreeable environment. Visits from extended family members may be required to demonstrate continued pleasant and noncontroversial relationships. If dissonance exists in any relationship with others, it is usually dealt with in culturally prescribed ways.

Imitative magic functions in other proscriptions in addition to food. Mexicans advise against pregnant women witnessing an eclipse of the moon because they believe it may cause a cleft palate in the infant. Snow (1974) noted that among some African-Americans a pregnant woman must not ridicule someone with an affliction for fear her child might be born with the same handicap; a mother should not hate a person lest her child resemble that person; and dental work should not be done during pregnancy because it may cause a baby to have a harelip. Carrington (1978) described a widely held folk belief in many cultures that includes refraining from raising one's arm above one's head and refraining from tying knots, so that the umbilical cord does not wrap around the baby's neck and become knotted.

Clothing

Although most cultural groups do not prescribe specific clothing for pregnancy, modesty is an expectation for many (Clark, 1970; Meleis, Sorrell, 1981). Spanish-speaking people of the Southwest may wear a cord beneath the breast and knotted over the umbilicus. This cord, called a *muneco*, is thought to prevent morning sickness and ensure a safe birth (Brown, 1976). Amulets, medals, and beads may be worn to ward off evil spirits.

Physical Activity and Rest

Norms that regulate physical activity of mothers during pregnancy vary tremendously. Many groups (Carrington, 1978; Horn, 1982; Lee, 1989) encourage women to be active, to walk, and to engage in normal although not strenuous activities to ensure that the baby is healthy and not too large. On the other hand, the Filipino woman is cautioned that any activity is dangerous, and others willingly take over work (Affonso, 1978; Stern, 1981). The belief among Filipinos is that inactivity constitutes a protection for mother and child. The mother is encouraged to simply produce the succeeding generation. Health care providers could misinterpret this behavior as laziness or noncompliance with the health regimen desired in prenatal care. Again, it is important for the nurse to find out the meaning of activity and rest for each culture.

Sexual Activity

In most cultures sexual activity is not prohibited until the end of pregnancy. Among African-Americans sexual relations are viewed as natural because pregnancy is a state of health (Carrington, 1978). Mexican-Americans view sexual activity as necessary to keep the birth canal lubricated (Kay, 1982). On the other hand, Vietnamese have definite proscriptions about sexual intercourse, requiring abstinence as early as the sixth month (Lee, 1989). Sexual taboos are more common after giving birth.

Diet

Nutritional information given by Western health care providers may be a source of conflict for many cultural groups. The conflict is commonly not known by the health care providers unless they have an understanding of dietary beliefs and practices of the persons for whom they are caring.

✦ EVALUATION

Maternal and fetal expected outcomes are continuously evaluated according to measurable, established criteria. The clinical findings that represent normal response are presented as plans/expected outcomes in the nursing care plans for each patient. These criteria are used as a basis for selecting appropriate nursing actions and evaluating their effectiveness (see Plan of Care).

SECOND TRIMESTER

By the second trimester the pregnancy usually has been positively diagnosed. The woman and her family have had time to adjust to the pregnancy, and the initial visit or two have been completed. For many women, discomforts common to the first trimester are resolving, but it is still too early to focus intently on the labor and birth.

For most women no apparent major problems are identified. For them, a common pattern for return visits is scheduled. Throughout the second trimester, monthly visits are sufficient, although additional visits may be warranted should the need arise.

Care Management

✦ ASSESSMENT

Maternal Assessment

Interview

Follow-up visits are less extensive than the initial prenatal visit. At each visit the woman is asked for a summary of events since the previous visit. She is asked about her general well-being, complaints or problems, and questions she may have. The interviewer can reinforce teaching about danger signs by inquiring about them at each visit. Personal and family needs are identified and explored. Success or failure of self-care measures is discussed; and learning needs and readiness for learning are assessed.

Careful, precise, and concise recording of patient responses and laboratory results contributes to the continuous supervision vital to the mother and fetus. A checklist of care needs during the second trimester of pregnancy is a valuable tool. It provides the team of care providers with a communication tool to prevent gaps and identify areas of repeated concern for patients. A sample checklist for the second trimester is shown in Box 7-4 .

BOX 7-4

Second-Trimester Checklist

Schedule and events of visits
Maternal assessment
Fetal growth and development
Diagnostic tests
  Specify
Counseling for self-care
  Birth plan
  Adaptations/discomforts
    Skin changes
    Palpitations
    Faintness
    Gastrointestinal distress
    Varicosities
    Neuromuscular and skeletal distress
  Safety (seat belts with shoulder harness and head rest)
  Exercise and rest
  Relaxation
  Nutrition
  Alcohol and other substances
  Sexuality
  Personal hygiene
  Warning signs of potential complications
Other

Physical Examination

Reevaluation is continuous. Each woman reacts differently to pregnancy. Careful monitoring of pregnancy and reactions to care is vital. A data base updated at each contact with a patient reveals patterns in movement and content.

At each visit temperature, pulse, and respirations are measured; blood pressure (right arm, woman sitting) is taken; weight and the determination of whether weight gain (or loss) is compatible with overall plan for weight gain are evaluated; and presence and degree of edema are noted. These findings reflect the status of maternal adaptations. When the interview or physical examination findings are suspicious, an in-depth examination is performed.

Careful interpretation of blood pressure is important in risk-factor analysis for all pregnant women. Blood pressure is evaluated on the basis of absolute values and length of gestation and is interpreted in the light of modifying factors. Pregnancy-induced hypertension (PIH) and *h*emolysis, *e*levated *l*iver enzyme, *l*ow *p*latelet count (HELLP) syndrome are serious complications of pregnancy and may be fatal.

Absolute values of a systolic blood pressure ≥ 140 mm Hg and a diastolic blood pressure ≥ 90 mm Hg are suggestive of hypertension. A rise in systolic blood pressure ≥ 30 mm Hg over baseline and in diastolic blood pres-

PLAN OF CARE

First Trimester—Discomforts of Pregnancy

Case History

Ruth has missed one period and suspects that she is pregnant. She tells you that she has been experiencing nausea and dry heaves in the morning and is extremely fatigued in the afternoon. She goes to bed early and is too tired to have sex with her husband. These changes are upsetting to Ruth, and she asks for help.

EXPECTED OUTCOMES	IMPLEMENTATION	RATIONALE	EVALUATION
Nursing Diagnosis: Altered nutrition, less than body requirements, related to nausea and dry heaves of early pregnancy			
Ruth will be free of nausea and dry heaves. Ruth will meet nutritional requirement and gain about 3 lb during the first trimester.	Discuss incidence, causes. Take a 24-hour diet history. Caution Ruth to avoid eating fried or greasy foods, or other offensive foods, especially before bedtime. Discuss eating small, frequent meals; avoid having an empty stomach. Advise Ruth to keep unsalted crackers (or other dry carbohydrate) at her bedside and to eat some on awakening, before getting out of bed. Advise her that if vomiting occurs and is severe, to call health care provider immediately.	Reassures that this is a common discomfort, can be treated, and is time limited. Establishes data base to identify foods that cause nausea. Removes potential causes. Food is essential to meet increased metabolic needs; it also helps to fend off fatigue. An empty stomach is associated with nausea. Increases ability to cope through self-care. Severe vomiting may indicate the complication of hyperemesis gravidarum (see Chapter 22).	Ruth verbalizes understanding of information. At next visit, Ruth reports occasional mild nausea but no dry heaves. Ruth gains 2.5 lb by the end of the first trimester.
Nursing Diagnosis: Fatigue related to early pregnancy and possibly to insufficient intake of calories			
Ruth will learn how to deal with the fatigue of early pregnancy. Ruth will be able to increase her activity level and resume activities of daily living without undue fatigue.	Discuss ways to deal with the fatigue of pregnancy: ▪ Adequate nutrition ▪ Rest periods while at work; nap after work, before supper ▪ Husband may be willing to prepare her favorite preferred foods and present them attractively Discuss resources to help with home maintenance. Reduce work hours for a few weeks.	Adequate nutrition is needed to meet increased metabolic demands and to prevent anemia. Participation in decision making has positive effect by lessening feeling of powerlessness. Increases ability to cope through self-care.	Ruth verbalizes understanding of information. At next visit, Ruth reports a lessening of fatigue and an increase in activity level. Her husband reports satisfaction with his ability to help out and contribute.

Continued.

PLAN OF CARE—con't.

First Trimester—Discomforts of Pregnancy

Nursing Diagnosis: Altered sexuality pattern related to discomforts of early pregnancy

Ruth will understand how physiology of pregnancy affects intercourse. Ruth will report satisfaction with sexual activities with her husband.	Ask appropriate questions and verbalize understanding and acceptance of information discussed. Discuss those symptoms Ruth is experiencing that affect foreplay and intercourse. Discuss sexuality and alternative sexual behaviors and positions that can be used during pregnancy.	Open discussion legitimizes this concern, which is shared by other pregnant couples. Open discussion demonstrates nurse's caring and ability to be a resource person. Alternative behaviors and positions are available for expression of sexuality. Presents possibility for enhancing couple's relationship and family coping.	Ruth verbalizes understanding of information. At the next visit, Ruth states that she and her husband had found mutually acceptable alternative behaviors and patterns. Ruth and her husband verbalize satisfaction with their sexual adaptation to pregnancy.

sure ≥15 mm Hg over baseline are also significant regardless of whether absolute values are less than 140/90. For example, if a woman's blood pressure normally is 105/60, a change to 120/75 must be viewed as potential for hypertension.

The *mean arterial pressure* (MAP) reaches its lowest point in the second trimester at about 22 weeks, then rises slowly to term (Page, Villee, Villee, 1981). A MAP of ≥90 in the second trimester is associated with an increase in the incidence of PIH in the third trimester.

Maternal anxiety can elevate blood pressure (BP) readings. If an elevated reading is found, the pregnant woman is given time to rest, and the reading is repeated.

The **roll-over test** is sometimes used as one predictor of a potential hypertensive problem in the third trimester. This test may be done at each visit after the twentieth week of gestation. The roll-over test can be done as follows (Fanaroff, Martin, 1992; Cunningham et al, 1993): position the woman on her side; determine the BP level in the upper arm once it is stable; roll her over onto her back, checking the pressure again; wait 5 minutes and check the BP level once again. An increase of 20 mm Hg in diastolic blood pressure from the side position to the back position indicates a *positive roll test*. The significance of a roll test is that, if negative, the chances are less than 1 in 100 that the pregnant woman will develop preeclampsia. If the test is positive, even though the BP level is within normal limits and the pregnant woman has no signs of fluid retention, full-blown PIH will develop at least 60% of the time. If the roll test is positive, it is imperative that home self-care measures be

instituted. The woman should spend more time in bed in the lateral recumbent position, stress in the home should be reduced, and her diet should be reviewed, and her BP should be monitored.

Laboratory Tests

Routine laboratory tests during the second trimester are limited. A clean-catch urine specimen is used to detect glucose, acetone, and albumin/protein. Glucose challenge is usually done between 24 and 28 weeks. Pregnant women may experience glycosuria. Urine for culture and sensitivity and blood samples are obtained only if signs and symptoms warrant. Hematocrit (HCT) or packed cell volume (PCV) may be done at each visit in some prenatal settings.

Fetal Assessment
Fundal Height

During the second trimester the uterus becomes an abdominal organ. Measurement of the height of the uterus above the symphysis pubis is used as one indicator of the progress of fetal growth. It also provides a gross estimate of the duration of pregnancy. Measurement of fundal height may aid in identification of high-risk factors: a stable or decreased fundal height may indicate intrauterine growth retardation; an excessive increase could mean multifetal gestation or hydramnios.

A paper tape measure or a pelvimeter may be used to measure **fundal height.** To increase measurement reliability, the same person can examine the pregnant woman at each of her prenatal visits, but often multiple

CLINICAL APPLICATION OF RESEARCH

EFFECTS OF MATERNAL POSITION ON FUNDAL HEIGHT MEASUREMENT

Fundal height measurements are useful in identifying many pregnancy complications involving errors in estimating gestational age, multiple gestation, and deviations from fetal growth. Engstrom et al. studied 192 women between 21 and 36 weeks' gestation. Fundal height measurements were taken with the women in four different positions—supine, trunk elevated, knees flexed, and both trunk elevated and knees flexed. All measurements were taken in the midline of the abdomen with a paper tape. The uterus was measured from the upper border of the symphysis pubis to the upper part of the fundus, with the tape in contact with the maternal abdomen during the measurement. The researchers found that measurements taken in the supine position were the largest and those taken with the trunk elevated and knees flexed were the smallest.

The researchers suggest that nurses and other clinicians should be consistent when they position pregnant women to measure fundal height. Nurses who are performing fundal height measurement during prenatal visits need to document the position the woman is in when the measurement is taken and what measurement technique is used.

Reference: Engstrom JL, Piscioneri LA, Low LK, et al: Fundal height measurement. Part 3. The effect of maternal position on fundal height measurement, *J Nurse Midwifery* 38(1):23, 1993.

clinicians see the woman for prenatal visits. All clinicians who examine pregnant women should be consistent in their measurement techniques. Ideally, a protocol is established for the health care setting that explicitly describes the measurement technique, including the woman's position on the examining table, the measuring device, and the method of measurement used. Conditions under which the measurements were taken can also be described, including whether the bladder was empty and whether the uterus was relaxed or contracted.

Various positions for fundal height measurement have been described in the literature. The woman can be supine, have her head elevated, have her knees flexed, or have both her head elevated and her knees flexed. Studies have shown that measurements are different in the various positions, making it even more important to standardize the fundal height measurement technique (see Clinical Application of Research).

Placement of the tape measure can also vary. The tape can be placed in the middle of the woman's abdomen and the measurement performed by measuring from the upper border of the symphysis pubis to the upper border of the fundus. The tape measure is held in contact with the skin for the entire length of the uterus (Fig. 7-7, *A*). Another measurement technique does not include the upper curve of the fundus in the measurement. One end of the tape measure is held at the upper border of the symphysis pubis with one hand; the other hand is placed at the upper border of the fundus. The tape is placed between the middle and index fingers and the measurement is taken at the point the hand intercepts the tape measure (Fig. 7-7, *B*) (Engstrom and Sittler, 1993).

McDonald's rule may be used by some examiners to add precision to the measurement of fundal height during the second and third trimesters. It is calculated as follows:

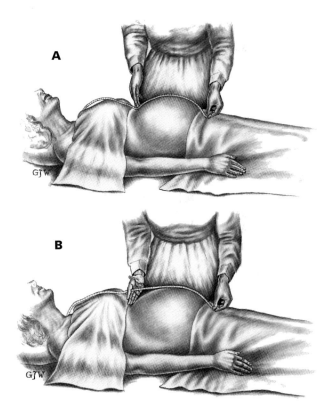

FIG. 7-7   A, Measurement of fundal height from symphysis that includes the upper curve of the fundus. **B,** Measurement of fundal height from the symphysis that does not include the upper curve of the fundus. Note position of hands and measuring tape.

Height of fundus (cm) $\times \frac{2}{7}$ (or $+ 3.5$) $=$
Duration of pregnancy in lunar months

Height of fundus (cm) $\times \frac{8}{7} =$
Duration of pregnancy in weeks

Gestational Age

In a normal pregnancy, fetal **gestational age** is estimated by determining the duration of pregnancy and estimated date of birth. Fetal gestational age is determined from the menstrual history, contraceptive history, pregnancy test, and clinical evaluation:

Menstrual history

First day of last normal menstrual period (LNMP): date, duration, amount

Last menstrual period (LMP): date, duration, amount

First day of previous menstrual period (before LMP) (PMP): date, duration, amount

Menarche: date, interval, duration

History of menstrual irregularity

Contraceptive history

Type of contraceptive

When stopped

Pregnancy test

Date

Type

Result

Clinical evaluation

First uterine size estimate: date, size

Fetal heart tone (FHT) first heard: Doptone, fetoscope

Date of quickening

Current fundal height, estimated fetal weight (EFW)

Current week of gestation

Ultrasound: date, week of gestation, biparietal diameter (BPD)

Reliability of dates

Health Status

Assessment of **fetal health status** includes consideration of fetal movement, fetal heart rate (FHR), and abnormal maternal or fetal symptoms.

The mother is instructed to note the extent and timing of fetal movements and to report immediately if the pattern changes or if movement ceases. Regular movement has been found to be a reliable determinant of fetal health (Cohen, 1985).

Fetal movement (quickening) is usually felt by the multigravida at approximately 16 weeks of pregnancy. The primigravida may not be able to identify the fluttering she is feeling as fetal movement until about 20 weeks.

The FHR is checked on routine visits once it has been heard (12 weeks by Doppler device; 18 to 20 weeks by fetoscope). Early in this trimester the FHR may be heard with the ultrasound stethoscope (Fig. 7-8, *B*) or the ultrasound fetoscope. Before the fetus can be palpated by Leopold's maneuvers, the scope is moved around the abdomen until the FHR is heard. Each nurse develops a set pattern for searching the abdomen, for example, starting first in the midline about 2 to 3 cm (1 in) above the symphysis followed by the left lower quadrant, and so on. The FHR is counted and the quality and rhythm noted (see Chapter 11). Later in the second trimester the FHR can be determined with the fetoscope or ultrasound stethoscope (Fig. 7-8, *A* to *C*). Normal rate and rhythm are other good indicators of fetal health. Absence of FHR, once noted, requires immediate investigation.

In some centers ultrasonography is used with all pregnancies, and a more exact estimation of gestational age can be made. Ultrasonography may be used to establish the duration of pregnancy if the woman is unable to give a precise date for her LMP or if the size of the uterus does not conform to the stated date of the LMP. Ultrasonography is not, however, a universally recommended procedure.

The second trimester is a period of rapid growth. Box 7-5 summarizes fetal development.

Intensive investigation of fetal health status is initiated if any maternal or fetal complications arise (e.g., maternal hypertension, growth lag, premature rupture of

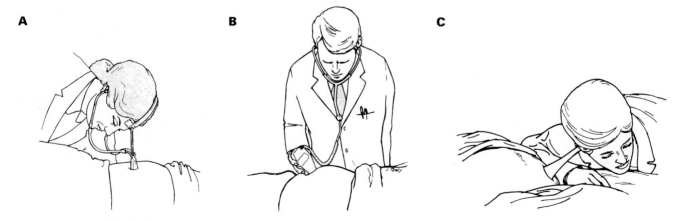

FIG. 7-8 Detecting fetal heartbeat. **A,** Fetoscope (18 to 20 weeks). **B,** Doppler ultrasound stethoscope (12 weeks). **C,** Pinard's stethoscope. *NOTE:* Hands should not touch stethoscope while nurse is listening.

membranes, or irregular or absent FHR). (See second and third trimester signs of potential complications below.)

✤ NURSING DIAGNOSES

Each individual is affected differently by pregnancy. Careful monitoring of the pregnancy and responses to care is of utmost importance. It is particularly difficult to distinguish discomforts of the second and third trimesters. Multiparous women tend to demonstrate some discomforts in pregnancy earlier than nulliparous women do. Continuous assessment, analysis, and formulation of diagnoses is imperative. The following are only a few examples of nursing diagnoses that can emerge from the data base.

Body image disturbance related to
- Anatomic and physiologic changes of pregnancy

Alteration in health maintenance related to knowledge deficit regarding self-care measures
- Rest and relaxation
- Personal hygiene (increased sweating, oily skin, leukorrhea)

Pain related to
- Discomforts of pregnancy

High risk for injury related to
- Nonuse of safety harness and head rest in automobiles
- Exposure to harmful chemicals

Altered family processes related to
- Lack of understanding of second trimester changes
- Changing sexual relationship or marital support

Anxiety related to
- Discomforts of pregnancy
- Changing family dynamics
- Fetal well-being

BOX 7-5

Fetal Development at 26 Weeks

Viable at week 24*
Fetal movements obvious
FHR readily heard
Scalp hair, eyebrows, eyelashes, fine downy lanugo and vernix cover the skin
Eyelids still fused
Skin is red, shiny, and thin
Face is wrinkled, giving an old man appearance
Length is 30 cm (12 in)
Weight is 600 g (1¼ lb)
Uterus at or just above level of umbilicus

*In Canada, viability is defined as 20 weeks' gestation and 500 g in weight.

✤ EXPECTED OUTCOMES

Planning care for patients during the second trimester of pregnancy is given direction from the nursing diagnoses. A plan is developed mutually with each patient to the extent possible. The plan is individualized, relating specifically to her needs. The information in this chapter is general; not all women experience all problems discussed or require all facets of care described.

Because of the high demand in most areas for prepared childbirth classes in the third trimester, it is recommended that those clients who are planning to attend these classes enroll early in the second trimester.

The nurse continues to foster the growing relation-

 SIGNS OF POTENTIAL COMPLICATIONS

SECOND AND THIRD TRIMESTERS

SIGN/SYMPTOM	POSSIBLE CAUSES
Persistent, severe vomiting	Hyperemesis gravidarum
Amniotic fluid discharge from vagina	Premature rupture of membranes (PROM)
Vaginal bleeding, severe abdominal pain	Miscarriage, placental separation
Chills, fever, burning on urination, diarrhea	Infection
Change in fetal movements: absence of fetal movements after quickening, any unusual change in pattern or amount	Fetal jeopardy or intrauterine fetal death
Uterine contractions	Preterm labor
Visual disturbances: blurring, double vision, or spots	Hypertensive conditions, PIH
Swelling of face or fingers and over sacrum	Hypertensive conditions, PIH
Headaches: severe, frequent, or continuous	Hypertensive conditions, PIH
Muscular irritability or convulsions	Hypertensive conditions, PIH
Epigastric pain (perceived as severe stomachache)	Hypertensive conditions, PIH
Glucosuria, positive glucose tolerance test reaction	Gestational diabetes mellitus

ship between care provider and patient. Expected outcomes are the same as those for the mother, fetus, and family given for the first trimester (p. 135).

✥ COLLABORATIVE CARE

The supportive and therapeutic nurse-patient relationship grows as the nurse implements the nursing process during the second trimester. The nausea often experienced in the first trimester has resolved. Nutrition counseling is offered at each visit, and the woman is complimented on her progress, as appropriate.

Education for Self-Care

Women experience several new discomforts or changes as maternal adaptations continue in the second trimester. Clear separation of discomforts and changes by trimester is impossible (Tables 7-2 and 7-3).

Counseling about sexuality and exposure to alcohol, cigarette smoke, and other substances is provided as necessary. It must be remembered that, although the consumption of three alcoholic drinks a day during the first trimester is associated with spontaneous abortion, as few as two drinks a day are associated with miscarriage during the second trimester (Cook, 1990).

Women who are prepared for the possibility of experiencing emotional changes are more likely to feel reassured that they are not unusual or unnatural and that it is acceptable to talk about their reactions. As pregnancy progresses, women become more open about their feelings toward themselves and others. Active listening by the nurse can help reassure women. If psychologic disturbance is severe, referral for appropriate treatment may be necessary.

Clothing

Comfortable loose clothing is best. Washable fabrics (e.g., cottons) are often preferred. Since maternity clothes are expensive and rarely wear out, hand-me-downs or used clothes from garage sales can suffice. Tight brassieres and belts, stretch pants, garters, tight-top knee socks, panty girdles, and other constrictive clothing should be avoided. Tight clothing over the perineum encourages vaginitis and miliaria (heat rash). Impaired circulation in the lower extremities favors varices.

Maternity brassieres are constructed to accommodate the increased breast weight, chest circumference, and size of breast tail tissue (under the arm). These brassieres have drop flaps over the nipples to facilitate breastfeeding. A good brassiere can help prevent neckache and backache.

Support hose may give considerable comfort to women with large varicose veins or swelling of the legs. Comfortable shoes that provide firm support and promote good posture and balance are advisable. Very high

heels and platform shoes are not recommended because of the woman's changed center of gravity. She tends to lose her balance. In the third trimester her pelvis tilts forward and her lumbar curve increases. Leg aches and leg cramps are aggravated by nonsupportive shoes.

Posture and Body Mechanics

Many maternal adaptations predispose the woman to backache and possible injury. The pregnant woman's center of gravity changes (Fig. 7-9). Pelvic joints soften and relax; stress is placed on abdominal musculature (see Figs. 5-10 and 5-11). Poor posture and body mechanics contribute to discomfort and potential for injury.

Women can acquire a kinesthetic sense for good body posture. In addition to fostering good posture, the activities in the Teaching Approaches box on p. 155 can be used.

Bathing and Swimming

Tub bathing is permitted even in late pregnancy, because water does not enter the vagina unless under pressure. However, tub bathing is contraindicated after rupture of the membranes. Baths and warm showers can be therapeutic because they relax tense tired muscles, help counter insomnia, and make the pregnant woman feel fresh. Physical maneuverability presents a problem (increased chance of falling) late in pregnancy due to the altered center of gravity. Swimming is also permitted during normal pregnancy, although diving is discouraged because of possible traumatic injury.

Physical Activity

Physical activity promotes a feeling of well-being in the pregnant woman. It improves circulation, assists relaxation and rest, and counteracts boredom as it does in the nonpregnant woman. Exercise tips for pregnancy are presented in detail in the Home Care box on p. 141. Suggestions for patient teaching of Kegel's exercises to strengthen the muscles around the reproductive organs and improve muscle tone are found on p. 137.

Rest and Relaxation

The pregnant woman is encouraged to plan regular rest periods particularly as pregnancy advances (Fig. 7-10). The side-lying position is recommended to promote uterine perfusion and fetoplacental oxygenation by eliminating pressure on the ascending vena cava (supine hypotension). During shorter rest periods the woman can assume the position in Fig. 7-12 to promote venous drainage from the legs and relieve leg edema and varicose veins. The mother is shown how to rise slowly from a side-lying position to avoid strain on the back and minimize the hypotension caused by changes in position common in the latter part of pregnancy. To stretch and rest back muscles at home or at work, the nurse can instruct the woman to do the following:

TABLE 7-3 Discomforts Related to Maternal Adaptations to Pregnancy

DISCOMFORT	PHYSIOLOGY	EDUCATION FOR SELF-CARE
Pigmentation deepens, acne, oily skin	Melanocyte-stimulating hormone (from anterior pituitary)	Not preventable; usually resolved during puerperium; reassurance given to women and their families
Spider nevi (telangiectasias) appear during trimesters 2 or 3 over neck, thorax, face, and arms	Focal networks of dilated arterioles (end arteries) from increased concentration of estrogens	Not preventable; reassurance that they fade slowly during late puerperium; rarely disappear completely
Palmar erythema occurs in 50% of pregnant women; may accompany spider nevi	Diffuse reddish mottling over palms and suffused skin over thenar eminences and fingertips may be caused by genetic predisposition or hyperestrogenism	Not preventable; reassurance that condition will fade within 1 week after giving birth
Pruritus (noninflammatory)	Unknown cause; various types as follows: Nonpapular; closely aggregated pruritic papules Increased excretory function of skin and stretching of skin possible factors	Keep fingernails short and clean; refer to health care provider for diagnosis of cause Not preventable; symptomatic: Keri baths; mild sedation Distraction; tepid baths with sodium bicarbonate or oatmeal added to water; lotions and oils; change of soaps or reduction in use of soap; loose clothing
Palpitations	Unknown; should not be accompanied by persistent cardiac irregularity	Not preventable; reassurance; refer to health care provider if accompanied by symptoms of cardiac decompensation
Supine hypotension (vena cava syndrome) and bradycardia	Posture induced by pressure of gravid uterus on ascending vena cava when woman is supine; reduces uterine-placental and renal perfusion	Side-lying position or semisitting posture, with knees slightly flexed (see supine hypotension, p. 131)
Faintness and, rarely, syncope (orthostatic hypotension) may persist throughout pregnancy	Vasomotor lability or postural hypotension from hormones; in late pregnancy may be caused by venous stasis in lower extremities	Moderate exercise, deep breathing, vigorous leg movement; avoid sudden changes in position* and warm crowded areas; move slowly and deliberately; keep environment cool; avoid hypoglycemia by eating 5 to 6 small meals per day; elastic hose; sit as necessary; if symptoms are serious, refer to health care provider
Food cravings	Cause unknown; cravings determined by culture or geographic area	Not preventable; satisfy craving unless it interferes with well-balanced diet; report unusual cravings to health care provider
Heartburn (pyrosis, or acid indigestion): burning sensation in lower chest or upper abdomen, occasionally with burping and regurgitation of a little sour-tasting fluid	Progesterone slows GI tract motility and digestion, reverses peristalsis, relaxes cardiac sphincter, and delays emptying time of stomach; stomach displaced upward and compressed by enlarging uterus	Limit or avoid gas-producing or fatty foods and large meals; maintain good posture; sips of milk for temporary relief; hot tea, chewing gum; health care provider may prescribe antacid between meals, refer to health care provider for persistent symptoms

*Caution woman to rise slowly and sit on edge of bed or to assume hands-and-knees posture before rising, and to get up slowly after sitting or squatting.

Continued.

TABLE 7-3 Discomforts Related to Maternal Adaptations to Pregnancy—cont'd

DISCOMFORT	PHYSIOLOGY	EDUCATION FOR SELF-CARE
Constipation	GI tract motility slowed because of progesterone, resulting in increased resorption of water and drying of stool; intestines compressed by enlarging uterus; predisposition to constipation because of oral iron supplementation	Six glasses of water per day; roughage in diet; moderate exercise; regular schedule for bowel movements; use relaxation techniques and deep breathing; *do not* take stool softener, laxatives, mineral oil, other drugs, or enemas without first consulting health care provider
Flatulence with bloating and belching	Reduced GI motility because of hormones, allowing time for bacterial action that produces gas; swallowing air	Chew foods slowly and thoroughly; avoid gas-producing foods, fatty foods, large meals; exercise; maintain regular bowel habits
Varicose veins: may be associated with aching legs and tenderness; may be present in legs and vulva; hemorrhoids are varicosities in the perianal area (Fig. 7-11)	Hereditary predisposition; relaxation of smooth muscle walls of veins because of hormones, causing pelvic vasocongestion; condition aggravated by enlarging uterus, gravity, and bearing down for bowel movements; thrombi from leg varices rare but may be produced by hemorrhoids	Avoidance of obesity, lengthy standing or sitting, constrictive clothing, and constipation and bearing down with bowel movements; moderate exercises; rest with legs and hips elevated (Fig. 7-12), support stockings; thrombosed hemorrhoid may be evacuated; relieve swelling and pain with warm sitz baths, local application of astringent compresses
Leukorrhea: often noted throughout pregnancy	Hormonally stimulated cervix becomes hypertrophic and hyperactive, producing abundant amount of mucus	Not preventable; *do not douche;* hygiene; perineal pads; reassurance; refer to health care provider if accompanied by pruritus, foul odor, or change in character or color
Headaches (through week 26)	Emotional tension (more common than vascular migraine headache); eye strain (refractory errors); vascular engorgement and congestion of sinuses from hormone stimulation	Emotional support; prenatal teaching; conscious relaxation; refer to health care provider for constant "splitting" headache, after assessing for PIH
Carpal tunnel syndrome (involves thumb, second and third fingers, lateral side of little finger)	Compression of median nerve from changes in surrounding tissues: pain, numbness, tingling, burning; loss of skilled movements (typing); dropping of objects	Not preventable; elevation of affected arms, splinting of affected hand may help; surgery is curative
Periodic numbness, tingling of fingers (acrodysesthesia) occurs in 5% of pregnant women	Brachial plexus traction syndrome from drooping of shoulders during pregnancy (occurs especially at night and early morning)	Maintain good posture; wear supportive maternity brassiere; reassurance that condition will disappear if lifting and carrying baby does not aggravate it
Round ligament pain (tenderness)	Stretching of ligament caused by enlarging uterus	Not preventable; reassurance, rest, good body mechanics to avoid overstretching ligament; relieve cramping by squatting or bringing knees to chest
Joint pain, backache, and pelvic pressure; hypermobility of joints	Relaxation of symphyseal and sacroiliac joints because of hormones, resulting in unstable pelvis; exaggerated lumbar and cervicothoracic curves caused by change in center of gravity from enlarging abdomen	Good posture and body mechanics; avoid fatigue; wear low-heeled shoes; conscious relaxation; firm mattress; local heat or ice and back rubs; pelvic rock exercise; rest; reassure that condition will disappear 6 to 8 weeks after birth

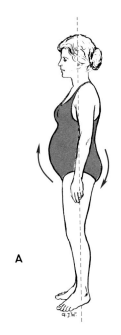

A

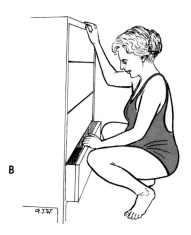

B

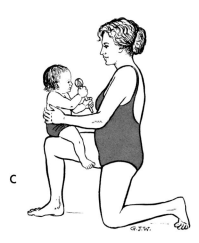

C

FIG. 7-9 Correct body mechanics. **A,** Standing. **B,** Stooping, **C,** Lifting.

 TEACHING APPROACHES

POSTURE AND BODY MECHANICS

To prevent or relieve backache
- Do pelvic tilt:
  —**Pelvic tilt (rock)** on hands and knees, and while sitting in straight-back chair (Fig. 7-6, *A*).
  —Pelvic tilt (rock) in standing position against a wall or lying on floor (Fig. 7-6, *B* and *C*).
  —Perform abdominal muscle contractions during pelvic tilt while standing, lying, or sitting to help strengthen rectus abdominis muscle (Fig. 7-6, *D*).
- Use good body mechanics:
  —Use leg muscles to reach objects on or near floor. Bend at the knees, not the back. Knees are bent to lower body to squatting position. Feet are kept 12 to 18 inches apart for a solid base to maintain balance (Fig. 7-6, *B*).
  —Lift with the legs. To lift heavy object (young child), one foot is placed slightly in front of the other and kept flat as woman lowers herself on one knee. She lifts the weight holding it close to her body and never higher than chest high. To stand up or sit down, one leg is placed slightly behind the other as she raises or lowers herself.

To restrict the lumbar curve:
- Wear a maternity girdle to support weak abdominal muscles.
- For prolonged standing (e.g., ironing, out-of-home employment), place one foot on low footstool or box: change positions often.
- Move car seat forward so that knees are bent and higher than hips. If needed, use a small pillow to support low back area.
- Sit in chairs low enough to allow both feet on floor and preferably with knees higher than hips.

To prevent round ligament pain and strain on abdominal muscles
- Implement suggestions given in Table 7-3.

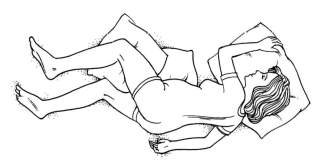

FIG. 7-10 Side-lying position for rest and relaxation. Some women prefer to support upper leg with pillows.

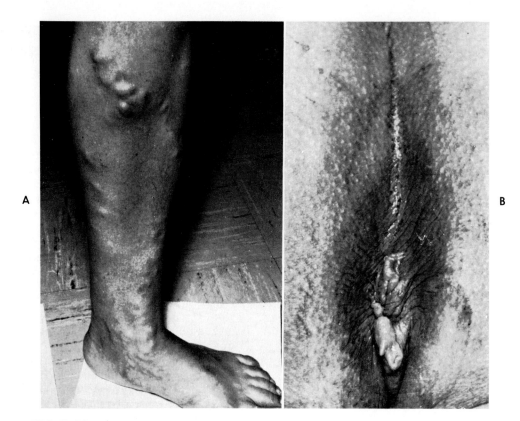

FIG. 7-11 **A,** Varicose veins of lower extremity. **B,** Varicosities of rectal area (hemorrhoids). (Courtesy Mercy Hospital and Medical Center, San Diego, CA.)

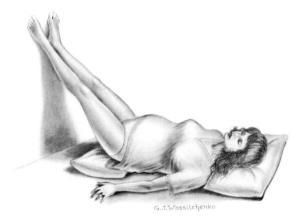

FIG. 7-12 Position for resting legs and for reducing swelling, edema, and varicosities. Encourage woman with vulvar varicosities to include pillow under her hips.

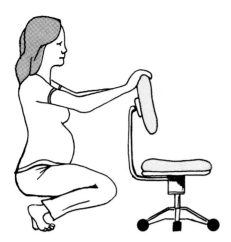

FIG. 7-13 Squatting for muscle relaxation and strengthening and for keeping leg and hip joints flexible.

Stand behind a chair. Support and balance self using the back of the chair (Fig. 7-13). Squat for 30 seconds; stand for 15 seconds. Repeat six times, several times per day, as needed.

While sitting in chair, lower head to knees for 30 seconds. Raise up. Repeat six times, several times per day, as needed.

Relaxation is the release of the mind and body from tension through conscious effort and practice. The ability to relax consciously and intentionally can be beneficial for the following reasons:

- Relief of normal discomforts related to pregnancy
- Reduction of stress and therefore diminished pain perception during the childbearing cycle
- Heightened self-awareness and trust in own ability to control one's responses and functions
- Coping with stress in everyday life situations, pregnant or not

The techniques for **conscious relaxation** are numerous and varied. The guidelines in the Teaching Approaches box can be used by anyone.

Preparation for Feeding the Newborn

Pregnant women are usually eager to discuss their plans for feeding the newborn. Breast milk is the food of choice, and breastfeeding is associated with a decreased incidence in perinatal morbidity and mortality. However, immaturity of the infant, deep-seated aversion to breastfeeding by mother or father, and certain medical complications, such as pulmonary tuberculosis, are contraindications to breastfeeding. The woman and her partner are encouraged to decide which method of feeding is suitable for them. Once the couple has been given information about the advantages and disadvantages of bottle-feeding and breastfeeding, they are in a position to make an informed choice. Nurses need only support their decisions.

Most women are motivated by the sixth or seventh

TEACHING APPROACHES

CONSCIOUS RELAXATION

Preparation: Loosen clothing, assume a comfortable sitting or side-lying position with all parts of body well-supported with pillows.

Beginning: Allow self to feel warm and comfortable. Inhale and exhale slowly, and imagine peaceful relaxation coming over each part of the body starting with the neck and working down to the toes. Often persons who learn conscious relaxation speak of feeling relaxed even if some discomfort is present.

Maintenance: Imagine (fantasize or daydream) to maintain the state of relaxation. With *active imagery* the person imagines herself moving or doing some activity and experiencing its sensations. With *passive imagery* one imagines watching a scene, such as a lovely sunset.

Awakening: Return to the wakeful state gradually. Slowly begin to take in the stimuli from the surrounding environment.

Further retention and development of the skill: Practice regularly for some periods of time each day, for example, at the same hour for 10 to 15 minutes each day to feel refreshed, revitalized, and invigorated.

---

month of pregnancy to learn about breast preparation and breastfeeding. The **pinch test** determines whether the nipple is erectile or retractile (Fig. 7-14). The nurse guides the woman through the pinch test. The woman places her thumb and forefinger on her areola and presses inward gently. This will cause her nipple to stand erect or to retract (invert). Most nipples will stand erect. Inverted nipples need more preparation time. Nipple preparation for these women can start during the last 2 months of pregnancy.

The woman learns that nipples are cleansed with warm water to prevent blocking of the ducts with dried colostrum. Soap is not used because it removes protective oils that keep nipples supple.

Some women obtain **nipple cups** designed specifically for correcting inverted nipples. Plastic doughnut-shaped cups are available for correcting inversions or retractions (Fig. 7-15). A continuous, gentle pressure exerted around the areola pushes the nipple through a central opening in the inner shield. Nipple cups should be worn during the last two months of pregnancy for 1 to 2 hours daily. The time for wearing them should be increased gradually. Brand names for these cups include Woolwich, Netsy, La Leche League Cups, Nurse-Dri, Free and Dry, and Hobbit Shields. These cups can also be worn after childbirth. However, because body warmth can foster

PLAN OF CARE

Second Trimester: Teaching about Warning Signs

Case History
Ruth has been regularly attending clinic. She is now 18 weeks pregnant. She states that she thinks she felt the baby move. She expresses concern that she does not know how to tell if something is wrong.

EXPECTED OUTCOMES	IMPLEMENTATION	RATIONALE	EVALUATION

Nursing Diagnosis: Knowledge deficit related to signs and symptoms of potential warning to self and fetus.

Ruth will verbalize knowledge about warning signs. Ruth calls promptly if any warning signs evolve.	Discuss warning signs with Ruth. Provide a written list of warning signs and symptoms. Include emergency phone number (e.g., prenatal clinic, hospital).	Medical conditions compromising Ruth or her fetus must be identified and treated promptly. The woman is often the first one to notice that something is wrong. Written material reinforces learning and gives the woman the opportunity to review information.	Ruth lists warning signs that should be reported. Ruth states she has taped the emergency number by her phone and will call if a warning sign appears.

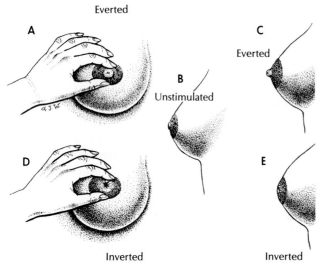

FIG. 7-14 Pinch Test. **A** and **C,** When stimulated, nipples evert (protract or become erect). **B,** Unstimulated, nipples look the same. **D** and **E,** When stimulated, nipples invert (retract).

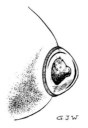

FIG. 7-15 Nipple cup in place.

rapid bacterial growth and contamination, milk that collects in the cup should be discarded and not fed to the infant.

Breast stimulation may produce uterine activity and should be avoided in women at risk for preterm labor if contractions are noted (Iams, Johnson, Creasy, 1988).

✦ EVALUATION

Maternal and fetal expected outcomes are continuously evaluated according to measurable, established criteria. The clinical findings that represent normal response are presented as plans/expected outcomes in the nursing care plans for each patient. These criteria are used as a basis for selecting appropriate nursing actions and evaluating their effectiveness.

THIRD TRIMESTER

The quiet period of the second trimester gives way to an active period, a trimester more oriented in reality for the expectant parents. Parental attachment to the fetus grows in the third trimester. Mixed among the daydreams about the coming baby are parental anxieties that focus on possible defects in mental and physical abilities of the child. The expectant mother's attention turns to thoughts of a safe passage for herself and her child. Fears of pain and mutilation and concerns about her behavior and possible loss of control during labor are important issues.

Physical discomforts and fetal movements often interrupt the expectant mother's rest. Dyspnea, return of urinary frequency, backache, constipation, and varicosities are experienced by most women in late pregnancy. Increased bulkiness and awkwardness affect the ability to perform activities of daily living. Positions of comfort are more difficult to achieve. Increasingly, the pregnant woman becomes more impatient to "get this over with."

For the expectant father the moratorium phase of the second trimester passes into the focusing phase (in Chapter 6 on p. 115). Activity and energy to create and achieve characterize this phase. Styles of involvement differ according to the man's perception of the male and fathering roles within his social group. Many expectant fathers become more involved with the pregnancy. They begin to redefine their relationship to the fetus and themselves as fathers. Role playing through daydreaming is common. The expectant father feels some of the same concerns as the expectant mother. Often, however, he does not share these concerns with anyone.

Expectant families approaching childbirth have many needs. Siblings and grandparents must be considered, too. Clearly the nurse is in a pivotal position within the team of health care providers to assist parents with these needs during the third trimester of pregnancy. The schedule of care reflects the increased need. Starting with week 28, visits are scheduled every 2 weeks until week 36, and then every week until birth.

Care Management

✤ ASSESSMENT

During the third trimester current family occurrences and their effect on the mother are assessed, for example, siblings' and grandparents' responses to the pregnancy and the coming child. In addition, the following questions are addressed:

- What anticipatory planning is in progress concerning new parenting responsibilities, sibling rivalry, recuperation from pregnancy and birth, and fertility management?
- What successes or frustrations is the mother experiencing with diet, rest and relaxation, sexuality, and emotional support?
- What is the mother's understanding of her family's needs in relation to the pregnancy and child?
- How well prepared are the parents in the event of emergency? That is, does the mother know and understand warning signs and how and to whom to report them?
- Does the mother know the signs of preterm and term labor?
- What is the mother's understanding of the labor process, expectations of herself and others during la-

---

BOX 7-6

Third Trimester Checklist

Schedule and events of visits
Counseling for self-care
  Adaptations/discomforts
    Dyspnea
    Insomnia
    Psychosocial responses and family dynamics
    Gingivitis and epulis
    Urinary frequency
    Perineal discomfort and pressure
    Braxton Hicks contractions
    Leg cramps
    Ankle edema
  Safety (balance)
  Exercise and rest
  Relaxation
  Nutrition
  Sexuality
  Warning signs of potential complications
  Warning signs—preterm labor
Fetal growth and development
Preparation for baby
  Feeding method
  Nipple preparation
Preparation for labor
  Recognition: false vs. true
  Prenatal classes
  Control of discomfort
  Hospital tour
  Provision for other family members
  Preparation for homecoming
Diagnostic tests
  Specify
Other

---

bor, and what to bring to the hospital?
- What plans have the mother and her family made for labor?
- What anxieties is the mother or her family experiencing regarding labor or child?
- What does the mother wish to know about control of discomfort during labor?
- Is the mother planning to attend any prebirth classes?
- Does the mother have questions about fetal development and methods to assess fetal well-being?

A checklist for third trimester assessment should be used to ensure that important areas are addressed (Box 7-6).

Maternal Assessment
Interview

The initial question in the third trimester interview is asked with the intent to identify the pregnant woman's main concern for the moment. Focusing on the woman takes advantage of her readiness to learn and affirms the caregiver's interest in her as a person. Based on the patient's expressed needs, her status to date, and generally accepted needs of most women in late pregnancy, the nurse's clinical judgment guides the content and direction of the interview.

A review of physical systems is appropriate at each meeting. Any suspicious signs or symptoms are assessed in depth. Discomforts reflecting pregnancy adaptations are identified. Special inquiries are made about possible infections (e.g., genitourinary tract, respiratory tract). Knowledge of and success with self-care measures and prescribed therapy are assessed. Psychosocial responses to the pregnancy and approaching parenthood are assessed.

Physical Examination

During the third trimester physical examination, temperature, pulse, respirations, blood pressure, and weight are assessed and noted. Suspicious signs and symptoms uncovered during the interview are assessed. Presence, location, and degree of edema are documented carefully. Gestational age is confirmed. In some clinics weekly pelvic examinations are begun at weeks 36 to 38 and are continued until term, primarily to confirm presenting part, corroborate station, and determine cervical dilatation and effacement. Risk assessment continues throughout pregnancy (see Signs of Potential Complications in second and third trimester on p. 151).

Laboratory Tests

At each visit urine is tested for glucose and albumin protein. A urine culture and sensitivity test is done as necessary. Hematocrit determination by finger stick is made at each visit in some facilities. Blood tests are repeated as necessary: test for syphilis; complete blood count (CBC) with hematocrit, hemoglobin, and differential values; antibody screen (Kell, Duffy, rubella, toxoplasmosis, anti-Rh, AIDS); sickle cell; and level of folacin when indicated. If not done earlier in pregnancy, a glucose challenge for women over 25 years of age is performed. Cervical and vaginal smears are repeated at 32 weeks or as necessary for *Chlamydia* organisms, gonorrhea, herpes simplex types 1 and 2, and group B streptococcus.

Fetal Assessment

Beginning at the thirty-second week, identification of fetal presentation, position, and station (engagement), with the aid of Leopold's maneuvers, is done weekly. This period of rapid fetal growth is summarized in Box 7-7.

Fundal height is measured at each visit. The method described on p. 148 is used. Uterine measurements and size (weight) of fetus are compared with supposed duration of pregnancy. Although some clinicians can estimate fetal weight with unbelievable accuracy, estimations are generally inconsistent and unreliable. Accuracy in esti-

---

BOX 7-7

Fetal Development at 40 Weeks

Nutrients and maternal immunoglobulins stored
Subcutaneous fat deposited
Dramatic storage of iron, nitrogen, and calcium
In male: testes are within well-wrinkled scrotum
In female: labia are well developed and cover vestibule
Lanugo shed, except for shoulders, generally
Body contours plump
Decreased vernix
Scalp hair 2 to 3 cm (1 in) long
Cartilage in nose and ears well developed
45 to 55 cm (18 to 22 in) in length
Weighs 3400 g (7½ lb) (average)
Fundal height below xiphoid after lightening

---

mating fetal weight improves with ultrasound determination of biparietal diameter (BPD). Possible growth retardation of fetus, multifetal pregnancy, and inaccuracy of EDB may be disclosed by ultrasound.

Fetal health status is evaluated at each visit. The mother is requested to describe fetal movements. She is asked if she has signs of potential complications (see p. 151) to report, for example, change in fetal movements, rupture of membranes.

❖ NURSING DIAGNOSES

Each pregnant woman and her family respond to and are affected by pregnancy in different ways. Careful monitoring of the pregnancy and responses to care is of the utmost importance. The following are representative of nursing diagnoses that can be formulated in the third trimester from the data base of a normal pregnancy.

Impaired individual coping related to knowledge deficit regarding
- Assessment for risks such as preterm labor
- Recognizing onset of true vs. false labor
- Self-care measures
- Emergency arrangements

Altered family processes related to
- Inadequate understanding of third trimester changes and needs
- Increased concern about labor
- Insomnia or sleep deficit

Sleep pattern disturbance related to
- Discomforts of late pregnancy
- Anxiety about approaching labor

Activity intolerance related to
- Increased weight and change in center of gravity
- Anxiety
- Sleep disturbances

✤ EXPECTED OUTCOMES

Planning care for patients and their families during the third trimester of pregnancy is given direction from identified nursing diagnoses and from a comprehensive view of the expectant family. A plan is developed mutually with the patient to the extent possible. The plan is individualized, relating specifically to the patient's needs and the needs of her family. Expected outcomes are similar to those of the first and second trimesters.

Expected outcomes related to physiologic care include the following:

1. Woman and her family will say they have pertinent information about maternal adaptations and fetal development as a basis for understanding the management of care during the third trimester.
2. Woman will demonstrate knowledge for self-care.
3. Woman will recognize symptoms that indicate deviations from normal progress and knows protocols for reporting them.

Expected outcomes related to psychosocial care include the following:

1. Woman will say she has learning needs.
2. Women and their families will be active participants in their care during the third trimester of pregnancy.
3. Woman will finalize the birth plan.
4. Woman's trusting relationship will continue to progress.

✤ COLLABORATIVE CARE

Esteem, affection, trust, concern, consideration of cultural and religious responses, and listening are components of emotional support. The woman's feelings of satisfaction with her relationships and support and of competence and sense of being in control are important issues to address in the third trimester. A discussion of parental awareness of the unborn child's responses to stimuli, such as sound, light, maternal posture or tension, and patterns of sleeping and waking can be helpful. Opportunities are also provided to discuss probable emotional tensions related to the following: childbirth experience such as fear of pain, loss of control, and possible birth of the child before reaching the hospital; responsibilities and tasks of parenthood; mutual parental concerns arising from anxiety for the safety of the mother and unborn child; mutual parental concerns related to siblings and their acceptance of the new baby; mutual parental concerns about social and economic responsibilities; and mutual parental concerns for cognitive dissonance arising from conflicts in cultural, religious, or personal value systems (Starn, 1991).

The father's commitment to the pregnancy, the couple's relationship, and their concerns about sexuality and sexual expression emerge as concerns for many expectant parents. An important support measure is to validate normalcy of their responses (if they fall within normal limits). Validation, feedback, and social comparison characterize appraisal support.

Providing opportunity to discuss concerns, providing a listening ear, and validating the normalcy of responses will meet the woman's needs to varying degrees. Nurses also need to implement specific "interventions targeted at improving expectant parents' partner support satisfaction, because this support constitutes the majority of their total support" (Brown, 1986).

Nurses need to recognize the increased vulnerability of men during pregnancy and implement anticipatory guidance and health promotion strategies to help them with their concerns. Nursing intervention may directly help fathers with concerns such as the need to share intimate feelings or may do so indirectly by education of mothers. Health care providers can stimulate and encourage open dialogue between the couple.

Education for Self-Care

Not only are some new discomforts seen in the third trimester, but also others seen previously in the first trimester (e.g., fatigue) recur. Women who are pregnant later in life may experience an aggravation of varicose veins or severe backache from postural changes associated with a heavy, pendulous abdomen and relaxed joints. Such symptoms are frightening and uncomfortable.

In Table 7-4 the physiology, prevention, and treatment of several discomforts are discussed. Relaxation, exercises, body mechanics, safety, and employment issues are described and discussed earlier in this chapter.

Review of Warning Signs

The nurse needs to answer questions honestly as they arise during pregnancy. It is often difficult for the pregnant woman to know when to report signs and symptoms. The mother is encouraged to refer to a printed list of potential complications (p. 151) and to listen to her body. If she senses that something is wrong, she should call her care provider. Several signs and symptoms need to be discussed more extensively. These include vaginal bleeding, alteration in fetal movements, symptoms of PIH, rupture of membranes, and preterm labor.

If *vaginal bleeding* occurs in the third trimester, it is important to rule out brownish spotting occurring 48 hours after vaginal examination or after intercourse and to rule out "show" of pinkish mucus. The woman is to come to the hospital's emergency area immediately for diagnosis and treatment if bleeding is other than one of the preceding types.

Should the pregnant woman notice cessation, noticeable diminution, or acceleration in the amount of *fetal movement,* she is to notify her health care provider.

Appearance of *edema* of the hands and around the eyes, severe *headaches, visual changes,* or feelings of *jitteriness* require immediate evaluation for PIH.

A gush or trickle of clear *watery discharge* that appears

TABLE 7-4 Discomforts Related to Maternal Adaptations During the Third Trimester

PROBLEM	PHYSIOLOGY	EDUCATION FOR SELF-CARE
Shortness of breath and dyspnea occur in 60% of pregnant women	Expansion of diaphragm limited by enlarging uterus; diaphragm is elevated about 4 cm (1½ in); some relief after lightening	Good posture; sleep with extra pillows; avoid overloading stomach; stop smoking; refer to health care provider if symptoms worsen to rule out anemia, emphysema, and asthma
Insomnia (later weeks of pregnancy)	Fetal movements, muscular cramping, urinary frequency, shortness of breath, or other discomforts	Reassurance; conscious relaxation; back massage or **effleurage** (Fig. 7-16); support of body parts with pillows; warm milk or warm shower before retiring
Psychosocial responses (Chapter 6): mood swings, mixed feelings, increased anxiety	Hormonal and metabolic adaptations; feelings about impending labor, birth, and parenthood	Reassurance and support from significant other and nurse; improved communication with partner, family, and others
Gingivitis and epulis (hyperemia, hypertrophy, bleeding, tenderness): condition will disappear spontaneously 1 to 2 months after birth	Increased vascularity and proliferation of connective tissue from estrogen stimulation	Well-balanced diet with adequate protein and fresh fruits and vegetables; gentle brushing and good dental hygiene; avoid infection
Urinary frequency and urgency return	Vascular engorgement and altered bladder function caused by hormones; bladder capacity reduced by enlarging uterus and fetal presenting part	Kegel's exercises; limit fluid intake before bedtime; reassurance; wear perineal pad; refer to health care provider for pain or burning sensation
Perineal discomfort and pressure	Pressure from enlarging uterus, especially when standing or walking; multifetal gestation	Rest, conscious relaxation and good posture; refer to health care provider for assessment and treatment if pain is present; rule out labor
Braxton Hicks contractions	Intensification of uterine contractions in preparation for work of labor	Reassurance; rest; change of position; practice breathing techniques when contractions are bothersome; effleurage; *rule out labor*
Leg cramps (gastrocnemius spasm) especially when reclining	Compression of nerves supplying lower extremities because of enlarging uterus; reduced level of diffusible serum calcium or elevation of serum phosphorus; aggravating factors: fatigue, poor peripheral circulation, pointing toes when stretching legs or when walking, drinking more than 1 L (1 qt) of milk per day	Rule out blood clot by checking for Homans' sign; if clot ruled out, use massage and heat over affected muscle; dorsiflex foot until spasm relaxes (Fig. 7-17); stand on cold surface; oral supplementation with calcium carbonate or calcium lactate tablets; aluminum hydroxide gel, 1 oz, with each meal removes phosphorus by absorbing it
Ankle edema (nonpitting) to lower extremities	Edema aggravated by prolonged standing, sitting, poor posture, lack of exercise, constrictive clothing (e.g., garters), or by hot weather	Ample fluid intake for natural diuretic effect; put on support stockings before arising; rest periodically with legs and hips elevated (see Fig. 7-12), exercise moderately; refer to health care provider if generalized edema develops; *diuretics are contraindicated*

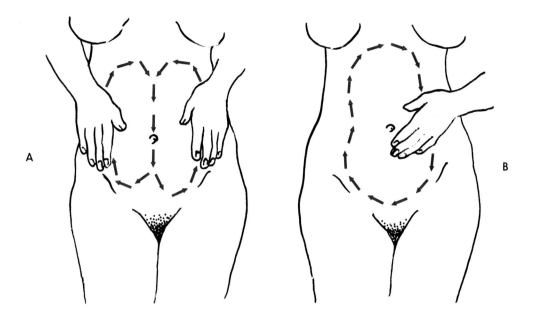

FIG. 7-16   Pattern for effleurage, a light, rhythmic stroking useful for inducing relaxation. **A,** Self-effleurage. **B,** Effleurage by another.

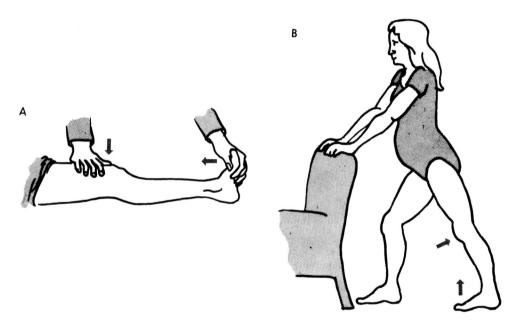

FIG. 7-17   Relief of muscle spasm (leg cramps). **A,** Another person dorsiflexes foot with knee extended. **B,** Woman stands and leans forward, thereby dorsiflexing foot of affected leg.

to come from the vagina may indicate rupture of membranes. The diagnosis requires a visit to the clinic or hospital for evaluation.

Recognizing Labor Symptoms

During the third trimester perhaps the most often asked question by pregnant women is "How will I know when I am in labor?" Educating women as to the signs and symptoms of labor serves two purposes. It decreases anxiety by providing information and it allows the woman

an active role in planning her labor and birth. Box 7-8 provides information on impending labor.

Recognizing Preterm Labor

Teaching each pregnant woman to recognize preterm labor is necessary (Johnson, 1989; Bonovich, 1990). Hospitals have developed pamphlets to help mothers remember what they learn. The Teaching Approaches box on p. 164 includes guidelines for recognizing preterm labor. Occasionally, birth occurs before the pregnant woman

BOX 7-8

Symptoms of Impending Labor

Uterine contractions: The woman is instructed to report the frequency, duration, and intensity of uterine contractions. True labor is characterized by an increase in frequency, strength, and duration of contractions. In true labor an increase in activity increases these symptoms. If the woman is in false labor, an increase in activity usually leads to a diminishing of the symptoms. Nulliparas are usually counseled to remain at home until contractions are regular and 5 minutes apart. Parous women are counseled to remain at home until contractions are regular and 10 minutes apart. If the woman lives more than 20 minutes from the hospital or has a history of rapid labors, these instructions are modified accordingly.

Rupture of the membranes.

Bloody show: The show is scant, pink, and sticky (contains mucus).

has access to professional attendants. Emergency childbirth is outlined in Chapter 12.

Prebirth Education

Prebirth education helps parents make the transition from the role of expectant parents to the role of parents responsible for their newborns.

This definition implies that childbirth education is *preparation for parenting*, not just preparation for labor and birth, which has traditionally been the focus of childbirth education. It is now being advocated that preparation for parenting begin as preconception counseling included in routine women's health care. Earlier education regarding exercise, nutrition, alcohol, smoking, and drugs in pregnancy, as well as reproductive choices, may lead to healthier and more satisfying outcomes.

Most childbirth educators would agree that expectant parents need a comprehensive education program to prepare them for the role and responsibilities of parenthood, but there are philosophic disagreements on when and how different topics should be taught. Many childbirth educators continue to focus almost exclusively on preparation for labor and birth in the third trimester because this seems to be the major concern of parents (Bliss-Holtz, 1988).

Previous pregnancy and childbirth experiences are important elements that influence a patient's and support person's current learning needs. The patient's (and support person's) age, cultural background, personal philosophy in regard to childbirth, socioeconomic status, spiritual beliefs, and learning styles all need to be assessed to develop the best plan to help the woman meet her needs.

TEACHING APPROACHES

HOW TO RECOGNIZE PRETERM LABOR

Because the onset of preterm labor is subtle and often hard to recognize, it is important to know how to feel your abdomen for uterine contractions. You can feel for contractions in the following way. While lying down, place your fingertips on the top of your uterus. A contraction is the periodic tightening or hardening of your uterus. If your uterus is contracting, you will actually feel your abdomen get tight or hard and then feel it relax or soften when the contraction is over.

If you think you are having any of the other signs and symptoms of preterm labor, empty your bladder, drink three to four glasses of water for hydration, lie down tilted toward your side, and place a pillow at your back for support.

Check for contractions for 1 hour. To tell how often contractions are occurring, check the minutes that elapse from the beginning of one contraction to the beginning of the next.

It is *normal* to have some uterine contractions throughout the day. They usually occur when a woman changes positions. These usually irregular and mild contractions are called Braxton Hicks contractions. They help with uterine tone and uteroplacental perfusion.

It is *not normal* to have frequent uterine contractions (every 10 minutes or more often for 1 hour).

Contractions of labor are regular, frequent, and hard. They also may be felt as a tightening of the abdomen or a backache. This type of contraction causes the cervix to efface and dilate.

Call your doctor, clinic, or labor and birth unit, or go to the hospital if any of the following signs occur:

- You have uterine contractions every 10 minutes or more often for 1 hour *or*
- You have any of the other signs and symptoms for 1 hour *or*
- You have any bloody spotting or leaking of fluid from your vagina

It is often difficult to identify preterm labor. Accurate diagnosis requires assessment by the health care provider, usually in the hospital or clinic.

Post these instructions where they can be seen by everyone in the family.

Parent Education Programs

Expectant parents and their families have different interests and information needs as the pregnancy progresses. A typical program is designed to meet the information needs of parents at the three major stages of pregnancy and after birth.

Early pregnancy ("early bird") classes provide fundamental information. Classes are developed around the following areas: (1) early fetal development, (2) physiologic and emotional changes of pregnancy, (3) human sexuality, and (4) the nutritional needs of the mother and fetus. Environmental and workplace hazards have become important concerns in recent years. Even though pregnancy is considered a normal process, exercises, warning signs, drugs, and self-medication are topics of interest and concern.

Midpregnancy classes emphasize the woman's participation in self-care. Classes provide information on preparation for breastfeeding and formula feeding, infant care, basic hygiene, common complaints and simple, safe remedies, infant health, and parenting.

Late pregnancy classes emphasize labor and birth. Different methods of coping with labor and birth have been developed and are often the basis for various prenatal classes. These include Lamaze, Bradley, and Dick-Read. The effectiveness of other methods such as hypnosis is being explored.

Throughout the series of classes there is discussion of support systems that people can use during pregnancy and after birth; such support systems help parents function independently and effectively. During all the classes the open expression of feelings and concerns about any aspect of pregnancy, birth, and parenting is welcomed.

Recent Trends in Parent Education

A variety of approaches to parent education have evolved as parent educators attempt to meet learning needs (Haire, 1991). In addition to classes designed specifically for pregnant adolescents, their partners, and/or parents, classes have begun for other groups with special learning needs such as first-time mothers over 35, single women, adoptive parents, and parents of twins. Refresher classes for parents with children not only review coping techniques for labor and birth but also help couples prepare for sibling reactions and adjustments to a new baby. Cesarean birth classes are offered for couples who have a scheduled cesarean birth because of breech position or some other predisposing factor. Another specialized class focuses on **vaginal birth after cesarean (VBAC).** This choice is supported by research and clinical trials indicating that many women successfully give birth vaginally after previously giving birth by cesarean (Safrin-Disler, 1990).

Because environmental influences and maternal behavior strongly affect newborn health, many programs encourage women to choose healthy lifestyles during pregnancy and early parenting. Preconception and early pregnancy classes support women to adopt nutrition and exercise behaviors that are closely associated with improved pregnancy outcomes and to avoid environmental hazards, smoking, alcohol, and drugs. Women with a developed sense of self-control tend to engage in health-promoting activities during pregnancy (Riesch, 1988;

Lewaller, 1989; Whitcher, 1989). Research supports that moderate exercise during the childbearing years has no adverse effects on women otherwise healthy but should be based on exercise guidelines for pregnancy and the postpartum period (ACOG, 1985, Fishbein and Phillips, 1990) (see Home Care box on p. 141).

Classes designed to meet the needs of America's growing multiethnic populations are also essential. Classes for new immigrants are particularly effective when taught in the first language (e.g., Spanish, Filipino, or Chinese). For classes to be meaningful parent educators must understand the value systems in other cultures and their influence on nutrition, valuing of early prenatal care, maternal weight gain, and infant feeding practices. Parent educators must establish rapport, be understood, and build on cultural practices, reinforcing the positive and promoting change only if a practice, such as pica, is directly harmful (USDA, USDHHS, 1990; Waxler-Morrison et al, 1990).

Most parent education classes are attended by the pregnant woman and her partner, although a friend, teenage daughter, or parent may be the designated support person. Because family-centered care has supported the presence of family members at birth, classes have also evolved for grandparents and siblings to prepare them for their attendance at birth and/or the arrival of the baby (Fig. 7-18). Siblings often see a birth film and learn ways they can help welcome the baby. They also learn to cope with the adjustment, including reduction in parental time and attention (Spadt et al, 1990). Grandparents learn about current child-care practices and how to help their adult children adapt to parenting without being perceived as interfering.

Birth Setting Choices

The concept of family-centered maternity care is implemented in birth rooms or **alternative birth centers (ABCs)** in the hospital. Hospital ABCs, as well as freestanding birth centers, are intended to offer families an alternative to home birth, providing a compromise between hospital and home. These birth setting choices have been shown to be safe alternatives to birth in a traditional delivery setting (Hutti, Johnson, 1988; Eakins et al, 1989). In addition, they can be designed to ensure quality control and to be cost effective, two significant issues in the birth of health care today. Women consider a variety of factors in choosing a setting for childbirth.

Alternative Birth Centers. ABCs usually are located in hospital suites away from the traditional obstetrics department. They are close to the delivery and operating rooms and medical or neonatal intensive care facilities for use when serious problems arise.

ABCs have homelike accommodations, including a double bed for the couple and a crib for the newborn.

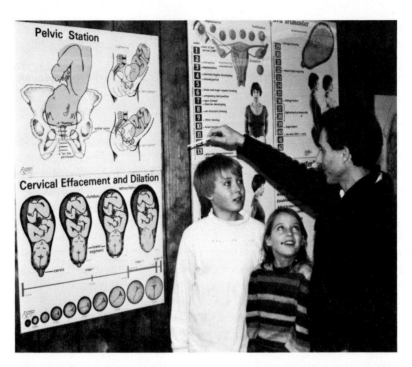

FIG. 7-18 Sibling preparation class. (Courtesy Community Birth Center, Community Hospital, Santa Cruz, CA.)

Emergency equipment and medications are discreetly stored within cupboards, out of view but easily accessible. Private bathroom facilities are incorporated into each birth center. There may be an early labor lounge or living room and small kitchen. There is careful screening of each applicant so that the ABC can rule out women with risk factors. Only low-risk and prepared women or couples are accepted.

The family is admitted to the ABC; the woman labors there and gives birth there. Members may remain there until discharge if the time interval and requirements for room use permit. If the family has to remain in the hospital for more than 24 hours after birth, the demand for use of the ABC by other families may require transfer of the first family to a regular postpartum room.

Labor, Delivery, Recovery, Postpartum (Birthing) Rooms. Labor, delivery, recovery (LDR) and labor, delivery, recovery, postpartum (LDRP) rooms offer families a comfortable, private space for childbirth. Unlike ABCs in hospitals, there are few admission or risk criteria for the use of these rooms.

Some hospitals incorporate labor support by highly trained nurses or monitrices. Women labor, give birth, and spend the first bonding time with their families in the LDR room. If they are not in an LDRP room, transfer to a postpartum room is usually the only room change they have to make.

Freestanding Birth Centers. Although most ABCs and LDR/LDRP rooms are located in hospitals, a growing number of **freestanding birth centers** are seen. These units, outside the hospital, are often close to a major hospital so that quick transfer to that institution is possible if necessary.

Most freestanding birth centers are staffed by physicians who have privileges at the local hospital and by certified nurse-midwives who are equipped to attend low-risk women through the puerperium. Ambulance service and emergency procedures are readily available. Fees vary with the services provided and the ability of the family to pay (reduced-fee sliding scale). Several insurance companies as well as Medicaid recognize and reimburse these clinics.

Services provided by the freestanding birth centers include those necessary for safe management during the childbearing cycle. There are some significant additions, however. Attendance at childbirth and parenting classes is required of all patients. Prenatal supervision of the woman, whose nutritional and health status must be good and who must be experiencing a low-risk pregnancy, begins in the first trimester. All patients must be familiar with situations requiring transfer to a hospital. Each expectant family identifies its *birth plan,* an explanation of practices and procedures they would like to include in or exclude from their childbirth experience.

Home Birth

Home birth has always been popular in certain advanced countries, such as Sweden and The Netherlands. In developing countries hospitals or adequate lying-in facilities often are unavailable to most pregnant women, and home birth is a necessity. In North America, home birth is gaining popularity.

National groups supporting home birth are the Home Oriented Maternity Experience (HOME) and the National Association of Parents for Safe Alternatives in Childbirth (NAPSAC). These groups support changes toward more humane childbearing practices at all levels, integrating the alternatives for childbirth to meet the needs of the total population.

The literature on childbirth contains excellent statistics on medically directed home birth services with skilled nurse-midwives and medical backup.

Selective home birth in uncomplicated pregnancies is feasible. However, those women at high risk must be identified during the prenatal period and referred for hospital birth. In addition, a transport system should be available for transfer of women with suddenly complicated labors to a nearby adequate medical facility.

Hospital Birth

If a hospital birth is planned, the woman is usually required to preregister at the hospital of choice. Most hospitals now provide pamphlets containing information such as where to report when labor begins and policies pertaining to visitors and visiting hours. Many facilities also conduct tours.

Counseling is provided to relieve emotional tensions, which often relate directly to the childbirth experience (e.g., anxiety about pain or possible birth of the child before reaching the hospital). Nursing strategies include providing an opportunity for discussing the woman's specific fears or anxieties, helping her make definite plans concerning what she will do when labor starts, repeating instructions willingly, and having sharing sessions with mothers who have recently given birth. If possible, involve significant others in preparation for the birth. Arrange to have them participate in a supportive way during labor and birth. These techniques may be effective in allaying or diffusing anxiety.

The families of women who are approaching labor may have their anxieties decreased through intervention before the event. Fantasies can be replaced by knowledge gained through activities such as the following:

- A hospital tour to enable visualization of the labor room and waiting areas
- A demonstration of helping and supportive measures to comfort the woman during labor
- A brief review of what to expect during the labor process
- A description of what to expect of the staff during labor

A realistic discussion of all known factors helps the father problem-solve more rationally and plan for the event. Such discussions are ego strengthening because they focus the father's energies toward more appropriate coping strategies by helping alleviate anxieties about the unknown. Today many fathers elect to participate actively during labor and the birth of their child. However, some men through personal or cultural concepts of the father role neither wish nor intend to participate. *The important concept is that the partners agree on the other's roles.* For nurses to advocate any changes in these roles may cause confusion or feelings of guilt.

Unfortunately many women who come to the hospital in labor still have not had any prenatal care. It is the responsibility of the nurse to provide this woman with the support and knowledge to successfully negotiate childbearing. A thorough assessment of immediate and long-term needs has to be done quickly. The clinician needs to provide information that includes the following:

1. Process of labor: examinations, care in labor, stages of labor
2. Methods to control pain: breathing and relaxation techniques, analgesia, and anesthesia
3. Responsibilities of the support person

It is often necessary to call on other members of the health care team, such as the social worker, to assist in financial or child care arrangements. It is not uncommon for a laboring woman with no prenatal care to come to the hospital accompanied by her young children with no one to care for them.

✤ EVALUATION

Evaluation is a continuous process as each intervention is assessed for effectiveness and an alternate intervention is used as necessary. Any change in patient condition or concern requires readjustment in the nursing care plan. The degree to which the expected outcomes for the mother, couple, or fetus are met is continuously evaluated according to measurable established criteria:

- The woman and her family have sufficient information about maternal adaptations and fetal development and say that they understand the management of care and self-care during the third trimester.
- The woman identified symptoms that could indicate deviations from normal progress and protocols for reporting them.
- The woman says that her need for information was met.
- The woman and her family were active participants in her care during the third trimester of pregnancy.
- The woman had formalized a birth plan.
- The woman's trusting relationship with caregivers continued to progress.

PLAN OF CARE

Third Trimester—Discomforts

Case History

Ruth is now 30 weeks pregnant. Her prenatal course has been uneventful except for the normal discomforts of pregnancy. She is experiencing insomnia, ankle edema, and Braxton Hicks contractions.

EXPECTED OUTCOMES	IMPLEMENTATION	RATIONALE	EVALUATION
Nursing Diagnosis: Sleep pattern disturbance related to discomforts of late pregnancy			
Ruth will learn and use self-care comfort measures and get a minimum of 7 hours restful sleep/night.	Reassure that insomnia is a common occurrence during late pregnancy. Teach rationale, demonstrate and observe return demonstration (where possible) of self-care measures: conscious relaxation; effleurage; support of body parts with pillows; warm milk or shower before retiring; whirlpool bath (jet hydrotherapy (Chapter 11) before retiring; avoidance of caffeine-containing fluids/foods late in day.	Validates normality of her "complaint." Knowledge and skill increase individual coping, self-esteem, and sense of power over situation. Measures utilize gate-control theory, normal physiologic function, and facilitate relaxation.	Ruth states she understands but she would feel better if she could sleep. At next visit Ruth states she is sleeping better, feels better, and both she and her husband are benefiting from the relaxation techniques; she states she and her husband are learning these same techniques in the parent education class.
Nursing Diagnosis: Leg pain related to ankle edema and compression of blood vessels and nerves supplying lower extremities because of enlarging uterus			
Ruth will experience less ankle edema and leg ache.	Explore possibility of her walking or stair climbing several times each day. Explore possibility of 15-20 min during morning, lunch, and afternoon breaks and after work to rest with legs and hips elevated (see Fig. 7-12) and to support arms and legs with pillows at night while in side-lying position. Suggest maternity girdle to help support heavy abdomen. Suggest maintaining water intake up to 8 glasses/day.	Standing and sitting for extended periods impairs peripheral circulation and causes fatigue and leg aches: Walking and climbing stairs stimulates circulation. Position uses gravity to help reduce ankle edema. Supporting and lifting heavy uterus facilitates venous/lymphatic drainage. Water intake and side-lying position aid in diuresis by improving renal perfusion.	At next visit Ruth reports she has noted less ankle edema and leg ache.

Continued.

PLAN OF CARE—con't
Third Trimester—Discomforts

EXPECTED OUTCOMES	IMPLEMENTATION	RATIONALE	EVALUATION
Nursing Diagnosis: Anxiety related to knowledge deficit regarding recognition of preterm labor			
Ruth will learn how to recognize preterm labor today. Ruth will put the pamphlet where family can see it, as soon as she gets home. Ruth will telephone her health care provider if she experiences any of the warning signs and symptoms of preterm labor.	Using written instructions* teach Ruth how to assess and time contractions. Suggest pamphlet/instructions be placed where husband/family can find them easily.	Knowledge permits Ruth to collaborate in her care; increases self-confidence. Ruth may be too anxious or unable to use them; family members may need to help with assessment and reporting to primary care provider.	Ruth demonstrates actions and states rationale correctly. At next visit 1 week later, Ruth states she posted instructions on the telephone after reviewing them with her husband/family.

*Nurse has determined that both Ruth and her husband can read the instructions.

KEY POINTS

- The prenatal period is a preparatory one both physically, in terms of fetal growth and maternal adaptations, and psychologically, in terms of anticipation of parenthood.
- The psychosocial aspects of care are paramount and may well affect the whole course of pregnancy, childbirth, and the adjustment of the new family.
- The woman's readiness to learn is at a high level, making this an excellent time to help her expand her self-care skills.
- Discomforts and changes of pregnancy can cause anxiety to the woman and her family and require sensitive attention and a plan for teaching self-care measures.
- Education about healthy ways of using the body (e.g., exercise, body mechanics) is essential given maternal anatomic and physiologic responses to pregnancy.
- Important components of the initial prenatal visit include detailed and carefully recorded findings from the interview, a comprehensive physical examination, and selected laboratory tests.
- Even in normal pregnancy the nurse must remain alert to hazards such as supine hypotension, warning signs and symptoms, and signs of potential parenting problems.

- Blood pressure is evaluated on the basis of absolute values and length of gestation and interpreted in the light of modifying factors; normal MAPs during the second trimester are <90 mm Hg.
- In the absence of factors that affect accuracy, measurement of fundal height is one of the indicators of the progress of fetal growth. Auscultation of fetal heart tones is another tool for assessing fetal health status.
- The quiet period of the second trimester gives way to an active period more oriented to the reality of impending childbirth and parenting responsibilities; attention to prebirth preparation is a necessary component of prenatal care.
- Each pregnant woman needs to know how to recognize and report preterm labor.
- Childbirth education is a process designed to help parents make the transition from the role of expectant parents to the role and responsibilities of parents of a new baby.
- Regardless of the pregnant woman's readiness to learn, attention to prebirth preparation is a necessary component of prenatal care.

CRITICAL THINKING EXERCISES

For each activity justify your claims, beliefs, conclusions, decisions, and actions.

1. In an actual or simulated clinical setting complete an initial prenatal interview and physical examination. Formulate at least two nursing diagnoses (one physical and one psychosocial). For each diagnosis develop at least one patient-centered expected outcome, intervention with rationale, and outcome evaluation criterion.

2. In a clinical setting interview a woman in her second trimester. Assess her discomforts and concerns. Differentiate normal from abnormal signs and symptoms. Develop a teaching plan to meet her learning needs. Refer abnormal findings for follow-up as appropriate.

3. Role play teaching a pregnant woman to recognize preterm labor.

4. Ms. Smith is pregnant with her first child. She confides in you that her mother-in-law is driving her crazy. She states that her mother-in-law is constantly telling her "When I had my children, we didn't do it that way." List three actions Mrs. Smith could take and why you would recommend them.

5. Ms. Warren arrives at the hospital in active labor. She has had no prenatal care. With her are her two children 10 months and 2 years old. She states that she has no one to care for them. Discuss what assessments need to be made and develop a plan of care for meeting her needs.

References

Affonso DD: The Filipino American. In Clark AL, editor: *Culture/childbearing/health professionals.* Philadelphia, 1978, FA Davis.

American College of Obstetricians and Gynecologists: *Home exercise program: exercise during pregnancy and the postnatal period,* Washington, DC, 1985, ACOG.

Barkauskas VH et al: *Health and physical assessment,* St Louis, 1994, Mosby.

Barry M, Bia F: Pregnancy and travel, *JAMA* 261:728, 1989.

Bernhardt TL et al: Hyperbaric oxygen treatment of cerebral air embolism from orogenital sex during pregnancy, *Crit Care Med* 16:729, 1988.

Bliss-Holtz VJ: Primiparas prenatal concern for learning infant care, *Nurs Res* 37:20, 1988.

Bonovich, L: Recognizing the onset of labor, *JOGNN* 19(2):141, 1990.

Boston Women's Health Book Collective: *The new our bodies, ourselves,* New York, 1992, Touchstone.

Brown MA: Marital support during pregnancy, *JOGNN* 15(6):475, 1986.

Brown MS: A cross-cultural look at pregnancy, labor, and delivery, *Obstet Gynecol Nurs* 5:35, 1976.

Bryant, H: Antenatal counseling for women working outside the homes, *Birth* 12:4, 1985.

Burgess MA: Rubella vaccination just before or during pregnancy, *Med J Aust* 152:507, 1990.

Carrington BW: The Afro-American. In Clark AL, editor: *Culture/childbearing/health professionals.* Philadelphia, 1978, FA Davis.

Clark M: *Health in the Mexican-American culture: a community study.* Berkeley, 1970, University of California Press.

Cohen A: Movement as a yardstick for fetal well-being, *Contemp OB/GYN* 26:61, 1985.

Cook PS, Petersen RC, Moore DT: *Alcohol, tobacco, and other drugs may harm the unborn.* US Department of Health and Human Services. DHHS Pub No (ADM)90-1711. Rockville, MD, 1990, Office for Substance Abuse Prevention.

Crosby, WM: Traumatic injuries during pregnancy, *Clin Obstet Gynecol* 26(4):902, 1983.

Culpepper L: Exercise during pregnancy. In Merkatz TR, Thompson JE, editors: *New perspectives on prenatal care,* New York, 1990, Elsevier.

Cunningham FG, MacDonald RC, Gant NF: *Williams obstetrics.* ed 19, Norwalk, CT, 1993, Appleton & Lange.

Dicke JM: Teratology: principles and practice, *Med Clin North Am* 73:567, 1989.

Eakins P, O'Reilly W, May L et al: Obstetric outcomes at the Birth Place in Menlo Park: the first seven years, *Birth* 16:123, 1989.

Engstrom JL, Sittler CP: Fundal height measurement. Part I. Techniques for measuring fundal height, *J Nurse Midwife,* 38(1):5, 1993.

Enkin M et al: *A guide to effective care in pregnancy and childbirth,* New York, 1989, Oxford University Press.

Fanaroff AA, Martin RJ, editors: *Neonatal-perinatal medicine: diseases of the fetus and infant,* ed 5, St Louis, 1992, Mosby.

Fishbein EG, Phillips M: How safe is exercise during pregnancy? *JOGNN* 19:45, 1990.

Goldsmith MF: Pregnancy Dx? Rx may now include condoms, *JAMA* 261(5):678, 1989.

Green NL: Stressful events related to childbearing in African-American women: a pilot study, *J Nurse Midwife* 35:231, 1990.

Haire D: Patient education in childbirth: a long way in forty years, *Int J Childbirth Educ* 6:7, 1991.

Hammond TL et al: The use of automobile safety restraint systems during pregnancy, *JOGNN* 19:339, 1990.

Horn BM: Northwest coast Indians: the Muckleshoot. In Kay MA, editor: *Anthropology of human birth,* Philadelphia. 1982. FA Davis.

Hutti M, Johnson J: Newborn Apgar scores of babies born in birthing rooms vs. traditional delivery rooms, *Appl Nurs Res* 1(2):68, 1988.

Iams JD, Johnson FF, Creasy RK: Prevention of preterm birth, *Clin Obstet Gynecol* 31:599, 1988.

Johnson FF: Assessment and education to prevent preterm labor, *MCN* 14:157, 1989.

Kay MA, editor: *Anthropology of human birth,* Philadelphia, 1982, FA Davis.

Kulig JC: Childbearing beliefs among Cambodian refugee women, *West J Nurs Res* 12:108, 1990.

Lazarus E, Philipson E: A longitudinal study comparing the prenatal care of Puerto Rican and white women, *Birth* 17(1):6, 1990.

Leatherman J, Blackburn D, Davidhizar R: How postpartum women explain their lack of obtaining adequate prenatal care, *J Adv Nurs* 15(3):256, 1990.

Lee RV: Understanding Southeast Asian mothers-to-be, *Childbirth Educ* 8:32, 1989.

Leviton A: Caffeine consumption and the risk of reproductive hazards, *J Reprod Med* 33:175, 1988.

Lewaller LP: Health beliefs and health practices of pregnant women, *JOGNN* 18:246, 1989.

McDonald A, Armstrong B, Sloan M: Cigarette, alcohol, and coffee consumption and congenital effects, *Am J Public Health* 82(1):91, 1992.

Meleis AI, Sorrell L: Bridging cultures: Arab American women and their birth experiences, *MCN* 6:171, 1981.

Mittelmark RA et al, editors: *Exercise in pregnancy,* ed 2, Baltimore, 1991, Williams & Wilkins.

NAACOG: Standards for the nursing care of women and newborns, ed 5, Washington, DC, 1985, NAACOG.

Nichols F, Humenick S: *Childbirth education: practice, research and theory.* Philadelphia, 1988, WB Saunders.

Page EW, Villee CA, Villee DB: *Human reproduction: essentials of reproductive and perinatal medicine,* ed 3, Philadelphia, 1981, WB Saunders.

Paglone A, Worthington S: Cautions and advice on exercise during pregnancy, *Contemp OB/GYN* 25:160, 1985 (special issue).

Peters H, Theorell C: Fetal and neonatal effects of maternal cocaine use, *JOGNN* 20(2):121, 1991.

Riesch SK: Changes in the exercise of self-care agency, *West J Nurs Res* 10:272, 1988.

Rynerson B, Lowdermilk D: Sexual intimacy in pregnancy. In

Knuppel R, Drukker J: *High-risk pregnancy: a team approach,* ed 2, Philadelphia, 1993, WB Saunders.

Safrin-Disler C: Vaginal birth after cesarean, *ICEA Rev* 14(3):9, 1990.

Scott JR et al: *Obstetrics and gynecology,* ed 6, Philadelphia, 1990, JB Lippincott.

Scupholme A, Robertson E, Kamons A: Barriers to prenatal care in a multiethnic, urban sample, *J Nurse-Midwife* 36(2):111, 1991.

Seidel HM et al: *Mosby's guide to physical examination,* ed 3. St Louis, 1995. Mosby.

Snow L: Folk medical beliefs and their implications for care of patients, *Ann Intern Med* 81:82, 1974.

Spadt SK, Martin KR, Thomas AM: Experiential classes for siblings-to-be, *MCN* 15:184, 1990.

Starn JR: Cultural childbearing: beliefs and practices, *Int J Childbirth Educ* 6:38, 1991.

Stern PM: Solving problems of cross-cultural health teaching: the Filipino childbearing family, *Image J Nurs Sch* 13:47, 1981.

USDA and USDHHA: *Cross-cultural counseling: a guide for nutrition and health counselors.* Washington, DC, 1990, US Government Printing Office.

Waxler-Morrison N, Anderson J, Richardson E, editors: *Cross-cultural nursing.* Vancouver, 1990, University of British Columbia Press.

Whitcher S: Preparation for pregnancy: a health promotion program, *Health Values* 13(5):32, 1989.

Wright LM, Leahey M: *Nurses and families: a guide to family assessment and interaction,* Philadelphia, 1984, FA Davis.

Bibliography

Burks J: Factors in the utilization of prenatal services by low-income Black women, *Nurse Pract* 17(4):34, 1992.

Chen S, Fitzgerald M, DeStefano L et al: Effects of a school nurse prenatal counseling program, *Public Health Nurs* 8(4):212, 1991.

Hillan E: Issues in the delivery of midwifery care, *J Adv Nurs* 17(3):274, 1992.

Lowe N: Maternal confidence in coping with labor: a self-efficacy concept, *JOGNN* 20(6):457, 1991.

Mackey M: Women's preparation for the childbirth experience, *Matern-Child Nurs J* 19(2):143, 1990.

Mattson S, Lew L: Culturally sensitive prenatal care for Southeast Asians, *JOGNN* 21(1):48, 1992.

Meister J, Warrick L, de Zapien J et al: Using lay health workers: case study of a community-based prenatal intervention, *J Community Health* 17(1):37, 1992.

Nichols F, editor: *Perinatal education: AWHONN's clinical issues in perinatal and women's health nursing,* Philadelphia, 1993, JB Lippincott.

Patterson E, Freese M, Goldenberg R: Seeking safe passage: utilizing health care during pregnancy, *Image J Nurs Sch* 22(1):27, 1990.

Warrick L, Wood A, Meister J et al: Evaluation of a peer health worker prenatal outreach and education program for Hispanic farmworker families, *J Community Health* 17(1):13, 1992.

8 Maternal and Fetal Nutrition

LINDA J. BOYNE

LEARNING OBJECTIVES

Define the key terms listed.

Explain optimum maternal weight gain during pregnancy, focusing on nutritional values of foods eaten to achieve recommended weight gain.

State recommended dietary allowances (RDAs) for energy, protein, and key vitamins and minerals during pregnancy.

Give examples of food sources of the nutrients required for optimum maternal nutrition during pregnancy.

Examine the need for nutritional supplements during pregnancy.

List five nutritional risk factors for problem pregnancies.

Give examples of cultural food patterns and possible dietary problems for two alternative eating patterns/ethnic groups.

Perform a nutritional assessment of a pregnant woman.

Apply the nursing process to maternal and fetal nutrition.

KEY TERMS

anemia
anthropometric measurements
body mass index (BMI)
diet history
energy (kcal)
food cravings
intrauterine growth retardation (IUGR)
lactose intolerance
low birth weight
pica
recommended weight gain
vegetarian diet

RELATED TOPICS

Basal metabolic rate *(Chap. 5)* • Cystic fibrosis *(Chap. 27)* • Exercise in pregnancy *(Chap. 7)* • Fetopelvic disproportion *(Chap. 24)* • Gestational diabetes *(Chap. 22)* • Phenylketonuria *(Chap. 27)* • Preconception counseling *(Chap. 4)* • Pregnancy-induced hypertension *(Chap. 21)*

Pregnancy is the initiating and sustaining of a new life—a time of growth. A woman's past health experiences join with her present condition to lay the foundation for a new life. Nutrition is one of the many factors that influence the outcome of a pregnancy (Fig. 8-1). Nutritional status is affected by the many factors that influence pregnancy outcome.

Factors that place a woman at nutritional risk, such as poverty, poor education, deprived environment, bizarre food habits, and poor health, will continue to affect her nutritional status and the growth and development of her fetus. Pregnant women with poor nutritional status need special care. Race can affect pregnancy outcome. The risk of delivering an infant of low birth weight is higher in African-American women of middle class than of white women of the same social class (Wegman,

1993). This might reflect the effects of previous generations of poverty and suggests the effects of long-term nutritional intake on pregnancy outcome (Collins, David, 1990).

The United States ranks twenty-second of 28 industrialized nations in infant mortality (Wegman, 1993). The major contributor in two thirds of all infant deaths is low birth weight (LBW). The most promising measure for preventing LBW is to provide high-quality prenatal care to all women. An important component of this quality care is appropriate, individualized nutritional counseling for the pregnant woman.

The importance of nutrition in a successful pregnancy was first realized during World War II when parts of Europe were blockaded and food supplies were depleted. The undernutrition that occurred greatly affected the

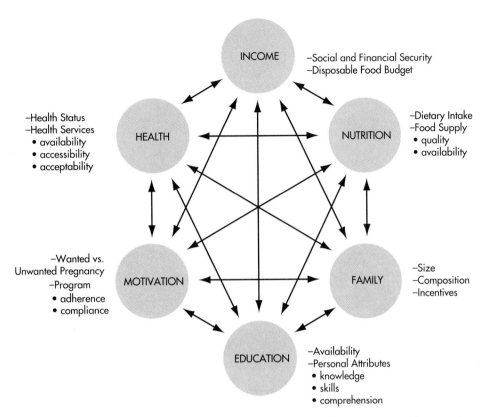

INCOME
–Social and Financial Security
–Disposable Food Budget

–Health Status
–Health Services
• availability
• accessibility
• acceptability

HEALTH

NUTRITION
–Dietary Intake
–Food Supply
• quality
• availability

–Wanted vs.
Unwanted Pregnancy
–Program
• adherence
• compliance

MOTIVATION

FAMILY
–Size
–Composition
–Incentives

EDUCATION
–Availability
–Personal Attributes
• knowledge
• skills
• comprehension

FIG. 8-1   Seamless web of influences that can affect outcome of pregnancy. Much more than luck goes into having a healthy baby. (From Wardlaw GM, Insel PM: *Perspectives in nutrition,* St Louis, 1993, Mosby.)

birth weight of infants whose mothers were in the second and third trimesters at the time of the blockade. Birth defects occurred more frequently and the number of conceptions decreased. After the blockades were lifted, birth weights increased, as did the number of pregnancies. It appeared that good maternal nutrition, not only during pregnancy but also prior to conception, affected both the mother's and the infant's health. Thus maternal nutrition is very important in all stages of reproductive life from childhood to menopause to help ensure that all women are in good health at the time of conception.

The importance of promoting healthful eating practices before conception is now well recognized. The Public Health Service Expert Panel on Prenatal Care recommends a preconceptional visit as part of routine prenatal care. During this visit the woman should be encouraged to follow the recommendations of the dietary guidelines or the food guide pyramid (Fig. 8-2).

One of the Year 2000 goals is to promote and achieve dietary adequacy by pregnant women (*Healthy People 2000,* 1990). This may be a bit ambitious considering recent data, which show that many women of childbearing age are consuming less than the **recommended dietary allowances** (RDAs) for many nutrients considered to be important during pregnancy (Brown and Story,

1990). Compounding this is the problem that dietary assessment and nutrition counseling are not, at this time, a routine part of prenatal care. Pregnancy is an especially good time to promote good nutrition, since most expectant women are highly motivated to change poor eating habits. Much valuable information and many resources are available to help women select foods and dietary patterns associated with a healthy pregnancy and a healthy outcome. Sources of written pamphlets include prenatal vitamin manufacturers, various infant formula manufacturers, the March of Dimes, and volunteer health-related organizations such as the American Dietetic Association.

WEIGHT GAIN

The importance of appropriate weight gain during pregnancy cannot be overemphasized. Weight gain during pregnancy makes an important contribution to the overall success of the pregnancy. However, weight gain alone should not be used to determine the adequacy of specific nutrient intakes; the quality of the gain may be a more important factor in overall fetal development. Fig. 8-3 shows the components of weight gain during pregnancy and how the gain is distributed between the de-

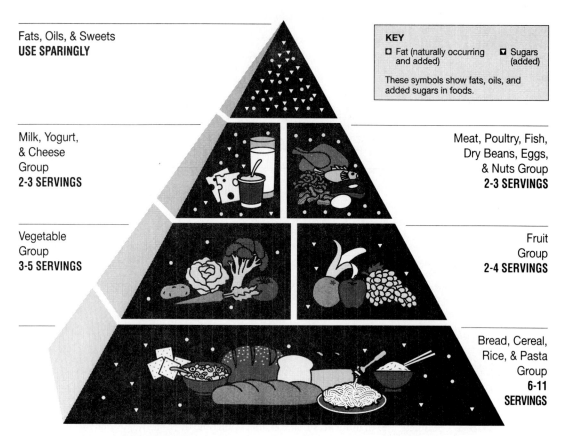

FIG. 8-2 Food guide pyramid, a guide to daily food choices.

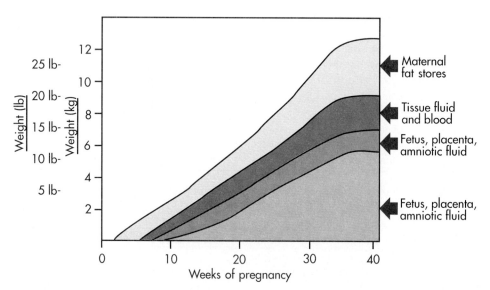

FIG. 8-3 Components of weight gain in pregnancy showing distribution of weight between maternal and fetal compartments. (From Wardlaw GM, Insel PM: *Perspectives in nutrition,* St Louis, 1993, Mosby.)

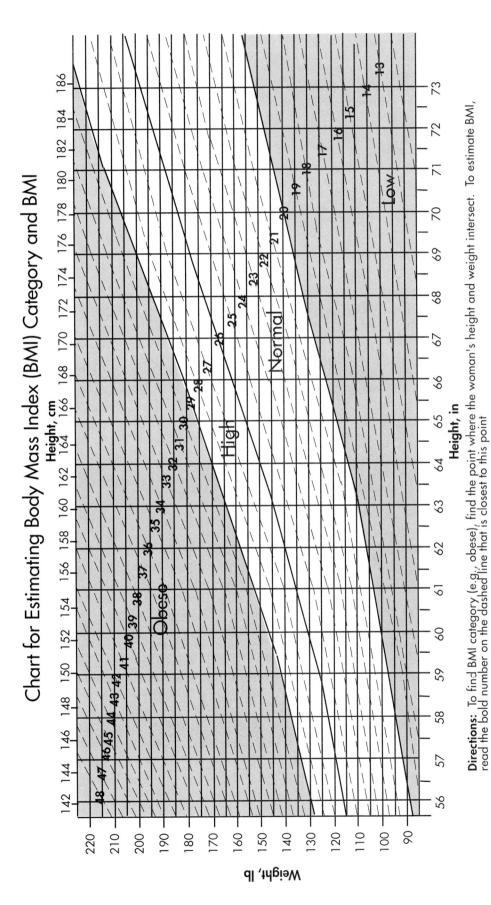

FIG. 8-4   Chart for estimating body mass index (BMI) category and BMI. To find BMI category (e.g., obese), find the point where height and weight intersect. To estimate BMI, read bold number on dashed line that is closest to this point. (Reprinted with permission from *Nutrition during pregnancy and lactation: an implementation guide.* Copyright 1992 by the National Academy of Sciences. Courtesy National Academy Press, Washington, D.C.)

veloping fetus and the mother's increase in body fluids and breast tissue. Note that some of the maternal weight gain is deposited as fat to provide for fetal growth during the last trimester and to use as a source of energy during the early part of lactation.

It is imperative that the pregnant woman does not use pregnancy as an excuse for dietary excesses. The woman who gains an excessive amount of weight (to more than 135% of *standard body weight*) is likely to retain much of this gain after birth. Chronic diseases associated with being overweight include hypertension, diabetes, and cardiovascular disorders. Dietary counseling during pregnancy should focus on improving the quality of the woman's overall dietary intake and avoiding unnecessary weight gain, which could pose health risks to the mother later in life.

Weight Gain and Fetal Growth

Weight gain during the second and third trimesters is an especially important determinant of fetal growth. Inadequate weight gain is associated with an increased risk of delivering a growth-retarded infant, commonly referred to as **intrauterine growth retardation (IUGR).** On the other hand, a very high gestational weight gain is associated with increased incidence of high birth weight, which is in turn associated with an increase in the risk of fetopelvic disproportion, operative delivery (use of forceps), birth trauma, asphyxia, and mortality. This problem is more pronounced in short women.

The relationship between gestational weight gain and fetal growth in part varies according to prepregnancy weight for height. An appropriate method for recommending a range of weight gain for a pregnant women is to use her preconception weight for height, or her **body mass index** (BMI) (Rosso, 1985). BMI is calculated by dividing the weight (in kilograms) by the height (in meters) squared. For example, a woman who weighs 54 kg (119 lb) before pregnancy and is 1.56 m (61.5 in) tall has a BMI of 22:

$$54 \div 1.56^2 = 22$$

Using the chart in Fig. 8-4, you can determine the woman's BMI. In the above example the BMI is in the normal range. Table 8-1 shows the recommended range of weight gain for each of the BMI categories (underweight, normal, overweight, and obese). Weight for height is the only anthropometric value necessary to use (Institute of Medicine, 1990) for making this recommendation. In some settings triceps skinfold (TSF) measurements could be used to assess obesity, but these measurements are difficult to replicate in a clinical setting, and there are no reference standards validated against fetal outcomes.

The new Institute of Medicine recommendations for weight gain are higher than earlier recommendations. This is motivated by the relationship between maternal weight gain and pregnancy outcome. This additional

TABLE 8-1 Recommended Total Weight Gain Ranges for Pregnant Women*

PREPREGNANCY WEIGHT-FOR-HEIGHT CATEGORY	RECOMMENDED TOTAL GAIN	
	LB	KG
Low (BMI <19.8)	28 to 40	12.5 to 18
Normal (BMI 19.8 to 26)	25 to 35	11.5 to 16
High (BMI >26.0 to 29.0)	15 to 25	7.0 to 11.5
Obese (BMI >29.0)	≥15	≥7.0

Reprinted with permission from *Nutrition during pregnancy and lactation: an implementation guide.* Copyright © 1992 by the National Academy of Sciences. Courtesy National Academy Press, Washington, D.C.
*For singleton pregnancies. The range for women carrying twins is 35 to 45 lb (16 to 20 kg). Young adolescents (<2 years after menarche) and African-American women should strive for gains at the upper end of the range. Short women (<62 in or <157 cm) should strive for gains at the lower end of the range.

gain does not appear to influence the amount of gain retained at 18 months postpartum (Keppel, Taffel, 1993).

Also, based on the woman's BMI, a graph has been developed for use in monitoring progression toward the mutually established goal (Fig. 8-5). This chart is a major improvement over the earlier commonly used chart, which did not take into account the relationship between a woman's weight and height.

Pattern of Weight Gain

The recommended rate of gain approximates 1 to 2 kg (2 to 4 lb) during the first trimester and 0.4 kg per week (0.8 lb) thereafter for a woman of standard weight for height (BMI 19.8 to 26). A smooth progressive weight gain in the last two trimesters generally represents a gain of lean and fat tissue. During the second trimester the gain is primarily in the mother, and in the third trimester it is mostly fetal growth. It is important to monitor the rate of gain to identify any abnormal pattern that may indicate a need for professional intervention. Weight gain should be assessed at each prenatal visit and plotted on the weight gain graph to monitor progress leading to the established goal. A variance in this rate (e.g., less than 0.5 kg [1 lb] per month for obese women or less than 1 kg [2 lb] per month in the last two trimesters for normal weight women) might indicate a need for intervention. Possible reasons for deviations from the expected rate of weight gain include measurement or recording errors, differences in weight of clothing, time of day, and accumulation of fluids, as well as inadequate or excessive dietary intake. An exceptionally high gain is likely to represent excessive fluid retention. A gain of more than 3 kg per month, especially after the twentieth week of gestation, may indicate a serious problem, such as pregnancy-induced hypertension (PIH).

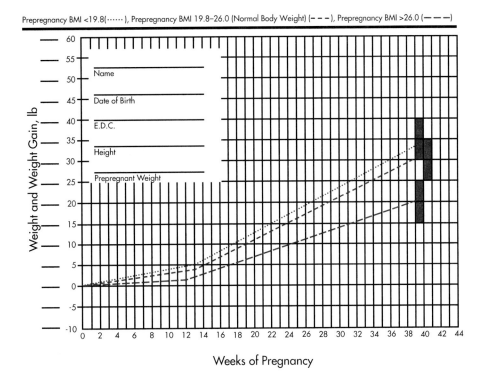

Prepregnancy BMI <19.8(······), Prepregnancy BMI 19.8–26.0 (Normal Body Weight) (– – –), Prepregnancy BMI >26.0 (— — —)

Date	Weeks of Gestation	Weight	Notes

FIG. 8-5   Prenatal weight gain chart. (Reprinted with permission from *Nutrition during pregnancy and lactation: an implementation guide.* Copyright 1992 by the National Academy of Sciences. Courtesy National Academy Press, Washington, D.C.)

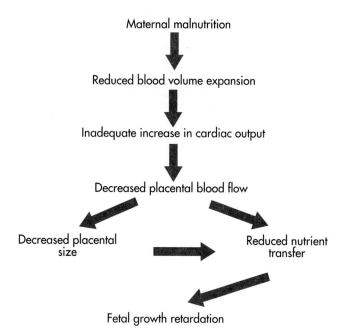

Maternal malnutrition

↓

Reduced blood volume expansion

↓

Inadequate increase in cardiac output

↓

Decreased placental blood flow

Decreased placental size

Reduced nutrient transfer

Fetal growth retardation

FIG. 8-6 Possible mechanism for fetal and placental growth retardation seen with maternal malnutrition in animal models and human subjects. (From Worthington-Roberts B, Williams SR: *Nutrition in pregnancy and lactation,* ed 5, St Louis, 1993, Mosby.)

Pregnancy is not the time for dieting. For the slender, figure-conscious woman (BMI < 19.8) weight gain may seem to be a real problem. The placenta of a poorly nourished mother often contains fewer and smaller cells and is less able to synthesize needed nutrients and facilitate the transport of the nutrients to the fetus (Fig. 8-6). The effects of undernutrition on fetal development should be pointed out to the mother. This counseling should include information on the components of the recommended gain and how much of this gain will be lost at the time of birth. Also, addressing the issue of how to lose the weight in the postpartum period helps relieve the mother's concerns. Ideally, the obese woman (BMI 26 to 29) or morbidly obese women (BMI >29) would undertake a weight reduction program prior to conception. However, all women need to gain some weight during gestation. The gain should at least equal the weight of the products of conception (fetus, placenta, amniotic fluid). The quality of the gain is important, and nutritional counseling for these women should stress nutrient-dense foods and the avoidance of empty calorie foods.

Low birth weight also correlates with maternal age. The highest percentage of low birth weight infants are born to teenagers and women over the age of 40. These women deserve special consideration when recommending weight gain ranges, particularly since the birth rates in both age groups have increased in the last 10 years

(Wegman, 1993). Teenagers often give birth to infants who weigh less, even with a comparable weight gain to an adult woman (Garn et al, 1984). This has been attributed to an immature reproductive system, which does not allow for a placental nutrient transfer as efficient as that of the more mature woman. The older woman may need fewer calories to support her pregnant state but have additional needs for specific nutrients. Nutritional counseling for each should focus on the necessity of supplying fetal nutritional needs by including nutrient-dense foods to promote the recommended weight gain. The main nutritional goal for these age groups is the same as for every pregnant woman: to produce a healthy baby while maintaining or improving the mother's health.

INCREASED NUTRIENT NEEDS OF PREGNANCY

To support these changes during gestation, many nutrients are needed in greater amounts than for normal adult maintenance. The changes occurring in all of the major organ systems in the mother allow for optimal fetal development as well as optimal maternal health.

During the latter part of the first trimester the blood volume of the mother increases rapidly—more rapidly than red blood cell (RBC) production. This is a normal event that causes a physiologic anemia of pregnancy, or *hemodilution*. It is not a serious problem unless the mother was iron deficient at the time of conception; if so, a true anemia could develop. Blood levels of many nutrients decrease or increase during pregnancy. Most lipid fractions rise (e.g., cholesterol), whereas other factors (e.g., total protein) decrease. At present there are no standards to use as a basis for evaluating blood nutrient levels for the pregnant woman.

The basal metabolic rate (BMR) increases about 20% during pregnancy. This increase includes the energy cost of tissue synthesis.

Recommendations for increased intake of specific nutrients during pregnancy have been made by the National Research Council (1989) in the form of RDAs (Table 8-2). The RDAs were developed for use with groups of people, and it is important that these recommendations *not* be confused with requirements. However, they do provide a *guideline* to begin individualized nutrition counseling. A margin of safety has been built into these allowances to cover a wide range of individual variations. For example, the reference woman in the typical RDA is age 18 to 24 years, weighs 58 kg (128 lb), is 164 cm (65 in) tall, lives in a temperate climate, and is a normally active, healthy woman. Variations from this state would need to be considered when doing individualized counseling. Age, activity level, and current weight are examples of variations that need to be considered.

TABLE 8-2 Nutritional Recommendations During Pregnancy and Lactation

NUTRIENT	RDA FOR NONPREGNANT FEMALE (25-50 YR)	RDA DURING PREGNANCY	RDA FOR LACTATION* (FIRST 6 MO/SECOND 6 MO)	REASONS FOR INCREASED NEED	FOOD SOURCES
Calories	2200	2200 (first trimester); 2500 (second and third trimesters)	2700/2700	Increased energy needs for fetal growth and milk production	Carbohydrate, fat, protein
Protein (g)	50	60	65/62	Synthesis of the products of conception: fetus, amniotic fluid, placenta; growth of maternal tissue: uterus, breasts, red blood cells, plasma proteins, secretion of milk protein during lactation	Meats, eggs, milk, cheese, legumes (dry beans and peas, peanuts), nuts, grains
Minerals					
Calcium (mg)	800	1200	1200/1200	Fetal skeleton and tooth bud formation; maintenance of maternal bone and tooth mineralization	Milk, cheese, yogurt, sardines or other fish eaten with bones left in, deep green leafy vegetables except spinach or Swiss chard,† tofu, baked beans
Phosphorus (mg)	800	1200	1200/1200	Fetal skeleton and tooth bud formation	Milk, cheese, yogurt, meats, whole grains, nuts, legumes
Iron (mg)	15	30	15/15	Increased maternal hemoglobin formation, fetal liver iron storage	Liver, meats, whole or enriched breads and cereals, deep green leafy vegetables, legumes, dried fruits
Zinc (mg)	12	15	19/16	Component of numerous enzyme systems; possibly important in preventing congenital malformations	Liver, shellfish, meats, whole grains, milk

Continued.

RDA, Recommended daily allowance.
*Milk production generally declines during the second 6 months of lactation as the infant's diet increasingly begins to include other foods. Thus maternal needs for many nutrients decrease.
†Spinach and chard contain calcium but also contain oxalin acid, which inhibits calcium absorption.

TABLE 8-2 Nutritional Recommendations During Pregnancy and Lactation—cont'd

NUTRIENT	RDA FOR NONPREGNANT FEMALE (25-50 YR)	RDA DURING PREGNANCY	RDA FOR LACTATION* (FIRST 6 MO/SECOND 6 MO)	REASONS FOR INCREASED NEED	FOOD SOURCES
Iodine (μg)	150	175	200/200	Increased maternal metabolic rate	Iodized salt, seafood, milk and milk products, commercial yeast breads, rolls, and donuts
Magnesium (μg)	280	320	355/340	Involved in energy and protein metabolism, tissue growth, muscle action	Nuts, legumes, cocoa, meats, whole grains
Selenium (mg)	55	65	75/75	Antioxidant (protects cell membranes), tooth component	Organ meats, seafood, whole grains, legumes, molasses
Fat-soluble vitamins					
A (RE)†	800	800	1300/1200	Essential for cell development, thus growth; tooth bud formation (development of enamel-forming cells in gum tissue); bone growth	Deep green leafy vegetables, dark yellow vegetables and fruits, chili peppers, liver, fortified margarine and butter
D (mg)‡	5	10	10/10	Involved in absorption of calcium and phosphorus, improves mineralization	Fortified milk, fortified margarine, egg yolk, butter, liver, seafood
E (μg)	8	10	12/11	Antioxidant (protects cell membranes from damage), especially important for preventing hemolysis of red blood cells	Vegetable oils, green leafy vegetables, whole grains, liver, nuts and seeds, cheese, fish
Water-soluble vitamins					
C (mg)	60	70	95/90	Tissue formation and integrity, formation of connective tissue, enhancement of iron absorption	Citrus fruits, strawberries, melons, broccoli, tomatoes, peppers, raw deep green leafy vegetables

*Milk production generally declines during the second 6 months of lactation as the infant's diet increasingly begins to include other foods. Thus maternal needs for many nutrients decreases.
†*RE*, Retinol equivalents. Replaces international units (IU). 1 RE = 5 IU.
‡As cholecalciferol. 10 μg cholecalciferol = 400 IU of vitamin D.

TABLE 8-2 Nutritional Recommendations During Pregnancy and Lactation—cont'd

NUTRIENT	RDA FOR NONPREGNANT FEMALE (25-50 YR)	RDA DURING PREGNANCY	RDA FOR LACTATION* (FIRST 6 MO/SECOND 6 MO)	REASONS FOR INCREASED NEED	FOOD SOURCES
Folic acid (µg)	180	400	280/260	Increased red blood cell formation, prevention of macrocytic or megaloblastic anemia	Green leafy vegetables, oranges, broccoli, asparagus, artichokes, liver
Thiamin (mg)	1.1	1.5	1.6/1.6	Involved in energy metabolism	Pork, beef, liver, whole or enriched grains, legumes
Riboflavin (mg)	1.3	1.6	1.8/1.7	Involved in energy and protein metabolism	Milk, liver, enriched grains, deep green and yellow vegetables
Pyridoxine (B$_6$) (mg)	1.6	2.2	2.1/2.1	Involved in protein metabolism	Meat, liver, deep green vegetables, whole grains
B$_{12}$ (µg)	2.0	2.2	2.6/2.6	Production of nucleic acids and proteins, especially important in formation of red blood cells and prevention of megaloblastic or macrocytic anemia	Milk, egg, meat, liver, cheese
Niacin (mg)	15	17	20/20	Involved in energy metabolism	Meat, fish, poultry, liver, whole or enriched grains, peanuts

*Milk production generally declines during the second 6 months of lactation as the infant's diet increasingly begins to include other foods. Thus maternal needs for many nutrients decrease.

Energy

Additional **energy (kcal)** needs during pregnancy are determined by changes in the woman's BMR, usual weight for height, physical activity, and age. This increase in basal needs plus the energy needed for new tissue metabolism is about 80,000 calories over the entire pregnancy. This means an additional 300 calories per day during the second and third trimesters for a woman of standard weight for height at the time of conception, or an increase in energy intake of 10% to 15% (see Table 8-1). For example, the additional 300 calories could be obtained by adding 1 cup of lowfat milk, two slices of bread, and an orange to a normal day's intake.

During the first trimester nutritional needs are more qualitative than quantitative. This means that the diet of the pregnant woman should be well balanced and include a variety of foods from the food guide pyramid (Fig. 8-2) but not necessarily be any higher in energy intake. The underweight woman (BMI <19) or the woman who participates in a high level of exercise during her pregnancy needs additional energy. The last trimester of pregnancy is the period when most fetal growth occurs, and fat, iron, and calcium stores are deposited for postnatal growth needs. The same recommendations for energy intake cannot be used for all pregnant women but *must* be individualized.

It is recommended that desirable body weight, or some weight between present and desirable weight— be used to calculate energy needs for the obese pregnant woman. A diet restrictive in energy intake also restricts the intake of specific nutrients needed to support a successful pregnancy. Optimum protein utilization in pregnancy apparently requires a minimum energy intake of 30 kcal per kilogram of body weight per day; otherwise dietary protein is used as an energy source rather than in tissue synthesis for fetal and maternal organs. Strict dietary restrictions could also result in the production of ketones because fat would be catabolized to produce needed energy. Fetal central nervous system development could be adversely affected by the resulting *ketosis*.

For older women a lower BMR affects nutritional needs. For each decade over the age of 20 the resting BMR decreases by about 2%. Energy needs for the pregnant woman over 35 may be about 4% less than for the younger woman. The recommended energy intake for these women may need to be less than for younger women but the need for specific nutrients may *not* be correspondingly lower.

Protein

Additional protein is needed during gestation to provide the essential nitrogen to meet the demands for fetal and maternal tissue growth. On average, 925 g of protein are deposited in the normal weight fetus and maternal accessory tissues. Thus the recommended intake is 60 g of protein each day. This recommendation assumes that the mother is consuming an adequate intake of energy to spare the protein for tissue synthesis. Achieving this intake is not difficult, since most women in the United States consume approximately 70 to 100 g of protein daily, or 10 to 40 g more than that needed during pregnancy. The additional protein should be of high biologic value, or proteins that contain all of the *essential amino acids*. Meat, fish, poultry, eggs, cheese, and milk are examples of proteins of high biologic value. Other important nutrients are also provided by these foods.

High-protein supplements are not recommended during pregnancy. These supplements have been associated with an increased number of prematurely born infants and an excessive number of neonatal deaths (Tierson, Olsen, Hook, 1986). It is believed that excessive protein intake may cause more rapid fetal maturation and bring about an earlier birth.

Recommendations for protein intake also vary with age. The following guidelines are suggested:
- Mature women (>18 years): 1.3 g protein per kilogram of pregnant weight
- Adolescent girls (15 to 18 years): 1.5 g protein per kilogram of pregnant weight
- Younger girls (<15 years): 1.7 g protein per kilogram of pregnant weight

The increased intake for adolescents and younger girls is based on the likelihood that their own bodies are continuing to develop. If a multifetal birth is expected, additional protein, as well as other nutrients, is needed in the mother's diet.

Fluid

Fluid is not often thought of as a nutrient, but water does play an important role during pregnancy. Water assists digestion by dissolving food and aiding its transport. Essential during the exchange of nutrients and waste products across cell membranes, water is the main substance of cells, blood, lymph, and other vital body fluids. It also aids in maintaining body temperature. A good fluid intake promotes good bowel function, which is sometimes a problem during pregnancy. The recommended daily intake is about 6 to 8 glasses (1500 to 2000 ml) of fluid. Water and fruit juices are two good sources. Caffeine-containing beverages, such as colas and some other soft drinks, and coffee should be consumed in limited quantities or avoided. Saccharin-containing beverages should be avoided altogether because it has been linked to bladder cancer in laboratory animals. Beverages containing aspartame (Equal, Nutrasweet), another alternate sweetener, should be consumed in moderate amounts. Aspartame has *not* been noted to have adverse effects on normal mothers carrying normal fetuses, but not enough evidence is available to recommend more than cautious use.

Vitamins and Minerals
Fat-Soluble Vitamins

There is an increased need for vitamins A, D, E, and K during pregnancy. However, symptoms of deficiencies of these vitamins are rarely seen during pregnancy. Vitamin E prevents the oxidation of vitamin A in the gastrointestinal tract, enabling more of the vitamin to be absorbed. A deficiency of vitamin K, known to be an essential factor in blood clotting, is extremely rare in adults. Vitamin K is produced by flora in the gastrointestinal tract. Transport across the placenta is so slow that most infants are born with a low level of this vitamin. They are usually several days old before their sterile gut can establish an effective microbe population. The recommendation is that all neonates receive an injection of vitamin K within 2 hours after birth to prevent the risk of intraventricular hemorrhage.

Because of the potential for toxicity, pregnant women are advised not to take fat-soluble vitamin supplements unless prescribed by a health care provider. Vitamins A and D are transported through the placenta by simple diffusion, and they will continue to accumulate in the fetus as long as maternal levels are high.

No increase is recommended in the daily intake of vitamin A. Doses larger than 25,000 IU a day have been found to cause problems with fetal development and liver damage in the mother. Routinely prescribed prenatal vitamins contain 8000 to 10,000 IUs and are not problematic. Increased intake of beta-carotene, a precursor of vitamin A, does not appear to cause problems. Special attention needs to be given to women who use the drug isotretinoin in the treatment of acne. The use of this product has been associated with fetal defects. This is more common when dealing with a pregnant teenager.

Vitamin D plays an important role in promoting positive calcium balance in pregnancy. It occurs naturally in fish oils, eggs, butter, and liver. It is also produced in the skin by the action of ultraviolet light (irradiation) on dehydrocholesterol. The daily consumption of a quart of milk provides the full recommended allowance of vitamin D, calcium, and protein for most women. An excessive intake of vitamin D by the mother may cause hypercalcemia in her infant, which could lead to neonatal seizures.

Water-Soluble Vitamins

An important function of thiamin, riboflavin, pyridoxine (B_6), and cobalamin (B_{12}) is that of coenzymes in energy metabolism. The need for these vitamins increases during the second and third trimesters of pregnancy when energy intake increases. This increased need is easily met from consuming a variety of foods including whole grains, organ meats, pork, dairy products, and leafy green vegetables. Low maternal levels of B_{12} are associated with prematurity and central nervous system abnormalities in the offspring. This occurs more often in women who are strict vegetarians (vegans) and is more pronounced if these infants are breastfed with B_{12}-deficient milk (Graham, Arvela, Wise, 1992).

Vitamin C (ascorbic acid) plays an important role in tissue formation and integrity and increases the absorption of iron, especially nonheme iron (iron from nonmeat sources). A slight increase in vitamin C intake is recommended during pregnancy. However, excessive doses may cause metabolic dependency in the fetus and lead to neonatal scurvy. The recommended daily intake of 70 mg is easily met by a normal diet that includes at least one serving of citrus fruit or juice.

Iron

The iron needed to support a normal single pregnancy is about 1000 mg (Institute of Medicine, 1990); 350 mg are for fetal and placental growth, 450 mg are for increased maternal red blood cell mass, and 240 mg for basal losses. This does not include the iron in the blood lost during birth. A healthy, full-term infant is born with iron stores of about 75 mg per kilogram of body weight, most of which is deposited during the last trimester of pregnancy. If adequate iron is not available to meet the needs of the mother, fetus, and placenta, this fetal reserve will not suffer but maternal iron stores will be depleted and maternal red blood cell mass will be reduced.

Iron deficiency, or frank anemia in the mother, can cause decreased oxygen for the fetus, leading to IUGR, and increased cardiac stress and complications during birth for the mother.

Iron is the one nutrient that cannot be obtained in adequate amounts from dietary sources during pregnancy. **Iron supplementation,** using a ferrous salt in a dose of 30 mg per day, is usually started at the first prenatal visit to maintain maternal reserves and to meet fetal requirements. For the woman who has used an intrauterine device (IUD) as a form of contraception, the need may be even greater because increased blood losses occur with the use of this device. The woman who has been taking oral contraceptives, however, may have good iron status at the time of conception because iron losses are reduced considerably by the decreased menstrual flow. Women who are at higher risk for iron deficiency, such as those just mentioned or those carrying multiple fetuses, may need a higher dose (e.g., 60 mg per day). Iron sulfate supplements may cause stool color to change to a grayish black. Some women experience nausea, vomiting, and even diarrhea or constipation. To reduce these symptoms, the supplemental iron should be taken between meals or at bedtime with a good source of vitamin C to promote absorption. The combination multivitamin/iron pill is not recommended because the calcium and magnesium salts present in the pill can interfere with iron availability (Teaching Approaches).

Calcium

The fetus draws about 250 to 300 mg of calcium per day from the maternal blood supply, primarily during the

TEACHING APPROACHES

IRON SUPPLEMENTATION

- It is difficult to consume enough iron in the diet to meet iron needs and prevent anemia during pregnancy.
- Vitamin C (in citrus fruits, tomatoes, melons, and strawberries) and heme iron (in meats) increase iron supplement absorption. Include these in the diet often.
- Bran, tea, coffee, milk, oxalates (in spinach and Swiss chard), and egg yolk decrease iron absorption. Avoid consuming them at the same time as the supplement.
- Iron is best absorbed if it is taken when the stomach is empty; that is, take it between meals with a beverage other than tea, coffee, or milk.
- Iron can be taken at bedtime if abdominal discomfort occurs when it is taken between meals.
- Keep the supplement in a child-proof container out of the reach of any children in the household.

third trimester. At birth the infant has deposited about 25 g for use in bone development. Maternal calcium metabolism undergoes changes during early pregnancy. These changes allow extra calcium to be stored in maternal bone to provide for the increased demands of the third trimester and of lactation. The recommended intake for calcium is 1200 mg per day (1600 mg if the pregnant woman is a teenager). This need of 1200 mg/day can easily be met by consuming 1 quart of milk daily (there are 300 mg of calcium in an 8-oz glass). This amount of milk also meets the need for extra protein and several other essential nutrients. Even in women who are somewhat **lactose (milk sugar) intolerant** (especially true of African-American and Hispanic women) there appears to be an increase in tolerance during pregnancy. Since dairy products provide the most available calcium, yogurt and cheese are recommended if milk cannot be used to meet calcium needs. Dark green, leafy vegetables such as kale, cabbage, collards, and turnip greens and calcium-fortified orange juice may also be used. Other dark green leafy vegetables such as spinach, chard, and beet greens contain calcium that is not available to the body. Some women must avoid all or most milk products. Some suggestions to increase the calcium intake of these women are listed in the Teaching Approaches box at right. If these suggestions prove unsuccessful, the use of a calcium supplement should be discussed with the health care provider. The type of supplement used should be carefully checked for lead content. Some "natural" calcium supplements contain excessive quantities of lead, which could potentially harm the developing fetus (Bourgoin et al, 1993).

The issue of calcium supplementation and its effect on pregnancy-induced hypertension (PIH) is still unresolved, although recent studies have demonstrated that calcium may play a role in its prevention (Knight, Keith, 1991).

Folate

Because folate is intimately involved in DNA synthesis and is also needed for the increased *erythropoiesis* (production of red blood cells), requirements are particularly high in rapidly growing cells such as fetal and placental tissues. The increased levels of steroid hormones during pregnancy may interfere with the utilization of folate. Women who have a history of using oral contraceptives may be marginal in folate status, since the steroid levels in these products also interfere with folate metabolism. Recently, diets deficient in folate have been implicated as a risk factor in the occurrence of neural tube defects (NTDs) in the offspring. The Centers for Disease Control and Prevention (1992) and the American Academy of Pediatrics (1993) have now recommended that all women of childbearing age who are capable of becoming pregnant receive a daily intake of 0.4 mg of folate. However, the minimal intake needed to prevent NTDs

TEACHING APPROACHES

WAYS TO INCREASE YOUR CALCIUM INTAKE IF YOU AVOID MOST MILK PRODUCTS

Choose more foods that provide calcium, such as the following:
- Foods equal to about 1 cup of milk in calcium content:
  3 oz of sardines (if the bones are eaten)
- Foods equal to about ½ cup of milk in calcium content:
  3 oz of canned salmon (if the bones are eaten)
  4 oz of tofu (if it has been processed with calcium sulfate)
  4 oz of collards
  1 waffle* (7 inches in diameter)
  4 corn tortillas (if processed with calcium salts)
- Foods equal to about ⅓ cup of milk in calcium content:
  1 cup of cooked dried beans
  4 oz of bok choy or turnip greens or kale
  1 medium square of cornbread* (2½ × 2½ × 1½ inches)
  2 pancakes* (4 inches in diameter)
  7 to 9 oysters
  3 oz of shrimp
- Foods that can be made high in calcium:
  Soups made from bones cooked with vinegar or tomato
  Macaroni and cheese* and other combination foods made with good sources of calcium
- Ask your health care provider about taking a calcium supplement.

Modified from Food and Nutrition Board, Institute of Medicine: *Nutrition during pregnancy and lactation: An implementation guide,* Washington, DC, 1992, National Academy Press.
*A dairy product is a major contributor to the calcium content of this food.

has not yet been established (Herbert, 1992). The chief dietary sources of folate are dark green leafy vegetables, oranges, bananas, whole wheat, liver, and potatoes. Supplements may be necessary for some individuals. The dangers of excess folate include masking symptoms of iron and vitamin B_{12} deficiencies.

Zinc

The metal zinc is a constituent of numerous enzymes involved in major metabolic pathways. Low maternal zinc levels are associated with more complications in the prenatal and intrapartum periods. Alcohol consumption is known to interfere with placental zinc transfer and may account for some of the anomalies noted in offspring with fetal alcohol syndrome. The RDA for zinc during pregnancy is 15 mg per day, which can readily be obtained from meat, shellfish, and whole grain breads and cereals. Caution must be taken regarding excess zinc supplementation because it could interfere with both iron and copper metabolism. High maternal zinc levels in midpregnancy are also associated with decreased fetal growth and may be associated with an inadequate zinc transfer to the fetus.

Sodium

Sodium metabolism is altered by the many hormonal interactions specific to the state of pregnancy. As the maternal fluid volume expands, the glomerular filtration rate of the kidneys increases to handle this greater fluid volume. Much of the weight gained during pregnancy is due to this increase in body fluid volume, which is primarily extracellular fluid (ECF). Sodium is a major constituent of ECF; therefore the need for sodium actually increases during pregnancy. The water-retaining effects of estrogen and the sodium-losing effect of progesterone produce a confusing picture of fluid and electrolyte balance during pregnancy. The practice of restricting dietary sodium was once used to help control the moderate peripheral edema of pregnancy caused by these hormones. Moderate edema is a normal phenomenon of pregnancy and should not be treated with diuretics or a restricted sodium intake. Sodium restriction may stress the body's ability to retain sodium, leading to a sodium depletion in the mother. Neonatal hyponatremia (low blood sodium) has been observed in infants born to women who severely restricted their intake of sodium prior to birth (Worthington-Roberts, Williams, 1993).

There is no RDA or estimated requirement for sodium during pregnancy, but a reasonable guideline is 2 to 3 gm per day unless the woman's medical condition contraindicates this amount. The use of high-sodium, low-nutrient foods is not recommended. This practice may lead to excessive fluid retention, causing a more generalized edema and perhaps predisposing the woman to PIH.

Fluoride

The role of fluoride in the prenatal development of teeth is not well understood. A long-term, prospective study is currently underway at the Eastman Dental Center in Rochester, in which the effectiveness of prenatal fluoride supplementation on the incidence of tooth decay in 5-year-old children is being evaluated (Worthington-Roberts, Williams, 1993). The final verdict on the effect of prenatal fluoride supplementation on the development of caries-resistant teeth in the infant is still out.

Nutrient Supplements

The indications for prescribing vitamin and mineral supplements for the pregnant woman appear in Table 8-3. The consensus of the 1990 Institute of Medicine committee is that food can and should be the normal ve-

hicle to meet the additional needs imposed by pregnancy, except for iron. Recall that a supplemental dose of 30 mg per day is recommended. For women who need a therapeutic dose of iron (60 mg per day or more) due to anemia, it is recommended that zinc and copper also be supplemented. The competition for binding sites for absorption of these nutrients could lead to a deficiency of the latter nutrients if supplements are not provided. However, some women chronically consume diets that are deficient in necessary nutrients and, for whatever reason, may be unable to change this intake. For these women a supplement should be considered. It is important that the pregnant woman understand that the use of a vitamin/mineral supplement does not lessen the need to consume a nutritious, well-balanced diet. Calcium supplementation may be recommended if daily intake falls below 600 mg. This supplement should be taken with meals to enhance absorption (Institute of Medicine, 1990).

Care Management

As stated earlier, maternal nutrition should be a focus during all phases of reproductive life, from childhood to menopause. Ideally, a nutritional assessment is performed before conception. This allows for any recommended changes in diet, lifestyle, and weight status to be undertaken before becoming pregnant. However, under usual circumstances this does not occur. Most women are highly motivated during pregnancy to do what is right for their baby and are very receptive to advice. Optimal nutrition cannot prevent all problems that might arise during pregnancy but does provide a sound basis for supporting the needs of the mother and her developing fetus.

✤ ASSESSMENT

The assessment and evaluation of nutritional status are generally made at the beginning of prenatal care, with continued follow-up throughout the pregnancy. The assessment consists of (1) an interview (background data including a diet history and evaluation, food practices, living situation), (2) a physical examination, including breast examination to identify potential problems with breastfeeding, and (3) laboratory tests.

The Interview

A woman's nutritional status can be affected by many nondietary factors (see Fig. 8-1). Thus diet and eating habits cannot be viewed in isolation from the rest of the woman's life situations. A good way to begin the nutritional assessment is to have the woman respond to a questionnaire that includes not only dietary intake information but available resources, commonly consumed beverages, and other eating behaviors. (Box 8-1 is an ex-

TABLE 8-3 Indications for Nutrient Supplementation

REPRODUCTIVE PERIOD AND CONDITION	LOW-DOSE (30 MG) IRON*,†	60-120 MG OF IRON†,‡	LOW-DOSE MULTIVITAMIN/ MINERAL PREPARATION	600 MG OF CALCIUM
Preconception, inter-conception				
Iron-deficiency anemia		✔	✔	
Pregnancy				
Normal	✔			
Complete vegetarian			✔	
Multiple gestation			✔	
Poor quality diet and resistant to change			✔	
Heavy cigarette smoking			✔	
Alcohol abuse			✔	
Under age 25, consuming no calcium-rich milk products, and resistant to change			✔§	✔
Iron-deficiency anemia		✔	✔	
Lactation				
Low energy intake			✔	
Low intake of milk products			✔§	✔
Iron-deficiency anemia		✔	✔	

Modified from Food and Nutrition Board, Institute of Medicine: *Nutrition during pregnancy and lactation: an implementation guide,* Washington, DC, 1992, National Academic Press.
*Begin routine iron supplementation for all pregnant women by the twelfth week of gestation.
†Iron should be taken with juice or water, apart from meals.
‡Therapeutic doses of iron should be taken apart from other supplements.
§The vitamin supplement is indicated to supply vitamin D. Regular exposure to sunshine reduces the need for this supplement.

ample of such a questionnaire.) If nutrition counseling is to be successful, it must be individualized for each woman based on information gathered during the interview. Whatever format is decided upon, the following information needs to be obtained:

- Dietary practices, including a *diet history* using a recall of the previous 24-hour intake and a review of foods typically consumed (food frequency)
- Analysis of intake using the food guide pyramid
- Screening for other problem areas: access to food, inclusion or exclusion of any foods that could be problematic, such as adherence to a strict vegetarian diet, cultural, ethnic, religious food practices, or fad diets
- Use of alcohol, illicit drugs, cigarettes (including exposure to passive smoke), caffeine

- Attitude regarding weight gain
- Pica (see p. 192 for a discussion of this practice)
- Emotional state regarding pregnancy
- Any recent major weight swings
- Early teenage pregnancy
- Multifetal pregnancy
- How the woman plans to feed her infant after birth

Laboratory Tests

Laboratory data provide vital baseline information for nutrition assessment at the beginning of pregnancy as well as a means of monitoring nutritional status throughout gestation. Hemoglobin and hematocrit are the only practical tests to administer in routine prenatal care. These values are normally lower in pregnant than in

BOX 8-1

Nutrition Questionnaire

What you eat and some of the lifestyle choices you make can affect your nutrition and health now and in the future. Your nutrition can also have an important effect on your baby's health. Please answer these questions by circling the answers that apply to you.

EATING BEHAVIOR

1. Are you frequently bothered by any of the following? (circle all that apply):

Nausea   Vomiting   Heartburn   Constipation

2. Do you skip meals at least 3 times a week?   No   Yes
3. Do you try to limit the amount or kind of food you eat to control your weight?   No   Yes
4. Are you on a special diet now?   No   Yes
5. Do you avoid any foods for health or religious reasons?   No   Yes

FOOD RESOURCES

1. Do you have a working stove?   No   Yes
   Do you have a working refrigerator?   No   Yes
2. Do you sometimes run out of food before you are able to buy more?   No   Yes
3. Can you afford to eat the way you should?   No   Yes
4. Are you receiving any food assistance now? (circle all that apply):   No   Yes

Food stamps   School breakfast   School lunch
WIC   Donated food/commodities   CSFP
Food from a food pantry, soup kitchen, or food bank

5. Do you feel you need help in obtaining food?   No   Yes

FOOD AND DRINK

1. Which of these did you drink yesterday?
   (circle all that apply):

Soft drinks	Coffee	Tea	Fruit drink
Orange juice	Grapefruit juice	Other juices	Milk
Kool-Aid	Beer	Wine	Alcoholic drinks
Water	Other beverages (list)_____

2. Which of these foods did you eat yesterday?
   (circle all that apply):

Cheese   Pizza   Macaroni and cheese
Yogurt   Cereal with milk
Other foods made with cheese (such as tacos, enchiladas, lasagna, cheeseburgers)

Corn	Potatoes	Sweet potatoes	Green salad
Carrots	Collard greens	Spinach	Turnip greens
Broccoli	Green beans	Green peas	Other vegetables
Apples	Bananas	Berries	Grapefruit
Melon	Oranges	Peaches	Other fruit
Meat	Fish	Chicken	Eggs
Peanut butter	Nuts	Seeds	Dried beans
Cold cuts	Hot dog	Bacon	Sausage
Cake	Cookies	Doughnut	Pastry
Chips	French fries		

Other deep-fried foods, such as fried chicken or egg rolls

| Bread | Rolls | Rice | Cereal |
| Noodles | Spaghetti | Tortillas | |

Were any of these whole grain?   No   Yes
3. Is the way you ate yesterday the way you usually eat?   No   Yes

LIFESTYLE

1. Do you exercise for at least 30 minutes on a regular basis (3 times a week or   No   Yes
   more)?
2. Do you ever smoke cigarettes or use smokeless tobacco?   No   Yes
3. Do you ever drink beer, wine, liquor, or any other alcoholic beverages?   No   Yes
4. Which of these do you take?
   (circle all that apply):

Prescribed drugs or medications
Any over-the-counter products (such as aspirin, Tylenol, antacids, or vitamins)
Street drugs (such as marijuana, speed, downers, crack, or heroin)

Modified from Food and Nutrition Board, Institute of Medicine: *Nutrition during pregnancy and lactation: an implementation guide,* Washington, DC, 1992, National Academic Press.

TABLE 8-4 Cutoff Values for Anemia for Women

PREGNANCY STATUS	HEMOGLOBIN (g/dl)	HEMATOCRIT (%)
Nonpregnant	12.0	36
Pregnant		
Trimester 1	11.0	33
Trimester 2	10.5	32
Trimester 3	11.0	33

nonpregnant women (Table 8-4). They are lowest during the second trimester of pregnancy, when the physiologic anemia of pregnancy occurs. Special cutoff values have been established for determining anemia in women who smoke cigarettes based on the number of cigarettes smoked per day. These cutoff points are higher than for the nonsmoking pregnant woman because of the decreased oxygen-carrying capacity of the mother's blood due to smoking. Altitude adjustments are also available in the Institute of Medicine Implementation Guide (1992). The effects of altitude and smoking are additive.

If desired, a serum ferritin test may also be performed to assess iron stores. Tests for blood levels of various vitamins and minerals are not considered valid because there are no pregnancy standards. Only nonpregnant standards are available, and these levels are affected by the stage of gestation. Universal screening for gestational diabetes is important for all pregnant women. This test is administered between the twenty-fourth and twenty-eighth week of pregnancy. Women who test positive should be referred to a registered dietitian for nutritional management.

Physical Examination

Anthropometry, the study of human body measurements, provides both short- and long-term indications of the level of nutrition and is therefore a valuable component of the nutrition assessment profile. Assessment of height and weight is performed and BMI is calculated. Care must be taken to ensure that proper equipment and techniques are used for anthropometric assessment; for example, the scale must be calibrated to zero before a weight is taken. Inaccurate measurements can lead to inappropriate conclusions. This could result in poor decisions followed by poor patient care management. Serial weight measurements give a reasonable indication of excessive weight gain and the possibility of obesity. Anthropometric data can be collected and plotted on an appropriate graph such as the one in Fig. 8-5.

The physical examination should include a breast examination to identify any problems, such as inverted nipples, which will need to be addressed if the mother wants to breastfeed her infant.

An obstetric health history includes the form of contraception used before conception, number of pregnancies and their outcomes, and interval between pregnancies. Any medical problems that may have nutritional implications, such as diabetes, cystic fibrosis, phenylketonuria, and lactose (milk sugar) intolerance, need to be identified. Information regarding the use of any medications and vitamin and mineral supplements should also be obtained.

General screening for dental health status provides helpful information on nutritional status. The most common clinical nutrition-related disorders likely to be encountered during the reproductive years are caries and periodontitis. These conditions cause mechanical and mastication difficulties that may interfere with the ingestion of certain types of foods, such as meats.

Each pregnant woman and her family present the nurse with a unique set of nutritional needs. The nurse formulates appropriate nursing diagnoses based on the identified needs from the assessment data. Box 8-2 provides a list of nutritional risk factors that might be encountered.

✤ NURSING DIAGNOSES

Nutrition-related nursing diagnoses that commonly arise from the assessment include the following:

Altered nutrition: less than body requirements related to

- A poor understanding of the nutritional needs and optimal weight gain during pregnancy, inadequate income, stress over an unwanted pregnancy, nausea and vomiting (either the mild to moderate effects of morning sickness or the more severe effects of hyperemesis gravidarum), cultural patterns of food intake, adherence to a therapeutic diet regimen, concurrent use of medications, drug or alcohol abuse, failure to take nutritional supplements as prescribed, smoking, multifetal gestation, or adolescent pregnancy, in which the increased needs of pregnancy are imposed on a girl whose own needs for growth and maturation are still high and whose eating habits are often poor.

Altered nutrition: more than body requirements related to

- A poor understanding of nutritional needs and optimal weight gain during pregnancy, with resultant overeating, cultural patterns that foster overeating, a decline in activity as pregnancy progresses, and use of unneeded dietary supplements (particularly supplements of fat-soluble vitamins).

Altered nutrition: high risk for more than body requirements related to

- The same factors as for preceding diagnosis.
- Constipation related to
- A decrease in activity with pregnancy, inadequate fiber or fluid intake, use of an iron supplement, displacement of the intestines by the enlarging uterus, and increased progesterone levels during pregnancy, which decrease the tone and motility of the intestinal musculature.

✤ EXPECTED OUTCOMES

The team approach has been devised as an attempt to meet some of the problems brought about by the rapid expansion of scientific knowledge, which in turn has brought an increasing complexity to health care. The rapid advance of science requires the cooperation of a team of specialists who share their special knowledge and learn from each other for the welfare of the patient.

Whether functioning in the hospital, the clinic, or the community, the registered dietitian (RD) and the nurse hold positions on the health team in a unique relationship with the patient. In certain respects they are closest to the pregnant woman and her family and have the opportunity to help determine many of the woman's needs, including basic nutritional needs. They must coordinate services and often are the only key professionals who can help the woman understand and participate in her own care. They have unparalleled opportunity to practice continuous patient-centered care that treats the whole person. Such practitioners realize that their most therapeutic contribution is their genuine involvement and concern. The nurse plays a critical role in providing individualized care by assessing the patient, consulting with other members of the health care team, and referring the patient as appropriate.

An individualized nursing care plan based on the nursing diagnoses should be developed with the patient. Some common nutrition-related expected outcomes are that the woman will take the following actions:

1. Achieve an appropriate weight gain during pregnancy. An appropriate goal for weight gain takes into account factors such as prepregnancy weight, presence of overweight/obesity or underweight, and whether the pregnancy is single or multifetal.
2. Consume adequate nutrients from the diet and supplements to meet estimated needs.
3. Cope with nutrition-related discomforts associated with pregnancy, such as pyrosis (heartburn), morning sickness, and constipation.
4. Avoid or reduce potentially harmful practices such as smoking, alcohol consumption, and caffeine intake.
5. Make an informed decision about the method of feeding her infant. This decision must be one with which the mother (and usually her family members or other members of her support system) is satisfied, and not necessarily the choice that would seem best to the health care team.
6. Return to prepregnancy weight (or an appropriate weight for height) within 6 months after giving birth.

✤ COLLABORATIVE CARE

Nutritional care and teaching generally involve (1) acquainting the woman with nutritional needs during pregnancy and the characteristics of an adequate diet, if necessary, (2) helping the woman to individualize her diet so that she achieves an adequate intake while satisfying her personal, cultural, financial, and health needs, (3) acquainting her with strategies for coping with the nutrition-related discomforts of pregnancy, (4) helping the woman to use nutrition supplements appropriately, (5) discussing with her the advantages and disadvantages of breastfeeding and formula feeding her infant and supporting her in her decision, and (6) consulting with and making referrals to other professionals or services as necessary.

Resources

Several helpful resources can provide nutrition information and guidance for the pregnant woman. These include the new food guide pyramid, a sample meal pat-

TABLE 8-5 Sample Daily Meal Patterns

FOOD GROUP	KEY NUTRIENTS SUPPLIED	NUMBER OF SERVINGS
Milk, yogurt, and cheese: 1 cup; 1½ ounces for cheese	Protein Riboflavin Calcium	3*
Meat, poultry, fish, dry beans, eggs, and nuts: 2-3 ounces meat; 1 cup beans; 2 eggs; ½ cup nuts	Protein Thiamin Vitamin B_6 Iron Zinc	3
Vegetables: ½ cup or ¾ cup raw	Vitamin A Vitamin C Folate Dietary fiber	3
Fruits: 1 piece generally	Vitamin C Folate Dietary fiber	2
Breads, cereals, rice, and pasta: 1 slice or ½-¾ cup cooked	B vitamins Iron Dietary fiber	6

Modified from Worthington-Roberts B and Williams SR: *Nutrition in pregnancy and lactation,* ed 5, St Louis, 1993, Mosby.
*Four servings if a teenager.

tern and sample menus, and information on cultural and ethnic food preferences and the vegetarian diet. Individuals with insufficient income to purchase foods may have a nutritionally inadequate diet. The nutrients that are most commonly deficient in this population are protein, iron, and folate. To help encourage a more adequate dietary intake, persons who have limited incomes should be referred to federal food programs such as the special supplemental food program for pregnant and lactating women and children (WIC) and the food stamp program. Nutrition education, counseling, and budgeting are also important to ensure the benefits of these programs.

In 1991 the basic 4 food groups, with which everyone was familiar, were replaced by the **food guide pyramid** (see Fig. 8-2). Each of the foods in the pyramid is a source of some, but not all, of the nutrients needed daily by all individuals. A diet consisting of a variety of foods from all levels of the pyramid can supply the needed nutrients to support pregnancy, except for iron. No one food group is more important than any other; for a nutritious diet all food groups should be included daily. The base of the pyramid emphasizes the importance of whole-grain breads and cereals, which are good sources of the B vitamins and fiber. The next level includes fruits and vegetables, also good sources of nutrients and fiber. Nearer the top are the meat, fish, poultry, and dairy product foods. These foods are good sources of protein, calcium, iron and zinc. At the top of the pyramid are fats, oils, and sweets. These items provide calories and also increase the palatability of some of the other foods on the pyramid. These items should be used sparingly. The appropriate number of servings from each of the five groups for pregnant women has not yet been determined.

It is necessary to show the pregnant woman how the food guide pyramid should be used. Sample daily meal patterns accompanied by sample menus can be very helpful (Table 8-5 and Box 8-3). A jointly developed plan, based on mutually acceptable goals, is more likely to be accepted and followed by the woman than one written by the nurse or dietitian alone.

Exercise

Exercise has an effect on the nutritional needs of the pregnant woman. Energy intake must be increased to support the recommended weight gain and allow for the energy expended during exercise. Providing additional protein could tax the already overworked renal system of the mother and is usually not recommended. Increased fluid intake is essential when exercising. About 5% to 10% of plasma volume can be lost during 30 minutes of strenuous exercise. Water is the recommended replacement for lost fluid.

Rigorous exercise, when the woman is not well conditioned, causes glucose to be diverted from the fetus and placenta to the mother's muscles for energy. This could also contribute to fetal hypoxia as the blood flow through the placenta is diverted to the mother, thus decreasing the supply of oxygen.

BOX 8-3

Sample Menu*

BREAKFAST

¾ cup raisin bran
4 ounces orange juice
½ cup 1% milk

SNACK

2 tablespoons peanut butter
1 slice whole-wheat toast
½ cup plain low-fat yogurt
½ cup strawberries

LUNCH

spinach salad with
2 tablespoons oil and vinegar dressing
½ sliced tomato
2 slices whole-wheat toast
1½ ounces of provolone cheese

DINNER

3 ounces lean ham
1 cup navy beans
1 cornbread muffin
¾ cup cooked broccoli
1 teaspoon corn oil margarine
iced tea or milk (if teenager)

SNACK

4 whole-wheat crackers
1 cup 1% milk

From Wardlaus GM and Insel PM: *Perspectives in nutrition,* St Louis, 1993, Mosby.
*This diet meets the RDA for pregnancy and lactation for only 1800 kcalories (34 mg of iron).

Nutrition-Related Discomforts of Pregnancy

As pregnancy progresses, general nutritional guidance may be needed for the more common gastrointestinal problems encountered. Most of these problems are normal, but individual counseling is needed. If the problems persist or become severe, medical care is advised.

Nausea and Vomiting

Nausea and vomiting of pregnancy, commonly referred to as morning sickness, were first described as far back as 2000 BC (Lucak, Lucak, 1991). To this day there is little documentation regarding the mechanisms responsible. Approximately 50% to 80% of pregnant women experience some degree of nausea and vomiting. The disorder usually disappears by the beginning of the second trimester, but in about 20% of those affected the problem persists throughout the pregnancy. It is of interest to note that a study of over 400 women (Tierson, Olsen, Hook, 1986) found that a significantly higher proportion of women who did not experience morning sickness had an increased number of fetal deaths and more low birth weight infants than women who did ex-

perience nausea and vomiting. Of the women who gave birth to live infants, those who experienced nausea and vomiting also had a higher weight gain. It seems that nausea and vomiting may be positively correlated with a successful pregnancy outcome, but further research using a broader socioeconomic level of subjects is needed.

Some strategies for dealing with the problem of nausea and vomiting are keeping crackers, melba toast, or dry cereal at the bedside to eat before getting up in the morning; eating smaller, more frequent meals; avoiding caffeine-containing beverages, consuming adequate quantities of fluids, but between meals rather than with meals; avoiding cooking or paint odors that cause nausea; and limiting intake of highly spiced foods. Antiemetics are not recommended. Hyperemesis gravidarum, a severe, prolonged, persistent vomiting, requires medical attention. Fluid and electrolyte replacement may be required to prevent complications of dehydration.

Heartburn

Heartburn, which is really the reflux of acidic gastric contents into the esophagus, is most commonly noted during the last trimester of pregnancy, when the fetus is competing with the gastrointestinal tract for abdominal space. The problem is called heartburn because of the proximity of the lower esophagus to the heart. Usually this problem can be controlled by slowly eating small, frequent, low-fat meals; drinking fluids between meals, rather than with meals; limiting spicy foods; avoiding lying down for 1 to 2 hours after eating; and wearing loose-fitting clothing.

Constipation

Constipation is a common problem during pregnancy. Progesterone, one of the placental hormones that plays an active role in pregnancy, causes smooth muscles to relax. This allows increased time for nutrient absorption to occur, an especially important factor for the woman who is of marginal nutritional status. However, it also invites constipation because the colon is more relaxed. In addition, late in pregnancy the enlarging uterus causes pressure on the lower portion of the intestine, making elimination difficult. Iron supplementation can also cause constipation. This problem can be helped by consuming adequate fluids daily, including water, juices, milk, and broth soups; eating high-fiber breads and cereals and generous amounts of fresh fruits and vegetables; and exercising. Laxatives should be avoided unless prescribed by the primary health care provider.

Enlarged veins in the anus caused by the increased fetal weight and downward pressure produced may contribute to *hemorrhoids,* which cause itching and burning. If rupture occurs and there is bleeding upon defecation, additional anxiety may be felt by the mother, and her health care provider should be contacted. Keeping regular bowel habits also helps prevent hemorrhoids and the problems accompanying them.

Leg Cramps

Leg cramps, which are particularly common in the latter stages of pregnancy, may be caused by a maternal imbalance between calcium and phosphorus levels. Limiting milk intake is not recommended. Rather, limiting the intake of phosphorus-containing foods such as soda, refrigerated bakery products, and processed cheese is recommended.

Food Beliefs, Cravings, Avoidances, and Aversions

During pregnancy most women experience aversions to what was once a favorite food. Others experience cravings ("pickles and ice cream"). These cravings and aversions are not necessarily bad. Many cravings result in increased calcium and energy intake. Aversions often result in a decreased alcohol and caffeine intake. Some aversions, however, result in a decreased intake of animal protein, which could be detrimental.

Consideration of a woman's cultural food preferences enhances communication, providing a greater opportunity for compliance with the agreed upon pattern of intake. Women in most cultures are encouraged to eat a diet typical for them. The nurse needs to be aware of what constitutes a typical diet for each cultural or ethnic group (Table 8-6). However, within one cultural group several variations may occur. Thus careful exploration of individual preferences is needed. Although ethnic and cultural food beliefs may seem, at first glance, to conflict with the dietary instruction provided by physicians, nurses, and dietitians, it is often possible for the empathic health care provider to identify cultural beliefs that are congruent with the modern understanding of pregnancy and fetal development. It is important to remember that many cultural food practices have some merit or the culture would not have survived. Food cravings during pregnancy are considered normal by many cultures, but the kinds of cravings often are culturally specific. In most cultures women crave acceptable foods, such as chicken, fish, and greens among African-Americans. Many of their cravings for cultural specialties cannot be completely ignored, even by the most educated women (Kruger, Maetzold, 1983).

Women in some cultures desire nonnutritive substances such as laundry starch, which contains silicone additives, or clay and dirt, which may contain parasites. Desiring or eating these substances is called **pica.** Pica has been attributed to a variety of factors and may be engaged in by children as well as pregnant women. Pica may be a psychologic response of someone needing attention, a truly cultural phenomenon, a response to hunger, or the body's response to needed nutrients. Scientific controversy exists about whether the iron deficiency observed in persons with pica is the cause or the effect of the anemia. Whatever the reason, according to Leiderman et al (1973) a documented result is increased iron-deficiency anemia because of interference with absorption of necessary nutrients when clay is eaten.

Any diet counseling must emphasize planning and implementing an adequate diet utilizing the woman's usual foods and food preferences. To do otherwise is to waste time and energy of both the woman and the nurse. Positive factors should be emphasized. For example, Southeast Asian tradition discourages alcohol consumption during pregnancy. Dietary instruction can reinforce and build on this prohibition. Also, positive teaching techniques should be used to correct problematic cultural or ethnic food habits.

Cultural and ethnic food *taboos* (foods that are forbidden) are more common than food *prescriptions* (foods that are acceptable). Food taboos often follow the principles of imitative magic, in which physical characteristics of food eaten by the mother may be transmitted to the child. Filipinos avoid eating prunes, and Chinese avoid eating soy sauce, in both instances to prevent a dark-skinned infant. Japanese women are cautioned

TABLE 8-6   Characteristic Food Patterns of Some Cultures

MILK GROUP	PROTEIN GROUP	FRUITS AND VEGETABLES	BREADS AND CEREALS	POSSIBLE DIETARY PROBLEMS
NATIVE AMERICAN (MANY TRIBAL VARIATIONS; MANY "AMERICANIZED")				
Fresh milk Evaporated milk for cooking Ice cream Cream pie	Pork, beef, lamb, rabbit Fowl, fish, eggs Legumes Sunflower seeds Nuts: walnut, acorn, pine, peanut butter Game meat	Green peas, beans Beets, turnips Leafy green and other vegetables Grapes, bananas, peaches, other fresh fruits Roots	Refined bread Whole wheat Cornmeal Rice Dry cereals "Fry" bread Tortillas	Obesity, diabetes, alcoholism, nutritional deficiencies expressed in dental problems and iron-deficiency anemia Inadequate amounts of all nutrients Excessive use of sugar
MIDDLE EASTERN* (ARMENIAN, GREEK, SYRIAN, TURKISH)				
Yogurt Little butter	Lamb Nuts Dried peas, beans, lentils Sesame seeds	Peppers, tomatoes, cabbage, grape leaves, cucumbers, squash Dried apricots, raisins, dates	Cracked wheat and dark bread	Fry many meats and vegetables Lack of fresh fruits Insufficient foods from milk group High consumption of sweetenings, lamb fat, and olive oil*
AFRICAN-AMERICAN				
Milk† Ice cream Cheese: longhorn, American	Pork: all cuts, plus organs, chitterlings Beef, lamb Chicken, giblets Eggs Nuts Legumes Fish, game	Leafy vegetables Green and yellow vegetables Potato: white, sweet Stewed fruit Bananas and other fresh fruit	Cornmeal and hominy grits Rice Biscuits, pancakes, white breads Puddings: bread, rice	Extensive use of frying, smothering in gravy, or simmering Fats: salt pork, bacon drippings, lard, and gravies High consumption of sweets Insufficient citrus Vegetables often boiled for long periods with pork fat and much salt Limited amounts from milk group†
CHINESE (CANTONESE MOST PREVALENT)				
Milk: water buffalo	Pork sausage‡ Eggs and pigeon eggs Fish Lamb, beef, goat Fowl: chicken, duck Nuts Legumes Soybean curd (tofu)	Many vegetables Radish leaves Bean, bamboo sprouts	Rice/rice flour products Cereals, noodles Wheat, corn, millet seed	Tendency of some immigrants to use large amounts of grease in cooking Limited use of milk and milk products Often low in protein, calories, or both Soy sauce (high sodium)

MSG, **Monosodium L-glutamate.**
*Religious holidays may involve fasting, which is believed to increase the likelihood of preterm labor. Fasting requirement may be waived during pregnancy.
†Lactose intolerance relatively common in adults.
‡Lower in fat content than Western sausage.

Continued.

TABLE 8-6 Characteristic Food Patterns of Some Cultures—cont'd

MILK GROUP	PROTEIN GROUP	FRUITS AND VEGETABLES	BREADS AND CEREALS	POSSIBLE DIETARY PROBLEMS
FILIPINO (SPANISH-CHINESE INFLUENCE)				
Flavored milk Milk in coffee Cheese: gouda, cheddar	Pork, beef, goat, rabbit Chicken Fish Eggs, nuts, legumes	Many vegetables and fruits	Rice, cooked cereals Noodles: rice, wheat	Limited use of milk and milk products Tendency to pre-wash rice Tendency to have only small portions of protein foods
ITALIAN				
Cheese Some ice cream	Meat Eggs Dried beans	Leafy vegetables Potatoes Eggplant, tomatoes, peppers Fruits	Pasta White breads, some whole wheat Farina Cereals	Prefer expensive imported cheeses; reluctant to substitute less expensive domestic varieties Tendency to overcook vegetables Limited use of whole grains High consumption of sweets Extensive use of olive oil* Insufficient servings from milk group
JAPANESE (ISEI, MORE JAPANESE INFLUENCE; NISEI, MORE WESTERNIZED)				
Increasing amounts being used by younger generations	Pork, beef, chicken Fish Eggs Legumes: soya, red, lima beans Tofu Nuts	Many vegetables and fruits Seaweed	Rice, rice cakes Wheat noodles Refined bread, noodles	Excessive sodium: pickles, salty crisp seaweed, MSG, and soy sauce Insufficient servings from milk group May use prewashed rice
HISPANIC, MEXICAN-AMERICAN				
Milk Cheese Flan, ice cream	Beef, pork, lamb, chicken, tripe, hot sausage, beef intestines Fish Eggs Nuts Dry beans: pinto, chickpeas (often eaten more than once daily)	Spinach, wild greens, tomatoes, chilies, corn, cactus leaves, cabbage, avocado, potatoes Pumpkin, zapote, peaches, guava, papaya, citrus	Rice, cornmeal Sweet bread, pastries Tortilla: corn, flour Vermicelli (fideo)	Limited meats primarily due to cost Limited use of milk and milk products Large amounts of lard Abundant use of sugar Tendency to boil vegetables for long periods

TABLE 8-6   Characteristic Food Patterns of Some Cultures—cont'd

MILK GROUP	PROTEIN GROUP	FRUITS AND VEGETABLES	BREADS AND CEREALS	POSSIBLE DIETARY PROBLEMS
POLISH				
Milk Sour cream Cheese Butter	Pork (preferred) Chicken	Vegetables—limited fresh Cabbage Roots—potatoes Fruits—limited fresh	Dark rye	Sodium in ham, sausage, pickles High consumption of sweets Tendency to over-cook vegetables Limited fruits, raw vegetables, meats
PUERTO RICAN				
Limited use of milk products Coffee with milk (café con leche)	Pork Poultry Eggs (Fridays) Dried codfish Beans (habichuelas)	Avocado, okra Eggplant Sweet yams Starchy vegetables and fruits (vian-das)	Rice Cornmeal	Small amounts of pork and poultry Extensive use of fat, lard, salt pork, and olive oil Lack of milk products
SCANDINAVIAN (DANISH, FINNISH, NORWEGIAN, SWEDISH)				
Cream Butter Cheeses	Wild game Reindeer Fish (fresh or dried) Eggs	Berries Dried fruit Vegetables: cole slaw, roots	Whole wheat, rye, barley, sweets (cookies and sweet breads)	Insufficient fresh fruits and veg-etables High consumption of sweets, pickled salted meats, and fish
SOUTHEAST ASIAN (VIETNAMESE, CAMBODIAN)				
Generally not taken Coffee with con-densed cow's milk Plain yogurt Ice cream (rare) Soybean milk	Fish (daily): fresh, dried, salted Poultry/eggs: duck, chicken Pork Beef (seldom) Dry beans Tofu	Seasonal variety: fresh or preserved Green, leafy veg-etables Yams Corn	Rice: grains, flour, noodles French bread "Cellophane" (bean starch) noodles	Fresh milk products generally not con-sumed Poultry/eggs may be limited Meat considered "unclean" is avoided Preference for a diet high in salt and pepper, as well as rice and pork High intake of MSG and soy sauce
JEWISH: ORTHODOX*				
Milk† Cheese†	Meat (bloodless; Ko-sher prepared): beef, lamb, goat, deer, poultry (all types), no pork Fish with fins and scales only No crustaceans	Wide variety	Wide variety	High intake of so-dium in meat products

*Religious holidays may involve fasting, which is believed to increase the likelihood of preterm labor. Fasting requirement may be waived during pregnancy.
†Milk and milk products not eaten with meat, milk may be taken before the meal or 6 hours after; different sets of dishes and silverware are used to serve milk and meat products.

TABLE 8-7 Complementary Plant Protein Combinations*

GENERAL GUIDELINES

1. Follow nutrition guide for regular food plan during pregnancy.
2. Eat a wide variety of foods, including milk and milk products and eggs.
3. If no milk is allowed, use a supplement of 4 µg of vitamin B_{12} daily. If goat and soymilk are used, partial supplementation may be needed.
4. If no milk is taken, also use supplements of 1200 mg of calcium and 10 mg of vitamin D daily. Partial supplementation will be necessary if less than four servings of milk and milk products are consumed.
5. Select a variety of plant foods (especially grains, legumes, nuts, and seeds) to obtain "complete" proteins by complementary combinations, as indicated in the list below.
6. Use iodized salt.

FOOD	AMINO ACIDS DEFICIENT	COMPLEMENTARY PROTEIN FOOD COMBINATIONS
Grains	Isoleucine Lysine	Rice + legumes Corn + legumes Wheat + legumes Wheat + peanuts + milk Wheat + sesame + soybean Rice + Brewer's yeast
Legumes	Tryptophan Methionine	Legumes + rice Beans + wheat Beans + corn Soybeans + rice + wheat Soybeans + corn + milk Soybeans + wheat + sesame Soybeans + peanuts + sesame Soybeans + peanuts + wheat + rice
Nuts and seeds	Isoleucine Lysine	Peanuts + sesame + soybeans Sesame + beans Sesame + soybeans + wheat Peanuts + sunflower seeds
Vegetables	Isoleucine Methionine	Lima beans Green beans Brussels sprouts } + Sesame seeds or Brazil nuts or mushrooms Cauliflower Broccoli Greens + millet or rice

*Modified from Lappé FM: *Diet for a small planet,* ed 2, New York, 1983, Friends of the Earth/Ballantine.

against hot, spicy, and salty foods, as are Filipino and Southeast Asian women. African-Americans in the southern United States, Guatemalans, Mexicans, and Mexican-Americans might not eat acid foods or certain other fresh fruits and vegetables.

Vegetarian Dietary Practices

Vegetarianism has gained popularity in recent years. Foods basic to almost all **vegetarian** diets are vegetables, fruits, legumes, nuts, and grains. There are several types of vegetarian diets, and some may not satisfy all nutrient requirements for the pregnant or lactating woman:

Semivegetarian: This is characteristic of many young vegetarians. Fish, poultry, eggs, and dairy products are consumed, but no red meat or pork. There are no nutritional problems with this type of vegetarian diet.

Lactoovovegetarian: Milk, eggs, and cheese are eaten in addition to the vegetable diet. There is no problem in obtaining adequate protein and other nutrients, except iron, due to the presence of milk in this diet. There are no nutritional problems with this type of vegetarian diet.

Lactovegetarian: The vegetable diet is supplemented with milk and cheese. Milk products also add complete protein to this diet. There is no problem in obtaining adequate protein and other nutrients, except iron, due to the presence of milk in this diet.

Case History

Marty Ellis, a 28-year-old woman in week 24 of her first pregnancy, comes to the clinic for a routine prenatal visit. Mary's height is 157.5 cm (5 ft, 2 in) and current weight is 70 kg (154 lb); her prepregnancy weight was 56 kg (123 lb). A review of her records reveals that her rate of weight gain has been high throughout pregnancy. She has no edema or proteinuria, and her blood pressure is 110/76. The nurse interviews Marty to update her diet history. Marty states that she especially craves ice cream and eats two or three servings most days. In addition, Marty complains that she is experiencing the need to defecate but has difficulty in doing so and that her stools have become infrequent (once or twice a week), hard, and small. She also reports that she is having heartburn (pyrosis).

EXPECTED OUTCOMES	IMPLEMENTATION	RATIONALE	EVALUATION
Nursing Diagnosis: Altered nutrition: more than body requirements			
Rate of weight gain will be reduced to no more than 2 kg (4.4 lb)/month for the remainder of pregnancy.	Discuss optimal weight gain for prepregnant weight. Review principles of a healthful diet.	Knowledge of optimal pattern of gain assists Marty to plan for weight gain during the remainder of pregnancy. A nutritious intake must be maintained, and no weight reduction diet should be begun during pregnancy to avoid ketonemia and to ensure that the diet is not so restricted that it becomes difficult to consume adequate nutrients.	Marty's gain slowed to 2.5 kg (5.5 lb) the first month. Although the goal was not completely achieved, Marty was pleased with her progress and wanted to continue with the plan.
	Review diet history with Marty and assist her to plan lower calorie menus.	Identification of excesses in her diet, especially excessive intake of fat, a major contributor to weight gain, can assist her to begin to develop new food habits.	
	Assist Marty to plan a regular exercise regimen using large-muscle groups.	Exercise increases energy expenditure.	
Nursing Diagnosis: Constipation			
Marty will have regular, soft, formed stools that are eliminated without discomfort.	Review diet history with Marty, identify fiber sources, and help her plan menus with increased raw fruits and vegetables, bran, and whole grains.	Identifies ways that fiber in the diet can be increased to produce bulky stools that stimulate peristalsis.	Marty's constipation resolves; she passes soft, formed stools daily.
	Encourage intake of 30 to 40 ml of fluid/kg daily (½ oz/lb) in water, fruit juices, decaffeinated tea, and milk.	Fluid helps to produce bulky stools.	
	Help Marty to devise a plan for regular exercise.	Exercise improves muscle tone, stimulates peristalsis.	

Continued.

PLAN OF CARE—con't

Nutrition in Pregnancy

EXPECTED OUTCOMES	IMPLEMENTATION	RATIONALE	EVALUATION
Nursing Diagnosis: Pain related to pyrosis (heartburn)			
Marty will experience no discomfort related to pyrosis.	Review diet history with Marty, with emphasis on time and type of foods/beverages consumed and the onset of discomfort.	Determining the relationship between food intake and onset of symptoms may assist the nurse and Marty in planning interventions.	Marty reports that pyrosis has resolved.
	Discuss with Marty the factors that can contribute to reflux of gastric fluid into the esophagus.	Understanding the physiologic basis of her discomfort will help Marty plan and implement interventions.	
	Recommend that Marty avoid lying down for at least 2 to 3 hours after eating.	The force of gravity helps reduce reflux when Marty is upright.	
	Help Marty plan her diet to include several small, nutritious meals daily, rather than two to three larger meals, and suggest that Marty consume most of her fluids between meals rather than with meals.	Reflux is more likely to occur when the stomach is very full; fluids, especially, can contribute to distention of the stomach.	

Strict vegetarian or vegan: This all-vegetable diet includes vegetables, fruits, legumes, nuts, and grains but is not supplemented with any animal foods or dairy products. This diet is deficient in vitamin B_{12}, and supplementation is encouraged. Vitamin B_6 may also be a problem. Iron, zinc, and calcium may not be present in adequate quantities because of the high phytate content of the vegetables, which interferes with absorption of these nutrients. Mothers following this diet need help achieving the right combination of plant protein sources to obtain adequate amounts of complete protein (Johnston, 1988). Table 8-7 provides guidelines for complementary plant protein combinations. Supplementation with a prenatal vitamin is recommended for the vegan mother.

Fruitarian: This diet consists of raw or dried fruits, nuts, honey, and olive oil. Potential inadequacy is greater in this diet than in any of the other diets. The woman who is a fruitarian should be referred to a registered dietitian for careful nutritional counseling.

Postpartum Nutrition

The need for a varied diet with representation from all food groups continues throughout lactation. Because of deposition of energy stores, the woman with optimal weight gain during pregnancy is heavier after birth than at the beginning of pregnancy. A weight reduction diet is not recommended during lactation inasmuch as it may interfere with milk production or impair maternal nutritional status. An intake of less than 1500 kcal can have adverse effects on milk volume. Additionally, the fatigue that commonly accompanies a rapid weight loss has a detrimental effect on the letdown reflex.

The woman who does not breastfeed will lose weight gradually if she consumes a balanced diet that provides slightly less than her daily energy expenditure. Fat is the most concentrated source of calories in the diet (9 kcal/g, vs. 4 kcal/g in carbohydrates and proteins), and fat calories are more efficiently converted into fat stores than are calories from carbohydrate or protein. Therefore the first step in weight reduction (or controlling excessive weight gain) is to evaluate sources of fat in the diet and explore with the woman ways of reducing them.

Even foods such as vegetables that are originally low in fat can become high in fat when fried or sauteed, served with excessive amounts of salad dressing, consumed with high-fat dips or sauces, or seasoned with butter or bacon drippings. A desirable rate of loss for the nonlactating mother is 1 to 2 pounds a week.

✤ EVALUATION

Evaluation is a continuous process that begins during prenatal assessment and continues throughout the pregnancy and postpartum period. Nurses are accountable for measuring and documenting patient outcomes. The criteria reflect the parameters used to measure the expected outcomes listed on p. 189. The case study and plan of care provide an example of expected outcomes, interventions, and evaluation for the pregnant woman with nutrition-related problems.

KEY POINTS

- A woman's nutritional status before, during, and after pregnancy contributes, to a significant degree, to her well-being and that of her developing fetus.
- Many physiologic changes occurring during pregnancy influence the need for additional nutrients and the efficiency with which the body utilizes them.
- Both the total maternal weight gain and the pattern of weight gain are important determinants of the outcome of pregnancy.
- The recommended weight gain during pregnancy is determined by the appropriateness of the mother's prepregnancy weight for height (BMI).
- Nutritional risk factors include adolescent pregnancy, bizarre or faddist food habits, abuse of nicotine, alcohol, or drugs, a low weight for height, and frequent pregnancies.

- Iron supplementation is recommended routinely during pregnancy because it is nearly impossible to obtain adequate intakes from dietary sources alone. Other supplements may be recommended when nutritional risk factors are present.
- The nurse and patient are influenced by cultural and personal values and beliefs during nutrition counseling.
- Pregnancy complications that may be nutrition related include anemia, pregnancy-induced hypertension, gestational diabetes, and intrauterine growth retardation.
- Dietary adaptation can be effective interventions for some of the common discomforts of pregnancy, including nausea and vomiting, constipation, and heartburn.

CRITICAL THINKING EXERCISES

1. At a prenatal clinic, assess the weight gain patterns of three different women. What advice is indicated based on the patterns seen?
2. Interview a pregnant woman at a prenatal clinic. Obtain a diet history using the nutrition questionnaire. With the woman's input, develop an appropriate meal pattern utilizing the food guide pyramid.
3. Keep a 4-day diet log including three weekdays and one weekend day for yourself. Assess your intake using the food guide pyramid. Answer the following questions: What cultural/ethnic influences affect your intake? What foods do you normally consume in less than the recommended amounts?
4. Develop an appropriate 1-day menu for a pregnant woman who chooses to use no dairy products or one who is a vegetarian.

References

Bourgoin BP et al: Lead content in 70 brands of dietary calcium supplements, *Am J Pub Health* 83:1155, 1993.

Brown JE, Story M: Let them eat cake or a prescription for improving the outcome of pregnancy? *Nutr Today* 25(6):18, 1990.

Centers for Disease Control: *MMWR* 41:1, 1992.

Collins JW Jr, David RJ: The differential effect of traditional risk factors on infant birthweight among blacks and whites in Chicago, *Am J Pub Health* 80:679, 1990.

Committee on Genetics, American Academy of Pediatrics: Folic acid for the prevention of neural tube defects, *Pediatrics* 92:493, 1993.

Food and Nutrition Board, National Academy of Sciences–National Research Council: *Recommended dietary allowances, revised 1989*, Washington, DC, 1989.

The food guide pyramid, Hyattsville, MD, 1992, US Department of Agriculture.

Garn SM et al: Are pregnant teenagers still in rapid growth? *Am J Dis Child* 138:32, 1984.

Graham SM, Arvela OM, Wise GA: Long-term neurologic consequences of nutritional vitamin B_{12} deficiency in infants, *J Pediatr* 121:710, 1992.

Healthy people 2000: national health promotion/disease prevention objectives, Washington, DC, 1990, US Government Printing Office.

Herbert V: Folate and neural tube defects, *Nutr Today* 27(6):30, 1992.

Johnston PK: Counseling the pregnant vegetarian, *Am J Clin Nutr* 48:901, 1988.

Keppel KG, Taffel SM: Pregnancy-related weight gain and retention: implications of the 1990 Institute of Medicine guidelines, *Am J Pub Health* 83:1100, 1993.

Knight KB, Keith RE: Calcium supplementation on normotensive and hypertensive women, *Am J Clin Nutr* 55:891, 1992.

Kruger S, Maetzold LD: Practices of tradition for pregnancy, *Matern Child Nurs J* 12:135, 1983.

Leiderman PH et al: *Culture and infancy,* New York, 1977, Academic Press.

Lucak SL, Lucak BK: The gastrointestinal tract in pregnancy, *Mediguide to GI diseases* 4(3):1, 1991.

National Academy of Sciences—Institute of Medicine: *Nutrition during pregnancy and lactation: an implementation guide,* Washington, DC, 1992, National Academy Press.

National Academy of Sciences—Institute of Medicine: *Nutrition during pregnancy,* Washington, DC, 1990, National Academy Press.

Rosso P: A new chart to monitor weight gain during pregnancy, *Am J Clin Nutr* 41:644, 1985.

Tierson FD, Olsen CL, Hook EB: Nausea and vomiting of pregnancy and association with pregnancy outcome. *Am J Obstet Gynecol* 155:1017, 1986.

Wegman ME: Annual summary of vital statistics—1992, *Pediatrics* 92:743, 1993.

Worthington-Roberts B, Williams SR: *Nutrition in pregnancy and lactation,* ed 5, St Louis, 1993, Mosby.

Bibliography

Czeizel AE, Dudas I: Prevention of the first occurrence of neural-tube defects by periconceptional vitamin supplementation, *N Engl J Med* 327:1832, 1992.

Eliades DC, Suitor CW, editors: *Nutrition in practice,* Arlington, VA, 1993, National Center for Education in Maternal and Child Health.

Executive summary—nutrition during pregnancy, *Nutr Today* 25(5):13, 1990.

Graham SM, Arvela OM, Wise GA: Long-term neurologic consequences of nutritional vitamin B_{12} deficiency in infants, *J Pediatr* 121:710, 1992.

Johnston CS, Christopher FS, Kandell LA: Pregnancy weight gain in adolescents and young adults, *J Am Coll Nutr* 10:185, 1991.

Lederman SA: Recent issues related to nutrition during pregnancy, *J Am Coll Nutr* 12(2):91, 1993.

Scholl RO, Hediger ML: A review of the epidemiology of nutrition and adolescent pregnancy: maternal growth during pregnancy and its effect on the fetus, *J Am Coll Nutr* 12:101, 1993.

Susser M: Maternal weight gain, infant birth weight, and diet: causal sequences, *Am J Clin Nutr* 53:1384, 1991.

Walker ARP, Walker BF, Domsci D et al: Nutritional needs in pregnancy: why is the state of knowledge still speculative? *Nutr Today* 26(6):18, 1991.

Three

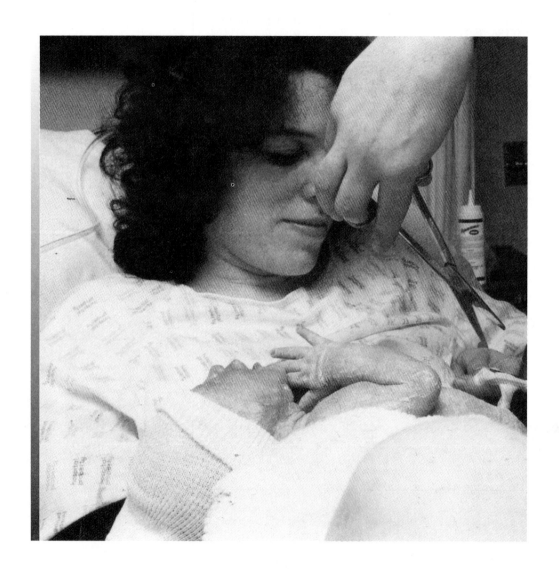

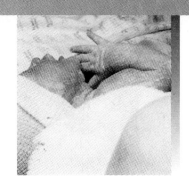

Childbirth

9 Essential Factors and Processes of Labor

10 Management of Discomfort

11 Fetal Assessment

12 Nursing Care during Labor and Birth

CHAPTER 9

Essential Factors and Processes of Labor

DEITRA LEONARD LOWDERMILK

During late pregnancy, the mother and the fetus prepare for the labor process. The fetus has grown and developed in preparation for extrauterine life. The mother has undergone various physiologic adaptations during pregnancy that prepare her for the process of birth and the role of motherhood. Labor and birth represent the end of pregnancy and the beginning of extrauterine life for the newborn infant.

Nurses must understand the essential factors of labor, the process involved, the normal progression of events, and the adaptations made by both the mother and fetus. Once this knowledge is mastered, nurses can proceed to apply the nursing process to each woman and family.

ESSENTIAL FACTORS IN LABOR

Five essential factors affect the process of labor and birth. These are easily remembered as the five *P*s: passenger (fetus and placenta), passageway (birth canal), powers, position of the mother, and psychologic response. The first four factors are presented here as the basis of understanding the physiologic process of labor. The fifth factor is discussed in Chapter 12.

Passenger

How the *passenger,* or fetus, moves through the birth canal is a result of several interacting factors: the size of the fetal head, fetal presentation, lie, attitude, and position.

Because the placenta must also pass through the birth canal, it may be considered a passenger along with the fetus. However, the placenta rarely impedes the process of labor in normal birth.

Size of Fetal Head

The fetal head, because of its size and relative rigidity, has a major effect on the birth process. The fetal skull is composed of two parietal bones, two temporal bones, the frontal bone, and the occipital bone (Fig. 9-1). These bones are united by membranous sutures: the sagittal, lambdoid, coronal, and frontal. Membrane-filled spaces called **fontanels** are located where the sutures intersect. During labor, after rupture of membranes, palpation of fontanels and sutures during vaginal examination identifies fetal presentation, position, and attitude. Assessment of their size reveals information about the age and well-being of the newborn.

The two most important fontanels are the anterior and posterior. The larger of these, the anterior fontanel, is diamond shaped and lies at the junction of the sagittal, coronal, and frontal sutures. It closes by 18 months of age. The posterior fontanel lies at the junction of the sutures of the two parietal bones and the one occipital bone and is triangular. It closes 6 to 8 weeks after birth.

The presence of sutures and fontanels gives the skull

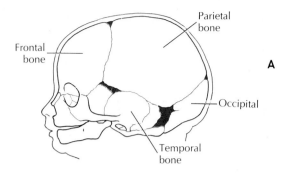
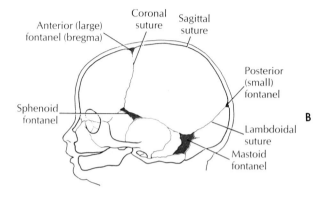
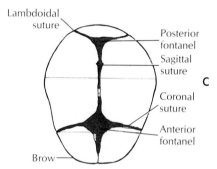

FIG. 9-1 Fetal head at term. **A,** Bones, **B** and **C,** Sutures and fontanels.

flexibility to accommodate the infant brain, which continues to grow for some time after birth. Because the bones are not firmly united, however, slight overlapping of the bones, or **molding** of the shape of the head, occurs during labor. Molding can be extensive, but with most newborns the head assumes its normal shape within 3 days of birth. This capacity of the bones to slide over one another also permits adaptation to the various diameters of the maternal pelvis.

Although the size of the fetal shoulders may affect passage, their position can be altered relatively easily during labor, so that one shoulder may occupy a lower level than the other. This creates a smaller shoulder diameter for negotiating the passageway. The circumference of the fetal hips is usually small enough not to create problems.

Fetal Presentation

Presentation refers to the part of the fetus that enters the pelvic inlet first and leads through the birth canal

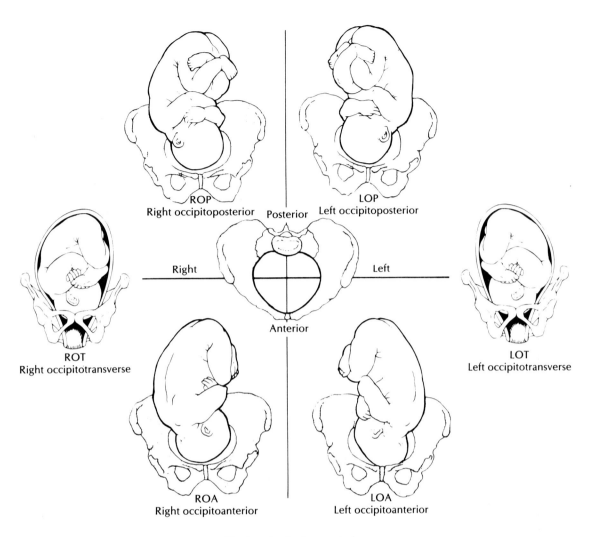

ROP
Right occipitoposterior

Posterior

LOP
Left occipitoposterior

Right

Left

Anterior

ROT
Right occipitotransverse

LOT
Left occipitotransverse

ROA
Right occipitoanterior

LOA
Left occipitoanterior

Lie: Longitudinal or vertical
Presentation: vertex
Reference point: occiput
Attitude: complete flexion

FIG. 9-2   Examples of fetal vertex (occiput) presentations in relation to front, back, and side of maternal pelvis.

during labor at term. The three main presentations are cephalic (head first), 96% (Fig. 9-2); breech (buttocks first), 3% (Fig. 9-3, *A* to *C*); and shoulders, 1% (Fig. 9-3, *D*). **Presenting part** refers to that part of the fetal body first felt by the examining finger during a vaginal examination. Factors that determine the presenting part include fetal lie, fetal attitude, and extension or flexion or the fetus's head.

Fetal Lie

Lie is the relationship of the long axis (spine) of the fetus to the long axis (spine) of the mother. There are two lies: (1) longitudinal, or vertical, in which the long axis of the fetus is parallel with the long axis of the mother; and (2) transverse, or horizontal, in which the long axis of the fetus is at a right angle to the long axis of the mother (Fig. 9-3, *D*). Longitudinal lies are either cepha-

lic or sacral(breech) presentations. These presentations depend on the fetal structure that first enters the mother's pelvis.

Fetal Attitude

Attitude is the relationship of the fetal body parts to each other. The fetus assumes characteristic posture (attitude) in utero partly because of the mode of fetal growth and partly because of accommodation to the shape of the uterine cavity. Normally the back of the fetus is markedly flexed; the head is flexed on the chest, the thighs are flexed at the knee joints. This attitude is called *general flexion.* The arms are crossed over the thorax, and the umbilical cord lies between the arms and the legs.

Deviations from the normal attitude may cause difficulties in childbirth. For example, in a cephalic presen-

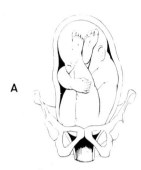

Frank breech

Lie: Longitudinal or vertical
Presentation: breech (incomplete)
Reference point: sacrum
Attitude: flexion, except for legs at knees

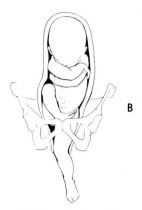

Single footling breech

Lie: Longitudinal or vertical
Presentation: breech (incomplete)
Reference point: sacrum
Attitude: flexion, except for one leg extended at hip and
knee

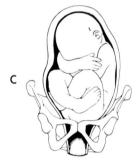

Complete breech

Lie: Longitudinal or vertical
Presentation: breech (sacrum and feet presenting)
Reference point: sacrum (with feet)
Attitude: general flexion

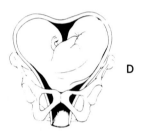

Shoulder presentation.

Lie: Transverse or horizontal
Presentation: shoulder
Reference point: scapula (Sc)
Attitude: flexion

FIG. 9-3 Fetal presentations. **A** to **C**, Breech (sacral) presentation. **D**, Shoulder presentation.

tation the fetal head may be extended or flexed in a manner that presents a head diameter unfavorable to the limits of the maternal pelvis.

The **biparietal diameter** is the largest transverse diameter of the fetal head (Fig. 9-4, *B*). Of the anteroposterior diameters shown, it can be seen that the attitudes of flexion or extension allow diameters of differing sizes to enter the maternal pelvis. With the head in complete flexion the **suboccipitobregmatic diameter** (the smallest diameter) enters the true pelvis easily (Figs. 9-4, *A* and 9-5, *A*).

Fetal Position

The presentation or presenting part indicates the portion of the fetus that overlies the pelvic inlet. In a **cephalic presentation** the presenting part is usually the occiput; in a **breech presentation** it is the sacrum; in the transverse lie the presenting part is the scapula of the shoulder. When the presenting part is the occiput, the pre-

sentation is noted as **vertex** (see Figs. 9-2, 9-4, and 9-5, *A*).

Position is the relationship of the presenting part (occiput, sacrum, mentum [chin], or sinciput [deflexed vertex]), to the four quadrants of the mother's pelvis (see Fig. 9-2). Position is described in abbreviated form determined by the first letter of each key word. For example, right occipitoanterior position is written as ROA; right occipitotransverse is abbreviated as ROT (see Fig. 9-2).

Engagement indicates that the largest transverse diameter of the presenting part has passed through the maternal pelvic brim or inlet into the true pelvis. In a well-flexed cephalic presentation the biparietal diameter (9.25 cm) is the widest (see Fig. 9-5, *B*). Engagement can be determined by abdominal or vaginal examination.

Station is the relationship of the presenting part of the fetus to an imaginary line drawn between the maternal ischial spines. Station is expressed in terms of centi-

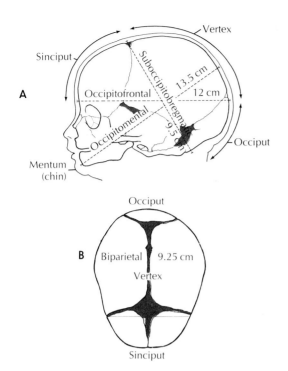

FIG. 9-4   Cephalic landmarks. **A,** Cephalic presentation: occiput, vertex, and sinciput; and cephalic diameters: suboccipitobregmatic, occipitofrontal, and occipitomental. **B,** Cephalic presentation and biparietal diameter.

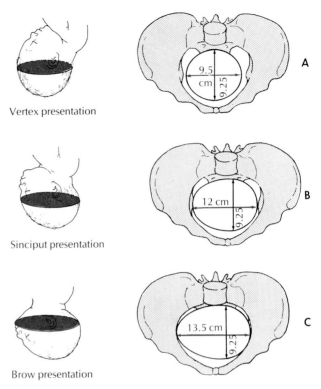

FIG. 9-5   Head entering pelvis. Biparietal diameter is indicated with *black arrow* (9.25 cm). **A,** Suboccipitobregmatic diameter: complete flexion of head on chest so that smallest diameter enters. **B,** Occipitofrontal diameter: moderate extension so that large diameter enters. **C,** Occipitomental diameter: marked extension so that largest diameter (which is too large to permit head to enter pelvis) is presenting.

meters above or below the spines. For example, when the presenting part is 1 cm above the spines, it is noted as being −1 (Fig. 9-6). At the level of the spines, the station is referred to as zero.

When the presenting part is 1 cm below the spines, however, the station is said to be +1. Birth is imminent when the presenting part is at +4 to +5 cm. For accurate documentation of the rate of descent of the fetus during labor the station of the presenting part should be determined when labor begins.

Passageway

The *passageway,* or birth canal, is composed of the mother's rigid bony pelvis and the soft tissues of the cervix, pelvic floor, vagina, and introitus (the external opening to the vagina). Although the soft tissues, particularly the muscular layers of the pelvic floor, contribute to birth of the fetus, the maternal pelvis plays a far greater role in the labor process. The fetus must successfully accommodate itself to this relatively rigid passageway. Therefore the size and shape of the pelvis must be determined before childbirth begins.

Bony Pelvis

The anatomy of the bony pelvis is detailed in Chapter 3. The following discussion focuses on the importance of pelvic configurations as they relate to the labor process. (It may be helpful to refer to Fig. 3-14.)

The bony pelvis is formed by the fusion of the ilium, ischium, pubis, and sacrum bones. The four pelvic joints are the symphysis pubis, the right and left sacroiliac joints, and the sacrococcygeal joint (Fig. 9-7). The bony pelvis is separated by the brim, or inlet, into two parts: the false pelvis and the true pelvis. The false pelvis is that part above the brim and has nothing to do with childbearing. The true pelvis is divided into three planes: the inlet, or brim; the midpelvis, or cavity; and the outlet.

The pelvic inlet, the upper border of the true pelvis, is formed anteriorly by the upper margins of the pubic bone, laterally by the iliopectineal lines along the innominate bones, and posteriorly by the anterior, upper margin of the sacrum and the sacral promontory.

The pelvic cavity, or midpelvis, is a curved passage having a short anterior wall and a much longer concave posterior wall. It is bounded by the posterior aspect of the symphysis pubis, the ischium, a portion of the ilium, the sacrum, and the coccyx.

The pelvic outlet is the lower border of the true pelvis. Viewed from below, it is ovoid, somewhat diamond shaped, bounded by the pubic arch anteriorly, the ischial tuberosities laterally, and the tip of the coccyx posteriorly. In the latter part of pregnancy the coccyx is mov-

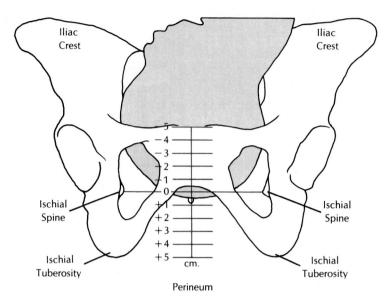

FIG. 9-6 Stations of presenting part or degree of descent. Silhouette shows head of infant approaching station −1. (Courtesy Ross Laboratories, Columbus, OH.)

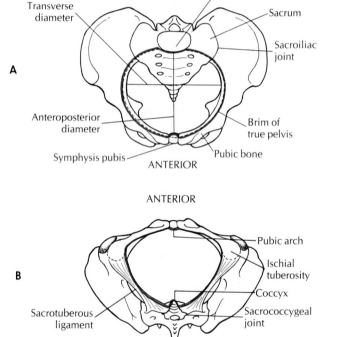

FIG. 9-7 Female pelvis. **A,** Pelvic brim from above. **B,** Pelvic outlet from below.

able (unless it has been broken in a fall during skiing or skating, for example, and has fused to the sacrum during healing).

The pelvic canal varies in size and shape at various levels. The diameters at the plane of the pelvic inlet, midpelvis, and outlet, plus the axis of the birth canal (Fig. 9-8), determine whether vaginal birth is possible and the

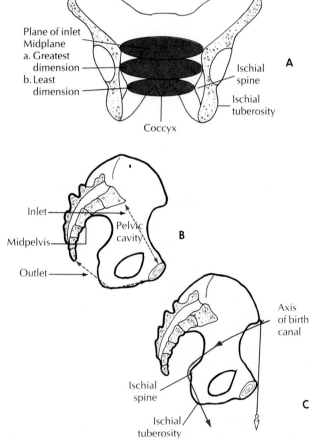

FIG. 9-8 Pelvic cavity. **A,** Inlet and midplane. Outlet not shown. **B,** Cavity of true pelvis. **C,** Note curve of sacrum and axis of birth canal.

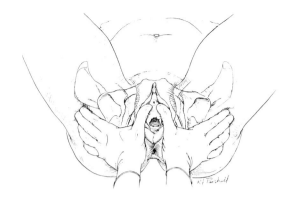

FIG. 9-9 Examination of angle of subpubic arch. Using both thumbs, examiner externally traces descending rami down to tuberosities. (From Barkauskas VH et al: *Health and physical assessment,* St Louis, 1994, Mosby.)

manner by which the fetus may pass down the birth canal (cardinal movements of the mechanism of labor).

The subpubic angle, which indicates the type of pubic arch, together with the length of the pubic rami and the intertuberous diameter, is of great importance. Because the fetus must first pass beneath the pubic arch, a narrow subpubic angle is less favorable than a rounded, wide arch. Measurement of the subpubic arch is shown in Fig. 9-9. A summary of obstetric measurements is given in Table 9-1.

The four basic types of pelvis are classified as follows:
1. Gynecoid (the classic female type)
2. Android (resembling the male pelvis)
3. Anthropoid (resembling the pelvis of anthropoid apes)
4. Platypelloid (the flat pelvis)

The **gynecoid pelvis** is the most common, with major gynecoid pelvic features present in 50% of all women. Examples of pelvic variations and their effects on the mode of birth are given in Table 9-2.

Assessment of the bony pelvis may be performed during the first prenatal evaluation and need not be repeated if the pelvis is of adequate size and suitable shape. In the third trimester of pregnancy the examination of the bony pelvis may be more thorough and the results more accurate because there is relaxation of the pelvic joints and ligaments. The hormones of pregnancy, especially the ovarian hormone progesterone, cause the development of considerable mobility in the pelvic joints. Widening of the joint of the symphysis pubis and instability may cause pain in any or all of the joints.

Because the examiner does not have direct access to the bony structures and because the bones are covered with varying amounts of soft tissue, estimates of size and shape are approximate. Precise bony pelvis measurements can be determined by use of computed tomography, ultrasound, or x-ray films. However, x-ray examination is rarely done because the x-rays may damage the developing fetus (see Appendix E).

Soft Tissues

The soft tissues of the passageway include the distensible lower uterine segment, cervix, pelvic floor muscles, vagina, and introitus (external opening to the vagina).

Before labor begins the uterus is composed of the uterine body (corpus) and cervix (neck). After labor has begun, uterine contractions cause the uterine body to change into a thick and muscular upper segment and a thin-walled passive muscular lower segment. A physiologic retraction ring separates the two segments (Fig. 9-10). The lower uterine segment gradually distends to accommodate the intrauterine contents as the wall of the upper segment becomes thick and its accommodating capacity is reduced. Contractions of the uterine body exert downward pressure on the fetus, pushing it against the cervix.

The cervix then effaces (thins) and dilates (opens) sufficiently to allow descent of the first fetal portion into the vagina. Actually the cervix is drawn upward and over this first part as it descends.

The pelvic floor is a muscular layer that separates the pelvic cavity above from the perineal space below. This structure helps the fetus rotate anteriorly as it passes through the birth canal. The vagina in turn distends to permit passage of the fetus into the external world. As noted earlier, the soft tissues of the vagina develop throughout pregnancy until at term the vagina can dilate to accommodate the fetus.

Powers

Involuntary and voluntary contractions by the mother combine to expel the fetus and the placenta out of the uterus. Involuntary uterine contractions, called the *primary powers,* signal the beginning of labor. Once the cervix has dilated, voluntary bearing-down efforts, called the *secondary powers,* augment the force of the involuntary contractions.

Primary Powers

The involuntary contractions originate at certain pacemaker points in the thickened muscle layers of the upper uterine segment. From the pacemaker points contractions move downward over the uterus in waves, separated by short rest periods. Terms used to describe these involuntary contractions include *frequency* (the time between contractions—specifically, the time between the beginning of one contraction and the beginning of the next); *duration* (length of contraction); and *intensity* (strength of contraction).

The primary powers are responsible for the effacement and dilatation of the cervix and descent of the fetus. **Effacement** of the cervix means the shortening and thinning of the cervix during the first stage of labor. The cer-

TABLE 9-1 Obstetric Measurements

PLANE	DIAMETER	MEASUREMENTS
Inlet (superior strait) 　Conjugates 　　Diagonal 　　Obstetric: measurement that determines whether presenting part can engage or enter superior strait	12.5 to 13 cm 1.5 to 2 cm less than diagonal (radiographic)	
True (vera) (anteroposterior)	≥11 cm (12.5) (radiographic)	Length of diagonal conjugate *(solid colored line)*, obstetric conjugate *(broken colored line)*, true conjugate *(black line).*
Midplane* 　Transverse diameter (interspinous diameter)	10.5 cm	Measurement of interspinous diameter. (From Malasanos et al: *Health assessment,* ed 4, St Louis, 1990, Mosby.)
Outlet† 　Transverse diameter (intertuberous diameter)	≥8 cm	Use of Thom's pelvimeter to measure intertuberous diameter. (From Malasanos et al: *Health assessment,* ed 4, St Louis, 1990, Mosby.)

*The midplane of the pelvis normally is its largest plane and the one of greatest diameter.
†The outlet presents the smallest plane of the pelvic canal.

TABLE 9-2 Comparison of Pelvic Types

	GYNECOID (50% OF WOMEN)	ANDROID (23% OF WOMEN)	ANTHROPOID (24% OF WOMEN)	PLATYPELLOID (3% OF WOMEN)
Brim	Slightly ovoid or transversely rounded	Heart shaped, angulated	Oval, wider antero-posteriorly	Flattened antero-posteriorly, wide transversely
	◯ Round	♡ Heart	⬭ Oval	⬭ Flat
Depth	Moderate	Deep	Deep	Shallow
Side walls	Straight	Convergent	Straight	Straight
Ischial spines	Blunt, somewhat widely separated	Prominent, narrow interspinous diameter	Prominent, often with narrow interspinous diameter	Blunted, widely separated
Sacrum	Deep, curved	Slightly curved, terminal portion often beaked	Slightly curved	Slightly curved
Subpubic arch	Wide	Narrow	Narrow	Wide
Usual mode of birth	Vaginal Spontaneous Occipitoanterior position	Cesarean Vaginal Difficult with forceps	Forceps/ spontaneous occipitoposterior or occipitoanterior position	Spontaneous

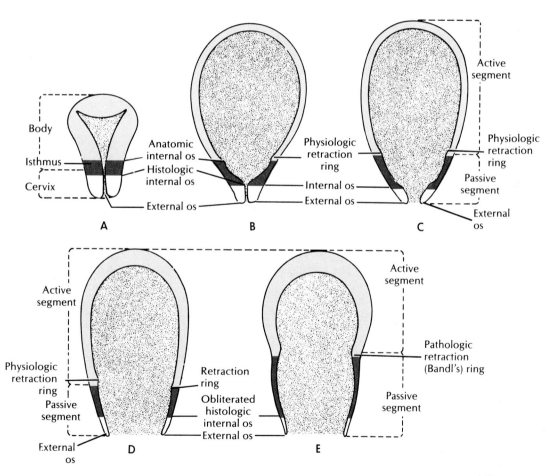

FIG. 9-10 Progressive development of segments and rings of uterus at term. Note differences in **A,** nonpregnant uterus, **B,** uterus at term, and uterus in normal labor in early first stage **C,** and second stage **D.** Passive segment is derived from lower uterine segment (isthmus) and cervix, and physiologic retraction ring is derived from anatomic internal os. **E,** Uterus in abnormal labor in second-stage dystocia. Pathologic retraction (Bandl's) ring that forms under abnormal conditions develops from physiologic ring. (Modified from Willson JR et al: *Obstetrics and gynecology,* ed 9, St Louis, 1991, Mosby.)

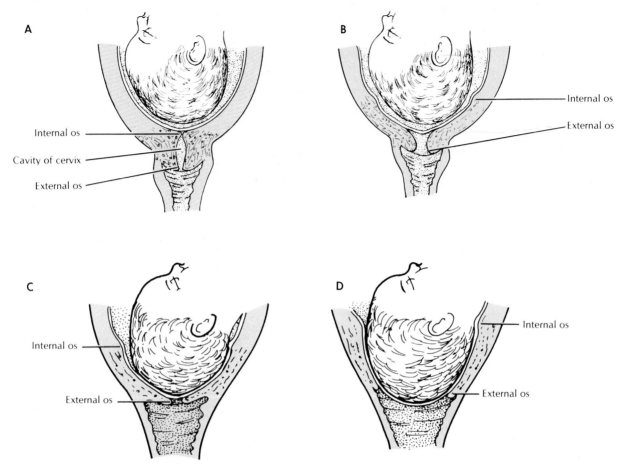

FIG. 9-11   Cervical effacement and dilatation. Note how cervix is drawn up around presenting part (internal os). Membranes are intact, and head is not well applied to cervix. **A,** Before labor. **B,** Early effacement. **C,** Complete effacement (100%). Head is well applied to cervix. **D,** Complete dilatation (10 cm). Some overlapping of cranial bones. Membranes still intact.

vix, normally 2 to 3 cm in length and about 1 cm thick, is obliterated or taken up by a shortening of the uterine muscle bundles during the thinning of the lower uterine segment in advancing labor. Eventually only a thin edge of the cervix can be palpated when effacement is complete. Effacement generally is advanced in first-time pregnancy at term before more than slight dilatation occurs. In subsequent pregnancies effacement and dilatation of the cervix tend to progress together. Degree of effacement is expressed in percentages from 0% to 100% (e.g., a cervix is 50% effaced) (Fig. 9-11).

Dilatation of the cervix is the enlargement or widening of the cervical opening and the cervical canal, which occurs once labor has begun. The diameter increases from perhaps less than 1 cm to full dilatation (approximately 10 cm) to allow birth of a term fetus. When the cervix is fully dilated (and completely retracted), it can no longer be palpated (Fig. 9-11). Full cervical dilatation marks the end of the first stage of labor.

Dilatation of the cervix occurs by the drawing upward of the musculofibrous components of the cervix with strong uterine contractions. Pressure exerted by the amniotic fluid while the membranes are intact or force applied by the presenting part also encourages cervical dilatation. Scarring of the cervix as a result of prior infection or surgery may retard cervical dilatation.

Secondary Powers

As soon as the presenting part reaches the pelvic floor the contractions change in character and become expulsive. The woman experiences an involuntary urge to push. The *bearing-down effort* (secondary powers) is aided by a voluntary effort similar to that used in the process of defecation. However, a different set of muscles is used for bearing down. The mother contracts her diaphragm and abdominal muscles and pushes out the contents of the birth canal. Bearing down results in increased intraabdominal pressure. The pressure compresses the uterus on all sides and adds to the power of the expulsive forces.

The secondary forces have no effect on cervical dilatation, but they are of considerable importance in the expulsion of the infant from the uterus and vagina after the cervix is fully dilated. Any voluntary bearing-down efforts by the woman earlier in labor are counterproductive to cervical dilatation. Straining will exhaust the woman and cause cervical trauma.

Position of the Mother

Maternal position affects her anatomic and physiologic adaptations to labor. An upright position offers a number of advantages. Frequent changes in position relieve fatigue, increase comfort, and improve circulation (Melzack et al, 1991). Upright positions include standing, walking, sitting, and squatting.

In an upright position gravity can assist in the descent of the fetus. Uterine contractions are generally stronger and more efficient in effacing and dilating the cervix, resulting in shorter labor. In addition, assuming an upright position reduces the incidence of umbilical cord compression.

An upright position is also beneficial to the mother's cardiac output, which normally increases during labor as uterine contractions return blood to the vascular bed. Increased cardiac output improves blood flow to the uteroplacental unit and the maternal kidneys. Cardiac output is compromised if the descending aorta and ascending vena cava are compressed during labor. Compression of these major vessels may result in supine hypotension and fetal heart rate deceleration or in hypertension that decreases placental perfusion. (For further discussion see p. 131). An upright position helps reduce pressure on the maternal vessels and prevents their compression.

As the fetus descends in the birth canal the pressure of the presenting part on stretch receptors of the pelvic floor stimulates the woman's bearing-down reflex. Stimulation of the stretch receptors in turn stimulates the release of oxytocin from the posterior pituitary **(Ferguson's reflex).** Oxytocin increases the intensity of the uterine contractions. In a sitting or squatting position abdominal muscles work in greater synchronicity with uterine contractions during bearing-down efforts.

PROCESS OF LABOR

Labor is the process of moving the fetus, placenta, and membranes out of the uterus and through the birth canal. Various changes take place in the woman's reproductive system in the days and weeks just before labor begins. Labor itself can be discussed in terms of the mechanisms involved in the process and the stages the woman moves through.

Reproductive System Changes

In first-time pregnancies the uterus sinks downward and forward about 2 weeks before term, when the fetus's presenting part (usually the head) descends into the true pelvis. This settling is called **lightening** or dropping and usually happens gradually (Fig. 9-12). After lightening, women feel less congested and breathe more easily. However, there is usually more bladder pressure as a result of this shift and consequently a return of urinary frequency. In a multiparous pregnancy lightening may not take place until after uterine contractions are established and true labor is in progress.

Persistent low backache and sacroiliac distress as a result of relaxation of the pelvic joints may be described. Occasionally the woman may identify strong, frequent, but irregular uterine (Braxton Hicks) contractions.

Prodromal labor events are signs and symptoms experienced before the onset of true labor. The vaginal mucus becomes more profuse in response to the extreme congestion of the vaginal mucous membranes. Brownish or blood-tinged cervical mucus may be passed **(bloody show).** The cervix becomes soft (ripens) and partially effaced and may begin to dilate. The membranes may rupture spontaneously.

Two other phenomena are common in the days preceding labor: (1) loss of 0.5 to 1.5 kg (1 to 3 lb) in weight, caused by water loss resulting from electrolyte shifts that in turn are produced by changes in estrogen and progesterone levels, and (2) a burst of energy. Women speak of a burst of energy that they often use to clean the house and put everything in order. This activity has been described as the "nesting instinct."

The onset of true labor cannot be ascribed to a single cause. Many factors, including changes in the maternal uterus, cervix, and pituitary gland, are involved. Hormones produced by the normal fetal hypothalamus, pituitary, and adrenal cortex probably contribute to the onset of labor. Progressive uterine distention, increasing intrauterine pressure, and aging of the placenta seem to be associated with increasing myometrial irritability. This is a result of increased concentrations of estrogen and

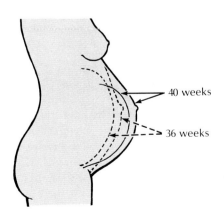

FIG. 9-12 Lightening.

prostaglandins, as well as decreasing progesterone levels. The mutually coordinated effects of these factors result in strong, regular, rhythmic uterine contractions that normally end with the birth of the fetus and the delivery of the placenta. It is still not completely understood how certain alterations trigger others and how proper checks and balances are maintained.

Afferent and efferent nerve impulses to and from the uterus alter its contractility. Although nerve impulses to the uterus will stimulate contractions, the denervated uterus still contracts well during labor because oxytocin in the circulating blood is a regulator of labor. Therefore some women who are paralyzed can still give birth vaginally.

Stages of Labor

Labor is considered "normal" when the woman is at or near term, no complications exist, a single fetus presents by vertex, and labor is completed within 24 hours. The course of normal labor, which is remarkably constant, consists of (1) regular progression of uterine contractions, (2) effacement and progressive dilatation of the cervix, and (3) progress in descent of the presenting part. *Four stages of labor* are recognized. These stages are discussed in greater detail, along with nursing care for the laboring woman and family, in Chapter 12.

The first stage of labor is considered to last from the onset of regular uterine contractions to full dilatation of the cervix. Commonly the onset of labor is difficult to establish; the woman may be admitted to the labor floor just before birth so that the beginning of labor may be only an estimate. The first stage is much longer than the second and third combined. Great variability is the rule, however, depending on the essential factors discussed earlier. Full dilatation may occur in less than 1 hour in some multiparous pregnancies. In first-time pregnancy complete dilatation of the cervix is seldom reached in less than 24 hours.

The first stage of labor has been divided into three phases: *a latent phase, an active phase, and a transition phase*. During the latent phase there is more progress in effacement of the cervix and little increase in descent. During the active phase and the transition phase there is more rapid dilatation of the cervix and descent of the presenting part. There are no absolute values for the normal length of the first stage of labor (Willson, Carrington, 1991). Variations may reflect differences in the client population or in clinical practice. The average total length of the first stage in a first-time pregnancy ranges from 3.3 hours to 19.7 hours; in subsequent pregnancies 0.1 to 14.3 hours.

The second stage of labor lasts from full dilatation of the cervix to birth of the fetus. Friedman (1978) provides statistical *upper limits* for the first and second stages of labor:

	Nulliparous	Multiparous
First stage		
Latent phase	20 hr	14 hr
Active phase	1.2 cm/hr	1.5 cm/hr
Second stage	2 hr	1.5 hr

The third stage of labor lasts from the birth of the fetus until the placenta is delivered. The placenta normally separates with the third or fourth strong uterine contraction after the infant has been born. Then it should be delivered with the next uterine contraction after placental separation. However, delivery of the placenta in 45 to 60 minutes is generally considered within normal limits.

The fourth stage of labor arbitrarily lasts about 2 hours after delivery of the placenta. It is the period of immediate recovery, when homeostasis is reestablished. It serves as an important period of observation for complications, such as abnormal bleeding.

Mechanism of Labor

The female pelvis has varied contours and diameters at different levels, and the presenting part of the passenger is large in proportion to the passage. For birth to occur, the fetus must adapt to the birth canal during the descent. The turns and other adjustments necessary in the human birth process are termed the mechanism of labor (Fig. 9-13). The seven **cardinal movements** of the mechanism of labor that occur in a vertex presentation are *engagement, descent, flexion, internal rotation, extension, external rotation (restitution),* and finally birth by *expulsion.* Although these phases are discussed separately, a combination of movements is occurring simultaneously. For example, engagement involves both descent and flexion.

Engagement

When the biparietal diameter of the head passes the pelvic inlet, the head is said to be engaged in the pelvic inlet (Fig. 9-13, *A*). In most nulliparous women this occurs before the onset of active labor because the firmer abdominal muscles direct the presenting part into the pelvis. In multiparous women, in whom the abdominal musculature is more relaxed, the head often remains freely movable above the pelvic brim until labor is established.

Descent

Descent refers to the progress of the presenting part through the pelvis. Descent depends on three forces: (1) pressure of the amniotic fluid, (2) direct pressure of the contracting fundus on the fetus, and (3) contraction of the maternal diaphragm and abdominal muscles in the second stage of labor. The effects of these forces are modified by the size and shape of the maternal pelvic planes and the size and capacity of the fetal head to mold.

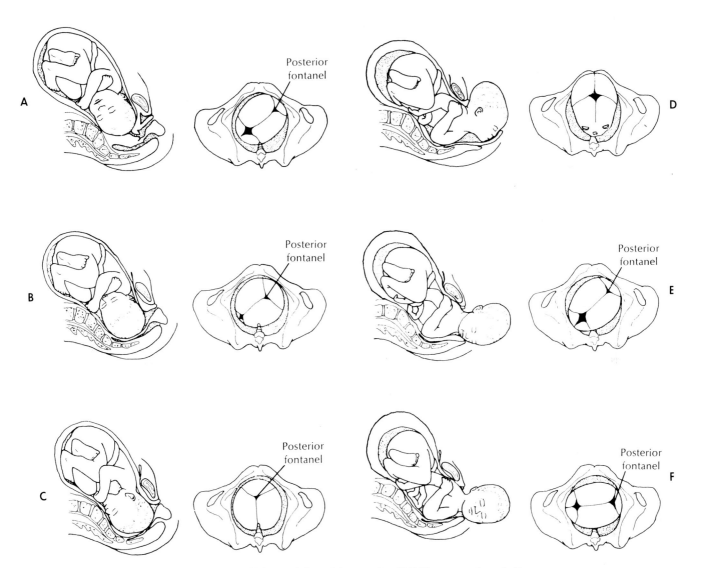

FIG. 9-13   Mechanism of labor in left occipitoanterior (LOA) presentation. **A,** Engagement and descent. **B,** Flexion. **C,** Internal rotation to OA. **D,** Extension. **E,** Restitution. **F,** External rotation.

The degree of descent is measured by the station of the presenting part (see Fig. 9-6). The speed of the descent increases in the second stage of labor. In first-time pregnancy this descent is slow but steady; in subsequent pregnancies the descent may be rapid. Progress in the descent of the presenting part is determined by abdominal palpation (Leopold's maneuvers) and vaginal examination until the presenting part can be seen at the introitus.

Flexion

As soon as the descending head meets resistance from the cervix, pelvic wall, or pelvic floor, flexion normally occurs and the chin is brought into close contact with the fetal chest (Fig. 9-13, *B*). Flexion permits the smaller suboccipitobregmatic diameter (9.5 cm) rather than the larger diameters to present to the outlet.

Internal Rotation

The maternal pelvic inlet is widest in the transverse diameter. Therefore the fetal head passes the inlet into the true pelvis in the occipitotransverse position. The outlet is widest in the anteroposterior diameter, however. To exit, the fetal head must rotate. Internal rotation begins at the level of the ischial spines but is not completed until the presenting part reaches the lower pelvis. As the occiput rotates anteriorly, the face rotates posteriorly. With each contraction the fetal head is guided by the bony pelvis and the muscles of the pelvic floor. Eventually the occiput is in the midline beneath the pubic arch. The head is almost always rotated by the time it reaches the pelvic floor (Fig. 9-13, *C*). Both the levator ani muscles and the bony pelvis are important for anterior rotation. Previous childbirth injury or regional anesthesia compromises the function of the levator sling.

Extension

When the fetal head reaches the perineum, it is deflected anteriorly by the perineum. The occiput passes under the lower border of the symphysis pubis first; then the head emerges by extension: first the occiput, then the face, and finally the chin (Fig. 9-13, *D*).

Restitution and External Rotation

After birth of the head, it rotates briefly to the position it occupied when it was engaged in the inlet. This movement is referred to as *restitution* (Fig. 9-13, *E* and *F*). The 45-degree turn realigns the infant's head with her or his back and shoulders. The head can then be seen to rotate further. External rotation occurs as the shoulders engage and descend in maneuvers similar to those of the head. As noted earlier, the anterior shoulder descends first. When it reaches the outlet, it rotates to the midline and is born from under the pubic arch. The posterior shoulder is guided over the perineum until it is free of the vaginal introitus.

Expulsion

After birth of the shoulders, the head and shoulders are lifted up toward the mother's pubic bone and the trunk of the baby is born by a movement of lateral flexion in the direction of the symphysis pubis. When the baby has completely emerged, birth is complete. *This* is the end of the second stage of labor, and the *time* is recorded on the records.

ADAPTATION TO LABOR

The mother and fetus must adapt anatomically and physiologically during the birth process. Accurate assessment of the mother and fetus requires a knowledge of expected adaptations.

Fetal Adaptation

The anatomic adaptations the fetus must undergo to pass through the birth canal have been discussed. Several important physiologic adaptations also occur. The nurse must be aware of what changes to expect in terms of fetal heart rate, fetal circulation, respiratory movements, and other behaviors.

Fetal Heart Rate

Fetal heart rate (FHR) monitoring provides reliable and predictive information about the condition of the fetus related to oxygenation. Stresses to the uterofetoplacental unit result in characteristic FHR patterns. It is important that the nurse have a basic understanding of the factors involved in fetal oxygenation and of the fetal responses that reflect adequate fetal oxygenation.

The average FHR at term is 140 beats/min. The normal range is 110 to 160 beats/min. Earlier in gestation the FHR is higher, with an average of approximately 160 beats/min at 20 weeks' gestation. The rate decreases progressively as the maturing fetus reaches term. However, temporary accelerations and slight early decelerations of the FHR can be expected in response to spontaneous fetal movement, vaginal examination, fundal pressure, uterine contractions, and abdominal palpation.

Fetal Circulation

Fetal circulation can be affected by many factors. These include maternal position, uterine contractions, blood pressure, and umbilical cord blood flow. Uterine contractions during labor tend to decrease circulation through the spiral arterioles and subsequent perfusion through the intervillous space. Most healthy fetuses are able to compensate for this stress. Usually umbilical cord blood flow is undisturbed by uterine contractions or fetal position.

Fetal Respiration and Behavior

Certain changes stimulate chemoreceptors in the aorta and carotid bodies to prepare the fetus for initiating respirations after birth. These changes include the following:

- 7 to 42 ml of amniotic fluid is squeezed out of the lungs (during vaginal birth).
- Fetal oxygen pressure (Po_2) falls.
- Arterial carbon dioxide pressure (Pco_2) rises.
- Arterial pH falls.

Fetal movement remains the same as in pregnancy, but decreases after membranes rupture.

Maternal Adaptation

A thorough understanding of maternal adaptations to pregnancy helps the nurse anticipate and meet the woman's needs during labor. Further changes occur as the woman progresses through the stages of labor. Various body systems adapt to the process of labor, exhibiting both objective and subjective symptoms.

Cardiovascular Changes

The nurse can expect some changes in the woman's cardiovascular system during labor. During each contraction 400 ml of blood is emptied from the uterus into the maternal vascular system. This increases *cardiac output* by about 10% to 15% in the first stage and by about 30% to 50% in the second stage.

The nurse can anticipate changes in *blood pressure*. Several factors alter blood pressure in the mother. Blood flow, reduced in the uterine artery by contractions, is redirected to peripheral vessels. Peripheral resistance occurs, blood pressure rises, and the *pulse rate* slows. During the first stage of labor, uterine contractions increase systolic readings by about 10 mm Hg. Therefore assessing blood pressure between contractions provides more accurate data. During the second stage, contractions may increase systolic pressures by 30 mm Hg and diastolic readings by 25 mm Hg. However, both systolic and diastolic pressures remain somewhat elevated even between contractions. The woman already at risk for hypertension is then placed at increased risk for complications such as cerebral hemorrhage.

The woman must be discouraged from using the **Valsalva maneuver** (holding one's breath and tightening abdominal muscles) for pushing during the second stage. This activity increases intrathoracic pressure, reduces venous return, and increases venous pressure. The cardiac output and blood pressure increase and pulse slows temporarily. During the Valsalva maneuver, fetal hypoxia may occur. The process is reversed when the woman takes a breath.

Supine hypotension occurs when the ascending vena cava and descending aorta are compressed. The mother is at greater risk for supine hypotension if the uterus is particularly large because of multifetal pregnancy, hydramnios, obesity, or dehydration and hypovolemia. In addition, anxiety and pain, as well as some analgesic and anesthetic medications, can cause hypotension.

White blood cells (WBCs) increase, often to $\geq 25,000/mm^3$. Although the mechanism leading to this increase in WBCs is unknown, it may be secondary to physical or emotional stress or to tissue trauma. Labor is strenuous. Physical exercise alone can increase WBC count.

Some peripheral vascular changes occur, perhaps in response to cervical dilatation or to compression of maternal vessels by the fetus passing through the birth canal. Malar flush (reddened cheeks), hot or cold feet, and eversion of hemorrhoids may result.

Respiratory Changes

Respiratory system adaptations also are seen. Increased physical activity with increased oxygen consumption is reflected in an increase in the respiratory rate. *Hyperventilation* may cause respiratory alkalosis (an increase in pH), hypoxia, and hypocapnia (decrease in carbon dioxide). In the unmedicated woman in the second stage, oxygen consumption almost doubles. Anxiety also increases oxygen consumption.

Renal Changes

In the second trimester the urinary bladder becomes an abdominal organ. When filling, it is palpable above the symphysis pubis. During labor spontaneous voiding may be difficult for various reasons: tissue edema caused by pressure from the presenting part, discomfort, sedation, and embarrassment. Proteinuria of 1+ is within normal limits inasmuch as the finding can occur in response to

the breakdown of muscle tissue from the physical work of labor.

Integumentary Changes

The integumentary system adaptations are evident especially in the great distensibility in the area of the vaginal introitus (opening). The degree of distensibility varies with the individual. Despite this ability to stretch, even in the absence of episiotomy or lacerations, minute tears in the skin around the vaginal introitus do occur.

Musculoskeletal Changes

The musculoskeletal system is stressed during labor. Diaphoresis, fatigue, proteinuria (1+), and perhaps an increased temperature accompany the marked increase in muscle activity. Backache and joint ache (unrelated to fetal position) occur as a result of increased joint laxity at term. The labor process itself and the woman's pointing her toes can cause leg cramps.

Neurologic Changes

The neurologic system reflects the stress and discomfort of labor. Sensorial changes occur as the woman moves through phases of the first stage of labor and as she moves from one stage to the next. Initially she may be euphoric. Euphoria gives way to increased seriousness, then to amnesia between contractions during the second stage, and finally to elation or fatigue after giving birth. Endogenous endorphins (morphinelike chemical produced naturally by the body) raise the pain threshold and produce sedation. In addition, physiologic anesthesia of perineal tissues, caused by pressure of the presenting part, decreases perception of pain.

Gastrointestinal Changes

Labor affects the woman's gastrointestinal system. Dry lips and mouth may result from mouth breathing, dehydration, and emotional response to labor. During labor, gastrointestinal motility and absorption are decreased and stomach emptying time is delayed. Nausea and vomiting of undigested food eaten after onset of labor are common. Nausea and belching also occur as a reflex response to full cervical dilatation. The mother may state that diarrhea accompanied the onset of labor, or the nurse may palpate hard or impacted stool in the rectum.

Endocrine Changes

The endocrine system is active during labor. The onset of labor may be attributed to decreasing levels of progesterone and increasing levels of estrogen, prostaglandins, and oxytocin. Metabolism increases, and blood glucose levels may decrease with the work of labor.

KEY POINTS

- Five essential factors affect the process of labor and birth.
- Because of its size and relative rigidity, the fetal head has a major effect on the birth process.
- The diameters at the plane of the pelvic inlet, midpelvis, and outlet, plus the axis of the birth canal, determine whether vaginal birth is possible and the manner by which the fetus may pass down the birth canal.
- The forces acting to expel the fetus and placenta are derived from involuntary uterine contractions during the first stage of labor, which are augmented by voluntary bearing-down efforts during the second stage.
- The mother's position affects her anatomic and physiologic adaptations to labor.
- The cardinal movements of the mechanism of labor are engagement, descent, flexion, internal rotation, extension, external rotation (restitution) and expulsion of the baby.
- Many factors, including changes in the maternal uterus, cervix, and pituitary gland, are involved in the initiation of labor.
- An understanding of maternal adaptations to pregnancy is fundamental to anticipating and meeting the mother's needs.
- A healthy fetus with an adequate uterofetoplacental circulation will respond in fairly predictable ways to stresses.

CRITICAL THINKING EXERCISES

1. You are assigned to a nulliparous woman who is in early labor. She is lying in bed on her back and says, "I sure hope the baby doesn't take all day to come."
   a. Discuss how the nurse can find out what the woman believes about the labor process.
   b. Formulate a plan of care for this woman that incorporates the theory of the labor process.
   c. What evaluation criteria would be appropriate?

References

Friedman EA: *Labor: clinical evaluation and management,* ed 2, New York, 1978, Appleton-Century-Crofts.

Melzack R, Belanger E, Lacroix R: Labor pain; effect of maternal position on front and back pain, *J Pain Symptom Manage* 6(8):476, 1991.

Paine LL, Tinker DD: The effect of maternal bearing-down efforts on the actual umbilical cord pH and length of second stage labor, *J Nurse Midwifery* 37(1):61, 1990.

Willson JR, Carrington ER: *Obstetrics and gynecology,* ed 9, St Louis, 1991, Mosby.

Bibliography

Barkauskas V et al: *Health and physical assessment,* St Louis, 1994, Mosby.

Cunningham FG et al: *Williams obstetrics,* ed 19, Norwalk, CT, 1993, Appleton & Lange.

Jones RE: *Human reproductive biology,* San Diego, 1991, Academic Press.

Scott JR et al: *Danforth's obstetrics and gynecology,* ed 6, Philadelphia, 1990, JB Lippincott.

10

Management of Discomfort

J E A N   A .   B A C H M A N

LEARNING OBJECTIVES

Define the key terms listed.

Compare childbirth preparation methods.

Describe the breathing and relaxation techniques used for each stage of labor.

Discuss the types of analgesic and anesthetic used during labor.

Compare types of pharmacologic control of discomfort by stage of labor and method of birth.

Discuss the use of naloxone (Narcan) and naltrexone (Trexan).

Relate each step of the nursing process to the pharmacologic management of labor discomfort.

Describe the nursing responsibilities for a woman receiving analgesia or anesthesia during labor.

KEY TERMS

agonist-antagonist compounds
allergic reaction
analgesia
anesthesia
ataractics
Bradley method
Dick-Read method
effleurage
endorphins
epidural block
epidural blood patch
gate-control theory
hyperventilation
Lamaze method
local infiltration anesthesia
low spinal (saddle) block
narcotic analgesics
narcotic antagonist
neonatal narcosis
paracervical block
psychoprophylaxis method
pudendal block
referred pain
somatic pain
subarachnoid (spinal) block
systemic analgesia
visceral pain

RELATED TOPICS

After-birth pains *(Chap. 18)* • Antenatal diagnostic studies *(Chap. 20)* • Augmentation of labor*(Chap. 24)* • Cesarean birth *(Chap. 24)* • Nonreassuring fetal heart rate *(Chap. 11)* • Substance abusing patient *(Chap. 23)* • Supine hypotension *(Chap. 7)*

Pregnant women commonly worry about the pain they will experience during labor and childbirth and how they will react to and deal with that pain. Interventions include a wide variety of childbirth preparation methods that help the woman or couple cope with the discomfort of labor. The interventions selected depend on the situation and the preference of both the woman and her health care provider. This chapter discusses discomfort during labor and presents nonpharmacologic and pharmacologic interventions throughout all stages of labor. This information provides the basis for understanding the nurse's role in management of maternal discomfort during labor.

DISCOMFORT DURING LABOR
Neurologic Origins

The discomfort experienced during labor has two origins (Hughs, 1992). During the *first stage of labor* uterine contractions cause (1) cervical dilatation and effacement and (2) uterine ischemia (decreased blood flow and therefore local oxygen deficit) from contraction of the arteries to the myometrium. Pain impulses during the first stage of labor are transmitted through the spinal nerve segment of T11-12 and accessory lower thoracic and upper lumbar sympathetic nerves. These nerves originate in the uterine body and cervix.

The discomfort from cervical changes and uterine ischemia is **visceral pain.** It is located over the lower portion of the abdomen and radiates to the lumbar area of the back and down the thighs. Usually the woman experiences discomfort only during contractions and is free from pain between contractions.

During the *second stage of labor,* the stage of expulsion of the baby, the woman experiences perineal or **somatic pain.** Perineal discomfort results from stretching of perineal tissues to allow passage of the fetus and traction on the peritoneum and uterocervical supports during contractions. Discomfort also can be produced by expulsion forces or from pressure by the presenting part on the bladder, bowel, or other sensitive pelvic structures. Pain impulses during the second stage of labor are carried through S1-4 and the parasympathetic system from perineal tissues. Pain experienced during the *third stage of labor,* as well as so-called afterpains, is uterine, similar to that experienced early in the first stage of labor. Areas of discomfort during labor are illustrated in Fig. 10-1.

Pain may be *local,* with cramps and a tearing or bursting sensation because of distention and laceration of the cervix, vagina, or perineal tissues. The discomfort is commonly perceived as an intense burning sensation that is felt as the tissue stretches. Pain also may be **referred,** in which the discomfort is felt in the back, flanks, and thighs.

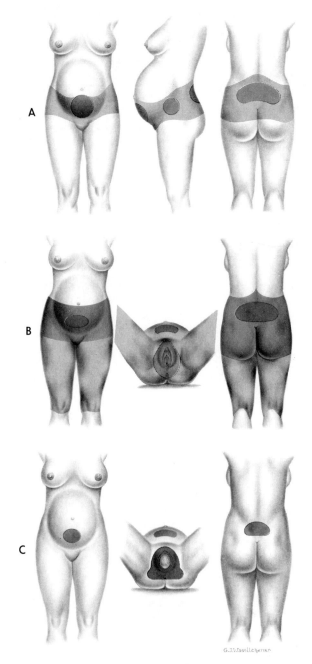

FIG. 10-1 Discomfort during labor. **A,** Distribution of labor pain during first stage. **B,** Distribution of labor pain during later phase of first stage and early phase of second stage. **C,** Distribution of labor pain during later phase of second stage and actual birth. (*Gray shading* indicates areas of mild discomfort; *light shading* indicates areas of moderate discomfort; *dark areas* indicate intense discomfort.)

Expression of Pain

Pain results in both psychic responses and reflex physical actions. The quality of physical pain has been described as prickling, burning, aching, throbbing, sharp, nauseating, and cramping. Pain in childbirth gives rise to symptoms that are identifiable. Increased activity of the sympathetic nervous system may occur in response to pain resulting in changes in blood pressure, pulse, respiration, and skin color. Pallor and diaphoresis may be seen (Potter and Perry, 1995). Bouts of nausea and vomiting and excessive perspiration also are common. Certain *affective expressions* of suffering are often seen. Affective changes include increasing anxiety with lessened perceptual field, writhing, crying, groaning, gesturing (hand clenching and wringing), and excessive muscular excitability throughout the body. Cultural expressions of pain may vary. For example, Native American women may endure pain quietly, whereas Hispanic women endure pain with patience but consider it acceptable to cry out (Mattson, Smith, 1993).

Perception of Pain

Although the pain threshold is remarkably similar in all persons regardless of sexual, social, ethnic, or cultural differences, these differences play a definite role in the individual's *perception of pain*. The effects of factors such as culture, counterstimuli, and distraction in coping with pain are not fully understood. The meaning of pain and the verbal and nonverbal expressions given to pain are apparently learned from interactions within the primary social group. Cultural influences may impose unrealistic expectations. For instance, Asian women believe it shameful to scream or show pain, and they avoid verbal expression (Mattson, Smith, 1993). Pain is personalized for each individual. As pain is experienced, people develop various coping mechanisms to deal with it. Emotional tension from anxiety and fear may increase pain and perception of pain during labor (see Dick-Read method, below). Pain, or the possibility of pain, can induce fear in which anxiety borders on panic. Fatigue and sleep deprivation magnify pain. Parity may affect perception of labor pain because primiparous women have longer labors and thus greater fatigue, causing a vicious circle of increased pain (Gatson-Johansson et al, 1988). Women with a history of substance abuse experience as much pain during labor as other women. It is usually unnecessary to withhold pain medications. However, close monitoring for complications associated with each substance is part of the nursing assessment.

At times pain stimuli that are particularly intense can be ignored. Certain nerve cell groupings within the spinal cord, brainstem, and cerebral cortex may have the ability to modulate the pain impulse through a blocking mechanism. This **gate-control theory** is helpful in understanding the approaches used in parent education for childbirth programs or the use of hypnosis in labor. According to this theory, pain sensations travel along sensory nerve pathways to the brain, and only a limited number of sensations or messages can travel through these nerve pathways at one time. By using distraction techniques such as massage or stroking, music, and imagery, the nerve pathways for pain perception are re-

duced or completely blocked. These distractors are thought to work by closing down a hypothetic gate in the spinal cord, thus blocking pain signals from reaching the brain. Perception of pain stimuli is diminished.

Also, when the laboring woman performs neuromuscular and motor skills, activity within the spinal cord itself further modifies the transmission of pain. Cognitive activities of concentration on breathing and relaxation require selective and directed cortical activity, which activates and closes the gating mechanism as well. The gate-control theory emphasizes the need for a supportive setting for birth. In such an environment the laboring woman may be able to relax and allow the various higher mental activities to be implemented.

At other times maternal fatigue, fetal size or position, or other factors require the use of medications in addition to comfort measures. Labor pain may result in physiologic responses that decrease uterine contractility and lengthen the labor. The nurse needs to understand that each woman experiences and perceives pain in her own unique way and that this pain needs to be acknowledged by the nurse as it is described by the woman. Concerns and anxieties can occur during later phases of labor and overcome the skills learned in parent education classes (Wuitchik et al, 1990).

NONPHARMACOLOGIC MANAGEMENT OF DISCOMFORT

The alleviation of pain is important. Commonly it is not the amount of pain the woman experiences, but *whether she meets her goals for herself in coping with the pain* that influences her perception of the birth experience as "good" or "bad." The observant nurse looks for cues to identify the woman's desired level of control in the management of pain and its relief.

Nonpharmacologic methods for relief of discomfort are taught in many different types of childbirth preparation classes. Whether or not a woman or couple has attended these classes or has read various books and magazines on the subject, the nurse can teach techniques to relieve discomfort during labor.

Childbirth Preparation Methods

Today most health care providers recommend or offer childbirth preparation classes to expectant parents. Major methods taught in the United States are (1) the **Dick-Read** or natural childbirth method, (2) the Lamaze or psychoprophylactic method (PPM), and (3) the Bradley method or husband-coached childbirth.

Dick-Read Method

Grantly Dick-Read was an English physician who published two books, *Natural Childbirth* (1933) and *Childbirth Without Fear* (1944), in which he theorized that pain in childbirth was the result of social conditioning and a fear-tension-pain syndrome.

According to Dick-Read (1959):

> Fear, tension, and pain are three veils opposed to the natural design which have been concerned with preparation for and attendance at childbirth. If fear, tension, and pain go hand in hand, then it must be necessary to relieve tension and to overcome fear in order to eliminate pain. The implementation of my theory demonstrates methods by which fear can be overcome, tension may be eliminated and replaced by physical and mental relaxation.

Dick-Read's work became the foundation for organized programs of childbirth preparation and teacher training throughout the United States, Canada, Great Britain, and South Africa. Nurses prepared in this method established the International Childbirth Education Association (ICEA) in 1960.

To replace fear of the unknown with understanding and confidence, Dick-Read's program includes information on labor and birth, as well as nutrition, hygiene, and exercise. Classes include practice in three techniques: physical exercise to prepare the body for labor; conscious relaxation; and breathing patterns.

Conscious relaxation involves progressive relaxation of muscle groups in the entire body. With practice, many women are able to relax on command, both during and between contractions. Some women actually sleep between contractions.

Breathing patterns include deep abdominal respirations for most of labor, shallow breathing toward the end of the first stage, and, until recently, breath holding for the second stage of labor. Teachers of the Dick-Read method contend that the weight of the abdominal musculature on the contracting uterus increases pain. The woman is taught to force her abdominal muscles to rise as the uterus rises forward during a contraction, thus lifting the abdominal muscles off the contracting uterus.

The Dick-Read method has been adapted to ensure that labor support provided in the past by the nursing staff is now provided by the father or a support person chosen by the mother.

Lamaze Method

During the 1960s the **Lamaze method** gained popularity in the United States after Marjorie Karmel introduced the **psychoprophylaxis method** (PPM) in her book, *Thank You, Dr. Lamaze*. The American Society for Psychoprophylaxis in Obstetrics (ASPO) was formed in 1960 and the National Association of Childbirth Education, Inc. (NACE) was formed in 1970 to promote the Lamaze method and prepare teachers in the method. In 1971 the national Council of Childbirth Education Specialists, Inc. (CCES) was founded to offer teacher training seminars.

The Lamaze method grew out of Pavlov's work on classical conditioning. According to Lamaze, pain is a conditioned response. Women can also be conditioned not to experience pain in labor; the Lamaze method conditions women to respond to mock uterine contractions with controlled muscular relaxation and breathing patterns instead of crying out and losing control (Lamaze, 1972). Coping strategies also include focusing on a focal point, such as a favorite picture or pattern, to keep nerve pathways occupied so they cannot respond to painful stimuli.

The woman is taught to relax uninvolved muscle groups while she contracts a specific muscle group. She applies this in labor by relaxing uninvolved muscles while her uterus contracts. Women who attended Lamaze-type childbirth preparation classes maintained a significantly higher level of neuromuscular control during the first stage of labor than women who were self-prepared (Bernardini, Maloni, Stegman, 1983). The perception of maintaining control is closely associated with satisfaction, according to studies by Cronenwett and Brickman (1983) and Mackey (1990).

Lamaze teachers believe that chest breathing lifts the diaphragm off the contracting uterus, thus giving it more room to expand. Chest breathing patterns vary according to the intensity of the contractions and the progress of labor. Teachers also seek to eliminate fear by increasing the understanding of how the body functions and the neurophysiology of pain. Support in labor is provided by the woman's husband or other support person or by a specially trained labor attendant termed a *monitrice*.

Bradley Method

Robert Bradley, a Denver obstetrician, published *Husband-Coached Childbirth* in 1965, advocating what he calls true natural childbirth, without anesthesia or analgesia and with a husband-coach and use of labor breathing techniques. The American Academy of Husband-Coached Childbirth (AAHCC) was founded to prepare teachers and make the method available.

The **Bradley method** is based on observations of animal behavior during birth and emphasizes working in harmony with the body, using breath control, abdominal breathing, and general body relaxation (Bradley, 1974). The technique stresses environmental factors such as darkness, solitude, and quiet to make childbirth a more natural experience. Women using the Bradley method often appear to be sleeping in labor, but they are actually in a state of deep mental relaxation.

Although the father's presence during labor seems to be very important to most women, the concept of the father as coach has been criticized by some (Klein et al, 1981). Some men are not comfortable with this role but can still be supportive of their wives during pregnancy and childbirth.

Comparison of Childbirth Methods

Most proponents of prepared childbirth agree that the major causes of pain in labor are fear and tension. All methods attempt to reduce these two factors and elimi-

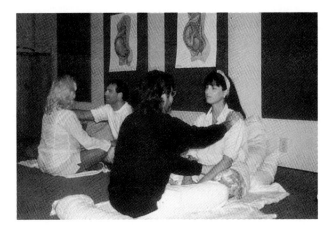

FIG. 10-2 Expectant parents learning relaxation techniques. (Courtesy Marjorie Pyle, RNC, *Lifecircle,* Costa Mesa, CA.)

nate pain by increasing the woman's knowledge of what to expect in labor and birth, enhancing her self-confidence and sense of control, preparing a support person (usually her husband), and training her in physical conditioning and relaxation breathing.

There are a few fine differences in approach. For example, Bradley teachers discourage the use of medication, encouraging the woman to focus inwardly and to take direction from her own body. Lamaze teachers believe that the judicious use of pain medication can be an appropriate adjunct to relaxation techniques and stress external focusing and distraction. In reality few instructors adhere strictly to one particular method but, instead, incorporate a variety of strategies aimed at increasing the woman's ability to cope with labor and minimize her need for medication.

Relaxation and Breathing Techniques
Focusing and Feedback Relaxation

Some women bring a favorite device for use in focusing attention. Others choose some fixed object in the labor room. As the contraction begins, they may focus on this object to reduce their perception of pain. This technique, coupled with feedback relaxation, helps the woman work with her contractions rather than against them. The coach monitors this process, giving the woman cues as to when to begin the breathing techniques (Fig. 10-2). A common feedback mechanism is for the woman and her coach to verbalize the word "relax" at the onset of each contraction and throughout it as needed. After the degree of relaxation has been assessed, relaxation techniques practiced in the prenatal period can be reviewed. The coach also keeps the woman from being disturbed by routine examinations for progress and checking of FHR. These procedures are postponed until the contraction is completed.

Breathing Techniques

Different approaches to childbirth preparation stress varying techniques for using breathing as a tool to help the woman maintain control through contractions. *In the first stage,* breathing techniques can promote relaxation of abdominal muscles and thereby increase the size of the abdominal cavity. This lessens friction and discomfort between the uterus and the abdominal wall. Because the muscles of the genital area also become more relaxed, they do not interfere with descent. *In the second stage,* breathing is used to increase abdominal pressure and thereby assist in expelling the fetus. It also is used to relax the pudendal muscles to prevent precipitate expulsion of the fetal head.

For those couples who have prepared for labor by practicing such techniques, occasional reminders may be all that is necessary. For those who have had no preparation, instruction in simple breathing and relaxation can be given early in labor and often is surprisingly successful. Motivation is high, and learning readiness is enhanced by the reality of labor.

There are varied approaches to breathing techniques during contractions. The nurse needs to ascertain what if any information the laboring couple has before providing them with instruction. Generally, slow abdominal breathing, approximately half the woman's normal breathing rate, is initiated when the woman can no longer walk or talk through contractions (Box 10-1). As contractions increase in frequency and intensity the woman may need to change to chest breathing, which is more shallow and approximately twice her normal rate of breathing.

The most difficult time to maintain control during contractions comes when the cervical dilatation reaches 8 to 10 cm. This period is also called the *transition period*. Even for the woman who has prepared for labor, concentration on breathing techniques is difficult to maintain. The type used may be the 4:1 pattern: breath, breath, breath, breath, puff (as though blowing out a candle). This ratio may increase to 6:1 or 8:1. These patterns begin with the routine cleansing breath and end with a deep breath exhaled to "blow the contraction away." An undesirable side effect of this type of breathing may be **hyperventilation.** The woman must be aware of the accompanying symptoms of the resultant *respiratory alkalosis:* lightheadedness, dizziness, tingling of fingers, and circumoral numbness. Alkalosis may be overcome by having the woman breathe into a paper bag that is tightly held around the mouth and nose. This enables her to rebreathe carbon dioxide and replace the bicarbonate ion. She can breathe into her cupped hands if no bag is available.

As the fetal head reaches the pelvic floor, the woman will experience the urge to push and will automatically begin to exert downward pressure by contracting her abdominal muscles. Descent cannot continue until the cervix is fully dilated and the presenting part is free to move

CLEANSING BREATH
Relaxed breath in through nose and out mouth. Used at the beginning and end of each contraction.
SLOW-PACED BREATHING (APPROXIMATELY 6-8 BREATHS PER MINUTE)
Not less than half normal breathing rate (No. breaths/min divided by 2)
IN-2-3-4/OUT-2-3-4/IN-2-3-4/OUT-2-3-4. . .
MODIFIED-PACED BREATHING (APPROXIMATELY 32-40 BREATHS PER MINUTE)
Not more than twice normal breathing rate (No. breaths/min × 2)
IN-OUT/IN-OUT/IN-OUT/IN-OUT/. . .
For more flexibility and variety, the woman may combine the slow and modified breathing by using the slow breathing for beginnings and ends of contractions and modified breathing for more intense peaks. This technique conserves energy and lessens fatigue.
PATTERNED-PACED BREATHING (SAME RATE AS MODIFIED)
Enhances concentration
a. 3:1 Patterned breathing
   IN-OUT/IN-OUT/IN-OUT/IN-BLOW
   (repeat through contraction)
b. 4:1 Patterned breathing
   IN-OUT/IN-OUT/IN-OUT/IN-OUT/IN-BLOW
   (repeat through contraction)

You may do any pattern desired, although ratios of 5:1 or higher tend to be very tiring. Some people like to do patterned breathing to a tune (Yankee Doodle, Old McDonald), to a repeated phrase (I think I can, I think I can), or in a pyramid pattern such as 1:1, 2:1, 3:1, 4:1, 5:1—5:1, 4:1, 3:1, 2:1, 1:1
c. *Coach call:* May be used when woman needs more distraction and concentration (e.g., during transition). The woman's coach signals the breathing ratio with his/her fingers or by verbal cues, changing the ratio after each "IN-BLOW."
Example:

IN-OUT/IN-OUT/IN-BLOW

IN-OUT/IN-OUT/IN-OUT/IN-OUT/IN-BLOW

IN-OUT/IN-BLOW

From Shapiro et al: *The Lamaze ready reference guide for labor and birth,* ed 2, Washington, DC, 1989, Chapter ASPO/Lamaze.

down the birth canal. Pushing before full dilatation is reached compresses the cervix between the fetal head and the pubic bone. This compression may result in a non-reassuring FHR, cervical edema, or cervical laceration. It may even slow the dilatation process. The woman can control the urge to push by taking panting breaths or by slowly exhaling through pursed lips. This is good practice for the type of breathing to be used as the fetal head is slowly born.

Effleurage and Sacral Pressure

Effleurage and sacral pressure, or massage, are two methods that have brought relief to many women during the first stage of labor. The gate-control theory may supply the reason for the effectiveness of these measures. **Effleurage** (see Fig. 7-16), which is a light stroking of the abdomen in rhythm with breathing during contractions, is used to distract the woman from contraction pain. The woman or her partner can perform effleurage on any area of her body. If a monitor belt makes it difficult to perform effleurage on the abdomen, a thigh or the chest may be used.

Jet Hydrotherapy

Jet hydrotherapy (whirlpool baths) is another nonpharmacologic method to use for increasing comfort and relaxation during labor although not universally accepted or implemented. Many new birthing units are installing baths with air jets. The buoyancy of the warm water, with or without air jets, provides support for tense muscles.

Several immediate benefits are seen. Relief from discomfort and general body relaxation reduce the woman's anxiety. Less anxiety decreases adrenalin production, which in turn allows an increase in levels of oxytocin (to stimulate labor) and endorphins (to reduce pain perception). In addition the bubbles and gentle lapping of the water stimulate the nipples (hyperstimulation of uterine contractions has not occurred [Aderhold, Perry, 1991]). Cervical dilatation of 2 to 3 cm in 30 minutes often is noted. Blood pressure readings decrease and diuresis occurs. If the woman is experiencing back labor secondary to occiput posterior or transverse presentation, she is encouraged to assume the hands and knees or the side-lying position in the tub (Fig. 10-3, *A* and *C*). Because this position decreases pain and increases relaxation and the

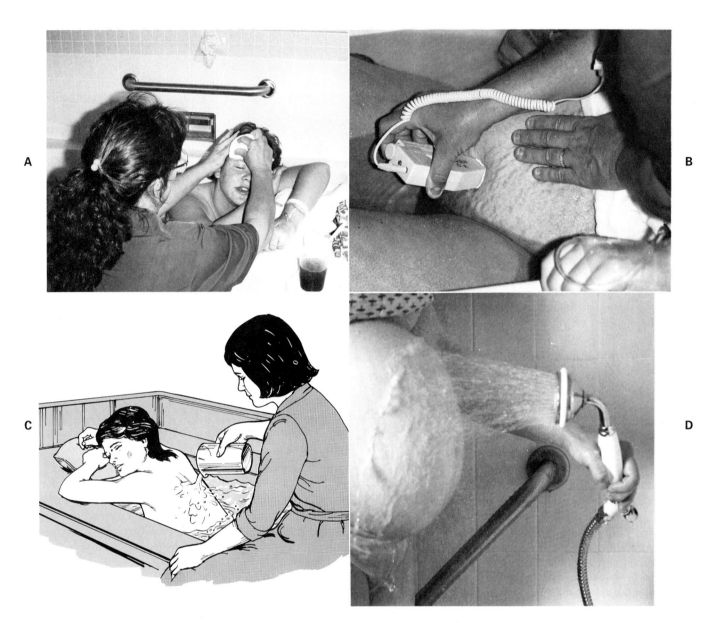

FIG. 10-3   Jet hydrotherapy during labor. **A,** Nurse provides comfort measures and ensures adequate hydration (note glass of clear fluid). **B,** Nurse assesses the FHR. **C,** Woman experiencing back labor, relaxing while nurse pours warm water over her back. **D,** Use of shower as one alternative to jet hydrotherapy during labor. (**A** and **B** courtesy Kathy Aderhold, CNM, Presbyterian/St. Luke's Medical Center, Denver; **D** courtesy Kathy Harold, RN, MS, Birth Place, Barnes Hospital at Washington University, Medical Center, St Louis.)

production of oxytocin, the fetus can rotate to the occiput anterior position spontaneously.

Jet hydrotherapy must be ordered by the primary health care provider. The mother's vital signs must be within normal limits, her cervix needs to be dilated 4 to 5 cm, and she must be in the active phase of the first stage of labor. If she is in the latent phase, her contractions may slow down. Fetal well-being must be established. Her membranes may be intact or ruptured. If ruptured, the fluid must be clear or only lightly stained with meconium (Aderhold, Perry, 1991). Heavy meconium

staining necessitates an internal electrode, in which case jet hydrotherapy would be contraindicated.

During the bath, if the woman's temperature and FHR increase, the water is cooled down or she is asked to step out of the bath to cool down. The bath water is kept between 96° and 98° F (35.6° and 36.7° C). The mother's temperature may remain slightly elevated for a short time after the bath. Fluids and ice chips and a cool face cloth are offered during the bath (Fig. 10-3, *A*). Maternal vital signs and labor and FHR are reassessed after the bath (Fig. 10-3, *B*).

The tub must be kept meticulously clean. Cleansing solutions vary with institution; however, household bleach (Clorox) is commonly used.

Transcutaneous Electrical Nerve Stimulation

Transcutaneous electrical nerve stimulation (TENS) may be effective because of the placebo effect, that is, confidence in TENS may stimulate the release of endogenous opiates (enkephalins) in the woman's body and thus alleviate the discomfort (Scott et al, 1990).

Two pairs of electrodes are taped on either side of the thoracic and sacral spine. Continuous mild electrical currents are applied from a battery-operated device. During a contraction the woman increases the stimulation by turning control knobs on the device. Women describe the sensation as a tingling or buzzing and pain relief as good or very good. The use of TENS poses no risk to the mother or fetus. TENS is credited with reducing or eliminating the need for analgesia and with increasing the woman's perception of control over the experience.

The nurse assists the mother who is using TENS by explaining the device and its use, by carefully placing and securing the electrodes, and by closely evaluating its effectiveness.

Other Nonpharmacologic Methods

Various other nonpharmacologic methods for control of discomfort are practiced. Many are learned in childbirth preparation classes. These include hypnosis, acupressure, yoga, biofeedback, and therapeutic touch (Lindberg, Lawlis, 1988; Nichols, Humenick, 1988; Kerschner, Scherck, 1991). Aromatherapy, the use of herbal teas or vapors, is reported to have good effects for some women (Valnet, 1990; Tesserand, 1990).

Women are being encouraged to *tune into their own body cues* and to incorporate natural responses. Techniques include vocalization, or sounding, to relieve tension, imagery-assisted relaxation (IAR), and visualization to guide women into positive spaces ("seeing" the vagina open up around the baby), hot compresses to the perineum, perineal massage, warm showers (Fig. 10-3, *D*) or bathing during labor, and relaxing music and subdued lighting.

PHARMACOLOGIC MANAGEMENT OF DISCOMFORT
Sedatives

Sedatives such as barbiturates relieve anxiety, promote relaxation, and induce sleep only in prodromal or early latent labor and in the absence of pain. If the woman has pain, sedatives given without an analgesic may increase apprehension and cause the mother to become hyperactive and disoriented. Undesirable side effects include re-

spiratory and vasomotor depression of both the mother and newborn. Because of these disadvantages, barbiturates are seldom used (Scott et al, 1990).

Analgesia and Anesthesia

The use of analgesia and anesthesia was not generally accepted as part of obstetric management until Queen Victoria used chloroform during the birth of her son in 1853. Since then much study has gone into the development of pharmacologic control of discomfort during the birth period. The goal of researchers is to develop methods that provide adequate pain relief to women without adding to maternal or fetal risk or affecting the progress of labor.

Nursing management of obstetric analgesia and anesthesia combines the nurse's expertise in maternity care with a knowledge and understanding of anatomy and physiology, and of medications and their desired and undesired side effects and methods of administration.

Anesthesia encompasses analgesia, amnesia, relaxation, and reflex activity. It is the abolition of pain perception by interrupting the nerve impulses going to the brain. Loss of sensation may be partial or complete, sometimes with the loss of consciousness.

The term **analgesia** is best reserved to describe only those states in which there is alleviation of the sensation of pain or the raising of one's threshold for pain perception. With analgesia there is no loss of consciousness.

Analgesia can be induced by positive conditioning (e.g., Lamaze method, imagery, relaxation) and analgesic drugs. A basic understanding of the normal course of labor and birth and proper physical and psychologic preparation by the pregnant woman may reduce perception of pain during childbirth. Especially important is good antenatal care in its broadest sense; reassurance and suggestion are beneficial. Participation in childbirth preparation classes such as those proposed by Dick-Read (1959) or psychoprophylaxis by Lamaze (1972) or Bradley (1974) should do much to alleviate distress.

The type of analgesic or anesthetic to be used is chosen in part by the stage of labor and by the method of birth (Box 10-2).

Systemic Analgesia

Systemic analgesia remains the major method of analgesia for women in labor when personnel trained in regional analgesia are not available (Scott et al, 1990). Systemic analgesics cross the blood-brain barrier to provide central analgesic effects. They also cross the placental barrier. Effects on the fetus depend on the maternal dosage, the pharmacokinetics of the specific drug, and the route and timing of administration. Intravenous (IV) administration is often preferred over intramuscular (IM) administration because the onset of the drug effect is faster and more reliable. Classes of analgesic drugs used include narcotic drugs, narcotic agonist-antagonist com-

---

BOX 10-2

Pharmacologic Control of Discomfort by Stage of Labor and Method of Birth

FIRST STAGE

Systemic analgesia
  Narcotic analgesic compounds
  Mixed narcotic agonist-antagonist compounds, analgesic potentiators
Nerve block analgesia/anesthesia
  Lumbar epidural analgesia
  Paracervical block

SECOND STAGE

Nerve block analgesia/anesthesia
  Local infiltration anesthesia
  Pudendal block
  Subarachnoid (spinal) anesthesia
  Epidural block
  Epidural and spinal narcotics
Inhalation analgesia/anesthesia
  Self-administered
  Nitrous oxide–oxygen
  General anesthesia

VAGINAL BIRTH

Local infiltration
Pudendal block
Lumbar epidural block
  Analgesia
  Anesthesia
Subarachnoid block
  Analgesia
  Anesthesia
Inhalation analgesia

CESAREAN BIRTH

Subarachnoid block
  Spinal
  Saddle block (low spinal)
Lumbar epidural block
  Anesthesia
Inhalation
  General anesthesia

---

pounds, and tranquilizers. Tranquilizers used are analgesic-potentiating drugs (ataractics).

Narcotic Analgesic Compounds

Narcotic analgesics, such as meperidine (Demerol) and fentanyl (Sublimaze), are especially effective for the relief of severe, persistent, or recurrent pain. They have no amnesic effect. Meperidine overcomes inhibitory factors in labor and may even relax the cervix.

Meperidine is the most commonly used narcotic for women in labor (Scott et al., 1990). After IV injection, onset is rapid (30 seconds), and maximum effect is reached in 5 to 10 minutes. Peak effect after IM injection is reached in 40 to 50 minutes, with a duration of about 3 hours. To minimize neonatal depression, birth should ideally occur less than 1 or more than 4 hours after IM injection. Since tachycardia is a possible side effect, meperidine is used cautiously for women with cardiac disease.

Fentanyl is a potent, short-acting narcotic analgesic. After IV injection, onset of the drug effect occurs within 2 minutes and lasts about 30 to 60 minutes. Onset of the drug effect after IM injection occurs in 7 to 15 minutes, reaches its peak effect in 20 to 30 minutes, and lasts for 1 to 2 hours. Additive central nervous system (CNS) and respiratory depression occurs if fentanyl is given with alcohol, antihistamines, antidepressants, or other sedatives/hypnotics.

Mixed Narcotic Agonist-Antagonist Compounds

An agonist is an agent that activates something; an antagonist is an agent that blocks something from happening. Mixed narcotic **agonist-antagonist compounds** such as butorphanol (Stadol) and nalbuphine (Nubain), in the doses used during labor provide analgesia without causing respiratory depression of the mother or neonate. Both IM and IV routes are used for administration. Butorphanol (1 to 3 mg IM; 0.5 to 2 mg IV) or nalbuphine (0.2 mg/kg SC/IM; 0.1 to 0.2 mg/kg IV) may be given during the first stage of labor. *If the woman has a preexisting narcotic dependency, the antagonist effect of these compounds will cause her to immediately exhibit symptoms of narcotic withdrawal.*

Analgesic Potentiators (Ataractics)

Phenothiazines, so-called tranquilizer drugs, have the property of augmenting most of the desirable but few of the undesirable effects of analgesics or general anesthetics. These **ataractics** do not relieve pain but decrease anxiety and apprehension, as well as potentiate narcotic effects. This potentiation effect causes two drugs to work together more effectively so that the addition of an ataractic allows the narcotic dosage to be reduced. Analgesic potentiators include compounds such as promethazine (Phenergan), propiomazine (Largon), hydroxyzine (Vistaril), and promazine (Sparine).

In addition to potentiating the effects of the analgesic, the ataractic (tranquilizer) also acts as an antinauseant and antiemetic. The combination can be administered safely until the end of the first stage of labor. Usual dosages include the following: promethazine 25 to 50 mg IM or 15 to 25 mg IV; promazine 50 mg IM or 5 to 10 mg IV; hydroxyzine 25 to 50 mg IM. Since hydroxyzine is given only by IM injection, onset of effect is slower and less predictable. Fetal or neonatal problems rarely develop with these dosages.

Narcotic Antagonists

Narcotics such as meperidine and fentanyl may cause too much CNS depression in the mother or the newborn. **Narcotic antagonists** such as naloxone (Narcan) and naltrexone (Trexan) promptly reverse the narcotic effects. In addition, the narcotic antagonist also counters the effect of stress-induced levels of endorphins. **Endorphins** are endogenous opioids secreted by the pituitary gland that act on the CNS and peripheral nervous system to reduce pain. Beta-endorphin is the most potent of the endorphins. The physiologic role of endorphins is not completely understood. It is thought that endorphins increase during pregnancy and birth in humans and may increase the ability of laboring women to tolerate acute pain.

A narcotic antagonist is especially valuable if labor is more rapid than expected and birth is anticipated when the narcotic is at its peak effect. The antagonist may be given through the woman's IV line or it may be administered IM into her gluteal muscle. Narcotic antagonists counteract maternal and neonatal narcotic effects. The mother needs to be told that with the administration of an antagonist the pain will return. *Narcotic antagonists must be administered cautiously to a substance-dependent woman because symptoms of narcotic withdrawal may occur.*

A narcotic antagonist can be given to the newborn. **Neonatal narcosis,** CNS depression in the newborn caused by a narcotic, may be exhibited by respiratory depression, hypotonia, lethargy, and a delay in temperature regulation. Alterations of neurologic and behavioral responses may be evident for 72 hours after birth. Meperidine may be present in the neonate's urine for up to 3 weeks. Some depression of attention and social responsiveness may be evident for up to 6 weeks (Briggs, Freeman, Yaffe, 1986).

Nerve Block Analgesia and Anesthesia

A variety of compounds are used in obstetrics to produce regional analgesia (minimal pain relief and motor block) and anesthesia (pain relief and motor block). Most of these drugs are related chemically to cocaine and carry the suffix -*caine.* This helps identify a local anesthetic.

The principal pharmacologic effect of local anesthetics is the temporary interruption of the conduction of nerve impulses, notably pain. Examples of common agents given in 0.5% to 1% solutions are lidocaine (Xylocaine), bupivacaine (Marcaine), chloroprocaine (Nesacaine), tetracaine (Pontocaine), and mepivacaine (Carbocaine).

Rarely, individuals are sensitive (allergic) to one or more local anesthetics. Sensitivity may be determined by testing with minute amounts of the drug to be used. Initially the CNS is stimulated when excessive amounts of anesthetic are injected. Stimulation may be followed by depression, hypotension, and other serious adverse effects. Atropine, antihistaminic drugs, oxygen, and supportive measures should bring relief.

As analgesia is established, a sympathetic blockage occurs, causing vasodilatation and pooling of blood in the lower extremities. Maternal hypotension also may occur. A fall of 20% to 30% in maternal blood pressure below the preblock average is regarded as hypotension and should be corrected promptly (Cheek and Gutsche, 1987). *Therefore adequate hydration for blood volume expansion is a prerequisite.* Hydration is achieved with a non–dextrose-containing balanced salt solution (e.g., Ringer's lactate or Plasma-Lyte). The mother is hydrated with 500 to 1000 ml intravenously within 20 minutes before the block. Facilities for cardiopulmonary resuscitation, including oxygen and suction, must be immediately available. If maternal and fetal resuscitation is needed, left uterine displacement must be maintained to optimize venous return and therefore perfusion of the uterus.

Local Infiltration Anesthesia

Local infiltration anesthesia of perineal tissue is commonly used when an episiotomy is to be done and when time or the fetal head position does not permit a pudendal block to be administered (Scott et al, 1990). Rapid anesthesia is produced by injecting an average of 10 to 20 ml of local anesthetic with 1% lidocaine or 2% chloroprocaine into the skin and then subcutaneously into the region to be anesthetized. Epinephrine often is added to the solution to intensify the anesthesia in a limited region and to prevent excessive bleeding and systemic effects by constricting local blood vessels (Clark et al, 1990). Repeated injection prolongs the anesthesia as long as needed.

Pudendal Block

Pudendal block is useful for the second stage of labor, episiotomy, and birth. Although a pudendal block does not relieve pain from uterine contractions, it does relieve pain in the clitoris, labia majora and minora, and the perineum.

Pudendal nerve block is administered 10 to 20 minutes before perineal anesthesia is needed. Once the presenting part descends through the cervix, vaginal and soon perineal distention occur. Vaginal and perineal pain

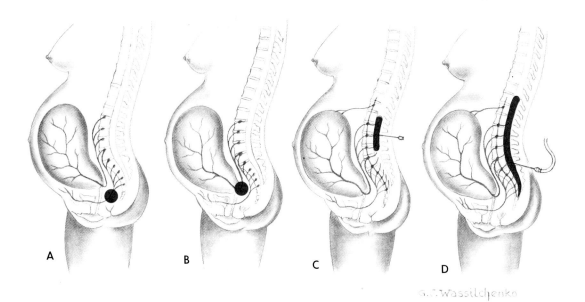

FIG. 10-4   Pain pathways and sites of pharmacologic nerve blocks. **A,** Pudendal block: suitable during second and third stages of labor and for repair of episiotomy. **B,** Paracervical (uterosacral) block: suitable during first stage of labor. **C,** Lumbar sympathetic block (one type of subarachnoid block): given as shown, suitable during first stage of labor. **D,** Epidural block: suitable during all stages of labor and for repair of episiotomy.

can be eliminated by a pudendal anesthetic block (Fig. 10-4, *A*). The pudendal nerve traverses the sacrosciatic notch just medial to the tip of the ischial spine on each side. Injection of an anesthetic solution at or near these points will anesthetize the pudendal nerves peripherally (Fig. 10-5). The transvaginal approach is generally used because it is less painful for the woman, has a higher success rate, and tends to cause fewer fetal complications (Scott et al, 1990). Pudendal block does not change maternal hemodynamic or respiratory functions, vital signs, or fetal heart rate (FHR). The bearing-down reflex is lessened or lost completely.

If all branches of the pudendal nerve are anesthetized, analgesia is sufficient for spontaneous vaginal birth or outlet (low) forceps-assisted birth. However, the anesthetic effect is insufficient to permit instrumental vaginal birth except for low forceps; and a pudendal block does not provide analgesia for uterine exploration or manual removal of the placenta (Scott et al, 1990).

Subarachnoid (Spinal) Anesthesia

In **subarachnoid (spinal) block,** local anesthetic is injected through the third, fourth, or fifth lumbar interspace into the subarachnoid space (Figs. 10-6 and 10-7), where the medication mixes with cerebrospinal fluid. This single-injection technique is useful for birth, but not for labor. For vaginal birth the anesthetic solution is administered during the second stage of labor when expulsion is imminent (e.g., fetal head is on the perineum.)

The **low spinal (saddle) block** injection is made with

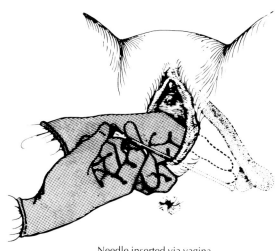

Needle inserted via vagina
through needle guide

FIG. 10-5   Pudendal block. Use of needle guide (Iowa trumpet) and Luer Lok syringe to inject medication. (Modified from Benson RC: *Handbook of obstetrics and gynecology,* ed 7, Los Altos, CA, 1980, Lange Medical Publications.)

the woman in a sitting position, her legs over the side of the delivery table, and her feet supported on a stool. The nurse stands in front of her. The woman rests her chin on her chest, arches her back, and leans on the nurse for support. The nurse comforts and coaches her. This posture is assumed to widen the intervertebral space for ease in inserting the spinal needle and to allow the heavy anesthetic solution to gravitate downward. The injection is

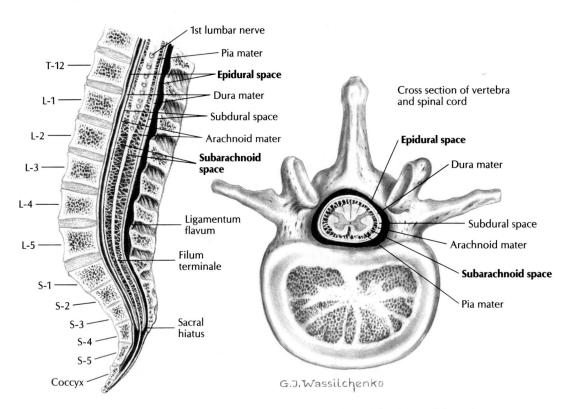

FIG. 10-6 Membranes and spaces of spinal cord; levels of sacral, lumbar, and thoracic nerves.

made between contractions to avoid an unexpectedly high block (medication rises above T10 with the potential of affecting the movement of diaphragm and muscles of respiration). Once the anesthetic has been injected, the woman remains upright for a period of 30 seconds to 2 minutes (as directed by the anesthesiologist) to permit downward diffusion. Then the woman is assisted to a supine position. She must remain supine with the head elevated slightly. Onset of anesthesia usually occurs within 1 to 2 minutes after injection. Duration of anesthesia is 1 to 3 hours, depending on the anesthetic used.

Marked hypotension, decreased cardiac output, and respiratory inadequacy tend to occur during any spinal anesthesia. Therefore the woman is hydrated with IV fluids before injection of anesthetic to decrease the potential for sympathetic blockade hypotension. After injection, maternal blood pressure, pulse, respirations, and FHR must be checked and recorded every 5 to 10 minutes. If signs of serious maternal hypotension or fetal distress develop, emergency care must be given (Emergency Box, p. 233).

Because the mother is not able to sense her contractions, she must be instructed when to bear down. If the birth occurs in a delivery room (rather than a labor-delivery-recovery room), the mother will need assistance to move back to her recovery bed after delivery of the placenta.

Advantages of spinal anesthesia include ease of administration and absence of fetal hypoxia with maintenance of normotension. Maternal consciousness is maintained, excellent muscular relaxation is achieved, and blood loss is not excessive. Maternal alertness enables the woman to participate in the birth process. Usually no other anesthetic agents (e.g., inhalation drugs) are required. If stirrups are used for birth, care must be taken to position them properly. Spinal anesthesia may be the method of choice for women with severe respiratory problems or with liver, kidney, or metabolic disease because it decreases the stress of labor and birth on these systems.

Disadvantages of spinal anesthesia include drug reactions (e.g., allergy), rare chemical myelitis or infection, hypotension, and high spinal anesthesia with respiratory paralysis; cardiopulmonary resuscitation (CPR) may be needed. When spinal anesthesia is given, the need for operative birth (episiotomy, low forceps extraction) tends to increase because of the elimination of voluntary expulsive efforts. After birth, there is an increased tendency for bladder and uterine atony as well as spinal headache.

Headache After Spinal (Lumbar) Puncture. Leakage of cerebrospinal fluid from the site of puncture of the *meninges* (membranous coverings of the spinal cord) is thought to be the major causative factor in post–lumbar puncture (postspinal) headache. Headache may be postural and occur only in the head-up or standing position. Presumably, with postural changes, the dimin-

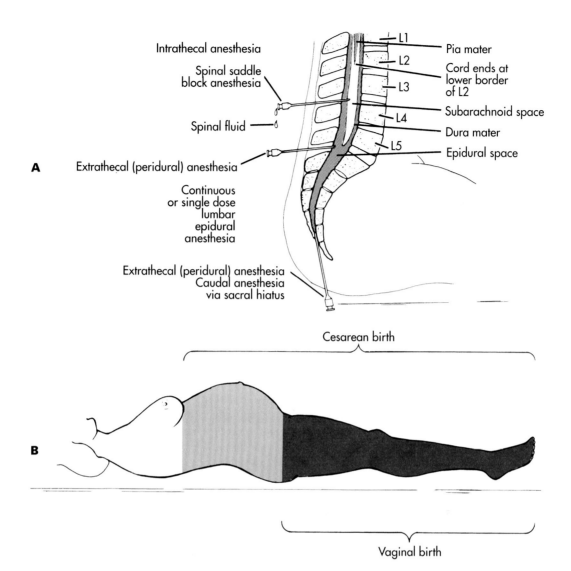

FIG. 10-7   A, Regional block anesthesia in obstetrics. **B,** Level of anesthesia necessary for cesarean birth and for vaginal birth. (Courtesy Ross Laboratories, Columbus, OH.)

EMERGENCY

MATERNAL HYPOTENSION WITH DECREASED PLACENTAL PERFUSION

SIGNS/SYMPTOMS

Maternal hypotension (20% drop from preblock level or less than 100 mm Hg systolic)
Fetal bradycardia
Decreased beat-to-beat FHR variability

INTERVENTIONS

Turn woman to lateral position or place pillow or wedge under right hip (see Fig. 12-8) to deflect uterus.
Maintain IV infusion at rate specified, or increase prn per hospital protocol.
Administer oxygen by face mask at 10 to 12 L/min.
Elevate the woman's legs.
Notify the physician/midwife/anesthesiologist/nurse anesthetist.
Administer IV vasopressor (e.g., ephedrine).
Remain with woman: continue to monitor maternal BP and FHR every 5 minutes until stable or per primary health care provider's order.

ished volume of cerebrospinal fluid creates traction on pain-sensitive CNS structures. Headache, auditory, and visual problems may persist for days or weeks.

However, the likelihood of this unpleasant complication can be reduced if the anesthesiologist uses a small-gauge spinal needle and avoids multiple punctures of the meninges. Positioning the woman absolutely flat in bed (with only a small, flat pillow for her head) for at least 8 hours has been recommended to prevent postspinal headache, but there is no definitive evidence that this procedure is effective. Positioning the woman on her abdomen is thought to decrease the loss of fluid through the puncture site. Hyperhydration has been claimed to be of value, but there is no compelling evidence to support its use (Cunningham et al, 1993). Initial treatment for postspinal headache usually includes analgesics, bed rest, caffeine, and increased fluid intake (i.e., 150 ml/hr IV) (Scott et al, 1990).

An autologous **epidural blood patch** (a patch repairing a tear or a hole in the dura mater around the spinal cord) has proven beneficial and may be considered if the headache does not resolve spontaneously (Scott et al, 1990). To form a patch, a few milliliters of the woman's blood without anticoagulant is injected epidurally at the site of the spinal tap (Fig. 10-8), forming a clot that covers the hole and prevents further fluid loss. Saline similarly injected in larger volumes has also been claimed to provide relief. Abdominal support with a girdle or abdominal binder seems to afford relief and is worth trying. For some women, the headache may be remarkably improved by the third day and absent by the fifth.

Epidural Block

Relief from the pain of uterine contractions and birth (vaginal and abdominal) can be accomplished by injecting a suitable local anesthetic into the epidural (peridural) space (see Figs. 10-6 and 10-7). The portal of entry into this space for obstetric analgesia and anesthesia is through either a lumbar intervertebral space or caudally through the sacral hiatus and sacral canal.

The caudal space is the lowest extent of the epidural, or peridural, space (see Figs. 10-6 and 10-7). Emerging from the dural sac a few inches higher, a rich network of sacral nerves passes downward through the caudal space. A suitable anesthetic solution filling the caudal canal may eliminate the sensation of pain carried via the sacral nerves to produce anesthesia suitable for vaginal birth. Higher levels with continuous caudal technique provide both analgesia in the first and second stages of labor and anesthesia for birth. Because of early analgesia, caudal epidural block is rarely used today (Writer, 1992). Specifics regarding this method are not presented. See medical texts listed in the bibliography for this information.

Complete lumbar **epidural block** for the discomfort of labor and vaginal birth requires a block from T10 to S5. For cesarean birth, a block is essential from at least

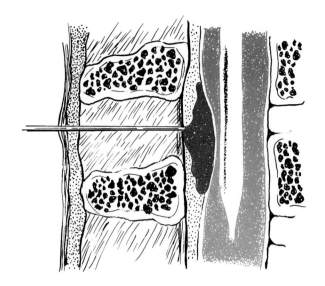

FIG. 10-8 Blood patch therapy for spinal headache.

T8 to S1. The diffusion of epidural anesthesia depends on the location of the catheter tip, the dosage and volume of anesthetic agent used, and the woman's position (e.g., horizontal or head up) (Cunningham et al, 1993).

For induction of lumbar epidural anesthesia, the woman is positioned as for a spinal injection (i.e., sitting) or in a modified Sims position (Fig. 10-9). For modified lateral Sims position the woman is placed on her side, shoulders parallel, legs slightly flexed, and back arched.

The woman is positioned preferably on her side to avoid weight of the uterus on the ascending vena cava and descending aorta, which can impair venous return and decrease placental perfusion. Oxygen is available should hypotension occur despite maintenance of IV fluid and displacement of the uterus to the side. The anesthesiologist may need to inject ephedrine (a vasopressor used to increase maternal blood pressure) and to accelerate IV fluid infusion (see Emergency Box, p. 233).

The FHR and progress in labor must be monitored carefully. The laboring woman will not be aware of changes in strength of uterine contractions or descent of the presenting part. Occasionally depression of contractions may result, necessitating augmentation of labor with oxytocin.

A single injection or continuous infusion (via pump) through an indwelling catheter results in excellent analgesia-anesthesia (Fig. 10-4, *D*). The *advantages* of continuous block are numerous: the mother remains alert and cooperative, good relaxation is achieved, airway reflexes remain intact, only partial motor paralysis develops, gastric emptying is not delayed, and blood loss is not excessive. Fetal distress is rare but may occur with rapid absorption or marked maternal hypotension. Dose, volume, and type of anesthetic can be modified quickly to allow the mother to push, to produce perineal anesthesia, and to permit forceps or even cesarean birth if required (Cunningham et al, 1993).

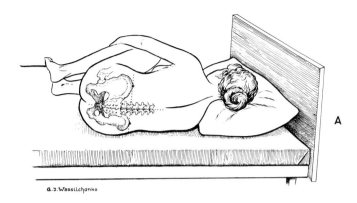

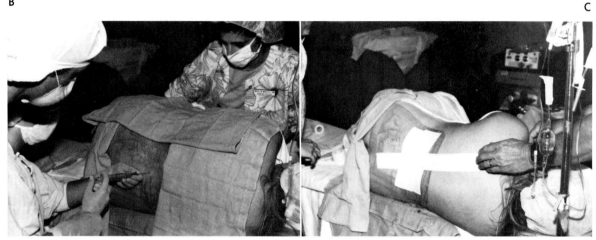

FIG. 10-9 A, Lateral decubitus position for epidural and subarachnoid block and anatomic landmarks to locate needle insertion site. **B,** Epidural anesthesia. Skin has been prepared with antiseptic solution (povidone-iodine [Betadine]). Area is draped with sterile towels. Nurse continues to support woman. **C,** Catheter is taped to woman's back; port segment is taped near her shoulder. (**B** and **C** courtesy Stanford University Hospital, Stanford, CA.)

The *disadvantages* of a continuous block for the woman include the need for an intravenous line, occasional dizziness, weakness of the legs, difficulty emptying the bladder, and shivering (Writer, 1992). Also, special training and experience are required by the anesthesiologist. Since a considerable amount of the drug must be used, reactions or rapid absorption of the anesthetic agent may result in hypotension, convulsions, or paresthesia. The incidence of operative birth (e.g., episiotomy, use of forceps) may be increased if the woman cannot bear down effectively. Occasionally accidental high spinal anesthesia (and later postspinal headache) may follow inadvertent perforation of the dural membrane when lumbar epidural anesthesia is administered.

For some women the anesthetic selected is not effective, and a second form of anesthesia is required. Establishment of effective pain relief with maximum safety takes time. Consequently, in case of rapid labor, the potential for pain relief during labor and for birth is not realized. For example, peridural anesthesia for women of higher parity in active labor is likely to prove not worth the bother, risk, and expense (Cunningham et al, 1993).

Epidural and Spinal Narcotics

There is a high concentration of narcotic receptors along the pain pathway in the spinal cord, in the brainstem, and in the thalamus. Because these receptors are highly sensitive to narcotics, a small quantity of narcotic produces marked analgesia lasting for several hours. Medication is injected through a catheter placed in the epidural or subarachnoid space, which reaches these narcotic receptors, and pain transmission is blocked.

Administration of epidural or spinal narcotics has several advantages. These narcotics do not cause maternal hypotension or affect vital signs. The woman feels contractions but not pain. Her ability to bear down during the second stage of labor is preserved because the pushing reflex is not lost and motor power remains intact.

Fentanyl may be used alone. Its effects last up to 90 minutes. When added to the local anesthetic at the time of epidural administration, it extends the duration of anesthesia. There are no cardiovascular effects. However, fentanyl does not provide adequate analgesia for second-stage labor pain, episiotomy, or birth (Cunningham et al, 1993).

The most common indication for the administration of epidural or spinal narcotics is for the relief of postoperative pain. For example, a woman who give birth by the abdominal route receives fentanyl (Innovar) or morphine after surgery through the catheter. The catheter may then be removed, and the woman is pain free for 24 hours. Occasionally the catheter is left in place in case another dose is needed.

Epidurally administered morphine allows the woman to be up with surprising ease and to care for her baby. Early ambulation and freedom from pain also facilitate bladder emptying. To women who have previously had a cesarean birth and have experienced the usual postoperative pain, the effects of this approach seem miraculous. However, nurses must utilize caution because the mother may not understand why she may experience pain after the narcotic wears off.

Side effects of morphine administered by the epidural or spinal route include nausea, vomiting, pruritus (itching), urinary retention, and delayed respiratory depression. Antiemetics, antipruritics, and narcotic antagonists are used to relieve symptoms. For example, naloxone or naltrexone, promethazine, or metoclopramide (Reglan) may be administered. Hospital protocols should provide specific instructions for treatment of these side effects. Some health care providers believe the risks of epidural or spinal injection are not sufficient to warrant its routine use. Respiratory depression is a serious concern; the woman's respiratory rate should be assessed and documented every hour for 24 hours.

Contraindications to Subarachnoid and Epidural Blocks

Some contraindications to epidural analgesia apply equally to caudal and subarachnoid blocks (Scott et al, 1990):

1. *Patient refusal.*
2. *Antepartum hemorrhage.* Acute hypovolemia leads to increased sympathetic tone to maintain the blood pressure. Any anesthetic technique that blocks the sympathetic fibers can lead to hypotension that can endanger the mother and baby.
3. *Anticoagulant therapy or bleeding disorder.* If a woman is receiving anticoagulant therapy or has a bleeding disorder, injury to a blood vessel may result in a hematoma. The hematoma may compress the cauda equina or the spinal cord and lead to serious CNS sequelae.
4. *Infection at the injection site.* Infection can be spread through the peridural or subarachnoid spaces if the needle traverses an infected area.
5. *Tumor at the injection site.* A tumor at the injection site is an unusual but definite contraindication.
6. *Allergy to anesthetic drug.*
7. *History of spinal injury, spinal surgery, or CNS disease.*
8. *Marked hypotension.*

Relative contraindications to intraspinal blocks include CNS disorders, extensive back surgery, morbid obesity or anatomic abnormality in which landmarks cannot be identified, and current or prior disease of the CNS (Scott et al, 1990).

Drug Effects on Neonate

Debate persists concerning the effects of epidural anesthesia on the neonate's neurobehavioral responses. Studies of associations between neurobehavioral outcome and epidural anesthesia are far from consistent (Avard, Nimrod, 1985). For example, neonatal neurobehavioral scores comparing infants born to mothers with and without epidural analgesia conflict between those showing no difference (Aboud et al, 1982; Marx, 1984) and those reporting that neonates did not score as well on neurobehavioral tests (Rosenblatt et al, 1981). Today, most believe this decreased muscle tone, if present, is temporary and of no clinical significance (Cheek, Gutsch, 1987).

Paracervical (Uterosacral) Block

Paracervical block is given to relieve pain from cervical dilatation and distention of the lower uterine segment in the first stage of labor during the active (acceleration) phase. For paracervical anesthesia a dilute local anesthetic drug (e.g., 5 ml of 1% procaine) is injected just beneath the mucosa adjacent to the outer rim of the cervix (9 and 3 o'clock positions) after the cervix is more than 5 cm dilated. A needle guide (e.g., the Iowa trumpet) is useful but not indispensable for transvaginal administration (Fig. 10-10). Relief from discomfort is noticed within approximately 5 minutes. Excellent pain relief lasts for at least 1 hour.

Anesthesia extends from the lower uterine segment and cervix to the upper one third of the vagina (see Fig. 10-4, *B*); there is no perineal anesthesia. Although there may be a transient depression of contractions, there is little or no effect on the labor. Repeat injections may be given until the cervix is dilated to 8 cm, whereupon another method, such as pudendal block, may be necessary.

Paracervical block anesthesia may cause fetal intoxication because of rapid absorption of the drug. When the anesthetic is injected into the tissues lateral to the cervix, it is picked up by the maternal circulation, which quickly involves the uterus and placenta. When overdosage occurs, the fetus may exhibit bradycardia because of the quinidine-like effect of the anesthetic on the myocardium or, because of a reduction in uterine blood flow. In addition, CNS medullary depression may develop, and the neonate may show vascular collapse and apnea at birth. Hematomas can develop at the site of injection if a uterine vessel is damaged.

Because of these potential complications, paracervical block may not be the method of choice for labor but remains an option for anesthesia during abortion or other gynecologic procedures.

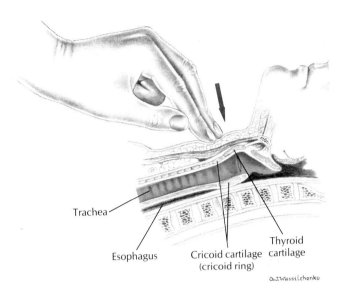

Trachea

Esophagus

Cricoid cartilage
(cricoid ring)

Thyroid
cartilage

G.J.Wassilchenko

FIG. 10-11   Technique of applying pressure on cricoid cartilage to occlude esophagus to prevent pulmonary aspiration of gastric contents during anesthesia induction.

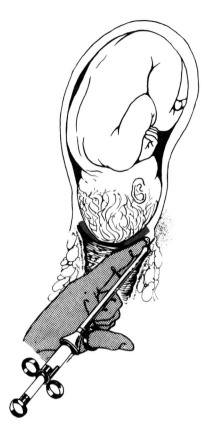

FIG. 10-10   Paracervical block. Note the position of the hand and fingers in relation to the cervix and fetal head and the shallow depth of the needle insertion. Note also that no undue pressure is applied at the vaginal fornix by the fingers or needle guide. (From Benson RC: *Handbook of obstetrics and gynecology,* ed 7, Los Altos, CA, 1980, Lange Medical Publications.)

General Anesthesia

General anesthesia is rarely indicated for uncomplicated vaginal birth. It may be necessary if there is a contraindication (including patient refusal) to nerve block analgesia/anesthesia, or if fetal indications necessitate rapid (STAT) birth (vaginal or abdominal). The woman is not awake with this method, and there is danger of respiratory depression and vomiting followed by aspiration. For women with hypovolemia, general anesthesia is safer than nerve block analgesia or anesthesia. Thiopental sodium (Pentothal) is commonly used for general anesthesia. Administered IV (4 mg per kilogram of body weight), thiopental sodium produces rapid induction of anesthesia and does not depress the fetus in this dosage (Scott et al, 1990).

If general anesthesia is being considered, the nurse gives the woman nothing by mouth and sees that an IV infusion is established. If time allows, the nurse premedicates the woman with a nonparticulate oral antacid such as sodium citrate (30 ml) to increase gastric pH to neutralize acid contents of the stomach. If there is sufficient time, some physicians also order a histamine blocker such as cimetidine to decrease production of gastric acid and

metoclopramide to increase gastric emptying (Scott et al, 1990). Before anesthesia a wedge should be placed under the woman's right hip to displace the uterus to the left to prevent aortal compression, which interferes with placental perfusion. Sometimes the nurse is asked to assist with *cricoid pressure* (Fig. 10-11) before intubation. Priorities for recovery room care are to maintain open airway, maintain cardiopulmonary functions, and prevent postpartum hemorrhage. Routine postpartum care is organized to facilitate parent-child attachment as soon as possible and to answer the mother's questions. When appropriate, the nurse assesses the mother's readiness to see the baby and her response to the anesthesia and to the event that necessitated general anesthesia (e.g., having a cesarean birth when vaginal birth was anticipated).

Combination Anesthesia for Cesarean Birth

Light general anesthesia, considered by many to be ideal for cesarean birth, is achieved with a combination of thiopental, nitrous oxide–oxygen, and succinylcholine. The woman is given 100% oxygen for 3 minutes, followed by almost simultaneous rapid administration of thiopental and succinylcholine. During intubation cricoid pressure is maintained, often by the nurse, to prevent aspiration of vomitus (Fig. 10-11). When the woman is somnolent, a nitrous oxide–oxygen mixture is given. Excellent tolerance of the anesthetic is widely reported.

Inhalation Analgesia

Self-administration of inhalation gases may be helpful, especially during the second stage of labor. The mother breathes subanesthetic concentrations of inhalation anesthetic such as methoxyflurane (Penthane). If these agents are given properly, the woman remains conscious but has profound pain relief. The anesthetic agent is usually self-administered from a capsule and mask strapped to the wrist. The health care provider sets the desired concentration and the woman inhales the drug during contractions. The goal of this method is for the woman to remain conscious while profound analgesia, as well as some amnesia for painful events, is achieved.

The nurse must stay with the woman and never administer the drug for her because overdose is a risk. The nurse must also monitor vital signs closely every 30 minutes and FHR every 15 minutes. The woman should remain conscious and not become delirious or excited. The nurse alerts the health care provider and removes the analgesic from the woman's hand if the mother has cardiac arrhythmia or loses consciousness or if FHR abnormalities occur. These inhalation analgesics are rarely used in the United States today.

Other inhalation agents include halothane (Fluothane) and nitrous oxide. Halothane inhalation relaxes the uterus quickly and facilitates intrauterine manipulation, version, and extraction. The desired effect is loss of sensitivity to touch, pain, and other stimulation.

A combination of 50% nitrous oxide (laughing gas) and 50% oxygen may be given for analgesic effect late in the first stage and with contractions during the period of expulsion in the second stage. Administered in low concentrations, nitrous oxide relieves the mother's pain but still allows her to bear down with her contractions during the second stage of labor. Care is needed to prevent maternal and neonatal respiratory depression when nitrous oxide is used as an analgesic/anesthetic.

Care Management

The choice of pain relief depends on a combination of factors: the woman's special needs and wishes, availability of the desired method of analgesia or anesthesia, the health care provider's preference and expertise, as well as the phase and stage of labor. The nurse is responsible for continuous maternal and fetal assessment and for establishing mutual goals with the woman (and her family), formulating nursing diagnosis, planning and implementing nursing care, and evaluating the effects of the plan of care.

✤ ASSESSMENT

The assessment of the laboring woman, her fetus, and her labor is a joint effort of the nurse and the primary health care providers, who then consult with the woman. The needs of each woman are different. Many factors enter into the nursing assessment to determine choice of analgesia and anesthesia (see Cultural Considerations).

CULTURAL CONSIDERATIONS

SOME CULTURAL BELIEFS ABOUT PAIN

The following are only examples of how women of different cultural backgrounds may react to pain. The nurse still needs to make assessments for each individual woman experiencing pain related to childbirth.

Chinese women may not exhibit reactions to pain. They consider it impolite to accept something when it is first offered; therefore, pain interventions may need to be offered more than once. Accupuncture may be used for pain relief.

Iranian women may be vocal with labor pain.

Japanese women may be stoic with labor pain.

Haitian women may demonstrate a high tolerance for pain.

Southeast Asian women may endure severe pain before requesting relief.

Mexican women may be stoic until late in labor, then they may become vocal and request pain relief.

History

The woman's prenatal record is read for relevant information. In addition to identifying data, the woman's parity, estimated date of birth, and complications and medications during pregnancy are noted. History of allergies is noted carefully and displayed prominently. History of smoking and neurologic and spinal disorders is noted.

Interview

Interview data establish time and type of food taken at the woman's last meal, existing respiratory condition (cold, allergy), and unusual reactions to medications, (e.g., allergy), cleansing agents, or tape. The woman is asked whether she attended parent education for childbirth. Her preparation and preferences for management of discomfort are noted. Her knowledge of choices for management of discomfort is assessed. The woman's perception of discomfort and her expressed need for pain medication add to the data base. The events since the woman's last contact with the primary health care provider are reviewed (e.g., infections, diarrhea, change in fetal behavior). If verbal and physical signs suggest current substance abuse, the nurse inquires about the type of drug used, time of last use, and method of administration.

Physical Examination

The character and status of this labor and fetal response are assessed (see Chapters 11 and 12). The nurse notes the degree of hydration by assessing intake and output, moisture of mucous membranes, and skin turgor. Bladder distention is noted. Evidence of skin infection near sites of possible needle insertion are recorded and reported. Signs of apprehension such as fist clenching and restlessness are noted.

If the woman is in labor, maternal and fetal vital signs, uterine contractions, and cervical effacement and dilatation, station, and anticipated time until birth are all considered. Length of labor and degree of fatigue are important considerations.

Laboratory Tests

Laboratory tests are reviewed for anemia (hemoglobin and hematocrit), coagulopathy (bleeding disorder), and infection (white cell count and differential). The prenatal record is reviewed for laboratory tests (e.g., blood, urine, amniotic fluid) related to disorders such as diabetes mellitus, cardiac disease, thyroid disease, infection, and current disorders such as preeclampsia or substance abuse. Antenatal diagnostic studies (ultrasound, nonstress test, contraction stress test, amniocentesis, and biophysical profile) and their findings are noted. The choice of analgesia and anesthesia varies by phase and stage of labor (see Box 10-2).

Signs of Potential Problems

Any medication can cause an **allergic reaction** that may be minor or as severe as anaphylaxis. Minor reactions can be characterized by development of a rash, rhinitis, fever, asthma, and pruritus. Management of the less acute allergic response is not an emergency. The nurse should monitor the vital signs, respiratory status, cardiovascular status, platelet count, and white blood cell count. The woman is observed for side effects of drug therapy, especially drowsiness; the fluid intake and output are monitored to determine urinary retention; and frequency of bowel movements is monitored to assess constipation (Clark et al, 1993).

Severe reactions may occur suddenly and produce shock. The most dramatic form of anaphylaxis is sudden severe bronchospasm, vasospasm, severe hypotension and death. Signs of anaphylaxis are largely caused by contraction of smooth muscles and may begin with irritability, extreme weakness, nausea, and vomiting. The reaction then proceeds to dyspnea, cyanosis, convulsions, and cardiac arrest. The acute allergic reaction—anaphylaxis—requires immediate diagnosis and treatment, usually 1:1000 epinephrine injected subcutaneously or intramuscularly, followed by parenteral antihistamines. Supportive care addresses symptoms and is based on rapid assessment of cardiovascular and respiratory response; CPR may be necessary. The nurse must also be alert to fetal well-being; FHR decelerations are noted and reported to the health care provider.

❖ NURSING DIAGNOSES

Nursing diagnoses vary from individual to individual. The following lists some examples of nursing diagnoses that are relevant to control of discomfort during the birth period:

High risk for altered tissue perfusion related to:
- Effects of analgesia or anesthesia
- Maternal position

Pain related to:
- The process of labor and birth

Situational low self-esteem related to:
- Negative perception of the woman's (or her family's) behavior

Anxiety or fear related to knowledge deficit of:
- Procedure for nerve block analgesia
- Expected sensation during nerve block analgesia
- Mother's role during nerve block analgesia
- Options for analgesia and anesthesia

High risk for maternal injury related to:
- Effects of analgesia and anesthesia on sensation and motor control

High risk for fetal injury related to:
- Maternal hypotension
- Maternal position (aortocaval compression)

❖ EXPECTED OUTCOMES

For each woman a plan is developed that relates specifically to her clinical and nursing problems. The plan involves the mother and family and incorporates their priorities and preferences. The nurse, in collaboration with the primary health care provider and laboring woman, selects those aspects of care relevant to the individual woman and her family.

The expected outcomes for nursing care related to control of discomfort include the following considerations:

1. The mother will achieve adequate pain relief without adding to maternal risk (e.g., through nonpharmacologic methods, appropriate medication, dosage, and timing and route of administration).
2. The fetus will maintain well-being, and the neonate will adjust to extrauterine life.
3. The family/significant others will know their needs and rights in relation to use of analgesia and anesthesia.

❖ COLLABORATIVE CARE

The woman's *perception* of her behavior during labor is of utmost importance. If she planned a nonmedicated birth but then needs and accepts medication, her self-esteem may falter. Verbal and nonverbal acceptance of her behavior is given (as necessary) and reinforced by visiting her the day after birth if possible. Explanations about fetal response to maternal discomfort, the effects of maternal fatigue, and the medication itself are supportive measures. Support may be needed by family/significant others if plans for a nonmedicated birth are altered.

Excessive stress (as yet undefined in perinatal medicine), causes increased maternal catecholamine production. Catecholamines have been linked to dysfunctional labor and fetal and neonatal distress and illness (Simkin, 1986a, b). Parents may feel reassured somewhat by hearing that medication is sometimes indicated for the baby's benefit.

Informed Consent

The primary health care provider and anesthesia care provider are responsible for informing women of the alternative methods of pharmacologic pain relief available in the hospital setting. The description of anesthetic techniques is essential to informed consent, even if the woman has received information about analgesia and anesthesia earlier in her pregnancy. This interview should take place just before or early in labor so the woman has time to consider the alternatives. Nurses play a part in the informed consent by clarifying and describing the procedures or by acting as a patient's advocate and asking the primary health care provider for further explanations. The procedure, its advantages, and its disadvantages must be thoroughly explained (Legal Tip).

LEGAL TIP: **Informed Consent for Anesthetic**

THE WOMAN RECEIVES (IN AN UNDERSTANDABLE MANNER):

Explanation of alternatives available for pain relief

Description of the anesthetic and the procedure for administration

Description of the benefits, discomfort, risks, and consequences for the mother and the fetus of the selected anesthetic

Explanation of how complications can be treated

Information that the anesthetic is not always effective

Indication that the woman may withdraw consent at any time

Opportunity to answer any questions

Opportunity to explain in the mother's own words components of the consent

CONSENT FORM:

Written in woman's primary language

Woman's signature

Date of consent

Signature of anesthetic caregiver certifying the woman has received an explanation and appears to understand the explanation

Timing of Administration

Orders are often written to dispense or administer medications on the basis of the nurse's clinical judgment. These orders require clinical knowledge and expertise. It is often the nurse who alerts the primary health care provider that the woman is in need of pharmacologic relief of discomfort. Box 10-2 lists pharmacologic control by stage of labor and method of birth.

Preparation for Procedures

The nurse reviews or validates the woman's choices for relief from discomfort and clarifies the mother's information as necessary. The woman needs an explanation of the procedure and what will be asked of her (e.g., to maintain flexed position during insertion of epidural medication). The woman benefits from knowing how the medication is to be given, the degree of discomfort to expect from administration of the medication, sensations she can expect, skin preparation, time requirement for administration, and the interval before the medication takes hold. The nurse explains the need for emptying the bladder before analgesic or anesthetic is given and for keeping the bladder empty. If an indwelling epidural catheter is threaded and the woman feels a momentary twinge down her leg, hip, or back, she is assured that it is not a sign of injury.

For paracervical and pudendal blocks a long needle is used (see Fig. 10-10). The sight of this needle may be frightening. The woman can be reassured that only the tip of the needle will be inserted.

Administration of Medication

Accuracy in the monitoring of the progress of labor is the basis for clinical judgment in the need for pharmacologic control of discomfort. Knowledge of the medications that are used during childbirth is essential. The most effective route of administration for each woman is selected. Then the medication is prepared and administered correctly.

Intravenous Route

The preferred route of administration of medications such as meperidine or fentanyl is through IV tubing. The infusion of IV solution is stopped while the medication is injected into the port nearest the woman. The medication is given slowly in small doses at the *beginning* of three to five consecutive contractions (Petree, 1983). Because uterine blood vessels are constricted during contractions, the medication stays within the maternal vascular system for several seconds before the uterine blood vessels reopen. The IV infusion is restarted slowly to prevent a bolus of medication. Through this method of injection the amount of drug crossing the placenta to the fetus is minimized. With decreased placental transfer the mother's degree of pain relief is maximized. The IV route has the following results:

Onset of pain relief is more predictable.

Pain relief is obtained with small doses of the drug.

Duration of effect is more predictable.

Intramuscular Route

IM injections of analgesics, although still used, are no longer the preferred route of administration for the laboring woman. Identified disadvantages of the IM route include the following:

Onset of pain relief is delayed.

Higher doses of medication are required.

Medication is released from the muscle tissue at an unpredictable rate and is available for transfer across the placenta to the fetus.

IM injections are given in the upper portion of the arm (deltoid site) if regional anesthesia is planned later in the labor. This is the preferred site because the autonomic blockage from the regional (e.g., epidural) anesthesia increases blood flow to the gluteal region and accelerates absorption of the drug. The maternal plasma level of the drug necessary to bring pain relief usually is reached 45 minutes after IM injection, followed by a decline in plasma levels. The maternal drug levels (after IM injections) are unequal because of uneven distribution (maternal uptake) and metabolism. The advantage of using the IM route is quick administration.

Nerve Blocks

An IV line is established before nerve blocks such as paracervical, epidural, subarachnoid spinal, and general anesthesia are introduced. Lactated Ringer's or Plasma-Lyte A and normal saline solutions are the preferred solutions. Infusion solutions without dextrose are preferred, especially when the solution needs to be infused rapidly (e.g., in the presence of severe dehydration or to maintain blood pressure). Solutions containing dextrose raise maternal blood glucose levels rapidly. The fetus responds to high blood glucose levels by increasing insulin production; fetal or neonatal hypoglycemia may result. In addition, dextrose changes osmotic pressure so that fluid is excreted from the kidneys more rapidly.

The woman needs assistance in assuming and maintaining the correct position for peridural and spinal anesthesia (see pp. 231 and 234).

Safety and General Care

After IV or IM injection or nerve block the woman is protected by raised side rails and a call bell within easy reach when the nurse is not in attendance. The woman must be protected from prolonged pressure on an anesthetized part (e.g., lying on one side with weight on one leg; tight bedclothes on feet). If stirrups are used, the nurse pads them, adjusts both stirrups at the same level and angle, places both of the woman's legs into them simultaneously to avoid pressure to the popliteal angle, and applies restraints without restricting circulation.

The nurse monitors and records the woman's response to medication: level of pain relief, level of apprehension, return of sensations and perception of pain, and allergic or untoward reactions (e.g., hypotension, respiratory depression). The nurse continues to monitor maternal vital signs, blood pressure, strength and frequency of uterine contractions, changes in the cervix and station of the presenting part, presence of the bearing-down reflex, bladder filling, and state of hydration. Determining the fetal response following administration of analgesia

---

 CLINICAL APPLICATION OF RESEARCH

EXPECTATIONS AND EXPERIENCES OF PAIN IN LABOR

Pain relief during labor is an important goal for mothers and their caregivers; other factors such as satisfaction and a sense of control are also important. In this study three questionnaires were sent to women who were to give birth at six maternity units in England. The questionnaires were sent between 28 and 32 weeks' gestation (825 responses), 4 weeks before their due dates (751 responses), and about 6 weeks after delivery (710 responses). The great majority of women expected labor to be "quite" or "very" painful, wanted the least amount of drugs to keep the labor bearable, and intended to use breathing and relaxation exercises in labor. There was little difference in expectations about pain based on educational level, and women who had previously given birth were less worried about pain in labor. Most of the women found labor less painful than they expected. Women whose expectations of pain were similar to what they experienced were most satisfied with their birth.

Some women felt pressure to use (or not use) pain-relieving drugs. Primiparas reported more use of pain-relieving medications. Women who used drugs were less satisfied with birth than women who did not. Breathing and relaxation exercises helped the majority of women who used them.

Nurses working with prenatal and laboring women need to be sensitive to the wishes and preferences of women when discussing the use of drugs in labor and respect their wishes and views. Since women who worried about pain consistently had worse outcomes on all measures, attention must be directed to reduction of anxiety in the prenatal period. Nurses are well qualified to work with women to reduce anxiety.

Reference: Green JM: Expectations and experiences of pain in labor: findings from a large prospective study, *Birth* 20(2):65, 1993.

PLAN OF CARE

Lumbar Epidural Block during Labor

Case History

Rose N. is a 24-year-old married woman with one child and is in her second pregnancy. Obstetric history includes a spontaneous vaginal birth of a healthy boy weighing 8 pounds 2 ounces after a 10-hour unmedicated labor. Rose's contractions began yesterday after supper 12 hours ago. She describes more discomfort than she had with her first labor. This morning at 7:00, assessment of Rose revealed that she was in active labor. Her vital signs, blood pressure, labor pattern, and FHR were stable and within normal limits. She was unable to sleep during the night. She felt she could no longer cope with the contractions and requested an epidural block. After Rose emptied her bladder, an IV infusion of lactated Ringer's solution was initiated and 1000 ml were infused. An epidural block was started 30 minutes ago. At this time Rose states she is comfortable. Rose is apologetic about wanting an epidural block; her husband comments that they had hoped she would not need any medication.

Rose's vital signs, blood pressure, labor pattern, and FHR remain stable and within normal limits. Her bladder is not palpable (distended) at this time. She is resting quietly. Her husband is at her side, holding her hand, and resting his head on his wife's pillow. The electronic fetal monitor is recording uterine contractions and FHR.

EXPECTED OUTCOMES	IMPLEMENTATION	RATIONALE	EVALUATION
Nursing diagnosis: High risk for maternal and fetal injury related to maternal hypotension secondary to effects of epidural block			
Rose will not experience hypotension: pulse and BP will remain WNL.	Place Rose in lateral position. Maintain IV infusion. Monitor maternal pulse and BP.	Avoids aortocaval compression; supports placental perfusion. Expands blood volume; increases cardiac output.	Rose does not experience hypotension: Her BP and pulse stay WNL.
FHR will remain WNL.	Monitor FHR. Be prepared to implement interventions for maternal hypotension (see Emergency Box, p. 233).	Allows early identification of maternal hypotension and its effect on the fetus. Corrects maternal hypotension and placental perfusion.	FHR remains WNL—no bradycardia or change in beat-to-beat variability.
Nursing diagnosis: Altered pattern of urinary elimination during labor related to effects of epidural block			
Rose's bladder does not become distended.	Palpate bladder superior to symphysis pubis and observe frequently for distention.	Rose received 1000 ml IV fluid before epidural block; IV is still infusing. Urinary retention is a side effect of epidural block: Rose may be unaware of the need to void. Rose may be unable to void spontaneously.	When Rose's bladder begins to fill, Rose is able to void spontaneously.
	Encourage frequent voiding. Catheterize if necessary.	Bladder distention may: Impede progress of fetus down birth canal. Increase the possibility of trauma to the bladder, especially during birth. Result in decreased bladder tone after giving birth.	Rose's bladder does not become distended.

PLAN OF CARE—con't

Lumbar Epidural Block during Labor

EXPECTED OUTCOMES	IMPLEMENTATION	RATIONALE	EVALUATION
Nursing diagnosis: Situational low self-esteem related to negative perception of behavior (asking for and accepting an epidural block)			
Rose and her husband maintain self-esteem.	Explain effect of pain on labor. Discuss pros/cons of medicated labor.	Increases their understanding of benefits of pain reduction in labor. Parents experience a heightened sensitivity to other's opinions during labor.	Rose and her husband state they feel good about their decision.

or anesthesia is vital. The woman is asked if she (or the family) has any questions. The nurse assesses the woman's and her family's understanding of the need for ensuring her safety (e.g., keeping side rails up, calling for assistance as needed).

The time between the administration of a narcotic and the time of the baby's birth are noted. The woman's record during childbirth serves as a documented means of communication among all members of the health care team. Documentation of the events is mandatory to meet legal requirements. Precise records also serve as a reservoir for research study (Clinical Application of Research, p. 241).

✦ EVALUATION

Evaluation is a continuous process. The nurse can be relatively assured that care was effective if the expected outcomes for care are met: the mother has adequate pain relief without risk; the unborn and newborn maintain well-being; and the family knows their needs and rights in relation to analgesia and anesthesia (see Plan of Care).

KEY POINTS

- The expected outcome of preparation for childbirth and parenting is "education for choice."
- Nonpharmacologic pain and stress management strategies are valuable for managing labor discomfort.
- The type of analgesic or anesthetic to be used is chosen in part by the stage of labor and the method of birth.
- Narcotic effects can be potentiated with ataractics.
- Naloxone and naltrexone are narcotic antagonists that can reverse narcotic effects, especially respiratory depression.
- Pharmacologic control of discomfort during labor requires collaboration among the health care providers and the laboring woman.
- The nurse must understand medications, their expected effect, potential side effects, and methods of administration.
- Placement of an IV line and maternal hydration are essential during regional nerve blocks.
- Maternal analgesia/anesthesia potentially affects neonatal neurobehavioral response.
- The use of narcotic agonist-antagonist compounds in women with preexisting narcotic dependency may cause symptoms of narcotic withdrawal.

CRITICAL THINKING EXERCISES

1. You are assigned to a woman in labor who feels strongly that medications are to be avoided, but she is now experiencing pain and wants relief. You are convinced that discomfort should be avoided if possible.
   a. Examine assumptions that both the nurse and the woman may have about pain relief.
   b. Analyze arguments for and against use of pharmacologic agents for control of discomfort.
   c. Formulate a plan of care for pain relief in this situation, and justify your choice of interventions.
2. Talk to a woman who has experienced childbirth previously. Ask her to describe her reactions to pain, the atmosphere of the childbirth setting, and the attitudes of the health care providers.
   a. Analyze how the atmosphere and the attitudes might have influenced the woman's perception of pain.
   b. Examine the childbirth setting in which you are now assigned.
      1) What is the atmosphere of the setting, and what are the attitudes of the health care providers regarding pain?
      2) Evaluate the impact of these factors on the setting.

References

Abboud TK et al: Maternal, fetal and neonatal responses after epidural anesthesia with bupivacaine, 2-chloroprocaine or lidocaine, *Anesth Analg* 61:638, 1982.

Aderhold KJ, Perry L: Jet hydrotherapy for labor and postpartum pain relief, *MCN* 16:97, 1991.

Avard DM, Nimrod CM: Risks and benefits of obstetric epidural analgesia: a review, *Birth* 12:215, 1985.

Bernardini JY, Maloni JA, Stegman CE: Neuromuscular control of childbirth-prepared women during the first stage of labor, *JOGNN* 2:105, 1983.

Bradley RA: *Husband-coached childbirth*, New York, 1974, Harper & Row.

Briggs GC, Freeman RK, Yaffe SJ: *Drugs in pregnancy and lactation*, ed 2, Baltimore, 1986, Williams & Wilkins.

Cheek TG, Gutsche BB: Epidural analgesia for labor and vaginal delivery, *Clin Obstet Gynecol* 30:515, 1987.

Clark JB, Queener SF, Karb VB: *Pharmacologic basis of nursing practice*, ed 4, St Louis, 1993, Mosby.

Cronenwett LR, Brickman P: Models of helping and coping in childbirth, *Nurs Res* 32:84, 1983.

Cunningham FG et al: *Williams obstetrics*, ed 19, Norwalk, CT, 1993, Appleton & Lange.

Dick-Read G: *Childbirth without fear*, ed 2, New York, 1959, Harper & Row.

Gatson-Johannsson F, Turner-Norvell K: Progression of labor pain in primiparas, *Nurs Res* 37:87, 1988.

Hughs SC: Analgesia methods during labour and delivery, *Can J Anaesth* 39:18, 1992.

Kershner J, Schenck V: Music therapy–assisted childbirth, *Int J Childbirth Educ* 6:32, 1991.

Klein RN et al: A study of father and nurse support during labor, *Birth* 8:161, 1981.

Lamaze F: *Painless childbirth*, New York, 1972, Pocket Books.

Lindberg C, Lawlis GF: The effectiveness of imagery as a childbirth preparatory technique, *J Ment Imagery* 12(1):103, 1988.

Mackey M: Women's preparation for the childbirth experience, *Matern Child Nurs J* 19:143, 1990.

Maloni J, McIndoe J, Rubenstein G: Expectant grandparents class, *JOGNN* 16:26, 1987.

Marx GF: Pain relief during labor—more than comfort, *J Calif Perinat Assn* 4:36, 1984.

Mattson S, Smith JE: *Core curriculum maternal-newborn nursing*, Philadelphia, 1993, WB Saunders.

Nichols F, Humenick S: *Childbirth education: practice, research and theory*, Philadelphia, 1988, WB Saunders.

Petree B: A nursing perspective of obstetrical analgesia/anesthesia, *NAACOG update series*, vol 1, lesson 12, 1983.

Potter PA, Perry AG: *Basic nursing: theory and practice*, ed 3, St Louis, 1995, Mosby.

Rosenblatt DB et al: The influence of maternal analgesia on neonatal behavior. II. Epidural bupivacaine, *Br J Obstet Gynaecol* 88:407, 1981.

Scott JR et al: *Danforth's obstetrics and gynecology*, ed 6, Philadelphia, 1990, JB Lippincott.

Simkin P: Stress, pain, and catecholamines in labor. I. A review, *Birth* 13:227, 1986a.

Simkin P: Stress, pain, and catecholamines in labor. II. A pilot survey of new mothers, *Birth* 13:234, 1986b.

Tisserand M: *Aromatherapy for women*, London, 1990, Thorsons.

Valnet J: *The practice of aromatherapy*, Rochester, VT, 1990, Healing Arts Press.

Writer D: Epidural analgesia for labor, *Anesth Clin North Am* 10:59, 1992.

Wuitchik M, Hesson K, Bakal DA: Perinatal predictors of pain and distress during labor, *Birth* 17:186, 1990.

Bibliography

Beal MW: Acupuncture and related treatment modalities. Part II. Applications to antepartal and intrapartal care, *J Nurse Midwifery* 37:260, 1992.

Berg TG, Rayburn WF: Effects of analgesia on labor, *Clin Obstet Gynecol* 35:457, 1992.

Bernat S et al: Biofeedback-assisted relaxation to reduce stress in labor, *JOGNN* 21:295, 1992.

Eakes M: Economic considerations for epidural anesthesia in childbirth, *Nurs Econ* 8:329, 1990.

Faut-Callahan M, Paice J: Postoperative pain control for the parturient, *J Perinat Neonat Nurs* 4:27, 1990.

Gordon SC, Gaines SK, Hauber RP: Self-administered versus nurse-administered epidural analgesia after cesarean section, *JOGNN* 23:99, 1994.

Harmon T, Hynan M, Tyre T: Improved obstetric outcomes using hypnotic analgesia and skill mastery combined with childbirth education, *J Consult Clin Psychol* 58(5):525, 1990.

Litwack K: Managing postanesthetic emergencies, *Nursing 91* 21:49, 1991.

Lowe NK: Maternal confidence in coping with labor: a self-efficacy concept, *JOGNN* 20:457, 1991.

Naulty JS, Becker RA: Neuraxial blockade for cesarean delivery, *Anesth Clin North Am* 10:103, 1992.

Nicholson C: Nursing considerations for the parturient who has received epidural narcotics during labor or delivery, *J Perinat Neonat Nurs* 4:14, 1990.

Ramanathan J: Pathophysiology and anesthetic implications in preeclampsia, *Clin Obstet Gynecol* 35:414, 1992.

Thorp JA, McNitt JD: Effects of epidural analgesia: some questions and answers, *Birth* 17:157, 1990.

Wright WC: Continuous epidural block for OB anesthesia, *Contemp OB/GYN* 36:89, 1991.

11

Fetal Assessment

KATHLEEN RICE SIMPSON

LEARNING OBJECTIVES

Define the key terms listed.

Explain baseline fetal heart rate and evaluate periodic changes.

Discuss fetal heart rate monitoring by periodic auscultation and electronic methods.

Identify typical nonreassuring fetal heart rate patterns and appropriate nursing interventions.

Review nursing standards for electronic fetal heart rate monitoring.

KEY TERMS

accelerations
amnioinfusion
baseline fetal heart rate (FHR)
bradycardia
decelerations
electronic fetal monitoring (EFM)
intrauterine pressure catheter (IUPC)
nonreassuring FHR patterns
prolonged decelerations
reassuring FHR patterns
spiral electrode
supine hypotension syndrome
tachycardia
tocotransducer
ultrasound transducer
uteroplacental insufficiency
variability

RELATED TOPICS

Conduction anesthesia *(Chap. 10)* • Diabetes mellitus, cardiac complications *(Chap. 22)* • Leopold's maneuvers *(Chap. 12)* • Nonstress test *(Chap. 20)* • Oxytocin challenge test *(Chap. 20)* • Oxytocin induction of labor *(Chap. 24)* • Placenta previa, abruptio placentae *(Chap. 21)* • Pregnancy-induced hypertension *(Chap. 21)* • Prolapsed cord *(Chap. 12)* • Supine hypotensive syndrome *(Chap. 7)*

HISTORY

In the seventeenth century the fetal heart tones were first heard and described. Several health care providers in France, Switzerland, and the United States made the discovery independently and reported their findings in obstetric literature. During the next 200 years, health care providers periodically described fetal heart tones and uterine souffle in medical journals. Much of the early data about the fetal heart rate concerned the ability to predict fetal sex and weight based upon the average beats per minute. In 1880 Paul Munde of the Maternity Hospital of New York identified a decrease in the fetal heart rate (FHR) after a contraction as a possibly ominous sign. He was, perhaps, the first health care provider to describe

this pattern, later known as late deceleration. In 1893 F. Winckel of Germany reported other possible signs of fetal distress such as tachycardia, bradycardia, and irregularities of the fetal heart rate. Knowledge concerning intrapartum fetal heart rate patterns stem from these early findings. Although the methods of evaluating the FHR have changed over the past century, this early research about nonreassuring fetal heart rate patterns continues to hold true in current perinatal practice.

In 1917 David Hillis, an obstetrician at Chicago Lying-In Hospital, reported on the use of a head stethoscope (fetoscope). In 1922 J.B. DeLee, the chief of staff at the same institution, published a report on use of a similar instrument. A controversy developed because

DeLee claimed to have had the idea before the Hillis report. The instrument eventually became known as the DeLee-Hillis stethoscope and has remained essentially unchanged in design and use.

In 1958 Edward Hon of the Yale University School of Medicine published a report on continuous fetal electrocardiographic (ECG) monitoring from the maternal abdomen. Obstetricians Caldeyro-Barcia of Uruguay, in 1966, and Hammacher in Germany, in 1967, reported their observations of FHR patterns associated with fetal distress. Based on their work, the first generation of commercially available fetal monitors was produced in the late 1960s. Technologic advances continue to improve the quality and accuracy of the tracings.

Some experts believe electronic fetal monitoring should be reserved only for high-risk patients in labor. These experts cite studies that compare the neonatal outcomes in women who were monitored electronically during labor to the neonatal outcomes in women monitored by auscultation of the FHR using a fetoscope during labor. No significant difference in the outcomes for infants of both groups were noted. Other experts believe the widespread use of electronic fetal monitoring has contributed to the rising cesarean birth rate in the United States and to the increase in obstetric malpractice suits. Despite these concerns, nearly every woman who gives birth in the United States today is monitored by an electronic fetal monitor at some point during her labor. Most health care providers and nurses consider the electronic fetal monitor to be a useful tool in evaluating fetal response to the labor and birth process.

FETAL RESPONSE TO THE INTRAPARTUM PERIOD

Since labor represents a period of stress for the fetus, continuous monitoring of fetal health is part of the nursing care during labor. The fetal oxygen supply must be maintained during labor to prevent severe, debilitating conditions after birth. Fetal stress can result in death in utero or shortly after birth. The fetal oxygen supply can be reduced in a number of ways:

1. Reduction of blood flow through the maternal vessels as a result of maternal hypertension or hypotension (systolic blood pressure of 100 mm Hg in brachial artery is necessary for placental perfusion).
2. Reduction of the oxygen content of the maternal blood as a result of hemorrhage or severe anemia.
3. Alterations in fetal circulation, occurring with compression of the cord, placental separation, or head compression (head compression causes increased intracranial pressure and vagal nerve stimu-

lation with slowing of the heart rate).

Fetal well-being during labor can be measured by the *response of the FHR to uterine contractions*. In general, a **reassuring FHR pattern** is characterized by a FHR between 110 and 160 beats/min with normal baseline variability, absence of nonreassuring changes, and accelerations of FHR with fetal movement.

Characteristically, a normal uterine activity pattern in labor includes contractions every 2 to 5 minutes, duration of contractions less than 90 seconds, intensity of contractions less than 100 mm Hg pressure, 30 seconds or more from the end of one contraction to the beginning of the next contraction, and an average intrauterine pressure of 15 mm Hg or less between contractions.

Baseline Fetal Heart Rate

The intrinsic rhythmicity of the fetal heart and the fetal autonomic nervous system control the FHR. An increase in sympathetic response results in acceleration of the FHR. An augmentation in parasympathetic response produces a slowing of the FHR. Usually, a balanced increase of sympathetic and parasympathetic response occurs during contractions, with no observable change in the FHR.

Baseline fetal heart rate is the average rate when the woman is not in labor or is between contractions. At term this average is about 135 beats/min, a decrease from 155 beats/min early in pregnancy. The normal range at term is 110 to 160 beats/min.

Tachycardia is a baseline FHR above 160 beats/min. It can be considered an early sign of fetal hypoxia and can result from maternal or fetal infection, such as prolonged rupture of membranes with amnionitis; maternal hyperthyroidism, or fetal anemia; as well as in response to drugs such as atropine, hydroxyzine (Vistaril), or ritodrine.

Bradycardia is a baseline FHR below 110 beats/min (Bradycardia should be distinguished from prolonged deceleration patterns, which are *periodic changes* described later in this chapter). It can be considered a later sign of fetal hypoxia and is known to occur before fetal demise. Bradycardia can result from placental transfer of drugs such as anesthetics, prolonged compression of the umbilical cord, maternal hypothermia, and maternal hypotension. Maternal **supine hypotensive syndrome,** caused by uterine pressure (the weight of the gravid uterus) on the vena cava, decreases the return of blood flow to the maternal heart, which then reduces maternal cardiac output and blood pressure. These responses in the mother subsequently result in a decrease in the FHR and fetal bradycardia. Table 11-1 contrasts tachycardia with bradycardia.

Variability of the FHR can be described as the normal irregularity of the cardiac rhythm. Variability is described as being either short-term or long-term. Short-term variability is the change in FHR from one beat to the next. Even though a fetal heart may beat 140 times over the course of a minute, there are moments in that minute when the heart rate is 134 or 146. This normal irregularity or unevenness from one heart beat to the next is termed *short-term variability*. Only the internal signal source from a **spiral electrode** can accurately assess short-term variability (Fig. 11-1). However, monitors with autocorrelation can closely approximate short-term variability when using the external signal source, the **ultrasound transducer**. *Long-term variability* appears as rhythmic cycles (or waves) from the baseline, and there are generally 3 to 5 cycles per minute. All monitors can present evidence of long-term variability whether the woman is monitored internally or externally.

Absence of variability or a *smooth (flat) baseline* is considered nonreassuring and a possible sign of fetal distress. Decreased variability can result from fetal hypoxia and acidosis, as well as from certain drugs that depress the

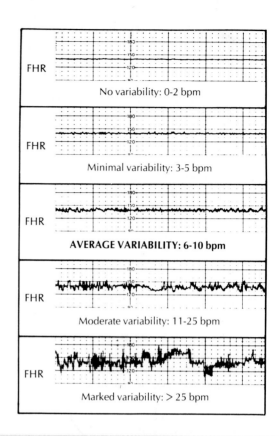

FIG. 11-1 Fetal heart rate variability. Short-term and long-term variability tend to increase and decrease together. (From Tucker SM: *Pocket guide to fetal monitoring*, ed 2, St Louis, 1992, Mosby.)

TABLE 11-1 Tachycardia and Bradycardia

	TACHYCARDIA	BRADYCARDIA
DEFINITION	FHR above 160 beats/min lasting longer than 10 min	FHR below 110 beats/min lasting longer than 10 min
CAUSE	Early fetal hypoxia Maternal fever Parasympatholytic drugs (atropine, hydroxyzine) Beta-sympathomimetic drugs (ritodrine, isoxsuprine) Amnionitis Maternal hyperthyroidism Fetal anemia Fetal heart failure Fetal cardiac arrhythmias	Late fetal hypoxia Beta-adrenergic blocking drugs (propranolol; anesthetics for epidural, spinal, caudal, and pudendal blocks) Maternal hypotension Prolonged umbilical cord compression Fetal congenital heart block
CLINICAL SIGNIFICANCE	Persistent tachycardia in absence of periodic changes does not appear serious in terms of neonatal outcome (especially true if tachycardia is associated with maternal fever); tachycardia is a nonreassuring sign when associated with late decelerations, severe variable decelerations, or absence of variability	Bradycardia with good variability and absence of periodic changes is not a sign of fetal distress if FHR remains above 80 beats/min; bradycardia caused by hypoxia is a nonreassuring sign when associated with loss of variability and late decelerations
NURSING INTERVENTION	Dependent on cause; reduce maternal fever with antipyretics as ordered and cooling measures; oxygen* at 10 to 12 L/min per face mask may be of some value; carry out health care provider's orders based on alleviating cause	Dependent on cause; intervention not warranted in fetus with heart block diagnosed by ECG; oxygen at 10 to 12 L/min per face mask may be of some value; carry out health care provider's orders based on alleviating cause

*Some hospital protocols specify oxygen rates of 7 to 8 L/min.

central nervous system (CNS), including analgesics, narcotics (meperidine [Demerol]), barbiturates (secobarbital [Seconal] and pentobarbital [Nembutal]), tranquilizers (diazepam [Valium]), ataractics (promethazine [Phenergan]), and general anesthetics. In addition, a temporary decrease in variability can occur when the fetus is in a sleep state. These sleep states do not usually last longer than 30 minutes before average variability resumes. Table 11-2 contrasts key differences between increased and decreased variability.

Periodic Changes in FHR

Periodic changes in the FHR are referred to as accelerations or decelerations. The latter are described as early, late, or variable depending on their characteristics of timing, shape, and repetitiveness in relation to uterine contractions.

Accelerations

Accelerations, caused by dominance of the *sympathetic* response, are usually encountered with breech presenta-

---

TABLE 11-2   Increased and Decreased Variability

INCREASED VARIABILITY	DECREASED VARIABILITY
CAUSE	
Early mild hypoxia	Hypoxia/acidosis
Fetal stimulation by the following:	CNS depressants
Uterine palpation	Analgesics/narcotics
Uterine contractions	Meperidine
Fetal activity	Alphaprodine (Nisentil)
Maternal activity	Morphine
	Pentazocine (Talwin)
	Barbiturates
	Secobarbital
	Pentobarbital
	Amobarbital (Amytal)
	Tranquilizers (diazepam)
	Ataractics
	Promethazine (Phenergan)
	Propiomazine (Largon)
	Hydroxyzine (Vistaril)
	Promazine (Sparine)
	Parasympatholytics (atropine)
	General anesthetics
	Prematurity
	Fetal sleep cycles
	Congenital abnormalities
	Fetal cardiac arrhythmias
CLINICAL SIGNIFICANCE	
Significance of marked variability not known; increased variability from a previous average variability, earliest FHR sign of mild hypoxia	Benign when associated with periodic fetal sleep states, which last 20 to 30 min; if caused by drugs, variability usually increases as drugs are excreted
	Decreased variability considered ominous if caused by hypoxia/asphyxia; occurring with late decelerations, decreased variability associated with fetal acidosis and low Apgar scores
NURSING INTERVENTION	
Observe FHR tracing carefully for any nonreassuring patterns including decreasing variability and late decelerations; if using external mode of monitoring, consider using internal mode (spiral electrode) for a more accurate tracing	Dependent on cause; intervention not warranted if associated with fetal sleep states or temporarily associated with CNS depressants; consider application of internal mode (spiral electrode); assist health care provider with fetal blood sampling for pH if ordered; prepare for birth if so indicated by health care provider

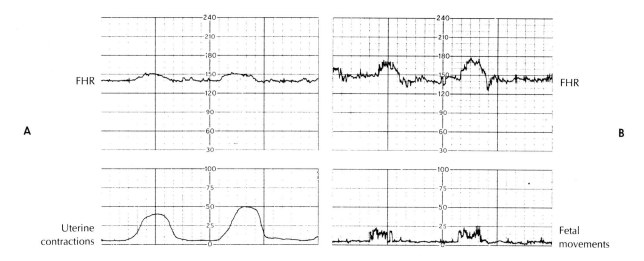

FIG. 11-2 **A,** Acceleration of FHR with uterine contractions. **B,** Acceleration of FHR with fetal movement. (From Tucker SM: *Pocket guide to fetal monitoring,* ed 2, St Louis, 1992, Mosby.)

tions (Fig. 11-2, *A*). Pressure applied to the infant's buttocks results in accelerations, whereas pressure applied to the head results in decelerations. Accelerations may occur, however, during the second stage of labor in cephalic presentations. Accelerations (Fig. 11-2, *B*) of the FHR occurring during fetal movement are indications of fetal well-being.

Decelerations

Decelerations, caused by dominance of *parasympathetic* response, may be benign or ominous. The three types of decelerations encountered during labor are early, late, and variable. FHR decelerations are described by their relation to the onset and the end of a contraction, as well as by their shape.

Early deceleration (slowing of heart rate) in response to compression of the fetal head is normal and usually a benign finding (Fig. 11-3, *A*). The deceleration is characterized by a uniform shape and an early onset corresponding to the rise in intrauterine pressure as the uterus contracts. It does not commonly occur. When present, early deceleration usually occurs during the first stage of labor when the cervix is dilated 4 to 7 cm. Early deceleration is sometimes seen during the second stage when the patient is pushing. Early decelerations as a response to fetal head compression can occur during vaginal examinations, as a result of fundal pressure, during placement of the internal mode for fetal monitoring, and during uterine contractions.

Since early decelerations are considered a benign pattern, interventions are not necessary. The value of identifying early decelerations is to be able to distinguish them from late or variable decelerations, which can be nonreassuring, and for which interventions are appropriate. Table 11-3 contrasts accelerations of FHR with early decelerations.

Uteroplacental insufficiency causes late decelerations. *Late decelerations* appear as a smooth, curvilinear, uniform heart rate pattern that mirrors the pattern of intrauterine pressure during a contraction. The deceleration necessarily begins *after* the contraction has been established and it consistently *persists into the interval after the contraction* (Fig. 11-3, *B*). Late deceleration patterns, when persistent or recurrent, usually indicate fetal hypoxia because of deficient placental perfusion. Persistent and repetitive late decelerations are associated with fetal hypoxia and acidosis. They should be considered an ominous sign when they are uncorrectable, especially if they are associated with decreased variability and tachycardia. Late decelerations caused by maternal supine hypotensive syndrome are usually correctable when the woman turns to her side to displace the weight of the gravid uterus off the vena cava. This allows a better return of maternal blood flow to the heart, which increases cardiac output and blood pressure.

Late decelerations caused by uteroplacental insufficiency can result from uterine hyperstimulation with oxytocin, pregnancy-induced hypertension (PIH), postmature syndrome, amnionitis, small-for-gestational-age (SGA) fetus, maternal diabetes, placenta previa, abruptio placentae, conduction anesthetics (producing maternal hypotension), maternal cardiac disease, and maternal anemia.

Variable decelerations occur anytime during the uterine contracting phase and are caused by compression of the umbilical cord. Table 11-4 contrasts late deceleration with variable deceleration. The appearance of variable deceleration patterns differs from the early and late decelerations, which mirror the uterine contraction. In contrast, variable decelerations are often a U or V shape characterized by a rapid descent and ascent to and from the nadir (or depth) of the deceleration (Fig. 11-3, *C*).

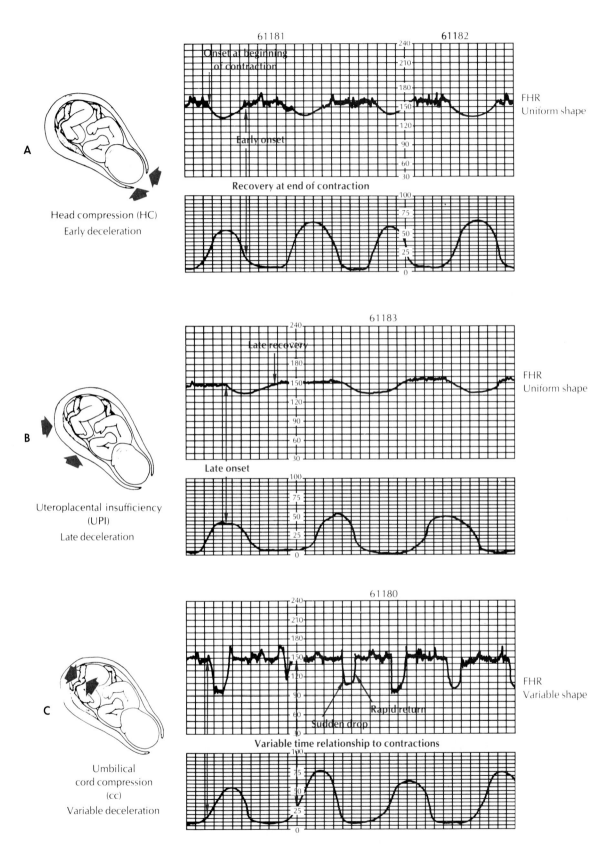

FIG. 11-3 **A,** Early deceleration caused by head compression. **B,** Late deceleration caused by uteroplacental insufficiency. **C,** Variable deceleration caused by cord compression.

TABLE 11-3 Acceleration and Early Deceleration

ACCELERATION	EARLY DECELERATION
DESCRIPTION	
Transitory increase of FHR above baseline (see Fig. 11-2)	Transitory decrease of FHR below baseline concurrent with uterine contractions (see Fig. 11-3, *A*)
SHAPE	
May resemble shape of uterine contraction	Uniform shape; mirror image of uterine contraction
ONSET	
Variable; often precedes or occurs simultaneously with uterine contraction	Early in contraction phase before peak of contraction
RECOVERY	
Variable	By end of contraction as uterine pressure returns to its resting tone
AMPLITUDE	
Usually 15 beats/min above baseline	Usually proportional to amplitude of contraction; rarely decelerates below 100 beats/min
BASELINE	
Usually associated with average baseline variability	Usually associated with average baseline variability
OCCURRENCE	
Variable; may be repetitive with each contraction	Repetitious (occurs with each contraction); usually between 4 and 7 cm dilatation and in second stage of labor
CAUSE	

Spontaneous fetal movement
Vaginal examination
Breech presentation
Occiput posterior position
Uterine contractions
Fundal pressure
Abdominal palpation
	Head compression resulting from following:
	    Uterine contractions
	    Vaginal examination
	    Fundal pressure
	    Placement of internal mode of monitoring

CLINICAL SIGNIFICANCE	
Acceleration with fetal movement signifies fetal well-being representing fetal alertness or arousal states	Reassuring pattern not associated with fetal hypoxia, acidosis, or low Apgar scores
NURSING INTERVENTION	
None required	None required

TABLE 11-4 Late Deceleration vs. Variable Deceleration

LATE DECELERATION	VARIABLE DECELERATION
DESCRIPTION	
Transitory decrease in FHR below baseline rate in contracting phase (see Fig. 11-3, *B*)	Abrupt transitory decrease in FHR that is variable in duration, intensity, and timing related to onset of contractions (Fig. 11-3, *C*)
SHAPE	
Uniform; mirror image of uterine contraction	Variable; characterized by sudden drop in FHR in V or U shape
ONSET	
Late in contraction phase; after peak of contraction; low point of deceleration occurs well after peak of contraction	Variable times in contracting phase; often preceded by transitory acceleration

TABLE 11-4   Late Deceleration vs. Variable Deceleration—cont'd

LATE DECELERATION	VARIABLE DECELERATION
RECOVERY	
Well after end of contraction	Return to baseline is rapid, sometimes with transitory acceleration or acceleration immediately preceding and following deceleration (shouldering or "overshoot"); slow return to baseline with severe variable decelerations
DECELERATION	
Usually proportional to amplitude of contraction; rarely decelerates below 100 beats/min	*Mild:* decelerates to any level, less than 30 sec with abrupt return to baseline *Moderate:* decelerates above 80 beats/min, any duration with abrupt return to baseline *Severe:* decelerates below 70 beats/min for greater than 30 sec with slow return to baseline
BASELINE	
Often associated with loss of variability and increasing baseline rate	Mild variables usually associated with average baseline variability; moderate and severe variables often associated with decreasing variability and increasing baseline rate
OCCURRENCE	
Occurs with each contraction; proportional to strength and duration of contractions	Variable; commonly observed late in labor with fetal descent and pushing
CAUSE	
Uteroplacental insufficiency caused by the following: Uterine hyperactivity or hypertonicity Maternal supine hypotension Epidural or spinal anesthesia Placenta previa Abruptio placentae Hypertensive disorders Postmaturity Intrauterine growth retardation (IUGR) Diabetes mellitus Amnionitis	Umbilical cord compression caused by the following: Maternal position with cord between fetus and maternal pelvis Cord around fetal neck, arm, leg, or other body part Short cord Knot in cord Prolapsed cord
CLINICAL SIGNIFICANCE	
Nonreassuring, worrisome pattern associated with fetal hypoxia, acidosis, and low Apgar scores; considered ominous if persistent and uncorrected, especially when associated with fetal tachycardia and loss of variability	Variable decelerations occur in about 50% of all labors and are usually transient, correctable, and not associated with low Apgar scores; mild variable decelerations reassuring; decelerations progressing from moderate to severe are associated with fetal acidosis, hypoxia, and low Apgar scores; severe variable decelerations with good baseline variability just before birth usually well tolerated
NURSING INTERVENTION	
Change maternal position Correct maternal hypotension Elevate legs Increase rate of maintenance IV Discontinue oxytocin if infusing Administer oxygen* at 10 to 12 L/min with tight face mask Assist with fetal blood sampling if ordered Prepare woman for cesarean birth if the cervix is not fully dilated and the pattern can not be corrected	Change maternal position; if decelerations do not yet meet criteria for mild variable deceleration, proceed with measures below: Discontinue oxytocin if infusing Administer oxygen* at 10 to 12 L/min with tight face mask Assist with vaginal or speculum examination, fetal blood sampling If cord is prolapsed, examiner will elevate fetal presenting part with cord between gloved fingers until cesarean birth is accomplished Assist with amnioinfusion if ordered Assist with birth

*Some hospital protocols specify 7 to 8 L/min.

Variable decelerations may be related to partial, brief compression of the cord. If encountered in the first stage of labor they can usually be eliminated by changing the mother's position, such as from one side to the other. Oxygen administration by face mask to the mother is sometimes helpful. Variable decelerations most often occur during the second stage of labor as a result of cord compression during fetal descent. Variable decelerations are associated with neonatal depression only when cord compression is severe or prolonged (e.g., tight nuchal cord, short cord, knot in cord, prolapsed cord). Variable decelerations occur in about half of all labors and are usually temporary and correctable by changing the mother's position. A nonreassuring sign is variable deceleration with a slow return to baseline and decreasing variability or deceleration below 70 beats/min for longer than 30 to 45 seconds. Some health care providers may consider **amnioinfusion** in women who have oligohydramnios (insufficient amniotic fluid). To add fluid around the umbilical cord and thereby prevent its compression during contractions, normal saline warmed to body temperature is infused into the uterine cavity via the intrauterine catheter (Devitt, 1992).

Prolonged Decelerations

Prolonged decelerations are difficult to classify, since they can occur in many situations.

Generally, the benign causes are pelvic examination, application of spiral electrode, rapid fetal descent, and sustained maternal Valsalva maneuver.

Progressive severe variable decelerations, sudden umbilical cord prolapse, and hypotension produced by spinal or epidural anesthesia cause other prolonged decelerations. Paracervical anesthesia, a tetanic contraction, and maternal hypoxia, which may occur during a seizure, often produce prolonged decelerations. When the duration of the deceleration is longer than 2 to 3 minutes, a loss of variability with rebound tachycardia usually occurs. Occasionally, a period of late decelerations follows. These responses normally clear spontaneously. However, when a prolonged deceleration is seen late in the course of severe variable decelerations or during a prolonged series of late decelerations, the prolonged deceleration may occur just before fetal death.

Nurses should notify the health care providers immediately and initiate appropriate treatment when they see a prolonged deceleration (see Nursing Intervention, Table 11-4).

MONITORING TECHNIQUES
Periodic Auscultation: FHR

Periodic auscultation of the fetal heart may reveal tachycardia, bradycardia, or arrhythmia that may occur during the brief examination (Fig. 11-4).

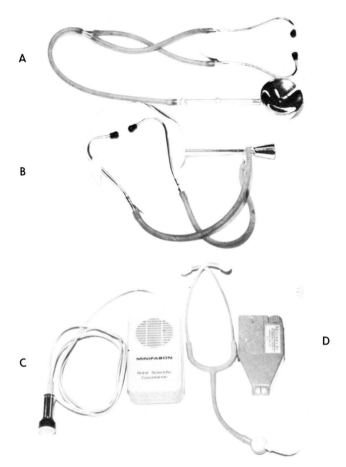

FIG. 11-4 **A,** Leffscope. **B,** DeLee-Hillis fetoscope. **C,** Ultrasound fetoscope; amplifies sound to those in immediate area. **D,** Ultrasound stethoscope; amplifies mechanical movement of fetal heart sound to listener by means of ear pieces. (From Ingalls AJ, Salerno MC: *Maternal and child health nursing*, ed 5, St Louis, 1983, Mosby.)

In low-risk women auscultation of the FHR may be done every 30 minutes in the active phase of the first stage of labor and every 15 minutes during the second stage of labor. In both instances auscultation is done during a uterine contraction and for a period of 30 seconds immediately after the end of the contraction (NAACOG, 1990). However, nonreassuring and potentially ominous FHR patterns may not occur during the periods of auscultation and may pass unrecognized by the examiner (AAP/ACOG, 1992; ACOG, 1989).

The counting of FHR during sequential contractions and for 3 minutes thereafter is an improved method that helps diagnose fetal compromise in high-risk pregnancies. Persistent, postcontraction bradycardia (e.g., FHR of 100 beats/min, or a persistent drop of 30 beats/min or more below baseline) or gross irregularity is a nonreassuring sign.

The woman becomes anxious if the nurse cannot locate the FHR. For the inexperienced listener, it often takes time to locate the heartbeat and find the point of

TABLE 11-5   External and Internal Modes of Monitoring

EXTERNAL MODE	INTERNAL MODE
FETAL HEART RATE (FHR)	
Ultrasound transducer: High-frequency sound waves reflect mechanical action of the fetal heart. Used during the antepartum and intrapartum period.	*Spiral electrode:* Electrode converts fetal ECG as obtained from the presenting part to FHR via a cardiotachometer. This method can only be used when membranes are ruptured and cervix sufficiently dilated during the intrapartum period. Electrode penetrates fetal presenting part 1.5 mm and must be on securely to ensure a good signal.
Phonotransducer: Microphone amplifies sound, reflects excessive noise when woman is in labor. Used infrequently for *antepartum monitoring.*	
Abdominal electrodes: Fetal ECG is obtained when electrodes are properly positioned. Used infrequently for antepartum monitoring because of ease and reliability of ultrasound transducer.	
UTERINE ACTIVITY	
Tocotransducer: This instrument monitors frequency and duration of contractions by means of pressure-sensing device applied to the maternal abdomen. Used during both the antepartum and intrapartum periods.	*Intrauterine pressure catheter (IUPC):* This instrument monitors frequency, duration, and *intensity of contractions.* There are two types of IUPCs. One is a fluid-filled system, and the other is a solid catheter. Both measure intrauterine pressure at the catheter tip and convert the pressure into millimeters of mercury on the uterine activity panel of the strip chart. Both can be used when membranes are ruptured and the cervix sufficiently dilated during the intrapartum period.

maximum intensity (PMI). The mother can be told that the nurse is "finding the spot where the sounds are loudest." If it has taken considerable time to locate this spot, reassure the mother by offering an opportunity to hear them too. If the nurse cannot locate the FHR, assistance should be requested.

Electronic Fetal Monitoring (EFM)

There are two modes of electronic monitoring. The external mode employs the use of external transducers placed on the woman's abdomen to assess heart rate and uterine activity. The internal mode uses a **spiral electrode** applied to the fetal presenting part to assess the fetal ECG, and the **intrauterine pressure catheter (IUPC)** to access uterine activity and pressure. A brief description contrasting the external and internal modes of **electronic fetal monitoring (EFM)** is provided in Table 11-5.

External EFM-FHR

Continuous EFM has a lower false-normal rate than intermittent auscultation of the FHR (Quirk, Miller, 1986). Separate transducers monitor the FHR and uterine contractions (Fig. 11-5). The *ultrasound transducer* acts through the reflection of high-frequency sound waves from a moving interface, in this case the fetal heart and valves. Therefore short-term variability and beat-to-beat changes in the FHR cannot be assessed by

this method. It is also difficult to reproduce a continuous and precise record of the FHR because of artifacts introduced by fetal and maternal movement. The FHR tracing is printed on a strip chart. Once the nurse locates the *point of maximum intensity of FHR,* conductive gel is applied to the surface of the ultrasound transducer, and the transducer is positioned over this area.

The **tocotransducer** (tocodynamometer) measures *uterine activity* transabdominally. Uterine contractions or fetal movement depress a pressure-sensitive surface on the side next to the abdomen. The device is placed over the fundus above the umbilicus. The tocotransducer can measure and record the frequency, regularity, and duration of uterine contractions but not their intensity. This method is especially valuable during the first stage of labor in women with intact membranes, or it can be used in the nonstress test (NST) or oxytocin challenge test (OCT).

The equipment is easily applied by the nurse, but must be repositioned as the mother or fetus changes position. The woman is asked to assume a semi-sitting position or lateral position (see Fig. 11-5, *B*). The equipment is removed periodically to wash the applicator sites and to give back rubs. This type of monitoring confines the woman to bed. Portable telemetry monitors allow observation of the FHR and uterine contraction patterns by means of centrally located electronic display stations. These portable units permit the woman to walk around during electronic monitoring.

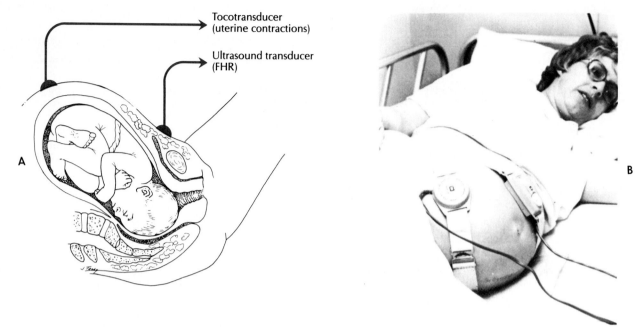

FIG. 11-5 Diagrammatic representation of external noninvasive monitoring with tocotransducer and ultrasound transducer. **A,** With ultrasound transducer placed below umbilicus and tocotransducer placed on uterine fundus. **B,** Note the woman is lying in left lateral position. (B from Tucker SM: *Fetal monitoring and fetal assessment in high risk pregnancy,* St Louis, 1978, Mosby.)

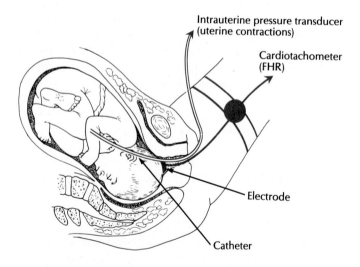

FIG. 11-6 Diagrammatic representation of internal invasive fetal monitoring with intrauterine catheter and spiral electrode in place (membranes ruptured and cervix dilated).

Internal EFM-FHR

The technique of continuous internal monitoring provides an accurate appraisal of fetal well-being during labor (Fig. 11-6). For this type of monitoring, the membranes must be ruptured, the cervix sufficiently dilated, and the presenting part low enough for placement of the electrode. A small electrode attached to the presenting part yields a continuous FHR on the fetal monitor strip.

A solid or fluid-filled catheter is introduced into the uterine cavity to monitor uterine activity. A solid catheter has a pressure-sensitive tip that measures changes in intrauterine pressure. A catheter filled with sterile water can also be used. As the uterus contracts, it compresses the fluid-filled catheter, placing pressure on the monitor strain gauge or pressure transducer. As a result, the fluid in the catheter acts as a transmitter of changes in uterine pressure. The pressures sensed by both types of catheters are then converted into a pressure reading in millimeters of mercury. The normal range during a contraction is 50 to 75 mm Hg. The display of FHR and uterine activity on the chart paper differs for the two modes of electronic monitoring (Fig. 11-7). *Note that each small square represents 10 seconds; each larger box of 6 squares equals 1 minute when the monitor is set to run at 3 cm/min.*

Patient Teaching

Before initiating fetal monitoring, the nurse should fully explain the procedure to the woman and her support person. When using external fetal monitoring, the nurse discusses how the monitor detects the FHR, and assures the woman that if the signal is temporarily lost and the FHR is not tracing, then the monitor needs to be readjusted. Women frequently worry that something is wrong with their baby when the external monitor is not tracing the FHR. The woman also needs to know that the external transducer detecting contractions does not accurately

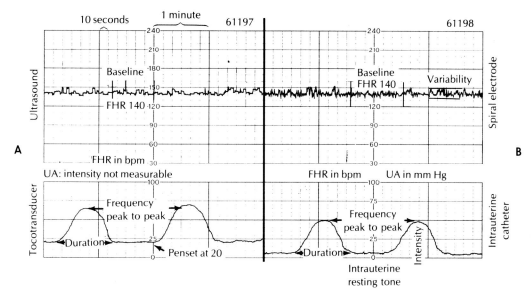

FIG. 11-7   Display of FHR and uterine activity on chart paper. **A,** External mode with ultrasound and tocotransducer as signal source. **B,** Internal mode with spiral electrode and intrauterine catheter as signal source. (From Tucker SM: *Pocket guide to fetal monitoring,* ed 2, St Louis, 1992, Mosby.)

sense the true intensity of contractions. Many times women in labor believe the monitor does not give them credit for the discomfort they experience, because the recording contractions appear to be mild.

Before inserting the internal monitor, the nurse explains how the scalp electrode is attached, and where the intrauterine pressure catheter is placed. These explanations give the woman reassurance and can prevent maternal anxiety concerning imagined fetal injury or pain related to internal leads.

The nurse initiating the fetal monitor may have an important impact on how the woman feels about her fetal monitoring experience. Women who believe the nurse fully explained how the monitor worked when it was first used report a more positive attitude about their fetal monitoring experience than women who think they did not receive a thorough explanation.

Troubleshooting EFM Equipment

A nurse who plans to work with electronic monitors requires additional education about their use. In addition to knowing how to apply the monitor and interpret tracings, the nurse needs to know troubleshooting techniques. A checklist for fetal monitoring equipment is presented in Box 11-1.

OTHER METHODS TO EVALUATE FETAL WELL-BEING

Fetal Blood Sampling

It is thought that fetal acidosis results from hypoxia. As a part of the intrapartum fetal monitoring process, it may be useful to determine the fetal capillary pH, although

the exact role of this procedure remains controversial (ACOG, 1989). Because blood gas values can vary so rapidly with transient circulatory changes, the use of fetal blood sampling during the intrapartum period is not routinely warranted. Some of the factors causing this variability include maternal acidosis or alkalosis, caput succedaneum, stage of labor, and time relationship of scalp sampling to uterine contraction (Tucker, 1992).

The procedure is performed by a health care provider who obtains the sample from the fetal scalp transcervically after rupture of membranes. The scalp is swabbed with a disinfecting solution before making the puncture. The sample is collected and sent to the laboratory for analysis.

Fetal Stimulation

Stimulation of the fetus, in order to elicit an acceleration of the FHR of 15 beats/min for at least 15 seconds, is sometimes used as an alternative to fetal blood sampling (Tucker, 1992). The two methods of fetal stimulation currently in practice include scalp stimulation, using digital pressure during a vaginal examination, and vibroacoustic stimulation, using an artificial larynx or fetal acoustic stimulation device over the fetal head for 1 to 2 seconds. Approximately 50% of stimulated fetuses will have an acceleration of the FHR of 15 beats/min for at least 15 minutes. Stimulation may be repeated at 1 minute intervals up to three times if acceleration does not occur. An FHR acceleration usually indicates fetal well-being. If the fetus does not have an acceleration, however, it does not necessarily indicate fetal compromise, but further evaluation of fetal well-being is needed. The advantage of fetal stimulation is that it does not require ruptured membranes.

BOX 11-1

Checklist for Fetal Monitoring Equipment

Name:_____   Evaluator:_____
Date:_____

Items to be Checked

Items to be Checked

PREPARATION OF MONITOR
1. Is the paper inserted correctly?
2. Are transducer cables plugged into the appropriate outlet of the monitor?

ULTRASOUND TRANSDUCER
1. Has transmission gel been applied to the ultrasound transducer?
2. Was the FHR tested and noted on the chart paper?
3. Does a signal light flash with each heart beat?
4. Is the strap secure and snug?

TOCOTRANSDUCER
1. Is the tocotransducer firmly strapped where the least maternal tissue is in evidence?
2. Has it been applied without gel or paste?
3. Was the pen-set knob adjusted between 20 and 25 mm marks and noted on chart paper?
4. Was this setting done between contractions?
5. Is the strap secure and snug?

SPIRAL ELECTRODE
1. Are the wires attached firmly to the posts on the leg plate?
2. Is the spiral electrode attached to the presenting part of the fetus?
3. Is the inner surface of the leg plate covered with electrode paste?
4. Is the leg plate properly secured to the woman's thigh?

INTERNAL CATHETER/STRAIN GAUGE*
1. Is the strain gauge located about half the height of the uterus (approximately at maternal xiphoid)?
2. Is the catheter filled with sterile water?
3. Is the black line on the catheter visible at the introitus?
4. Is it noted on the chart paper that the stopcock was opened to room air (reading 0 on paper)?
5. Was the uterine activity (UA) tested for 10 seconds?
6. Is the stopcock turned off to the syringe during monitoring?

DOCUMENTATION
1. Are testings of FHR and UA written on chart paper at least every 4 hours?
2. Is the chart paper properly labeled with the following:
   a. Woman's name
   b. Identification number
   c. Date
   d. Time monitor attached and mode
   e. High-risk conditions (pregnancy-induced hypertension, diabetes, etc.)
   f. Membranes intact or ruptured
   g. Gestational age
   h. Dilatation and station
3. Are the following noted?
   a. Maternal position and repositioning in bed
   b. Vaginal examinations
   c. Epidural anesthesia
   d. Medication given
   e. BP and temperature, pulse, respiration (TPR)
   f. Voidings
   g. O$_2$ given
   h. Emesis
   i. Pushing
   j. Fetal movement
   k. Notations of baseline or periodic changes
   l. Any change in mode of monitoring
   m. Adjustments of equipment, i.e.
      (1) Relocation of transducers
      (2) Flushing catheter
      (3) Replacement of electrode
      (4) Replacement of catheter
      Time lapse when changing recording paper

---

*New internal catheters are solid, without syringes or stopcocks.

From Tucker SM: *Pocket guide to fetal monitoring,* St Louis, 1992, Mosby.

EFM PATTERN RECOGNITION
Reassuring and Nonreassuring FHR Patterns

Nurses must evaluate many factors to determine if an FHR pattern is reassuring or nonreassuring. This includes a systematic assessment and evaluation of baseline rate and variability, identification of accelerations and decelerations, and consideration of the frequency and strength of uterine contractions. Nurses evaluate these factors based on other obstetric complications, progress in labor, and analgesia or anesthesia. They must also consider the estimated time interval until birth. Interventions are, therefore, based on clinical judgment of a complex, integrated process.

The maternity nurse must assess FHR patterns, perform independent nursing interventions, and report nonreassuring patterns to the health care provider in a timely manner (Box 11-2).

Labor and birth FHR monitoring is expected to detect early occurrences of mild fetal hypoxia and to prevent severe fetal hypoxia. Nurses must continually think about whether the FHR pattern is reassuring and whether the fetus has enough oxygen.

Reassuring FHR Patterns

1. Baseline FHR in the normal range of 110 to 160 beats/min with average baseline variability
2. Accelerations
3. Early decelerations
4. Mild variable decelerations

Nonreassuring FHR Patterns

1. Progressive increase or decrease in baseline FHR
2. Tachycardia above 160 beats/min
3. Progressive decrease in baseline variability
4. Severe variable decelerations (FHR less than 70 beats/min lasting longer than 30 to 60 seconds with rising baseline, decreasing variability, and/or slow return to baseline)
5. Late decelerations of any magnitude, especially repetitive and uncorrectable decelerations with a decreasing variability and rising baseline
6. Absence of variability
7. Prolonged deceleration
8. Severe bradycardia

Nursing Interventions

Nursing interventions for nonreassuring FHR patterns include changing maternal position, discontinuing oxytocin, increasing parenteral fluid infusion rate, and administering oxygen with a face mask according to protocols or orders from the health care provider for fetal monitoring (see Box 11-3). The nursing intervention is based on the presenting FHR pattern and clinical situation. Appropriate nursing interventions for each type of nonreassuring FHR pattern have been described in this chapter and are summarized in Table 11-6. Only the health care provider can make the decision for medical intervention by expeditious vaginal or cesarean birth.

BOX 11-2

Fetal Heart Rate Assessment Checklist

Patient's name_____Date/time_____

1. What is the baseline fetal heart rate (FHR)?
   _____Beats per minute (bpm)
   Check one of the following as observed on the monitor strip:
   _____Average baseline FHR (110 to 160 beats/min)
   _____Tachycardia (>160 bpm or >30 beats/min from normal/previous baseline)
   _____Bradycardia (<110 bpm or <30 beats/min from normal/previous baseline)
2. What is the baseline variability?
   _____Average short-term variability (6 to 10 beats/min)
   _____Average long-term variability (3 to 5 cycles/min)
   _____Minimal variability
   _____Absence of variability
   _____Marked variability
3. Are there any periodic changes in FHR?
   _____Accelerations with fetal movement
   _____Repetitive accelerations with each contraction
   _____Early decelerations (head compression)
   _____Late decelerations (uteroplacental insufficiency)
   _____Variable decelerations (cord compression)
   _____Mild
   _____Moderate
   _____Severe
4. What does the uterine activity panel show?
   _____Frequency (peak to peak)
   _____Duration (beginning to end)
   _____Intensity (in mm Hg only with intrauterine catheter)
   _____Resting time at least 30 seconds
   _____Resting tone (<15 mm Hg pressure)
   COMMENTS:_____
   PANEL NUMBER   WHAT CAN BE OR
                         SHOULD HAVE
                         BEEN DONE

Modified from Tucker SM: *Pocket Guide to fetal monitoring*, St Louis, 1992, Mosby.

BOX 11-3

Protocol For Fetal Heart Rate Monitoring

PATIENT/FAMILY TEACHING

Explain purpose of monitoring

Explain procedure

Provide rationale for maternal position other than supine

CARE

Assist woman to a comfortable position other than supine

Change maternal position at least every 2 hours

Change placement of monitor belts every 2 hours when possible

Provide perineal care as needed when internal monitoring is implemented

MATERNAL/FETAL ASSESSMENTS

Obtain a 20-minute strip by EFM on all patients admitted to labor unit

Low-risk Patient:

Auscultate or assess tracing every 30 minutes in active phase of stage one labor

Auscultate or assess tracing every 15 minutes in second stage

High-risk Patient:

Auscultate or assess tracing every 15 minutes in active phase and every 5 minutes in second stage

Auscultation—All Patients:

Count baseline FHR in between contractions

Assess FHR during the contraction and for at least 30 seconds after the contraction

Note presence or absence of decelerations

Assess FHR before ambulation

EFM—All Patients:

Assess and interpret FHR baseline, variability (long-term for external, long-term and short-term for internal), presence or absence of decelerations and accelerations

Assessments for all Patients:

Assess uterine activity for frequency, duration, intensity of contractions and uterine resting tone

Assess FHR immediately after rupture of membranes, vaginal examinations, any invasive procedure

REPORTABLE CONDITIONS

Presence of nonreassuring patterns

Worsening of any patternPresence of any fetal arrhythmias

Difficulty in obtaining adequate FHR tracing or inadequate audible FHR

EMERGENCY MEASURES

Implement immediately for nonreassuring patterns:

Reposition patient in lateral position to increase uteroplacental perfusion or relieve cord compression

Administer oxygen at 10 to 12 L/min or per hospital protocol via face mask

Discontinue oxytocin if infusing

Correct maternal hypovolemia by increasing IV rate per protocol or as ordered

Assess for bleeding or other cause of pattern change, such as maternal hypotension

Notify health care provider

Anticipate emergency preparation for surgical intervention if nonreassuring pattern continues despite interventions

DOCUMENTATION

Patient Record - Auscultation:

FHR baseline, rate and rhythm, presence of decelerations, and uterine activity data

Patient Record - EFM:

Method of monitoring, change in method, and adjustments to equipment

FHR range, variability, presence of decelerations, and presence of accelerations

Uterine activity by palpation, external, and/or internal monitoring

Interpretation of FHR data, nursing interventions, and patient responses

Notification of health care provider

Patient identification data per hospital procedure

Monitor Strip:

Patient identification data

Assessments, procedures, and interventions (medications, etc.)

Notification of health care provider

Significant occurrences such as sterile vaginal examination, rupture of membranes, etc.

Monitor adjustments

TABLE 11-6 Nonreassuring FHR Patterns and Nursing Interventions

NONREASSURING FHR PATTERNS	NURSING INTERVENTION

Severe variable deceleration; definition: FHR below 70 beats/min lasting longer than 30 to 60 sec with any of the following:
Rising baseline FHR
Decreasing variability
Slow return to baseline; may be with "overshoot" (FHR goes above baseline then returns immediately to baseline)
	With severe variable deceleration:
	  Change maternal position
	  Perform vaginal or speculum examination or both
	  Discontinue oxytocin if infusing
	  Administer oxygen at 10 to 12 L/min (or per hospital protocol) by tight face mask
	  Birth considered by health care provider if pattern cannot be corrected to meet criteria of mild variable deceleration

Late decelerations of any magnitude—more serious if associated with decreasing variability or rising baseline	Intervene in step-by-step approach, proceeding to next step *only* if pattern is uncorrected Keep woman on her side Correct maternal hypotension; elevate legs or change bed position, increase rate of maintenance IV infusion Discontinue oxytocin if infusing Administer oxygen at 10 to 12 L/min by tight face mask Assist health care provider with fetal pH sampling, if done; pH if done; pH >7.2; repeat pH in 10 to 15 min: pH <7.2; prepare for immediate birth Expeditious birth considered by health care provider if pattern cannot be corrected
Absence of variability	Correct identifiable cause; if uncorrectable, assist health care provider with birth
Prolonged deceleration	As above
Severe bradycardia	As above

GUIDELINES AND STANDARDS OF NURSING CARE RELATED TO EFM

The Association of Women's Health, Obstetric, and Neonatal Nurses (AWHONN) has established guidelines for didactic content and clinical experiences for FHR monitoring. The organization periodically issues statements to update practice (see Appendix C). The Joint Commission on Accreditation of Healthcare Organizations (JCAHO) also established guidelines for education of nurses who use monitoring equipment. The responsibility of nurses who work with electronic fetal monitoring is to be familiar with published educational and practice guidelines and to practice accordingly. Becoming a member of the nursing specialty organization is one way to keep informed about new practice guidelines.

NURSING LIABILITY

Nurses who care for women during the labor and birth process may be more likely to become involved in a lawsuit than nurses in less litigious nursing specialties. Prospective risk management includes careful documentation, both in the medical record and on the monitor strip, and establishment of a good nurse-patient relationship.

LEGAL TIP: **Fetal Monitoring Standards**

 Nurses who work with women during the childbirth process are legally responsible for correctly interpreting FHR patterns, initiating appropriate nursing interventions based on that pattern, and documenting the outcome of the interventions. Labor nurses are also responsible for timely notification of the physician or nurse-midwife in the case of nonreassuring FHR patterns.

KEY POINTS

- Fetal well-being during labor is measured by the response of the FHR to uterine contractions.
- FHR characteristics include the baseline FHR and periodic changes in FHR.
- Monitoring techniques of fetal well-being include FHR assessment and fetal stimulation.
- It is the responsibility of the labor nurse to assess FHR patterns, perform independent nursing interventions, and report nonreassuring patterns to the health care provider.
- The Association of Women's Health, Obstetrics and Neonatal Nurses (AWHONN) and Joint Commission on Accreditation of Health Care Organizations (JCAHO) have established educational guidelines for EFM.

CRITICAL THINKING EXERCISES

1. Study at least 10 actual or sample fetal monitor strips and determine:
   a. FHR baseline
   b. Variability
   c. Contraction interval, duration, intensity, and resting tone
   d. Periodic changes, if any
2. For activity 1, describe the appropriate nursing actions for each sample in writing; exchange and compare their descriptions with those developed by other students.
3. Role-play a mother in the first stage of labor who is upset and unknowledgeable of the uses of the fetal monitor, and a nurse who is using the equipment in an actual case for the first time. Make suggestions concerning actions that would be supportive and reassuring.

References

American Academy of Pediatrics/American College of Obstetricians and Gynecologists: *Guidelines for perinatal care*, Elk Grove Village, IL, 1992, AAP/ACOG.

American College of Obstetricians and Gynecologists: *Intrapartum fetal heart rate monitoring* (ACOG Technical Bulletin No 132), Washington, DC, 1989, ACOG.

Devitt N: Saline amnioinfusion for relief of variable decelerations, *American Family Physician*, 46:778, 1992.

NAACOG: *Fetal heart rate auscultation* (OGN Practice Resource), Washington, DC, 1990, NAACOG.

Quirk JG, Miller FC: FHR tracing characteristics that jeopardize the diagnosis of fetal well-being, *Clin Obstet Gynecol* 29(1):12, 1986.

Tucker SM: *Pocket guide to fetal monitoring*, ed 2, St Louis, 1992, Mosby.

Bibliography

Eganhouse DJ: Electronic fetal monitoring: education and quality assurance, *JOGNN* 20(1):16, 1991.

Eganhouse DJ: Fetal monitoring of twins, *JOGNN* 21(1):17, 1992.

Eganhouse DJ: Nursing assessment and responsibilities in monitoring the preterm pregnancy, *JOGNN* 21(5):355, 1992.

Ellison PH et al: Electronic fetal heart monitoring, auscultation, and neonatal outcome, *Am J Obstet Gynecol* 164(5):1281, 1991.

Goodwin L: Home fetal assessment, *J Perinat Neonat Nurs*, 5(4):33, 1992.

Gregor C, Paine L: Antepartal fetal assessment techniques: an update for today's perinatal nurse, *J Perinat Neonat Nurs*, 5(4):1, 1992.

Mandeville L, Troiano N: Protocol for fetal heart rate monitoring. In Mandeville L, Troiano N, editors: *High risk intrapartum nursing*, Philadelphia, 1992, JP Lippincott.

Sarno AP et al: Fetal acoustic stimulation in the early intrapartum period as a predictor of subsequent fetal condition, *Am J Obstet Gynecol* 162(3):762, 1990.

Schifrin BS, Clement D: Why fetal monitoring remains a good idea, *Contemp OB/GYN* Feb:70, 1990.

Plate 1 Normal Vaginal Labor

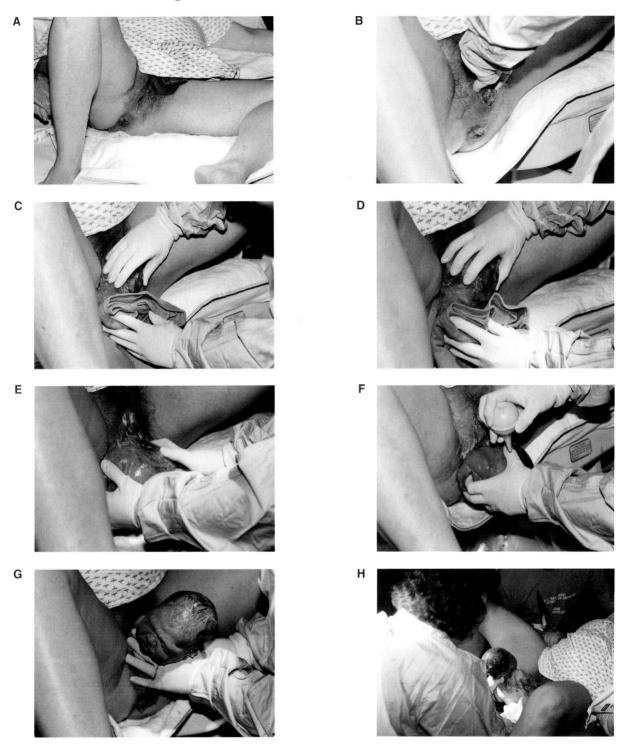

A, Anteroposterior slit. Vertex visible during contraction. Note fetal monitor. **B,** Oval opening. Vertex presenting. **C,** Circular shape. Midwife using Ritgen maneuver. **D,** Crowning. Midwife continues with Ritgen maneuver as head is born by extension. **E,** After checking for nuchal cord, midwife supports head during external rotation and restitution. **F,** Use of bulb syringe to suction mucus. **G,** Birth of posterior shoulder. **H,** Birth by slow expulsion of fetus/newborn.

Plate 1 Normal Vaginal Labor—cont'd

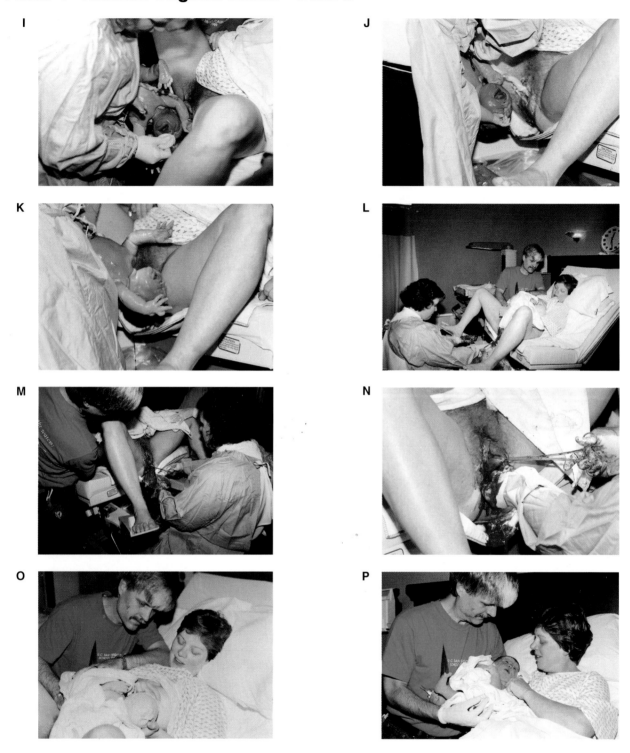

I, Second stage is complete. Newborn is supported in the head-down position while nasal and oral mucus is removed with bulb syringe. Note that newborn is not completely pink yet. J, Cutting of the umbilical cord. K, Newborn is completely pink. Note increased vaginal bleeding as the placenta separates. L, Newborn suckling at breast while midwife begins to deliver placenta. Note the intensity of the parents' gaze and their attentiveness to the newborn. M, Delivery of the placenta is complete, marking the end of the third stage of labor. N, Assessment of the cervix for birth trauma. O, Parents are engrossed in their newborn, who is actively suckling at the breast. P, Father taking newborn to hold (newborn's cap fell off briefly).

Plate 2 Cesarean Birth

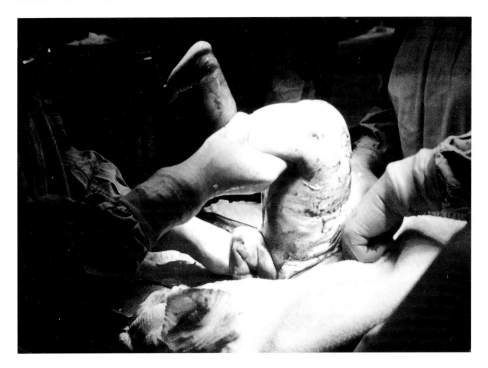

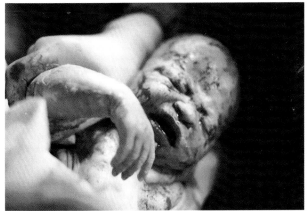

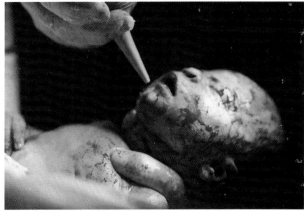

Plate 2 Family Dynamics after Childbirth—cont'd

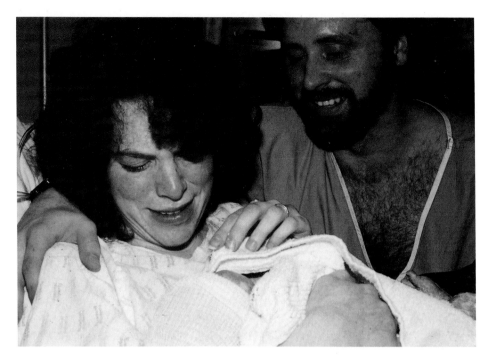

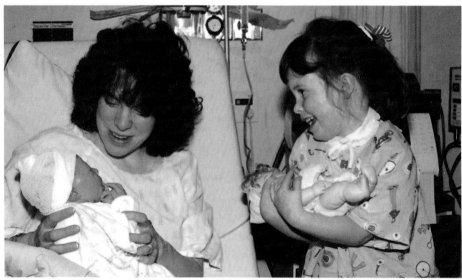

Plate 3 Newborn Assessment Techniques

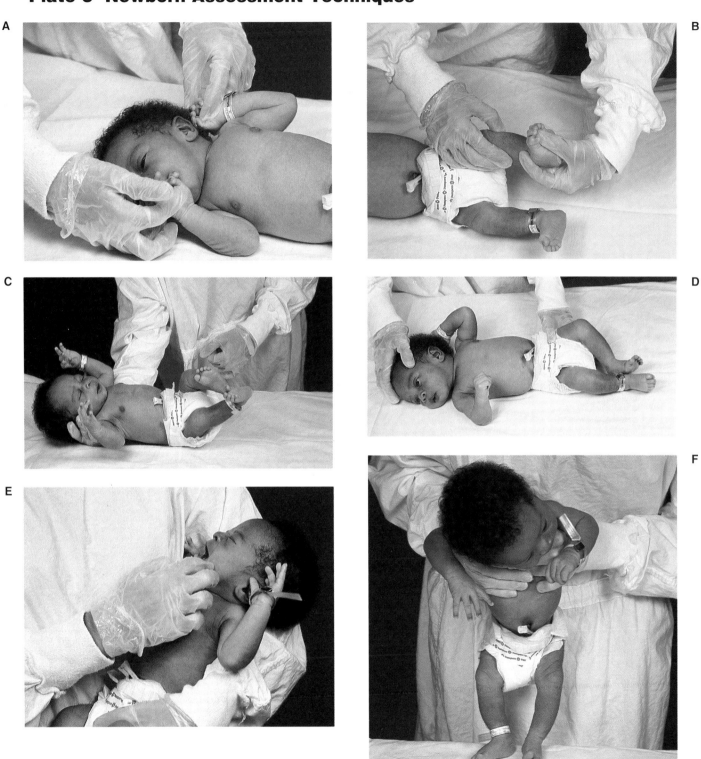

Assessment of reflexes. **A,** Palmar grasp. **B,** Plantar grasp. **C,** Moro reflex. **D,** Tonic neck reflex. This illustration shows proper positioning of the head and neck, but this infant is too young for the reflex to be present. **E,** Rooting reflex. **F,** Stepping reflex.

Plate 3 Newborn Assessment Techniques—cont'd

G

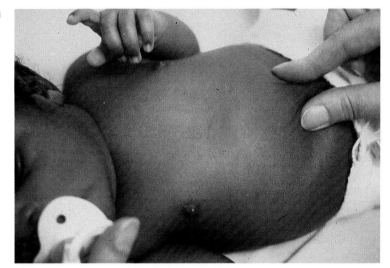

Ha

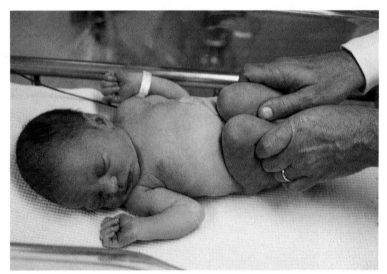

Hb

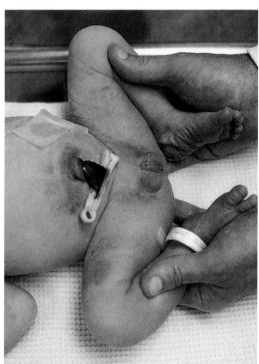

I

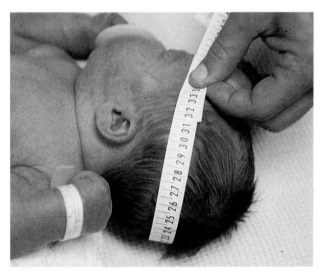

G, Testing skin turgor in infant. H, Barlow-Ortolani maneuver to detect congenital hip dislocation. a, Phase I, adduction. b, Phase II abduction. I, Appropriate placement of the measuring tape to obtain the head circumference.

Plate 4 Common Variations in the Newborn

A
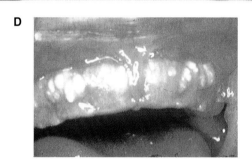

B
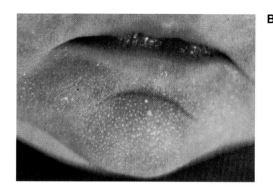

C
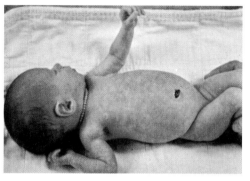

D

E
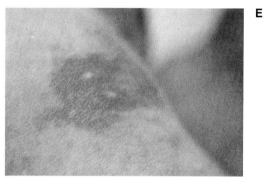

A, Mongolian spots are common in babies with dark skin. B, Milia. C, Ruddy color of newborn. D, Epstein pearls. E, Erythema toxicum.

Plate 4 Common Variations in the Newborn—cont'd

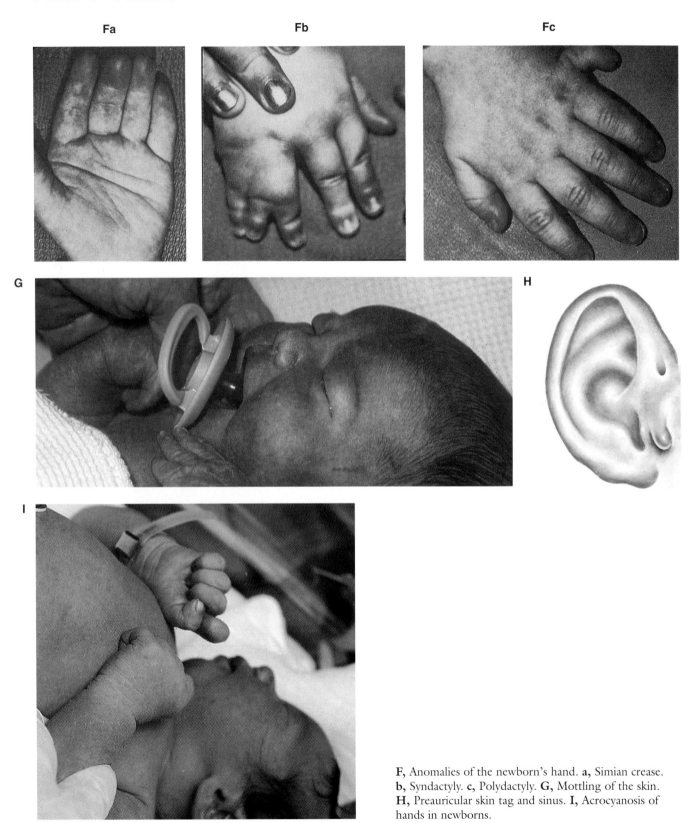

F, Anomalies of the newborn's hand. a, Simian crease.
b, Syndactyly. c, Polydactyly. G, Mottling of the skin.
H, Preauricular skin tag and sinus. I, Acrocyanosis of
hands in newborns.

12 Nursing Care during Labor and Birth

DEITRA LEONARD LOWDERMILK

LEARNING OBJECTIVES

Define the key terms listed.

Review the factors involved in the initial assessment of the woman in labor.

Identify beliefs/practices of selected cultures about labor and birth.

Summarize the subsequent assessment of progress during the four stages of labor.

Identify nursing diagnoses, and develop an appropriate plan of care throughout the four stages of labor.

Describe the role of the woman's supportive persons/family members during the four stages of labor.

Summarize the nurse's role in supporting the woman and her supportive persons/family during the four stages of labor.

Discuss assessment of the fetus during the first and second stages of labor.

Outline nursing actions in preparation for birth.

Describe the role and responsibilities of the nurse in emergency birth.

Outline the nurse's role in the care of the new mother who experienced an episiotomy or a laceration.

Identify priorities of maternal care immediately after the birth.

Discuss the maternal fluid balance and nutritional needs in the fourth stage of labor.

Prioritize measures to prevent hemorrhage.

Formulate measures to prevent bladder distention.

Explain measures to facilitate parent-infant interaction.

KEY TERMS

afterpains
atony
bearing down
bloody show
caul
crowning
duration (of contractions)
episiotomy
Ferguson's reflex
fourth stage of labor
frequency (of contractions)
Hawthorne effect
hematoma
hemorrhage
intensity (of contractions)
interval (between contractions)
lithotomy position
nuchal cord
orthostatic hypotension
placental separation
prolapse of the umbilical cord
resting tone (of contractions)
ring of fire
Ritgen maneuver
splanchnic engorgement
Valsalva's maneuver

RELATED TOPICS

Abruptio placentae *(Chap. 21)* • Birth plan *(Chap. 7)* • Cardinal movements of labor *(Chap. 9)* • Cephalopelvic disproportion *(Chap. 9)* • Cesarean birth *(Chap. 24)* • Deep tendon reflex assessment *(Chap. 21)* • Estimated date of birth (EDB) *(Chap. 7)* • Fetal monitoring *(Chap. 11)* • Hemorrhage *(Chap. 21)* • Immediate newborn assessments *(Chap. 14)* • Immediate postpartum care *(Chap. 18)* • Infection *(Chap. 21)* • Nonreassuring fetal status *(Chap. 11)* • Pain management *(Chap. 10)* • Pelvic support injuries *(Chap. 30)* • Prodromal labor *(Chap. 9)* • Universal precautions *(Chap. 21)* • Uterine dystocia *(Chap. 24)*

The labor process is an exciting and anxious time for the woman and her family. For most women, labor begins with the first uterine contraction, continues with hours of hard work during dilatation and birth, and ends as the woman and her family begin the attachment process with the infant. Nursing care focuses on supporting the woman and her family throughout the labor process in order to ensure the best possible outcome for all involved.

FIRST STAGE OF LABOR

The first stage of labor begins with the onset of regular uterine contractions and ends with full cervical dilatation. Care begins when the woman reports one or more of the following:

- onset of progressive, regular uterine contractions that increase in frequency, strength, and duration
- blood-tinged vaginal discharge (**bloody show**)
- fluid discharge from the vagina (spontaneous rupture of membranes)

Care Management

✦ ASSESSMENT

Assessment begins at the first contact with the woman, whether by telephone or in person. Many women will call the hospital or birthing center first to receive validation that it is all right for them to come to the hospital. The manner in which the nurse communicates with the woman during this first contact can set the tone for a positive birth experience. If possible, the nurse needs to have the woman's prenatal record in hand when speaking to her or admitting her for evaluation of labor.

Certain factors are initially assessed to determine if the woman is in *true labor* and should come to the hospital or be admitted (Cunningham, MacDonald, Gant 1993) (see Teaching Approaches). If a patient calls and there is any doubt about admitting her, the nurse should suggest that she either call her health care provider or come to the hospital.

When the woman arrives at the perinatal unit, assessment is top priority. The nurse will perform a detailed systems assessment by using interview, physical assessment, and laboratory findings to determine the woman's labor status (Fig. 12-1).

Admission Forms

The admission forms can provide a guideline for important assessment information when a woman in labor is being evaluated or admitted. Additional sources include (1) the prenatal record, (2) initial interview, (3) physical examination to determine baseline physiologic parameters, (4) laboratory results, (5) expressed psychosocial and cultural factors, and (6) the clinical evaluation of labor status in progress. It is preferable to have a form that integrates admission and labor data as shown in Fig. 12-2.

Prenatal Record

The admitting nurse reviews the prenatal record to identify the woman's individual needs and risks. If the woman

---

TEACHING APPROACHES

HOW TO DISTINGUISH TRUE LABOR FROM FALSE LABOR

TRUE LABOR
Contractions
- Occur regularly, becoming stronger, lasting longer, occurring closer together
- Increase in intensity with walking
- Are felt in lower back, radiating to lower portion of abdomen
- Continue despite use of comfort measures

Cervix
- Shows progressive change (softening, effacement, and dilatation signaled by the appearance of bloody show)
- Moves to an increasingly anterior position; cannot be determined without vaginal examination

Fetus
- Presenting part usually becomes engaged in the pelvis, often referred to as the fetus "dropping" (lightening). This results in increased ease of breathing; at the same time the bladder is compressed from the downward pressure exerted by the presenting part.

FALSE LABOR
Contractions
- Occur irregularly or become regular only temporarily
- Often stop with walking or position change
- Are felt in the back or abdomen above the navel
- Often can be stopped with use of comfort measures

Cervix
- May be soft but there is no significant change in effacement or dilatation or evidence of bloody show
- Is often in a posterior position; cannot be detected without vaginal examination

Fetus
- Presenting part is usually not engaged in the pelvis

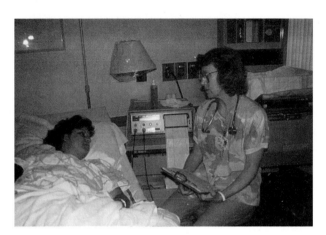

FIG. 12-1 Woman being admitted. (Courtesy Marjorie Pyle, RNC, *Lifecircle,* Costa Mesa, CA.)

has not had any prenatal care, certain baseline information needs to be obtained. If the woman experiences discomfort, the nurse attempts to ask questions between contractions when the woman can concentrate better.

It is important to know the woman's *age* so that the plan of care can be tailored to her age-group. For example, a 14-year-old and a 40-year-old have different but specific needs, and their ages place them at risk for different problems. *Height and weight* relationships are important to identify the potential risk for cephalopelvic disproportion (CPD). Other factors to consider are *general health,* any current *medical conditions or allergies, respiratory status,* the type and time of the last solid food taken, and previous *surgeries.*

Past and present *obstetric and pregnancy history* are carefully assessed. Important *obstetric history* includes the following: pregnancies (gravidity), births over the age of viability (about 22 weeks' gestation), preterm labors and births, spontaneous and elective abortions, and number of living children (parity). Other *obstetric problems* to consider include history of the following: vaginal bleeding, pregnancy-induced hypertension, anemia, gestational diabetes, infections (bacterial or sexually transmitted), and immunodeficiencies.

If this is not the woman's first labor and birth experience, it is important to note the characteristics of her previous experiences. Their duration, the type of anesthesia used, and the kind of birth (spontaneous vaginal, forceps, vacuum- or cesarean-assisted birth) are important historic factors. While assessing past births, the nurse collects data related to the condition of the babies (their weight, *Apgar scores,* and general health at and following birth). It is important to confirm that the expected date of birth (EDB) is as accurate as possible. Other data in the prenatal record include patterns of maternal weight gain, physiologic measurements such as blood pressure, baseline fetal heart rate, and laboratory test re-

sults. These tests include blood type and Rh factor, complete or partial blood count (CBC or hemoglobin and hematocrit), rubella titer, serologic findings (VDRL or rapid plasma reagin [RPR]), hepatitis B surface antigen (HB_{SAG}), group B streptococcus status, and urinalysis. Additional tests may include tuberculosis screen with purified protein derivative (PPD), human immunodeficiency virus (HIV), sickle cell trait, or other genetic screening.

Interview

The woman's chief complaint or reason for coming to the hospital is determined in the interview. Her primary complaint may be that her "bag of waters" broke with or without contractions. In this case she came in for an *obstetric check* (or period of observation). The obstetric check is reserved for women who are unsure about onset of labor. This designation allows time on the unit for diagnosis of labor without official admission, which minimizes or avoids cost to the patient.

Even the experienced mother may have difficulty determining the onset of labor. The woman is asked to recall the events of the previous days. She is assessed for the prodromal signs of labor and for the onset of regular contractions. She is asked to describe the following:
1. Frequency and duration of contractions
2. Location and character of discomfort from contractions (i.e., back pain, suprapubic discomfort)
3. Persistence of contractions despite changes in maternal position when walking or lying down
4. Presence and character of vaginal discharge or show
5. Status of amniotic membranes such as gush or seepage of fluid. If there is a discharge that may be amniotic fluid, she is asked the date and time the fluid was first noted and the fluid's color. In many instances a sterile speculum examination and a nitrazine (pH) or fern test confirm that the membranes are ruptured (p. 277).

These descriptions also help the nurse assess the degree of progress by determining the character of the contractions and the nature of the vaginal discharge. **Bloody show** is distinguished from bleeding in that it is pink in color and feels sticky because of its mucoid nature. It is scant to begin with and increases with effacement and dilatation of the cervix. A woman may report a scant brownish discharge that may be attributed to cervical trauma as a result of vaginal examination or coitus within the last 48 hours.

In case general anesthesia may be required at a moment's notice, it is important to know about the woman's respiratory status. The nurse asks if the woman has a "cold" or related symptoms, "stuffy nose," sore throat, or cough. Allergies are rechecked, including allergies to drugs routinely used such as meperidine (Demerol) or lidocaine (Xylocaine). Some allergic responses cause swelling of mucous membranes of the respiratory

Labor and Delivery Screening Summary

PRENATAL CARE:
- ☐ UNC OB Faculty   UNC Resident
- ☐ FPC   (Name: _____)
- ☐ OCCHS   (Specify: _____)
- ☐ Other   (Specify: _____)

DATE: _____   TIME: _____

CHIEF COMPLAINT: _____

MATERNAL HISTORY: Serology: _____ Rubella titer: _____ Blood group: _____
Age: _____   G: _____   Para: _ _ _ _   LMP: _____   EDC: _____   Gestation: _____ (wks)

OB HISTORY: (Specify)
    Current: _____   Previous: _____

MEDICAL HISTORY: _____
    Medication: _____   Last dose: _____

SUBSTANCE USE:
    ☐ None
    ☐ Drugs (Specify: _____)   ☐ ETOH (Specify: _____)
                                             ☐ Smoking (Specify: _____)

ALLERGIES: ☐ None   ☐ Yes: _____   Type reaction: _____

MATERNAL ASSESSMENT:
T: _____ P: _____ R: _____ BP: _____   Left side: _____ Right side: _____
Ht: _____   Wt: _____   Edema: _____   Vag. discharge: _____

MEMBRANES: ☐ Intact   ☐ Ruptured at _____ on _____

FLUID: ☐ Clear ☐ Meconium stained ☐ Other: _____ ☐ Nitrazine: _____ ☐ Fern: _____

URINALYSIS: Sugar: _____   Acetone: _____   Protein: _____   LE: _____

UTERINE CONTRACTIONS: ☐ None   Onset: _____ Interval: _____ Duration: _____ Quality: _____

SVE: _____   by: _____

CULTURES: ☐ Chlamydia ☐ Beta Strep   ☐ GC   ☐ Other _____

BLOOD DRAWN: ☐ CBC ☐ Hold ☐ Type & screen ☐ Adm. panel ☐ LFTs ☐ Clotting studies ☐ Other: _____

RISK FACTORS: _____

FETAL ASSESSMENT: ☐ EFM (____ ext. ____ int.) ☐ Auscultation   Fetal movement: _____
    BASELINE: Rate _____   Variability _____
    Periodic/Nonperiodic changes: ☐ None ☐ Acceleration (15 beats x 15 sec) ☐ Decelerations _____
                                           ☐ Fetal Arrythmias _____ ☐ Other _____

    OTHER (Specify): _____

PATIENT/S.O. TEACHING & UNDERSTANDING: _____

PHYSICIAN: _____   Notified @ _____   Arrived @ _____

DISPOSITION: ☐ Home @ _____ ☐ Walking @ _____ ☐ Reevaluated @ _____ ☐ Adm @ _____

COMMENTS: _____
_____
_____
_____
_____
_____

_____   SIGNATURE: _____

FIG. 12-2 Admission labor record. (Courtesy University of North Carolina Hospitals, Chapel Hill, NC.)

system. Because vomiting and subsequent aspiration into the respiratory tract can complicate an otherwise normal labor, the nurse records the type and time of the woman's last solid food.

Any information not found in the prenatal record is requested on admission. If the woman has prepared a formal birth plan, a copy will usually be in the prenatal record. The nurse reviews it before the woman arrives in the birthing unit. If no written plan has been made, the nurse discusses the woman's wishes and preferences when she arrives and informs her of any institutional policies that might prevent granting some of the requests. The nurse also prepares the woman for the possibility of the need to make changes in her plan as labor progresses, and assures her that information will be provided so that she can make informed decisions. Requests in a birth plan may include choosing her birth companions, wearing her own clothes, bringing her own pillow, using music, videotaping labor and birth, walking, mode of fetal monitoring, position for birth, choosing pain relief methods, having the father cut the umbilical cord, and breastfeeding immediately after birth (Myles, 1989). The nurse uses the birth plan information to plan individualize care for the woman's labor.

Psychosocial Factors

The woman's general appearance and behavior (and that of her partner) provide valuable clues to the type of supportive care she will need. Factors to assess include the following:

Verbal interactions. Does the woman ask questions? Can she ask for what she needs? Does her partner do all the talking? Does she talk to her support person(s)? Does she talk freely with the nurse or respond only to questions?

Body language. Is she relaxed or tense? What is her anxiety level? How does she react to being touched by the nurse? Support person? Does she change position or lie rigidly still? Does she avoid eye contact? Where does her partner sit? Does she look tired? How much rest has she had during the last day?

Perceptual ability. Does she understand what the nurse says? Is there a language barrier? Does her anxiety level require repeated explanations? Can she repeat what she has been told or demonstrate understanding?

Discomfort level. To what degree does the woman express what she is experiencing? How does she react to a contraction? Are there any nonverbal pain messages seen? Does she complain to the nurse? To her partner? Can she ask for comfort measures?

Stress in Labor

Usually women in labor have a variety of concerns that they voice if asked, but rarely volunteer. It is, therefore, important for the nurse to ask the woman what she expects in order to clear up misinformation or suggest that the woman ask her health care provider about an issue. The following are common concerns that women in labor have: Will my baby be all right? Will I be able to stand labor? Will my labor be long? How will I act? Will I need medication? Will it work for me? Will my partner/someone be there to support me? Do I have to have an IV, an enema, etc.?

The nurse's responsibility to the woman in labor is to answer her questions or find out the answers, to provide support to her and her family/significant others, to take care of her in a partnership with those persons the woman wants as her support team, and to be her advocate. The nurse communicates to the woman that she is not expected to act in any particular way and that the process will yield the birth of her baby, which is the only expectation she should have.

The father, coach, or significant other also experiences stress during labor. The nurse can assist and support by identifying needs and expectations and by helping that person meet them. What role does this person expect to play? Is he or she nervous, anxious, aggressive, or hostile? Does he or she watch television, sleep, or stay out of the room instead of paying attention to the woman? Does he or she touch the woman? Has the couple attended childbirth classes? The nurse ascertains what role the support person intends to fulfill and whether he or she is prepared. The nurse must be sensitive to needs and provide teaching support as appropriate.

 CULTURAL CONSIDERATIONS

BIRTH PRACTICES IN DIFFERENT CULTURES

South Korea—Stoic response to labor pain; fathers usually not present

Japan—Natural childbirth methods practiced; may labor silently; father may be present; may eat during labor

China—Stoic response to pain; fathers not present; side-lying position preferred for labor and birth, because this position is thought to reduce infant trauma

India—Natural childbirth methods preferred; father usually not present; female relatives usually present

Iran—Father not present; prefers female support and female caregivers

Mexico—May be stoic about discomfort until second stage, then may request pain relief; fathers and female relatives may be present

Laos—May use squatting position for birth; fathers may or may not be present; prefer female attendants

From Geissler E: *Pocket Guide to Cultural Assessment,* St Louis, 1994, Mosby.

TABLE 12-1 Sociocultural Basis of Pain Experience

WOMAN IN LABOR	NURSE
PERCEPTION OF MEANING	
Origin: Cultural concept of and personal experience with pain; for example: Pain in childbirth is inevitable, something to be borne Pain in childbirth can be avoided completely Pain in childbirth is punishment for sin Pain in childbirth can be controlled	Origin: Cultural concept of and personal experience with pain; in addition, nurse becomes accustomed to working with certain "expected" pain trajectories. For example, in obstetrics, pain is expected to increase as labor progresses, be intermittent in character, and have end point; relief can be derived from drugs once labor is well established and fetus or newborn can cope with amount and elimination of drug; relief can also come from woman's knowledge, attitude, and support from family or friends.
COPING MECHANISMS	
Woman may exhibit the following behaviors: Be traditionally vocal or nonvocal; crying out or groaning or both may be part of ritual of her response to pain Use counterstimulation to minimize pain; for example, rubbing, applying heat, or counterpressure Use relaxation, distraction, autosuggestion as pain-countering techniques Resist any use of "needles" as modes of administering pain relief	Nurse may respond by: Using self effectively; for example, tone of voice, closeness in space, and touch as media for message of interest and caring Using avoidance, belittling, or other distracting actions as protective device for self Using pharmacologic resources at hand judiciously Using comfort measures Assuming accountability for control and management of pain.
EXPECTATIONS OF OTHERS	
Nurse may be seen as someone who will accept woman's statement of pain and act as her advocate Medical personnel may be expected to relieve woman of all pain sensations Nurse may be expected to be interested, gentle, kind, and accepting of behavior exhibited	Only certain verbal or nonverbal behaviors as responses to pain may be accepted Couple that is prepared for childbirth may be expected to refuse medication and to wish to "do everything on their own" Woman's definition of pain may not be accepted; that is, woman may wish to experience and participate in controlling pain or may not be able to accept any pain as reasonable

Cultural Factors

It is important to note the woman's ethnic/cultural background to anticipate nursing interventions that may need to be added or deleted from the individualized plan of care. If a special request contradicts observed protocol, the woman should be encouraged to ask her health care provider to write an order for the special request. For example, in some cultures it is traditional to take the placenta home; in others the woman is given only certain nourishments during labor (see Cultural Considerations).

Women are culturally taught the "right" way to behave while in labor. These behaviors can range from total silence to moaning or screaming. If the woman's coach is her mother, she may perceive the need to "behave" more strongly than if her coach is the father of the baby. She will perceive herself as failing or succeeding on the basis of her ability to adhere to these "standards" of behavior. A woman who moans with contractions may not be in as much physical pain as a woman who remains silent and winces during contractions (see Table 12-1).

The Non–English-Speaking Woman in Labor

A woman's level of anxiety in labor rises when she does not understand what is happening to her or what is being said. This can and does happen to English-speaking women (Bentz, 1980), causing some level of stress. The toll on non–English-speaking women is significantly more dramatic because they often feel a complete loss of control over their situation. They can panic and withdraw or become physically abusive to anyone who tries to do something they perceive might harm them or their babies. Sometimes they bring a support person with them who is able to communicate in English. However, this arrangement is not always an improvement because the "translator" friend may misrepresent what the nurse or others are saying and raise the woman's stress level even more.

If there is a list of employee translators, one may be contacted for help. If no one in the hospital is able to translate, a bilingual employee can be called so that a telephone translation can take place. A female interpreter may be more acceptable to the woman. If no translator is available, a set of cards with graphics illustrating common situations the nurse will need to communicate to non–English-speaking patients can be generated to assist in the process. Even if the nurse is able to verbally communicate only marginally with the woman, in most cases it is meaningful to the woman that the nurse is making an effort to communicate with her. This attempt may initiate a nonverbal bond between the nurse and the woman/support persons.

When to Admit

The first-time mother, because of eagerness to complete labor, may come to the hospital early in the first stage. If she lives near the hospital, she may be asked to return home to wait for further progress, that is either in frequency and strength of contractions or in amount of show. She is encouraged to walk about but is asked to restrict ingestion to clear fluids. Clear fluids are advised because digestion slows significantly during labor and any food taken is liable to be vomited during transition or second stage. Examples of clear liquids are tea with sugar and juices such as apple or cranberry. Liquids should be sipped slowly and continuously during early labor to avoid nausea and to provide the woman with a source of nutrition inasmuch as labor burns extra calories.

It can be disheartening for the woman and her partner to find out that the contractions that feel strong and regular to her are not true labor contractions because they are not causing cervical dilatation. However, the woman who lives a considerable distance from the hospital may be admitted in early labor.

Physical Examination

The initial examination confirms the onset of true labor. The findings serve as a baseline for assessing the woman's progress from that point. Knowledge of pregnancy, careful initial assessment, and follow-up of progress are necessary during labor. The initial physical examination includes general systems assessment, performance of Leopold's maneuvers to determine fetal presentation, fetal position, and points of maximum intensity (PMI) for auscultating the fetal heart rate (FHR); assessment of uterine contractions; and vaginal examination to assess cervical dilatation and effacement, fetal descent, and status of membranes/amniotic fluid. Patients often focus on contractions as the clearest indicator of how far advanced their labor is. However, the nurse considers the

TABLE 12-2	Example of Minimum Assessment of the Low-risk Patient in the First Stage of Labor
ASSESSMENT	**FREQUENCY**
Blood pressure	every 1 hour
Pulse	every 1 hour
Temperature	every 4 hours; every 2 hours if membranes are ruptured
Uterine activity	every 1 hour until active; every 30 minutes when active
Intake and output	every 8 hours; dipstick urine for protein and ketones every voiding
Bladder distention	every 1 hour
Show	every 1 hour
Fetal heart rate	every hour in latent phase, every 30 minutes in active phase; when membranes rupture
Vaginal examination	as necessary to identify progress of labor: 1. To confirm change when symptoms indicate (e.g., strength, duration, or frequency of contractions; increase in amount of bloody show; membranes rupture; or woman feels pressure on her rectum) 2. To determine whether dilatation and descent are sufficient for administration of analgesic or anesthetic 3. To reassess progress if labor takes longer than expected 4. To determine station of presenting part

Modified from NAACOG: *Fetal heart rate auscultation, OGN Practice Resource,* Washington, DC, 1990, NAACOG; University of North Carolina Hospitals Department of Nursing: *Care of patient in labor protocol,* Chapel Hill, NC, 1990.

vaginal examination more conclusive, especially for first-time mothers, in estimating the woman's phase of labor. In addition, the presence of ruptured membranes significantly effects the woman's care plan. The most vital aspect of assessment is that of fetal status.

Assessment is continuous throughout labor. The routine for assessment of progress and of the continued well-being of the mother and fetus is usually set on a minimum level by hospital policy (Table 12-2). Any unusual findings would prompt more frequent performance of assessment procedures.

TABLE 12-3 Maternal Progress in First Stage of Labor Within Normal Limits

CRITERION	PHASES MARKED BY CERVICAL DILATATION*		
	0 TO 3 CM	4 TO 7 CM	8 TO 10 CM (TRANSITION)
Duration	About 8 to 10 hr	About 3 hr	About 1 to 2 hr
Contractions			
Strength	Mild	Moderate	Strong to expulsive
Rhythm	Irregular	More regular	Regular
Frequency	5 to 30 min apart	3 to 5 min apart	2 to 3 min apart
Duration	10 to 30 sec	30 to 45 sec	45 to 60 (few to 90) sec
Descent			
Station of presenting part	Nulliparous: 0 Multiparous: 0 to −2 cm	About +1 to +2 cm About +1 to +2 cm	+2 to +3 cm +2 to +3 cm
Show			
Color	Brownish discharge, mucous plug or pale, pink mucus	Pink to bloody mucus	Bloody mucus
Amount	Scant	Scant to moderate	Copious
Behavior and Appearance†	Excited; thoughts center on self, labor, and baby; may be talkative or mute, calm or tense; some apprehension; pain controlled fairly well; alert, follows directions readily; open to instructions	Becoming more serious, doubtful of control of pain, more apprehensive; desires companionship and encouragement; attention more inner directed; fatigue evidenced; malar flush; has some difficulty following directions	Pain described as severe; backache common; feelings of frustration, fear of loss of control, and irritability surface; vague in communications; amnesia between contractions; writhing with contractions; nausea and vomiting, especially if hyperventilating; hyperesthesia; circumoral pallor, perspiration on forehead and upper lips; shaking tremor of thighs; feeling of need to defecate, pressure on anus

*In the nullipara, effacement is often complete before dilatation begins; in the multipara, it occurs simultaneously with dilatation.
†Women who have epidural analgesic for pain relief may not demonstrate these behaviors.

The signs of progress in labor are well defined (Table 12-3). The character of the woman's uterine contractions, her behavior, and her appearance correlate with the phase of labor she is experiencing. The woman's culture, fatigue, and other factors may affect how she deals with labor.

Careful assessment provides the cues for selection and implementation of nursing actions. *The nurse assumes much of the responsibility for making the assessment of progress. It is the nurse's responsibility to keep the health care provider informed about progress and any deviations from normal findings.*

General Systems Assessment

A brief systems assessment needs to be performed by the nurse, including heart, lungs, and skin; presence of edema of the legs, face, hands or sacrum; and deep tendon reflexes and clonus.

Vital signs and blood pressure (BP) are assessed on the woman's admission to the hospital. Findings are assessed for normality and are used for comparison with future values. If the BP is elevated, it should first be determined whether the correct size of BP cuff has been used; then BP should be reassessed 30 minutes later to obtain a reading after the woman has relaxed. The

PROCEDURES 12-1

Leopold's Maneuvers and Determination of the Points of Maximum Intensity of the Fetal Heart Rate

Leopold's maneuvers
Wash hands.
Ask woman to empty bladder.
Position woman supine with one pillow under her head and with her knees slightly flexed.
Place small rolled towel under woman's right hip to displace uterus to left off major blood vessels (avoids supine hypotensive syndrome, Fig. 12-8).
If right-handed, stand on woman's right, facing her:

1. Identify fetal part that occupies the fundus. The head feels round, firm, freely movable, and palpable by ballottement; the breech feels less regular and softer (identifies fetal lie [vertical or horizontal] and presentation [vertex or breech]; Fig. 12-3).
2. Using palmar surface of one hand, locate and palpate the smooth convex contour of the fetal back and the irregularities that identify the small parts (feet, hands, elbows). This assists in identifying fetal presentation (Fig. 12-3).
3. With the right hand, determine which fetal part is presenting over the inlet to the true pelvis. Gently grasp the lower pole of the uterus between the thumb and fingers, pressing in slightly (Fig. 12-3). If the head is presenting and not engaged, determine the attitude of the head.
4. Turn to face the woman's feet. Using two hands, outline the fetal head (Fig. 12-3) with palmar surface of fingertips.
   When presenting part has descended deeply, only a small portion of it may be outlined.
   Palpation of cephalic prominence assists in identifying attitude of head.

If the cephalic prominence is found on the same side as the small parts, the head must be flexed, and the vertex is presenting (Fig. 12-3). If the cephalic prominence is on the same side as the back, the presenting head is extended (Fig. 12-3).
Determination of PMI of FHR:
Wash hands.
Perform Leopold's maneuvers.
Auscultate FHR (Fig. 12-4).
Chart fetal presentation, position, and lie; whether presenting part is flexed or extended, engaged or free floating. Use hospital's protocol for charting (e.g., "Vtx, LOA, floating").
Chart PMI of FHR using a two-line figure to indicate the four quadrants of the maternal abdomen, right upper quadrant (RUQ), left upper quadrant (LUQ), left lower quadrant (LLQ), and right lower quadrant (RLQ):

RUQ	LUQ
RLQ	LLQ

The umbilicus is the point where the lines cross. The PMI for the fetus in vertex presentation, in general flexion with the back on the mother's right side, commonly is found in the mother's right lower quadrant and is recorded with an "x" or with the FHR as follows:

or

x | 140 |

---

woman should also be encouraged to lie on her side and not in a supine position in order to avoid supine hypotension and fetal distress (see Fig. 12-8). Her temperature is monitored for signs of infection.

Leopold's Maneuvers (Abdominal Palpation)

After the woman is in bed, the nurse asks her to lie on her back momentarily so that the nurse can perform Leopold's maneuvers (Procedure 12-1 above and Fig. 12-3). These maneuvers provide information about (1) the number of fetuses, (2) the identity of presenting part, the fetal lie, and attitude, (3) the degree of descent into the pelvis, and (4) the location of the PMI of FHR in relation to the woman's abdomen.

Auscultation of Fetal Heart Rate

It is important for the nurse to understand the relationship of location of the PMI of FHR to fetal presentation, lie, and position. Assessment of high risk for birth complications may be diagnosed by variations in these factors. The PMI of the FHR is the location on the maternal abdomen where the FHR is heard the loudest. This place is usually directly over the fetal back. The PMI is also an aid in determining the fetal position (Fig. 12-4). In a vertex presentation the FHR is heard *below* the mother's umbilicus in either the right or left lower quadrant of the abdomen. In a breech presentation, the FHR is heard *above* the mother's umbilicus (Fig. 12-4). As fetal descent and internal rotation occur, the FHR is heard lower and closer to the midline of the maternal abdo-

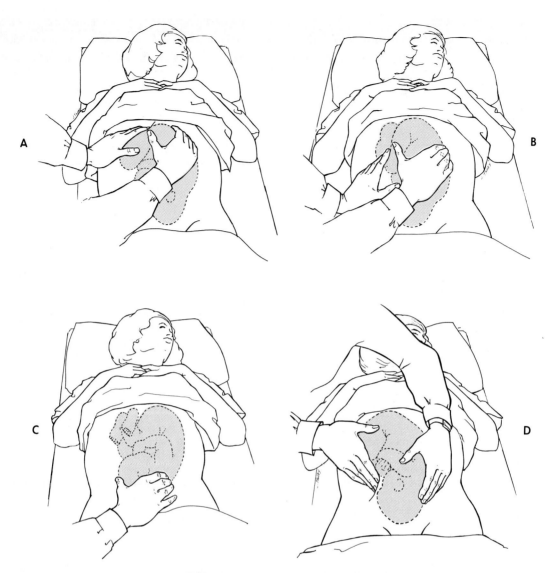

FIG. 12-3 Leopold's maneuvers.

men. Fig. 12-4 presents diagrams of PMI for different presentations and positions. Table 12-2 notes the recommended assessment of fetal status during labor. *In addition, the FHR must be assessed immediately after rupture of membranes, because this is the most common time for prolapse of the umbilical cord (p 282).*

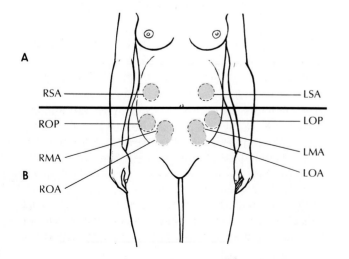

FIG. 12-4 Points of maximum intensity of FHR for differing positions: *RSA*, right sacrum anterior; *ROP*, right occipitoposterior; *RMA*, right mentum anterior; *ROA*, right occipitoanterior; *LSA*, left sacrum anterior; *LOP*, left occipitoposterior; *LMA*, left mentum anterior; and *LOA*, left occipitoanterior; **A,** Presentation is usually *breech* if FHR is heard *above* umbilicus. **B,** Presentation is usually *vertex* if FHR is heard *below* umbilicus.

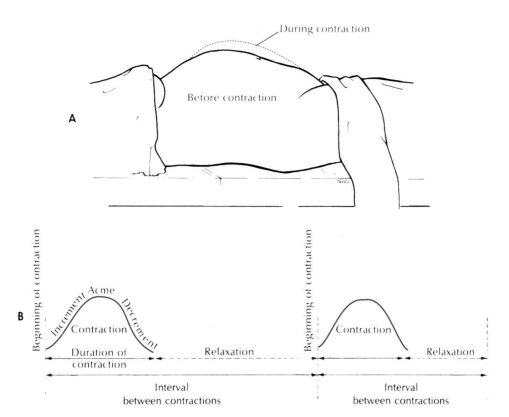

FIG. 12-5   Assessment of uterine contractions. **A,** Abdominal contour before and during uterine contraction. **B,** Wavelike pattern of contractile activity.

Assessment of Uterine Contractions

A general characteristic of effective labor is regular uterine activity. Uterine activity is not directly related to labor progress. Several methods are used to evaluate uterine contractions. These include the woman's subjective description, palpation and timing of the contraction by a clinician, and electronic monitoring devices.

Each contraction exhibits a wavelike pattern. Contractions begin with a slow *increment* (the "building up" of a contraction from its onset), gradually reaching an *acme* (the peak), and then diminishes rather rapidly (*decrement,* the "letting down" of the contraction). An **interval** of rest follows (intrauterine pressure is 8 to 15 mm Hg), which is broken when the next contraction begins (Fig. 12-5 diagrams a typical uterine contraction).

The following characteristics describe a uterine contraction:

frequency how often uterine contractions occur; the period of time from the beginning of one contraction to the beginning of the next or from peak to peak
intensity the strength of a contraction at its peak
duration the period of time that elapses between the onset and the end of a contraction
resting tone the tension in the uterine muscle between contractions

The most common ways to measure uterine contractions are by palpation or by external or internal electronic monitor. When the woman is admitted, a 20- to 30-minute baseline monitoring of uterine contractions and the FHR usually is done (Scott et al, 1990). Table 12-3 describes the progress to expect as labor advances.

Frequency and duration can be determined by all three methods of uterine activity monitoring. Palpation is a less precise method of determining the intensity of uterine contractions. The following terms are used to describe what is felt on palpation:

mild slightly tense fundus that is easy to indent with fingertips
moderate firm fundus that is difficult to indent with fingertips
strong rigid, boardlike fundus that is almost impossible to indent with fingertips

Women in labor tend to describe the pain of contractions in terms of their sensations in the lower uterine segment or in the back, which may be unrelated to the firmness of the uterine fundus. Thus their report of the strength of their contractions can be less reliable than that assessed by a health care provider.

External electronic monitoring provides information about the relative strength of the contractions. Internal electronic monitoring is the most reliable method of assessment of uterine contractions.

When uterine activity is discussed, it must be related to its effect on cervical effacement and dilatation and on the degree of descent of the presenting part. The effect

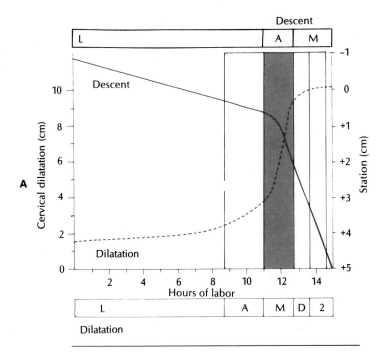

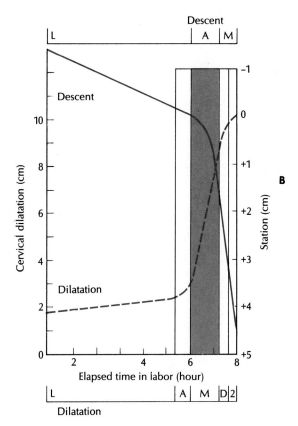

FIG. 12-6 Partogram showing relationship between cervical dilatation and descent of presenting part. **A,** Nulliparous labor. **B,** Multiparous labor. The phases of cervical dilatation are identified by the letters L, A, M, and D. A number, for example, "2" refers to the stage of labor. The latent phase *(L)* of the first stage of labor is that time between the onset of labor and the onset of acceleration. The active phase begins with the acceleration phase *(A)* and spans the time between the onset of the upward curve of cervical dilatation and full dilatation of the cervix. Friedman (1978) divides the active phase into three parts: (1) *acceleration phase (A)*, (2) *phase of maximum slope (M)*, and (3) *deceleration phase (D)*. The dotted line denotes cervical dilatation. The phases of descent are identified by the letters L, A, and M, located over the graph. The L refers to the latent phase of minimum descent. Active descent *(A)* generally begins when the cervical dilatation curve reaches its phase of maximum slope. The rate of descent reaches its maximum at the beginning of the deceleration phase of cervical dilatation. Maximum descent *(M)* continues in a linear manner until the perineum is reached. The solid line shows the rate of descent.

on the fetus also must be considered. Labor progress is effectively verified by the use of graphic charts *(partograms)* on which cervical dilatation and station (descent) are plotted. This assists in early identification of deviations from normal labor patterns. Fig. 12-6 shows the normal pattern of cervical dilatation and descent for both nulliparous labor and multiparous labor. Fig. 12-7 is one example of a partogram; however, hospitals often develop their own graphs for recording assessments. This example charts cervical dilatation and descent. Other graphs may also include vital signs, fetal heart rate, and uterine activity.

Vaginal Examination

The vaginal examination reveals whether the woman is in true labor, and enables the examiner to determine if the membranes have ruptured. Labor is initiated by *spontaneous rupture of the membranes (SROM)* in almost 25% of pregnant women at term. The lag period, rarely exceeding 24 hours, precedes the onset of labor.

The vaginal examination includes the following steps:
1. The nurse assembles all the equipment needed, including single sterile glove, antiseptic solution or soluble gel, and a light source.
2. The nurse prepares the woman by explaining the procedure and by draping her to prevent chill and protect privacy. She is positioned to prevent supine hypotensive syndrome (Fig. 12-8).
3. The nurse washes her hands and puts on the sterile glove by following aseptic technique. The nurse explains to the woman that she will feel the nurse inserting the first and middle fingers into the her vagina.
4. The woman is assessed for the following (Fig. 12-9):
   a. Dilatation and effacement of cervix
   b. Presenting part, position, station, and if vertex, any molding of the head
   c. Status of membranes, intact or ruptured
   d. Presence of stool in rectum
5. The woman is helped to a comfortable position, and the nurse reports and records all these data.

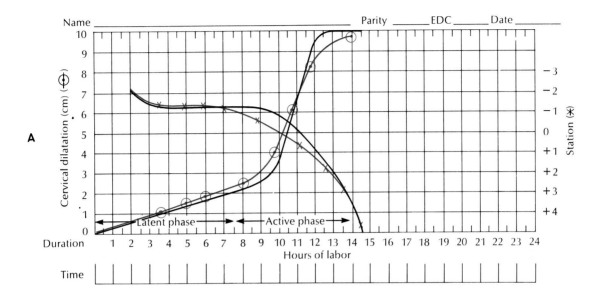

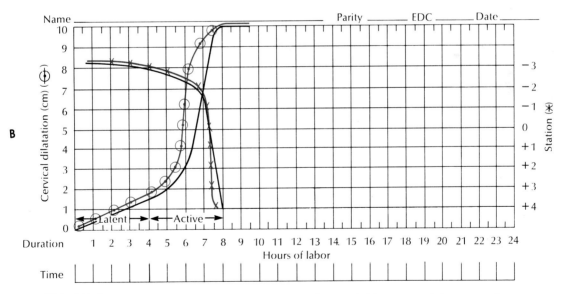

FIG. 12-7 Partogram for assessment of patterns of cervical dilatation and descent. Individual woman's labor pattern *(colored)* superimposed on prepared labor graph *(black)* for comparison. **A,** Nulliparous labor. **B,** Multiparous labor. The rate of cervical dilatation is indicated by the symbol "O." A line drawn through the symbols depicts the slope of the curve. Station is indicated with an X. A line drawn through the Xs reveals the pattern of descent.

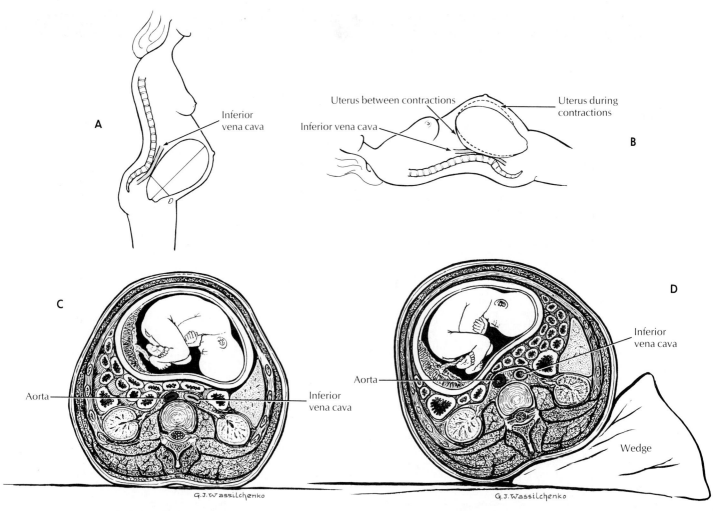

FIG. 12-8   Supine hypotension. Note relationship of pregnant uterus to ascending vena cava in standing posture. **A,** and in supine posture **B. C,** Compression of aorta and inferior vena cava with woman in supine position. **D,** Relieved by use of a wedge pillow placed under woman's right side.

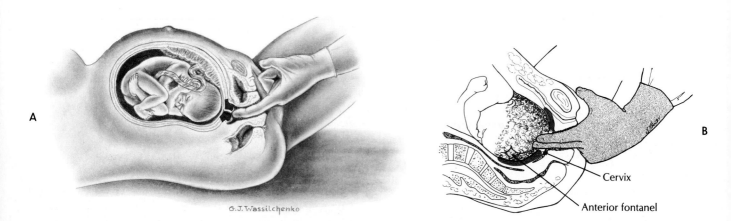

FIG. 12-9   Vaginal examination. **A,** Undilated, uneffaced cervix. Membranes intact. **B,** Palpation of sagittal suture line. Cervix effaced and partially dilated.

PROCEDURES 12-2

Tests for Rupture of Membranes

NITRAZINE TEST FOR pH

Explain procedure to woman/couple.

Procedure

Use **Nitrazine test** paper, a dye 1-1—impregnated test paper for pH. (Differentiates amniotic fluid, which is slightly alkaline, from urine and purulent material [pus], which are acidic.)

Wearing a sterile glove lubricated with water, place a piece of test paper at the cervical os

OR

Use a sterile, cotton-tipped applicator to dip deep into vagina to pick up fluid; touch applicator to test paper. This procedure may be done during a speculum examination.

Read Results:

Membranes probably intact: identifies vaginal and most body fluids that are acidic

Yellow	pH 5.0
Olive yellow	pH 5.5
Olive green	pH 6.0

Membranes probably ruptured: identifies amniotic fluid that is alkaline.

Blue-green	pH 6.5
Blue-gray	pH 7.0
Deep blue	pH 7.5

Realize that false test results are possible because of presence of bloody show, insufficient amniotic fluid, or semen.

Remove gloves and wash hands.

Chart Results: positive or negative

TEST FOR FERNING OR FERN PATTERN

Explain procedure to woman/couple.

Wash hands, apply sterile gloves, obtain specimen of fluid (usually with sterile speculum examination).

Spread a drop of fluid from vagina on a clean glass slide with a sterile, cotton-tipped applicator.

Allow fluid to dry.

Assess slide under microscope: observe for appearance of ferning, a frondlike crystalline pattern (do not confuse with cervical mucus test, when high levels of estrogen are responsible for the ferning).

Observe for absence of ferning (alerts staff to possibility that specimen was inadequate or that specimen was urine, vaginal discharge, or blood).

Remove gloves and wash hands.

Chart Results: either a positive or negative fern test finding

TEST FOR LANUGO HAIRS OR FETAL SQUAMOUS CELLS

Explain procedure to woman/couple.

Wash hands and apply sterile gloves.

Aspirate fluid from posterior vaginal vault with sterile aspiration syringe.

Place on clean glass slide.

Observe under microscope for presence of fetal lanugo hairs or fetal squamous cells.

Stain with Nile blue stain to identify fetal cells because some squamous cells that contain lipids stain yellow; other squamous cells and hairs stain blue.

Assess findings.

Remove gloves and wash hands.

Chart Results: Nile blue stain shows some squamous cells and some blue squamous cells and hair.

Laboratory and Diagnostic Tests

The nurse can anticipate the need for urinalysis and tests for blood values and rupture of membranes.

Urine Specimen

A urine specimen is obtained to gather data about the pregnant woman's health. It is a convenient and simple procedure that can provide information about her hydration status (specific gravity, color, amount), nutritional status (ketones), or possible complications, for example, pregnancy-induced hypertension (protein). The results can be obtained quickly and will help the nurse determine appropriate interventions.

Blood Tests

Blood tests vary with hospital protocol and patient history. An example of minimum assessment is a hematocrit determination, in which the specimen is processed by using a centrifuge on the perinatal unit. This can be accomplished with blood from a finger stick or the hub of a catheter used to start an intravenous (IV) line. More comprehensive blood assessments include hemoglobin and hematocrit values and a complete blood cell count (CBC).

If the woman's blood type has not been verified, blood will be drawn to establish type and Rh factor. If blood typing was previously done, the health care provider may choose to repeat the test. If obvious signs of immunocompromise are present, other diagnostic blood tests may be ordered by the health care provider.

Rupture of Membranes

Membranes (the bag of waters) can rupture spontaneously any time during labor. It is the nurse's responsibility to monitor FHR for several minutes immediately after *rupture of membranes (ROM)*, to ascertain fetal well-being, and to document findings. Tests for assessing ROM are discussed in Procedure 12-2. *Artificial rupture of membranes (AROM)* sometimes is done to augment or induce labor, or to place internal monitors because fetal status is difficult to maintain by external means. Assessment of amniotic fluid includes the following routine measures.

Amniotic Fluid

Color. Amniotic fluid is normally pale and straw-colored, and may contain flecks of vernix caseosa. If the amniotic fluid is greenish-brown, the fetus has probably undergone a hypoxic episode causing relaxation of the anal sphincter and the passage of by-products of fetal ingestion in utero called *meconium.* Yellow-stained amniotic fluid may indicate fetal hypoxia that occurred 36 hours or more before ROM, fetal hemolytic disease (Rh or ABO incompatibility), or intrauterine infection. Meconium-stained amniotic fluid may be a normal finding in a breech presentation, resulting from pressure on the fetal rectum during descent. Amniotic fluid that is port-wine colored may indicate premature separation of the placenta (abruptio). Although it is thought that meconium-stained amniotic fluid is an ominous finding in labor, it is not always associated with fetal hypoxia and must be viewed in the context of the total clinical picture of labor (Scott et al, 1990). The nurse's responsibility is to report the findings promptly to the health care provider and to record them in the labor record and on the monitor strip. After this finding, continuous electronic monitoring usually is used for the duration of labor. The presence of meconium-stained amniotic fluid alerts the nurse to observe fetal status more closely. After birth the newborn may be at high risk for alteration in respiratory status.

Character. Amniotic fluid normally has a watery consistency and lacks a strong odor. If fluid is thick or has an unpleasant odor, infection is suspected.

Amount. The normal amount of amniotic fluid ranges from 500 to 1200 ml. Most of the amniotic fluid originates from the maternal blood stream with additions of fetal urination.

Hydramnios (>2000 ml) often is associated with congenital anomalies of the fetus, resulting from the inability of the fetus to drink the fluid or for fluid to be trapped in the fetal body. *Oligohydramnios* (<500 ml) is an abnormally small amount of amniotic fluid and can be associated with incomplete formation or absence of the kidneys or obstruction of the urethra. If the fetus is unable to secrete and excrete urine, the volume of amniotic fluid decreases. Fetal surgery can now correct some obstructive conditions.

Infection. When membranes rupture, microorganisms from the vagina can ascend into the amniotic sac. Amnionitis and placentitis may develop. Even when membranes are intact, microorganisms may ascend and

SIGNS OF POTENTIAL COMPLICATIONS

LABOR

Intrauterine pressure >75 mm Hg (by IUPC)
Contractions consistently lasting ≥90 sec
Contractions consistently occurring ≤2 min
Fetal bradycardia, tachycardia, or persistent decreased variability
Irregular FHR; suspected fetal arrhythmias
Absence of fetal heart beat
Appearance of fluid from the vagina that is meconium stained or bloody
Prolapsed umbilical cord
Arrest in progress of cervical dilatation/effacement and/or descent of the fetus
Maternal temperature ≥100.4° F (38° C)
Foul-smelling vaginal discharge
Persistent bright or dark-red vaginal bleeding

directly cause premature ROM. There is a controversy regarding whether prophylactic antibiotic therapy protects against the infection known as chorioamnionitis, which involves both the maternal and fetal sides of the membrane. Maternal temperature and vaginal discharge are assessed frequently (every 1 to 2 hours) for early identification of a developing infection after ROM.

Signs of Potential Problems

Assessment findings serve as a baseline for evaluation of the woman's progress during the first stage of labor. Although some complications of labor are anticipated, others appear only in the clinical course of labor. Knowledge of pregnancy, careful initial assessment, and follow-up of progress are necessary during normal labor, as well as during a labor in which complications arise (see Signs of Potential Complications).

✦ NURSING DIAGNOSES

Nursing diagnoses provide direction to types of nursing actions needed to implement a plan of care. When establishing nursing diagnoses, the nurse analyzes the significance of findings collected during assessment.

Initial Assessment

Impaired verbal communication related to
- Foreign language barrier

Anxiety related to
- Knowledge deficit related to physical examination procedures
- Lack of previous experiences or preparation-for-parenthood classes

High risk for injury related to

- Lack of prenatal testing of blood and urine

Subsequent Assessments

Pain related to
- Intense contractions

Fluid volume deficit related to
- Decreased fluid intake

Impaired physical mobility related to
- Station of fetal presenting part
- Status of fetal membranes
- Fetal monitoring

Altered patterns of urinary elimination related to
- Reduced fluid intake
- IV fluids
- Bed rest
- Lack of privacy
- Analgesia
- Anesthesia

Assessment of Stress During Labor

Impaired gas exchange, fetal, related to
- Maternal position
- Hyperventilation

Spiritual distress, maternal, related to
- Inability to meet self-expectations

Ineffective family coping: compromised, related to
- Knowledge deficit of comfort measures that can be used for the laboring woman

✥ EXPECTED OUTCOMES

The nurse and patient set and prioritize expected outcomes, which focus on the patient. Appropriate nursing and patient actions are determined to meet these expected outcomes. Planning with the patient is essential for the implementation of these expected outcomes. Throughout the first stage of labor the woman will:

1. Demonstrate normal progression of labor
2. Express satisfaction with the assistance of her support person and nursing staff
3. Verbalize her desires for participation in labor and participate as tolerated throughout labor
4. Continue normal progression of labor while the FHR remains within normal range without distress signs
5. Maintain adequate hydration status through oral or intravenous intake
6. Void at least every 2 hours to prevent bladder distention
7. Encourage participation of support person by verbalizing discomfort and indicating measures that help reduce discomfort and promote relaxation

✥ COLLABORATIVE CARE

Standards of Care

Standards of care guide the nurse in preparing for and implementing procedures with the expectant mother (see

Appendix A). Protocols for care include the following:
1. Check the health care provider's orders.
2. Assess the health care provider's orders for appropriateness and correctness; for example, enema, and when not to carry out the procedure.
3. Check labels on IV solutions, drugs, and other materials used for nursing care.
4. Check expiration date on any packs of supplies used for ordered procedures.
5. Ensure that information on the woman's identification band is correct (also check that identification band is accurate; e.g., if she has allergies, the band is the appropriate color).
6. Employ an empathic approach when giving care;
   a. Use words the woman can understand when explaining procedures.
   b. Establish a rapport with the woman and her support person(s).
   c. Be kind, caring, and competent when performing necessary procedures.
   d. Acknowledge that pain and discomfort are as the woman describes.
   e. Repeat instructions as necessary and ensure the woman understands.
   f. Carry out appropriate comfort measures, for example, mouth care and back care of the woman and ensure that support person is coping.
7. Use universal precautions, including precautions for invasive procedures, as needed (see Chapter 21).
8. Document care according to hospital guidelines and communicate information to the health care provider when indicated (see Box 12-1 for an example of care plan using protocols and standards of care).

LEGAL TIP: **Standards of Care for Labor**

1. Provide explanations to patient for all procedures
2. Assess maternal and fetal status, as well as progress of labor
   a. continue to monitor fetal status until birth
3. Intervene based on analysis of assessment data
   a. Carry out all orders/protocols for care
   b. Notify health care provider of assessments and outcomes of interventions
   c. Protect patient from injury
   d. Maintain competency and currency of skills to uphold standard of care
4. Evaluate care given and revise care based on assessment
5. Document all care and patient response to interventions

BOX 12-1

Patient Care Plan Using Protocols and Nursing Standards

PATIENT CARE PLAN FOR LABOR   Paula Jones
                                 Unit No. 4587024

Date Initiated:_____   Time:_____   RN:_____

OUTCOME STANDARDS:

1. Patient will demonstrate normal labor progress while the fetus tolerates the labor process without demonstrating nonreassuring signs. Date met:_____
2. Patient will participate as desired in decisions about her care. Date met:_____
3. Patient and her partner will verbalize knowledge of labor process and their expectations for the birth experience. Date met:_____

INITIATED Date/RN	PROBLEM	NURSING INTERVENTIONS	DISCONTINUED Date/RN
	Alteration in maternal/fetal gas exchange	Implement fetal monitoring per protocol or orders from health care provider (Chapter 11, p. 260)	
	Risk related to labor progress:	Provide nursing care per hospital procedure manual	
	▪ altered pattern of urinary elimination	Implement labor care per protocol (see Table 12-2)	
	▪ tissue trauma related to birth	Notify health care provider of problems (see Signs of Potential Complications, p. 278)	
		Provide care for vaginal birth per hospital procedure manual	
		Provide immediate care for newborn per hospital procedure manual	
		Implement protocol for fourth stage of labor (see Procedure 12-3 on p. 307)	
	Anxiety related to maternal/fetal status	Encourage patient and her partner to express their concerns	
		Keep couple informed of labor progress	
		Involve patient in decision-making regarding her care	
	Knowledge deficit about labor/procedures	Explain procedures in terms patient can understand	
	Pain associated with labor	Promote use of relaxation techniques	
		Provide comfort measures	
		Offer pain medications as ordered	
		Evaluate response to pain relief measures	
	Other problems:		

Physical Nursing Care during Labor

Physical nursing care of the woman in labor is an essential function. Physical needs, nursing actions, and rationale for care are presented in Table 12-4.

Ambulation and Positioning

Ambulation ad lib may be encouraged if membranes are intact, if the fetal presenting part is engaged after ROM, and if the woman has not received medication for pain (Fig. 12-10). Sitting or standing during early labor has been shown to be more comfortable than lying down (Melzack, Belanger, Lacroix, 1991).

Ambulation may be contraindicated because of mater-

nal and/or fetal status. When the woman lies in bed, she is encouraged to lie on her side in order to promote optimal uteroplacental and renal blood flow. If the woman wants to lie supine, the nurse can place a pillow under one side as a wedge to achieve the same result. If the fetus is in the occiput-posterior position, it may be helpful to encourage the woman to squat or use the hands and knees position during contractions. These positions increase pelvic diameter, allowing rotation of the fetus' head to a more anterior position.

Much research is being directed toward a better understanding of the physiologic and psychic effects of maternal position in labor. Fetal presentations or mecha-

TABLE 12-4 Physical Nursing Care during Labor

NEED	NURSING ACTIONS	RATIONALE
GENERAL HYGIENE		
Showers/bed baths jacuzzi bath	Assess for progress in labor	Determines appropriateness for the activity
	Supervise showers closely if woman is in true labor	Prevents injury from fall; labor may accelerate
	Suggest allowing warm water to strike lower back	Aids relaxation; increases comfort
Vulva	Mini-prep if ordered	Facilitates cutting and repair of episiotomy, however, may increase risk of infection
Oral hygiene	Offer toothbrush, mouthwash, or wash the teeth with an ice-cold, wet washcloth as needed	Refreshes mouth; improves morale; helps counteract dry, thirsty feeling
Hair	Brush, braid per woman's wishes	Improves morale
Hand washing	Offer washcloths before and after voiding and as needed	Maintains cleanliness; improves morale and comfort
Face	Offer cool washcloth	Improves morale; relief from diaphoresis
Gowns/linens	Change prn; fluff pillows	Improves morale and comfort; probably through the Hawthorne effect (p. 284)
FLUID INTAKE		
Oral	Per health care provider's orders, offer clear fluids, small amounts of ice chips, hard candy, or lollipops	Meets standard of care; provides hydration; provides calories; absorbs quickly and is less likely to be vomited; provides positive emotional experience
IV	Establish and maintain IV as ordered	Maintains hydration; provides venous access for medications
Nothing by mouth (NPO)	Inform family of NPO and rationale	A precautionary measure if anesthesia is a possibility; deters vomiting and its possible sequelae
	Provide mouth care	Promotes comfort
ELIMINATION		
Voiding	Encourage voiding at least every 2 hours	A full bladder may impede descent of presenting part; overdistention may cause bladder atony and injury as well as postnatal voiding difficulty
Ambulatory	Allow ambulation to bathroom per health care provider's orders, *if:*	Reinforces normal process of urination
	The presenting part is engaged	Precautionary measure against prolapse of umbilical cord
	The membranes are not ruptured	
	The woman is not medicated	Precautionary measure against injury
Bed rest	Offer bedpan	Prevents hazards of bladder distention and ambulation
	Turn on the tap water to run; pour warm water over the vulva; and give positive suggestion	Encourages voiding
	Provide privacy	Shows respect for woman
	Put up side rails on bed	Prevents injury from fall
	Place call bell within reach	
	Offer washcloth for hands	Maintains cleanliness and comfort
	Wash vulvar area	Maintains standard of care
Catheterization	Catheterize per health care provider's order or per hospital protocol	Prevents hazards of bladder distention
	Insert catheter between contractions	Minimizes discomfort
	Avoid force if obstacle to insertion is noted	"Obstacle" may be caused by compression of urethra by presenting part
	If presenting part is low, introduce two fingers of free hand into introitus to apply upward pressure on presenting part while other hand inserts the catheter	Minimizes potential for injury and subsequent infection to urethra
Bowel elimination	After careful assessment ambulate the woman to bathroom or offer her a bedpan	Avoids misinterpretation of rectal pressure from the presenting part as the need to defecate

nisms of labor may be helped or hindered by maternal posture (see Fig. 12-11; Liu, 1989; McKay, Roberts, 1989; Andrews, Chrzanowski, 1990; Biancuzzo, 1991).

Emergency Interventions

Emergency conditions can arise with startling speed and require immediate nursing intervention.

Prolapsed Umbilical Cord

Prolapse of the umbilical cord occurs when the cord lies below the presenting part of the fetus. Umbilical cord prolapse may be occult (hidden, not visible) at any time during labor whether or not membranes are ruptured (Fig. 12-12, *A* and *B*). It is most common to see

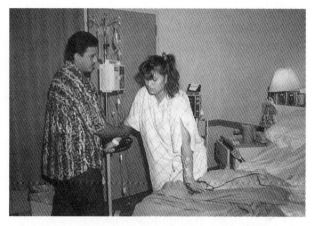

FIG. 12-10 Woman walking with husband. (Courtesy Marjorie Pyle, RNC, *Lifecircle*, Costa Mesa, CA.)

frank (visible) prolapse directly after ROM, when gravity washes the cord in front of the presenting part (Fig. 12-12, *C* and *D*). This occurs in one of 400 births. Contributing factors are a long cord (>100 cm or 40 inches), malpresentation (breech), transverse lie, or unengaged presenting part.

When the presenting part does not fit snugly into the lower uterine segment, as in hydramnios or when the membranes rupture, a sudden gush of amniotic fluid may cause the cord to be displaced downward. Similarly the cord may prolapse during AROM if the presenting part is high. A small fetus also may not fit snugly into the lower uterine segment; as a result, cord prolapse is more likely to occur.

Other predisposing factors in cord prolapse that are associated with a high presenting part are multiparity, cephalopelvic disproportion, and placenta previa. Prolapse of the cord is difficult to diagnose; however, an alert nurse or health care provider may make the diagnosis on vaginal examination after a sudden gush of fluid. Prompt recognition is important because fetal hypoxia from prolonged cord compression (occlusion of blood flow to and from the fetus for more than 5 minutes) usually results in central nervous system (CNS) damage or demise of the fetus (see Emergency box) Pressure on the cord is relieved by the examiner putting a sterile gloved hand into the vagina and holding the presenting part off of the umbilical cord (Fig. 12-13, *A, B,*). The woman is assisted into a position such as a modified Sims' (Fig. 12-13, *C*), Trendelenburg's, or knee-chest (Fig. 12-13, *D*), where gravity keeps the presenting part off of the cord. If the cervix is fully dilated, forceps or vacuum-assisted birth can be performed for the fetus in a cephalic presentation; otherwise a cesarean birth is likely to be performed. Nonreassuring fetal status, inadequate uterine

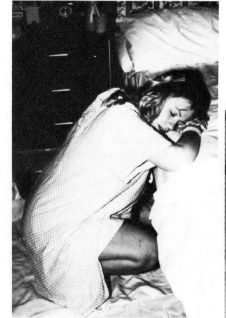

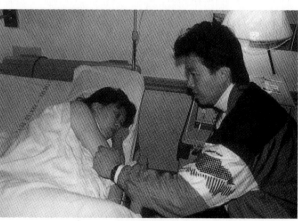

FIG. 12-11 Maternal positions for labor. **A,** Squatting. **B,** Woman using focusing and breathing with coaching from husband. (Courtesy Marjorie Pyle, RNC, *Lifecircle*, Costa Mesa, CA.)

A

B

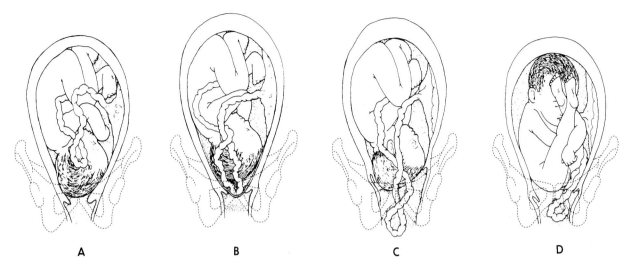

FIG. 12-12   Prolapse of umbilical cord. Note pressure of presenting part on umbilical cord, which endangers fetal circulation. **A,** Occult (hidden) prolapse of cord. **B,** Complete prolapse of cord. Note membranes are intact. **C,** Cord presenting in front of fetal head and may be seen within vagina. **D,** Frank breech presentation with prolapsed cord.

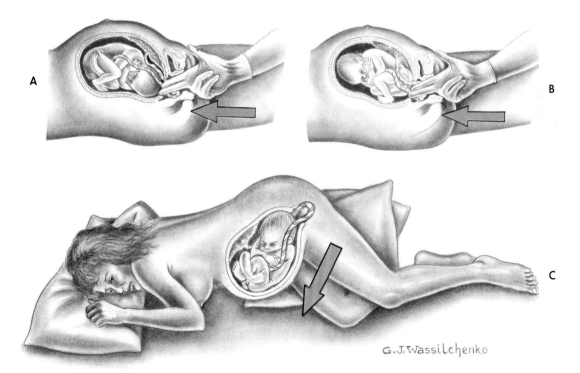

FIG. 12-13   Arrows indicate direction of pressure against presenting part to relieve compression of prolapsed umbilical cord. Pressure exerted by examiner's fingers in **A,** vertex presentation, and **B,** in breech position. **C,** Gravity relieves pressure with a woman in modified Sims position with hips elevated as high as possible with pillows.   *Continued*

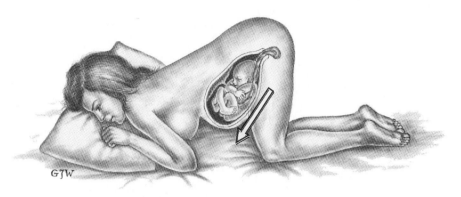

FIG. 12-13, cont'd D, Knee-chest position.

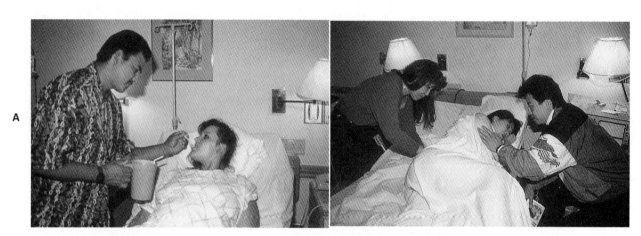

FIG. 12-14 **A,** Father-to-be providing comfort measures. **B,** Support person applying sacral pressure while father-to-be provides encouragement. (Courtesy Marjorie Pyle, RNC, *Lifecircle*, Costa Mesa, CA.)

relaxation, and bleeding can also occur as a result of a prolapsed umbilical cord. Indications for immediate interventions are presented in the Emergency box.

Support Measures

Nursing care for a woman in labor includes (1) helping the woman participate to the extent she wishes in the birth of her infant, (2) meeting the woman's expected outcomes for herself, (3) helping the woman conserve her energy, and (4) helping the woman control her discomfort.

The nurse acts as an advocate for the woman and her family. Couples who have attended parenthood education programs using the psychoprophylactic approach will know something about the labor process, coaching techniques, and comfort measures. The staff should play a supportive role and keep the couple informed of progress. Even if the expectant parents have not attended classes, the various techniques may be taught, to a degree, during the early phase of labor. In this case the

nurse will be expected to do more of the coaching and give supportive care.

The nurse serves as a coach to the woman in the absence of other support persons or as an assistant coach to the support persons present. The nurse must have a thorough knowledge of breathing and relaxation techniques in order to assist the woman and her partner in coping with labor. The nurse needs to provide comfort measures, such as warmth to the lower back in the case of back labor, a cool cloth to the forehead (Fig. 12-14), and room temperature controlled for the laboring woman's comfort. The **Hawthorne effect** is the "phenomenon that occurs when a person in pain begins to feel more comfortable as the nurse talks soothingly, fluffs a pillow, and promises to stay nearby. Positive support, especially by one in authority, enhances the ability to cope with stress" (Jimenez, 1983).

Comfort measures vary with the situation. The nurse can draw on the couple's repertoire of comfort measures learned during the pregnancy. Comfort measures include maintaining a comfortable, supportive atmosphere in the

EMERGENCY

INTERVENTIONS FOR EMERGENCIES

SIGNS	INTERVENTIONS
Nonreassuring Fetal Heart Rate Fetal bradycardia (FHR <110 beats/min for >2 min Fetal tachycardia (if term, FHR is >160 beats/min for >2 min) Irregular FHR, abnormal sinus rhythm with internal monitor Persistent decrease in FHR variability Absence of FHR	Notify health care provider Change maternal position to side-lying Increase IV fluids, if infusing Start an IV if one is not in place Administer oxygen at 10 to 12 L/min by tight face mask
Inadequate Uterine Relaxation Intrauterine pressure >75 mm Hg (by IUPC) Contractions consistently lasting >90 sec Contraction interval <2 min	Notify health care provider Discontinue oxytocin (Pitocin) if infusing Position woman on left side Increase infusion rate of IV fluids Administer oxygen at 10 to 12 L/min by tight face mask If no IV is in place, start IV now Palpate and evaluate contractions Give tocolytics (terbutaline, ritodrine) as ordered
Vaginal Bleeding Vaginal bleeding (bright red, dark red, or in an amount in excess of that expected during normal cervical dilation) Continuous vaginal bleeding with FHR changes Pain: may or may not be present	Notify health care provider Anticipate emergency (crash) cesarean birth
Infection Foul-smelling amniotic fluid Maternal temperature >100.4° F (38° C) in presence of adequate hydration (straw-colored urine) Fetal tachycardia >160 beats/min for >2 min	Notify health care provider Institute cooling measures for laboring woman Start IV hydration Send catheterized urine specimen to the laboratory for urinalysis and amniotic fluid sample for culture
Prolapse of Cord Fetal bradycardia with variable deceleration during uterine contraction Woman reports feeling the cord after membranes rupture Cord is seen or felt in or protruding from the vagina	Call for assistance Notify health care provider immediately Glove the examining hand quickly and insert two fingers into the vagina to the cervix. With one finger on either side of the cord or both fingers to one side, exert upward pressure against the presenting part to relieve compression of the cord (Fig. 12-13, A and B). Apply a rolled towel under the woman's right hip Place woman into extreme Trendelenburg's or modified Sims' position (Fig. 12-13, C), or knee-chest position (Fig. 12-13, D). If cord is protruding from vagina, wrap loosely in a sterile towel wet with warm sterile normal saline Administer oxygen to the woman by mask, 10 to 12 L/min, until birth is accomplished Start IV fluids or increase existing drip rate Continue to monitor fetal heart rate by internal fetal scalp electrode if possible Explain to woman and support person what is happening and how it is being managed

TABLE 12-5 Woman's Expected Responses and Support Person's Actions during Labor

WOMAN	SUPPORT PERSON
DILATATION OF CERVIX 0 TO 3 CM (contractions 10 to 30 sec long, 5 to 30 min apart, mild to moderate)	

Mood: alert, happy, excited, mild anxiety
Settles into labor room; selects focal point
Rests or sleeps, if possible
Uses breathing techniques
Uses effleurage, focusing, and relaxation techniques
	Provides encouragement, feedback for relaxation, companionship
	Assists with contractions
	  Uses focusing techniques
	  Concentration on breathing technique
	Uses comfort measures
	  Position most comfortable for woman
	  Keeps woman aware of progress, explains procedures and routines
	  Gives praise
	  Offers ataractics as ordered

DILATATION OF CERVIX 4 TO 7 CM (contractions 30 to 40 sec long, 3 to 5 min apart, moderate to strong)	

Mood: seriously labor oriented, concentration and energy needed for contractions, alert, more demanding
Continues relaxation, focusing techniques
Uses breathing techniques
	Acts as buffer, limits assessment techniques to between contractions
	Assists with contractions
	  May need to encourage woman to help her maintain breathing techniques
	Uses comfort measures
	  Positions woman on side
	  Encourages voluntary relaxation of muscles of back, buttocks, thighs, and perineum; effleurage
	  Uses counterpressure to sacrococcygeal area
	  Encourages and praises
	  Keeps woman aware of progress
	  Offers analgesics and anesthetics as ordered
	  Checks bladder, encourages to void
	  Gives mouth care, ice chips

DILATATION OF CERVIX 8 TO 10 CM (TRANSITION) (contractions 45 to 90 sec long, 2 to 3 min apart, strong)	

Mood: irritable, intense concentration, symptoms of transition
Continues relaxation, needs greater concentration to do this
Breathing techniques
  Uses 4:1 breathing pattern if possible
  Uses panting to overcome response to urge to push
	Stays with woman, provides constant support
	Assists with contractions
	  Probably will need to remind, reassure, and encourage to reestablish breathing pattern and concentration
	  If sedated or drowsy, woman needs warning to begin breathing pattern before contraction becomes too intense
	  If woman begins to push, institutes panting respirations
	Uses comfort measures
	  Accepts woman's inability to comply with instructions
	  Accepts irritable response to helping, such as counterpressure
	  Supports woman who has nausea and vomiting, gives mouth care as needed, gives reassurance regarding signs of end point of first stage
	Uses countertension techniques (effleurage and voluntary relaxation)
	Keeps woman aware of progress, and assists with pushing when appropriate time to push

labor and birth area; using touch therapeutically; providing nonpharmacologic management of discomfort; and administering analgesics when necessary; but, most of all, just *being there* (Table 12-5).

Labor rooms need to be light and airy; however, the bright overhead lights are turned off when not needed. The area should be large enough to accommodate a comfortable chair for the woman's partner as well as the monitoring equipment and hospital personnel. In some hospitals, couples are urged to bring extra pillows to help make the hospital surrounding more homelike.

The Father/Partner during Labor

The father of the baby is usually the woman's partner who supports her in labor. Throughout the last 20 years childbirth preparation has been widely practiced. The ideal father's role was thought to be that of labor coach. Fathers were expected to actively help the woman cope with labor. This expectation may be unrealistic for all men, because some men have concerns about their labor coaching abilities (Berry, 1988). Chapman (1992) reported at least three roles adopted by men during labor and birth—coach, teammate, and witness. As the *coach*, the father actively assists the woman during and after labor contractions. Coaches express a strong need to be in control of themselves and of the labor experience. Women express a high desire for the father to be physically involved in labor. The father acting as the *teammate* assists the woman during labor and birth by responding to requests for physical or emotional support or both. Teammates usually adopt the follower or helper role and look to the woman or nurse to tell them what to do. Women express a strong desire to have the father present and willing to help in any way. In the role of *witness*, the father acts as a companion and gives emotional and moral support. He watches the woman labor and give birth, but he often sleeps, watches television, or leaves the room for long periods of time. Witnesses believe there is little they can do to physically help the woman and look to the nurses and health care providers to be in charge of the experience. Women do not expect the father to do more than be present.

The degree of mutuality (level of interdependency and sharing) and understanding (the ability to know each other's needs) in a couple's relationship determines which role the father adopts. The coach and teammate roles are often adopted by men in couples with a high degree of mutuality. Men in relationships where mutuality is low tend to adopt the witness role.

Since a father can participate in labor and birth in different ways, nurses need to encourage him to adopt the role most comfortable for him and for the woman, rather than an artificial role.

Supporting both the father and the mother in labor elevates the nurse's role. It is another step forward from merely providing custodial care to enacting a therapeutic role. Support of the father reflects the nurse's orientation and commitment to each person, the family, and the community. Therapeutic nursing actions convey several important concepts to the father.

First, the father is of value as a person. He is not a comic-strip character, inept and bungling or idle, nervous, and inconsequential. Secondly, he can learn to be a partner in the mother's care. Finally, childbearing is a partnership.

The nurse can support the father/partner in the following ways:

1. Regardless of the degree of involvement desired, orient him to the maternity unit, and what he can do there (sleep, telephone), rest room, cafeteria, waiting room, nursery, visiting hours, and names and functions of personnel present. Also include the woman's labor room and show him what he can do there (i.e., sleep, telephone).

2. Respect his or the couple's decisions as to his degree of involvement, whether the decision is active participation in the birth room or just being kept informed. When appropriate, provide data on which he or they can base decisions; offer freedom of choice as opposed to coercion one way or another. This is *their* experience and *their* baby.

3. Indicate to him when his presence has been helpful and continue to reinforce this throughout labor.

4. Offer to teach him comfort measures to the degree he wants to know them. Reassure him that he is not assuming the responsibility for observation and management of his partner's labor, rather his responsibility is to support her as she progresses.

5. Communicate with him frequently regarding the woman's progress and his needs. Keep him informed of procedures to be performed, what to expect from procedures, and what is expected of him.

6. Prepare him for changes in the woman's behavior and physical appearance.

7. Remind him to eat; offer snacks and fluids if possible.

8. Relieve him as necessary; offer blankets if he is to sleep in a chair by the bedside. Acknowledge the stress of the situation on each partner, and identify normal responses. The nonjudgmental attitude of staff members helps the father and mother accept their own and the other parent's behavior.

9. Attempt to modify or eliminate unsettling stimuli such as extra noise, extra light, and chatter.

Culture and Father's Participation

Many hospitals encourage the father's presence during labor and birth. If the father is unable to attend, another significant person may be present. In some cultures the father may be available, but his presence with the mother may not be appropriate and he may resist involvement. His behavior could be misunderstood by the nursing staff as lack of concern, caring, or interest. Lantican and Corona (1992) identify the importance of the affectional bond between Mexican-American and Filipino women and their female relatives, in regard to home-related activities like childbearing. This is also true for many other cultural groups. The presence of another woman or women is highly desired for these activities. Among some cultures, if childbearing occurs in the hospital, at least one woman is desired to be present for assistance. Often women from Southeast Asia (Hollingsworth et al, 1980), African American (Carrington, 1978; Johnson, Snow, 1978), Native American (Farris, 1978; Horn, 1982), and Arab American (Meleis, Lipton, Paul, 1981) cultures prefer female assistance during childbearing.

According to Pillsbury (1978), the Chinese husband is not allowed in the birth room, lest he become polluted by the woman's blood. A nurse from a different culture might think it odd that a Chinese husband does not seem to give any emotional support to his wife during labor and birth. However, Chinese women have significant others who can provide the necessary emotional support—mothers, in-laws, cousins, other members of the extended family, or close friends.

Due to the variation in the choice of the preferred person or persons, it is critical for the nurse to determine from the woman and her family what persons are wanted during labor and birth.

Support of the Grandparents during Labor

Especially in situations in which the grandparents take the place of the husband as a labor coach, it is important to support them and treat them with respect. They may have a way to deal with pain relief based on their experience. They need to be given a chance to help if their actions will not compromise the status of the mother or the fetus. The nurse acts as a role model for parents by treating grandparents with dignity and respect, by acknowledging the value of their contributions to parental support, and by recognizing the difficulty parents have in witnessing their child's discomfort or crisis, regardless of the child's age.

Of particular value is the availability of grandparents or another person or persons to relieve the father/coach. This may be necessary to assist the woman in labor with walking, especially if IV poles need to be pushed, as well as to help the woman when she needs two tasks performed simultaneously.

Whenever possible the nurse offers grandparents emotional support. A nurse can show support by providing liquid refreshment, even if unsolicited, and by initiating discussion with open-ended questions or statements, such as "It is sometimes hard to watch a daughter in labor."

Siblings during Labor

Preparation for acceptance of the new child helps with the attachment process. Preparation for and participation during pregnancy and labor may help older children accept this change. The older child or children become *active* participants who are important to the family (Bliss, 1980). Rehearsal for the event before labor is essential. Preparation for the entire family includes the additional support person who will be responsible for the older children throughout the childbirth process.

The age and developmental level of children influence their responses; therefore preparation should meet each child's needs. Children younger than 2 years old show little interest in pregnancy and labor; for older children, the experience may reduce fears and misconceptions. Most parents have a "feel" for their children's maturational level and ability to cope. Preparation includes description of anticipated sights and sounds. Children must learn that their mother will be working hard. She will not be able to talk to them during contractions. She may groan and pant. Labor is uncomfortable, but their mother's body is made for the job. The sights, sounds, smells, and behavior of participants are experiences for which fathers are prepared. Films are available for preparing older preschool and school-age children for participating in the birth experience (see Appendix H).

Preparation for Giving Birth

The first stage of labor ends with the complete dilatation of the cervix. For many multiparous women, birth usually occurs within minutes of complete dilatation, perhaps only one push later. Nulliparous women usually push for 1 to 2 hours before giving birth. If the woman has epidural anesthesia, pushing can last more than 2 hours. The nurse begins preparation for birth when a multiparous woman is 6 to 7 cm dilated, because progression through the last few centimeters of dilatation can occur any time from a few minutes to hours. Factors that influence the process are fetal position (e.g., occiput posterior) and size in relation to previous babies.

Birth Setting

Significant changes have occurred in the location where birth takes place. A 1991 survey reported that more than half of all pregnant women give birth somewhere other than the traditional labor and delivery room (American College of Obstetricians and Gynecologists, 1993). The most common change in birth settings is the labor, delivery, recovery, postpartum (LDRP) room where the woman stays during her entire hospitalization (see Fig. 12-15). This avoids the confusion of multiple transfers of the woman from the labor room to delivery room to recovery room. Another option is the labor, delivery, and recovery (LDR) room, in which the woman stays during her labor and immediate postpartum recovery period (1 to 2 hours) and then transfers to a "postpartum"

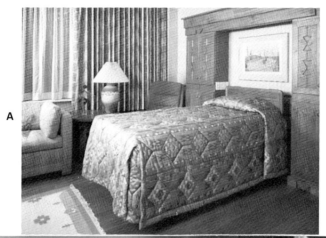

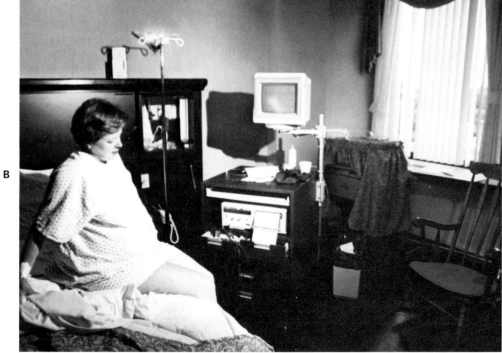

FIG. 12-15   Examples of a labor, delivery, recovery, postpartum (LDRP) room. (**A,** Courtesy Vogler/Perinatal Healthcare Consultants, Kailua, HI. **B,** Courtesy Kathy Hanold, RN, MS, Birth Place, Barnes Hospital at Washington University Medical Center, St Louis.)

room. Here she stays for the duration of her hospitalization. Some hospitals, however, lack birthing rooms, and transfer during second stage is required. If birth is to occur in the delivery room, it is best to transfer the woman early enough to avoid a last-minute rush. For nulliparous women transfer can take place when the presenting part begins to distend the perineum. For multiparous women transfer should take place in the first stage, when the cervix is dilated 8 to 9 cm.

✤ EVALUATION

Evaluation of progress and outcomes is a continuous activity during the first stage of labor. The nurse must care-

fully evaluate each interaction with the mother-to-be and her family, and critically appraise how well the formulated expected outcomes for care are being met. The following results reflect effective care:

- The woman demonstrates normal labor progress while the FHR remains within normal range without signs of distress.
- She expresses satisfaction with the assistance of her support person and nursing staff.
- She verbalizes her desire for participation in her care during labor and participates as tolerated throughout labor.
- She maintains adequate hydration and empties her bladder as needed.

PLAN OF CARE

Needs during Active Labor

Case History

Paula Jones, a 24-year-old, gravida 2, para 1-0-0-1 at 39 weeks' gestation, is admitted to the birthing unit. The assessment data include cervical dilatation 5 cm, effacement 60%, station −2. Uterine contractions occur every 4 to 5 min, last 40 to 60 sec, and are of moderate intensity. Maternal vital signs are within normal limits, and the fetus is active with a fetal heart rate of 132 beats/min. Paula says she feels anxious about this birth, and feels uncomfortable during contractions.

EXPECTED OUTCOMES	IMPLEMENTATION	RATIONALE	EVALUATION
Nursing Diagnosis: Fear/anxiety related to maternal/fetal well-being during labor			
Paula will identify sources of fear and anxiety Paula will express concerns about labor and birth Paula will verbalize that she feels less anxious and fearful	Promote an open, trusting relationship with Paula Communicate an acceptance of her fears and anxieties Encourage Paula to differentiate between real and imagined threats to personal or fetal well-being	Verbalizing fears and concerns will help Paula to deal with them. It is important to decrease fear and anxiety because they can interfere with labor progress	Paula says she is afraid of being left alone during labor and worries that if she takes medication for pain, it will hurt the fetus The nurse acknowledges her fears, and provides her with information about effects of pain medication on the fetus and the chances of problems actually occurring. The nurse also assures Paula that she will not be left alone because she is in active labor Paula says she is less fearful after discussing these concerns with the nurse
Nursing Diagnosis: Pain related to increasing frequency and intensity of uterine contractions			
Paula will report increased comfort	Assess Paula's verbal and nonverbal communication. Promote the use of focused breathing techniques Offer massage and other therapeutic touch techniques (Chapter 10) Involve her in decision-making regarding comfort measures she prefers Explain all procedures in simple language Provide her with choices regarding administration of ordered medications Inform her regarding progress in labor	Reduction of perception of pain increases woman's ability to cope with labor. Focused breathing distracts Improves morale and comfort (Hawthorne effect) Knowledge provides basis for decision-making	Paula reports increased comfort Paula is able to use relaxation techniques and does not request pain medication

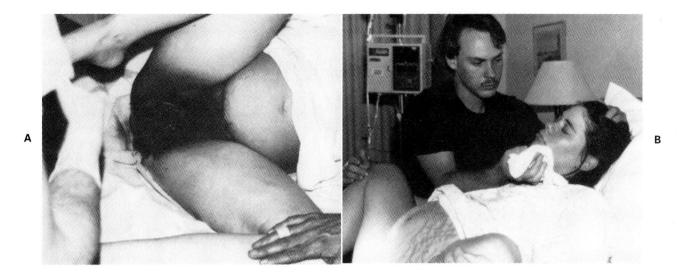

FIG. 12-16   A, Pushing, side-lying position, perineal bulging. **B,** Pushing, semi-sitting. Husband wiping woman's face with cool cloth between contractions. (Courtesy Marjorie Pyle, RNC, *Lifecircle,* Costa Mesa, CA.)

- She indicates those measures that help to reduce her discomfort and promote relaxation to her support person or nurse.

If the evaluation process identifies that results fall short of achieving an expected outcome, further assessment, planning, and implementation are imperative to attain the correct nursing care for the woman and her family (see Plan of Care on p. 290).

SECOND STAGE OF LABOR

The second stage of labor is the stage where the fetus is born. This stage begins with full cervical dilatation (10 cm) and ends with the baby's birth. This stage has been described as having two or three phases. These phases are characterized by maternal verbal and nonverbal behaviors, the status of uterine activity, the urge to bear down, and fetal descent. Phase one begins when the woman expresses the urge to push, usually at the peak of a contraction. The woman may complain of increased discomfort, but in between contractions she is quiet and often has her eyes closed. In the second phase, the woman becomes more focused on pushing and changes positions frequently to find a more comfortable pushing position. Bearing-down efforts become rhythmic. The woman frequently announces the start of contractions and becomes more vocal as she bears down (Fig. 12-16). In the third phase, the presenting part is on the perineum, and bearing-down efforts are most effective for birth. The woman may be more verbal about pain, may scream or swear, and may act out of control (Aderhold, Roberts, 1991). The woman needs to be encour-

aged to listen to her body as she progresses through the second stage of labor.

✛ ASSESSMENT

The only certain objective sign that the second stage of labor has begun occurs when, upon vaginal examination, the examiner cannot feel the cervix (Myles, 1989). Other signs that suggest the onset of the second stage include the following:*

1. Sudden appearance of sweat on upper lip
2. An episode of vomiting
3. An increased bloody show
4. Shaking of extremities
5. Increased restlessness; verbalization that "I can't go on"
6. Involuntary bearing-down efforts

These signs commonly appear at the time the cervix reaches full dilatation (Myles, 1989; Scott et al, 1990). Other indicators for assessing progress during each phase of the second stage can be found in Table 12-6.

Assessment is continuous during the second stage of labor. Hospital protocol determines the specific type and timing of assessments.

Duration of Second Stage

Considerable controversy exists over the precise duration of the second stage and the time limits that should be regarded as normal. The Friedman curves for nulliparous

---

*If the woman has an epidural block, she may not exhibit signs of being in the second stage.

TABLE 12-6 Maternal Progress in Second Stage of Labor

CRITERION	PHASE 1	PHASE 2	PHASE 3

CONTRACTIONS
  Magnitude (intensity)
  Frequency
	Period of physiologic lull
	  for all criteria
	2 to 3 min
		Significant increase
		
		2 to 2½ min
			Overwhelmingly strong
			Expulsive
			1 to 2 min

DESCENT		Increases and **Ferguson's reflex*** activated	Rapid
STATION	0 to +2	+2 to +4	+4 to birth
SHOW: COLOR AND AMOUNT		Significant increase in dark red bloody show	Fetal head visible at introitus; bloody show accompanies birth of head
SPONTANEOUS BEARING-DOWN EFFORTS	Slight to absent except with peaks of strongest contractions	Increased urgency to bear down	Greatly increased
VOCALIZATION	Quiet Concern over progress	Grunting sounds or expiratory vocalization; announces contractions	Grunting sounds and expiratory vocalizations continue; may scream or swear
MATERNAL BEHAVIOR	Experiences sense of relief that transition to second stage is finished Feels fatigued and sleepy Feels a sense of accomplishment and optimism, since the "worst is over" Feels in control	Senses increased urgency to push Alters respiratory pattern: has short 4 to 5 sec breathholds with regular breaths in between, 5 to 7 times per contraction Makes grunting sounds or expiratory vocalizations Frequent repositioning	Expresses sense of extreme pain Expresses feelings of powerlessness Shows decreased ability to listen or concentrate on anything but giving birth Describes the **"ring of fire"**† Often shows excitement immediately following birth of head

Based on data from Aderhold, Roberts, 1991; Mahan, McKay, 1984.

*Ferguson's reflex. Pressure of presenting part on stretch receptors of pelvic floor stimulates release of oxytocin from posterior pituitary, resulting in more intense uterine contractions.

†Ring of fire. Burning sensation of acute pain as vagina stretches and fetal head crowns.

and multiparous women are commonly used to assess the progress of the second stage. A second stage of more than 2 hours in a first pregnancy and 1½ hours in subsequent pregnancies is considered abnormal and must be reported to a health care provider. Other factors that must be considered are the FHR pattern, the descent of the presenting part, the quality of the uterine contractions, and the fetal scalp blood pH (Mahan, McKay, 1984). On the basis of Friedman's data, the range and average duration of the second stage of labor vary with parity.*

Parity	Range (min)	Average (min)
First pregnancy	25 to 75	57
Subsequent pregnancy	13 to 17	14.4

*Duration of second stage may be prolonged for the woman who has had an epidural block, which causes loss of the bearing-down reflex.

Signs of Potential Problems

Prolonged second stage (see discussion above) is reported to the health care provider. Signs and symptoms of impending birth (Table 12-6) may appear unexpectedly, requiring immediate action by the nurse.

❖ NURSING DIAGNOSES

Nursing diagnoses lend direction to the nursing action needed to implement care. Before establishing diagnoses, the nurse analyzes the significance of the findings collected during assessment. The following are some nursing diagnoses indicating potential areas for concern during the second stage:

High risk for injury to mother and fetus related to
  • Persistent use of Valsalva's maneuver
Situational low self-esteem related to

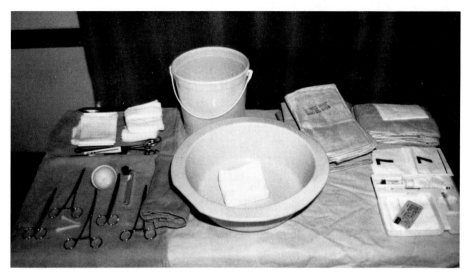

FIG. 12-17 Instrument Table.

- Knowledge deficit of normal, beneficial effects of vocalization during bearing-down efforts
- Inability to carry out birth plan for birth without medication

Ineffective individual coping related to
- Coaching that contradicts woman's physiologic urge to push

Pain related to
- Bearing-down efforts and distention of the perineum

Anxiety related to
- Inability to control defecation with bearing-down efforts

Anxiety related to knowledge deficit regarding
- Inexperience with reasons for perineal sensation

High risk for injury to mother related to
- Inappropriate positioning of mother's legs in stirrups

Situational low-self-esteem of father related to
- Inability to support mother in final stage of labor

❖ EXPECTED OUTCOMES

Planning for the second and third stages of labor done during the first stage. Previously determined expected outcomes may be modified as these stages progress.

Expected outcomes for the woman in the second stage of labor may include that the woman will:
1. Actively participate in the labor process
2. Sustain no injury during the labor process (nor will the fetus)
3. Obtain comfort and support from family members

❖ COLLABORATIVE CARE

The nurse implements plans to monitor constantly the events of the second stage and mechanism of birth, ma-ternal physiologic and emotional responses to the second stage, the partner's response to the second stage, and fetal response to the stress of the second stage.

The nurse continues to provide comfort measures for the mother such as positioning, mouth care, maintaining clean, dry bedding, and avoiding extraneous noise, conversation, or other distractions (e.g., laughing, talking of attending personnel in or outside the labor area). The woman is encouraged to indicate other support measures she would like.

If the mother is to be transferred to another area for birth, the nurse makes the transfer early enough to avoid rushing the patient. The birth area also is readied for the birth.

Prebirth Considerations

Supplies, Instruments, and Equipment

To prepare for birth in any setting, the birthing table or case cart is usually set up during the transition phase for nulliparous women and during the active phase for multiparous women.

The birthing table is prepared, and instruments are arranged on the instrument table (Fig. 12-17). Standard procedures are followed for gloving, identifying and opening sterile packages, adding sterile supplies to the instrument table, and unwrapping and handing sterile instruments to the health care provider. The crib and equipment are readied for the support and stabilization of the infant (Fig. 12-18).

The following are suggestions for preparation for birth. These items may vary among different facilities, therefore the protocols from each facility's procedure manual should be consulted.
1. Scrubbing facilities, scrub brushes, cuticle sticks, cleaning agent, and masks with shield or protective glasses/goggles are available.

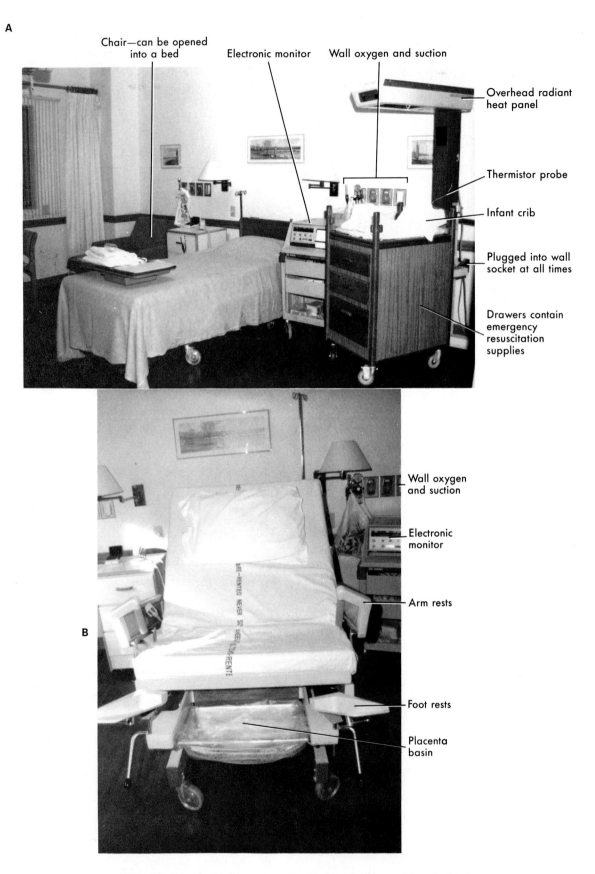

FIG. 12-18 **A,** Birthing room. **B,** Birthing bed in position for birth.

2. The following tasks have been done:
   a. Sterile gowns and gloves for the health care provider, sterile drapes and towels for draping the woman, and sterile instruments and other supplies (such as bulb syringes, sutures, and anesthetic solutions) are arranged on a sterile table for convenient use.
   b. Sterile basin and water for hand washing during birthing process are readied for use.
   c. Supplies for cleansing vulva are available (sterile basin, sterile water, and cleaning solution).
   d. Birth area is warmed and free of drafts.
   e. Infant identification materials have been readied.
   f. Infant receiving blankets and heated crib are readied. Material for prophylactic care of infant's eyes and vitamin K injection are available (see p. 393-394).
3. Equipment is in working order; birthing table (bed or chair), overhead lights, and mirror.
4. Emergency equipment, anesthesia, laryngoscope, and supplies are available and in working order if needed for emergency situations such as control of maternal hemorrhage or fetal respiratory distress.
5. Additional supplies (anesthetics, oxytocics for injection, and obstetric forceps) are available.
6. Woman's record is up-to-date and ready for use in birth area. In areas such as the labor unit, recordings are made as symptoms are noted, assessments are made, and care is given. It is imperative to have recordings complete at all times.

Maternal Position

The woman may want to assume various positions such as squatting (Scherer, 1989; Gardosi, Sylvester, Lynch, 1989; Andrews, Chrzanowski, 1990; McKay, Roberts, 1990). For this position a firm surface is required, and the woman will need side support. In a birthing bed a squat bar is available to assist (Fig. 12-19). Another position is the side-lying position with the upper part of the leg held by the nurse or coach or placed on a pillow. Some women prefer Fowler's position (can be attained with the support of a wedged pillow or with the father/partner supporting the woman). Others prefer the hands-and-knees or standing position when bearing down. When a woman is in the standing position, with weight being borne on both femoral heads, the pressure in the acetabulum will increase the transverse diameter of the pelvic outlet by up to 1 cm. This can be helpful if descent of the head is delayed as a result of failure of the occiput to rotate from the lateral (transverse diameter of pelvis) to the anterior position (Liu, 1989). The woman also may want to sit on the toilet to push because many women are concerned about stool incontinence during this stage. These women must be closely monitored and removed from the toilet before birth becomes imminent.

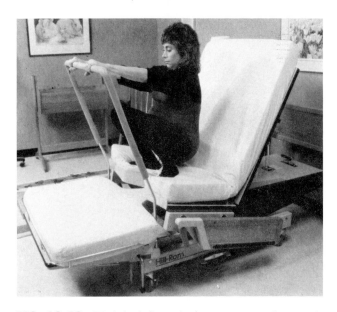

FIG. 12-19 Birth bed for a single-room maternity care in labor, delivery, recovery, and postpartum room (LDRP) (Courtesy The Borning Corp, Spokane, WA.)

Birthing Beds and Chairs

The birthing bed (Fig. 12-20) changes shape according to the mother's needs. The woman can squat, kneel, recline, or sit, choosing the position most comfortable for her. At the same time, there is excellent exposure for examination, electrode placement, fetal scalp sampling, and birth. Birthing chairs also may be used and may provide women with a better physiologic position during childbirth, although some women feel restricted by a chair. Potentially there is both a physiologic and psychologic advantage to the upright position. The mother can see the birth as it occurs and also maintain *en face* contact with the attendant. Most chairs are designed so that if an emergency occurs, the chair can be adjusted to the horizontal or the Trendelenburg position. Some evidence is offered for a higher incidence of postpartum hemorrhage when a chair is used. Birthing stools can also be used (Waldenstrom, Gottvall, 1991).

Bearing-Down Efforts

As the fetal head reaches the pelvic floor, most women experience the urge to push. Automatically the woman will begin to exert downward pressure by contracting her abdominal muscles while relaxing her pelvic floor. This **bearing down** is an involuntary reflex response to the pressure of the presenting part on stretch receptors of pelvic musculature. A strong expiratory grunt may accompany the push (McKay, Roberts, 1990). When coaching women to push, the nurse encourages them to push as *they* feel like pushing, rather than giving a prolonged push on command (Thompson, 1993). The nurse monitors the woman's breathing so that the woman does not hold her breath more than 5 seconds

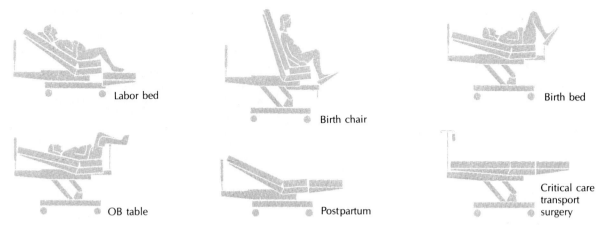

FIG. 12-20 The versatility of today's birthing bed makes it practical in a variety of settings. (Courtesy Hill-Rom.)

at a time. Prolonged breath-holding may trigger **Valsalva's maneuver,** which results from the woman's closing the glottis, thereby increasing intrathoracic and cardiovascular pressure (Metzer, Therrien, 1990). In addition, holding the breath for more than 5 seconds diminishes the perfusion of oxygen across the placenta and results in fetal hypoxia. The nurse reminds the woman to take deep breaths to refill her lungs after each contraction.

To ensure slow birth of the fetal head, the nurse encourages the woman to control her urge to push. The urge to push is controlled by coaching the woman to take panting breaths or to exhale slowly through pursed lips as the baby's head crowns. The woman needs simple, clear directions from *one* coach.

Amnesia between contractions often is pronounced in the second stage, and the woman may have to be roused to cooperate in the bearing-down process.

Fetal Heart Rate

FHR must be checked as noted previously. If the rate begins to drop or if there is a loss of variability, prompt treatment must be initiated. The woman can be turned on her side to reduce the pressure of the uterus against the ascending vena cava and descending aorta (see Fig. 12-8), and oxygen can be administered by mask at 10 to 12 L/min. This is often all that is required to restore the normal rate. If the FHR does not return to normal immediately, the health care provider should be quickly notified because medical intervention to hasten the birth may be necessary.

Support of the Father/Coach

During the second stage the woman needs continuous support and coaching. Since the coaching process can be physically and emotionally tiring for the father/coach (Jordan, 1990; Malestic, 1990; Queenan, 1990), the nurse can offer nourishment, fluids, and short breaks. The support person who attends the birth in a delivery

room follows instructions as to donning a cover gown or scrub suit, mask, hat, and shoe covers. Other information includes specifying support measures for the laboring woman and pointing out areas of the room in which the partner can move freely. If birth occurs in a labor, delivery, recovery room (LDR) or a labor, delivery, recovery, postpartum room (LDRP), the partner usually can remain in street clothes.

Partners are encouraged to be present at the birth of their infants, if this is in keeping with their cultural expectations. The psychologic closeness of the family unit is maintained, and the partner can continue the supportive care given in labor. The mother and her partner need an equal opportunity to initiate the attachment process with the baby.

Birth in a Delivery Room or Birthing Room

If the woman must move from the labor bed to the delivery table, she will need assistance. If this is done between contractions, the mother can help, but because of her awkwardness, she cannot be rushed.

The position assumed for birth may be *Sims' position* (if this is the case, the attendant will need to support the upper part of the leg), dorsal position, or lithotomy position.

The **lithotomy position** is the position most commonly used for birth in Western cultures, although this is changing slowly. The lithotomy position makes it more convenient for the health care provider to deal with any complications that arise (Fig. 12-20). The buttocks are brought to the edge of the table, and the legs are placed in stirrups. Care must be taken to pad the stirrups, raise and place both legs simultaneously, and adjust the shanks of the stirrups so that the calves of the legs are supported. There should be no pressure on the popliteal space. If the stirrups are not the same height, strained ligaments can develop in the woman's back as she bears down. This

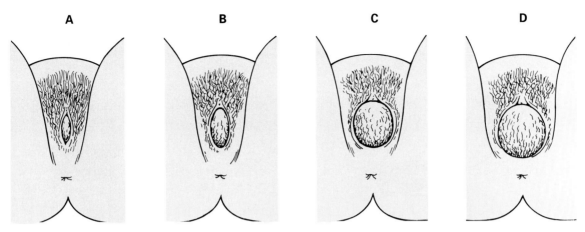

FIG. 12-21   Beginning birth with vertex presenting. **A,** Anteroposterior slit. **B,** Oval opening. **C,** Circular shape. **D,** Crowning.

strain causes considerable discomfort in the postbirth period. The lower portion of the table may be dropped down and rolled back under the table.

Positions for birth in an LDR or LDRP vary from that of lithotomy with legs in stirrups, feet resting on foot rests, squat bar, or a side-lying position with legs propped up on a squat bar. The foot of the bed can be removed. This is done when the health care provider assisting with the birth specifies the need for better perineal access in order to perform episiotomy (p. 302). Otherwise the foot of the bed is left in place and lowered slightly to form a ledge providing access for birth and a place to set the newborn infant.

Once the woman is positioned for birth, the vulva is washed thoroughly with soap and water or sprayed with disinfectant to prevent bacterial contamination. The health care provider puts on a cap and mask that has a shield or protective eyewear, and shoe covers. Nurses attending the birth may also need to wear protective eyewear, gowns, and gloves. Then the mother may be draped with sterile towels and sheets.

The circulating nurse continues to coach and encourage the woman. The nurse auscultates FHR every 5 to 15 minutes or continues electronic monitoring, and notifies the health care provider as to the rate and regularity. The equipment for taking the blood pressure should be readied for instant use if signs of shock develop. As the woman pushes, BP readings will be distorted (increased) by the increase in thoracic and abdominal pressures. A reading will be taken after birth before transferring the woman to the recovery room. An oxytocic medication such as Pitocin may be prepared for administration after delivery of the placenta. The nurse records all observations and procedures on the woman's chart.

Contact with parents is maintained by touch, verbal comforting, instructions as to reasons for care, and sharing in the parents' joy at the birth of their child. The

nurse notes and records the time of birth (i.e., when the infant is born completely).

Mechanism of Birth: Vertex Presentation

Most of the time the birth remains in the hands of the obstetrician or certified nurse-midwife. The time may come, however, when the nurse must assist the woman to give birth (p. 300). The nurse's knowledge of the birth process provides a basis for patient preparation before and during birth.

The nurse reviews with the woman or couple the cardinal movements of labor. Once the cervix is fully dilated, descent occurs. The vertex advances with each contraction and recedes slightly as the contraction wanes; descent is constant, and late in the second stage the head reaches the pelvic floor. *Bulging of the perineum* occurs during the *descent phase,* when the fetal presenting part is distending the perineum but is not yet visible at the introitus. The occiput generally rotates anteriorly, and with voluntary bearing-down efforts, the head appears at the introitus (Fig. 12-21 and Plate 1, *A-C*). Although more and more head may be seen with each push, **crowning** occurs when the head's widest part (the biparietal diameter) distends the vulva just before birth (Plate 1, *D*). Immediately before birth, the perineal musculature becomes greatly distended. If an **episiotomy** is necessary, it is done at this time to minimize soft tissue damage (p. 302). The head is born by extension and after birth restitutes with the shoulders (Plate 1, *E*). Interiorly the shoulders rotate into the anteroposterior diameter of the pelvis; external rotation of the head is observed. The body is born by lateral flexion.

The three phases of a spontaneous birth of the fetus in a vertex presentation are (1) birth of the head, (2) birth of the shoulders, and (3) birth of the body and extremities.

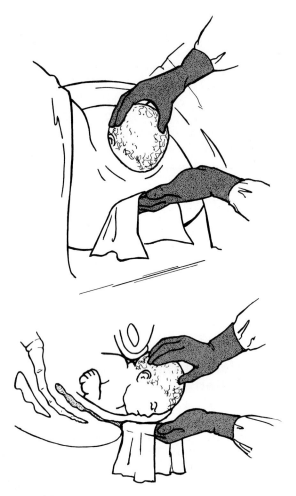

FIG. 12-22 Birth of head by modified Ritgen maneuver. Note control to prevent rapid birth of head.

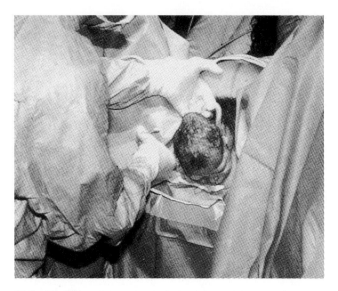

FIG. 12-23 Loosening nuchal cord (umbilical cord around neck). (Courtesy Marjorie Pyle, RNC, *Lifecircle*, Costa Mesa, CA.)

Birth of Head

The vertex first appears, followed by the forehead, face, chin, and neck. The speed of the birth of the head must be controlled, because sudden birth of the head may cause severe lacerations through the anal sphincter or even into the mother's rectum. The health care provider controls the birth of the head by (1) applying pressure against the rectum, drawing it downward to aid in flexing the head as the back of the neck catches under the symphysis pubis; (2) then applying upward pressure from the coccygeal region (modified **Ritgen maneuver;** Fig. 12-22 and Plates 1, *C and D*) to extend the head during the actual birth, thereby protecting the musculature of the perineum; and (3) assisting the mother with voluntary control of the bearing-down efforts by coaching her to pant. In addition to protecting the maternal tissues, gradual birth is imperative to prevent fetal intracranial injury.

The membranes may not be ruptured before birth. During birth of the head these membranes look like a hood covering the head. This hood of intact amniotic membranes covering the head during birth is known as

a **caul.** In Scotland a child born with a caul is thought to be gifted with "second sight."

The umbilical cord often encircles the neck (**nuchal cord**), but rarely so tightly as to cause hypoxia. The health care provider should slip the cord gently over the head (Fig. 12-23). If the loop is tight, or if there is a second loop, then the cord is clamped twice, severed between the clamps, and unwound from around the neck before the birth continues. Mucus, blood, or meconium in the nasal or oral passages may prevent the newborn from breathing. Moist gauze sponges are used to wipe the nose and mouth. A bulb syringe is inserted into the mouth and oropharynx to aspirate contents (Plate 1, *F*). Next, the nares are cleared while supporting the head.

During labor, if meconium has been present in the amniotic fluid, a DeLee suction apparatus is placed on the sterile field and wall suction is prepared. Thus when the health care provider prepares for birth of the head, the DeLee device is connected to the suction tubing. The health care provider should refrain from using the DeLee device and oral suction to withdraw fluid from the infant unless the suction device isolates the mucus from the user's airway (see Fig. 14-5, p. 371). Perinatal infections most often are transmitted through contact with body fluids. Thus it is important for any health care worker to wear gloves when coming in contact with body fluids from the woman giving birth or when touching her baby.

Birth of Shoulders

Before the shoulders can be born, they must engage in the pelvic inlet. Internal rotation of the shoulders occurs, accompanied by restitution and external rotation of the head, and the shoulders now lie in the anteroposterior diameter of the inlet (see also Fig. 9-13, *E* and *F*). The shoulders can now pass through the pelvic cavity.

The head is drawn downward and backward by the health care provider to help the anterior shoulder impinge beneath the arch of the symphysis and slide beneath the pubic arch. Normally the anterior shoulder is delivered with this slight downward traction toward the perineum. The posterior shoulder distends the perineum, and to prevent perineal trauma the head is lifted toward the symphysis pubis, resulting in the birth of the shoulder over the perineum (Myles, 1989; Plate 1, *G*).

Use of Fundal Pressure. The increased use of alternative positions for pushing has decreased the use of fundal pressure. Alternative positioning assists in fetal descent. In some cases in which regional or conduction anesthesia (epidural) is used, fundal pressure may be needed because of decreased maternal expulsive power. If fundal pressure is needed, a *skilled* nurse in collaboration with the health care provider, performs the procedure. Fundal pressure is used most often when there is slight shoulder dystocia (Kline-Kaye, Miller-Slade, 1990).

Birth of Body and Extremities

Expulsion is controlled so that it occurs slowly. As lateral flexion is continued, the health care provider's lower hand supports the weight of the baby, in order to prevent perineal trauma. Slight rotation of the body to the right or left may be used to facilitate the birth. The time of birth is the precise time when the entire body is out of the mother.

The cord may be clamped at this time, and the health care provider may ask if the woman's partner would like to cut the cord (Plate 1, *J*). If so, the health care provider provides a clean pair of scissors and gives instructions to cut the cord 1 inch above the clamp.

Siblings during the Second Stage

A young child may become frightened by the intensity of the second stage. Sights such as rupture of the membranes and sounds such as their mother's moans, screams, and grunts can be unsettling. It is not uncommon for a woman to say things during the second stage and birth that she would not say otherwise and that might scare her child, for example "I can't take any more, take this baby out of me" or "This pain is killing me. I'm going to die." The child present during birth needs someone to be close and give explanations in a simple and calm manner. The child may want to be held.

Hospitals are now more supportive of siblings' participation in the birth experience than in previous years. Organized sibling preparation classes now provide orientation to the birth environment and is required for a sibling to attend the birth. Although the set age limits

vary, most hospitals will not allow children younger than 3 years old to attend the birth. Many hospitals deal with sibling attendance on an individual basis, taking into consideration the child's age, maturity, and preparation. Long-term effects on young children witnessing birth are not yet known.

An alternative to sibling presence at birth is for a trusted person to remain with the child in the waiting area until after the birth. At that time the child can be brought into the room and see the baby being held by the mother, who has become her "normal" self again.

Emergency Childbirth

Even under the best of circumstances there probably will come a time when the perinatal nurse will be required to assist with the birth of an infant without medical assistance. Consider the multiparous woman who arrives at the community hospital fully dilated in the middle of the night. Since it is impossible to prevent an impending birth, the perinatal nurse needs to be able to function independently and be skilled in safe birth of a vertex fetus (Box 12-2).

✤ EVALUATION

Evaluation of outcomes is an ongoing activity. During each encounter with the woman and her family during the second stage of labor the nurse evaluates the degree to which the expected outcomes are being met. For example, the woman has actively participated in the labor process, neither she nor her fetus has sustained any injury during the labor process, and she has been able to obtain comfort and support from family members of choice. If the evaluation shows that results fall short of achieving an expected outcome, further assessment and collaborative care are warranted.

THIRD STAGE OF LABOR

The third stage of labor lasts from the birth of the baby until the birth of the placenta. The goal in the management of the third stage of labor is the prompt separation and expulsion of the placenta, achieved in the easiest, safest manner.

The placenta is attached to the decidual layer of the basal plate's thin endometrium by numerous, randomized, fibrous anchor villi—much like a postage stamp is attached to a sheet of postage stamps. After the birth of the fetus, in the presence of strong uterine contractions, the placental site becomes noticeably smaller. This reduced size causes the anchor villi to break and the placenta to separate from its attachments. Normally the first few strong contractions, 5 to 7 minutes after the baby's birth, shear the placenta from the basal plate. A placenta does not easily detach itself from a flaccid (relaxed)

BOX 12-2

Guidelines for Assistance for an Emergency Birth of a Fetus in the Vertex Position

1. The woman usually assumes the position most comfortable for her.
2. Reassure the woman verbally. Use eye-to-eye contact and a calm, relaxed manner. If there is someone else available (e.g., the partner), that person could help support the woman in position, assist with coaching, and compliment her efforts.
3. Wash your hands and put gloves on, if possible.
4. Place under woman's buttocks whatever clean material is available.
5. Avoid touching the vaginal area to decrease the possibility of infection.
6. As the head begins to crown, the birth attendant should do the following:
   a. Tear the amniotic membrane (caul) if it is still intact.
   b. Instruct the woman to pant or pant-blow, thus avoiding the urge to push.
   c. Place the flat side of the hand on the exposed fetal head and apply *gentle* pressure toward the vagina to prevent the head from "popping out." NOTE: Rapid birth of the fetal head must be prevented because a rapid change of pressure within the molded fetal skull follows, which may result in dural or subdural tears, and may cause vaginal or perineal lacerations.
7. After the birth of the head, check for an umbilical cord. If the cord is around the neck, try to slip it over the baby's head or pull *gently* to get some slack so that it can slip over the shoulders.
8. Support the fetal head as restitution (external rotation) occurs. After restitution, with one hand on each side of the baby's head, exert *gentle* pressure downward so that the anterior shoulder emerges under the symphysis pubis and acts as a fulcrum; then as *gentle* pressure is exerted in the opposite direction, the posterior shoulder, which has passed over the sacrum and coccyx, emerges.
9. Be alert! Hold the baby securely because the rest of the body may emerge quickly. The baby will be slippery!
10. Cradle the baby's head and back in one hand and the buttocks in the other. Keeping the head down to drain away the mucus (Plate 1, *I*). Use a bulb syringe to remove mucus if one is available.
11. Dry the baby rapidly to prevent rapid heat loss. Keep the baby at the same level as the mother's uterus until the end of the cord stops pulsating. NOTE: Keep the baby at the same level to prevent gravity flow of baby's blood to or from the placenta and the resultant hypovolemia or hypervolemia. Also, do not "milk" the cord.
12. Place the baby on the mother's abdomen, cover the baby (remember to keep the head warm too) with the mother's clothing, and have her cuddle the baby. Compliment her (them) on a job well done, and on the baby, if appropriate.

13. *Wait* for the placenta to separate; *do not* tug on the cord.
    NOTE: Injudicious traction may tear the cord, separate the placenta, or invert the uterus. Signs of placental separation include a slight gush of dark blood from the introitus, lengthening of the cord, and change in uterine contour from discoid to globular shape.
14. Instruct the mother to push in order to deliver the separated placenta. Gently ease out the placental membranes using an up-and-down motion until they are removed. If birth occurs outside the hospital setting, to minimize complications, do not cut the cord without proper clamps and a sterile cutting tool. Inspect the placenta for intactness. Place the baby on the placenta and wrap the two together for additional warmth.
15. Check the firmness of the uterus. Gently massage the uterus and demonstrate to the mother how she can massage her own uterus properly.
16. If supplies are available, clean the mother's perineal area and apply a peripad.
17. In addition to gentle massage, the following measures can be taken to prevent or minimize hemorrhage:
    a. The baby can be put to the breast as soon as possible (Plate 1, *L*). Sucking or nuzzling and licking the breast stimulates the release of oxytocin from the posterior pituitary.
    NOTE: If the baby does not or cannot nurse, manually stimulate the mother's breasts.
    b. Expel any clots from the mother's uterus (see Procedures 12-3 on p. 307 and Fig. 12-28 on p. 308).
18. Comfort or reassure the mother and her family or friends. Keep the mother and the baby warm. Give her fluids if available and tolerated.
19. Make notations on the birth.
    a. Fetal presentation and position
    b. Presence of cord around neck (nuchal cord) or other parts and number of times cord encircles part
    c. Color, character, and amount of amniotic fluid, if rupture of membranes (ROM) occurs immediately before birth
    d. Time of birth
    e. Estimated time of Apgar score, resuscitation efforts, and ultimate condition of baby
    f. Sex of baby
    g. Time of placental expulsion, its appearance, and completeness
    h. Maternal condition: affect, amount of bleeding, and status of uterine tonicity
    i. Any unusual occurrences during the birth (i.e., maternal or paternal response, verbalizations, or gestures to birth or newborn)

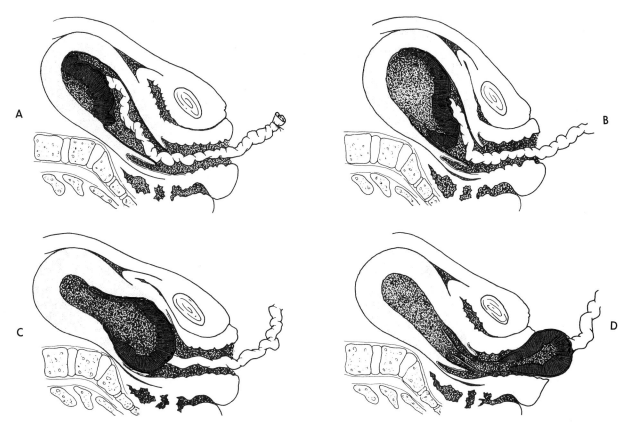

FIG. 12-24   Third stage of labor. **A,** Placenta begins the separating in central portion with retroplacental bleeding. Uterus changes from discoid to globular shape. **B,** Placenta completes separation and enters lower uterine segment. Uterus is globular in shape. **C,** Placenta enters vagina, cord is seen to lengthen, and there may be increase in bleeding. **D,** Expulsion (birth) of placenta and completion of third stage.

uterus because the placental site is not reduced in size.

Placental separation is indicated by the following signs (Fig. 12-24):

1. A firmly contracting fundus
2. A change in the uterus from a discoid to a globular ovoid shape, as the placenta moves to the lower segment
3. A sudden gush of dark blood from the introitus
4. Apparent lengthening of the umbilical cord as the placenta gets closer to the introitus
5. A vaginal fullness (the placenta) noted on vaginal or rectal examination, or fetal membranes seen at the introitus

Whether the placenta first appears by its shiny fetal surface (Schultze's mechanism) or turns to show its dark roughened maternal surface (Duncan's mechanism) is of no clinical importance. After the placenta and its membranes emerge, the nurse examines it for intactness to ensure that no portion remains in the uterine cavity (i.e., no retained fragments of the placenta or membranes).

Signs of Potential Problems

Even as the health care provider completes the birth of the placenta, the nurse observes the mother for signs of an altered level of consciousness (LOC) or alteration in respirations. Because of the rapid cardiovascular changes (e.g., the increased intracranial pressure during pushing and the rapid increase in cardiac output), this period represents the risk *of rupture of a preexisting cerebral aneurysm and of pulmonary emboli.* The risk of *pulmonary amniotic fluid emboli* arises from another source as well. As the placenta separates, there is a possibility of amniotic fluid entering the maternal circulation if the uterine musculature does not contract rapidly and well. The incidence of these possible complications is small; however, the alert nurse can contribute to their immediate recognition and promptly initiate therapy.

Nursing Considerations

To assist the mother in the birth of the placenta, the nurse or health care provider instructs the woman to push when signs of separation have occurred. If possible, the placenta should be expelled by maternal effort during a uterine contraction, but assistance such as *alternate compression* and *elevation of the fundus*, plus *minimum*, controlled traction on the umbilical cord may be used to facilitate the delivery of the placenta and membranes. If an oxytocic medication is ordered, the nurse administers the medication in the dosage and by the route indicated by the health care provider after the placenta has been expelled. When the third stage of labor is complete, and lacerations are repaired or an episiotomy is sutured, the vulvar area is gently cleansed with sterile water, and a sterile peripad is applied to the perineum.

The Family during the Third Stage

Most parents enjoy being able to handle, hold, explore, and examine the baby immediately after birth. Both parents can assist with the thorough drying of the infant. The infant may be wrapped in a receiving blanket and placed on the mother's abdomen. If skin-to-skin contact is desired, the unwrapped infant may be placed on the mother's abdomen and then covered with a warm blanket.

Holding the newborn next to her skin helps maintain the baby's body heat; care must be taken to keep the head warm as well. Stockinette caps are sometimes used to cover the newborn's head (Plate 1, *O*). It is the nurse's responsibility to make sure the infant stays warm and is in no danger of slipping from the parent's grasp.

Many women wish to begin breastfeeding their newborns at this time to take advantage of the infant's alert state (first period of reactivity) and to stimulate the production of oxytocin that promotes contraction (Plates 1, *L and O*) of the uterus. Others wish to wait until the newborn, parents, and older siblings are together in the recovery room.

While the health care provider carries out the postbirth vaginal examination (Plate 1, *K*), the mother usually feels discomfort. Therefore while the process is being completed, the nurse can assess the newborn's physical condition; the baby can be weighed and measured, wrapped in warm blankets, and then given to the partner to hold (Plate 1, *P*).

Parent-Newborn Relationships

The mother's reaction to the sight of her newborn may range from excited outbursts of laughing, talking, and even crying to apparent apathy. A polite smile and nod may acknowledge the comments of nurses and health care providers. Occasionally the reaction is one of anger or indifference; the mother turns away from the baby, concentrates on her own pain, and sometimes makes hostile comments. These varied reactions can arise from pleasure, exhaustion, or deep disappointment. Whatever the reaction and cause may be, the mother needs con-

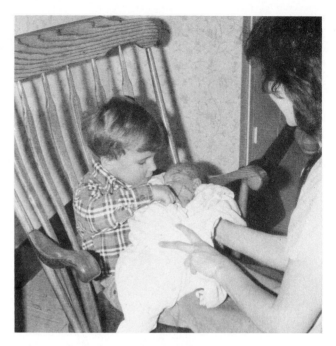

FIG. 12-25 Nurse helps big brother become acquainted with new baby sister.

tinuing acceptance and support from all staff. Notation regarding the parents' reaction to the newborn can be made in the recovery record. How do parents *look*? What do they *say*? What do they *do*?

Siblings, who may have appeared only remotely interested in the final phases of the second stage, tend to experience renewed interest and excitement and can be encouraged to hold the new family member (Fig. 12-25).

Parents are usually responsive to praise of their newborn. Many require reassurance that the dusky appearance of their baby's extremities immediately after birth is normal until circulation is well established (Plate 1, *I*). If appropriate, nurses should explain the reason for the molding of their newborn's head. Information about hospital routine can be communicated. Hospital staff members, by their interest and concern, can do much to make this a satisfying experience for parents, family, and significant others.

INTERRUPTION IN SKIN INTEGRITY RELATED TO CHILDBIRTH
Episiotomy

An **episiotomy** is an incision made in the perineum to enlarge the vaginal outlet. Episiotomies are performed more commonly in the United States and Canada than in Europe. The use of the side-lying position for birth is used routinely in Europe, whereas the position with legs

CLINICAL APPLICATION OF RESEARCH

MIDLINE EPISIOTOMY AND THE RISK OF THIRD-DEGREE AND FOURTH-DEGREE LACERATIONS

Researchers have found that midline episiotomies are associated with lacerations of the perineum and rectum. Even with mediolateral episiotomies, rectal lacerations can occur. Helwig and associates studied whether midline episiotomies and operative births (forceps or vacuum) influence the incidence of perineal trauma. Using a retrospective chart review, 392 operative vaginal births were examined. Variables considered included first vaginal births, fetal size, fetal heart rate abnormalities, meconium-stained fluid and shoulder dystocia. The researchers found that more third- and fourth-degree perineal lacerations occurred when an episiotomy was performed, the baby was over 3500 grams, or the birth was the first vaginal one. Episiotomies were more common when the infant weighed more than 3500 grams, when faculty (rather than residents) were attending the birth, when forceps were used, with epidural anesthesia, and with Asian mothers. In this setting, 11% of the women had operative vaginal births and 15% had episiotomies. Episiotomy is the most common operative procedure in the United States; the serious consequences of this procedure may not always be considered. In childbirth classes, nurses can inform expectant parents about indications for, and risks of, episiotomy and operative birth. Labor and birth nurses can work with mothers to push effectively during labor, thereby decreasing the need for operative birth. Parents can make more informed choices when selecting type of analgesia during labor, and they may opt for more discomfort in order to retain the ability to push effectively. In turn, this may decrease the need for episiotomy and operative births and also reduce the incidence of perineal trauma.

Reference: Helwig JT, Thorp JM, Bowes WA: Does midline episiotomy increase the risk of third- and fourth-degree lacerations in operative vaginal deliveries? *Obstetrics & Gynecology* 82:276, 1993.

---

in stirrups is more commonly used in the United States and Canada. With the side-lying position there is less tension on the perineum and a gradual stretching of the perineum is possible. As a result the indications for use of episiotomies are fewer.

The proponents for using the episiotomy say it serves the following purposes:

1. Prevents tearing of the perineum. The clean and properly placed incision heals more properly than does a ragged tear. Some conditions that predispose a woman to perineal tearing and are, therefore, indications for episiotomy are a large infant, rapid labor in which there is not sufficient time for stretching of the perineum to take place, a narrow subpubic arch with a constricted outlet, and malpresentations of the fetus (e.g., the face).

2. Possibly minimizes prolonged and severe stretching of the muscles supporting the bladder or rectum, which may later lead to stress incontinence or to vaginal prolapse.

3. Reduces duration of the second stage, which may be important for maternal reasons (e.g., a hypertensive state) or fetal reasons (e.g., persistent bradycardia).

4. Enlarges the vagina in case manipulation is needed for the infant's birth, for example, in a breech presentation or for application of forceps (see Clinical Application of Research).

Those opposed to the *routine* use of episiotomies maintain the following:

1. The perineum can be prepared for birth through use of the Kegel exercises and massage in the prenatal period. Use of Kegel exercises in the postpartum period improves and restores the tone of the perineal muscles.

2. Lacerations may occur even with the use of an episiotomy.

3. Pain and discomfort from episiotomies can interfere with mother-infant interactions and the reestablishment of parental sexual intercourse.

4. Episiotomies *are indicated* (a) if the well-being of the mother or fetus is in jeopardy, to shorten the second stage of labor, (b) if the infant is preterm and cerebral hemorrhage is a possibility because of capillary fragility, (c) if the infant is large (more than 4000 g [9 lb]), or (d) in most forceps and breech births (Pernoll, Benson, 1987).

The type of episiotomy is designated by site and direction of the incision (Fig. 12-26).

Midline episiotomy is most commonly used. It is effective, easily repaired, and generally the least painful. Occasionally there may be an extension through the rectal sphincter (third-degree laceration) or even into the anal canal (fourth-degree laceration). Fortunately primary healing and a good repair usually lead to restored sphincter tone.

Mediolateral episiotomy is employed in operative birth when posterior extension is likely. Although a fourth-degree laceration may thus be avoided, a third-degree laceration may occur. Moreover, as compared with a mid-

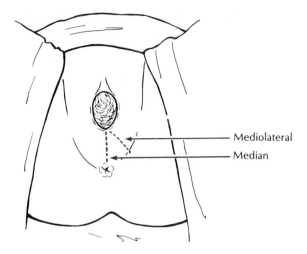

Mediolateral
Median

FIG. 12-26 Types of episiotomies.

line episiotomy, blood loss is greater and repair is more difficult and painful.

Lacerations

Most acute injuries and laceration of the perineum, vagina, uterus, and their support tissues occur during childbirth, and their management is an obstetric problem. Some injuries to the supporting tissues, whether they were acute or nonacute and whether they were repaired or not, may become gynecologic problems later in life.

The soft tissues of the birth canal and adjacent structures suffer some damage during every birth. Damage usually is more pronounced in nulliparous women because the tissues are firmer and more resistant than in multiparous women. Perineal skin and vaginal mucosa may appear intact, obscuring numerous small lacerations in underlying muscle and its fascia. Damage to pelvic supports usually is readily apparent and repaired after birth.

The individual woman's tendency to sustain lacerations varies; that is, the soft tissue in some women may be less capable of distention. Heredity may be a factor. For example, the tissue of very light-skinned women, especially those with reddish hair, is not as readily distensible as that of a darker-skinned woman. Women whose tissues show a tendency to lacerate also may have varicose veins and diastasis recti abdominis. In addition, healing may occur less efficiently in these women.

Immediate repair promotes healing and limits residual damage, as well as decreases the possibility of infection. Immediately after every birth the cervix, vagina, and perineum are inspected. During the early postpartum days, the nurse and health care provider carefully inspect the perineum and evaluate lochia and symptoms to identify any previously missed damage.

Perineal Lacerations

Perineal lacerations usually occur as the fetal head is being born. The extent of the laceration is defined on the basis of depth:

1. *First-degree.* Laceration extends through the skin and structures superficial to muscles.
2. *Second-degree.* Laceration extends through muscles of perineal body.
3. *Third-degree.* Laceration continues through anal sphincter muscle.
4. *Fourth-degree.* Laceration also involves the anterior rectal wall.

Immediate repair with absorbable suture is necessary. Third- and fourth-degree lacerations require special attention so that the woman retains fecal continence. The woman's comfort increases and healing is promoted by measures taken to ensure soft stools for a few days. Antimicrobial therapy may be used in some cases.

Vaginal Lacerations

Vaginal lacerations often accompany perineal lacerations. Vaginal lacerations tend to extend up the lateral walls (sulci) and, if deep enough, involve the levator ani. Additional injury may occur high in the vaginal vault near the level of the ischial spines. Vaginal vault lacerations may result from forceps rotation, rapid fetal descent, and precipitous birth (Wheeler, 1991).

The location of lacerations and the rapid and profuse bleeding make it difficult to expose and repair these types of tears.

Cervical Injuries

Cervical injuries may occur when the cervix retracts over the advancing fetal head. Obstetrically acquired *cervical lacerations* occur at the lateral angles of the external os; most are shallow and bleeding is minimal. More extensive lacerations may extend to the vaginal vault or beyond the vault into the lower uterine segment; serious bleeding may occur. Extensive lacerations may follow hasty attempts to enlarge the cervical opening artificially or to deliver the fetus before full cervical dilatation is achieved.

FOURTH STAGE OF LABOR

The fourth stage of labor, the stage of recovery, is a critical period for the mother and newborn. They not only are recovering from the physical process of birth but also are initiating new relationships.

During the first 2 hours after the birth, maternal organs undergo their initial readjustment to the nonpregnant state, and body systems begin to stabilize. For several hours the newborn continues the transition from intrauterine to extrauterine existence. Many parents choose early discharge from the hospital; others must leave because of diagnosis-related group (DRG) and insurance requirements. The health care team must be reasonably assured that no potential for disruption in these normal processes for the mother or newborn exists. The nurse's skills can make a critical difference during the fourth stage (see Chapter 14 for newborn care).

Care Management

✤ ASSESSMENT

If the nurse has not previously cared for the new mother, assessment begins with review of the prenatal and labor record. In many institutions the labor nurse now follows the woman through the initial 2 hours after birth. Of primary importance are conditions that could predispose the mother to hemorrhage (such as precipitous labor, large baby, grand multiparity, or induced labor), which is a potential danger during the fourth stage of labor.

To help the nurse provide comprehensive care, a worksheet or recovery record is suggested (Fig. 12-27). During the first hour in the recovery room, physical assessment of the mother is frequent. All factors except temperature are assessed every 15 minutes for 1 hour. After the fourth 15-minute assessment, if all parameters have stabilized within the normal range, assessment is repeated two more times at 30-minute intervals. The physical assessment of the mother during the fourth stage of labor is given in Procedure 12-3. The area of examination and purpose, the method of assessment, and findings within normal limits are discussed briefly.

Signs of Potential Problems

Because hemorrhage is a significant potential complication, it is discussed extensively. The nurse must always be alert for potential complications including hypertensive states, infections, endocrine disorders, psychosocial disorders, and loss and grief (see Related Topics).

✤ NURSING DIAGNOSES

Nursing diagnoses lend direction to the type of nursing action needed to implement a plan of care. Before establishing nursing diagnoses, the nurse analyzes the significance of findings collected during assessment. Examples of nursing diagnoses include the following:

High risk for fluid volume deficit (hemorrhage) related to
  • Uterine atony after childbirth
Urinary retention related to
  • Effects of labor/birth on urinary tract sensation
Pain related to
  • Interruption in skin integrity secondary to the process of childbirth

High risk for injury related to
  • Early ambulation
High risk for altered parenting related to
  • Postpartum pain or fatigue
  • Disappointment in sex or appearance of newborn
Altered family processes related to
  • Addition of new member
Ineffective breastfeeding related to
  • Lack of experience

✤ EXPECTED OUTCOMES

During the planning step, *expected outcomes* are set in patient-centered terms and prioritized. Expected outcomes for the fourth stage of labor may include that the woman will:

1. Saturate no more than one pad per hour
2. Void spontaneously in amounts greater than 300 ml within 6 to 8 hours after birth
3. Verbalize acceptance of labor process after expressing concerns
4. Exhibit initial bonding/attachment behaviors with infant
5. Verbalize increased comfort after initiation of comfort measures

✤ COLLABORATIVE CARE

During the fourth stage of labor, the nurse must organize care to include observation of vital signs, provision of comfort measures, education of the mother, and care of the infant. Nursing concerns include prevention of hemorrhage, prevention of urinary bladder distention, maintenance of comfort, maintenance of cleanliness, maintenance of fluid balance and nutrition, support of parental emotional needs, and promotion of maternal and infant care education.

During the fourth stage of labor, the nurse uses every opportunity to teach the new mother. Regardless of parity, new mothers can benefit from explanations for the various nursing actions during the immediate postpartum period. Teaching is correlated with goals, assessment findings, nursing actions, and evaluation.

Prevention of Hemorrhage

Assessments are designed for early identification of events that may lead to **hemorrhage.** Postpartum hemorrhage is considered to be the loss of 500 ml of blood or more within the first 24 hours after birth. The mother's temperature, pulse, and blood pressure (BP) are assessed and recorded and should be within normal limits. The pulse rate will generally be between 60 and 70 beats/min. If the pulse rate is more than 90 beats/min, investigation and continued supervision are necessary. The temperature may be below normal because of

DELIVERY/RECOVERY RECORD

[ ] SVD   [ ] VACUUM   [ ] FORCEPS outlet low mid   [ ] ROTATIONS _____

[ ] Cesarean   [ ] low cervical/transverse   [ ] classical   [ ] primary   [ ] repeat X

Indications for Operative Delivery: _____   CATH IN DR ____ cc @ _____

Pres: [ ] Vtx   [ ] Breech [ ] Other _____ Rom _____ hrs.[ ] Mec. _____ [ ] Elevated maternal temp _____ F @ _____

Episiotomy: [ ] midline [ ] mediolateral [ ] episoproctotomy [ ] lacerations (type + grade) _____ [ ] Repaired

Type & Rh ____ EBL [ ] Aver. [ ] ____ cc [ ] Transfusion _____ (amt.) [ ] Type: ____

Anesthesia: [ ] local [ ] pudendal [ ] epidural [ ] spinal [ ] general

Physician: _____   Anesthesia: _____

Assistant: _____   Pediatrician: _____

Nurse(s): _____   Others: _____

MEDICATIONS IV# _____

In Labor	In Delivery
☐ Demerol ____ mg IV/IM @ ___	☐ Pitocin ___ units @ ___
☐ ____	☐ IV in ___ cc/ IM ☐
☐ Stadol ____ mg IV/IM @ ___	☐ ____ mg IV/IM @ ___
☐ ____ mg IV/IM @ ___	☐ ____ mg IV/IM @ ___

INFANT

DATE: _____ TIME: _____ SEX: [ ] male [ ] female [ ] alive [ ] stillborn [ ] multiple _____

WEIGHT: ____ lbs. ____ oz. ____ ____ gm Electrode [ ] removed intact [ ] Cord blood to lab

CORD: [ ] 3 vessels [ ] nuchal X ____ [ ] abnormalities _____ MR# _____

[ ] Voided [ ] Meconium [ ] Resuscitated _____ I.D. band# _____

APGAR	0	1	2	1'	5'
Heart rate	Absent	<100	>100		
Resp Effort	Absent	Slow Irreg.	Good Cry		
Reflex Irrit	None	Grimace	Cry		
Tone	Limp	Some Flexion	Active Motion		
Color	Blue	Blue Extreme.	Pink		

Scored By: _____

KEY:
V=Void
S=Stool E=Emesis
LOCHIA:
Sm=Small
Mod=Moderate
Lg=Large
PERINEUM:
Cl=Clear
RI=Repair intact
Sw=Swollen
I=Ice applied
UTERUS:
FF=Fundus firm
B=Boggy
MF=Massaged firm
@ U=at umbilicus
1/u = 1 finger above
u/1 = 1 finger below
the umbilicus

NEWBORN   POST-DELIVERY ASSESSMENT   MATERNAL

NEWBORN							MATERNAL
Time							Time
Temp							Temp
Pulse							Pulse
Resp.							Resp.
Br. Fd.							I & O
RN Initial							BP
Latch-on good = L+ Nutritive Sucking = N+							Uterus
Comments:							Perineum
							Lochia
							Meds Dose Route
RN Init/Signature							R.N. Initital
RN Init/Signature							

RESUSCITATION

[ ] bulb syringe

[ ] gastric aspir./amt ____ cc
     color _____

Intubated X _____

[ ] Cords Clear [ ] Mec below

[ ] Suctioned amt. ____ cc
     color _____

[ ] Free-flow Oxygen ____ %

[ ] mask [ ] tube for ____ min.

[ ] Pos. pressure ventilation:
     # ____ ETT [ ] bag & mask.

Resus. by _____

NEWBORN ASSESSMENT RECORD

Admission date and time: _____   Admission weight: _____ lbs. _____ oz. _____ gms.

Length ____ in. ____ cm. Vital Signs ____ temp ☐ Axillary ☐ Rectal   **Admission Meds**

Head ____ in. ____ cm.   BP ____ pulse (AP) ____ resp.   Vit. K in L/R anterior thigh @ ____ by ____

Chest ____ in. ____ cm. BLD. GLUC. ____ @ ____ by ____   Eye prophylaxis OU @ ____ by ____

Abd. ____ in. ____ cm. ☐ Chemstrip ☐ Accucheck ☐ D-stix   Agent: ☐ Silver Nitrate* ☐ Other

Admission R.N. Sign/Init. _____   ☐ Erythromycin/Ilotycin

Other comments: _____

INITIAL SYSTEMS ASSESSMENT

RN Init = item observed   * = see nurses notes or comments

CNS: [ ] moves extremities, muscle tone good
[ ] reflexes present/strong
     suck, root, Moro, step, grasps
[ ] symmetrical features, movements

CARD: [ ] ant. font. soft/flat
[ ] pulses strong/equal bilat.
[ ] heart ausc. strong/reg.
[ ] Ø murmur ausc.

SKIN: Color: [ ] pink [ ] acrocyanosis
[ ] Ø lesions, abrasions, rash
Peeling [ ] yes [ ] no
[ ] birthmarks _____

RESP: [ ] lungs ausc. clear bilat.
[ ] Ø upper airway congestion
[ ] resp. rate <60/min
[ ] chest expansion symmetrical

GU: [ ] Ø bleeding/discharge
Male: [ ] testes descended bilat.

GI: [ ] abd. soft/Ø dist
[ ] bowel sounds active

RN Init. Signature

ENT: [ ] eyes clear
[ ] mouth clear
[ ] palates intact
[ ] nares patent

Birth Inj./Variation
[ ] caput/molding
[ ] vacuum "cap"
[ ] forceps marks
[ ] other _____

Comments/Transition Vital Signs: _____

ADDRESSOGRAPH

© 1990 Vogler/Perinatal Healthcare Consultants   OB4791

* Silver nitrate has been banned in Canada; its use is declining in the United States.

FIG. 12-27 An example of a birth/recovery record. (Courtesy Joyce Vogler/Perinatal Healthcare Consultants, Kailua, HI.)

PROCEDURES 12-3

Assessment during Fourth Stage of Labor

Assemble equipment.
Explain procedure.
Wash hands.

Blood pressure
Measure per assessment schedule.

Pulse
Count pulse, assess rate, amplitude (indicating volume), rhythm and symmetry, regularity.

Temperature
Determine temperature.

Fundus
Apply gloves, when needed
Position woman with knees flexed.
Just below umbilicus, cup hand, press firmly into abdomen.
If fundus is firm (and bladder is empty), with uterus in midline, measure its position relative to woman's umbilicus. Lay fingers flat on abdomen under umbilicus; measure how many fingerbreadths fit between umbilicus and top of fundus.
If fundus is *not* firm, stimulate "living ligature" to regain tone and expel any clots before measuring distance from umbilicus.
Place hands appropriately, massage gently only until firm.
Expel clots while keeping hands placed as in Fig. 12-28. With upper hand, firmly apply pressure downward toward vagina; observe perineum for amount/size of expelled clots. Measure height of firm fundus.

Bladder
Assess distention by noting location and firmness of uterine fundus and by observation and palpation of bladder. Distended bladder is seen as a suprapubic rounded bulge that is dull to percussion and fluctuates like a water-filled balloon. When bladder is distended, uterus may be boggy, well above umbilicus, and usually to woman's right side.
Assess bladder function. Ask woman to void; measure amount of urine voided.
Catheterize as needed.
Reassess and compare findings with signs of an empty bladder: fundus firm, in midline; bladder nonpalpable.

Lochia
Observe lochia on perineal pads and on linen under mother's buttocks. Determine amount and color; note size and number of clots; note odor.
Observe perineum for source of bleeding (e.g., episiotomy, lacerations).

Perineum
Ask or assist woman to turn on her side and flex upper leg on hip.
Lift upper buttock.
Observe perineum in good lighting.

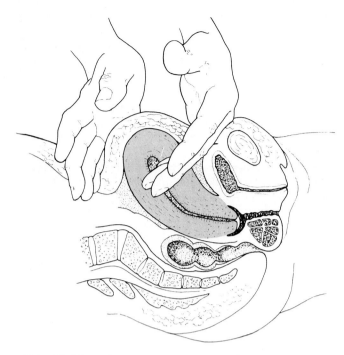

FIG. 12-28 Palpating fundus of uterus during first hour after birth. Note that upper hand is cupped over fundus; lower hand dips in above symphysis pubis and supports uterus while it is massaged gently.

loss of body heat. On occasion it may be higher than 37.2° C (99° F) because of dehydration or long labor. After a difficult labor, systolic BP less than 110 mm Hg, accompanied by a pulse over 100 beats/min, usually results from hemorrhage or shock.

The uterus must be palpated at frequent intervals to ascertain that it is not filling with blood (Fig. 12-28). The pad must be checked frequently to ensure that blood is not excessive (Fig. 12-29). Lochia may be described as scant, light, moderate, or heavy (profuse). Normally the fundus is firm or may be returned to a state of firmness with intermittent gentle massage. As noted earlier, **atony** *(relaxation) of the uterine musculature* may occur. As the relaxed uterus distends with blood and clots, blood vessels in the placental site are not clamped off and bleeding results. The uterus is unable to function as the "living ligature" that promotes sustained uterine contraction.

As the effect of the oxytocic medication administered after the birth wears off, the amount of lochia will increase because the myometrium relaxes somewhat. The nurse *always checks* under the mother's buttocks, as well as on the perineal pad. Bleeding may flow between the buttocks onto the linens under the mother while the amount on the perineal pad is slight. A perineal pad that is soaked through from tail to tail contains approximately 68 to 80 ml of blood (Luegenbiehl et al, 1990). When hemorrhage is suspected, the nurse should save all peripads and underpads for the health care provider to as-

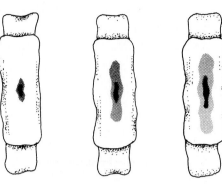

FIG. 12-29 Peripad saturation volumes.

sess. If a pad is found to be soaked through in 15 minutes, or if blood is seen pooled under the buttocks, continuous observation of blood loss, vital signs, and maternal color and behavior is essential.

Another potential source of hemorrhage is the development of a **hematoma** under the vaginal mucosa or in the connective tissue of the vulva. This may occur as a result of injury to a blood vessel during the birth or in repairing the laceration/episiotomy. The bleeding may be slow but continuous as the blood oozes from the vessel and distends the surrounding tissue. In many cases this distention of the tissue may not be visualized by the nurse. The woman's initial complaint is severe and intense pressure and/or pain in the perineal or rectal area. The nurse should carefully inspect the perineum, monitor vital signs, and report all findings to the health care provider immediately, with emphasis placed on the woman's complaint and the location of pain.

A vulvar hematoma may be visualized as the swelling increases. It usually is unilateral and becomes purplish. A vaginal hematoma is usually found only through manual examination. A soft mass may be palpated during a vaginal or rectal examination. The blood loss with this type of hematoma may be excessive. A loss of 500 ml or more is not unusual.

The hematoma continues to be evaluated, and if it remains small, treatment is unnecessary or limited to ice packs because the hematoma will reabsorb. Many times it is necessary for the nurse to prepare the woman for surgical incision and evacuation of the hematoma. The procedure is performed with general anesthesia or regional anesthesia in the area from which the clots are removed and ligation of the blood vessel is necessary. Nursing care after the procedure includes careful monitoring of the perineum and blood loss, maintenance of intravenous (IV) fluids, monitoring of vital signs and laboratory work, preparing for a possible blood transfusion, and administering prescribed antibiotics as prophylaxis against infection.

If bleeding is in the form of a continuous trickle or seen to come in spurts, *lacerations* of the vagina or cer-

EMERGENCY

HYPOVOLEMIC SHOCK

SIGNS/SYMPTOMS

Persistent significant bleeding—perineal pad soaked within 15 min; *may not be accompanied by a change in vital signs or maternal color or behavior*

Woman states she feels light-headed, "funny," "sick to my stomach," or sees "stars"

Woman begins to act anxious or exhibits air hunger

Woman's color turns ashen or grayish

Temperature of skin feels cool and clammy

Increasing pulse rate

Falling BP

Intense perineal pain (possible hematoma)

INTERVENTIONS

Notify health care provider

If uterus is atonic, massage gently and expel clots to allow uterus to contract; compress uterus manually, as needed, using two hands. Add oxytocic to IV drip, as ordered

Give oxygen by face mask or nasal prongs at 8 to 10 L/min.

Tilt the woman to her side or elevate the right hip; elevate her legs to at least a 30-degree angle

Provide additional or maintain existing IV of lactated ringer's solution or normal saline to restore circulatory volume

Monitor vital signs

Indwelling urinary catheter may be inserted to monitor perfusion of kidneys

Administer emergency drugs as ordered

Prepare for possible incision and evacuation of hematoma

Chart incident, medical and nursing interventions employed, and results of treatments

---

vix or the presence of an unligated vessel in the episiotomy are suspected and surgical correction is likely.

Hypovolemic Shock

Hypovolemic shock as a result of hemorrhage may occur in an otherwise normal fourth stage of labor. Prompt identification, diagnosis, and intervention usually result in rapid stabilization of the woman's BP, pulse, and other signs. This occurs if adequate circulating blood volume to assist the body to compensate for the loss is available or is infused intravenously. If compensatory mechanisms become ineffective, shock may ensue. The woman will experience symptoms that include light-headedness, pallor, air hunger, and cool clammy skin. These are caused by sympathetic nervous system stimulation and hypoxia of both brain and tissue cells.

Beta-adrenergic receptors are stimulated and the circulatory system attempts to compensate for tissue hypoxia and metabolic acidosis. The BP falls, and in response, the pulse increases. Measures such as uterine massage and IV administration of oxytocin are implemented to prevent further blood loss. It is important for the nurse to stay with and reassure the woman and family to decrease their anxiety. The nurse then documents all nursing and medical interventions that have been employed and their results (Luegenbiehl, 1991). The Emergency box (above) provides a quick reference for danger signs and symptoms, as well as interventions for hypovolemic shock.

Prevention of Bladder Distention

Palpation to determine the amount of *bladder distention* should accompany palpation of the fundus. The full bladder forces the uterus upward and to the right of the midline. This position causes uterine relaxation. Hemorrhage results. Distention of the bladder can result in atony of the bladder wall. Atony leads to urinary retention, which provides a favorable environment for infection.

A nurse encourages the woman to void naturally, employing one or more of the following methods: placing a bedpan under the mother, giving her water to drink (if fluids have been ordered), turning on the water faucet, pouring warm water over the perineum, helping her walk to the bathroom (if ordered), and providing privacy. If after these measures the woman still cannot void, most health care providers write an order for catheterization.

Maintenance of Safety

The mother is settled comfortably in bed. A woman who has just given birth may need to remain in bed for a period of time to allow her body systems to adjust to fluid volume changes. The nurse caring for the woman will decide the appropriate time for the first ambulation. The nurse takes several things into consideration when making this decision: baseline BP, the amount of blood loss, type and amount of analgesic or anesthetic medications administered during labor and birth, the level of pain evident in the woman's movements, and the woman's desire to ambulate. The rapid decrease in intraabdominal pressure after birth results in a dilation of blood vessels supplying the intestines, which is known as **splanchnic engorgement,** causing blood to pool in the viscera. This contributes to **orthostatic hypotension,** which tends to occur when a woman who has recently given birth stands up; consequently she may faint or feel light-headed.

It is imperative to keep within the nurse's reach aromatic ammonia ampules, which can be easily broken, to receive the woman who is ambulating for the first time.* The nurse must caution the woman to use her call bell to summon help before she attempts to get out of bed. The nurse will assess her color, pulse, and level of consciousness (LOC) in response to conversation, and then assist her in ambulating to the bathroom. Once the woman has reached the bathroom, the nurse should remain outside the door and inquire as to her well-being every minute or so. If there is no answer, the nurse enters the bathroom to assess the woman's condition. A wheelchair should be handy in the room or just outside in case the woman feels too weak to walk back to bed. She is encouraged to rest after the ambulation, so that she can regain her strength.

The woman who has received conduction anesthesia (epidural block) is kept in bed until she is able to fully move and feel sensation in her legs and her BP and pulse are within normal limits. Ambulation can occur within the first 2 hours, depending on whether the last dose was administered just before birth. If the woman had local anesthesia and some intravenously or intramuscularly administered analgesic shortly before birth, the nurse will need to assess her ability to communicate, her LOC, and her vital signs for stability (within normal limits) before allowing the woman to get out of bed. Other types of anesthesia consist of saddle block, spinal block, and paracervical block (see Chapter 10). The nurse will check that the woman is wearing shoes before she ambulates.

The woman who has received analgesics needs to be watched until she is fully recovered from the medication (i.e., vital signs are stable within her normal range, and she is fully awake).

Maintenance of Comfort

Uterine contractions may result in discomfort known as **afterpains.** After birth the volume within the uterus decreases. The force of the myometrial contractions is considerable; the intrauterine pressure is much greater than that during labor, reaching 150 mm Hg or more.

During the first 2 hours after birth, uterine contractions become regular and strong, especially in multiparous women. The nurse adds to the woman's comfort by performing the following measures:
1. Explaining the normal physiology of afterpains
2. Helping the mother keep her urinary bladder empty

3. Placing a warmed blanket on the mother's abdomen
4. Administering analgesics ordered by the health care provider
5. Encouraging relaxation and breathing exercises

As the bladder fills, it presses against the uterus, causing it to relax. The uterus attempts to stay firm by increasing the force of contractions, thereby increasing the discomfort of afterpains. Gentle massage of the fundus increases uterine contractions, thereby intensifying afterpains. To help the new mother cope with the discomforts of assessment measures, the nurse first explains what is being done and why, and then encourages the woman to perform the procedure.

The episiotomy site or hemorrhoids often contribute to a new mother's discomfort. Immediately after the birth, cold therapy such as ice packs are applied to the perineum directly over the episiotomy to minimize edema formation. Edema adds to perineal discomfort. After the first 2 hours, ice packs have little effect on minimizing edema; they are used to increase comfort by numbing the area. Chemical ice packs attached to sanitary pads are used if available, but they are expensive.

Disposable ice packs are easily made from rubber examining gloves filled with ice chips and covered with something clean such as a disposable wash cloth or one of the disposable towels. Commercial disposable ice packs may be used if available. The health care provider may order any one of several antiseptic or anesthetic ointments or sprays to ease discomfort in the perineal area. A side-lying position relieves direct pressure on the area.

If the woman has had a saddle block or other regional anesthetic, the nurse's description of sensations to expect as the anesthetic wears off can be reassuring. Women describe the sensation as tingling or prickly, much like that experienced after sitting cross-legged for a long time and the legs have "gone to sleep."

Some women experience intense postpartum tremors that resemble the shivering of a chill. The chilling may be related to the sudden release of pressure on pelvic nerves. According to another theory, chilling may be symptomatic of a fetus-to-mother transfusion that sometimes occurs during placental separation. The feeling of a chill may be a reaction to epinephrine (adrenaline) production during birth. The nurse can help the woman relax or feel comforted by providing her with warm blankets and an explanation that the tremors are commonly seen after birth and are not related to infection. Some women experience the tremors without any feeling of chill; these women also should be covered with a blanket, preferably warm if tolerated. The tremors usually are self-limiting and last only a short while. The warm blanket also provides a means of "mothering the mother." This helps restore her energy so she can move from a focus on herself to a focus on her baby as she moves from "taking-in" to "taking-hold" (Chapter 17).

---

*No aromatic spirits should be used if the woman has a heart condition.

If the nurse administers analgesics, the sedating effect of these analgesics necessitates such protective care as raising side rails, placing the call bell within reach, and cautioning about remaining in bed. The woman must be warned about any expected dizziness or drowsiness resulting from the medications.

Maintenance of Cleanliness

Perineal care increases the mother's comfort and safety (prevention of infection). A clean perineal pad is placed in position, buttocks dried, and any wet linen removed so the woman will be warm and comfortable. The nurse wears clean gloves before touching the mother's linens, soiled perineal pad, or perineal area. The nurse instructs the mother first to wash her hands, then cleanse the vulvar area from front to back, using a separate tissue for each wipe, and end by rewashing her hands. A woman who has had a repair to her perineum may be encouraged not to use tissue to wipe her vulva after voiding but to use the hospital's available perineal cleansing alternatives. The woman is instructed to change her pad each time she uses the bathroom.

Maintenance of Fluid Balance and Nutrition

Restriction of food and fluid intake and the loss of fluids (blood, perspiration, or emesis) during labor cause many women to express a sudden desire to eat and drink soon after they give birth. The type of nourishment the nurse offers depends on several factors, including type of anesthetic used and the amount of blood loss after the birth. If local or pudendal anesthetic was used in preparation for episiotomy or for perineal repair and if lochia flow is small to moderate, the woman usually can have sips of a drink of her choice followed by a regular diet. She is cautioned to drink *small* amounts of fluid initially. Rapid drinking, especially of large amounts, can lead to nausea and possibly vomiting.

If the woman had another type of anesthetic, the anesthesiologist decides when the effect of the anesthetic has worn off significantly and she can resume oral intake. Heavy bleeding may signal retained placental fragments which may require the administration of general anesthetic to remove the placental fragments and stop the bleeding. Thus the woman with heavy bleeding is usually given nothing by mouth (NPO) until the bleeding is controlled. The IV line is maintained, and the fluid is usually switched to a solution that contains dextrose to provide some calories until oral feedings resume. The nurse monitors the IV line and notes in the chart the type, amount, and tolerance of any oral intake.

Support of Parental Psychosocial Needs

It is acceptable for the nurse to share openly in the excitement and emotion of birth. The nurse assists the parents by accepting any expressions of disappointment about the child's sex or appearance and reassures them that these feelings are normal. The nurse may reassure the mother that her behavior during labor was acceptable if she appears worried about this. The new mother may need to talk about her labor and may endeavor to fill in gaps ("missing pieces") that she cannot remember, particularly if the birth was hurried (Affonso, 1977).

Psychologic states of new mothers range from euphoria and a feeling of well-being to a sleepy state marked by an unawareness of surroundings. As noted earlier, first reactions of new mothers and fathers to their newborns vary greatly. These reactions give the perinatal team cues to use in individualizing plans of care. Women who have experienced long, difficult labors or who are in pain are commonly too exhausted to extend interest to the child. The nurse can offer to take the baby to the nursery, if available, until the mother is rested. The father/coach/partner may be invited to accompany the nurse to the nursery at this stage. After sufficient rest a mother's attitude can be surprisingly different. The child unwanted for diverse reasons may continue to be rejected or be viewed with only mild interest. The attitude of the father is often reflected in the mother. His pleasure arouses a responsive pleasure, or his disappointment arouses corresponding disappointment.

Ethnic or cultural origins dictate behaviors that are deemed appropriate for special occasions. Some parents may not be able to express their delight openly; others wish to welcome the newcomer noisily. For example, some Southeast Asians may not want to hold the baby immediately after birth, and may consider compliments about the baby bad luck (Geissler, 1994).

The single or teenage mother may express mixed emotions at the baby's birth. The nurse can help her express her emotions, involve any significant other family/friends, or refer her to a social worker, if appropriate.

Some mothers, particularly with their firstborn, are surprised and disturbed by the passivity or disinterest they experience on seeing their long-awaited infant. The nurse can reassure the mother of the normality of these feelings. The idealized "mother love" does not necessarily appear right after birth. The gradual growth of such love comes to some as they assume the care of and responsibility for their child.

Some interventions can facilitate parent-infant acquaintance and beginning bonding or attachment. The father/partner can be encouraged to hold the baby in the birth room or the recovery area (Fig. 12-30). In a warm, quiet, dimly lighted environment, an infant responds by opening the eyes. Parents are encouraged to hold the infant *en face*. In the en face position, parents and newborns gaze into each other's eyes (Tomlinson, Rothenberg, Carver, 1991). Newborns focus best at about 20.3 cm (8 in) distance. Body odor can be noticed (mothers have remarked that each child smells dif-

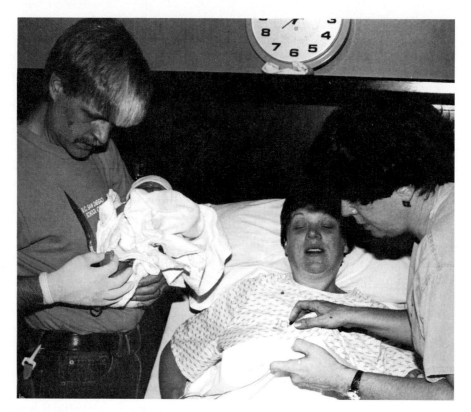

FIG. 12-30 Father engrossed in examining newborn as nurse prepares for mother's fourth-stage care. (Courtesy Kathy Hanold, RN, MS, Birth Place, Barnes Hospital at Washington University Medical Center, St Louis.)

ferent). Skin contact between mother and baby should be encouraged during this time. Neonatal temperatures remain stable if mother and newborn are placed chest-to-chest and covered by a blanket. The mother is encouraged to explore her baby and put her baby to the breast if she plans to breastfeed. Immediately after birth the baby has a strong desire to suck; thus this early feed is most encouraging for the mother and bonding is prompted.

Transfer from the Recovery Area

During the recovery period of 1 to 2 hours, the recovery nurse (who often functions as the birth nurse) completes any required paperwork while performing the frequent postpartum assessments. After the initial recovery period has passed (per hospital protocol), the woman may be transferred to a postpartum room in the same or another nursing unit. In labor, delivery, recovery, postpartum room (LDRP) settings the nurse who has provided care during the recovery period usually continues caring for the woman. In the labor, delivery, recovery room (LDR) or traditional setting the woman is transferred to a "postpartum" area where the postpartum nursing staff cares for her. In some settings, nurses are responsible for both members of the mother-baby couple.

In preparing the transfer report, the recovery nurse uses information from the admission record, the birth record, and the recovery record. Information that needs to be communicated to the postpartum nurse includes identity of the health care provider, gravidity and parity, age, anesthetic used, duration of labor and rupture of membranes, type of birth and repair, blood type, the state of rubella immunity, VDRL and hepatitis serology test results, the IV infusion of any fluids, physiologic status since birth; description of fundus, lochia, bladder, perineum, and hemorrhoids; sex and weight of infant, time of birth, pediatrician, chosen method of feeding, any abnormalities noted; and assessment of initial parental-infant interaction (Table 12-7).

This information also must be documented for the nursing staff in the newborn nursery. In addition, specific information should be provided regarding the infant's Apgar scores, weight, voiding, and feeding since the birth. Nursing interventions that have been completed (e.g., eye prophylaxis, vitamin K injection) also should be recorded (Table 12-7).

✦ EVALUATION

Evaluation of progress and outcomes continues throughout the fourth stage of labor. The nurse evaluates the

TABLE 12-7   Recovery Nurse's Report

ITEM	EXAMPLE OF DOCUMENTATION OF MOTHER	EXAMPLE OF DOCUMENTATION OF NEWBORN
Type of labor and birth; unusual observations, if any, of the placenta	Spontaneous or assisted (forceps) vaginal birth; vertex presentation	Spontaneous or assisted (forceps, vacuum extractor) vaginal birth in vertex presentation
Gravidity and parity, age	GI, PI, 22 years old	GI, PI, 22 years old
Anesthesia and analgesia used	None; epidural, low spinal, local	None; epidural, low spinal, or local
Condition of perineum	Episiotomy; repair of lacerations	
Events since birth	Vital signs, BP, fundus, lochia, intake and output, medications (dosage, time of administration, and results), response to newborn, observation of family interactions, including siblings, if present	Nursed at breast; took nipple well Voided ×1; meconium ×1 Eye prophylaxis Vitamin K injection Held by siblings who are happy (or have other response) to newborn
Condition and sex of newborn; other information	Apgar at 1 and 5 min; time of birth; eye prophylaxis given; weight; whether breastfeeding or bottle feeding; if breastfeeding, whether newborn was at breast; name of pediatrician; sex of the baby	Apgar scores at 1 and 5 min Male; 3400 g (7 lb 8 oz); name of pediatrician; breastfeeding or bottle-feeding; mother's hepatitis B status
Relevant information from prenatal record	Need for rubella vaccination; presence of infections; hepatitis B status blood type; Rh status	Unremarkable pregnancy
Miscellaneous information		
IV drip	If IV drip is infusing, rate of infusion, medications added (e.g., Pitocin), whether to keep open or discontinue after completion of bag that is hung	
Social factors	If woman is releasing baby for adoption, whether she wants to see baby, breastfeed, allow visitors, or other preferences she may have	

physiologic recovery from pregnancy and labor, as well as development of parent-infant attachment and new family interrelationships. The degree to which expected outcomes of care are being met must be critically appraised in terms of the following factors:

- The new mother does not saturate more than one perineal pad per hour.
- She voids if her bladder is filling during the fourth stage.
- She verbalizes acceptance of the labor process after expressing concerns.
- She (and other family members, if present) exhibit bonding/attachment behaviors.
- She verbalizes increased comfort after initiation of comfort measures.

If the evaluation process identifies that results fall short of achieving any expected outcome further assessment, planning and collaborative care are imperative to attain the correct nursing care for the woman and her family.

KEY POINTS

- The onset of labor may be difficult to determine even for the experienced pregnant woman.
- Although some complications of labor are anticipated, others appear only in the clinical course of labor.
- The nurse assumes much of the responsibility for making the assessment of progress and keeping the health care provider informed about that progress and any deviations from normal findings.

- Although meconium-stained fluid may be noted with fetal asphyxia, its presence is not always diagnostic of prospective fetal distress.
- The woman's level of anxiety may rise when she does not understand what is being said to her about her labor because of the medical terminology used or because of a language barrier.
- Prolapsed umbilical cord requires prompt recognition and intervention to prevent fetal hypoxia.
- Coaching, support, and comfort measures help the woman use her energy constructively in relaxing and working with the contractions.
- The nurse can be a positive influence in promotion of family integration of the birth process.
- The nurse who is aware of the sociocultural aspects of childbirth is able to incorporate those expectations into the plan of care.
- The woman needs continuous monitoring, support, and coaching during the second stage of labor.
- If any laboring woman states that "the baby is coming," immediate birth should be anticipated.

- There are five signs that placental separation has occurred and the placenta is ready to be expelled; before placental separation, excessive traction can result in immediate or delayed injury to the mother.
- Most parents (families) enjoy being able to handle, hold, explore, and examine the baby immediately after birth. The nurse should assist in this process and be alert for warning signs of an impaired relationship.
- The fourth stage of labor, the stage of recovery, is a critical period for the mother and newborn.
- The primary nursing concern during the fourth stage of labor is the prevention of hemorrhage. Other concerns include bladder distention, safety, comfort, and nutrition.
- The nurse can facilitate mother-infant attachment by meeting the new mother's physical, support, and teaching needs.
- Regardless of parity, marital status, or age, new mothers can benefit from explanations for the various nursing actions during the immediate postpartum period.

CRITICAL THINKING EXERCISES

1. Compare the cervical dilatation and station of the fetal presenting part of a multiparous woman and a nulliparous woman during the first stage of labor.
    a. Examine how findings differ, whether they follow the normal labor curve, and how you account for any deviations.
    b. Identify nursing diagnoses and prepare a plan of care for each woman. Justify differences and similarities in the plans.
2. You are assigned to a laboring woman and her family who are culturally different from you.
    a. Compare their perceptions and beliefs about labor to your own.
    b. Analyze how these factors might affect the behavior of the woman, her family, and the nurse during the first stage of labor.
    c. How would you incorporate this knowledge into your plan of care?
3. You are assigned to a woman and her family during the second and third stages of labor.
    a. Develop assumptions about the behaviors observed among the family members.
    b. Examine your response to and feelings about the birth. Identify your positive or negative feelings, and explore their causes.
    c. Examine the birth setting and the procedures performed during these stages, and assess their potential effect on parent-infant attachment.
    d. Observe parent-infant interactions.
        1. Identify any behaviors that make you uncomfortable.
        2. Explore the cause of those behaviors.
        3. What impact could these feelings have on your ability to facilitate parent-infant interactions?
4. The nurse has just received a postpartum mother and her husband in the recovery area. They are expressing disappointment over the sex of their child, and the father is hinting that it is his wife's fault.
    a. Identify the assumptions of the father.
    b. Analyze the significance of these assumptions for the family and the nurse.
    c. Formulate a plan of care that provides the family with information about sex determination.

References

Aderhold KJ, Roberts JE: Phases of second stage labor: four descriptive care studies, *J Nurse Midwife* 36(5):267, 1991.

Affonso D: Missing pieces: a study of postpartum feelings, *Birth Fam J* 4:159, 1977.

American College of Obstetricians and Gynecologists: More women now deliver in alternative birth sites, *ACOG Newsletter* 37(1):8, 1993.

Andrews CM, Chrzanowski M: Maternal position, labor, and comfort, *Appl Nurs Res* 3:7, 1990.

Bentz JM: Missed meanings in nurse/patient communications, *MCN* 5:55, 1980.

Berry LM: Realistic expectations of the labor coach, *JOGNN* 17:354, 1988.

Biancuzzo M: The patient observer: does the hands and knees position during labor help to rotate the occiput posterior fetus? *Birth* 18(1):40, 1991.

Bliss J: New baby in the family, *Can Nurse* 76:42, 1980.

Carrington BW: The Afro-American. In Clark AL, editor: *Culture/childbearing/health professionals*, Philadelphia, 1978, FA Davis Co.

Chapman LL: Expectant fathers' roles during labor and birth, *JOGNN* 21(2):114, 1992.

Cunningham FG, MacDonald PC, Gant NF: *Williams obstetrics*, ed 19, Norwalk, CT, 1993, Appleton & Lange.

Farris L: The American Indian. In Clark AL, editor: *Culture/childbearing/health professionals*, Philadelphia, 1978, FA Davis Co.

Friedman EA, Sachtleben MR: Station of the presenting part, *Am J Obstet Gynecol* 93:522, 1965.

Gardosi J, Sylvester SB, Lynch C: Alternative positions in the second stage of labour: a randomized controlled trial, *Br J Obstet Gynecol* 96:1290, 1989.

Geissler E: *Pocket guide to cultural assessment*, St Louis, 1994, Mosby.

Hollingsworth AD et al: The refugees and childbearing: what to expect, *RN* 43:45, 1980.

Horn BM: Northwest coast Indians: the Muckleshoot. In Kay MA, editor: *Anthropology of human birth*, Philadelphia, 1982, FA Davis Co.

Jimenez SL: Application of the body's natural pain relief mechanisms to reduce discomfort in labor and delivery, *NAACOG Update Series* lesson 1, vol 1, 1983.

Johnson SM, Snow LF: Profile of some unplanned pregnancies. In Bauwens EE, editor: *The anthropology of health*, St Louis, 1978, Mosby.

Jordan PL: Laboring for relevance: expectant and new fatherhood, *Nurs Res* 39:11, 1990.

Kline-Kaye V, Miller-Slade D: The use of fundal pressure during the second stage of labor, *JOGNN* 19(6):511, 1990.

Lantican S, Corona D: Comparison of the social support networks of Filipinos and Mexican American primigravidas, *Health Care Women Int* 13:329, 1992.

Liu YC: Effects of the upright position during childbirth, *Image J Nurs Sch* 21:14, 1989.

Luegenbiehl DL et al: Standarized assessment of blood loss, *MCN* 15:241, 1990.

Luegenbiehl DL: Postpartum bleeding, *NAACOG's Clinical Issues in Perinatal and Women's Health Nursing* 2(3):402, 1991.

Mahan CS, McKay S: Are we overmanaging second stage labor? *Contemp OB/GYN* 24:37, 1984.

Malestic SL: Fathers need help during labor, too, *RN* 53:23, 1990.

McKay S, Roberts J: Maternal position during labor and birth: what have we learned? *IJCE, ICEA Rev* 13:19, 1989.

McKay S, Roberts J: Obstetrics by ear. Maternal and caregiver perceptions of the meaning of maternal sounds during second stage labor, *J Nurse Midwife* 35:266, 1990.

Meleis A, Lipson J, Paul S: Ethnicity and health among five middle-eastern immigrant groups, *Nurs Res* 41(2):98, 1981.

Melzak R, Belanger E, Lacroix R: Labor pain: effects of maternal position on front and back pain, *J Pain Symptom Manage* 6(8):476, 1991.

Metzer BL, Therrien B: Effect of position on cardiovascular response during the Valsalva maneuver, *Nurs Res* 39:198, 1990.

Myles M: *Textbook for midwives*, ed 11, Edinburgh, 1989, Churchill Livingstone.

Pernoll ML, Benson RC: *Current obstetric and gynecologic diagnosis and treatment*, ed 6, Los Altos, CA, 1987, Appleton & Lange.

Pillsbury BLK: "Doing the month": confinement and convalescence of Chinese women after birth, *Soc Sci Med* 12:11, 1978.

Queenan JT: Partners in the delivery room: a natural evolution, *Contemp OB/GYN* 35:8, 1990.

Scherer P: Supported squatting enhances the second stage of labor, *AJN* 89:1266, 1989.

Scott JR et al: *Danforth's obstetrics and gynecology*, ed 6, Philadelphia, 1990, JB Lippincott Co.

Tomlinson PS, Rothenberg MA, Carver LD: Behavioral interaction of fathers with infants and mothers in the immediate postpartum period, *J Nurs Midwife* 36:232, 1991.

Thomson AM: Pushing techniques in the second stage of labour, *J Adv Nurs* 18:171, 1993.

Waldenstrom U, Gottvall K: A randomized trial of birthing stool or conventional semirecumbent position for second-stage labor, *Birth* 18(1):5, 1991.

Wheeler DG: Intrapartum bleeding, *NAACOGs Clin Issu Perinat Womens Health Nurs* 2(3):381, 1991.

Bibliography

Begley CM: A comparison of "active" and "physiological" management of the third stage of labour, *Midwif* 6:3, 1990.

Bergstrom L et al: "You'll feel me touching you, sweetie": vaginal examinations during the second stage of labor, *Birth* 19(1):10, 1992.

Bonovich L: Recognizing the onset of labor, *JOGNN* 19:141, 1990.

Gannon JM: Delivery on the hands and knees, *J Nurse Midwife* 37(1):48, 1992.

Lowe NK: Maternal confidence in coping with labor: a self-efficacy concept, *JOGNN* 20(6):457, 1991.

Marcelin CF: Men in ob-gyn nursing: a student's enlightenment or nightmare? *Imprint* 39(3):33, 1992.

McKay S, Barrows T, Roberts J: Women's views of second stage labor as assessed by interviews and videotapes, *Birth* 17:192, 1990.

Moon JM, Smith CV, Rayburn WF: Perinatal outcome after a prolonged second stage of labor, *J Reprod Med* 35:299, 1990.

Paine LL, Tinker DD: The effect of maternal bearing-down efforts on the arterial umbilical cord pH and length of second stage labor, *J Nurse Midwife* 31(1):61, 1992.

Varney H: *Nurse-midwifery*, ed 3, Boston, 1991, Blackwell Scientific.

Willson JR, Carrington ER: *Obstet Gynecol*, ed 9, St Louis, 1991, Mosby.

U N I T
Four

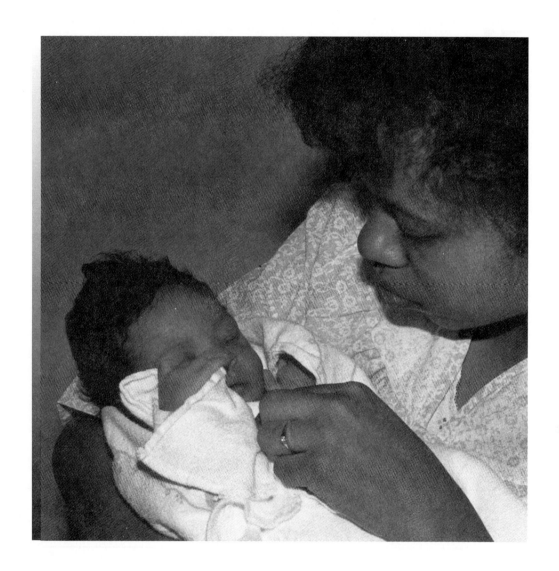

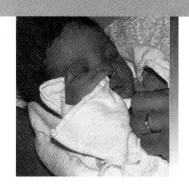

The Newborn

13 **The Newborn**

14 **Nursing Care of the Newborn**

15 **Newborn Nutrition and Feeding**

13 The Newborn

S H A N N O N   E .   P E R R Y

LEARNING OBJECTIVES

Define the key terms listed.
List characteristics of the biologic systems of the newborn.
Describe behavioral characteristics of the newborn.
Outline essential components of a newborn assessment.
Describe reflexes of a newborn.

KEY TERMS

Brazelton Neonatal Behavioral Assessment
  Scale (NBAS)
cold stress
hyperbilirubinemia
sensory behaviors
sleep-wake cycles
state-related behaviors
surfactant
thermogenesis
transition period

RELATED TOPICS

Fetal lung maturity tests *(Chap. 20)* • Gestational assessment *(Chap. 14)* • Kernicterus *(Chap. 27)* • Newborn nutrition *(Chap. 15)* • Parent-infant interaction *(Chap. 17)* • Phototherapy *(Chap. 14)* • Respiratory distress syndrome (RDS) *(Chap. 27)*

The newborn infant must accomplish a number of developmental tasks to establish and maintain a physical existence apart from the mother. The profound biologic adaptations that occur at birth make the newborn infant's transition from intrauterine to extrauterine life possible. These adaptations set the stage for future growth and development.

Nurses play a vital role during this transition period. They help the newborn infant make a safe transition to extrauterine life and assist the mother and her significant others throughout their transition to parenthood. Nurses perform the initial assessment of the newborn infant, provide a physical environment conducive to adaptation, and monitor the newborn infant's condition during the early adaptation phases.

BIOLOGIC CHARACTERISTICS

By term gestation the fetus' various anatomic and physiologic systems have reached a level of development and functioning that permits a separate existence from the mother. At birth the newborn infant manifests behavioral competencies and a readiness for social interaction. The neonatal period, from birth through day 28, represents a time of dramatic physical change for the newborn infant.

Cardiovascular System

The cardiovascular system changes markedly after birth. The foramen ovale, ductus arteriosus, and ductus venosus close. The umbilical arteries, umbilical vein, and hepatic arteries become ligaments (Fig. 13-1).

The infant's first breath inflates the lungs and reduces pulmonary vascular resistance to the pulmonary blood flow. The pulmonary artery pressure drops. This sequence is the major mechanism by which pressure in the *right atrium declines*. The increased pulmonary blood flow returned to the left side of the heart *increases* the pressure in the *left atrium*. This change in pressures causes a functional closure of the foramen ovale. During the first few days of life, crying may reverse the flow through the foramen ovale temporarily and lead to mild cyanosis.

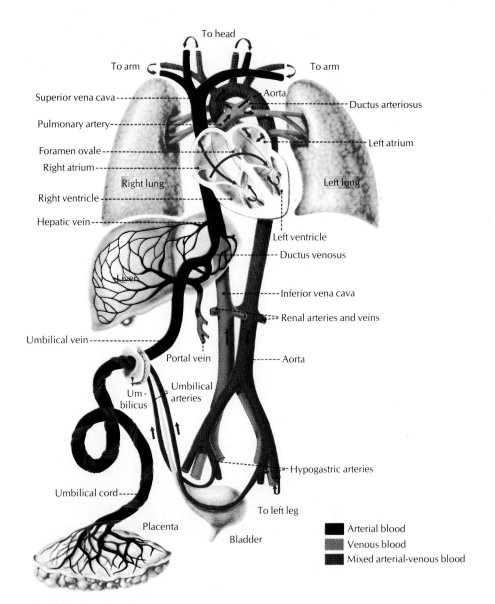

FIG. 13-1 Fetal circulation. *Before birth.* Arterialized blood from the placenta flows into the fetus through the umbilical vein and passes rapidly through the liver into the inferior vena cava; it flows through the foramen ovale into the left atrium, soon to appear in the aorta and arteries of the head. A portion bypasses the liver through the ductus venosus. Venous blood from the lower extremities and head passes predominantly into the right atrium, the right ventricle, and then into the descending pulmonary artery and ductus arteriosus. Thus the foramen ovale and the ductus arteriosus act as bypass channels, allowing a large part of the combined cardiac output to return to the placenta without flowing through the lungs. Approximately 55% of the combined ventricular output flows to the placenta; 35% perfuses body tissues; and the remaining 10% flows through the lungs (Behrman, Vaughan, 1987). *After birth.* The foramen ovale closes, the ductus arteriosus closes and becomes a ligament, the ductus venosus closes and becomes a ligament, and the umbilical vein and arteries close and become ligaments. (Courtesy Ross Laboratories, Columbus, OH.)

When the Po_2 level in the arterial blood approximates 50 mm Hg, the ductus arteriosus constricts (fetal $Po_2 \cong$ 27 mm Hg). Later, the ductus arteriosus occludes and becomes a ligament. With the clamping and severing of the cord, the umbilical arteries, umbilical vein, and ductus venosus close immediately and are converted into ligaments. The hypogastric arteries also occlude and become ligaments.

Heart Rate and Sound

The heart rate averages 140 beats/min at birth, with variations from 120 to 160 beats/min noted during sleeping and waking states. At 1 week of age the mean heart rate is 128 beats/min asleep and 163 beats/min awake; at 1 month of age it is 138 beats/min asleep and 167 beats/min awake. Sinus arrhythmia (irregular heart rate) may be considered a physiologic phenomenon in infancy and an indication of good heart function (Lowrey, 1986).

Heart sounds after birth reflect the series action of the heart pump. They are described as the familiar "lub, dub, lub, dub" sound. The "lub" is associated with closure of the mitral and tricuspid valves at the beginning of systole and the "dub" with closure of the aortic and pulmonic valves at the end of systole. The "lub" is the first heart sound and the "dub" the second heart sound. The normal cycle of the heart starts with the beginning of systole (Guyton, 1991). Heart sounds during the neonatal period are higher pitched, shorter in duration, and of greater intensity than those of adults. The first sound is typically louder and duller than the second sound, which is sharp in quality. Most heart murmurs heard during the neonatal period have no pathologic significance, and more than half disappear by 6 months.

By term gestation the infant's heart lies midway between the crown of the head and the buttocks. The point of maximum impulse (PMI) in the newborn infant is at the fourth intercostal space and to the left of the midclavicular line. The PMI is often visible.

Blood Pressure and Volume

The newborn infant's average systolic blood pressure is 78, and the average diastolic pressure is 42. The blood pressure varies from day to day during the first month of life. A drop in systolic blood pressure (about 15 mm Hg) the first hour after birth is common. Crying and moving usually cause increases in the systolic blood pressure.

Blood volume in the newborn ranges from 80 to 110 ml/kg during the first several days and doubles by the end of the first year. Proportionately, the newborn has approximately 10% greater blood volume and nearly 20% greater red blood cell mass than the adult. However, the newborn's blood is about 20% less plasma volume when compared by kilogram of body weight with the adult. The infant born prematurely has a relatively greater blood volume than the term newborn. This is because the preterm infant has a proportionately greater plasma volume, not a greater red blood cell mass.

Early or late clamping of the cord changes circulatory dynamics of the newborn. Late clamping expands the blood volume from the so-called placental transfusion. This, in turn, causes an increase in the heart's size, increased systolic blood pressure, and a higher respiratory rate.

Hematopoietic System

Hematopoietic characteristics of the newborn include certain variations from the hematopoietic system of the adult. There are differences in red blood cells (RBCs) and leukocytes and relatively few differences in platelets.

At birth the average values of hemoglobin, hematocrit, and RBCs are higher than those values found in adults. Newborn hemoglobin ranges from 14.5 to 22.5 g/dl, the hematocrit ranges from 44% to 72%, and the RBC count ranges from 5 to 7.5 million/mm^3. The hemoglobin and RBC count fall and reach the average levels of 11 to 17 g/dl and 4.2 to 5.2/mm^3 respectively by the end of the first month.

The newborn infant's blood contains about 80% fetal hemoglobin. The percentage of fetal hemoglobin falls to 55% by 5 weeks and falls to 5% by 20 weeks of age. The fall occurs because of the shorter life span of the cells containing fetal hemoglobin. Iron stores generally are sufficient to sustain normal RBC production for 5 months, and as a result the slight, brief anemia is not serious. Delayed clamping of the cord increases available iron, as 80 ml of placental blood yields 50 mg of iron (Cunningham, MacDonald, Gant, 1993).

The values may be affected by several factors. Delayed clamping of the cord causes a rise in hemoglobin, hematocrit, and RBC count. Capillary blood will give higher values than venous blood. The time after birth when the blood sample is obtained is important; there is a slight rise in RBCs after birth, followed by a substantial drop.

Leukocytosis, with the white blood cell (WBC) count approximately 18,000/mm^3, is normal at birth. The number, largely polymorphs, increases to between 23,000 and 24,000/mm^3 during the first day after birth. A level of 11,500/mm^3 normally is maintained during the neonatal period. In contrast to adults, the WBC count of the newborn does not increase markedly in infections. In most instances sepsis is accompanied by a decline in WBCs, particularly in neutrophils.

Platelet count and aggregation are essentially the same in newborn infants as in adults. Bleeding tendencies in the newborn are rare, and unless there is a marked vitamin K deficiency, clotting is sufficient to prevent hemorrhage.

The infant's blood group is established early in fetal life. However, during the neonatal period there is a gradual increase in the strength of the agglutinogens present in the RBC membrane.

Respiratory System

The most critical adjustment a newborn must make at birth is the establishment of respirations. At term the lungs hold approximately 20 ml fluid/kg (Blackburn, Loper, 1992). Air must be substituted for fluid that filled the respiratory tract to the alveoli. During the course of normal vaginal birth, some fluid is squeezed or drained from the newborn's trachea and lungs.

During the first hour of life the pulmonary lymphatics continue to remove large amounts of fluid. Removal of fluid is also a result of the pressure gradient from alveoli to interstitial tissue to blood capillary. Reduced vascular resistance accommodates this flow of lung fluid.

Abnormal respiration and failure to completely expand the lungs retard the movement of fetal lung fluid from alveoli and interstices into the pulmonary circulation. Retention of fluid interferes with the infant's ability to maintain adequate oxygenation.

Initial breathing is probably the result of a reflex triggered by pressure changes, chilling, noise, light, and other sensations related to the birth process. In addition, the chemoreceptors in the aorta and carotid bodies initiate neurologic reflexes when arterial oxygen pressure (Po_2) falls from 80 to 15 mm Hg, arterial carbon dioxide pressure (Pco_2) rises from 40 to 70 mm Hg, and arterial pH falls below 7.35. When these changes are extreme, respiratory depression can occur. In most cases an exaggerated respiratory reaction follows within 1 minute of birth, and the infant takes a first gasping breath and cries.

Certain respiratory patterns are characteristic of the normal term newborn. After respirations are established, breaths are shallow and irregular, ranging from 30 to 60 breaths per minute, with short periods of apnea (less than 15 seconds). These short periods of apnea occur most often during the active (rapid eye movement [REM]) sleep cycle and decrease in frequency and duration with age. Apneic periods over 15 seconds in duration should be evaluated.

Newborn infants are preferential nose breathers. The reflex response to nasal obstruction is to open the mouth to maintain an airway. This response is not present in most infants until 3 weeks after birth. Therefore cyanosis or asphyxia may occur with nasal blockage.

The chest circumference is approximately 30 to 33 cm (12 to 13 inches) at birth. Auscultation of the chest of a newborn infant reveals loud, clear breath sounds that seem very near, because little chest tissue intervenes. The ribs of the infant articulate with the spine at a horizontal rather than a downward slope; consequently the rib cage cannot expand with inspiration as readily as an adult's. Neonatal respiratory function is largely a matter of diaphragmatic contraction. The negative intrathoracic pressure is created by the descent of the diaphragm, much

like negative pressure is created in the barrel of a syringe when medication is drawn up by retracting the plunger. The newborn infant's chest and abdomen rise simultaneously with inspiration. Seesaw respirations are not normal (Fig. 13-2).

The alveoli of the infant's lungs are lined with **surfactant.** Lung expansion augments surfactant secretion. Surfactant functions (1) to lower surface tension, therefore, requiring less pressure to keep the alveolus open and (2) to maintain alveolar stability by changing surface tension as the size of the alveolus changes. The surfactant system develops as the infant develops in utero. Fetal pulmonary maturity can be determined by examining amniotic fluid for lecithin/sphingomyelin ratio (L/S) and other phospholipid levels. Phosphatidylglycerol appears at 35 to 36 weeks; its presence is a more predictable indicator of lung maturity.

The concentration of lecithin and sphingomyelin increases with gestational age. Mature fetal lungs have an L/S ratio greater than 2:1. Infants born before the L/S ratio is 2:1 will have varying degrees of respiratory distress. Characteristics of the respiratory system of the neonate and the effects of these characteristics on respiratory function are listed in Table 13-1.

Renal System

By the fourth month of fetal life the kidneys are formed. In utero, urine forms in the kidneys and is excreted into the amniotic fluid.

At term gestation the kidneys occupy a large portion of the posterior abdominal wall. The bladder lies close to the anterior abdominal wall and is partially an abdominal, as well as a pelvic, organ. In the newborn almost all palpable masses in the abdomen are renal in origin.

Kidney function similar to that of an adult is not approached until the second year of life. The newborn has a narrow range of chemical balance and safety. Diarrhea, infection, or improper feeding can lead rapidly to acidosis and fluid imbalances such as dehydration or edema. Renal immaturity also limits the newborn infant's ability to excrete drugs.

Small amounts of urine are usually present in the bladder at birth; however, the newborn may not void for 12

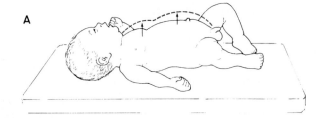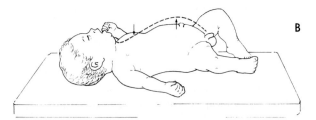

FIG. 13-2 Comparison of normal and seesaw respirations. **A,** Normal respiration. Chest and abdomen rise with inspiration. **B,** Seesaw respiration. Chest wall retracts and abdomen rises with inspiration. (Courtesy Mead Johnson & Co., Evansville, IN.)

TABLE 13-1   Characteristics of the Respiratory System of the Neonate

CHARACTERISTIC	EFFECT ON FUNCTION
Lung elastic tissue and recoil is decreased	Lung compliance is decreased; more work and higher pressure are required to expand; risk of atelectasis
Limited movement of diaphragm	Respiratory movement less effective; risk of atelectasis
Preferential nose breather; larynx and epiglottis high	Can breathe and swallow at the same time; risk of airway obstruction; difficulty intubating
Airway passages small and compliant; high airway resistance; weak cough reflex	Risk of obstruction of the airway and apnea
Surfactant system altered in immature infants	Atelectic areas; work of breathing increased; risk of respiratory distress syndrome (RDS)
Respiratory control immature	Respirations irregular; unable to increase rate and depth of respirations rapidly

Modified from Blackburn S: Alterations of the respiratory system in the neonate: implications for clinical practice, *J Perinat Neonat Nurs* 6(2):46, 1992.

to 24 hours. Voiding after this period is frequent. Six to 10 voidings a day of pale, straw-colored urine are indicative of adequate fluid intake. Generally, term infants void 15 to 60 ml of urine per kilogram per day (Blackburn, Loper, 1992; Fanaroff, Martin, 1992). Sometimes pink-tinged stains ("brick dust") appear on the diaper. These stains are caused by urate crystals and are normal.

Differences in newborn's fluid and electrolyte balance from adult physiologic response include the following:

1. The distribution of extracellular and intracellular fluid differs from that of the adult. About 40% of the body weight of the newborn is extracellular fluid, whereas in the adult it is 20%.
2. The rate of exchange of extracellular fluid differs. Each day the newborn takes in and excretes 600 to 700 ml of water, which is 20% of the total body fluid, or 50% of the extracellular fluid. In contrast, the adult exchanges 2000 ml of water, which is 5% of the total body fluid and 14% of the extracellular fluid.
3. The composition of body fluids shows variations. There is a higher concentration of sodium, phosphates, chloride, and organic acids and a lower

concentration of bicarbonate ions in the newborn. These findings mean that the newborn is in a compensated acidotic state.

4. The glomerular filtration rate is about 30% in the newborn, in contrast to 50% of that of the adult. This results in a decreased ability to remove nitrogenous and other waste products from the blood. However, the newborn's ingested protein is almost totally metabolized for growth.
5. The decreased ability to excrete excessive sodium results in hypotonic urine compared to plasma.
6. The sodium reabsorption decreases as a result of lowered sodium-potassium-activated adenosine-triphosphatase (ATPase) activity.
7. The newborn can dilute urine down to 50 milliosmols (mOsm). The capacity to dilute urine exceeds the capacity to concentrate it. There is some limitation in the ability to increase urinary volume.
8. The newborn can concentrate urine from 600 to 700 mOsm compared with the adult's capacity of 1400 mOsm. The inability to concentrate urine is not absolute, but in terms of adult function, it is somewhat limited. The newborn's specific gravity ranges from 1.005 to 1.015.
9. The newborn has a higher renal threshold for glucose.

Comparative laboratory values for newborns and adults appear in Appendix F.

Gastrointestinal System

The term newborn is capable of swallowing, digesting, metabolizing, and absorbing proteins and simple carbohydrates, and emulsifying fats. With the exception of pancreatic amylase, the characteristic enzymes and digestive juices are present even in low-birth weight infants.

In the adequately hydrated newborn infant the mucous membrane of the mouth is moist and pink. Pallor and cyanosis of the mucous membrane are normally not present. Drooling of mucus is common in the first few hours after birth. Retention cysts, small whitish areas (Epstein's pearls), may be found on the gum margins and at the juncture of the hard and soft palate. The hard and soft palates are intact. The cheeks are full because of well-developed sucking pads. These, like the labial tubercles (sucking calluses) on the upper lip, disappear when the sucking period is over. Occasionally an infant may be born with one or more teeth; this occurs more often among Native American infants.

A special mechanism, present in normal newborns weighing more than 1500 g, coordinates the breathing, sucking, and swallowing reflexes necessary for oral feeding. Sucking in the newborn takes place in small bursts of three or four sucks at a time. In the term newborn, longer and more efficient sucking attempts occur after only a few hours. The newborn infant is unable to move food from the lips to the pharynx making it necessary to place the nipple (breast or bottle) well inside the baby's mouth. Peristaltic activity in the esophagus is uncoordinated in the first few days of life. It quickly becomes a coordinated pattern in normal infants, and they swallow easily.

Bacteria are not present in the infant's gastrointestinal tract at birth. Soon after birth, oral and anal orifices permit entrance of bacteria and air. Bowel sounds can be heard 1 hour after birth. Generally the highest bacterial concentration is found in the lower portion of the intestine, particularly in the large intestine. The normal intestinal flora help synthesize vitamin K, folic acid, and biotin.

The capacity of the stomach varies from 30 to 90 ml depending on the size of the infant. Emptying time for the stomach varies greatly. Several factors, such as time and volume of feedings, type and temperature of food, and psychic stress, may affect the emptying time. This can range from 1 to 24 hours. Regurgitation may be noted during the neonatal period. The cardiac sphincter and nervous control of the stomach are still immature.

Digestion

The infant's gastric acidity at birth normally equals the adult level but is reduced within a week and may remain reduced for 2 to 3 months. The reduction in gastric acidity may lead to "colic." Infants with colic usually remain awake, crying in apparent distress between feedings, often between the same two feedings every day. Nothing seems to appease them. They appear to "grow out" of this behavior by 3 months of age.

Further digestion and absorption of nutrients occur in the small intestine. Pancreatic secretions, secretions from the liver through the common bile duct, and secretions from the duodenal portion of the small intestine make this complex process possible.

The newborn infant's ability to digest carbohydrates, fats, and proteins is regulated by the presence of certain enzymes. Most of these enzymes are functional at birth. One exception is *amylase,* produced by the salivary glands after about 3 months and by the pancreas at about 6 months of age. This enzyme is necessary to convert starch into maltose. The other exception is *lipase,* also secreted by the pancreas, which is necessary for the digestion of fat. Thus the normal newborn is capable of digesting simple carbohydrates and proteins but has a limited ability to digest fats.

Stools

At birth the lower intestine is filled with *meconium.* Meconium is formed during fetal life from the amniotic fluid and its constituents, intestinal secretions, and cells shed from the mucosa. Meconium is greenish-black and viscous, and it contains occult blood. The first meconium passed is sterile, but within hours all meconium passed contains bacteria. About 69% of normal term infants pass

meconium within 12 hours of life, 94% by 24 hours, and 99.8% in 48 hours (Blackburn, Loper, 1992).

The number of newborn stools varies considerably during the first week and are most numerous between the third and sixth days. Transitional stools (thin, slimy, and brown to green in color because of the continued presence of meconium) are passed from the third to sixth day. Newborns fed early pass stool sooner than those fed later (Boyer, Vidyasagar, 1987). The stools of the breast-fed babies and bottle-fed babies differ. The stools of the breastfed baby are loose, golden yellow in color, and nonirritating to the infant's skin. It is normal for the baby to have a bowel movement with each feeding or a bowel movement every 3 to 4 days. Even if the latter is the case, the stools remain loose and unformed. The stools of the bottle-fed baby are formed but soft, are pale yellow, and have a typical stool odor. Also, they tend to irritate to the baby's skin. The number of stools decreases in the first 2 weeks from five or six stools daily (one after every feeding) to one or two per day.

Distention of the stomach muscles causes a corresponding relaxation and contraction of the muscles of the colon. As a result, infants often have bowel movements during or just after a feeding. Stooling at these times has been attributed to the gastrocolic reflex.

The infant develops an elimination pattern by the second week of life. With the addition of solid food, the infant's stool gradually assumes the characteristics of an adult's stool.

Feeding Behaviors

Variations occur among infants regarding interest in food, symptoms of hunger, and amount ingested at any one time. The amount that the infant takes at any one feeding depends, of course, on the size of the infant, but other factors seem to play a part as well. For example, if put to breast, some infants nurse immediately, whereas others require a learning period of up to 48 hours before nursing can be said to be effective. Random hand-to-mouth movement and sucking of fingers have been seen in utero. These actions are well developed at birth and intensify with hunger.

Hepatic System

The liver and gallbladder are formed by the fourth week of gestation. In the newborn the liver can be palpated about 1 cm below the right costal margin, because it is enlarged and occupies about 40% of the abdominal cavity.

Iron Storage

The fetal liver (which serves as the site for production of hemoglobin after birth) begins storing iron in utero. If the mother had adequate iron intake during pregnancy, the infant will have an iron store that will last until the fifth month of life.

Conjugation of Bilirubin

The liver controls the amount of circulating unbound bilirubin. Bilirubin is a yellow pigment derived from the hemoglobin released with the breakdown of RBCs and the myoglobin in muscle cells. The hemoglobin is phagocytized by the reticuloendothelial cells, converted to bilirubin, and released in an unconjugated form. Unconjugated bilirubin, termed *indirect bilirubin,* is relatively insoluble in water and is almost entirely bound to circulating albumin, a plasma protein. The unbound bilirubin can leave the vascular system and permeate other extravascular tissues (e.g., the skin, sclera, and oral mucous membranes). The resultant yellow coloring is termed *jaundice.*

In the liver the unbound bilirubin is conjugated with glucuronide in the presence of the enzyme glucuronyltransferase. The conjugated form of bilirubin is excreted from liver cells as a constituent of bile. It is termed *direct bilirubin* and is soluble in water. Along with other components of bile, direct bilirubin is excreted into the biliary tract system that carries the bile into the duodenum. Bilirubin is converted to urobilinogen and stercobilin within the duodenum through the action of the bacterial flora. Urobilinogen is excreted in urine and feces; stercobilin is only excreted in the feces (Fig. 13-3). Total serum bilirubin is the sum of conjugated (direct) and unconjugated (indirect) bilirubin.

Adequate serum albumin-binding sites are available unless the infant experiences asphyxia neonatorum, cold stress, or hypoglycemia. Maternal prebirth ingestion of drugs, such as sulfa drugs and aspirin, can reduce the amount of serum albumin–binding sites in the newborn. Although the newborn has the functional capacity to convert bilirubin, physiologic hyperbilirubinemia occurs in most infants.

Physiologic Hyperbilirubinemia

Physiologic **hyperbilirubinemia,** or neonatal jaundice, is a normal occurrence in 50% of full-term and in 80% of preterm newborns. Korones (1986) noted that neonatal jaundice occurs because:

1. The newborn has a higher rate of bilirubin production. The number of fetal red blood cells per kilogram of weight is greater than the adult. The fetal red blood cells have a shorter survival time, 40 to 90 days compared to 120 days in the adult.
2. There is considerable reabsorption of bilirubin from the neonatal small intestine.

Although neonatal jaundice is considered benign, bilirubin may accumulate to hazardous levels and become pathologic. Linn et al (1985) reported ethnic differences in the rate of hyperbilirubinemia. They reported that 49.2% of Asian, 20% of white, and 12.1% of African-American newborns had bilirubin levels of 10 mg/dl or more. Asian and Native American newborns appear to have increased physiologic jaundice regardless of feeding

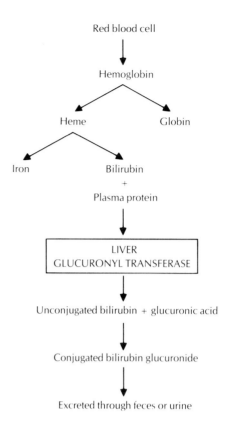

FIG. 13-3 Formation and excretion of *bilirubin.* (From Whaley, Wong: *Essentials of pediatric nursing,* ed 4, St Louis, 1993, Mosby.)

method (Auerbach, Gartner, 1987). The risk of hyperbilirubinemia increases with delayed clamping of the cord. Physiologic jaundice fulfills the following specific criteria (Korones, 1986):

(1) The infant is otherwise well; (2) in term infants, jaundice first appears after 24 hours and disappears by the end of the seventh day; (3) in premature infants, jaundice is first evident after 48 hours and disappears by the ninth or tenth day; (4) serum unconjugated bilirubin concentration does not exceed 12 mg/100 ml, either in term or preterm infants; (5) hyperbilirubinemia is almost exclusively of the unconjugated variety, and conjugated (direct) bilirubin should not exceed 1 to 1.5 mg/100 ml; (6) daily increments of bilirubin concentration should not surpass 5 mg/100 ml. Bilirubin levels in excess of 12 mg/100 ml may indicate either an exaggeration of the physiologic handicap or the presence of disease. *At any serum bilirubin level, the appearance of jaundice during the first day of life or persistence beyond the ages previously delineated usually indicates a pathologic process.*

Several nursery practices may influence the appearance and degree of physiologic hyperbilirubinemia. *Early feeding* tends to keep the serum bilirubin level low by stimulating intestinal activity and the passage of meconium and stool. Removal of intestinal contents prevents the reabsorption (and recycling) of bilirubin from the gut.

Cold stress of the newborn may result in acidosis and raise the level of free fatty acids. In the presence of acidosis, albumin binding of bilirubin is *weakened* and bilirubin is freed. *Kernicterus,* the most serious complication of neonatal hyperbilirubinemia, is caused by the precipitation of bilirubin in neuronal cells, resulting in their destruction. Cerebral palsy, mental retardation, or other neurologic problems may occur in survivors.

There is an increase in the number of mothers and infants being discharged from the hospital between 2 and 48 hours after birth, and others who elect to give birth at home. As a result, the professional attendant may not be available to assess pathologic rises in circulating unbound bilirubin. *Therefore all parents need instruction in how to assess jaundice and to whom to report the findings.*

Jaundice Associated with Breastfeeding

Two types of jaundice are associated with breastfeeding: breast*feeding* jaundice and breast *milk* jaundice. Breastfeeding jaundice is associated with the breastfeeding pattern and occurs earlier than breast milk jaundice. Breast milk jaundice is thought to be caused by the presence of an enzyme in the milk and lasts longer than breastfeeding jaundice.

Breastfeeding Jaundice

Breastfeeding jaundice usually becomes apparent about the third day of life. There is no other clinical cause. Dehydration, lack of fluid, and weight loss are not causes (Lascari, 1986; Lawrence, 1994). Recent research has documented that the number of breastfeedings during the first 3 days of life relates to bilirubin levels (Lascari, 1986). The greater the number of feedings, the lower the bilirubin level (Lascari, 1986; Lawrence, 1994). The newborn should be fed eight or more times per day. The mother is encouraged to feed her infant around the clock. Colostrum (a precursor to milk) is a natural laxative that helps promote passage of meconium. Consequently early, frequent nursings will enhance meconium excretion and decrease bilirubin levels (Lawrence, 1994).

Breast Milk Jaundice

Breast milk jaundice is defined as increasing indirect hyperbilirubinemia after the first week of life. Jaundice from ingestion of breast milk occurs in 0.5% to 2% of full-term newborns (Wilkerson, 1988). It is thought that an enzyme present in the milk of some women inhibits the enzyme glucuronyl transferase, which is necessary for the conjugation of bilirubin. Although breast milk jaundice is a form of physiologic jaundice, it occurs after the mature milk has come in, usually about the fifth or sixth day of life in a thriving infant whose mother is lactating well. This type of jaundice usually persists longer (up to 6 weeks) than breastfeeding jaundice. Unconjugated bilirubin rises beyond physiologic limits (15 to 20 mg/dl) by the seventh day. The levels subside by 5 to 10 mg if breastfeeding is discontinued for 12 to 24 hours. Usu-

ally 3 to 5 days pass before the previous high level is again reached. Mothers are encouraged to maintain their milk supply during this test period by pumping or manually expressing the milk. Mothers need reassurance that nothing is wrong with their milk (Brovten et al, 1985; Lascari, 1986; Locklin, 1987).

Immune System

The cells that supply the infant's immunity develop early in fetal life; however, they are not activated for several months. For the first 3 months of life, the infant is protected by passive immunity received from the mother. Natural barriers such as the stomach's acidity or the production of pepsin and trypsin, which maintain sterility of the small intestine, do not fully develop until 3 to 4 weeks of age (Medici, 1983). The membrane-protective IgA is missing from the respiratory and urinary tracts, and unless the newborn is breastfed, it is absent from the gastrointestinal tract as well. The infant begins to synthesize IgG, and about 40% of adult levels are reached by 1 year of age. Significant amounts of IgM are produced at birth, and adult levels are reached by 9 months of age. The production of IgA, IgD, and IgE is much more gradual, and maximum levels are not attained until early childhood. The infant who is breastfed receives passive immunity through the colostrum and the breast milk. The protection provided varies with the infant's age and maturity as well as the mother's own immune system (Lawrence, 1994)

Integumentary System

All the skin structures are present at birth but are immature. The epidermis and dermis are loosely bound and very thin. Vernix caseosa is also fused with the epidermis and serves as a protective covering. The infant's skin is very sensitive and can be easily damaged. The term infant has an erythematous skin (beefy red) for a few hours after birth, after which the skin fades to its normal color. The skin often appears blotchy or mottled, especially over the extremities. The hands and feet appear slightly cyanotic. This bluish discoloration, *acrocyanosis,* is caused by vasomotor instability, capillary stasis, and a high hemoglobin level. This is normal, transient in occurrence, and persists over the first 7 to 10 days, especially with exposure to the cold.

The healthy term newborn is plump. Subcutaneous fat accumulated during the last trimester acts to insulate the infant. The skin may be slightly tight, suggesting fluid retention. Fine *lanugo hair* may be seen on the face, shoulders, and back. Actual edema of the face and *ecchymosis* (bruising) may have resulted from face presentation or forceps birth. Petechiae may be present if increased pressure was applied to an area. Petechiae scattered over the infant's body should be reported to the pediatrician because their presence may indicate underlying problems such as low platelet count or infection.

Caput Succedaneum

Caput succedaneum is an easily identifiable edematous area of the scalp (Fig. 13-4, *A*). The sustained pressure of the presenting vertex against the cervix results in compression of local vessels, thus slowing venous return. The slower venous return causes an increase in tissue fluids within the skin of the scalp, and an edematous swelling develops. This boggy edematous swelling, present at birth, extends across suture lines of the skull and disappears spontaneously within 3 to 4 days.

Cephalhematoma

Cephalhematoma is a collection of blood between a skull bone and its periosteum. Therefore a cephalhematoma never crosses a cranial suture line (Fig. 13-4, *B*). Bleeding may occur with spontaneous birth from pressure against the maternal bony pelvis. Low forceps birth, as well as difficult forceps rotation and extraction, may also cause bleeding. This soft, fluctuating, irreducible fullness does not pulsate or bulge when the infant cries. It appears several hours after birth, the day after birth, or becomes apparent following absorption of a caput succedaneum (Fig. 13-4, *A*). It is usually largest on the second or third day, by which time the bleeding stops. The fullness of cephalhematoma spontaneously resolves in 3 to 6 weeks. It is not aspirated because infection may develop if the skin is punctured.

As the hematoma resolves, the hemolysis of RBCs occurs. Hyperbilirubinemia may result after the newborn is home. Therefore the parents are instructed to observe the newborn for jaundice and may be asked to bring the infant back to the hospital to be rechecked before the usual 4-week visit.

Desquamation

Desquamation (peeling) of the infant's skin does not occur until a few days after birth. Its presence at birth is an indication of postmaturity.

Sweat and Oil Glands

Sweat glands are present at birth but do not respond to increases in ambient or body temperature. There is some fetal *sebaceous* (oil) *gland* hyperplasia and secretion of sebum as a result of the hormonal influences of pregnancy. Vernix caseosa, a cheeselike substance, is a product of the sebaceous glands. Distended sebaceous glands, noticeable in the newborn, particularly on the chin and nose, are known as *milia*. Although sebaceous glands are well developed at birth, they are only minimally active during childhood. They become more active as androgen production increases before puberty.

Mongolian Spots

Mongolian spots, bluish-black areas of pigmentation, may appear over any part of the body's surface, including the extremities. They are more commonly noted on the back and buttocks. These pigmented areas are noted in babies whose origins are from the shores of the Mediterranean, Latin America, Asia, Africa, or a number of other areas in the world. They are more common in dark-skinned individuals regardless of race. They fade gradually over a period of months or years.

Nevi

Known as "stork bites," telangiectatic nevi are pink and easily blanched (Fig. 13-5, *A*). They appear on the upper eyelids, nose, upper lip, lower occiput bone, and nape

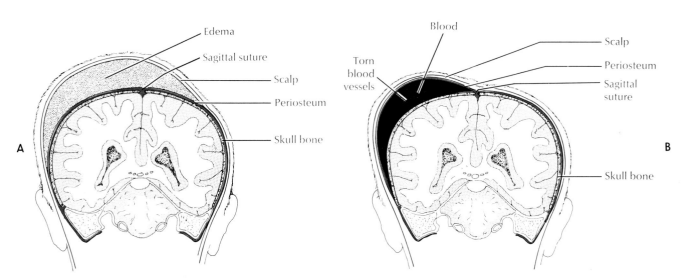

FIG. 13-4 Differences between caput succedaneum and cephalhematoma. **A,** Caput succedaneum: edema of scalp noted at birth; crosses suture line. **B,** Cephalhematoma: bleeding between periosteum and skull bone appearing within first 2 days; does not cross suture lines.

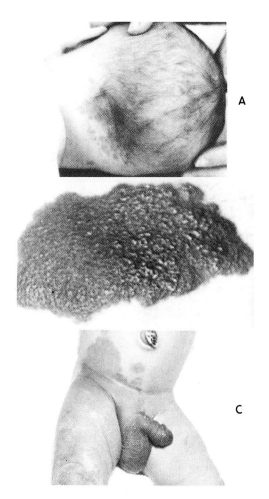

FIG. 13-5 Nevi. **A,** Telangiectatic nevi (stork bite). **B,** Strawberry mark, or nevus vasculosus. **C,** Port-wine stain, or nevus flammeus. (Courtesy Mead Johnson & Co., Evansville, IN.)

of the neck. They have no clinical significance and fade between the first and second years.

The strawberry mark, or nevus vasculosus, is the second most common type of capillary hemangioma (Fig. 13-5, B). It consists of dilated, newly formed capillaries occupying the entire dermal and subdermal layers with associated connective tissue hypertrophy. The typical lesion is a raised, sharply demarcated, bright or dark red, rough-surfaced swelling that resembles a strawberry. Lesions are usually single but may be multiple; 75% occur in the head region. These lesions can remain until the child is of school age or sometimes even longer.

A port-wine stain, or nevus flammeus, is usually observed at birth and is composed of a plexus of newly formed capillaries in the papillary layer of the corium. It is red to purple; varies in size, shape, and location; and is not elevated (Fig. 13-5, C). True port-wine stains do not blanch on pressure and do not disappear spontaneously.

Erythema Toxicum

A transient rash, erythema toxicum is also called *erythema neonatorum,* or "flea-bite" dermatitis. It has lesions in different stages, erythematous macules, papules, or small vesicles, and it may appear suddenly anywhere on the body. The rash is thought to be an inflammatory response. Eosinophils, which help decrease inflammation, are found in the vesicles. The rash is found only in term infants during the first 3 weeks after birth (Medici, 1983). Although the appearance is alarming, it has no clinical significance and requires no treatment.

Reproductive System
Female

At birth the ovaries contain thousands of primitive germ cells. These represent the full complement of potential ova, since no oogonia form after birth in term infants. The ovarian cortex, which is primarily made up of primordial follicles, forms a thicker portion of the ovary in the newborn than it does in the adult. The number of ova decreases from birth to maturity by approximately 90%.

An increase of estrogen during pregnancy followed by a drop after birth results in a mucoid vaginal discharge and even some slight bloody spotting (pseudomenstruation). External genitals are usually edematous with increased pigmentation. In term newborn infants, the labia majora and minora cover the vestibule (Fig. 13-6, A). In preterm infants, the clitoris is prominent and the labia majora are small and widely separated. Vaginal or hymenal tags are common findings and have no clinical significance.

Male

The testes descend into the scrotum in 90% of newborn boys. Although this percentage drops with preterm birth, by 1 year of age the incidence of undescended testes in all boys is less than 1%. Spermatogenesis does not occur until puberty.

A tight prepuce (foreskin) is common in newborns. The urethral opening may be completely covered by the prepuce, which may not be retractable for 3 to 4 years.

In response to maternal estrogen, external genitals in the term newborn may be increased in size and pigmentation. Rugae cover the scrotal sac (Fig. 13-6, B). Hydroceles (accumulation of fluid around the testes) are common and usually decrease in size without treatment.

Swelling of Breast Tissue

Swelling of the breast tissue in newborn infants of both sexes is caused by the increase in estrogen during pregnancy. In a few newborns a thin discharge (witch's milk) can be seen. The finding has no clinical significance, requires no treatment, and will subside as the maternal hormones are eliminated from the newborn infant's body. Breast tissue and areola size increase with gestation.

Skeletal System

The cephalocaudal direction of development is evident in total body growth. The head at term is one fourth of the body length. The arms are slightly longer than the legs.

The face is small in relation to the skull, which is comparatively larger and heavier. Cranial size and shape can be distorted by molding (shaping of the fetal head by overlapping of the cranial bones; Fig. 13-7, A).

There are two curvatures in the vertebral column: thoracic and sacral. When the infant gains head control, another curvature occurs in the cervical region.

In newborn infants there is a significant separation of the knees when the ankles are held together, which results in an appearance of bowlegs. At birth, there is no apparent arch to the foot.

The extremities should be symmetric. Fingernails and toenails should be present. There are creases on the palms of the hand. Creases cover the soles of term infants' feet, too.

Neuromuscular System

Before the late 1950s the human newborn was thought to be immature and disorganized, as well as able to function only at a brainstem level. Neurobehavioral assessment of the neonate was primarily an evaluation of primitive reflexes and muscle tone. Today the term newborn is recognized as a vital, responsive, and reactive being. The newborn's sensory development and capacity for social interaction and self-organization are remarkable (Fanaroff, Martin, 1992).

Growth of the brain after birth follows a predictable pattern of rapid growth during infancy and early childhood. This growth becomes more gradual during the remainder of the first decade and minimal during adolescence. The cerebellum ends its growth spurt, which be-

gan at about 30 weeks of gestation, by the end of the first year. Perhaps this is why the brain is vulnerable to nutritional trauma or other trauma during early infancy.

The brain requires glucose as a source of energy and a large supply of oxygen for adequate metabolism. Such requirements signal a need for careful assessment of the newborn's ability to maintain an open airway and assessment of respiratory conditions requiring oxygen therapy. The necessity for glucose requires careful monitoring of those newborn infants who may have hypoglycemic episodes (see Clinical Application of Research).

Spontaneous motor activity may be seen in transient tremors of mouth and chin, especially when crying, and of extremities, notably the arms and hands. These tremors are normal. Persistent tremors or tremors involving the total body, however, may be indicative of pathologic conditions. Marked tonicity, clonicity, and twitching of facial muscles are signs of convulsions. There is a need to distinguish normal tremors from tremors of hypoglycemia and central nervous system (CNS) disorders so that corrective care can be initiated as necessary (Parker et al, 1990).

Neuromuscular control in the newborn, although still very limited, can be noted. If newborns are placed facedown on a firm surface, they will turn their heads to the side to maintain an airway. They attempt to hold their heads in line with their bodies if they are raised by their arms.

Newborn Reflexes

The normal infant has many primitive reflexes. The times at which these newborn reflexes appear and disappear reflect the maturity and intactness of the developing nervous system.

The most common reflexes found in the normal newborn are described in Table 13-6.

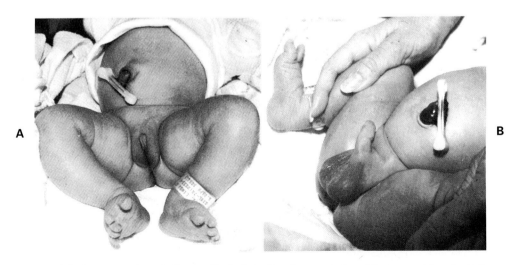

FIG. 13-6 External genitalia. **A,** Genitals in female term infant. Note mucoid vaginal discharge. **B,** Genitals in male infant. Uncircumcised penis. Rugae cover scrotum, indicating term gestation. Cord has been swabbed with ethylene blue to prevent infection.

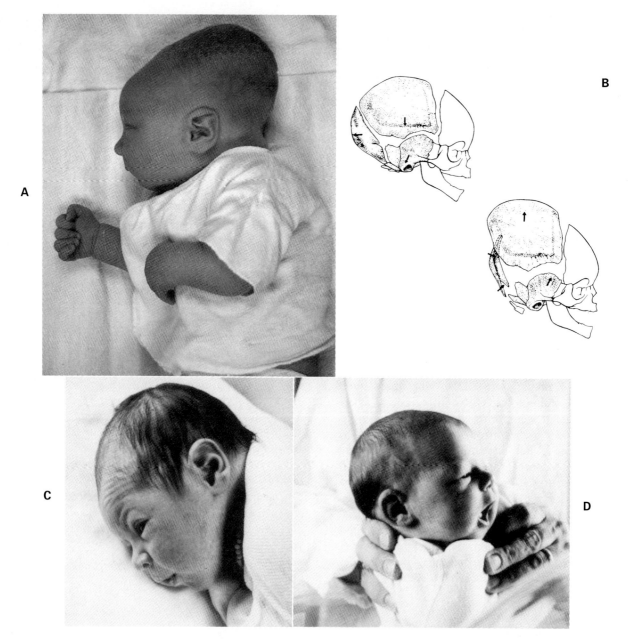

FIG. 13-7 Molding. **A,** Significant molding, soon after birth. **B,** Schematic of bones of skull when molding is present. **C,** Some resolution of molding on second or third day of life, **D,** Molding resolved.

Thermogenic System

Thermogenesis means the production of heat (thermo = heat, genesis = origin). Effective neonatal care is based on the maintenance of an optimum thermal environment. The narrow limits of normal body temperature are maintained by producing heat in response to its dissipation. Hypothermia from excessive heat loss is a prevalent and dangerous problem in newborn infants. The newborn's ability to produce heat often approaches the capacity of an adult. However, the tendency toward rapid heat loss in a cool, thermal environment increases and often becomes hazardous to the newborn (Table 13-2).

Heat Production

The shivering mechanism of heat production is rarely operable in the newborn. Nonshivering thermogenesis is accomplished primarily by *brown fat* which is unique to the newborn (Blackburn, Loper, 1992; Fanaroff, Martin, 1992), and secondarily accomplished by increased metabolic activity in the brain, heart, and liver. Brown fat is located in superficial deposits in the interscapular region and axillae, as well as in deep deposits at the thoracic inlet, along the vertebral column, and around the kidneys. Brown fat has a richer vascular and nerve supply than ordinary fat. Heat produced by intense lipid

CLINICAL APPLICATION OF RESEARCH

FACTORS ASSOCIATED WITH HYPOGLYCEMIA

Hypoglycemia in a newborn is usually considered to be a mild condition that can easily be treated by feeding. However, if hypoglycemia is not recognized or remains untreated, then serious problems, including death, can result. The incidence of hypoglycemia is usually reported as 4%. This retrospective study was conducted by identifying infants who were hypoglycemic and then reviewing the charts of the infants and their mothers. The purpose of the study was to (a) determine the incidence of hypoglycemia, (b) identify antenatal factors associated with hypoglycemia, and (c) describe symptoms in healthy term newborns. The sample included 168 infants, 101 born vaginally and 57 by cesarean birth. Hypoglycemia occurred in 17 (10.7%) of the infants, and this rate was higher in infants born by cesarean (15.7%) than in those born by the vaginal route (7.9%).

The most significant factor associated with hypoglycemia was the infusion of 3000 ml or more of lactated Ringer's solution intravenously during labor. The major symptoms that nurses observed in hypoglycemic newborns were jitteriness, tachypnea, and hypotonia. Nurses working with newborn infants should be familiar with signs of hypoglycemia in the neonate. Infants born by cesarean birth, or of mothers who received large amount of intravenous fluids during labor, should be closely observed. Nurses can prevent adverse sequelae by careful observation and treatment of newborn infants who experience hypoglycemia.

Reference: Cole MD: New factors associated with the incidence of hypoglycemia: a research study, *Neonatal Network* 10(4):47, 1991.

metabolic activity in brown fat can warm the newborn by increasing heat production as much as 100%. Reserves of brown fat, usually present for several weeks after birth, are rapidly depleted with cold stress. The less mature the infant, the less reserve of this essential fat is available at birth.

Temperature Regulation

Anatomic and physiologic differences between the newborn and an adult are notable:

1. The newborn's thermal insulation is less than an adult's. Blood vessels are closer to the surface of the skin. Changes in environmental temperature alter blood temperature, thereby influencing temperature-regulating centers in the hypothalamus.
2. The newborn has a larger body surface to body weight (mass) ratio. The flexed position assumed by the newborn safeguards against heat loss, because it substantially diminishes the amount of body surface exposed to the hostile thermal environment
3. The newborn's vasomotor control is not as well developed, however, the ability to constrict subcutaneous and skin vessels is as efficient in preterm infants as it is in adults.
4. The newborn produces heat primarily by nonshivering thermogenesis.
5. The newborn's sweat glands have little function until the fourth week or more of extrauterine life.

In response to the discomfort of lower environmental temperature, the normal term infant may try to increase body temperature by crying or by increased mo-

TABLE 13-2	Mechanisms of Heat Loss in the Newborn	
DEFINITION	**NURSING IMPLICATION**
CONVECTION	
Flow of heat from the body surface to cooler ambient air	Maintain nursery ambient temperature at 24° C (75° F). Wrap the newborn to protect from the cold.
RADIATION	
Loss of heat from the body surface to cooler solid surfaces that are not in direct contact with each other, but in relative proximity to each other	Place nursery cribs and examining tables away from outside windows.
EVAPORATION	
Loss of heat that occurs when a liquid is converted to a vapor (e.g., vaporization of moisture from the skin); invisible vapor, also known as insensible water loss (IWL)	Dry infant after birth. Bathe and dry infant rapidly in a warm environment.
CONDUCTION	
Loss of heat from the body surface to cooler surfaces that are in direct contact with each other	At birth wrap the newborn in a warmed blanket. Place the infant in a warmed bed.

tor activity. Crying increases the work load, and the cost of energy (calories) may be expensive, particularly in a compromised infant.

Cold Stress

Cold stress imposes metabolic and physiologic problems on all newborn infants, regardless of gestational age and condition (see Fig. 13-8). The respiratory rate increases as a response to the increased need for oxygen when the oxygen consumption increases significantly in cold stress. Oxygen consumption and energy in the cold-stressed newborn are diverted from maintaining normal brain cell and cardiac function and growth to thermogenesis for survival.

If the newborn infant cannot maintain an adequate oxygen tension, vasoconstriction follows and jeopardizes pulmonary perfusion. As a consequence, arterial blood gas levels of Po_2 decrease, and the blood pH drops. These changes may cause respiratory distress or aggravate existing respiratory distress syndrome (RDS), also known as hyaline membrane disease (HMD). Moreover, decreased pulmonary perfusion and oxygen tension may maintain or reopen the right-to-left shunt across the patent ductus arteriosus.

The basal metabolic rate increases with cold stress. If cold stress is prolonged, anaerobic glycolysis occurs, resulting in increased production of acids. Metabolic acidosis develops, and if there is a defect in respiratory function, respiratory acidosis also develops. Excessive fatty acids displace the bilirubin from the albumin-binding sites. The resulting increased level of circulating unbound bilirubin increases the risk of kernicterus even at serum bilirubin levels of 10 mg/dl or less.

BEHAVIORAL CHARACTERISTICS

The healthy newborn infant must achieve both biologic and behavioral tasks to develop normally. Behavioral characteristics form the basis of the newborn's social capabilities. Through the first half of this century the focus of developmental research was on how the environment affected the newborn. Infants were considered to have been born with neither personality nor the ability to interact.

Today it is recognized that newborns are well equipped to begin social interactions with their parents immediately after birth. Research indicates that individual personalities and behavioral characteristics of newborn infants play a major role in the ultimate relationship between infants and their parents.

Brazelton (1984) noted the importance of the newborn's behavioral states. They believe that the behavioral responses of newborn infants are indicative of cortical control, responsiveness, and eventual management of the infant's environment. They emphasize the importance of infant-parent interaction. By their responses infants act to either consolidate relationships or alienate the people in their immediate environment. By their actions they encourage or discourage attachment and caregiving activities. The development of parent-child love does not occur without feedback. The absence of feedback, because of separation or incorrectly interpreted feedback, can impair the growth of parental love.

One of the first tasks parents must accomplish is to become aware of the unique behavioral responses of their newborn infant. Brazelton (1969) demonstrated that

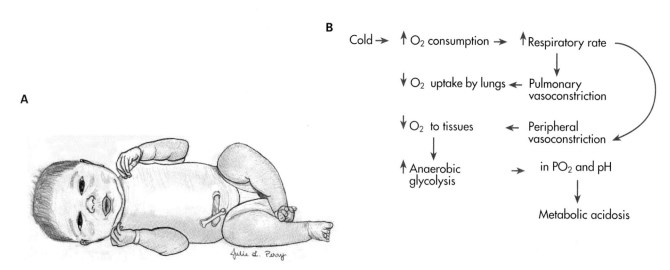

FIG. 13-8 Effects of cold stress. When an infant is stressed by cold, oxygen consumption increases, pulmonary and peripheral vasoconstriction occur, thereby decreasing oxygen uptake by the lungs and oxygen to the tissues; anaerobic glycolysis increases, and there is an increase in Po_2 and pH leading to metabolic acidosis. (**A**, courtesy Julie L. Perry.)

normal newborns differ from one another in such things as activity (active, average, quiet), feeding patterns, sleeping patterns, and responsiveness from the moment of birth. The **Brazelton Neonatal Behavioral Assessment Scale (NBAS)** is used to rate the newborn's unique characteristics, dependent, in part, on the newborn's sleep-wake state. Brazelton suggested that the parents' reaction to their newborn infant is partially determined by these differences.

Behavioral characteristics, like physical characteristics, change during the **transition period.** This period is made up of phases of instability through which the infant passes during the first 6 to 8 hours after birth. Knowledge of these phases and the parents presence during the infant's reactive phases help promote attachment and successful feeding.

The newborn is in a state of quiet alertness during the *first period of reactivity.* The eyes are open and alert. The newborn can focus attention on the parents' faces and attend to voices, especially the voice of the mother. This phase lasts about 15 minutes and is followed by a phase of *active alertness.* During this active alert period, the newborn has frequent bursts of movement and may cry. The infant demonstrates a strong sucking reflex and may appear hungry. This is a good time to initiate breastfeeding.

The first period of reactivity facilitates attachment. Parents should have time to hold and talk to their newborn. Eye-to-eye contact can be fostered by delaying eye treatment so the baby can interact with the parents.

After this first 30 minutes the newborn becomes drowsy and falls asleep. The newborn appears relaxed and is unresponsive and difficult to awaken during this period. This period of *inactivity* may last from 2 to 4 hours.

After the rest period the newborn enters the *second period of reactivity.* Once again the newborn is awake and alert and demonstrates states of quiet alertness, active alertness, and crying. This period may last 4 to 6 hours in a normal newborn. Feeding may be initiated if it was not begun during the first period of reactivity. The newborn sucks, roots, and swallows during this second period of reactivity and becomes interested in feeding.

Sleep-Wake Cycles

Variations in *state of consciousness* of newborn infants are called the **sleep-wake cycles** (Brazelton, 1984). These cycles form a continuum with deep sleep, narcosis, or lethargy at one end and extreme irritability at the other end. There are two sleep states: deep sleep and light sleep, and four wake states: drowsiness, quiet alert, active alert, and crying. The ability of infants to control or modify their responses varies as they move from a particular sleep or wake state to another. Their reactions to external and internal stimuli reflect their potential for organization of behavior.

Organization of behavior refers to integrated functioning of an infant's physiologic and behavioral systems (D'Apolito, 1991). Organized infants can process external events without disrupting their physiologic and behavioral functioning. Table 13-3 compares the physiologic and behavioral responses of an infant in organized and disorganized states. As shown in Table 13-4, each state has its own distinguishing characteristics and **state-related behaviors.** The quiet alert state is also known as the optimum state of arousal. During this state newborn infants may be observed smiling, vocalizing, or moving in synchrony. Even during the first day of life, smiling is evident in a surprising number of infants (Bamford et al, 1990). Newborn infants seem to watch their parents' faces carefully and respond to other persons talking to them. They move their bodies in coordination with voices and movement of the speaker's body (Condon, Sander, 1974). Brazelton (1969) noted that this synchronous movement gives feedback to the speaker and encourages more interaction. Infants imitate facial gestures (tongue protrusion, opening the mouth) by 2 weeks of age. Also by 2 weeks of age, many infants begin a type of vocalizing by making small, cooing, throaty noises while feeding.

The infant uses purposeful behavior to maintain the optimum state of arousal, for example: (1) active withdrawal by increasing physical distance, (2) a rejecting motion of pushing away with hands and feet, (3) decreasing sensitivity by falling asleep or breaking eye contact by turning the head, or (4) use of signaling behavior, fussing, or crying (Brazelton, 1984). Use of such behaviors permits infants to quiet themselves and reinstate readiness to interact.

The newborn sleeps a total of about 17 hours a day, with the periods of wakefulness gradually increasing. By the fourth week of life, some infants stay awake from one feeding session to the next.

Other Factors Influencing Neonatal Behavior

Several other variables, in addition to sleep-wake state, affect the newborn's responses. These are discussed below.

The *gestational age* of the infant and level of central nervous system (CNS) maturity will affect observed behavior. An infant with an immature CNS will have an entire body response to a pinprick of the foot. The mature infant will withdraw the foot. CNS immaturity will also be reflected in reflex development and sleep-wake cycles.

Length of *time* to recuperate from labor and birth will affect the behavior of newborn infants as they attempt to become organized. The time since the last feeding and the time of day may influence newborns' responses, too.

Environmental events and *stimuli* will have an effect on the behavioral responses of newborn infants. Nurses in intensive care nurseries observe that infants respond to loud noises, bright lights, monitor alarms, and tension in the unit. It has been well documented that new-

TABLE 13-3 Infant Responses that Depict Organization and Disorganization

ORGANIZATION	DISORGANIZATION
PHYSIOLOGIC FUNCTIONING	**PHYSIOLOGIC FUNCTIONING**
1. Stable heart and respiratory rates	1. Fluctuations in heart and respiratory rates that may result in apnea or bradycardia
2. Stable color	2. Color changes from pink to pale or dusky
3. Tolerance of feedings	3. Increased stooling and inability to tolerate feedings
	4. Hiccoughs or sneezing
	5. Gagging or yawning
	6. Blood pressure instability
BEHAVIORAL FUNCTIONING	**BEHAVIORAL FUNCTIONING**
1. Smooth and synchronous body movements	1. Frantic body movements and jitteriness, changes in muscle tone to flacid or limp
2. Smooth transitions between sleep and wake states	2. Inability to modulate state, sudden state changes, and/or prolongation of the alert state
3. Utilization of self-consoling behaviors such as finger sucking, hand-to-face maneuvers, position changes, and anchoring of extremities against animate or inanimate objects	3. Limited use of self-consoling behaviors
4. Consolable from an external source when upset	4. Inability to be consoled
5. Ability to "shut out" or habituate to noxious or repetitive stimuli by decreasing body movements and/or modulating from an awake to a sleep state	5. Inability to habituate or decrease motor and state responses to noxious or repeated stimuli

From D'Apolito K: What is an organized infant? *Neonatal Network* 10(1):24, 1991.

born infants of mothers who are tense have more muscle activity and their heart rates change to become parallel to their mothers' during feeding. In addition, the newborn responds differently to animate and inanimate stimulation.

There is controversy concerning the effects on newborn infant behavior of *maternal medication* (analgesia, anesthesia) during labor. Some researchers have noted that infants of mothers who were given medications may continue to demonstrate poor state organization beyond the fifth day (Kangas-Saarela et al, 1989). Others believe that the effect can be beneficial or that no effect exists.

Some of the most interesting research findings have been the ethnic differences in infant behavior (Chitty, Winter, 1989; Freedman, 1979). Freedman and Freedman (1969) found that Chinese-American infants had more self-quieting activities, fewer state changes, and more rapid responses to consoling activities than did white American infants. A study of Navajo newborns paralleled the stereotype of the stoic, impassive Native American (Freedman, 1979). Among Navajo babies, crying was rare, limb movements were reduced and calming was almost immediate after tests for Moro's reflex. In Freedman's study (1979), Japanese newborns were more sensitive and irritable than either the Chinese or Navajo newborns. Mexican mothers use tactile stimulation more often than vocalization to quiet their newborns (Garcia Coll, 1990). The Zincanteco Indians in southern Mexico demonstrated greater motor maturity and increased ability to maintain quiet alert states for longer times than American infants (Brazelton, 1969).

These studies suggest that neonatal behavior represents a behavioral phenotype, which expresses a complex relation among genetic endowment, intrauterine environment, and maternal obstetric history.

Sensory Behaviors

From birth, infants possess **sensory behaviors** that indicate a state of readiness for social interaction. Infants are able to use behavioral responses effectively in establishing their first dialogues. These responses, coupled with the newborns' "baby appearance" (the face is proportioned so that the forehead and eyes are larger than the lower portion of the face) and their smallness and helplessness, rouse feelings of wanting to hold, protect, and interact with them.

Vision

At birth the pupils react to light and the blink reflex is easily elicited. Tear glands usually do not begin to function until the infant is 2 to 4 weeks old. The clearest visual distance is 17 to 20 cm (7 to 8 in), which is about the distance the newborn infant's face is from the mother's face as she breastfeeds or cuddles. Newborn infants are sensitive to light. They will frown if a bright light is flashed in their eyes and will turn toward a soft red light. If the room is darkened, they will open their eyes widely and look about. This is noticeable when the birth area is darkened after birth.

Response to movement is noticeable. If a bright object is shown to newborns (even at 15 minutes of age), they will follow it with their eyes, and some will even

TABLE 13-4 Behavioral States and State Behavior

STATE	BODY ACTIVITY	EYE MOVEMENTS	FACIAL MOVEMENTS	RESPIRATORY PATTERN	LEVEL OF RESPONSE
			CHARACTERISTICS OF STATE		
SLEEP STATES					
Deep sleep	Nearly still, except for occasional startle or twitch	None	Without facial movements, except for occasional sucking movement at regular intervals	Smooth and regular	Threshold to stimuli is very high so that only very intense and disturbing stimuli will arouse infants.
Light sleep	Some body movements	Rapid eye movements (REM), fluttering of eyes beneath closed eyelids	May smile and make brief fussy or crying sounds	Irregular	More responsive to internal and external stimuli. When these stimuli occur, infants may remain in light sleep, return to deep sleep, or arouse to drowsy.
AWAKE STATES					
Drowsy	Activity level variable, with mild startles interspersed from time to time. Movements usually smooth	Eyes open and close occasionally, are heavy-lidded with dull, glazed appearance	May have some facial movements; often there are none, and face appears still	Irregular	Infants react to sensory stimuli although responses are delayed. State change after stimulation frequently noted.
Quiet alert	Minimal	Brightening and widening of eyes	Faces have bright, shining, sparkling looks	Regular	Infants attend most to environment, focusing attention on any stimuli that are present. Optimum state of arousal.
Active alert	Much body activity; may have periods of fussiness	Eyes open with less brightening	Much facial movement; faces not as bright as quiet alert state	Irregular	Increasingly sensitive to disturbing stimuli (hunger, fatigue, noise, excessive handling).
Crying	Increased motor activity, with color changes	Eyes may be tightly closed or open	Grimaces	More irregular	Extreme response to unpleasant external or internal stimuli.

From Barnard KE et al: Behavioral states and state behaviors. In *Early parent-infant relationships*, White Plains, NY, 1978, March of Dimes Birth Defects Foundation. Reprinted by permission.

turn their heads to do so. Because human eyes are bright shiny objects, newborns will track them.

Visual acuity is surprising; even at 2 weeks of age infants can distinguish patterns with stripes 3 mm (⅛ in) apart. They prefer to look at black and white patterns rather than plain surfaces, even if the latter are brightly colored (Luddington-Hoe, 1983). They also prefer more complex patterns to simple ones. They prefer novelty (changes in pattern) by 2 months of age. This is significant knowledge, since it means the infant of a few weeks of age is capable of responding actively to an enriched environment.

From birth onward, infants are able to fix their eyes and gaze intently at objects. They gaze at their parents' faces and respond to changes in them. This ability permits parents and children to gaze into each other's eyes, and a subtle communication pattern results. Eye contact is very important in parent-infant interactions. Children of blind parents and parents who have blind children must circumvent this obstacle for the formation of a relationship.

Hearing

As soon as the amniotic fluid drains from the ear, the infant's hearing is similar to an adult's. This may occur as early as 1 minute of age. Loud sounds of about 90 decibels cause the infant to respond with a startle reflex. The newborn responds to low-frequency sounds, such as a heartbeat or a lullaby, by decreasing motor activity or crying. The response to a high-frequency sound elicits an alerting reaction (Barr, 1990). Screening for hearing impairment can occur in the newborn using auditory brainstem response (Letko, 1992).

The infant responds readily to the mother's voice (Brazelton, 1984; Curnock, 1989; Redshaw, Rivers, Rosenblatt, 1985). This may be a response to having heard or felt sound waves from the mother's voice while the infant was in utero.

All these studies indicate a selective listening to the maternal voice sounds and rhythms during intrauterine life that prepares newborns for recognition and interaction with their primary caregivers—their mothers. Fetuses are accustomed in the uterus to hearing the regular rhythm of the mother's heartbeat. As a result newborns respond by relaxing and ceasing to fuss and cry if a regular heartbeat simulator is placed in their cribs.

Touch

The infant is responsive to touch on all parts of the body. The face, especially the mouth, the hands, and the soles of the feet appear to be the most sensitive. Reflexes can be elicited by stroking the infant. The newborn's responses to touch suggest this sensory system is well prepared to receive and process tactile messages. Touch and motion have been reported as being essential to normal growth and development (Gunzenhauser, 1990). However, each infant is unique, and variations can be seen in newborns' responses to touch.

The new mother uses touch as one of the first interaction behaviors: fingertip touch, soft stroking of the face, and gentle massage of the back. Birth trauma or stress and depressant drugs taken by the mother decrease the infant's sensitivity to touch or painful stimuli.

Taste

The newborn has a well-developed taste system, and different solutions elicit different facial expressions. A tasteless solution produces no response whereas a sweet solution causes eager sucking. A sour solution results in puckering of the lips, and a bitter solution causes anger. Newborns have been reported to prefer glucose water over sterile water (Pete, 1989). These studies demonstrate not only the newborn's response to various tastes but also the strength of the taste response and its independence from cortical levels of the nervous system.

It is generally accepted that young infants are oriented toward the use of their mouths both for meeting their nutritional needs for rapid growth and for releasing tension through sucking. The early development of circumoral sensation, muscle activity, and taste would seem to be preparation for survival in the extrauterine environment.

Smell

The newborn's sense of smell is well developed at birth. Newborns appear to react similarly to adults when exposed to strong or pleasant odors. Breastfed infants are able to smell breast milk and can differentiate their mothers from other lactating women (Lawrence, 1994). Bottle-fed female babies prefer the breast odor of a nursing woman to the breast odor from a nonlactating woman (Makin, Porter, 1989). These maternal odors are believed to influence bonding and adequate feeding (Porter, Cernoch, Perry, 1983).

The significance of smell in maternal identification of offspring and vice versa in the animal world is well documented. Human mothers are also able to distinguish between the odors of shirts worn by their own infant, and those worn by an unfamiliar infant (Porter, Cernoch, McLaughlin, 1983). Stainton (1985) noted that mothers notice their infants smell different from other infants from birth onward.

Response to Environmental Stimuli

Infants respond to the environment in a number of ways. Classic studies have identified individual variations in the primary reaction pattern of newborns and described them as *temperament* (Thomas, 1961, 1970).

Temperament

There are individual differences in behavioral styles of infants during the first few weeks of life. These differences are not related to the personalities of their parents or how the infants are handled. The characteristic temperament style persists in most infants.

Chess's work (1969) led to the recognition of three major behavioral styles or temperament patterns:

1. The easy child who demonstrates regularity in bodily functions, readily adapts to change, has a predominantly positive mood, a moderate sensory threshold, and approaches new situations or objects with a response of moderate intensity.
2. The slow-to-warm-up child who has a low activity level, withdraws on first exposure to new stimuli, is slow to adapt, low in intensity of response, and is somewhat negative in mood.
3. The difficult child who is irregular in bodily functions, intense in reactions, generally negative in mood, resistant to change or new stimuli, and often cries loudly for long periods.

The human newborn possesses sensory receptors capable of responding selectively to various stimuli present in the internal and external environment. Infants also possess individual characteristics that define them as unique personalities.

Habituation

Habituation is a protective mechanism. It allows the infant to become accustomed to environmental stimuli. Habituation is a psychologic and physiologic phenomenon whereby the response to a constant or repetitive stimuli decreases. The term newborn demonstrates this in several ways. Shining a bright light into a newborn's eyes will cause a startle or squinting the first two or three times. The third or fourth flash will elicit a diminished response and by the fifth or sixth flash, the infant ceases to respond (Brazelton, 1984). The same response pattern holds true for the sounds of a rattle or a pinprick to a heel. Newborns presented with new stimuli become wide-eyed and alter their gaze for a time but eventually will show a diminished interest.

The ability to habituate also allows the newborn to select stimuli that promote continued learning about the social world, thus avoiding overload. The intrauterine experiences seem to have programmed the newborn to be especially responsive to human voices, soft lights, soft sounds, and sweet tastes.

Consolability

Korner (1971) reported studies that describe variations in the ability of newborns to console themselves or to be consoled. In the crying state, most initiate one of several ways to reduce their distress. Hand-to-mouth movements are common, with or without sucking, as well as alerting to voices, noises, or visual stimuli.

Cuddliness

Cuddliness is especially important to new parents because they gauge their ability to care for the newborn by the newborn's responses to their actions. The degree to which newborns will mold into the contours of the person holding them varies. Barr (1990) tested the effect of body contact and vestibular stimulation in both soothing babies and creating alertness. The vestibular stimulation of being picked up and moved had the greater effect on newborns.

Irritability

Some newborns cry longer and harder than others do. For some the sensory threshold seems low. They are readily upset by unusual noises, hunger, wetness, or new experiences, and they respond intensely. Others with a high sensory threshold require a great deal more stimulation and variation to reach the active, alert state (Barr, 1990).

Crying

Crying in an infant is a means of communication and may signal hunger, pain, desire for attention, or fussiness. Some mothers say that they can distinguish the reasons for crying. A hunger cry is often loud and prolonged, not ceasing until the infant is fed. A pain cry is higher pitched and piercing. A fussy cry may be lower pitched and varying in its intensity.

PHYSICAL ASSESSMENT

The nurse uses knowledge of the biologic and behavioral characteristics of the newborn as a basis for the care of the infant and the teaching and counseling of the parents.

Biologic characteristics are demonstrated through physical assessment. Average findings, normal variations, and deviations from normal range are all displayed in Table 13-5. These findings provide a data base for implementing the nursing process with newborns (and their families) discussed in Chapter 14.

The physical assessment given by nurses includes a neurologic assessment of the newborn's reflexes. This provides useful information about the infant's nervous system and state of neurologic maturation. Many of the reflex behaviors are important for survival, for example, sucking and rooting. Other reflex behaviors such as gagging, coughing, and sneezing act as safety mechanisms. The assessment needs to be carried out as early as possible because abnormal signs present in the early neonatal period may disappear. These signs may reappear months or years later as abnormal functions. Table 13-6 gives the techniques for eliciting significant reflexes and characteristic responses.

The assessment should be conducted in a warm, well-lit environment. Performing the assessment in the presence of the parents provides the opportunity to incorporate teaching about normal responses and behaviors into the assessment.

TABLE 13-5 Physical Assessment of Newborn

AREA ASSESSED AND APPRAISAL PROCEDURE	NORMAL FINDINGS		DEVIATIONS FROM NORMAL RANGE: POSSIBLE PROBLEMS (ETIOLOGY)
	AVERAGE FINDINGS	NORMAL VARIATIONS	
POSTURE			
Inspect newborn before disturbing for assessment Refer to maternal chart for fetal presentation, position, and type of birth (vaginal, surgical), since newborn readily assumes prenatal position	Vertex: arms, legs in moderate flexion; fists are clenched Newborn resists having extremities extended for examination or measurement and may cry when this is attempted Crying ceases when allowed to reassume curled-up fetal position Normal spontaneous movement is bilaterally asynchronous (legs move in bicycle fashion) but equally extensive in all extremities	Frank breech: legs are straighter and stiff; newborn will assume intrauterine position in repose for a few days Prenatal pressure on limb or shoulder may cause temporary facial asymmetry or resistance to extension of extremities	Hypotonia, relaxed posture while awake (prematurity or hypoxia in utero, maternal medications) Hypertonia (drug dependence, CNS disorder) Opisthotonos (CNS disturbance) Limitation of motion in any of extremities (see Extremities, p. 350-351)
VITAL SIGNS			

Heart rate and pulses
  Thorax (chest)
    Inspection
    Palpation
    Auscultation
    Apex: mitral valve
    Second interspace, left of sternum: pulmonic valve
    Second interspace, right of sternum: aortic valve
    Junction of xiphoid process and sternum: tricuspid valve
	Pulsations visible in left midclavicular line; fifth intercostal space
	Apical pulse; fourth intercostal space 120 to 160 beats/min
	Quality: *first sound* (closure of mitral and tricuspid valves) and *second sound* (closure of aortic and pulmonic valves) should be sharp and clear
		100 (sleeping) to 160 (crying); may be irregular for brief periods, especially after crying
		Murmurs, especially over base or at left sternal border in interspace 3 or 4 (foramen ovale anatomically closes at about 1 year)
			Tachycardia: persistent; ≥160 (RDS)
			Bradycardia: persistent: ≤120 (congenital heart block)
			Murmurs (may be functional)
			Arrhythmias: irregular rate
			Sounds
			  Distant (pneumomediastinum)
			  Poor quality
			  Extra
			  Heart on right side of chest: dextrocardia; often accompanied by reversal of intestines

Femoral pulse palpation: place fingers along inguinal ligament about midway between symphysis pubis and iliac crest; feel bilaterally simultaneously	Femoral pulses should be equal and strong		Weak or absent femoral pulses (hip dysplasia, coarctation of aorta, thrombophlebitis)

Temperature
  Axillary: method of choice until 6 years of age
  Electronic: thermistor probe (avoid taping over bony area)
	Axillary: 37° C (98.6° F)
	Temperature stabilized by 8 to 10 hours of age
	Shivering mechanism undeveloped
		36.5° to 37.2° C (97.6° to 99° F)
		Heat loss: 200 kcal/kg/min from evaporation, conduction, convection, radiation
			Subnormal (prematurity, infection, low environmental temperature, inadequate clothing, dehydration)

TABLE 13-5   Physical Assessment of Newborn—cont'd

AREA ASSESSED AND APPRAISAL PROCEDURE	NORMAL FINDINGS		DEVIATIONS FROM NORMAL RANGE: POSSIBLE PROBLEMS (ETIOLOGY)
	AVERAGE FINDINGS	NORMAL VARIATIONS	
VITAL SIGNS—cont'd			
			Increased (infection, high environmental temperature, excessive clothing, proximity to heating unit or in direct sunshine, drug addiction, diarrhea and dehydration)
			Temperature not stabilized by 10 hours after birth (if mother received magnesium sulfate, newborn is less able to conserve heat by vasoconstriction; maternal analgesics may reduce thermal stability in newborn)

Respiratory rate and effort
Observe respirations when infant is at rest
Count respirations for full minute
Apnea monitor
Listen for sounds audible without stethoscope
Observe respiratory effort
	40/min
	Tend to be shallow, and when infant is awake, irregular in rate, rhythm, and depth
	No sounds should be audible on inspiration or expiration
	Breath sounds: bronchial; loud, clear, near
		30 to 60/min
		May appear to be Cheyne-Stokes with short periods of apnea and with no evidence of respiratory distress
		First period (reactivity): 50 to 60/min
		Second period: 50 to 70/min
		Stabilization (1 to 2 days): 30 to 40/min
			Apneic episodes: ≥15 sec (preterm infant: "periodic breathing," rapid warming or cooling of infant)
			Bradypnea: ≤25/min (maternal narcosis from analgesics or anesthetics, birth trauma)
			Tachypnea: ≥60/min (RDS, aspiration syndrome, diaphragmatic hernia; (TTN transient tachypnea of newborn)
			Sounds
			  Crackles, rhonchi, wheezes (fluid in lungs)
			  Expiratory grant (narrowing of bronchi)
			Distress evidenced by nasal flaring, retractions, chin tug, labored breathing (RDS, fluid in lungs)

Blood pressure (BP) (usually assessed only if a problem is suspected)
Electronic monitor
BP cuff: BP cuff width affects readings; use cuff 2.5 cm (1 in) wide and palpate radial pulse
	78/42 (approximately)
	At birth
	  Systolic: 60 to 80 mm Hg
	  Diastolic: 40 to 50 mm Hg
	At 10 days
	  Systolic: 95 to 100 mm Hg
	  Diastolic: slight increase
		Varies with change in activity level: awake, crying, sleeping	Difference between upper and lower extremity pressures (coarctation of aorta)
			Hypotension (sepsis, hypovolemia)
			Hypertension (coarctation of aorta)

Continued.

TABLE 13-5 Physical Assessment of Newborn—cont'd

AREA ASSESSED AND APPRAISAL PROCEDURE	NORMAL FINDINGS		DEVIATIONS FROM NORMAL RANGE: POSSIBLE PROBLEMS (ETIOLOGY)
	AVERAGE FINDINGS	NORMAL VARIATIONS	
WEIGHT*			
Put protective liner cloth or paper in place and adjust scale to 0 (Fig. 13-9) Weigh at same time each day Protect newborn from heat loss	Female 　3400 g (7 lb 8 oz) Male 　3500 g (7 lb 11 oz) Regain birth weight within first 2 weeks	2500 to 4000 g (5 lb 8 oz to 8 lb 13 oz) Acceptable weight loss: 10% or less White baby generally weighs ½ lb more than infants of other races Second baby weighs more than first	Weight ≤2500 g (prematurity, small for gestational age, rubella syndrome) Weight ≥4000 g (large for gestational age, maternal diabetes, heredity: normal for these parents) Weight loss over 10% (dehydration)
LENGTH			
Measure length from top of head to heel; difficult to measure in term infant because of presence of molding, incomplete extension of knees (Fig. 13-10, *C*)	50 cm (20 in)	45 to 55 cm (18 to 22 in)	<45 or >55 cm (chromosomal aberration, heredity: normal for these parents)
HEAD CIRCUMFERENCE			
Measure head at greatest diameter: occipitofrontal circumference (Fig. 13-10, *A*) May need to remeasure on second or third day after resolution of molding and caput succedaneum	33 to 35 cm (13 to 14 in) Circumference of head and chest may be about the same for first 1 or 2 days after birth	32 to 36.8 cm (12½ to 14½ in)	Small head ≤32 cm: microcephaly (rubella, toxoplasmosis, cytomegalic inclusion disease) Hydrocephaly: sutures widely separated, circumference ≥4 cm more than chest Increased intracranial pressure (hemorrhage, space-occupying lesion)
CHEST CIRCUMFERENCE			
Measure at nipple line (Fig. 13-10, *B*)	2 cm (¾ in) less than head circumference; averages between 30 to 33 cm (12 to 13 in)		≤30 cm (prematurity)
ABDOMINAL CIRCUMFERENCE			
Measure below umbilicus (Fig. 13-10, *D*) (not usually measured unless specific indication)	Abdomen enlarges after feeding because of lax abdominal muscles Same size as chest		Enlarging abdomen between feedings (abdominal mass or blockage in intestinal tract)

*NOTE: Weight, length, and head circumference should all be close to same percentile for any child.

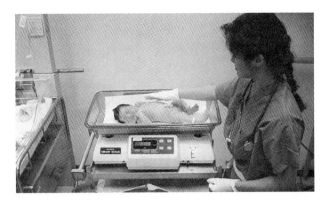

FIG. 13-9 Weighing infant. Note hand is held over infant as a safety measure. Scale is covered to protect against cross-infection.

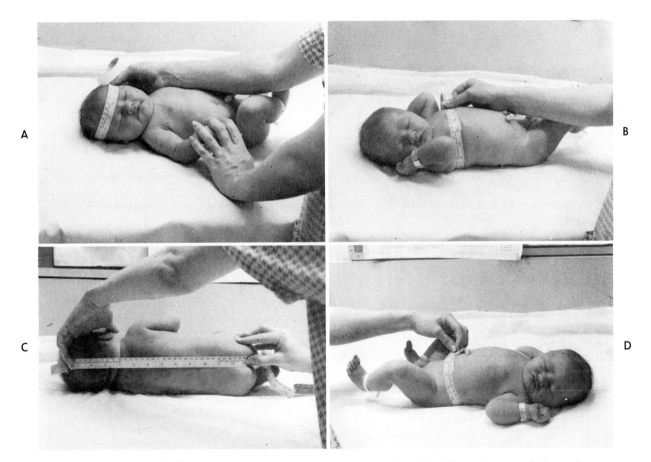

FIG. 13-10 Measurements. **A,** Circumference of head. **B,** Circumference of chest. **C,** Length, crown to rump. To determine total length, length of legs is included. **D,** Abdominal circumference.

TABLE 13-5 Physical Assessment of Newborn—cont'd

AREA ASSESSED AND APPRAISAL PROCEDURE	NORMAL FINDINGS		DEVIATIONS FROM NORMAL RANGE: POSSIBLE PROBLEMS (ETIOLOGY)
	AVERAGE FINDINGS	NORMAL VARIATIONS	
INTEGUMENT			
Color	Generally pink	Mottling	Dark red (prematurity, polycythemia)
Inspection and palpation	Varies with ethnic origin; skin pigmentation begins to deepen right after birth in basal layer of epidermis	Harlequin sign	Pallor (cardiovascular problem, CNS damage, blood dyscrasia, blood loss, twin transfusion, nosocomial infection)
Inspect naked newborn in well-lit, warm area without drafts; natural daylight provides best lighting	Acrocyanosis, especially if chilled	Plethora	
		Telangiectases ("stork bites" or capillary hemangiomas)	Cyanosis (hypothermia, infection, hypoglycemia, cardiopulmonary diseases, cardiac, neurologic, or respiratory malformations)
Inspect newborn when quiet and when active		Erythema toxicum/neonatorum ("newborn rash")	
		Milia	
		Petechiae over presenting part	Petechiae over any other area (clotting factor deficiency, infection)
		Ecchymoses from forceps in vertex births or over buttocks and legs in breech births	Ecchymoses in any other area (hemorrhagic disease, traumatic birth)
Check for jaundice	None at birth	Physiologic jaundice occurs in 50% of term infants	Gray (hypotension, poor perfusion)
			Jaundice within first 24 hr (Rh isoimmunization)
Birthmarks	Transient hyperpigmentation	Mongolian spotting	Hemangiomas
Inspect and palpate for location, size, distribution, characteristics, color	Areolae	Infants of black, Asian, and Native American origin; 70%	Nevus flammeus: port-wine stain (Fig. 13-5, C)
	Genitals	Infants of white origin: 9%	Nevus vasculosus: strawberry mark (Fig. 13-5, B)
	Linea nigra		Cavernous hemangiomas
Condition	No skin edema	Slightly thick; superficial cracking, peeling, especially of hands, feet	Edema on hands, feet; pitting over tibia
Inspect and palpate for intactness, smoothness, texture, edema	Opacity: few large blood vessels seen indistinctly over abdomen	No blood vessels seen; a few large vessels clearly seen over abdomen	Texture thin, smooth, or of medium thickness; rash or superficial peeling seen
		Some fingernail scratches	Numerous vessels easily seen over abdomen (prematurity)
			Texture thick, parchment-like; cracking, peeling (postmaturity)
			Skin tags; webbing
			Papules, pustules, vesicles, ulcers, maceration (impetigo, candidiasis, herpes, diaper rash)

TABLE 13-5   Physical Assessment of Newborn—cont'd

AREA ASSESSED AND APPRAISAL PROCEDURE	NORMAL FINDINGS		DEVIATIONS FROM NORMAL RANGE: POSSIBLE PROBLEMS (ETIOLOGY)
	AVERAGE FINDINGS	NORMAL VARIATIONS	
INTEGUMENT—cont'd			
Hydration and consistency Weigh infant routinely Inspection and palpation Gently pinch skin between thumb and forefinger over abdomen and inner thigh to check for turgor Check subcutaneous fat deposits (adipose pads) over cheeks, buttocks	Dehydration: best indicator is loss of weight After pinch is released, skin returns to original state immediately	Normal weight loss after birth is up to 10% of birth weight May feel puffy Amount of subcutaneous fat varies	Loose, wrinkled skin (prematurity, postmaturity, dehydration: fold of skin persists after release of pinch) Tense, tight, shiny skin (edema, extreme cold, shock, infection) Lack of subcutaneous fat, clavicle or ribs prominent (prematurity, malnutrition)
Check voiding	Voids within 24 hours of birth Voids 6 to 10 times per day		
Vernix caseosa Observe amount		Amount varies; usually more is found in creases, folds	Absent or minimal (postmaturity) Excessive (prematurity)
Observe its color and odor before bath or wiping If not readily apparent over total body, check in folds of axilla and groin	Whitish, cheesy, odorless		Yellow color (possible fetal anoxia 36 hours or more before birth, Rh or ABO incompatibility) Green color (possible in utero release of meconium or presence of bilirubin) Odor (possible intrauterine infection)
Lanugo Inspect for this fine, downy hair; amount, distribution	Over shoulders, pinnas of ears, forehead	Amount varies	Absent (postmaturity) Excessive (prematurity, especially if lanugo is abundant and long and thick over back)
HEAD			
Palpate skin	See Integument, p. 328	Caput succedaneum; may show some ecchymosis	Cephalhematoma
Inspect shape and size	Makes up one fourth of body length Molding (Fig. 13-7)	Slight asymmetry from intrauterine position Lack of molding (prematurity, breech presentation, cesarean birth)	Molding Severe molding (birth trauma)

Continued.

TABLE 13-5 Physical Assessment of Newborn—cont'd

AREA ASSESSED AND APPRAISAL PROCEDURE	NORMAL FINDINGS		DEVIATIONS FROM NORMAL RANGE: POSSIBLE PROBLEMS (ETIOLOGY)
	AVERAGE FINDINGS	NORMAL VARIATIONS	
HEAD—cont'd			
Palpate, inspect, measure fontanels	Anterior fontanel 5 cm diamond; increases as molding resolves Posterior fontanel triangle; smaller than anterior	Fontanel size varies with degree of molding Fontanels may be difficult to feel because of molding	Fontanels Full, bulging (tumor, hemorrhage, infection) Large, flat, soft (malnutrition, hydrocephaly, retarded bone age, hypothyroidism) Depressed (dehydration)
Palpate sutures	Sutures palpable and not joined	Sutures may overlap with molding	Sutures Widely spaced (hydrocephaly) Premature closure
Inspect pattern, distribution, amount of hair; feel texture	Silky, single strands, lies flat; growth pattern is toward face and neck	Amount varies	Fine, wooly (prematurity) Unusual swirls, patterns, hairline or coarse, brittle (endocrine or genetic disorders)
EYES			
Placement on face	Eyes and space between eyes each ⅓ the distance from outer-to-outer canthus		
Symmetry in size, shape Eyelids: size, movements, blink	Symmetric in size, shape Blink reflex Epicanthal folds: normal racial characteristic	Edema if silver nitrate instilled	Epicanthal folds when present with other signs (chromosomal disorders such as Down syndrome, cri-du-chat syndrome)
Discharge	None	Some discharge if silver nitrate used	
Eyeballs: presence, size, shape	No tears Both present and of equal size; both round, firm	Occasionally has some tears Subconjunctival hemorrhage	Agenesis or absence of one or both eyeballs Small eyeball size (rubella syndrome) Lens opacity or absence of red reflex (congenital cataracts, possibly from rubella) Lesions: coloboma, absence of part of iris (congenital) Pink color of iris (albinism) Jaundiced sclera (hyperbilirubinemia) Discharge: purulent (infection)

TABLE 13-5   Physical Assessment of Newborn—cont'd

AREA ASSESSED AND APPRAISAL PROCEDURE	NORMAL FINDINGS		DEVIATIONS FROM NORMAL RANGE: POSSIBLE PROBLEMS (ETIOLOGY)
	AVERAGE FINDINGS	NORMAL VARIATIONS	
EYES—cont'd			
Pupils	Present, equal in size, react to light		Pupils: unequal, constricted, dilated, fixed (intracranial pressure, medications, tumors)
Eyeball movement	Random, jerky, uneven, can focus briefly, can follow to midline	Transient strabismus or nystagmus until third or fourth month	Persistent strabismus Doll's eyes (increased intracranial pressure) Sunset (increased intracranial pressure)
Eyebrows: amount, pattern	Distinct (not connected in midline)		Connected in midline (Cornelia de Lange's syndrome)
NOSE			
Observe shape, placement, patency, configuration of bridge of nose	Midline Apparent lack of bridge, flat, broad Some mucus but no drainage Preferential nose breather Sneezes to clear nose	Slight deformity from passage through birth canal	Copious drainage, with or without regular periods of cyanosis at rest and return of pink color with crying (choanal atresia, congenital syphilis) Malformed (congenital syphilis, chromosomal disorder) Flaring of nares (respiratory distress)
EARS			
Observe size, placement on head, amount of cartilage, open auditory canal	Correct placement: line drawn through inner and outer canthi of eye should come to top notch of ear (at junction with scalp) Well-formed, firm cartilage	Size: small, large, floppy Darwin's tubercle (nodule on posterior helix)	Agenesis Lack of cartilage (prematurity) Low placement (chromosomal disorder, mental retardation, kidney disorder) Preauricular tags Size: may have overly prominent or protruding ears
Hearing	Responds to voice and other sounds	State influences response	Deaf: no response to sound
FACIES			
Observe overall appearance of face	Infant looks "normal"; features are well placed, proportionate to face, symmetric	Positional deformities	Infant looks "odd" or "funny" Usually accompanied by other features, such as low-set ears and other structural disorders (hereditary, chromosomal aberration)

Continued.

TABLE 13-5   Physical Assessment of Newborn—cont'd

AREA ASSESSED AND APPRAISAL PROCEDURE	NORMAL FINDINGS		DEVIATIONS FROM NORMAL RANGE: POSSIBLE PROBLEMS (ETIOLOGY)
	AVERAGE FINDINGS	NORMAL VARIATIONS	
MOUTH			
Inspection and palpation Placement on face Lips: color, configuration, movement	Symmetry of lip movement	Transient circumoral cyanosis	Gross anomalies in placement, size, shape (cleft lip and/or palate, gums) Cyanosis; circumoral pallor (respiratory distress, hypothermia) Asymmetry in movement of lips (seventh cranial nerve paralysis)
Gums	Pink gums	Inclusion cysts (Epstein's pearls)	Teeth: predeciduous or deciduous (hereditary)
Tongue: attachment, mobility, movement, size	Tongue does not protrude, is freely movable; symmetric in shape, movement	Short frenulum	Macroglossia (prematurity, chromosomal disorder)
Cheeks	Sucking pads inside cheeks		Thrush: white plaques on cheeks or tongue that bleed if touched (*Candida albicans*)
Palate (soft, hard) Arch Uvula	Soft and hard palates intact Uvula in midline	Anatomic groove in palate to accommodate nipple; disappears by 3 to 4 years of age Epstein's pearls (Bohn's nodules): whitish, hard nodules on gums or roof of mouth	Cleft hard or soft palate
Chin	Distinct chin		Micrognathia (Pierre Robin or other syndrome)
Saliva: amount, character			Excessive saliva (esophageal atresia, tracheoesophageal fistula)
Reflexes Rooting Sucking Extrusion	Reflexes present	Reflex response dependent on state of wakefulness and hunger	Absent (prematurity)
NECK			
Inspection and palpation Length	Short, thick, surrounded by skinfolds; no webbing		Webbing (Turner's syndrome)
Sternocleidomastoid muscles; movement and position of head	Head held in midline, i.e., sternocleidomastoid muscles are equal; no masses Freedom of movement from side to side and flexion and extension; cannot move chin past shoulder	Transient positional deformity apparent when newborn is at rest: head can be moved passively	Restricted movement; head held at angle (torticollis [wryneck], opisthotonos) Absence of head control (prematurity; Down syndrome)
Trachea: position; thyroid gland	Thyroid not palpable		Masses (enlarged thyroid) Distended veins (cardiopulmonary disorder) Skin tags

TABLE 13-5 Physical Assessment of Newborn—cont'd

AREA ASSESSED AND APPRAISED PROCEDURE	NORMAL FINDINGS		DEVIATIONS FROM NORMAL RANGE: POSSIBLE PROBLEMS (ETIOLOGY)
	AVERAGE FINDINGS	NORMAL VARIATIONS	
CHEST			
Inspection and palpation Shape	Almost circular; barrel-shaped	Tip of sternum may be prominent	Bulging of chest, unequal movement (pneumothorax, pneumomediastinum) Malformation (funnel chest—pectus excavatum)
Respiratory movements	Symmetric chest movements; chest and abdominal movements synchronized during respirations	Occasional retractions, especially when crying	Retractions with or without respiratory distress (prematurity, RDS)
Clavicles			Fracture of clavicle (trauma)
Ribs			Poor development of rib cage and musculature (prematurity)
Nipples: size, placement, number	Nipples prominent, well formed; symmetrically placed		Nipples Supernumerary, along nipple line Malpositioned or widely spaced
Breast tissue	Breast nodule: approximately 6 mm in term infant	Breast nodule: 3 to 10 mm Secretion of witch's milk	Lack of breast tissue (prematurity)
Auscultation Heart tones and rate and breath sounds (see Vital signs, p. 340)			Sounds: bowel sounds (see Abdomen, below)
ABDOMEN			
Inspect, palpate, and smell umbilical cord	Two arteries, one vein (AVA) Whitish-gray Definite demarcation between cord and skin; no intestinal structures within cord Dry around base; drying Odorless Cord clamp in place for 24 hr		One artery (internal anomalies) Meconium stained (intrauterine distress) Bleeding or oozing around cord (hemorrhagic disease) Redness or drainage around cord (infection, possible persistence of urachus)
		Reducible umbilical herniation	Hernia: herniation of abdominal contents into area of cord (e.g., omphalocele); defect covered with thin, friable membrane, may be extensive Gastroschisis: fissure of abdominal cavity

Continued.

TABLE 13-5 Physical Assessment of Newborn—cont'd

AREA ASSESSED AND APPRAISAL PROCEDURE	NORMAL FINDINGS		DEVIATIONS FROM NORMAL RANGE: POSSIBLE PROBLEMS (ETIOLOGY)
	AVERAGE FINDINGS	NORMAL VARIATIONS	
ABDOMEN—cont'd			
Inspect size of abdomen and palpate contour (Fig. 13-10, *D*)	Rounded, prominent, dome shaped because abdominal musculature is not fully developed Liver may be palpable 1 to 2 cm below right costal margin No other masses palpable No distention	Some diastasis of abdominal musculature	Distention at birth (ruptured viscus, genitourinary masses or malformations: hydronephrosis; teratomas, abdominal tumors) Mild (overfeeding, high gastrointestinal tract obstruction) Marked (lower gastrointestinal tract obstruction, imperforate anus) Intermittent or transient (overfeeding) Partial intestinal obstruction (stenosis of bowel) Malrotation of bowel or adhesions Sepsis (infection)
Auscultate bowel sounds and note number, amount, and character of stools, and behavior—crying, fussiness—before or during elimination Color	Sounds present within 1 to 2 hours after birth Meconium stool passes within 24 to 48 hours after birth	Linea nigra may be apparent; possibly caused by hormone influence during pregnancy	Scaphoid, with bowel sounds in chest and respiratory distress (diaphragmatic hernia)
Movement with respiration	Respirations primarily diaphragmatic; abdominal and chest movement synchronous		Decreased abdominal breathing (intrathoracic disease, diaphragmatic hernia) "Seesaw" (respiratory distress)
GENITALS (SEE FIG. 13-6) Girl Inspection and palpation General appearance Clitoris Labia majora	Female genitals Usually edematous Usually edematous; cover labia minora in term newborns	Increased pigmentation caused by pregnancy hormones Edema and ecchymosis following breech birth	Ambiguous genitals— enlarged clitoris with urinary meatus on tip; fused labia (chromosomal disorder; maternal drug ingestion)
Labia minora	May protrude over labia majora	Blood-tinged discharge from pseudomenstruation caused by pregnancy hormones	Stenosed meatus
Discharge	Smegma		

TABLE 13-5 Physical Assessment of Newborn—cont'd

AREA ASSESSED AND APPRAISAL PROCEDURE	NORMAL FINDINGS		DEVIATIONS FROM NORMAL RANGE: POSSIBLE PROBLEMS (ETIOLOGY)
	AVERAGE FINDINGS	NORMAL VARIATIONS	
GENITALS—cont'd			
Vagina	Orifice open. Mucoid discharge. Hymenal/vaginal tag present	Some vernix caseosa may be between labia	Labia majora widely separated and labia minora prominent (prematurity). Absence of vaginal orifice or imperforate hymen. Fecal discharge (fistula)
Urinary meatus	Beneath clitoris; hard to see—watch for voiding	Rust-stained urine (uric acid crystals) (to determine whether rust color is caused by uric acid or blood, wash under running warm tap water; uric acid washes out, blood does not)	
Boy			
Inspection and palpation			
General appearance	Male genitals	Increased size and pigmentation caused by pregnancy hormones	Ambiguous genitals
Penis	Meatus at tip of penis		Urinary meatus not on tip of glans penis (hypospadias, epispadias)
Urinary meatus seen as slit			
Prepuce	Prepuce (foreskin) covers glans penis and is not retractable	Prepuce removed if circumcised. Size of genitals varies widely	
Scrotum	Large, edematous, pendulous in term infant; covered with rugae	Scrotal edema and ecchymosis if breech birth. Hydrocele, small, noncommunicating	Scrotum smooth and testes undescended (prematurity, cryptorchidism). Hydrocele. Inguinal hernia. Round meatal opening
Rugae (wrinkles)			
Testes	Palpable on each side	Bulge palpable in inguinal canal	Undescended (prematurity)
Urination	Voiding within 24 hours, stream adequate, amount adequate	Rust-stained urine (uric acid crystals)	
Reflexes			
Erection	Erection may occur spontaneously and when genitals are touched		
Cremasteric	Testes are retracted, especially when newborn is chilled		
EXTREMITIES			
General			
Inspection and palpation	Assumes position maintained in utero	Transient (positional) deformities	Limited motion (malformations). Poor muscle tone (prematurity, maternal medications, CNS anomalies). Positive scarf sign
Degree of flexion	Attitude of general flexion		
Range of motion	Full range of motion, spontaneous movements		
Symmetry of motion			
Muscle tone			
Clavicles	Intact		Crepitus/fracture (trauma)

Continued.

TABLE 13-5 Physical Assessment of Newborn—cont'd

AREA ASSESSED AND APPRAISAL PROCEDURE	NORMAL FINDINGS		DEVIATIONS FROM NORMAL RANGE: POSSIBLE PROBLEMS (ETIOLOGY)
	AVERAGE FINDINGS	NORMAL VARIATIONS	
EXTREMITIES—cont'd			
Arms and Hands			
Inspection and palpation	Longer than legs in newborn period	Slight tremors may be seen at times	Asymmetry of movement (fracture/crepitus, brachial nerve trauma, malformations)
Color	Contours and movement are symmetric	Some acrocyanosis, especially when chilled	
Intactness			Asymmetry of contour (malformations, fracture)
Appropriate placement			
Number of fingers	Five on each hand	Single palmar crease on one hand common in Asian babies	Amelia or phocomelia (teratogens)
Palpate humerus	Fist often clenched with thumb under fingers		Webbing of fingers: syndactyly
			Absence or excess of fingers
Joints	Full range of motion; symmetric contour		Palmar creases
Shoulder			Simian line seen with short, incurved little fingers (Down syndrome)
Elbow			
Wrist			
Fingers			Strong, rigid flexion; persistent fists; fists held in front of mouth constantly (CNS disorder)
Reflex: grasp			
			Increased tonicity, clonicity, prolonged tremors (CNS disorder)
Legs and Feet			
Inspection and palpation	Appear bowed since lateral muscles more developed than medial muscles	Feet appear to turn in but can be easily rotated externally, also positional defects tend to correct while infant is crying	Amelia, phocomelia (chromosomal defect, teratogenic effect)
Color			
Intactness			Webbing, syndactyly (chromosomal defect)
Length—in relation to arms and body and to each other		Acrocyanosis	Absence or excess of digits (chromosomal defect, familial trait)
Major gluteal folds	Major gluteal folds even		Femoral fracture (difficult breech birth)
Number of toes	Five on each foot		
Femur	Femur should be intact		Congenital hip dysplasia/dislocation
Head of femur as legs are flexed and abducted; placement in acetabulum	No click should be heard; femoral head should not override acetabulum		Soles of feet
			Few lines: (prematurity)
Soles of the feet	Soles well lined (or wrinkled) over two thirds of foot in term infants		Covered with lines (postmaturity)
	Planter fat pad gives flatfooted effect		Congental clubfoot
Joints	Full range of motion; symmetric contour		Hypermobility of joints (Down syndrome)
Hip			Yellowed nail beds (meconium staining)
Knee			
Ankle			Temperature of one leg differs from that of the other (circulatory deficiency, CNS disorder)
Toes			
Reflexes			Asymmetric movement (trauma, CNS disorder)

TABLE 13-5 Physical Assessment of Newborn—cont'd

AREA ASSESSED AND APPRAISAL PROCEDURE	NORMAL FINDINGS		DEVIATIONS FROM NORMAL RANGE: POSSIBLE PROBLEMS (ETIOLOGY)
	AVERAGE FINDINGS	NORMAL VARIATIONS	
BACK			
Anatomy			
Inspection and palpation	Spine straight and easily flexed	Temporary minor positional deformities, which can be corrected with passive manipulation	Limitation of movement (fusion or deformity of vertebra)
Spine	Infant can raise and support head momentarily when prone		Pigmented nevus with tuft of hair when located anywhere along the spine is often associated with spina bifida occulta
Shoulders			
Scapulae	Shoulders, scapulae, and iliac crests should line up in same plane		
Iliac crests			
Base of spine— pilonidal area			Spina bifida cystica (meningocele, myelomeningocele)
Reflexes (spinal related)			
Test reflexes			
ANUS			
Inspection and palpation	One anus with good sphincter tone	Passage of meconium within 48 hours after birth	Low obstruction: anal membrane
Placement			
Number	Passage of meconium within 24 hours after birth		High obstruction: anal or rectal atresia
Patency			
Test for sphincter response (active "wink" reflex)	Good "wink" reflex of anal sphincter		Drainage of fecal material from vagina in female or urinary meatus in male (rectal fistula)
Observe for following:			
Abdominal distention			
Passage of meconium			
Passage of fecal drainage from surrounding orifices			
STOOLS	Meconium followed by transitional and soft yellow stools (see p. 326)		No stool (obstruction)
			Frequent watery stools (infection, phototherapy)

TABLE 13-6 Assessment of Newborn's Reflexes

REFLEX	ELICITING THE REFLEX	CHARACTERISTIC RESPONSE	COMMENTS
Sucking and rooting	Touch infant's lip, cheek, or corner of mouth with nipple	Infant turns head toward stimulus, opens mouth, takes hold, and sucks	Difficult if not impossible to elicit after infant has been fed; if weak or absent, consider prematurity or neurologic defect
			Parental guidance
			Avoid trying to turn head toward breast or nipple; allow infant to root
			Disappears after 3 to 4 months but may persist up to 1 year

Continued.

TABLE 13-6 Assessment of Newborn's Reflexes

REFLEX	ELICITING THE REFLEX	CHARACTERISTIC RESPONSE	COMMENTS
Swallowing	Feed infant; swallowing usually follows sucking and obtaining fluids	Swallowing is usually co-ordinated with sucking and usually occurs without gagging, coughing, or vomiting	If weak or absent, may indicate prematurity or neurologic defect Suck and swallow often uncoordinated in preterm infant
Grasp Palmar Plantar	 Place finger in palm of hand Place finger at base of toes	 Infant's fingers curl around examiner's fingers; toes curl downward	Palmar response lessens by 3 to 4 months; parents enjoy this contact with infant; plantar response lessens by 8 months
Extrusion	Touch or depress tip of tongue	Newborn forces tongue outward	Disappears about fourth month
Glabellar (Myerson's)	Tap over forehead, bridge of nose, or maxilla of newborn whose eyes are open	Newborn blinks for first 4 or 5 taps	Continued blinking with repeated taps is consistent with extrapyramidal disorder

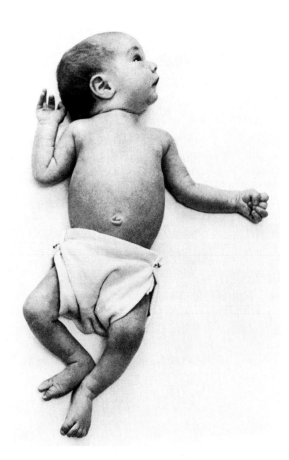

FIG. 13-11 Classic pose in spontaneous tonic neck reflex. (Courtesy Mead Johnson & Co., Evansville, IN.)

TABLE 13-6   Assessment of Newborn's Reflexes

REFLEX	ELICITING THE REFLEX	CHARACTERISTIC RESPONSE	COMMENTS
Tonic neck or "fencing" (Fig. 13-11)	With infant falling asleep or sleeping, turn head quickly to one side	With infant facing left side, arm and leg on that side extend; opposite arm and leg flex (turn head to right, and extremities assume opposite postures)	Responses in leg are more consistent Complete response disappears by 3 to 4 months; incomplete response may be seen until third or fourth year After 6 weeks persistent response is sign of possible cerebral palsy
Moro (Fig. 13-12)	Hold infant in semisitting position; allow head and trunk to fall backward to an angle of at least 30 degrees Place infant on flat surface; strike surface to startle infant	Symmetric abduction and extension of arms; fingers fan out and form a **C** with thumb and forefinger; slight tremor may be noted; arms are adducted in embracing motion and return to relaxed flexion and movement Legs may follow similar pattern of response Preterm infant does not complete "embrace," instead, arms fall backward because of weakness	Present at birth; complete response may be seen until 8 weeks* of age; body jerk only, between 8 to 18 weeks; absent by 6 months if neurologic maturation is not delayed; may be incomplete if infant is deeply asleep; give parental guidance about normal response Asymmetric response; possible injury to brachial plexus, clavicle, or humerus Persistent response after 6 months: possible brain damage
Stepping or "walking"	Hold infant vertically, allowing one foot to touch table surface	Infant will simulate walking, alternating flexion and extension of feet; term infants walk on soles of their feet, and preterm infants walk on their toes	Normally present for 3 to 4 weeks
Crawling	Place newborn on abdomen	Newborn makes crawling movements with arms and legs	Should disappear about 6 weeks of age
Deep tendon	Use finger instead of percussion hammer to elicit patellar, or knee jerk, reflex; newborn must be relaxed	Reflex jerk is present; even with newborn relaxed, nonselective overall reaction may occur	
Crossed extension (Fig. 13-13)	Infant should be supine; extend one leg, press knee downward, stimulate bottom of foot; observe opposite leg	Opposite leg flexes, adducts, and then extends	
Startle	Loud noise of sharp hand clap elicits response; best elicited if newborn is 24 to 36 hr old or older	Arms abduct with flexion of elbows; hands stay clenched	Should disappear by 4 months Elicited more readily in preterm newborn (inform parents of this characteristic)

*All durations for persistance of reflexes are based on time elapsed since 40 weeks' gestation, that is, if this newborn was born at 36 weeks' gestation, add 1 month to all time limits given.   *Continued.*

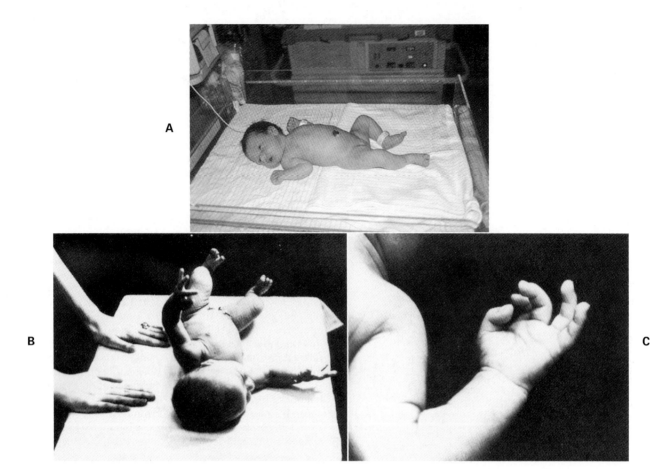

FIG. 13-12 Moro's reflex. **A,** Position of rest. **B,** Moro's reflex consists predominantly of abduction and extension of arms. **C,** Interesting subtlety of Moro's response in newborn infants is **C** position of fingers: digits extend, except finger and thumb, which are often semi-flexed, forming shape of **C.** (**A** courtesy Marjorie Pyle, RNC, *Lifecirle*, Costa Mesa, CA. **B** and **C** courtesy Mead Johnson & Co., Evansville, IN.)

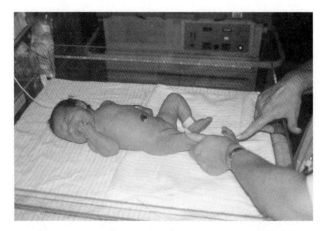

FIG. 13-13 Crossed extension reflex. With infant in supine position, examiner extends one of infant's legs and presses knee down. Stimulation of sole of foot of fixated limb should cause *free* leg to flex, adduct, and extend as if attempting to push away stimulating agent. This reflex should be present during newborn period. Absence of response suggests a spinal cord lesion; weak response suggest peripheral nerve damage. (Courtesy Marjorie Pyle, RNC, *Lifecircle*, Costa Mesa, CA.)

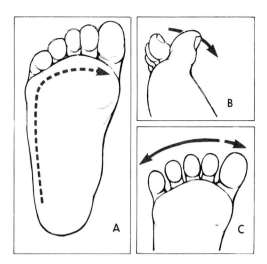

FIG. 13-14 Babinski's reflex. **A,** Direction of stroke. **B,** Dorsiflexion of big toe. **C,** Fanning of toes. (From Whaley LF, Wong DL: *Nursing care of infants and children,* ed 4, St Louis, 1995, Mosby.)

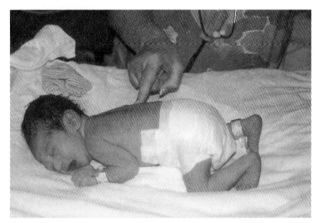

FIG. 13-15 Trunk incurvation reflex. In prone position, infant responds to linear skin stimulus (blunt end of pin or finger) along paravertebral area by flexing trunk and swinging pelvis toward stimulus. With transverse lesions of cord, there will be no response below that level. Complete absence of response suggests general depression or nervous system abnormality. Response may vary but should be obtainable in all infants, including preterm ones. If not seen in the first few days, it is usually apparent by 5 to 6 days. (Courtesy Marjorie Pyle, RNC, *Lifecircle,* Costa Mesa, CA.)

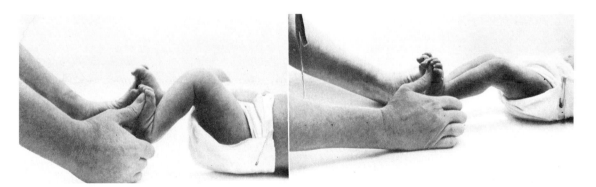

FIG. 13-16 Magnet reflex. With child in supine position and lower limbs semiflexed, light pressure is applied with fingers to both feet. Normally, while examiner's fingers maintain contact with soles of feet, lower limbs extend. Absence of this reflex suggests damage to spinal cord or malformation. Weak reflex may be seen following breech presentation *without* extended legs or may indicate sciatic nerve stretch syndrome. Breech presentation *with* extended legs may evoke an exaggerated response. (Courtesy Mead Johnson & Co., Evansville, IN)

TABLE 13-6 Assessment of Newborn's Reflexes—cont'd

REFLEX	ELICITING THE REFLEX	CHARACTERISTIC RESPONSE	COMMENTS
Babinski's sign (plantar) (Fig. 13-14)	On sole of foot, beginning at heel, stroke upward along lateral aspect of sole, then move finger across ball of foot	All toes hyperextend, with dorsiflexion of big toe—recorded as a positive sign	Absence requires neurologic evaluation; should disappear after 1 year of age
Pull-to-sit (traction)	Pull infant up by wrists from supine position with head in midline	Head will lag until infant is in upright position; then head will be held in same plane with chest and shoulder momentarily before falling forward; infant will attempt to right head	Depends on general muscle tone and maturity and condition of infant
Trunk incurvation (Galant) (Fig. 13-15)	Infant should be prone on flat surface, run finger down back about 4 to 5 cm (1½ to 2 in) lateral to spine, first on one side, and then down other	Trunk is flexed and pelvis is swung toward stimulated side	Response disappears by fourth week
Magnet (Fig. 13-16)	Infant should be supine; partially flex both lower extremities and apply pressure to soles of feet	Both lower limbs should extend against examiner's pressure	
Additional newborn responses			
Yawn, stretch, burp, hiccup, sneeze	Spontaneous behaviors	May be slightly depressed temporarily because of maternal analgesia or anesthesia, fetal hypoxia, or infection	Parental guidance Most of these behaviors are pleasurable to parents Parents need to be assured that behaviors are normal Sneeze is usually response to lint, etc., in nose and not an indicator of a cold No treatment is needed for hiccups; sucking may help

KEY POINTS

- By term the infant's various anatomic and physiologic systems have reached a level of development and functioning that permit a physical existence apart from the mother and sensory capabilities that indicate a state of readiness for social interaction.

- There are several significant differences between the respiratory, renal, and thermogenic systems in the newborn and those of the adult.

- At any serum bilirubin level, the appearance of jaundice during the first day of life or persistence of jaundice usually indicates a pathologic process.

- Chilling (cold stress) of a newborn, even a healthy term newborn, may result in acidosis and raise the level of free fatty acids.

- Many reflex behaviors are important for the newborn's survival.

- The individual personalities and behavior characteristics of infants play a major role in the ultimate relationship between infants and their parents.

- Behavioral responses of infants are indicative of cortical control, responsiveness, and eventual ability to manage their environment.

- The development of parent-child love does not occur without feedback.
- Sleep-wake cycles and other factors influence the newborn's behavior.
- Each newborn has a predisposed capacity to handle the multitude of stimuli in the external world.

CRITICAL THINKING EXERCISES

1. Observe and record findings of a normal newborn immediately after birth and in follow-up periods for several days thereafter. Include both physiologic and behavioral data; compare data, and identify questions for further research.

2. Prepare teaching materials that could be used for a new-parent class on changes and challenges to one of the newborn's body systems. Justify selections.

References

Auerbach KG, Gartner LM: Breastfeeding and human milk: their association with jaundice in the neonate, *Clin Perinatol* 14(1):89, 1987.

Bamford FN et al: Sleep in the first year of life, *Dev Med Child Neurol* 32:718, 1990.

Barr RG: The normal crying curve: what do we really know? *Dev Med Child Neurol* 32:356, 1990.

Blackburn ST, Loper DL: *Maternal, fetal and neonatal physiology: a clinical perspective*, Philadelphia, 1992, WB Saunders.

Boyer DB, Vidyasagar D: Serum indirect bilirubin levels and meconium passage in early fed normal newborns, *Nurs Res* 36:174, 1987.

Brazelton TB: *Infants and mothers*, ed 1, New York, 1969, Dell Publishing Co.

Brazelton TB: *Neonatal behavioral assessment scale*, ed 2, Philadelphia, 1984, JB Lippincott Co.

Brovten D et al: Breastmilk jaundice, *JOGNN* 14:220, May/June 1985.

Chess S: Individuality and baby care, *Dev Med Child Neurol* 11:749, 1969.

Chitty LS, Winter RM: *Perinatal mortality in different ethnic groups*, *Arch Dis Child* 64:1036, 1989.

Condon WS, Sander LW: Neonate movement is synchronized with adult speech: interactional participation and language acquisition, *Science* 183:99, 1974.

Cunningham FG, MacDonald PC, and Gant NF: *Williams Obstetrics*, ed 19, Norwalk, CT, 1993, Appleton & Lange.

Curnock DA: The senses of the newborn: tests for hearing and vision have improved, *BMJ* 299:1478, 1989.

D'Apolito K: What is an organized infant? *Neonatal Network* 10(1):23, 1991.

Fanaroff AA, Martin RJ: *Neonatal-perinatal medicine: diseases of the fetus and infant*, ed 5, St Louis, 1992, Mosby.

Freedman DG: Ethnic differences in babies, *Hum Nature*, p 36, Jan 1979.

Freedman DG, Freedman N: Behavioral differences between Chinese-American and European-American newborns, *Nature* 224:1227, 1969.

Garcia Coll CT: Developmental outcome of minority infants: a process-oriented look into our beginnings, *Child Dev* 61:270, 1990.

Gunzenhauser N, editor: *Advances in touch: new implications in human development*, Skillman, NJ, 1990, Johnson & Johnson Consumer Products.

Guyton A: *Textbook of medical physiology*, Philadelphia, 1991, WB Saunders.

Kangas-Saarela T et al: The effect of lumbar epidural analgesia on the neurobehavioural responses of newborn infants, *Acta Anaesthesiol Scand* 33:320, 1989.

Korner AF: Individual differences at birth: implications for early experiences and later development, *Am J Orthopsychiatry* 41:608, 1971.

Korones SB: *High-risk newborn infants: the basis for intensive nursing care*, ed 4, p. 321, St Louis, 1986, Mosby.

Lascari AD: "Early" breast-feeding jaundice: clinical significance, *J Pediatr* 108:156, 1986.

Lawrence RA: *Breastfeeding: a guide for the medical profession*, ed 4, St Louis, 1994, Mosby.

Letko MD: Detecting and preventing infant hearing loss, *Neonatal Network* 11(5):33, 1992.

Linn S et al: Epidemiology of neonatal hyperbilirubinemia, *Pediatrics* 75(4):770, 1985.

Locklin M: Assessing jaundice in full-term newborns, *Pediatr Nurs* 13:15, Jan 1987.

Lowrey G: *Growth and development of children*, ed 8, Chicago, 1986, Year Book Medical Publishers.

Luddington-Hoe SM: What can newborns really see? *Am J Nurs* 83:1286, 1983.

Makin JW, Porter RH: Attractiveness of lactating females' breast odors to neonates, *Child Dev* 60:803, 1989.

Medici MA: The fight against infection: neonatal defense mechanisms, *J Calif Perinat Assoc* 3(2):25, 1983.

Parker S et al: Jitteriness in full-term neonates: prevalence and correlates, *Pediatrics* 85:17, 1990.

Pete J: Newborn infant's preference for sterile water versus five-percent glucose and water, *J Pediatr Nurs* 4:263, 1989.

Porter RH, Cernoch JM, McLaughlin FJ: Maternal recognition of neonates through olfactory cues, *Physio Behav* 16:75, 1983.

Porter RH, Cernoch JM, Perry S: The importance of odors in mother-infant interactions, *Matern Child Nurs J* 12:147, 1983.

Redshaw ME, Rivers RPA, Rosenblatt DB: *Born too early: special care for preterm baby*, New York, 1985, Oxford University Press.

Stainton C: *Origins of attachment, culture, and cue sensitivity*, doctoral dissertation, San Francisco, 1985, University of California.

Thomas A et al: Individuality in responses of children to similar environmental situations, *Am J Psychiatry* 117:798, 1961.

Thomas A et al: The origin of personality, *Sci Am* 223:102, 1970.

Wilkerson N: A comprehensive look at hyperbilirubinemia, *Matern Child Nurs J* 13:360, 1988.

Bibliography

Barkauskas VH et al: *Health and physical assessment,* St Louis, 1994, Mosby.

Feeg VD: New legislative efforts to improve child health and decrease infant mortality, *Pediatr Nurs* 15(2):145, 1989.

NAACOG: *Neonatal skin care* (OGN Nursing Practice Resource), Washington, DC, Jan 1992, NAACOG.

NAACOG *Physical assessment of the neonate* (OGN Nursing Practice Resource), Washington, DC, Aug 1991, NAACOG.

Seidel HM et al: *Mosby's guide to physical examination, ed 5,* St Louis, 1995, Mosby.

CHAPTER 14

Nursing Care of the Newborn

SHANNON E. PERRY

LEARNING OBJECTIVES

Define key terms.
List relevant prenatal and intrapartal health history information.
Identify a systematic way to assess a newborn.
Describe Apgar scoring and the purpose of this Apgar score.
Describe gestational assessment of a newborn.
Explain what is meant by a safe environment.
Discuss methods to maintain a newborn's temperature.
Compare methods of maintaining an adequate oxygen supply.
Outline the procedures for cardiopulmonary resuscitation and for relieving airway obstruction.
Describe precautions in administering an intramuscular injection to a newborn.
Discuss phototherapy and guidelines for teaching parents about this treatment.
Explain the purpose and methods of circumcision, postoperative care, and relevant parent teaching.
Review procedures for heel stick, collection of urine specimen, assisting with venipuncture, and restraining the newborn.
Describe criteria for early discharge.
Describe home care of a newborn.

KEY TERMS

Apgar score
bulb syringe
cardiopulmonary resuscitation (CPR)
circumcision
clovehitch restraint
cold stress
DeLee mucus-trap suction apparatus
heel stick
hyperbilirubinemia
hypocalcemia
hypoglycemia
hypothermia
mummy restraint
phototherapy
physiologic jaundice
prepuce
protective environment
thermoregulation

RELATED TOPICS

ABO incompatibility *(Chap. 27)* · congenital anomalies *(Chap. 27)* · Combs' test *(Chap. 27)* · exchange blood transfusion *(Chap. 27)* · fourth stage of labor *(Chap. 12)* · hemolytic disease of newborn *(Chap. 27)* · high-risk newborn *(Chap. 26)* · kernicterus *(Chap. 27)* · meconium aspiration syndrome *(Chap. 27)* · perinatal asphyxia *(Chap. 26)* · respiratory distress syndrome *(Chap. 27)*

BOX 14-1

Initial Physical Assessment by Body System

CNS [ ] moves extremities, muscle tone good
[ ] symmetrical features, movement
[ ] suck, rooting, Moro response, grasp
reflexes good
[ ] anterior fontanel soft and flat

CV [ ] heart auscultation, strong and regular
[ ] no murmurs heard
[ ] pulses strong/equal bilaterally

RESP [ ] lungs auscultated, clear bilaterally
[ ] respiratory rate <60 breaths/min
[ ] chest expansion symmetrical
[ ] no upper airway congestion

GU [ ] male: urethral opening at tip of penis
testes descended bilaterally
female: vaginal opening apparent

GI [ ] abdomen soft, no distention
[ ] cord attached and clamped
[ ] anus appears patent

ENT [ ] eyes clear
[ ] palates intact
[ ] nares patent

SKIN Color [ ] pink [ ] acrocyanotic
[ ] no lesions or abrasions
[ ] no peeling
[ ] birthmarks _____
[ ] caput/molding
[ ] vacuum "cap"
[ ] forceps marks
[ ] other _____
Comments: _____
_____
_____
_____

Newborn infants undergo numerous biologic changes during the first hours and days after birth. Although most infants make the necessary adjustments to extrauterine existence without undue difficulty, their well-being depends on the care they receive from others. The nursing care described in this chapter is based on careful assessment of biologic and behavioral responses and formulation of nursing diagnoses. It includes planning and implementing appropriate nursing actions and evaluating their effectiveness.

Care Management

✦ ASSESSMENT

Initial Assessment

The first assessment of the infant is done at birth, using the Apgar score (Table 14-1) and a brief physical assessment (Box 14-1). The nurse or the birth attendant may assign the Apgar score. An assessment of gestational age may be done within the first 2 hours after birth (Fig. 14-1). A more comprehensive physical examination is completed within 24 hours (see Table 13-5).

The **Apgar score** permits a rapid assessment of the need for resuscitation based on five signs that indicate the physiologic state of the neonate (Table 14-1): *heart rate*, based on auscultation with a stethoscope; *respiration*, based on observed movement of the chest wall; *muscle tone*, based on degree of flexion and movement of the extremities; *reflex irritability*, based on response to gentle slaps on the soles of the feet; and *color*, described as pallid, cyanotic, or pink. Each item is scored as a 0, 1, or 2. Evaluations are made 1 and 5 minutes after birth. Scores of 0 to 3 indicate severe distress, scores of 4 to 6 indicate moderate difficulty, and scores of 7 to 10 indicate that the infant will have no difficulty adjusting to extrauterine life. Apgar scores do not predict future neurologic outcome.

The *initial physical assessment* includes a brief review of systems (Box 14-1). For this initial brief examination, the nurse assesses the following:

1. *External:* notes skin color, staining, peeling, or wasting (dysmaturity); length of nails and creases on soles

TABLE 14-1 Apgar Score

SIGN	SCORE		
	0	1	2
Heart rate	Absent	Slow (<100)	Over 100
Respiratory rate	Absent	Slow, weak cry	Good cry
Muscle tone	Flaccid	Some flexion of extremities	Well-flexed
Reflex irritability	No response	Grimace	Cry
Color	Blue, pale	Body pink, extremities blue	Completely pink

NEWBORN MATURITY RATING and CLASSIFICATION

ESTIMATION OF GESTATIONAL AGE BY MATURITY RATING
Symbols: X - 1st Exam   O - 2nd Exam

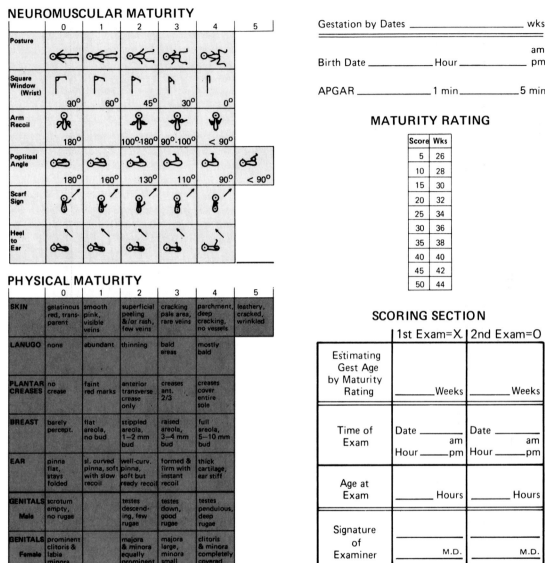

FIG. 14-1 Newborn maturity rating and classification. (Mead Johnson & Co., Evansville, IN. Scoring section adapted from Ballard JL et al: *Pediatr Res* 11:374, 1977. Figures modified from Sweet AY: Classification of the low-birth-weight infant. In Klaus MH, Fanaroff AA: *Care of the high-risk infant*, Philadelphia, PA, 1977, WB Saunders Co.)

of feet; checks for presence of breast tissue; assesses nasal patency by covering one nostril at a time while observing respirations and color; notes meconium staining of cord, skin, fingernails, or amniotic fluid (staining may indicate fetal hypoxia; offensive odor may indicate intrauterine infection)

2. *Chest:* palpates for site of point of maximal impulse, and auscultates for rate and quality of heart tones and murmurs; notes character of respirations and presence of rales or rhonchi; note equality of breath sounds on each side of chest by holding stethoscope in each axilla

3. *Abdomen:* verifies presence of a domed abdomen and absence of anomalies; notes number of vessels in cord

4. *Neurologic:* checks muscle tone and reflex reaction; palpates anterior fontanel for fullness or bulge; notes by palpation the presence and size of the fontanels and sutures

5. *Other observations:* notes gross structural malformations obvious at birth

The nurse responsible for the care of the newborn immediately after birth verifies that respirations have been established, dries the infant, assesses temperature, and places identical identification bracelets on the infant and the mother. In some settings, the father also wears an identification bracelet (see Legal Tip). The infant may be wrapped in a warm blanket and placed in the arms of the mother, given to the father to hold, or kept undressed under a radiant warmer. In some settings, immediately after birth, the infant is placed on the mother's abdomen to allow skin to skin contact, which contributes to maintenance of the infant's optimum temperature and parental bonding. The infant may be admitted to a nursery or remain with the parents throughout the hospital stay.

The initial examination of the newborn can occur while the nurse is drying and wrapping the infant, or observations can be made while the infant is lying on the mother's abdomen or in her arms immediately after birth. Efforts should be directed to minimizing interference in the initial parent-infant acquaintance process. If the infant is breathing easily, has good color, and is normal in appearance, then further examination can be delayed until after the parents have had an opportunity to interact with the infant.

Routine procedures and the admission process can be carried out in the mother's room or in a separate nursery. Box 14-2 shows an example of newborn routine orders.

LEGAL TIP: **Infant Identification**

Identical identification bands should be placed on the mother and infant while they are still in the birthing room. Each time the infant is taken to the mother the bands should be checked to be sure that the numbers match.

Gestational Assessment

Assessment of physical and neurologic findings to determine gestational age is based on the method devised by Dubowitz et al (1970). Ideally, the tests are performed between 2 and 8 hours of age. If the tests are done earlier while the infant is recovering from the stress of birth, muscle movements may reflect fatigue; for example, the arm recoil is slower. After 48 hours, some responses change significantly. The plantar creases on the soles of the feet appear to increase in number and become visible as the skin loses fluid and dries. The commonly used gestational assessment scale is the Simplified Assessment of Gestational Age (Ballard, Novak, Driver, 1979; Fig. 14-1). This scale is a modified form of the Dubowitz scale. It is composed of six external physical and six neuromuscular signs. A score is assigned to each sign. The maturity rating of 26 to 44 weeks is derived from the

---

BOX 14-2

Routine Admission Orders

Vital signs: on admission and q 30 min × 2, q1h × 2, then q8h

Weight, length, and head and chest circumference on admission; then weigh daily

Tetracycline or erythromycin ophthalmic ointment 5 mg/g 1 line each eye (ou)

Vitamin K 1 mg IM

Hematocrit by warm heel stick within 3 to 8 hours of age; call health care provider if <44 or >72

Dextrostix prn; notify health care provider if <40 mg/dl; offer early D_5W po

Feedings: sterile water × 1 by nurse within first 4 hours of life; if tolerated, begin formula q3 to 4 hours on demand. Breastfeeding on demand may be initiated immediately after birth

Rooming in as desired and infant's condition permits

Newborn screen for phenylketonuria (PKU), thyroxine (T_4), and galactosemia on day of discharge (see Table 14-4).

---

cumulative score and is accurate within ±2 weeks. The rating is valid for infants of all races (Stevens-Simon et al, 1989).

Ongoing Assessment

Whenever a newborn receives care, observations and recordings of the infant's progress are made. During each 8-hour period the following assessments are made, compared with the norm, and recorded:

- Axillary temperature
- Respiratory rate, rhythm, and effort
- Breath sounds
- Heart rate and rhythm
- Skin color
- Activity level and muscle tone
- Feeding and elimination
- Fontanels
- Parent-infant interaction

When deviations from the norm are noted, interventions and notification of the pediatrician may be necessary.

Physical Examination

A thorough physical examination is done within 24 hours after birth, when the newborn's temperature stabilizes. Reviewing the maternal history and the prenatal and intrapartal records provides a background for any potential problems. Knowing the type of analgesic and anesthetic the mother received in labor helps explain the infant's current status and alerts the nurse to potential problems. Pertinent information from the mother's prenatal record and the record of events during the mother's labor and the newborn's birth may be recorded on a

Neonatal Health History

Date _____ Infant _____
Date of birth _____ Sex _____
Time of birth _____ Age (in hours) now _____

Prenatal data
Maternal age _____ Blood type and Rh _____
Indirect Coombs' _____ EDB via dates _____

Previous obstetric history
Parity (explain all items) _____
Previous pregnancies:
Date _____ Gestational age _____ Sex _____ Weight _____ Delivery _____ Complications _____

Complications of this pregnancy
Preeclampsia _____ Hypertension _____
Diabetes (class) _____ Bleeding _____
Viral/bacterial infection _____
Environmental teratogens _____
Drug use _____
　　Over-the-counter _____ Alcohol _____
　　Prescription _____ Cocaine _____
　　Heroin _____ Methadone _____
Other _____

Results of fetal testing
AFP assay _____
Ultrasound _____ Amniocentesis _____
NST _____ BPS _____

Intrapartum data
Onset of contractions _____
Rupture of membranes (ROM) _____ When? _____
Bloody _____ Meconium stained _____ Foul smell _____
Abnormalities of maternal vital signs _____
Medications during labor _____
Anesthesia/analgesia _____ Time last administered _____
Fetal monitoring (external/internal) _____
Fetal distress _____ Fetal pH _____
Length of stages of labor: 1st _____ 2nd _____ 3rd _____

Birth
Time _____ Route _____
Reason for operative birth _____

Resuscitation
Apgar score: 1 minute _____ 5 minute _____
Suction _____ Whiffs of O_2 _____
Positive pressure _____ via mask/endotracheal tube _____
Length _____
Time of first spontaneous breath _____
Medications _____

Other
Voided _____ Stool _____
Breastfed _____ Bonding time _____
Observations of bonding behavior _____

In nursery
Time of transfer to nursery if applicable _____
First temperature _____ Placed in warmer/Isolette _____
Eye prophylaxis _____
Vitamin K _____ Time _____ Location _____

FIG. 14-2 Neonatal health history. (From Dickason EJ, Schult MO, Silverman BL: *Maternal-infant nursing care,* ed 2, St Louis, 1994, Mosby.)

form such as the one in Fig. 14-2. At a glance, this form shows significant data from the antenatal period through birth. The nurse can use these data to plan care for the newborn.

Having the parents present during the examination permits prompt discussion of parental concerns and actively involves the parents in the health care of their child from birth. Parental interactions with the infant can be observed. This aids in early diagnosis of concerns in the parent-infant relationship and the identification of learning needs.

The area used for the examination should be well-lit, warm, and free of drafts. The infant is undressed as needed and placed on a firm, flat surface. The infant may need to be picked up and cuddled at times for reassurance. The examination is carried out in a systematic manner. It begins with a general evaluation of such characteristics as appearance, maturity, nutritional status, activity, and state of well-being. More specific observations follow this general evaluation (see Tables 13-5 and 13-6).

Data are recorded as descriptive notes or are summarized on standard forms. Identifying data are entered first: name; hospital number; birthdate; weight; length; chest and head circumferences; race; sex; mother's and infant's blood type and Rh; Coombs' test results; and time of examination.

The *general appearance* (posture, maturity, activity, tone, cry, color, edema) and *sleep-wake state* (see Table 13-4) of the infant are assessed before disturbing the infant. These observations aid in the interpretation of the findings. Each examiner has a preferred pattern for assessment. Blood pressure (BP) is not assessed routinely. *Heart and respiratory rates* are easiest to assess when the newborn is quiet. Respirations are counted by observing the chest wall, noting whether the sternum retracts or nares flare and chin lags on inspiration. The examiner notes whether the infant is a nose breather (i.e., sleeps with mouth closed, does not have to interrupt feedings

to breathe), assesses breath sounds, and notes abnormal sounds—grunting or wheezing—during inspiration or expiration.

The examiner notes the efficiency of the gagging, sneezing, and swallowing reflexes. The examiner watches for bouts of rapid and irregular respirations, gagging, and regurgitation of mucus during "reactivity" periods following birth and after 4 to 6 hours of life.

The infant's *color* is assessed for cyanosis. A pink color over head and trunk and mucous membrane is indicative of adequate oxygenation. Feet and hands may remain slightly cyanotic (acrocyanosis) for 48 hours, especially when they are cold.

On admission and each time the *skin* is exposed while giving care, the infant's skin is assessed for rashes, excoriations (e.g., from fingernails), color (e.g., petechiae, ecchymosis, jaundice, general color, mottling), wounds (e.g., internal fetal monitoring, forceps, scalpel during cesarean birth, circumcision, cord, heel sticks, injections), vernix caseosa, and lanugo. The axillary *temperature* is measured. Taking the temperature rectally is ordinarily contraindicated. A well-lubricated rectal thermometer may be inserted up to 0.5 inches to assess patency of the anus. Waiting for the first stool to appear, however, is the preferable means of assessing anal patency.

The baby's *head* is assessed for skin, hair pattern and distribution, molding, fontanels and sutures, size, shape, symmetry, eyes, nose, mouth, ears, and facies. (see Clinical Application of Research) The neck is inspected and palpated. *Chest assessment* includes measuring the chest circumference and noting the shape of the thorax, the breasts and nipples, and chest movement with respirations. The rate and rhythm of the heart and presence or absence of murmurs are noted. Lung fields are auscultated. The shape of the *abdomen* and the condition of the umbilical cord are assessed. Abdominal circumference may be measured. Bowel sounds and record of stooling behavior are noted. The newborn's *genitals, uri-*

CLINICAL APPLICATION OF RESEARCH

MEASUREMENT OF NEWBORN HEAD CIRCUMFERENCE

Head circumference is used to make inferences about the size and growth of the brain. Clinical decisions may be made based on serial measurements of head circumference (HC). Most clinical studies do not discuss measurement errors of HC. Bhushan and Paneth studied whether the HC of low-birth-weight (LBW) infants can clinically be measured reliably. Measurements of the HC of 927 infants by pediatricians and ultrasound (US) technologists trained to measure HC were compared. The average of the measurements of the pediatricians was 27.66 cm and of the US technologists was 27.64. The average

difference was 0.0185 cm, a difference that was neither statistically nor clinically significant. However, in 5% of the cases, there were differences of more than 1.4 cm, which may be a substantial difference in LBW infants. Nurses and others who measure HC as part of newborn assessment must be trained in the technique of accurate measurement; periodic reliability checks should be made to ensure that accuracy of measurements continues.

Reference: from Bhushan V, Paneth N: The reliability of neonatal head circumference measurement, *J Clin Epidemiol* 44:1027, 1991.

nary meatus, and *anus* are assessed carefully. The *skeletal system* is also inspected.

Neonatal *reflexes* are assessed. The responses reveal the status of the neuromuscular and skeletal systems. State-related behaviors (Table 13-4 and 14-2) are assessed and documented.

❖ NURSING DIAGNOSES

Analysis of the significance of the assessment's findings leads to the establishment of nursing diagnoses. Possible nursing diagnoses for the *newborn* are as follows:

Ineffective breathing pattern related to
- Obstructed airway

Impaired gas exchange related to
- Hypothermia (cold stress)

High risk for ineffective thermoregulation related to
- Heat loss to environment

High risk for infection related to
- Environmental factors

High risk for pain related to
- Circumcision

TABLE 14-2   Infant State-Related Behavior Chart

BEHAVIOR/DESCRIPTION OF BEHAVIOR	INFANT STATE CONSIDERATION	IMPLICATIONS FOR CAREGIVING
ALERTING Widening and brightening of the eyes. Infants focus attention on stimuli, whether visual, auditory, or objects to be sucked.	From drowsy or active alert to quiet alert.	Infant state and timing are important. When trying to alert infants, try to: 1. Unwrap infant (arms out at least). 2. Place infant in upright position. 3. Talk to infant, putting variation in your pitch and tempo. 4. Show your face to infant. 5. Elicit the rooting, sucking, or grasp reflexes.
VISUAL RESPONSE Newborns have pupillary responses to differences in brightness. Infants can focus on objects or faces about 7 to 8 inches away. Newborns have preferences for more complex patterns, human faces, and moving objects.	Quiet alert.	Newborn's visual alertness provides opportunities for eye-to-eye contact with caregivers, an important source of beginning caregiver-infant interaction.
AUDITORY RESPONSE Reaction to a variety of sounds, especially in the human voice range. Infants can hear sounds and locate the general direction of the sound, if the source is constant.	Drowsy, quiet alert, active alert.	Enhances communication between infants and caregivers. Crying infants can often be consoled by voice.
IRRITABILITY How easily infants are upset by loud noises, handling by caregivers, temperature changes, removal of blankets or clothes, etc.	From deep sleep, light sleep, drowsy, quiet alert, or active alert to fussing or crying.	Irritable infants need more frequent consoling and more subdued external environments. Parents can be helped to cope with more irritable infants.
READABILITY The cues infants give through motor behavior and activity, looking, listening, and behavior patterns.	All states.	Parents need to learn that newborns' behaviors are part of their individual temperaments and not reflections on their parenting abilities. By observing and understanding an infant's characteristic pattern, parents can respond more appropriately.

Modified from Barnard KE et al: Infant state-related behavior chart. In *Early parent-infant relationships*, White Plains, NY, 1978 March of Dimes Birth Defects Foundation.   *Continued.*

TABLE 14-2 Infant State-Related Behavior Chart—cont'd

BEHAVIOR/DESCRIPTION OF BEHAVIOR	INFANT STATE CONSIDERATION	IMPLICATIONS FOR CAREGIVING
SMILE Ranging from a faint grimace to a full-fledged smile. Reflexive.	Drowsy, active alert, quiet alert, light sleep.	Initial smile in the neonatal period is the forerunner of the social smile at 3 to 4 weeks of age. Important for caregivers to respond to it.
HABITUATION The ability to lessen one's response to repeated stimuli. This is seen where the Moro response is repeatedly elicited. If a noise is continually repeated, infants will usually cease to respond.	Deep sleep, light sleep, also seen in drowsy.	Because of this ability, families can carry out normal activities without disturbing infants. Infants who have more difficulty with this will probably not sleep well in active environments.
CUDDLINESS Infants' response to being held. Infants nestle and work themselves into the contours of caregivers' bodies.	Primarily in awake states.	Cuddliness is usually rewarding behavior for the caregivers. If infants do not nestle and mold, show the caregivers how to position infants to maximize this response.
CONSOLABILITY Measured when infants have been crying for at least 15 sec. The ability of infants to bring themselves or to be brought by others to a lower state.	From crying to active alert, quiet alert, drowsy, or sleep states.	Crying is the infant behavior that presents the greatest challenge to caregivers. Parents' success or failure in consoling their infants has a significant impact on their feelings of competence as parents.
SELF-CONSOLING Maneuvers used by infants to console themselves and move to a lower state: 1. Hand-to-mouth movement. 2. Sucking on fingers, fist, or tongue. 3. Paying attention to voices or faces. 4. Changes in position.	From crying to active alert, quiet alert, drowsy, or sleep states.	If caregivers are aware of these behaviors, they may allow infants the opportunity to gain control of themselves. This does not imply that newborns should be left to cry. Once newborns are crying and do not initiate self-consoling activities, they may need attention from caregivers.
CONSOLING BY CAREGIVERS After crying for longer than 15 sec the caregivers may try to: 1. Show face to infant. 2. Talk to infant in a steady, soft voice. 3. Hold both infant's arms close to body. 4. Swaddle infant. 5. Pick up infant. 6. Rock infant. 7. Give a pacifier or feed.	From crying to active alert, quiet alert, drowsy, or sleep states.	Often parental initial reaction is to pick up infants or feed them when they cry. Parents could be taught to try other soothing maneuvers, after ascertaining that the diaper is clean and dry.
MOTOR BEHAVIOR AND ACTIVITY Spontaneous movements of extremities and body when stimulated vs. when left alone. Smooth, rhythmical movements vs. jerky ones.	Quiet alert, active alert.	Smooth, nonjerky movements with periods of inactivity seem most natural. Some parents see jerky movements and startles as negative response to their caregiving and are frightened.

Possible nursing diagnoses *for the parent or parents* are as follows:

Family coping, potential for growth related to
- Knowledge of newborn's social capabilities
- Knowledge of newborn's dependency needs
- Knowledge of biologic characteristics of the newborn

Situational low self-esteem related to
- Misinterpretation of newborn's responses

The nursing plan of care on p. 402 provides examples of formulating nursing diagnoses from specific assessment findings.

✤ EXPECTED OUTCOMES

Plans for care of the newborn reflect the rapid growth and development during the neonatal period. Changes in biologic and behavioral states are measured in minutes and hours since birth. The neonatal period extends through the first 28 days after birth. By that time the rate of change has slowed enough so that the child's appearance and needs can be referred to in terms of weeks and months.

The focus of care changes between birth and 28 days. During the first 2 hours of life (HOL) the main focus is on the infant's physiologic adaptation. By the end of the neonatal period the infant's socialization needs assume equal importance with physiologic needs.

The care given the neonate during the first 2 HOL is part of the care given parents and newborns in the fourth stage of labor. Care related to nutritional needs of infants, including techniques of feeding, is presented in Chapter 15. Parent-infant interactions are discussed in detail in Chapter 17.

The information in this section pertains to the maintenance of vital functions, the daily care of infants, and the forms of general therapy carried out routinely in the newborn period. Parental education is outlined.

The *expected outcomes* for newborn care relate to the infant and parents. The expected outcomes for the infant include that the infant will:

1. Make the transition from intrauterine to extrauterine life
2. Maintain effective breathing patterns
3. Maintain effective thermoregulation
4. Remain free from infection

For the parents, expected outcomes will include:

1. Attain knowledge, skill, and confidence relevant to infant-care activities
2. State understanding of biologic and behavioral characteristics of their newborn
3. Demonstrate interactional/lifestyle behaviors that promote healthy family functioning
4. Have opportunities to intensify their relationship with the infant
5. Begin to integrate the infant into the family

✤ COLLABORATIVE CARE

Neonatal care includes techniques for health maintenance, detection of disability, and institution of remedial measures. These techniques can be used for teaching purposes. Careful and concise recording of the infant responses or laboratory results contribute to the continuous supervision vital to mother, newborn, and family. The nurse's ease in handling and caring for the infant encourages new parents and serves as a role model for them.

Protective Environment

The provision of a **protective environment** is basic to the care of the newborn. The construction, maintenance, and operation of nurseries in accredited hospitals are directed by national professional organizations, such as the American Academy of Pediatrics, and local or state governing bodies. Prescribed standards cover areas such as the following:

1. *Environmental factors:* provision of adequate lighting, elimination of potential fire hazards, safety of electric appliances, adequate ventilation, and controlled temperature (warm and free of drafts) and humidity (lower than 50%).
2. *Measures to control infection:* adequate floor space to permit positioning bassinets at least 60 cm (24 in) apart, hand-washing facilities, and an area for the cleaning of equipment and the storing of supplies. Good handwashing between handling of infants is the single most important measure to prevent neonatal infection (Larson, 1987).

In response to the acquired immunodeficiency syndrome (AIDS) epidemic, the Centers for Disease Control and Prevention (CDC) in Atlanta recommends the following practice (NAACOG, 1986a): *health care workers must wear gloves when touching mucous membranes or nonintact skin of all patients.* In addition, masks, eye coverings, and gowns must be used when indicated. Health care personnel *must wear gloves and gowns when handling the infant until blood and amniotic fluid have been removed from the infant's skin, when drawing blood (e.g., heel stick), and when caring for a fresh wound (e.g., circumcision).*

Persons coming from "outside" are expected to wash their hands before coming in contact with infants or equipment. Such people include nurses, other health care providers, parents, brothers and sisters, department supervisors, electricians, and housekeepers. Cover gowns are not necessary (Rush et al, 1990).

Individuals with infectious conditions are excluded from contact or must take special precautions when working with newborns. This includes people with upper respiratory tract infections, gastrointestinal tract infections, and infectious skin conditions. Most agencies have now coupled this day-to-day self-screening of personnel with yearly health examinations.

Health care workers should wear gloves when caring for people with herpes. Good hand-washing techniques are required at all times. Visitors usually are not restricted.

3. *Safety factors.* Security measures have been implemented in many agencies in response to kidnappings from nurseries. Identical identification bracelets are placed on infants and their parents. Infants are footprinted and/or have identification pictures taken after birth before they leave the mother's side. Personnel wear picture identification badges or other badges that identify them as newborn personnel. Mothers are instructed to be certain they know the identity of anyone who cares for the infant and never to release the infant to anyone who is not wearing the appropriate identification.

Supporting Adaptation to Extrauterine Life

Body Temperature

During all procedures heat loss must be avoided or minimized for the newborn. **Cold stress** is detrimental to the newborn. It increases the need for oxygen and can upset the acid-base balance. The infant may react by increasing its respiratory rate and may become cyanotic. An axillary temperature should be taken every hour until the newborn's temperature stabilizes. Initial temperatures as low as 96.8°F (36°C) are not uncommon. By the twelfth hour, the newborn's temperature should stabilize within the normal range **(thermoregulation).**

The nurse can help stabilize the newborn's body temperature in several ways. The ambient temperature of the nursery unit should be 75° F (24° C). The newborn should be dried and wrapped in warmed blankets immediately after birth, taking care to keep the head well covered while the parent holds the newborn. The infant may be placed directly on the mother's abdomen or chest, dried, and covered with a warm blanket (Clinical Application of Research). If the infant does not remain with the parents during the first 1 to 2 hours after birth, the thoroughly dried, unclothed baby can be placed under a radiant heat panel or warmer until the body temperature stabilizes. The infant's skin temperature is used as the point of control when using a warmer with a servocontrol mechanism. The control panel usually is maintained between 96.8° and 98.6° F (36° and 37° C). This setting should maintain the infant's skin temperature around 97.6° F (36.5° C). A thermistor probe (automatic sensor) is taped to the right upper quadrant of the abdomen immediately below the right intercostal margin, never over a bone. This will ensure detection of minor changes resulting from peripheral vasoconstriction, dilatation, or increased metabolism long before a change in deep (core) body temperature develops. The other end of the probe cord is attached to the control panel. The sensor needs to be checked periodically to make sure it is securely attached to the infant's skin. The temperature of the newborn is checked by axilla every hour with a thermometer.

Other examinations and activities are performed with the newborn under a heat panel. The initial bath is postponed until the newborn's skin temperature reaches 97.6° F (36.5° C) and is maintained for at least for 2 hours.

CLINICAL APPLICATION OF RESEARCH

THERMOREGULATION IMMEDIATELY AFTER BIRTH

Immediately after birth, infants are often placed under a radiant warmer, dried, and observed until they are ready to be admitted to a nursery. Sometimes the unclothed infant is immediately placed on the mother's chest, dried, and the mother and infant are covered with a warmed blanket. Is there a difference in the infant's ability to maintain a normal temperature related to these two practices? In a replication of a previous study, Vaughans (1990) assessed 20 infants who were divided into two groups; 11 infants were dried and placed on the mother's chest and covered with a warmed blanket immediately after birth; nine infants were dried and placed under a radiant warmer. The range of axillary temperatures assessed after 10 minutes for the group given to mothers immediately was 96.3° to 98.4° F and for the group placed under the radiant warmer, 96.7° to 98.5° F. The

average axillary temperature for each group was 97.7° F. Therefore no statistical differences between the two groups existed. Some temperatures in both groups fell below an acceptable minimum temperature. Further research is indicated to determine why some temperatures fall, and what factors contribute to the fall in temperature. This study supported the findings of other researchers that newborn infants are able to maintain their temperatures when placed in skin-to-skin contact with their mothers immediately after birth. Thus this practice is safe and can be incorporated into family-centered care. Continued monitoring of the neonate's temperature in the early newborn period is essential.

Reference: Vaughans, B: Early maternal-infant contact and neonatal thermoregulation, *Neonat Netw* 8(5):19, 1990.

Warming Infant with Hypothermia

Even a normal full-term infant in good health can become hypothermic. Birth in a car on the way to the hospital, a cold birthing room, or inadequate drying and wrapping immediately after birth may cause the infant's temperature to fall below the normal range (**hypothermia**). Warming the hypothermic baby is accomplished with care. Rapid warming or cooling may cause apneic spells and acidosis in an infant. Therefore the warming process is monitored to progress slowly over a period of 2 to 4 hours.

Adequate Oxygen Supply

Establishing a patent airway is a primary objective during birth. Four conditions are essential for maintenance of an adequate oxygen supply:
- A clear airway
- Respiratory efforts
- A functioning cardiopulmonary system
- Heat support (exposure to cold stress increases oxygen needs)

Signs of potential complications related to abnormal breathing are shown in the box on p. 372.

Maintenance of Clear Airway

Generally the normal full-term infant born vaginally has little difficulty clearing the air passages. Most secretions are moved by gravity and brought to the oropharynx by the cough reflex to be drained or swallowed. The infant is maintained in a side-lying position with a rolled blanket at the back to facilitate drainage (Fig. 14-3). If excessive mucus is present, the foot of the crib may be slightly elevated, and the oropharynx is suctioned with a bulb syringe (Fig. 14-4) or a DeLee mucus-trap suction

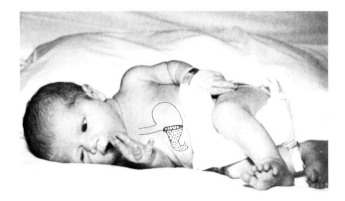

FIG. 14-3 Side-lying position. Infant is turned to right side and supported in this position to facilitate drainage from mouth and to promote emptying into the small intestine.

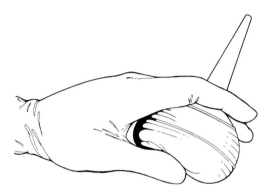

FIG. 14-4 Bulb syringe. Bulb must be compressed before insertion. (From Smith DP et al: *Comprehensive child and family nursing*, St Louis, 1991, Mosby.)

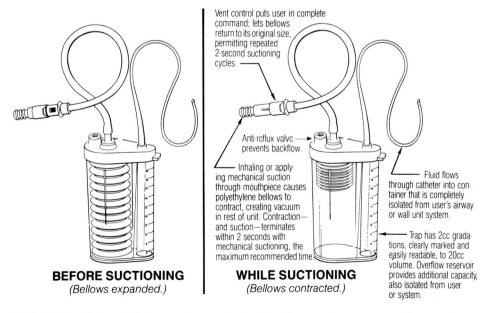

Vent control puts user in complete command; lets bellows return to its original size, permitting repeated 2-second suctioning cycles.

Anti reflux valve prevents backflow.

Inhaling or applying mechanical suction through mouthpiece causes polyethylene bellows to contract, creating vacuum in rest of unit. Contraction—and suction—terminates within 2 seconds with mechanical suctioning, the maximum recommended time.

Fluid flows through catheter into container that is completely isolated from user's airway or wall unit system.

Trap has 2cc gradations, clearly marked and easily readable, to 20cc volume. Overflow reservoir provides additional capacity, also isolated from user or system.

BEFORE SUCTIONING
(Bellows expanded.)

WHILE SUCTIONING
(Bellows contracted.)

FIG. 14-5 (Isolated) DeLee suction method with catheter and mucus trap. (Courtesy Busse Hospital Disposables, Hauppauge, NY.)

SIGNS OF POTENTIAL COMPLICATIONS

ABNORMAL NEWBORN BREATHING

1. Bradypnea: respirations ≤ 25/min
2. Tachypnea: respirations ≥ 60/min
3. Abnormal breath sounds: crackles (rales), rhonchi, wheezes, expiratory grunt
4. Respiratory distress: nasal flaring, retractions, chin tug, labored breathing

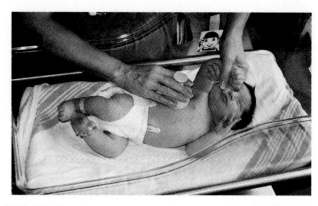

FIG. 14-6   Chest percussion. Nurse performs gentle percussion over the chest wall using a percussion cup to aid in loosening secretions before suctioning.

catheter (Fig. 14-5). The nurse may perform gentle percussion over the chest wall using a soft circular mask or a percussion cup to aid in loosening secretions before suctioning (Whaley, Wong, 1995) (Fig. 14-6). "Milking" the trachea is ineffective, may injure cartilage, and often delays effective suctioning.

Suctioning of Upper Airway

If the infant has excess mucus in the respiratory tract, the mouth and nasal passages may be suctioned with a **bulb syringe.** The infant who is coughing and choking on the secretions should be supported with its head downward. The infant should never be suspended by the ankles. First suction the mouth. This prevents the infant from inhaling pharyngeal secretions by gasping as the nares are touched. The bulb is compressed and inserted into one side of the mouth. The center of the infant's mouth is avoided because this could stimulate the gag reflex. The nasal passages are suctioned one nostril at a time. When the infant's cry does not sound as though it were through mucus or a bubble, suctioning can be stopped. The bulb syringe should always be kept in the infant's crib. The parents should be given demonstrations on how to use the bulb syringe and asked to perform a return demonstration.

A **DeLee mucus-trap suction apparatus** may be needed to remove secretions. The catheter tip should be lubricated with sterile water before it is inserted through the nares. A 120 ml (4 oz) bottle of sterile water for feeding is convenient for this purpose, already in a sterile container, and decreases risk of contamination possible with large stock bottles. The suction apparatus is placed in the user's mouth or attached to a wall suction, and gentle suction is applied as the tube is rotated and removed from the infant's nose. The procedure also can be performed by inserting the tube through the infant's mouth along the base of the tongue. To prevent tissue trauma, forcing the catheter should be avoided. Correct placement is determined by the stimulation of the infant's gagging reflex, which indicates entrance into the esophagus, or coughing, which indicates entrance into the trachea. Suctioning should be discontinued when the cry is clear. The mucus obtained may be sent to the laboratory for examination and cultures if necessary.

The DeLee mucus-trap suction apparatus is used most commonly during the birth process. The isolated DeLee suction method (Busse bac/shield) provides safe oral or mechanical suctioning of newborns while preventing the transmission of bacteria, viruses, and other infectious material from the newborn to the user (Fig. 14-5).

Use of a Nasopharyngeal Catheter with Mechanical Suction Apparatus

Deeper suctioning may be necessary to remove excessive or tenacious mucus from the infant's nasopharynx. The same procedure is followed for deep suctioning as just described with the DeLee device. Proper tube insertion and suctioning 10 seconds or less per tube insertion will help prevent laryngospasms and oxygen depletion. If wall suction is used, the pressure should be adjusted to less than 80 mm Hg. The catheter is lubricated in sterile water. The catheter is inserted either orally along the base of the tongue or horizontally through the nose into the nares. Then it is raised to advance it beyond the bend at the back of nares. After the catheter is properly placed, suction is created by placing a thumb over the control as the catheter is carefully rotated and gently withdrawn. This procedure may need to be repeated until the infant's cry sounds clear and air entry into the lungs is heard by stethoscope.

Relieving Airway Obstruction

A choking infant needs immediate attention. The infant is placed face down over the rescuer's arm with the head lower than the trunk and the head supported. Four quick, sharp back blows are delivered between the infant's shoulder blades with the heel of the rescuer's hand (Fig. 14-7, *A*). After delivery of the back blows, the rescuer's free hand is placed flat on the infant's back so that the infant is "sandwiched" between the two hands, making certain the neck and chin are well supported. While the rescuer maintains support with the infant's head lower than the trunk, the infant is turned

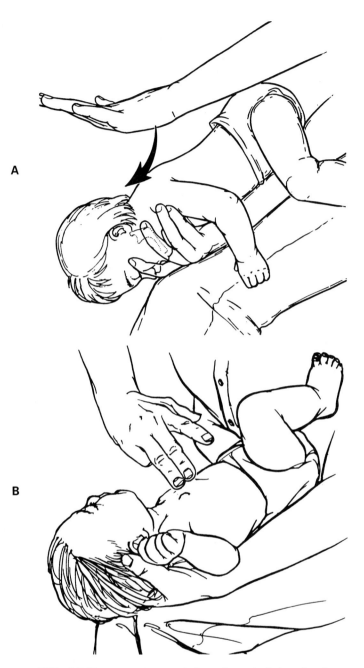

FIG. 14-7   Back blows and chest thrust in infant for clearing airway obstruction. **A,** Back blow. **B,** Chest thrust. (From Emergency Cardiac Care Committee and Subcommittees, American Heart Association: Guidelines for cardiopulmonary resuscitation and emergency cardiac care, V, pediatric basic life support, *JAMA* 268(16):2251, 1991.)

and placed supine on the rescuer's thigh, where four chest thrusts are applied in rapid succession (Fig. 14-7, *B*) in the same place as external chest compressions described for **cardiopulmonary resuscitation (CPR)** (see Emergency Boxes).

All personnel working with infants must have current infant CPR certification. Many institutions offer infant CPR courses to new parents (Donaher-Wagner, Braun, 1992). Cardiac and respiratory arrest can occur in in-

fants. Careful monitoring is necessary so that rapid treatment can be given.

Common Problems in the Newborn
Physical Injuries

Birth trauma includes any physical injury sustained by a newborn during labor and birth. Many injuries are minor and readily resolved in the neonatal period without treatment. Other traumas require some degree of intervention. A few are serious enough to be fatal.

Several factors predispose an infant to birth trauma (Fanaroff, Martin, 1992). *Maternal factors* include uterine dysfunction that leads to prolonged or precipitous labor, preterm or postterm labor, and cephalopelvic disproportion. Injury may result from dystocia caused by *fetal* macrosomia, multifetal gestation, abnormal or difficult presentation, and congenital anomalies. *Intrapartum events* that can result in scalp injury include the use of intrapartum monitoring of FHR and fetal scalp sampling. *Obstetric birth techniques* can also cause injury. Forceps birth, vacuum extraction, version and extraction, and cesarean birth are all potential contributory factors.

Soft Tissue Injuries

Caput succedaneum and *cephalhematoma* are described in Chapter 13 (see Fig. 13-4).

Subconjunctival and retinal hemorrhages result from the rupture of capillaries because of increased intracranial pressure during birth. The capillaries clear within 5 days after birth and usually present no further problems. Parents need explanation and reassurance that these injuries are harmless.

Erythema, ecchymoses, petechiae, abrasions, lacerations, and edema of buttocks and extremities may be present. Localized discoloration may appear over presenting or dependent parts and from application of forceps or the vacuum extractor. Ecchymoses and edema may appear anywhere on the body. Petechiae, or pinpoint hemorrhagic areas, acquired during birth may extend over the upper trunk and face. These lesions are benign if they disappear within 2 days of birth and no new lesions appear. Ecchymoses and petechiae may be signs of a more serious disorder, such as *thrombocytopenic purpura*. To differentiate hemorrhagic areas from skin rashes and discolorations, try to blanch the skin with two fingers. Petechiae and ecchymoses do not blanch because extravasated blood remains within the tissues.

Trauma secondary to dystocia occurs over the presenting part. Forceps injury and bruising from the vacuum cup occur at the site of application of the instruments. Forceps injury commonly has a linear configuration across both sides of the face outlining the blades of the forceps. The affected areas are kept clean to minimize risk of infection. The increased use of the vacuum extractor and use of padded forceps blades may significantly

E M E R G E N C Y

CARDIOPULMONARY RESUSCITATION (CPR)

Wash hands before and after touching infant and equipment. Wear gloves, if possible.

RESUSCITATION
Assess Responsiveness:

Observe color; tap or gently shake shoulders.

Yell for help; if alone, perform CPR for 1 min before calling for help again.

Position Infant:

Turn the infant on to back, supporting the head and neck.

Place the infant on firm, flat surface.

Airway:

Open the airway with the head tilt–chin lift method (Fig. 14-8).

Place one hand on the infant's forehead and tilt the head back.

Place the fingers of other hand under the bone of the lower jaw at the chin.

Breathing:

Assess for evidence of breathing:
  Observe for chest movement.
  Listen for exhaled air.
  Feel for exhaled air flow.

To breathe for infant:
  Take a breath.
  Place mouth over the infant's nose and mouth to create a seal.
  Note: When available, a mask with a one-way valve should be used.
  Give two slow breaths (1 to 1.5 sec/breath), pausing to inhale between breaths.
  Note: Gently puff the volume of air in your cheeks into infant. Do not force air.

The infant's chest should rise slightly with each puff; keep fingers on the chest wall to sense air entry.

Circulation:

Assess circulation:

Check pulse of the brachial artery (Fig. 14-9) while maintaining the head tilt.

If the pulse is present, initiate rescue breathing. Continue at a rate of once every 3 seconds or 20 times/min until spontaneous breathing resumes.

If the pulse is absent, initiate chest compressions and coordinate them with breathing.

Chest compression. There are two systems of chest compression. Nurses should know both methods.

Maintain the head tilt and:

1. Place thumbs side-by-side in the middle third of the sternum with fingers around the chest and supporting the back (Fig. 14-10).
   —Compress the sternum ½ to ¾ inch.

2. Place index finger of hand just under an imaginary line drawn between the nipples. Place the middle and ring fingers on the sternum adjacent to the index finger.
   —Using the middle and ring fingers, compress the sternum approximately ½ to 1 inch.

Avoid compression of the xiphoid process.

Release the pressure without moving the thumbs/fingers from the chest.

Repeat at a rate of at least 100 times/min; five compressions in 3 seconds or less.

Perform 10 cycles of 5 compressions and 1 ventilation. After the cycles, check the brachial artery to determine presence of the pulse.

Discontinue compressions when the infant's spontaneous heart rate reaches or exceeds 80 beats/min.

Record the time and duration of the procedure and the effects of intervention.

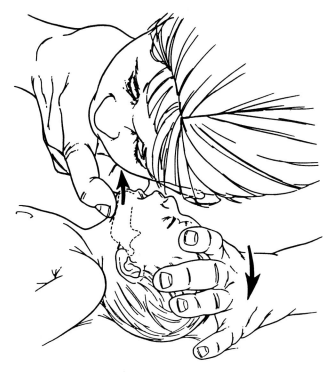

FIG. 14-8 Opening airway with head tilt–chin lift method. (From Emergency Cardiac Care Committee and Subcommittees, American Heart Association: Guidelines for cardiopulmonary resuscitation and emergency cardiac care, V, pediatric basic life support, *JAMA* 268(16):2251, 1991.)

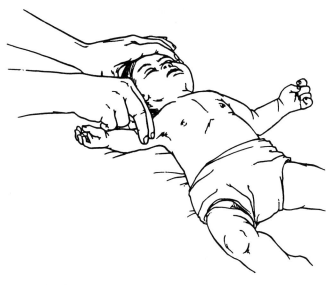

FIG. 14-9 Checking pulse of brachial artery. (From Emergency Cardiac Care Committee and Subcommittees, American Heart Association: Guidelines for cardiopulmonary resuscitation and emergency cardiac care, V, pediatric basic life support, *JAMA* 268(16):2251, 1991.)

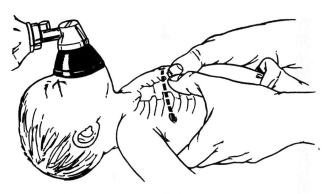

FIG. 14-10 Side-by-side thumb placement for chest compressions in newborns. (From Emergency Cardiac Care Committee and Subcommittees, American Heart Association: Guidelines for cardiopulmonary resuscitation and emergency cardiac care, V, pediatric basic life support, *JAMA* 268(16): 2251, 1991.)

E M E R G E N C Y

RELIEVING AIRWAY OBSTRUCTION

Back blow and chest thrusts are used to clear an airway obstructed by a foreign body.

BACK BLOWS (Fig. 14-7, A):
Position the infant prone over forearm with the head down and with the infant's jaw firmly supported.
Rest the supporting arm on the thigh.
Deliver four back blows forcefully between the infant's shoulder blades with the heel of the free hand.

TURN INFANT:
Place the free hand on the infant's back to sandwich the baby between both hands; one hand supports the neck, jaw, and chest while the other supports the back.
Turn the infant over and place the head lower than the chest, supporting the head and neck.
Alternative position: Place the infant face down on your lap with the head lower than the trunk; firmly support the head. Apply back blows and then turn the infant as a unit.

CHEST THRUSTS (FIG. 14-7, B):
Provide four downward chest thrusts on the lower third of the sternum.
Remove foreign body, if it is visible.

E M E R G E N C Y

RELIEVING AIRWAY OBSTRUCTION— cont'd

OPEN AIRWAY
Open airway with the head-tilt/chin-lift maneuver and attempt to ventilate.
Repeat the sequence of back blows, turn, and chest thrusts.
Continue these emergency procedures until signs of recovery occur:
Palpable peripheral pulses return.
The pupils become normal size and are responsive.
Mottling and cyanosis disappear.
Record the time and duration of the procedure and the effects of this intervention.

reduce the incidence of these lesions (Fanaroff, Martin, 1992).

Accidental lacerations may be inflicted with a scalpel during cesarean birth. These cuts may occur on any part of the body but are most often found on the scalp, buttocks, and thighs. Usually they are superficial, needing only to be kept clean. Butterfly adhesive strips will hold together the edges of more serious lacerations. Rarely are sutures needed.

Skeletal Injuries

The *clavicle* is the bone most often fractured during birth. Usually the break is in the middle third of the bone. Dystocia, particularly shoulder dystocia, may be the predisposing problem. Limitation of motion of the arm, crepitus of the bone, and no Moro reflex on the affected side are diagnostic. Except for use of gentle rather than rigorous handling, there is no accepted treatment for fractured clavicle. The infant may be positioned in bed with the fractured side up. The figure-of-eight bandage, which is appropriate for the older child, should not be used for the newborn. The prognosis is good.

The *humerus* and *femur* are other bones that may be fractured during a difficult birth. Fractures in newborns generally heal rapidly. Immobilization is accomplished with slings, splints, swaddling, and other devices.

The infant's immature, flexible skull can withstand a great deal of molding before fracture results. Location of the fracture determines whether it is insignificant or fatal. Unless a blood vessel is involved, linear fractures heal without special treatment. These fractures account for 70% of all fractures in this age group. Depressed skull fractures may occur without laceration of either the skin or the dural membrane. These fractures may occur during difficult births from pressure of the head on the bony pelvis or from injudicious application of forceps.

Congenital dislocation of the hip or *congenital hip dysplasia* is often a hereditary disorder and occurs more commonly in girls because of the structure of the pelvis. In this condition, the acetabulum is abnormally shallow. The head of the femur becomes dislocated upward and backward to lie on the dorsal aspect of the ilium. The pressure of the displaced femoral head may form a false acetabulum on the ilium. A stretched joint capsule results, and ossification of the femoral head is delayed.

Before dislocation occurs, reduced movement, splinting of the affected hip, limited abduction, and asymmetry of the hip may be noted. After dislocation, all of these signs are present, together with external rotation and shortening of the leg. A clicking sound may be heard on gentle forced abduction of the leg (Ortolani's sign, Fig. 14-11), and a bulge of the femoral head is felt or seen (Fig. 14-11, *B*). The deformity in congenital dysplasia of the hip can be seen on x-ray examination.

Treatment involves pressing the femoral head into the acetabulum to form an adequate socket before ossification is complete. Thick diapers may be applied to abduct and externally rotate the leg and flex the hip; anterior flaps of the diapers are pinned under the posterior flaps. Alternatively, a Frejka pillow may be applied over a diaper and plastic pants. A Pavlik Harness is also frequently used in treatment of congenital hip dislocation (Fig. 14-

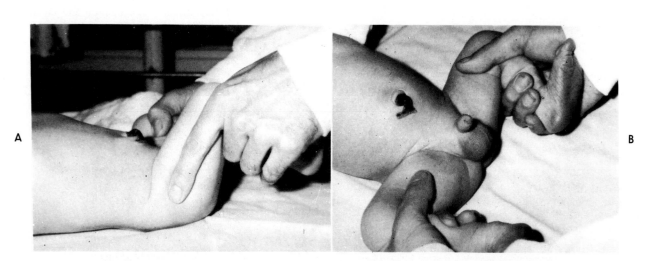

FIG. 14-11 Method of assessing for hip dysplasia using Ortolani's maneuver. **A,** Examiner's middle fingers are placed over greater trochanter and thumbs over inner thigh opposite lesser trochanter. **B,** Gentle pressure is exerted to further flex thigh on hip, and thighs are rotated outward. If hip dysplasia is present, head of femur can be felt to slip forward in acetabulum and slip back when pressure is released and legs returned to their original position. A click is sometimes heard (Ortolani's sign).

12). Later a spica cast is usually applied to maintain abduction, extension and internal rotation, usually with the infant in a "frog-leg" position.

Parents need support in handling an infant with skeletal injuries because they are often fearful of hurting their newborn. Parents are encouraged to practice handling, changing, and feeding the injured newborn under the guidance of the nursing staff. This increases the parents' knowledge and confidence, in addition to facilitating attachment. A plan for follow-up therapy is developed with the parents so that the times and arrangements for therapy are convenient for them.

Physiologic Problems

Physiologic Jaundice. Approximately 50% of all full-term newborns are visibly jaundiced (yellowish in color) during the first 3 days of life. Serum bilirubin levels less than 5 mg/dl usually are not reflected in visible skin jaundice. **Physiologic jaundice** is characterized by a progressive increase in serum levels of unconjugated bilirubin from 2 mg/dl in cord blood to a mean peak of 6 mg/dl by 72 hours of age, followed by a decline to 5 mg/dl by day 5, and not exceeding 12 mg/dl. These serum values are within the normal physiologic limitations of the healthy term newborn who was not exposed to perinatal complication (such as hypoxia). No bilirubin toxicity develops. For the normal full-term newborn, serum bilirubin of 12 to 15 mg/dl is the cut-off point

for use of phototherapy and 20 mg/dl for exchange transfusion.

Every newborn is assessed for jaundice. The *blanch test* assists in the differentiation of cutaneous jaundice from skin color. To do the test, apply pressure with a finger over a bony area (e.g., nose, forehead, sternum) for several seconds to empty all the capillaries in that spot. If jaundice is present, the blanched area will look yellow before the capillaries refill. The conjunctival sacs and buccal mucosa are assessed, especially in darker-skinned infants. It is preferable to assess for jaundice in daylight, because there is possible distortion of color from artificial lighting, reflection from nursery walls, and the like.

Jaundice is noticeable first in the head and then progresses gradually toward the abdomen and extremities because of the newborn infant's circulatory pattern (cephalocaudal developmental progression). The appearance of jaundice in the various body locations gives a rough estimate of the circulating levels of unbound bilirubin. For example, when jaundice appears over the nose, the circulating level of unbound bilirubin is approximately 3 mg; levels at which other body areas appear jaundiced are as follows:

Approximate Level of Hyperbilirubinemia by Cephalocaudal Distribution

Nose: 3 mg/dl   Abdomen: 10 mg/dl
Face: 5 mg/dl   Legs: 12 mg/dl
Chest: 7 mg/dl   Palms: 20 mg/dl

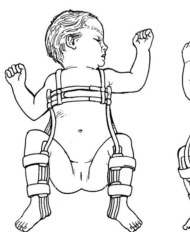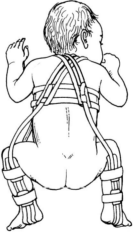

FIG. 14-12   Treatment for congenital hip dislocation by application of the Pavlik Harness. 1. Position the infant in a relaxed supine position. 2. The shoulder straps on the chest halter should cross in the back to prevent slippage down the shoulders. 3. The buckles for the anterior (flexor) stirrup-straps should be placed at the anterior line. 4. The buckles for the posterior (abduction) stirrup-straps should be placed over the scapula. 5. The Velcro® straps for the proximal part of the leg should be placed just below the popliteal fossa. 6. Place the feet into the stirrups and secure the straps. 7. The posterior straps should already be attached and should not need to be unfastened when the harness is removed. 8. Secure the straps attached to the stirrups to the anterior buckles positioning the hips at 90 degree flexion and 70 degree abduction.

Hypoglycemia. Hypoglycemia during the early newborn period is defined as a blood glucose concentration of less than 35 mg/dl or as a plasma concentration of less than 40 mg/dl in the term newborn. At birth when the cord is cut, the newborn abruptly loses its glucose supply. Glucose levels fall normally over the first hours after birth. Since hypoglycemia may be asymptomatic, a blood-glucose test is often done soon after birth and repeated at 4 hours of age. More frequent monitoring is required if the newborn is in an at-risk group [i.e., large or small for gestational age or low-birth-weight (LBW)] or has been exposed to stressors such as cold, perinatal asphyxia, or tocolysis for preterm labor.

Signs of hypoglycemia include jitteriness, irregular respiratory effort; cyanosis; apnea; weak, high-pitched cry; feeding difficulty; hunger; lethargy; twitching; eye-rolling; and seizures. The signs may be transient and recurrent.

Hypoglycemia in the low-risk term infant is usually resolved by feeding the infant. Occasionally administration of intravenous glucose is required.

Hypocalcemia. Hypocalcemia (less than 7 mg/dl) is strongly associated with newborns of diabetic mothers, perinatal asphyxia, trauma, LBW, and preterm birth. Early-onset hypocalcemia occurs within the first 72 hours after birth. Signs of hypocalcemia include jitteriness, edema, apnea, intermittent cyanosis, and abdominal distention.

In most instances, early-onset hypocalcemia is self-limiting and resolves within 1 to 3 days. Treatment includes early feeding and, occasionally, administration of calcium supplements.

Jitteriness is a symptom of both hypoglycemia and hypocalcemia. Hypocalcemia must be considered if therapy for hypoglycemia is ineffective. In many newborns, jitteriness remains despite therapy and cannot be explained by hypoglycemia or hypocalcemia (Fanaroff, Martin, 1992)

Supporting Parents in the Care of Their Infant

The sensitivity of the caregiver to the social responses of the infant is basic to the development of a mutually satisfying parent-child relationship. Sensitivity increases over time as parents' awareness of their infant's social capabilities becomes more acute (see Cultural Considerations).

Social Interactions

The activities of daily care during the neonatal period offer the best times for infant and family interaction. While caring for their baby, mother and father can talk to the infant, play baby games, and caress and cuddle the child. In Fig. 14-13, mother, father, and infant engage in arousal, imitation of facial expression, and smiling. Older

CULTURAL CONSIDERATIONS

SOME CULTURAL BELIEFS ABOUT NEWBORNS

Mexican women may wish to place belly bands or coins over the infant's navel.

Muslim (Saudi Arabia) women may wish to say a prayer in the newborn's ear at the time of birth. Some groups still practice female circumcision.

Iranian male infants are usually circumcised.

Southeast Asians usually do not circumcise males. The infant should not be complimented because it is believed to cause the infant to be captured by evil spirits.

The birth of male Indian infants is celebrated, while female births are not.

Haitian infants are usually not named until they are 1 month old.

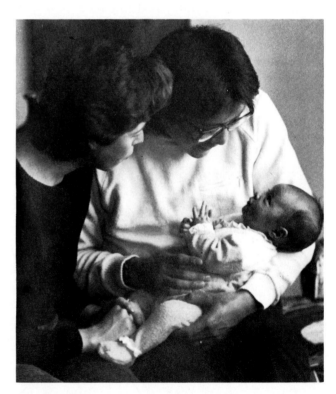

FIG. 14-13 Mother-father-baby interactions. (Courtesy Colleen Stainton.)

children's contact with a newborn needs to be supervised for strength of hugs, exploring of eyes and nose, and attempts to feed the baby. Parents often keep baby books that record their infant's progress.

Caregiving activities for the newborn are shared by the nurse and the parents. The nurse acts as teacher and sup-

Infant Care Teaching Record

INFANT CARE	DATE	INITIALS	TEACHING/ LEARNING CODE
Using/reading thermometer			
Temperature regulation			
Cord care*			
Dressing, wrapping, comforting*			
Voiding/stool			
Diapering*			
Bulb syringe*			
Car seat			
Circumcision			
Newborn screening			
Birth certificate			
INFANT FEEDING			
Frequency of feeding			
Positions for feeding			
Burping*			
INFANT FEEDING – BREAST			
Length of feedings			
Colostrum/ when milk comes in			
Breaking suction*			
Milk supply			
Engorgement			
Hand expression			
Breast pump and milk storage			
INFANT FEEDING - BOTTLE			
Amount of feedings			
Formula preparation and storage			
Warming formula			
Don't use honey [†]			

Teaching/Learning Code:

VT = videotape   V = verbal instruction

D   = demonstration   R = return demonstration

VU = verbalizes understanding   P = printed material given

NA = not applicable

*Return demonstration required before discharged at 24 hours.

[†] Honey contains botulism spores. Children under the age of 12 months should not be given
   honey (Turick-Gibson, 1988).

FIG. 14-14 Infant care teaching record.

port person. As soon as the mother feels physically able, she is encouraged to participate in her child's care. The mother's need for knowledge and the factors that may hinder her learning are determined through questioning and observation. The content taught and teaching aids used should reflect the mother's level of understanding. Films and tapes can be valuable timesavers in teaching. Most hospitals provide parents with written instructions for infant care. The care given the infant is supervised, and the parents are encouraged to ask questions. The in-

fant care teaching record (Fig. 14-14) can serve as a guideline for teaching parents.

Infant Feeding

The infant may be put to breast shortly after birth or at least within 4 hours of birth. If the infant is to be bottle-fed, a nurse may offer a few sips of sterile water to be certain that the infant's sucking and swallowing reflexes are intact and that there are no anomalies such as tracheoesophageal fistula before the mother feeds the baby. Most infants are on *demand feeding schedules* and are allowed to feed when they awaken. Ordinarily feedings are encouraged every 3 to 4 hours during the day and only when the infant awakens during the night in the first few days after birth. Breastfed babies will nurse more often than bottle-fed babies since human breast milk is digested faster than formulas made from cow's milk, and because the stomach will empty sooner. Water supple-

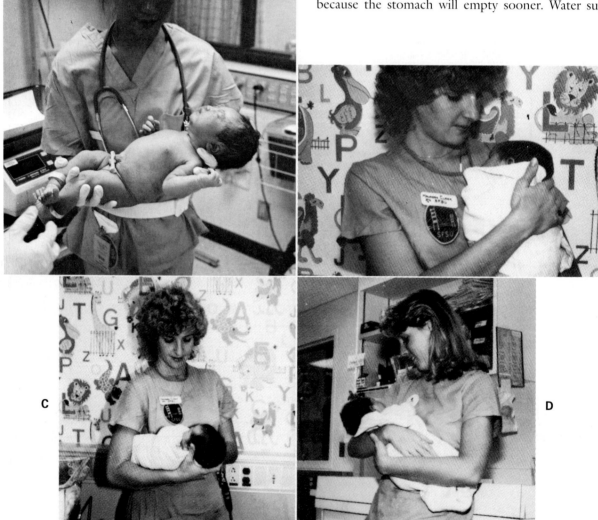

FIG. 14-15 Holding baby securely with support for head. **A,** Holding infant while moving infant from one place to another. Baby (whose temperature is well stabilized in a warm nursery) is undressed to show posture. Note lack of curvature in normal infant's spine and flexion of extremities. **B,** Holding baby upright in "burping" position. **C,** "Football" hold. **D,** Cradling hold. (**A,** Courtesy Kim Molloy, San Jose, CA.)

ments are usually not recommended. For a thorough discussion of infant feeding, see Chapter 15.

Holding and Positioning

The infant is held securely with support for the head because newborns are unable to maintain an erect head posture for more than a few moments. Fig. 14-15 illustrates various positions for holding an infant with adequate support. Too much stimulation is avoided after feeding and before a sleep period.

After feeding, positioning the infant on the right side promotes gastric emptying into the small intestine (see Fig. 14-3). Placing the infant in the crib in a side-lying position also permits drainage of mucus from the mouth and applies no pressure to the cord or the sensitive circumcised penis. The infant's position is changed from side to side to help develop even contours of the head and to ease pressure on the other parts of the body (see Clinical Application of Research).

Anatomically the infant's shape—barrel chest and flat, curveless spine—makes it easy for the child to roll and startle. A folded or rolled blanket against the spine will prevent rolling to the supine position and will promote a feeling of security. Care must be taken to prevent the infant from rolling off flat, unguarded surfaces. The parent or nurse who must turn away from the infant even for a moment keeps one hand securely on the infant. If left on the parent's bed, the infant is walled in with pillows.

Umbilical Cord Care

The care of the umbilical cord is the same as that for any surgical wound. The goal of care is prevention and early identification of hemorrhage or infection. If bleeding from the blood vessels of the cord is noted, the nurse checks the clamp (or tie) and applies a second clamp next to the first one. If bleeding is not stopped immediately, the nurse calls for assistance.

Hospital protocol directs the time and technique for routine cord care. The nurse cleanses the cord and skin

area around the base of the cord with the prescribed preparation (e.g., erythromycin solution, triple blue dye, or alcohol) and checks daily for signs of infection. The cord clamp is removed after 24 hours when the cord is dry (Fig. 14-16).

Bathing

Bathing serves a number of purposes. It provides opportunities for (1) a complete cleansing of the infant, (2) observing the condition, (3) promoting comfort, and (4) parent-child-family socializing. The initial bath is postponed until the infant's skin temperature stabilizes at 36.5° C (97.6° F) or until the core temperature stabilizes at 37° C (98.6° F) for 2 hours. Until the initial bath

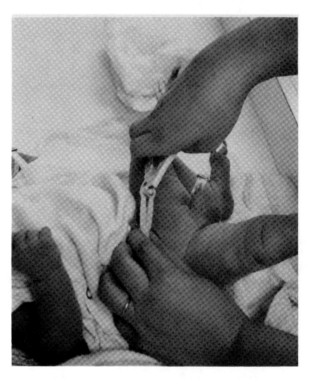

FIG. 14-16   Removal of cord clamp when cord is dry.

 CLINICAL APPLICATION OF RESEARCH

SLEEPING PRONE AND THE RISK OF SUDDEN INFANT DEATH SYNDROME

Researchers from Great Britain, Australia, New Zealand, and the Netherlands have documented an association with the incidence of Sudden Infant Death syndrome (SIDS) and sleeping in the prone position. After publicity in these countries advising against using the prone position, the incidence of SIDS decreased significantly. Guntheroth and Spiers (1992) advise against the prone position for the first 6 months of life, suggesting that side-lying or back-lying is preferable. This research has

been criticized for ignoring the effects of soft mattresses, pillows, and other variables that may affect the incidence of SIDS. The American Academy of Pediatrics now advises against the use of the prone position in the first few months of life.

Reference: Guntheroth WG; Spiers PS: Sleeping prone and the risk of sudden infant death syndrome, *JAMA* 267(17):2359, 1992.

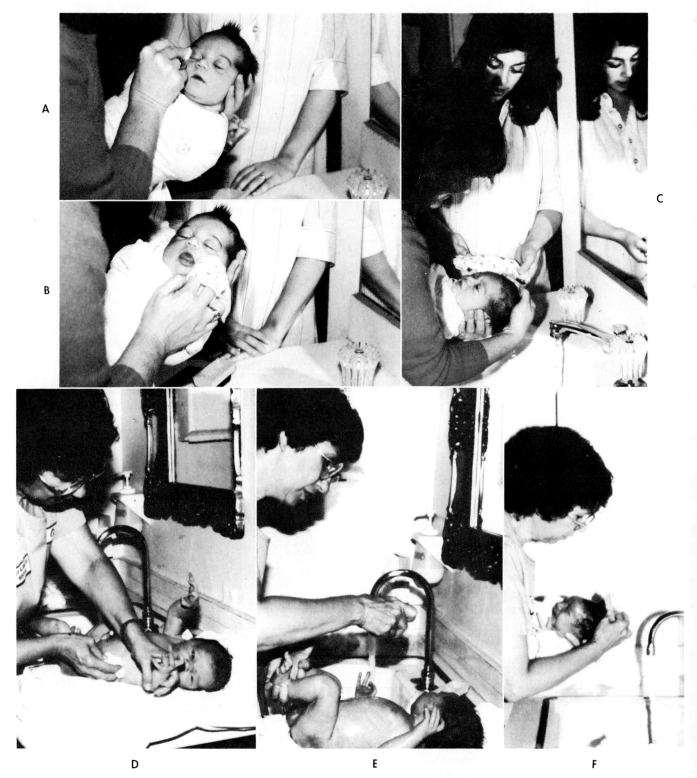

FIG. 14-17 Bathing baby. **A,** Eyes. **B,** Face. **C,** Head and hair. **D,** Sponge-bathing baby. **E,** Rinsing baby. **F,** Brushing hair. Mother in **A, B,** and **C** is being supervised. Note in **D, E,** and **F** that nurse keeps one hand on baby. No gloves required since this is not the first bath. (Courtesy Marjorie Pyle, RNC, *Lifecircle,* Costa Mesa, CA.)

is completed, personnel must wear gloves when handling the newborn. In some hospitals the infant is given the initial bath with mild soap to remove blood and amniotic fluid. Cleansing of the genitals as necessary is deemed sufficient for the first 3 to 4 days. Bathing with warm water is sufficient for the first week. Then a mild soap may be used (NAACOG, 1992). A newborn may not need a bath every day. Creases under the neck and arms and in the diaper area need more attention. If a documented staphylococcal skin infection outbreak occurs in a nursery, the newborn is bathed with dilute hexachlorophene detergent (pHisoHex) (less than 3%), followed by thorough rinsing of the skin. As pHisoHex is a potential neurotoxin, particularly for infants weighing less than 2000 g, it is no longer used in many nurseries. (see Home Care Boxes). The nurse does not need to wear gloves during the bath demonstration (Fig. 14-17).

Questions have arisen about some routine practices: use of soap, oils, powder, lotion, and sponging. One of the most important considerations in skin cleansing is a preservation of the skin's *acid mantle*, which is formed from the uppermost horny layer of the epidermis, sweat, superficial fat, metabolic products, and external substances such as amniotic fluid, microorganisms, and cosmetics. At birth the skin pH is less acidic than that of older infants and adults. Within 4 days the pH of the newborn's skin surface falls to within the bacteriostatic range (pH < 5) (NAACOG, 1992). Consequently, only plain, warm water should be used for the bath (NAACOG, 1992). Alkaline soaps such as Ivory, oils, powder, and lotions are not used because they alter the acid mantle and provide a medium for bacterial growth. The sponging technique generally is used; however, bathing the newborn by immersion has been found to cause less heat loss and less crying, but should not be done until the umbilical cord falls off (about 10 days to 2 weeks).

Rashes

Diaper Rash. Treatment of diaper rash involves exposing the rash to warmth and air. Immediately washing and drying the wet and soiled area and changing the diaper after voiding or defecating prevent and help treat diaper rash. The warmth can be achieved with a 25-watt bulb placed 45 cm (18 in) from the affected area. Disposable diapers and plastic pants may aggravate the rash and should be avoided until healing occurs.

The most severe type of diaper rash occurs when the area becomes infected, indurated (hardened), and tender. Medical advice should be sought and a specifically ordered medication applied.

Other Rashes. A rash on the face may result from the infant's scratching (excoriation) or from rubbing the face against the sheets, particularly if regurgitated stom-

ach contents are not washed off promptly. Newborn rash or erythema toxicum is a common finding.

Clothing

Parents commonly ask how warmly they should dress their infant. A simple rule of thumb is to dress the child as the parents would dress themselves, adding or subtracting clothes and wraps for the infant as necessary. A shirt and diaper may be sufficient clothing for the young infant. A bonnet is needed to protect the scalp and to minimize heat loss if it is cool or to protect against sunburn and to shade the eyes if it is sunny and hot. Wrapping the infant snugly in a blanket maintains body temperature and promotes a feeling of security. Overdressing in warm temperatures can cause discomfort and prickly heat. Underdressing in cold weather also can cause discomfort; cheeks, fingers, and toes can easily become frostbitten.

Care of the Infant's Linens

Care of the infant's clothes and bedding is directed toward minimizing cross infection and removing residue from soap, feces, or urine that may irritate the infant's skin. In the hospital, clothing and bedding are washed separately from other linens and are autoclaved. Some hospitals use disposable shirts and diapers. At home the baby's clothes should be washed with a mild detergent and hot water. A double rinse usually removes traces of the potentially irritating cleansing agent or acid residue from the urine or stool. If possible, the clothing and bedding are dried in the sun to neutralize residue. Parents who have to use coin-operated machines to wash and dry clothes may find it expensive or impossible to wash and rinse the baby's clothes well.

Bedding requires frequent changing. The top of a plastic-coated mattress should be washed frequently, and the crib or bassinet should be damp dusted. The infant's toilet articles may be kept convenient for use in a box or basket.

Home Care

With the trend toward shorter hospital stays after low-risk childbirth, the focus and place of infant care may change. In the in-patient setting, priorities of care must be established and a systematic teaching plan for infant care devised. One way to achieve this end is to use critical path case management for delivery of nursing care (Zander, 1989). *Critical paths or care paths* are defined as shortened case management plans (Gillerman, Beckham, 1991). The care path clearly delineates what teaching/discharge planning should occur within specified times. This ensures that essential topics are addressed and that repetition is avoided. The infant must meet criteria for early discharge (see Box 14-3). A care path may also be developed for the changes expected in the infant over the first several days. The Care Path on p. 387 is an ex-

HOME CARE

SPONGE BATHING (see Fig. 14-17)

FITTING BATHS INTO FAMILY'S SCHEDULE

Give a bath at any time convenient to you but not immediately after a feeding period because the increased handling may cause regurgitation of the feeding.

PREVENTING HEAT LOSS

The temperature of the room should be 75° F (24° C), and the bathing area should be free of drafts.

Control heat loss during the bath period to conserve the infant's energy. Bathing the infant quickly, exposing only a portion of the body at a time, and thorough drying are all parts of the bathing technique.

GATHERING SUPPLIES AND CLOTHING BEFORE STARTING

Clothing suitable for wearing indoors: diaper, shirt; stretch suit or nightgown optional

Unscented, mild soap

Pins, if needed for diaper, closed and placed well out of baby's reach

Cotton balls

Towels for drying infant and a clean washcloth

Receiving blanket

Tub for water or use a sink

BATHING THE BABY

Bring infant to bathing area when all supplies are ready. *Never leave the infant alone on bath table or in bath water, not even for a second!* If you have to leave, take the infant with you or put back into crib.

Test temperature of the water. It should feel pleasantly warm to the inner wrist (about 98° to 99° F).

Do not hold infant under running water—water temperature may change, and infant may be scalded or chilled rapidly.

Wash infant's head before unwrapping and undressing to prevent heat loss.

Cleanse the eyes from the inner canthus outward, using separate parts of a clean washcloth for each eye. For the first 2 to 3 days a discharge may result from the reaction of the conjunctiva to the substance (erythromycin) used as a prophylactic measure against infection. Any discharge should be considered abnormal and reported to the health care provider.

Wash the *scalp* with water and mild soap; rinse well and dry thoroughly. Scalp desquamation, called cradle cap, often can be prevented by removing any scales with a fine-toothed comb or brush after washing. If condition persists, the health care provider may prescribe an ointment to massage into the scalp.

Creases under the chin and arms and in the groin may need daily cleansing. The crease under the chin may be exposed by elevating the infant's shoulders 5 cm (2 in) and letting the head drop back.

Cleanse *ears* and *nose* with twists made of moistened cotton or a corner of the washcloth.

Do not use cotton-tipped swabs as these may cause injury.

Undress baby and wash body and arms and legs. Pat dry gently. Baby may be tub bathed after the cord drops off and umbilicus and circumcised penis are completely healed.

PREVENTING SKIN TRAUMA

The fragile skin can be injured by too vigorous cleansing.

If stool or other debris has dried and caked on the skin, soak the area to remove it. Do not attempt to rub it off, because abrasion may result. Gentleness, patting dry rather than rubbing, and use of a mild soap without perfumes or coloring are recommended. Chemicals in the coloring and perfume can cause rashes in sensitive skin.

CARE OF THE CORD

Use a cotton swab. Dip swab in solution the health care provider has ordered and cleanse around base of the cord, where it joins the skin. Notify the health care provider of any odor, discharge, or skin inflammation around the cord. The clamp is removed when the cord is dry (about 24 hours; see Fig. 14-16). The diaper should not cover the cord. A wet or soiled diaper will slow or prevent drying of the cord and foster infection. When the cord drops off after a week to 10 days, small drops of blood may be seen when the baby cries. This will heal itself. It is not dangerous.

CARE OF HANDS AND FEET

Wash and dry between the fingers and toes.

Do not cut fingernails and toenails immediately after birth. The nails have to grow out far enough from the skin so that the skin is not cut by mistake. If the baby scratches himself or herself, apply loosely fitted mitts over each of the baby's hands. Do so as a last resort, however, because it interferes with the baby's ability for self-consolation. When the nails have grown, the *fingernails* and *toenails* can be cut more easily with manicure scissors (preferably scissors with rounded tips) when the infant is asleep. Nails should be kept short.

HOME CARE

SPONGE BATHING—cont'd

CLEANSING GENITALS

Cleanse the *genitals* of infants daily and after voiding and defecating. For girls, cleansing of the genitals may be done by separating the labia and gently washing from the pubic area to the anus. For uncircumcised boys, gently pull back (retract) the foreskin. Stop when resistance is felt. Wash the tip (glans) with soap and warm water and replace the foreskin. The foreskin must be returned to its original position to prevent constriction and swelling. In most newborns the inner layer of the foreskin adheres to the glans and the foreskin cannot be retracted. By the age of 3 years, in 90% of boys the foreskin can be retracted easily without pain or trauma. For others, the foreskin is not retractable until the teens. As soon as the foreskin is partly retractable, and the child is old enough, he can be taught self-care.

DRESSING THE INFANT

When dressing the child, bunch up the shirt in both hands and expand the neck opening before placing the neck opening over the face; then slip the shirt over the rest of the head. Do not pull shirts roughly over the face or catch fingers in shirt sleeves.

If cloth diapers are used, absorbency can be increased by bringing the bulk of the diaper in the front for a boy and in the back for a girl. This will help absorb urine so that skin is protected. The diaper between the infant's legs should not be bulky because it can cause outward displacement of the hips. A soaker pad can be placed under the infant as a protection for the blanket. The continued use of plastic or rubber pants may lead to diaper rash.

Store infant's towels, washcloths, and supplies apart from the family for 2 to 4 months to prevent infection.

HOME CARE

TUB BATHING

See guidelines for sponge bathing.

Place liner on bottom of tub to prevent infant from slipping.

Add 3 inches of comfortably warm water (98° to 99° F—pleasantly warm to your inner wrist).

Wash face and shampoo hair as for sponge bath. Undress baby. Lower infant slowly into water.

Hold baby safely with fingers under the baby's armpit, with your thumb around the shoulder. The other hand supports the baby's bottom and legs.

Wash the front of the baby.

Go from front to back between the legs. Rinse with the wet washcloth.

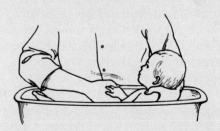

Wash the baby's back with your free hand lathered with soap.

Rinse well with the wet washcloth.

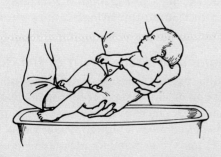

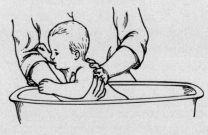

Remove infant from the water and gently pat dry.

BOX 14-3

Criteria for Early Discharge

Term infant (38 to 41 weeks of gestation) with birth weight of 2500 to 4500 g*

Normal findings on physical assessment performed by health care provider*

Normal laboratory data, including negative Coombs' test result and hematocrit 40% to 65%*

Stable vital signs*

Temperature stability*

Successful feeding (normal sucking and swallowing)*

Apgar score > 7 at 1 and 5 min

Normal voiding and stooling

PKU and thyroid screening tests completed; repeat of PKU test scheduled for 2 weeks of age*

Demonstration of skill by mother in feeding, providing skin and cord care, measuring temperature with a thermometer, assessing infant well-being and signs of illness, and providing emergency care*

PKU, Phenylketonuria.

*Recommendations of American Academy of Pediatrics: Criteria for early infant discharge and follow-up evaluation, *Pediatrics* 65:651, 1980.

BOX 14-4

Standard Laboratory Values in a Term Newborn

Hemoglobin	14.5 to 22.5 g/dl
Hematocrit	44% to 72%
Glucose	40 to 60 mg/dl
Bilirubin, direct	0 to 1 mg/dl
Blood gases	
Arterial	pH 7.31 to 7.45
	P_{CO_2} 33 to 48 mm Hg
	P_{O_2} 50 to 70 mm Hg
Venous	pH 7.28 to 7.42
	P_{CO_2} 38 to 52 mm Hg
	P_{O_2} 20 to 49 mm Hg

ample of a care path for infant adaptation to extrauterine life. When variations from the care path occur, further assessment and intervention may be necessary.

Parents need the reassurance of knowing when and where to direct calls for questions about newborn adaptation and care. Some agencies have established "warm lines" for such purposes. Others incorporate follow-up telephone calls 24 hours after discharge, especially for those mothers who were discharged early.

When problems are anticipated, referral to a social worker or visiting nurse is appropriate. Other referrals may be to groups such as the La Leche League to assist with breastfeeding questions and problems, parent support groups to provide emotional and practical assistance in parenting, and support groups for parents of twins. Nurses should obtain or compile a list of relevant community agencies and groups so that appropriate referrals may be made in a timely fashion. In some settings, referral to a social worker or visiting nurse must be approved by a physician.

Home care may be provided by a nurse as part of the follow-up of patients in an early discharge program or through a visiting nurse or community health nurse referral. When care moves to the home, environmental factors, in addition to infant development and parenting skills, are considered. For example, the nurse observes the location of the bassinet or crib; placement along an inside wall is preferred. This is recommended because the infant's body heat can be lost by radiation to the outside if the bed is placed near an outside wall. Room temperature and appropriateness of clothing is noted. The examination of the infant is directed to ascertaining the infant's adjustment to extrauterine life as age appropriate. Color, presence of jaundice, skin turgor, and the umbilical stump and circumcision site, if appropriate, are inspected. The mouth is inspected for signs of thrush; the scalp for cradle cap; and the skin for excoriation, diaper rash, and cleanliness. The heart and lungs are auscultated. The parent is asked about the infant's eating pattern, voiding, and stooling. The parent is reminded, as necessary, about the need for repeat laboratory tests such as the one for phenylketonuria (PKU), for well-baby checkups, and immunizations. The physiologic rise of phenylalanine in infants with PKU may not occur by the time of discharge from the hospital. Therefore many screening programs recommend a repeat of the PKU screen at 2 weeks of age (Wright, Brown, Davidson-Mundt, 1992).

The parents' skill in infant care activities is observed as opportunities arise. If knowledge deficits are ascertained, then instruction and supervised practice can be provided. Parent-infant interaction and sibling relations are noted. The nurse provides positive reinforcement for parents in their infant caregiving activities whenever appropriate.

Environmental Assessment of the Home

In addition to the assessments described above, the "quantity and quality of support for cognitive, social and emotional development available to a child in the home environment" (Bradley, Caldwell, 1988) can be assessed with the Home Observation for Measurement of the Environment (HOME) inventory. A sample of categories of items assessed on this inventory includes the emotional and verbal responsiveness of the parents, parents' involvement with the child, opportunities for stimulation, and organization of the environment. Combining

CARE PATH

Neonatal Adaptation to Extrauterine Life

	Day 1	Day 2	Day 3	Day 4	Day 7	Day 14
WEIGHT		Loss of 5% to 10% of birth-weight	Gain of 150 to 300 g per day			Birth-weight regained
TEMPERATURE	Stabilized at (37° C)					
FEEDINGS Volume Frequency	15 to 60 ml 6 to 10 times/24 hours	60 to 90 ml	60 to 90 ml 6 to 10 times/24 hours	60 to 90 ml	60 to 90 ml 6 to 10 times/24 hours	60 to 90 ml
VOIDING	At least 1 time in first 24 hours	2 to 6 times/24 hours	6 to 10 times/24 hours			6 to 10 times/24 hours
STOOLS		Meconium; at least 1 time in first 48 hours	Transitional stool; 1 to 5/day	Yellow stool; 1 to 5/day		Yellow stool; 1 to 2/day
SLEEP	16 to 20 hours/24 hours					16 to 20 hours/24 hours
UMBILICAL CORD	Moist; clamped	Dry; clamp removed				Cord off
CIRCUMCISION	Red; sore	Yellow exudate covers glans	Healing	Healing		Healed
COLOR	Pink; acrocyanosis	Pink; slight jaundice	Peak of jaundice		Pink	
BILIRUBIN LEVEL	0 to 6 mg/dl	≤8 mg/dl	≤12 mg/dl		2 mg/dl	
LABORATORY TESTS	Glucose when required; HCT	PKU, T_4; galactose				repeat PKU, if needed
MEDICATIONS	Eye prophylaxis and Vitamin K within 2 hours of birth; HBV within 12 hours of birth					

TABLE 14-4 Newborn Screening Summary

DISORDER	BASIC DEFECT	SYMPTOMS	+ SCREENING INCIDENCE	CRITERIA	TREATMENT	FOLLOW-UP NEEDS
PKU (Classic)	Lack of enzyme to properly convert the amino acid phenylalanine to tyrosine.	Severe mental retardation, eczema, seizures, behavior disorders, decreased pigmentation, distinctive "mousey" odor.	1:10,000 to 1:15,000 More common in whites	Elevated phenylalanine	Low phenylalanine diet; possible tyrosine supplementation	Lifelong dietary management; careful monitoring of hyperphe variants; careful management and preconception counseling and intervention for PKU women in the reproductive years.
Congenital hypothyroidism (primary)	Absent or hypoplastic gland; dysfunctional gland.	Mental and motor retardation, short stature, coarse, dry skin and hair, hoarse cry, constipation.	Overall 1:4,000 with ethnic variation 1:12,000 Black 1:1,000 Indian	Low T$_4$, Elevated TSH	Replacement of L-thyroxine	Maintain L-thyroxine levels in upper half of normal range; Periodic bone age to monitor growth.
Galactosemia (transferase deficiency)	Absent or low activity of enzyme to convert galactose into glucose.	Neonatal death from severe dehydration, sepsis or liver pathology; mental retardation, jaundice, blindness, cataracts.	1:10,000 to 1:90,000	Elevated galactose (Hill); low or absent fluorescence (Beutler)	Eliminate galactose and lactose from the diet; soy formulas in infancy; lactose-free solid foods.	Provide early monitoring for speech and neurological problems; educate parents about hidden sources of lactose; monitor females for secondary ovarian failure; avoid medications with lactose fillers.

Disorder	Description	Incidence	Finding	Treatment	Nursing Care
Maple syrup urine disease (MSUD)	Absent or low activity of enzyme needed to metabolize leucine, isoleucine, and valine.	1:90,000 to 1:200,000	Elevated leucine	Diet low in leucine, isoleucine, and valine; thiamine supplement if responsive.	Educate family and friends regarding strict dietary regimen; social and education evaluation; behavioral counseling; neurological monitoring; prompt treatment of illness to minimize acidosis.
	Acidosis; hypertonicity and seizures, vomiting, drowsiness, apnea, coma; infant death or severe mental retardation and neurological impairment; behavioral disorders.				
Homocystinuria	Deficiency of enzyme cytothianine synthase which is needed for homocystine metabolism	1:200,000	Elevated methionine	Methionine-restricted diet; cystine supplement; B_6 supplement if responsive.	Maintain lifelong low methionine diet; monitor for thrombosis (check pulses, etc); ophthalmological care; educational and psychological evaluation; avoid unnecessary surgery.
	Mental retardation, seizures, behavior disorders, early onset thromboses, dislocated lenses, tall lanky body habitus.				
Congenital adrenal hyperplasia (CAH)	Defect in the enzyme-21-hydroxylase	1:15,000 to 1:3,000 native Eskimos	Elevated 17-hydroxy progesterone; abnormal electrolytes	Replace corticosteroids; plastic surgery to correct ambiguous genitalia.	Maintain adequate corticosteroids; elevate doses or give injectable doses in times of stress; periodic bone age to monitor adequate treatment; maintain pediatric endocrinology follow-up appointments.
	Hyponatremia, hypokalemia, hypoglycemia, dehydration and early death; ambiguous genitalia in females; progressive virilization in both sexes.				
Biotinidase deficiency	Low activity of the enzyme biotinidase; biotin deficiency	1:60,000 to 1:100,000	Deficient or absent activity of biotinidase on calorimetric assay.	10 mg biotin daily	Monitor compliance; periodic follow-up and evaluation.
	Mental retardation, seizures, ataxia, skin rash, hearing loss, alopecia, optic nerve atrophy, coma, and death.				

From Wright L, Brown A, Davidson-Murdt A: Newborn screening: the miracle and the challenge, *J Pediatr Nurs* 7:26, 1992. Used with permission.

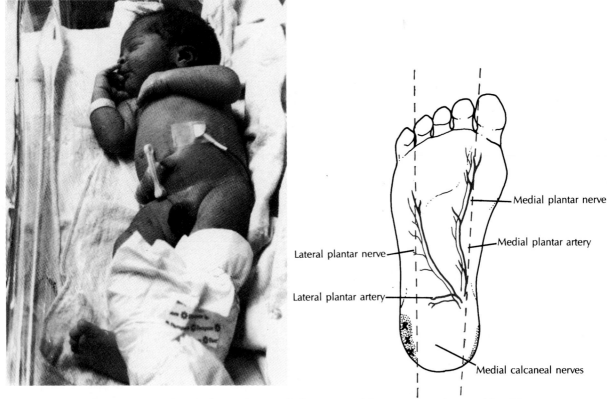

FIG. 14-18 Heel stick. **A,** Newborn with foot wrapped for warmth to increase blood flow to extremity before heel stick. **B,** Puncture sites *(x)* on infant's foot for heel stick samples of capillary blood.

the HOME with other developmental measures, such as the Bayley Scales of Infant Development, assists in establishing the degree of risk in an infant for developmental problems and can provide useful information to the nurse.

Collection of Specimens

Ongoing evaluation of a newborn requires obtaining blood and urine specimens. The following procedures are used for collecting those specimens: **heel stick** venipuncture, and collection of urine specimen. Nurses should wear gloves when collecting any specimen.

Heel Stick

Capillary blood is used for determination of blood glucose level, hematocrit (Box 14-4) and to test for PKU, galactosemia, hypothyroidism, and other inborn errors of metabolism. Table 14-4, a summary of newborn screening, includes the major disorders for which infants are checked, the basic defects, symptoms, incidence, criteria for diagnosis, treatment, and follow-up needs. The nurse or laboratory technician draws blood for these tests.

Before the sample is taken, it is helpful to warm the heel in order to help dilate the vessels in the area. A cloth soaked with warm water and wrapped loosely around the foot for 5 to 10 minutes provides effective warming (Fig. 14-18, *A*). Covering the foot in plastic prevents dissipation of heat and can cause thermal burns (NAACOG, 1992). Second- and third-degree burns have been reported from inappropriate heel warming techniques.

To identify the appropriate puncture sites, the nurse draws an imaginary line between the fourth and fifth toes that runs parallel to the lateral aspect of the heel, or a line running from the great toe that runs parallel to the medial aspect of the heel (Fig. 14-18, *B*).

To perform a heel stick, the infant's foot is restrained, cleansed with alcohol, allowed to dry, and then the selected site is punctured with a No. 11 scalpel blade or a lancet.

After the specimen has been collected, pressure is applied with a dry gauze square. Reapplying alcohol will cause the site to continue bleeding. The site is covered with an adhesive bandage. The nurse ensures proper disposal of the equipment used, reviews the laboratory slip for correct identifications, and checks the specimen for adequate labeling and routing.

A heel stick causes pain. After several heel sticks infants have been observed to withdraw their foot when it is touched. Pain pathways are present and functional in the infant (Shapiro, 1989). To reassure the infant and promote feelings of safety, the newborn should be

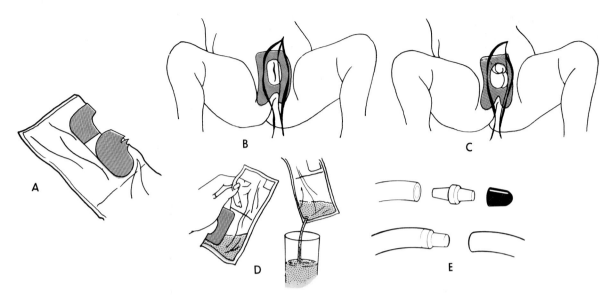

FIG. 14-19   Pediatric urine collection bag. **A,** Protective paper is being removed from the adhesive surface. **B,** Applied to girl. **C,** Applied to boy. **D,** Cut to drain urine. **E,** Collection tube. (Courtesy Hollister, Inc., Chicago, IL.)

cuddled and comforted when the procedure is completed.

The most serious complication of infant heel stick is necrotizing osteochondritis from lancet penetration of the bone. To avoid this, the stick should be no deeper than 2.4 mm and should be made at the outer aspect of the heel (Whaley, Wong, 1995). Repeated trauma to the walking surface of the heel can cause fibrosis and scarring that may lead to problems with walking (Reiner, Meltes, Hayes, 1990; Whaley, Wong, 1995).

Obtaining Urine Specimen

Examination of urine is a valuable laboratory tool for infant assessment. The way in which the specimen is collected may influence the results. The urine sample should be fresh and examined within 1 hour of collection.

A variety of urine collection bags are available, including the Hollister U-Bag (Fig. 14-19). These bags are clear plastic, single-use bags with self-adhering material around the opening at the point of attachment.

To prepare the infant, the nurse removes the diaper and places the infant in a supine position. The genitalia, perineum, and surrounding skin are washed and thoroughly dried because the adhesive of the bag will not stick to moist, powdered, or oily skin surfaces. The protective paper is removed to expose the adhesive (Fig. 14-19, *A*). For girls, the perineum is stretched to flatten skin folds. Then the adhesive is pressed firmly to the skin all around the urinary meatus and vagina. (NOTE: Start with the narrow portion of the butterfly-shaped adhesive patch.) The nurse must be sure to start at the bridge of skin separating the rectum from the vagina and work upward (Fig. 14-19, *B*). For boys, the penis and scrotum are tucked through the aperture of the collector before the nurse removes the protective paper from the adhesive. The bag is fitted over the penis, and the flaps are pressed firmly to the perineum, making sure the entire adhesive coating is firmly attached to the skin with no puckering of the adhesive (Fig. 14-19, *C*). This helps ensure a leak-proof seal and decreases the chance of contamination from stool. Cutting a slit in the diaper and pulling the bag through the slit also may help prevent leaking.

The diaper is carefully replaced, and the bag is checked frequently. When 1 to 2 ml of urine have been obtained, the bag is removed. The infant's skin is observed for signs of irritation. The specimen can be aspirated with a syringe or drained directly from the bag. For draining, the bag is held in one hand and tilted to keep urine away from the tab. The tab is removed, and the urine is drained into a clean receptacle (Fig. 14-19, *D*).

Collection of a 24 hour specimen can be a challenge. The infant may need to be restrained. The 24-hour U-Bag is applied in the manner just described, and the drainage is directed into a receptacle. The collection tube can be shortened or capped (Fig. 14-19, *E*). The infant's skin is watched closely for signs of irritation and lack of a proper seal.

For some types of urine testing, urine can be aspirated directly from the diaper by means of a syringe without a needle. If the diaper has absorbent gelling material that traps urine, a small-gauge dressing or some cotton balls are placed inside the diaper and the urine is aspirated from them (Whaley, Wong, 1995).

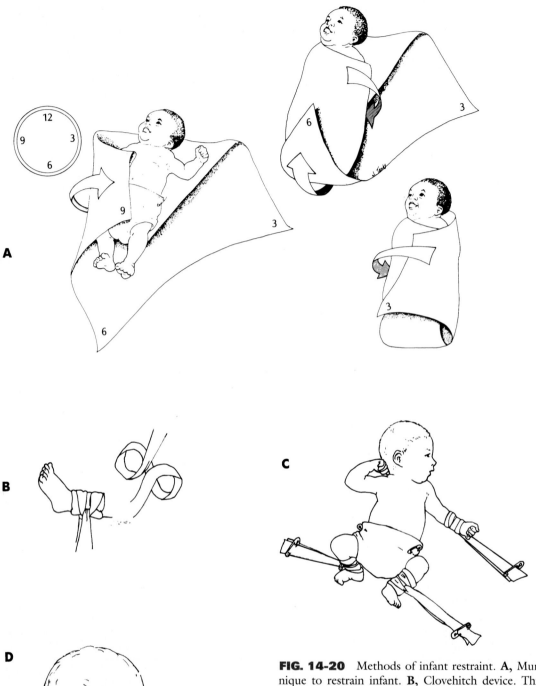

FIG. 14-20 Methods of infant restraint. **A,** Mummy technique to restrain infant. **B,** Clovehitch device. This restraint does not tighten after its application. Apply padding before applying device. **C,** Clovehitch restraints in place. **D,** Position for lumbar puncture.

Venipuncture

Venous blood samples can be drawn from veins on the back of the hand, the antecubital space, or the jugular or femoral veins. If an intravenous (IV) site is used to obtain a blood specimen, it is important to consider the type of infusion fluid to determine whether it is appropriate to draw blood from that site. Small veins punctured by small needles yield slow blood return, and patience must be exercised during the procedure.

The **mummy restraint** is used frequently to secure the infant (Fig. 14-20, *A*). If the radial vein is used, the infant's arm is exposed and held securely in place. For external jugular venipuncture, the infant is mummied, and the infant's head is lowered over a rolled towel or the edge of a table and stabilized. For femoral venipuncture, the infant is positioned in a "frog posture." The hands are placed over the infant's knees. Pressure of fingers over the inner aspect of the thigh is avoided. These positions ensure safety and exposure of the puncture sites. When the procedure is completed, firm pressure is applied over the area with sterile gauze for 1 to 3 minutes. The infant should be cuddled and comforted when the procedure is completed.

For an hour after any venipuncture, the nurse should observe the infant frequently for evidence of bleeding or hematoma at the puncture site. Determination of the infant's tolerance of the procedure should be made and recorded.

Crying, fear, and agitation will affect the values when venipuncture or arterial puncture is performed for blood gas studies. Efforts should be made to keep the infant quiet during the procedure. For blood gas studies the blood sample tubes are packed in ice to reduce blood cell metabolism and are taken immediately to the laboratory for analysis. If arterial puncture is used to collect the specimen, firm pressure over the puncture site for at least 5 minutes is required to prevent bleeding from the site.

Therapeutic Interventions
Intramuscular Injection

Administering vitamin K intramuscularly is routine in the newborn period. A single parenteral dose of 0.5 to 1 mg of vitamin K soon after birth is given to prevent hemorrhagic disorders. Vitamin K is produced in the gastrointestinal tract starting soon after microorganisms are introduced. By day 8, normal newborns are able to produce their own vitamin K.

Hepatitis B vaccination is recommended for all infants. Infants at highest risk of contracting hepatitis B are those born of women who come from Asia, Africa, South America, the South Pacific, and southern and eastern Europe. If the infant is born to an infected mother or to a mother who is a chronic carrier, hepatitis vaccine and Hepatitis B Immune Globulin (HBIG) should be given within 12 hours of birth. The hepatitis vaccine is given in one site and the HBIG in another site. For infants born to healthy women, the first dose of the vaccine may be given at birth or at 1 to 2 months of age. Parental consent should be obtained before administering these medications.

For the injection of vitamin K and hepatitis vaccine, a 25-gauge, 5/8-inch needle should be used. For the injection of thicker medications, a 22-gauge needle may be required. The preferred site for injection in the newborn is the vastus lateralis muscle (Fig. 14-21), although the rectus femoris muscle also can be used. Gloves are worn for injections.

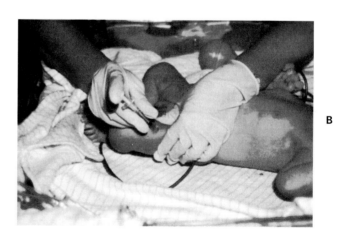

FIG. 14-21 Intramuscular injection sites. **A,** Acceptable intramuscular injection sites for children. *X,* preferred injection site; *Y,* alternate injection site. **B,** Infant's leg stabilized for intramuscular injection. Nurse is wearing gloves to give injection. (**A,** From Whaley LF, Wong DL: *Nursing care of infants and children,* ed 5, St Louis, 1995, Mosby. **B,** Courtesy Marjorie Pyle, RNC, *Lifecircle,* Costa Mesa, CA.)

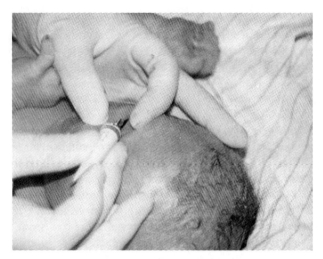

FIG. 14-22 Instillation of medication into eye of newborn. Thumb and forefinger are used to open the eye; medication is placed in the lower conjunctiva from the inner to the outer canthus. (From Dickason E et al: *Maternal-Infant Nursing Care,* ed 2, St Louis, 1994, Mosby.)

Newborn infants offer little, if any resistance to injections. Although infants squirm and may be difficult to hold in position when they are awake, they usually can be restrained without assistance from a second person.

The nurse should always remember to comfort the infant after an injection. Then equipment should be properly discarded. It is important to record medication, amount, route, site of injection, and infant's tolerance of injection.

Eye Prophylaxis

Erythromycin or tetracaine ophthalmic ointment is instilled into the lower conjunctiva of each eye within 2 hours after birth to prevent ophthalmia neonatorum, an infection caused by *Neisseria gonorrhoeae* and inclusion conjunctivitis, an infection caused by *Chlamydia trachomatis.* The infant may be exposed to these bacteria when passing through the vaginal canal.

Opening the eyelids to instill medications into the conjunctiva of the newborn requires practice. The thumb and forefinger are placed on the upper and lower lids, close to the eyelashes (Fig. 14-22). The eyelids are gently but firmly separated, and the medication is immediately placed in the lower conjunctiva, moving from the inner canthus to the outer canthus of the eye. After instillation of the medication, the eyelids are massaged gently to ensure spread of the medication. Excess medication may be wiped off with sterile cotton, but flushing the eye is not recommended.

Therapy for Hyperbilirubinemia

The expected outcome of treatment for **hyperbilirubinemia** is to help the newborn's body reduce serum lev-

---

Effects of Phototherapy

Phototherapy causes reversible isomerization of unconjugated bilirubin in the skin (NAACOG, 1986b; Valman, 1989). During phototherapy, infants form a substance called *lumirubin,* a water-soluble product. Lumirubin is formed slowly and excreted rapidly both in the urine and feces. Because infants excrete lumirubin efficiently, increasing the formation of lumirubin improves the effectiveness of phototherapy in the treatment of neonatal jaundice.

Traditional phototherapy consists of a light source (e.g., four special blue and four daylight bulbs) that will most effectively accomplish the isomerization process. The light source is placed about 18 to 20 inches from the newborn in an incubator. The fluorescent bulbs currently used (daylight, cool light, blue, and special blue bulbs) have different distribution points on the light spectrum and different peaks of maximal emission. The generally accepted light range for maximum absorption by bilirubin is 400 to 500 nanometers. Blue or special blue lights are considered to be more specific and effective. Blue lights can make the detection of cyanosis in the infant difficult and may strain the nursery staff's eyes (NAACOG, 1986b). The side effects of phototherapy do not appear to produce any long-term effects (Tan, 1989).

Bronze baby syndrome has occurred in some newborns receiving phototherapy. The serum, urine, and skin turn bronze (brown-black). The cause is unclear. Almost all newborns recover from bronze baby syndrome without sequelae.

---

els of unconjugated bilirubin. As fetal RBCs disintegrate, the amount of bilirubin increases. Serum levels of unconjugated bilirubin may rise beyond normal limits (hyperbilirubinemia). If untreated, the levels can continue to rise, and the risk of kernicterus increases. Feeding of the newborn soon after birth stimulates the gastrocolic reflex and the passage of meconium. Because bilirubin is excreted in meconium, early feeding may help prevent jaundice.

The two principal methods for reducing serum bilirubin levels are phototherapy and exchange blood transfusion. Exchange blood transfusion is used to treat infants whose levels of bilirubin cannot be controlled by phototherapy (Box 14-5).

Phototherapy

During **phototherapy** the unclothed infant is placed approximately 18 to 20 inches under a bank of lights for several hours or days until the serum bilirubin level drops to an acceptable range. The decision to discontinue

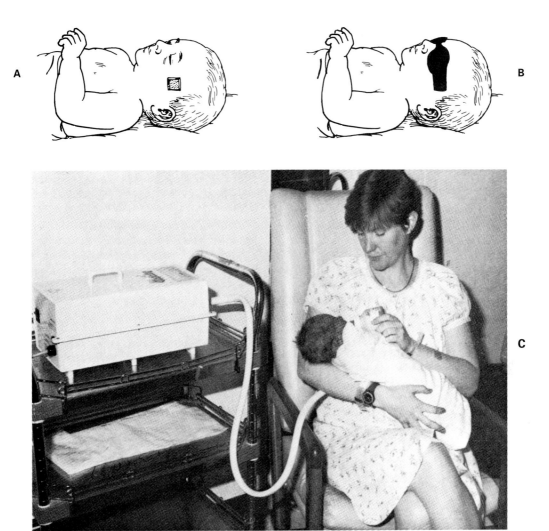

FIG. 14-23 Eye patches for newborn receiving phototherapy. **A,** Small Velcro patch stuck to both sides of head. **B,** Eye cover sticks to Velcro patch, which reduces movement of eye cover and facilitates removal for feedings. **C,** Fiberoptic phototherapy blanket permits baby to be fed, held, and changed without the need for eye patches. (From Rosenfeld W, Twist P, Conception L: A new device for phototherapy treatment of jaundiced infants, *J Perinat* 10:243, 1990.)

therapy is based on a definite downward trend in bilirubin values. After therapy has been terminated, the infant should be retested several hours later to ascertain whether rebound occurs (NAACOG, 1986b).

Several precautions need to be taken while the infant is under phototherapy. The infant's eyes must be protected by an opaque mask to prevent overexposure to the light. The eye shield should be the correct size to completely cover the eyes but not occlude the nares. Before the mask is applied, the infant's eyes should be closed gently to prevent excoriation of the corneas. The mask should be removed during infant feedings so that the eyes can be checked and the infant can receive visual contact with the parents (Fig. 14-23, *A* and *B*).

Often a "string bikini" made from a disposable face mask is used. This allows optimum skin exposure, yet sufficient protection to the genitals. The metal strip must be removed from the mask to prevent its overheating and burning the infant. Lotions and ointments also should be avoided because they too can cause the infant to become burned.

Because the infant is unclothed and the lights produce heat, the infant's temperature needs to be monitored. The lights also increase the rate of insensible water loss (NAACOG, 1992). Therefore fluid loss and dehydration also can occur. The infant should be turned every 2 hours to expose all body surfaces to the lights.

Phototherapy may cause the infant to sleep for longer than the usual 4-hour periods. The infant should be kept on a regular feeding schedule. The number and consistency of stools should be monitored. Bilirubin breakdown increases gastric motility, which results in loose

DEFINITIONS

Hyperbilirubinemia: higher levels of bilirubin than normal

Bilirubin: end product of RBCs when they mature and break down

RBCs: red blood cells

Jaundice: yellow skin tone, whites of eyes, and mucous membranes caused by circulating bilirubin

Phototherapy: the use of fluorescent light to break down the bilirubin in the skin into substances that can be excreted in the feces (stool) and urine

Bililites: fluorescent lights used for phototherapy

HOW JAUNDICE HAPPENS

- When RBCs break down, they release bilirubin. Bilirubin circulates in the blood. The bilirubin combines with another substance in the liver. This combined substance moves through the blood to the kidneys and the intestines where it is eliminated in the urine and the stool. The bilirubin gives the yellow color to urine and the brown color to the stool.

- Before birth, babies have more RBCs in each ounce of blood than adults have. The RBCs of the unborn infant have a shorter life span (70 to 90 days) than RBCs formed after birth (120 days). When the RBCs of a fetus break down, the bilirubin produced by this is carried by the fetus' blood, through the placenta, and to the mother's liver to be excreted.

- After birth, the infant's liver must get rid of the bilirubin. Even though a baby's liver functions well, it may not be able to get rid of all the bilirubin produced by break down of RBCs. Bilirubin seeps out of the blood and into the tissues, coloring them yellow (jaundice). The blood level of bilirubin rises quickly up to the fifth day, and then it goes down; the jaundice usually clears up by the end of the week.

THE DANGER OF EXCESS BILIRUBIN

Some newborns seem to have extra bilirubin to excrete. The amount in the tissues becomes too great when the blood level reaches 12 mg/dl. Bilirubin at high levels may cause damage to the brain. Consequently, the health care provider requests that the infant be placed under the Bililite for phototherapy. This will help the infant eliminate the extra bilirubin and prevent damage to the brain.

CARING FOR THE INFANT

The newborn is placed in an incubator to keep it warm and so that the nurse can observe it.

The infant wears an eye mask to keep the light out of the eyes.

The baby is undressed so that as much light as possible can reach the skin.

The newborn wears a "string bikini," which is made out of a paper diaper or a face mask, as a small diaper.

The baby's temperature is taken often so that any changes in temperature can be noted and to prevent the infant from becoming too hot or too cold.

The baby is given extra water to drink because infants have watery, green stools from the excretion of the extra bilirubin.

The newborn is taken out from under the lights for feedings and cuddling. The nurse tells the mother when it is time for her to come for feedings and hold her baby.

The nurse takes blood tests to check the amount of bilirubin still in the newborn's blood and updates the parents about the results.

AFTER THE NEWBORN GOES HOME

The parents should be encouraged to ask any questions that they might have. The nurse gives them a telephone number to call at any hour with their questions.

BOX 14-6

American Academy of Pediatrics Report of the Task Force on Circumcision

Newborn circumcision, when properly performed, prevents phimosis, paraphimosis, and inflammation of the glands and prepuce and may reduce the incidence of infections of the urinary tract. The incidence of penile cancer is lower in American men who have been circumcised than in American men who are uncircumcised. There is conflicting evidence regarding the association between circumcision and sexually transmitted diseases. The partners of uncircumcised men infected with human papillomavirus have an increased incidence of cancer of the cervix.

Newborn circumcision is an elective, rapid, and usually safe procedure that should be performed only if the infant is healthy and stable. The infant experiences pain with the procedure that is manifested by physiologic and behavioral changes. Local anesthesia may reduce the physiologic responses of the newborn infant to circumcision. However, local anesthesia has some risks. There is a lack of follow-up reports of the procedure conducted under local anesthesia.

Potential medical benefits and advantages exist with newborn circumcision, as well as disadvantages and risks. Parents of newborn males should receive an explanation of the procedure's benefits and risks. Informed parental consent must be obtained before performing this procedure.

Reference: Task Force on Circumcision: Report of the task force on circumcision, *Pediatrics* 84(4):388, 1989.

stools that can cause skin excoriation and breakdown. The infant's buttocks should be cleaned after each stool to help maintain skin integrity.

A new device for phototherapy consisting of a fiberoptic panel attached to an illuminator was compared with traditional phototherapy (Rosenfeld, Twist, Conception, 1990). The researchers found no complications of therapy; the fiberoptic panel proved effective and safe. This new fiberoptic blanket, which wraps light around the newborn's torso, delivers continuous phototherapy. The newborn can remain in the mother's room in an open crib or in her arms during treatment without the need for eye patches (Fig. 14-23, C) (Murphy, Oellrich, 1990; Rose, 1990).

The time therapy begins, the times the infant is removed for care, and the time when the therapy ends are all recorded. The infant's response (i.e., stools, temperature, intake) is noted.

Parent Education

Serum levels of bilirubin in the newborn continue to rise until the fifth day of life. Most parents leave the hospital by the second or third day and some as early as 2 hours after birth. Therefore parents must be able to assess the newborn's degree of jaundice. They should have written instructions that include the contact person to whom the infant's condition should be reported. A nurse may make a home visit to evaluate the infant's responses (see Teaching Approaches for parental guidelines concerning hyperbilirubinemia). Determination of bilirubin level may be necessary after discharge from the hospital. The nurse may draw the blood for the specimen, or the parents may go to a laboratory for the determination.

Circumcision

Circumcision is a matter of parental choice. The parents' decision to have their newborn circumcised usually is based on one or more of the following factors: hygiene, religious conviction, tradition, culture, or social norms (see Box 14-6). Some people do not like to touch their infant's genitals, so circumcision may be the wisest choice for these parents. Regardless of the reason for the decision, it should be made only after parents have the available facts and sufficient time to review their options.

Parents need to begin learning about circumcision during the prenatal period (Lund, 1990). However, circumcision often is not discussed with the parents before labor. In many instances, it is during admission to the hospital or labor unit that the mother confronts the decision regarding circumcision. The stress of the intrapartal period makes this a difficult time for parental decision making, although consenting to their son's circumcision is ultimately the parents' choice. The mother may be asked to sign a circumcision permit form during this admission procedure. Some hospitals require parents to sign a different form stating that they do not want their son to be circumcised, if that is their desire.

Procedure

In **circumcision** the **prepuce** (foreskin) of the glans is removed. The operation is performed in the hospital before the infant's discharge. However, the circumcision of a Jewish male is performed on the eighth day after birth and is done at home unless the infant is unwell. The procedure is not done immediately after birth because of the danger of cold stress. Clotting factors drop somewhat immediately after birth and return to prebirth levels by the end of the first week. Therefore performing the circumcision after the baby is a week old is logical from a physiologic standpoint.

Feedings are withheld for 4 hours before the circumcision. For the circumcision procedure the infant is positioned on a plastic restraint form to restrict his movements (Fig. 14-24). The penis is cleansed with soap and

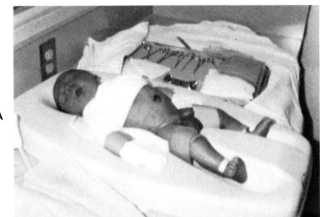
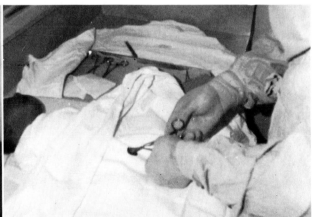

FIG. 14-24   Circumcision. **A,** Proper positioning of infant in Circumstraint. **B,** Physician performing circumcision. Baby is completely covered to prevent cold stress.

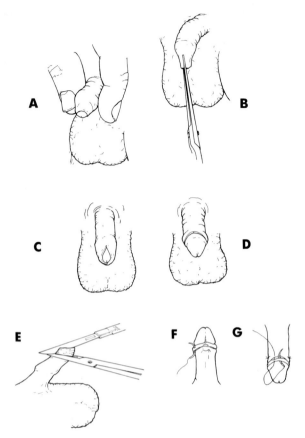

FIG. 14-25 Technique of circumcision. **A** to **D,** Prepuce is stripped and slit to facilitate its retraction behind glans penis. **E,** Prepuce is now clamped and excessive prepuce cut off. **F** and **G,** Suture material used is plain 00 or 000 catgut in a very small needle; some physicians prefer silk suture.

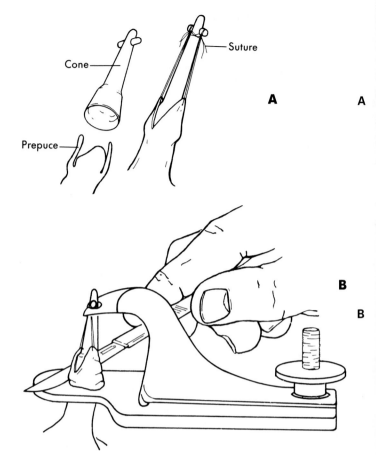

FIG. 14-26 Circumcision with Yellen clamp. **A,** Prepuce drawn over cone. **B,** Yellen clamp is applied, hemostasis occurs, then prepuce (over cone) is cut away.

water or Betadine. The infant is draped to provide warmth and a sterile field. The sterile equipment is readied for use.

Some techniques do not require special equipment or appliances (Fig. 14-25). However, numerous instruments have been designed for circumcision. The Yellen clamp (Fig. 14-26) may make this an almost bloodless operation. The procedure takes only a few minutes. After it is completed, a small petrolatum gauze dressing may be applied for the first day to prevent a cloth diaper from adhering. If a Plastibell is used, the bell applies constant direct pressure to prevent hemorrhage. It also protects against infection, sticking to the diaper, and pain with urination. The bell fits over the glans. The suture is tied around the rim of the bell. Excess prepuce is cut away. The plastic rim remains in place for about a week until it falls off, after healing has taken place (Fig. 14-27). Petrolatum gauze is not needed when the bell is used.

Discomfort

Circumcision is painful. If the infant has undergone this surgery without anesthetic, he is comforted until he qui-

ets (Campos, 1989; Marchette et al, 1991). Then he is returned to his mother. These infants usually are fussy for about 2 to 3 hours and may refuse a feeding. It is not uncommon for the infant to have a loose, green stool after the circumcision.

In the Jewish ritual the newborn is given a few drops of wine to relax him in preparation for the surgery. Dorsal penile nerve blocks may reduce pain and stress during newborn circumcision. Reported use of local anesthesia for circumcision is limited and needs further study. Pain may not end when the operation is over because the wound requires as long as a week to heal.

Care of the Newly Circumcised Penis

The nurse observes the infant for bleeding and voiding. If bleeding results from the circumcision, the nurse applies gentle pressure to the site of bleeding with a folded sterile gauze pad (4 × 4 inches) or sprinkles on powdered gel foam. If bleeding is not easily controlled, a blood vessel may need to be ligated. One nurse notifies the health care provider and prepares the equipment (circumcision tray and suture) while another nurse maintains

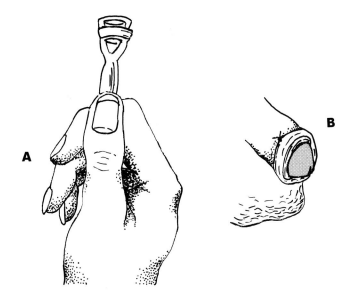

FIG. 14-27   Circumcision using the Plastibell.

pressure *intermittently* until the health care provider arrives. The penis is checked hourly for bleeding for 12 hours. If the parents take the baby home before the end of 12 hours, they have to be taught the preceding actions. Ordinarily the infant must void before leaving the hospital. Before the infant leaves the hospital, the nurse checks to see that the parents have the health care provider's telephone number.

Nursing actions are planned and implemented to prevent infection. Prepackaged wipes should be avoided because they contain alcohol. The nurse washes the penis gently with water to remove urine and feces and reapplies fresh sterile petrolatum around the glans after each diaper change. The glans penis, normally dark red in appearance during healing, becomes covered with a yellow exudate in 24 hours. This is part of the normal healing process, not an infective process. No attempt is made to remove the exudate, which persists for 2 to 3 days. Parents should be taught to fanfold the diaper so that it does not press upon the circumcised area. They should be encouraged to change the diaper at least every 4 hours to prevent it from sticking to the penis.

Restraining the Newborn

The infant may be restrained in order to (1) protect him from injury, (2) facilitate examinations, and (3) limit discomfort during tests, procedures, and specimen collections. When restraining an infant, nurses must keep in mind the following special considerations:

- Apply restraints and check them to prevent skin irritation and circulatory impairment.
- Maintain proper body alignment.
- Apply restraints without use of knots or pins if possible. If knots are necessary, make the kind that can be released quickly. Use pins with care to prevent puncture wounds and pressure areas, and to prevent

the infant from swallowing one of them.
- If the infant is an incubator, secure the infant to the mattress to protect the extremities, especially when the lid is raised or the mattress moved.
- Check the infant hourly, more frequently if indicated.

Mummy Restraint

The **mummy restraint** is used with the stronger, more vigorous neonate. It is used during examinations, treatments, or specimen collections that involve the head and neck.

Equipment includes a blanket and one or two large safety pins (see Fig. 14-20, *A*). The procedure is as follows:

1. Spread the blanket on a flat surface; a crib could suffice.
2. Fold over one corner (12 o'clock position).
3. Lay the newborn on the blanket so that the neck is at the fold.
4. Fold the corner at the 9 o'clock position over the right shoulder; tuck this corner securely under the infant's left side.
5. Bring the corner at the 6 o'clock position up over the feet, and either tuck it under the infant's left side or, if it is long enough, fold it over blanket, crossing it under the infant's chin.
6. Swing the corner of the 3 o'clock position snugly over the infant, and fold under the infant's right side. Pin this corner into place. When tucked tightly, it is not always necessary to use a pin.

Extremity Restraints

This type of restraint is used to control movements of the infant's arms or legs. It is used during many procedures, such as intubating or gavage (gravity) feedings or (IV) infusion. If one extremity is restrained, all four extremities must be restrained.

Equipment includes gauze strips or wide strips of soft material and cotton wadding. Pins are optional.

The procedure depends on which type of extremity restraint is used. The following are examples:

1. *Pad extremity with cotton wadding.* Fold one end of gauze strip over the extremity and pin. Pin the other end to the mattress.
2. *Clovehitch restraint.* To make a **clovehitch restraint** arrange a long strip of material that is 5 cm (2 inches) wide as shown in Fig. 14-20, *B*. Loop this device over the extremity, which has been padded with cotton; pin the loose ends to mattress (Fig. 14-20, *C*). The clovehitch does not tighten even when the infant's movements tug on the restraint.

Towel Support

Although the towel support is not a true restraint, it controls the infant's position and movement. The towel may be rolled and placed at the infant's back or sides, or it may be folded and placed under the neck or upper back. A towel support has the following advantages:

1. It provides comfort and security by stabilizing the infant's position.
2. It maintains positioning to assist respiratory effort and gastrointestinal functions, and it prevents skin break down.
3. It prevents the infant from rolling against the side of the crib, where the child may lose heat by convection.

Restraint without Appliances

The nurse may restrain the infant by using the hands and body. Fig. 14-20, *D*, illustrates restraint of the infant in position for lumbar puncture.

Anticipatory Guidance in Infant Care

For the new parent, infant-care activities can cause much anxiety. Support from nurses in the mother's beginning efforts can be an important factor in her seeking and accepting help in the future. Whether or not this is the couple's first baby, parents appreciate anticipatory guidance in the care of their infant. The following topics can be included in discussions with parents. Knowledge deficits of the parents should be ascertained before beginning to teach. Avoid covering everything at once because the parents can be overwhelmed and become anxious. Follow parental cues to set priorities for teaching. Normal growth, development, and changing needs of the infant (e.g., for stimulation, exercise, and social contacts), as well as the following topics should all be included in discussions with parents. The pediatrician and neonatal nurse can give the parents printed directions regarding how they can make their house safe for an infant.

Temperature

Review the following topics:

1. The causes of elevation in body temperature (such as crying, cold stress with resultant vasoconstriction, and minimal response to infection) and the body's response to extremes in environmental temperature.
2. Signs that need to be reported, such as high or low temperatures with fussiness, stuffy nose, lethargy, irritability, poor feeding, and crying.
3. Ways to lower body temperature, such as giving a lukewarm tub bath, dressing the infant appropriately for the temperature of the air, and protecting the infant from long exposure to sunlight.
4. The importance of using of warm wraps or extra blankets in cold weather.
5. How to read a thermometer and take the baby's axillary temperature.

> ### BOX 14-7
> #### Baby Powder Aspiration Pneumonia
>
> Although the use of talc has been discouraged, it is a common baby-care product and can cause severe and often fatal aspiration pneumonia. One of the factors involved in talc aspiration is the similar appearance of baby powder containers and nursing bottles. Talc containers often become favorite playthings and are placed in the mouth. Improper use of powder by sprinkling it directly on the skin creates a cloud of talc dust that is easily inhaled.

Respirations

Review the following points:

1. What normal variations in rate and rhythm are.
2. What reflexes are demonstrated by the infant, such as sneezing to clear the air passages.
3. The need to protect the infant from the following:
   a. People with upper respiratory tract infections
   b. Pollution from a smoke-filled environment
   c. Suffocation from loose bedding, water beds, and bean bag chairs, drowning (bath water), entrapment under excessive bedding, anything tied around the infant's neck, poorly constructed playpens, bassinets, or cribs (see Clinical Application of Research, p 381, for a discussion of sleeping positions)
   d. Aspiration pneumonia that can develop after use of such substances as baby powder, which is usually a mixture of talc (hydrous magnesium silicate) and other silicates (Whaley, Wong, 1995; Box 14-7). Advise parents of the danger of baby powder and discourage them from using it. If a powder is used, it should be placed in the caregiver's hand and then applied to the skin, never shaken directly from the container to the skin. The container is kept closed and immediately stored in a safe place, especially away from curious toddlers who often imitate caregiving activities and may shake it on the infant.
4. What signs indicate the common cold. Parents need to watch for nasal congestion, coughing, sneezing, difficulty in swallowing (sore throat), and low-grade fever. Advise the parents on measures to help their infant, for example:
   a. Feed the infant smaller amounts but more frequently in order to avoid overtiring the infant.
   b. Hold the baby in an upright position to feed.
   c. Offer extra sterile water or nursing time.
   d. For sleeping, raise the infant's head and chest by raising the mattress 30 degrees (do not use pillow).

PLAN OF CARE—CONT'D

Parent's Care of Newborn: Gagging, Circumcision Care, and Crying

EXPECTED OUTCOMES	IMPLEMENTATION	RATIONALE	EVALUATION
	Position Ernest on his side (not abdomen):	Prevents pressure on the penis and promotes comfort.	
	▪ Caution about the use of alcohol.	Alcohol delays healing and causes discomfort.	
	▪ Demonstrate, and ask for a return demonstration for controlling possible hemorrhage.	Increases Karen's skill and self-confidence; teaches accepted therapy for hemorrhage.	
	▪ Describe the yellow exudate that normally forms in 24 hours.	Provides anticipatory guidance about normal healing process; allays parental anxiety.	
	▪ Explain indications for calling the health care provider.	Provides signs of problems.	

Nursing diagnosis: Family coping, potential for growth, related to anticipatory guidance regarding responses to son's crying

Parents will learn how to cope effectively with Ernest's crying.	Alert parents to crying as a child's form of communication and that soon they will be able to differentiate the cries: hunger, wet, pain, loneliness.	Provides reassurance that crying is not a sign of the infant's rejection of them and that they will soon be able to interpret the different cries.	Karen states she understands about crying and methods to cope with it.
	Differentiate self-consoling behaviors from fussing/crying.	Presents parents with concrete examples of interventions.	
	Discuss methods of consoling infant who has been crying:	Reassures parents that no one intervention works all the time.	At next visit, Karen
	▪ Check his diaper and change as necessary.	Anticipating a problem and considering a number of options increases self-confidence.	▪ States she/they are "getting better" in coping with Ernest's crying.
	▪ Show face to the infant.		▪ Relates the techniques that work the best.
	▪ Talk to the infant in a steady, soft voice.		▪ Describes some successes in accurately interpreting Ernest's cries.
	▪ Hold both of the infant's arms close to body.		
	▪ Swaddle him.		
	▪ Pick up the infant.		
	▪ Rock him.		
	▪ Give him a pacifier or feed him.		

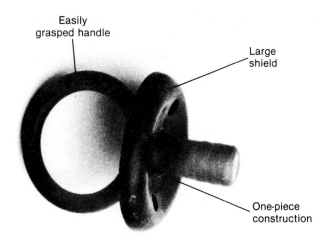

Easily grasped handle

Large shield

One-piece construction

FIG. 14-29 Design of a safe pacifier. (From Whaley LF, Wong DL: *Nursing care of infants and children,* ed 5, St Louis, 1995, Mosby.)

months of age, then every 3 months until 18 months, at 2 years, 3 years, preschool, and every 2 years thereafter.

The newborn's record serves as a documented means of communication among all members of the health care team. The record contains accurate and complete recordings of the history, physical examination, and laboratory test results, sequential observations, goals, interventions, and the newborn's responses. The record should be readily accessible to the health care professionals caring for the infant and family. Documentation of the parent's health education, counseling, and responses to information are included. These data provide valuable information for the pediatrician and nurse for the infant's follow-up care and serve as a reservoir for data for future research.

✦ EVALUATION

The nurse can be reasonably assured that care was effective to the degree that the expected outcomes of care were achieved. For the infant this includes the following:

- Successful transition from intrauterine to extrauterine life
- Maintenance of effective breathing patterns and thermoregulation
- Freedom from infection

The mother/parent has achieved the following outcomes:

- Attained knowledge, skill, and confidence relevant to infant care activities
- Can state understanding of biologic and behavioral characteristics of the newborn
- Has demonstrated behavioral/life style changes to reduce potential for development of problems
- Has taken the opportunity to intensify relationships with the newborn
- Has begun to integrate the infant into the family

KEY POINTS

- Assessment of the newborn requires data from the prenatal, intranatal, and postnatal periods.
- Knowledge of the biologic and behavioral characteristics is essential for guiding assessment and interpreting data.
- Providing a protective environment is a key role for the nurse that includes such actions as careful identification procedures, restraining techniques, measures to prevent infection, and support of physiologic functions.
- Maintenance of adequate ventilation includes ensuring an adequate airway and body temperature.

- Each nurse must develop skill in CPR and relieving airway obstruction.
- Parent education is a major role for the nurse and includes involving parents in all phases of the nursing process.
- Circumcision is an elective surgical procedure.
- The newborn has social, as well as physical, needs.
- Whether or not this is the couple's first baby, parents appreciate anticipatory guidance in the care of their child.
- The focus of care changes when the home becomes the locus of care.

CRITICAL THINKING EXERCISES

1. Examine the Case Study included in this chapter (p. 402). To what racial/ethnic group do you think Karen belongs? What clues in the description led to your conclusion? Select another racial/ethnic group and modify the case study to fit a mother of this background. Were your modifications based on facts or stereotypes?

2. Interview three mothers in the postpartum period. How soon after birth did they hold their babies? If they did not hold their babies immediately, what was the reason for the delay? Interview three labor and birth unit nurses. How soon after birth do they give the baby to the mother to hold? If they do not give the baby to the mother immediately, what is the reason for the delay? Are the reasons the mothers and the nurses gave the same? Can these delays be avoided?

REFERENCES

Anderson G: Pacifiers: the positive side, *MCN* 11:122, 1986.

Ballard JL, Novak KK, Driver M: A simplified score for assessment of fetal maturation of newly born infants, *J Pediatr* 95(5):769, 1979.

Bradley RJ, Caldwell BM: Using the HOME inventory to assess the family environment, *Pediatr Nurs* 14(2):97, 1988.

Campos RG: Soothing pain-elicited distress in infants with swaddling and pacifiers, *Child Dev* 60:781, 1989.

Donaher-Wagner BM, Braun DH: Infant cardiopulmonary resuscitation for expectant and new parents, *MCN* 17:27, 1992.

Dubowitz LMS et al: Gestational age of the newborn, *J Pediatr* 77:1, 1970.

Fanaroff AA, Martin RJ: *Neonatal-perinatal medicine: diseases of the fetus and infant,* ed 5, St Louis, 1992, Mosby.

Gillerman H, Beckham MH: The postpartum early discharge dilemma: an innovative solution, *J Perinat Neonat Nurs* 5:9, 1991.

Larson E: Rituals in infection control: what works in the newborn nursery: *JOGNN* 16:411, 1987.

Lund MM: Perspectives on newborn male circumcision, *Neonat Netw* 9(3):7, 1990.

Marchette L et al: Pain reduction interventions during neonatal circumcision, *Nurs Res* 40:241, 1991.

Millunchick E, McArtor R: Fatal aspiration of a make-shift pacifier, *Pediatrics* 77(3):369, 1986.

Murphy MR, Oellrich RG: (1990), A new method of phototherapy: nursing perspectives, *J Perinat* 10:249, 1990.

NAACOG: CDC reports caution about AIDS virus, *NAACOG Newsletter* 13(6):1, 1986a, NAACOG.

NAACOG: Neonatal skin care, *OGN Nursing Practice Resource,* Jan 1992, NAACOG.

NAACOG: Phototherapy and nursing care of the newborn with hyperbilirubinemia, *OGN Nursing Practice Resource* 15 July, 1986b, NAACOG.

Reiner CB, Meltes S, Hayes JR: Optimal sites and depths for skin puncture of infants and children as assessed from anatomical measurements, *Clin Chem* 36:547, 1990.

Rose BS: Phototherapy: all wrapped up? *Pediatr Nurs* 16(1): 57, 1990.

Rosenfeld W, Twist P, Conception L: A new device for phototherapy treatment of jaundiced infants, *J Perinat* 10:243, 1990.

Rush J et al: A randomized trial of a nursery ritual: wearing cover gowns to care for healthy newborns, *Birth* 17(1):25, 1990.

Shapiro C: Pain in the neonate: assessment and intervention, *Neonat Netw* 8:7, 1989.

Stevens-Simon C et al: Effects of race on the validity of clinical estimates of gestational age, *J Pediatr* 115(6):1000, 1989.

Tan KL, Efficacy of fluorescent daylight, blue, and green lamps in the management of nonhemolytic hyperbilirubinemia, *J Pediatr* 114:132, 1989.

Turick-Gibson T: Infant botulism, *Pediatr Nurs* 14(4):280, 1988.

Valman HB: Jaundice in the newborn, *BMJ* 299:1272, 1989.

Whaley LF, Wong DL: *Nursing care of infants and children,* ed 5, St Louis, 1995, Mosby.

Wright L, Brown A, Davison-Mundt A: Newborn screening: the miracle and the challenge, *J Pediatr Nurs* 7(1):26, 1992.

Zander K: Second generation critical paths, *Definition* 4(4):1, 1989.

BIBLIOGRAPHY

Blackburn ST, Loper DL: *Maternal, fetal and neonatal physiology: a clinical perspective,* Philadelphia, 1992, WB Saunders Co.

Lester P, Partridge JC, Cooke M: Postnatal human immunodeficiency virus antibody testing: the effects of current policy on infant care and maternal informed consent, *West J Med* 156(4):371, 1992.

Long CA: Teaching parents infant CPR—lecture or audiovisual tape? *MCN* 17:30, 1992.

NAACOG: Physical assessment of the neonate, *OBN Nursing Practice Resource,* Aug 1991.

Phillips CR: Single-room maternity care for maximum cost efficiency, *Perinat Neonat* 12:22, 1988.

Stang HJ et al: Local anesthesia for neonatal circumcision, *JAMA* 260:637, 1988.

Wong DL et al: Diapering choices: a critical review of the issues, *Pediatr Nurs* 18(1):41, 1992.

Newborn Nutrition and Feeding

SHANNON E. PERRY

LEARNING OBJECTIVES

Define the key terms.

Identify factors that affect parent and newborn readiness for feeding.

Evaluate nutrient needs in relation to an infant's growth and development.

Compare the composition and nutritional value of breast milk and infant formula.

Review the physiology of lactation.

Formulate nursing diagnoses relative to the infant's nutritional status and the parents' needs and preferences.

Examine breastfeeding in relation to advantages, care of breasts, diet and fluids, infant responses, secretion of drugs in milk, maintaining a job, and infant-related and maternal-related concerns.

Discuss formula-feeding in relation to advantages, care of breasts, diet and fluids, infant responses, and formula preparation.

Develop guidelines for teaching self-care for breastfeeding, formula-feeding, and formula preparation.

Explore cultural aspects of breastfeeding.

Describe the nurse's role in identifying and reducing barriers to successful breastfeeding.

Compare nutrition supplements recommended for the breastfed and formula-fed infant.

KEY TERMS

colostrum
demand feeding
engorgement
extrusion reflex
formula-feeding
formula preparation
growth pattern
lactation
lactoferrin
lactogenesis
let-down reflex
manual expression of milk
milk ejection
milk secretion
nipple erection reflex
nursing bottle caries
plugged ducts
sore nipples
weaning

RELATED TOPICS

Gastrointestinal anomalies *(Chap. 27)* • Infant of a diabetic mother *(Chap. 27)* • Jaundice *(Chap. 13 and 26)* • Reflexes (root, suck, swallow) *(Chap. 13)* • Immunoglobulins *(Chap. 3 and 13)*

Good nutrition in infancy fosters good health and optimal growth and development during the first few months of life and also establishes a basis for lasting good eating habits. Moreover, the feeding process is an important mechanism in the formation of a close, trusting relationship between the infant and primary caregiver(s), a key step in the infant's emotional development. Skillful health supervision of infants requires knowledge of their nutritional needs. This chapter focuses on nutritional needs for normal growth and development from birth to 3 months. Breastfeeding and formula-feeding are addressed.

INFANT DEVELOPMENT AND NUTRITIONAL NEEDS

Discussion of the child's **growth pattern** is often the starting point for effective communication with parents regarding proper nutrition for their child.

The full-term infant generally doubles the birth weight by 4 to 5 months of age and triples it in 1 year. Most newborn infants experience a 5% to 10% weight loss during the first few days of life due to excretion of urine, stool, and fluid through the lungs and the small amount of intake. Full-term infants usually regain this weight within 10 days.

Length increases about 50% during the first year. Doubling of birth length does not occur until about 4 years of age. Head circumference also increases rapidly during the first year in conjunction with rapid growth of the brain.

At birth the term infant's body is composed of about 16% fat (by weight). Between 2 and 6 months of age the increase in adipose tissue is more than twice as great as the increase in muscle mass; fat deposition occurs at a steady pace until about 9 months of age. Throughout infancy girls add a greater percentage of weight as fat than boys do; this trend continues throughout the remaining developmental years.

In the United States growth standards, or norms, have been developed for height or length, body weight, and head circumference. Children may differ in the rate of growth on the basis of race, socioeconomic status, and geography. Inadequate or excessive rates of growth may indicate nutritional problems.

Readiness for Feeding

At birth and for several months thereafter all the secretions of the infant's digestive tract contain enzymes especially suited to the digestion of human milk. The ability to handle foods other than milk depends on the physiologic development of the infant. The capacities for salivary, gastric, pancreatic, and intestinal digestion increase with age, indicating what may be a natural pattern for introduction of various solid foods.

At birth the infant produces little salivary or pancreatic amylase and thus is poorly prepared to digest the complex carbohydrates found in solid foods. Lipase production by the pancreas is lower than in older children or adults. Human milk fat and the vegetable oils used in commercial formulas are fairly well digested, but significant malabsorption of butterfat and other fats occurs. During the first few months of life rapid maturation occurs, so digestion of the starches found in cereals and vegetables is adequate by about 4 months of age. Therefore introduction of solid foods is practical after this age.

Kidney function of the full-term infant is not completely mature. Well-developed glomeruli satisfactorily filter the blood presented to the kidneys. The tubules, which are functionally less mature, are somewhat limited in their ability to reabsorb water and some solutes. Therefore it is important that the kidneys not be presented with excess solutes (renal solute load) to excrete. For this reason infants should receive only the protein needed for growth and no extra sodium, which is sometimes added to baby foods as sodium chloride (NaCl, or table salt).

The percentage of body water decreases from 75% at birth to 60% at 1 year of age. This reduction is almost entirely in extracellular water. The ability to retain body water through kidney function improves in the early months of life. To the infant this means that risk of dehydration decreases as renal concentrating capacity increases.

The newborn's development of feeding behavior depends on the maturation of the central nervous system (CNS). The rooting, sucking, and swallowing reflexes are present in the term newborn. The infant also has an **extrusion reflex** that automatically pushes food out of the mouth when it is placed on the tongue. Between 3 and 6 months of age the extrusion reflex becomes less pronounced.

Early emotional, psychologic, and social attachment of parents to the infant may influence the infant's personality. Feeding is the principal means by which the newborn establishes a human relationship with the parents. Development of trust is built on the close relationship between parents and infant. If the infant's needs are satisfied through food and love, a sense of trust is developed between the child and the parents. Food becomes the means by which infants bring together their parents and their own world. The newborn communicates by vigorous and sustained crying to express hunger, thirst, pain, and discomfort.

Feeding practices from birth, whether by breast or bottle, influence the infant's exposure to tactile stimulation. Tactile stimulation is essential to the infant's physical and emotional growth.

Nutrient Needs
Energy (Calories or kcal)

The energy needs of the infant may be considered in terms of three areas: (1) the basal energy requirement that sustains organ metabolic function, (2) the energy needed for physical activity and digestion of food, and (3) the energy needed for growth. During the first 4 months of life, 50% to 60% of the infant's energy is expended for basal metabolism, 25% to 40% for growth, and approximately 10% to 15% for activity and other needs.

The recommended daily dietary allowance (RDA) for energy for the first year is approximately 108 kcal per kilogram of body weight (49 kcal/lb) for the first 6 months and 98 kcal per kilogram (44.5 kcal/lb) for the second half of the year (Food and Nutrition Board, 1989). Both human milk and infant formulas supply approximately 67 kcal per deciliter (20 kcal/oz); thus 720 ml (24 oz) of human milk or formula supply about 480 kcal, sufficient for an infant weighing approximately 4.2 kg (9¼ lb).

Carbohydrate

There is no absolute requirement for carbohydrate. However, newborns have only small hepatic glycogen stores. Moreover, they may have limited ability for gluconeogenesis (formation of glucose from amino acids and other substrates) and ketogenesis (formation of ketone bodies from fat), which are mechanisms that provide alternative energy sources. Thus carbohydrates should provide at least 40% to 45% of the calories in the newborn's diet.

Lactose is the primary carbohydrate of milk. It also is the most abundant carbohydrate in the diet of infants to 6 months of age. Lactose provides calories in an easily available form. Its slow breakdown and absorption probably benefit calcium absorption. Lactose is added to formulas made from cow milk. Other commercial formulas may contain other forms of carbohydrates if they are soy based or are casein hydrolysate formulas.

Fat

For infants to acquire adequate calories from the limited amount of breast milk or formula they are able to consume, at least 50% of the calories provided must come from fat (triglycerides). The fat must be easily digested. Fat in human milk is easier to digest and absorb than that in cow milk. This is caused in part by the arrangement of fatty acids on the glycerol molecule. It also is related to the natural lipase activity present in human milk. Fecal loss of fat and therefore loss of energy may be excessive if whole or evaporated milk without added carbohydrate is fed to infants. Cow milk is used in preparing most commercial formulas, but the milk fat is removed, and a fat source such as corn oil, which is well digested and absorbed by the infant, is added.

In addition to the energy contributions made by fat, certain fats—the essential fatty acids (EFAs)—are required for growth and tissue maintenance. EFAs are components of cell membranes and precursors of some hormones. Inadequate intake of EFAs results in eczema and growth failure. Infants should not be fed skim or low-fat milk, since these products do not contain EFAs.

Protein

The protein requirement is greater per unit of body weight in the newborn than at any other time of life. The RDA for protein during the first 6 months is 2.2 g per kilogram.

The protein content of human milk, lower than that of unmodified cow milk, is sufficient for the newborn. Human milk contains far more lactalbumin in relation to casein, and lactalbumin is more easily digested than casein. In addition, the amino acid composition of human milk is ideally suited to the newborn infant's metabolic capabilities. For example, phenylalanine and methionine levels are low and cystine and taurine levels are high. The protein in some commercial formulas is modified to increase the amount of lactalbumin, or whey protein, and to decrease the relative proportion of casein. The amino acid composition of these formulas more closely resembles that of human milk than unmodified cow milk.

Fluids

The fluid requirement for normal infants is about 150 to 180 ml per kilogram per 24 hours (Hoekelman et al, 1992). This usually is consumed from the breast or in properly prepared formulas. Infants receiving this amount of water have approximately 100 ml per 24 hours available for secretion of urine.

Water intoxication resulting in hyponatremia, weakness, restlessness, nausea, vomiting, diarrhea, polyuria or oliguria, and convulsions can result from excessive feeding of water to infants (Hoekelman et al, 1992). Diluting formula to make it last longer has been observed as a cause of water intoxication.

Minerals and Vitamins

Most of the recommended minerals and vitamins are present in appropriate amounts in human milk and formula feedings. In contrast, unmodified cow milk is much higher in mineral content than is human milk, which is one important reason why it is unsuitable for the feeding of infants. The minerals and vitamins most likely to be a problem in various types of infant feedings are discussed next.

Human milk is low in calcium in comparison with cow milk and formulas, but the ratio of calcium to phosphorus is 2:1, which is optimal for bone mineralization. As a result, breastfed term infants receive ample calcium. Cow milk is very rich in calcium, but the calcium to phosphorus ratio is low. Because of the imbalance, hypocalcemia, tetany, and seizures frequently develop in young infants fed unmodified cow milk. The calcium to phosphorus ratio in commercial formulas is midway between human and cow milk.

Milk of all types is low in iron. However, iron from human milk is better absorbed (50%) than that from cow milk (10%), iron-fortified formula, or infant cereals (5%). Moreover, the fetus and the newborn infant deposit iron stores to draw upon for the first few months of life. Therefore the infant who is entirely breastfed normally maintains adequate hemoglobin levels for the first 6 months of life. After that time, iron-fortified infant cereals and other iron-containing foods are increasingly included in the diet so that dietary intake usually is sufficient. Formula-fed infants (and infants who are initially breastfed but then are weaned from the breast) should receive an iron-fortified formula until 12 months of age. Even though only a small percentage of the iron is absorbed from formulas, fortified formulas contain so much iron that the amount absorbed is sufficient.

Fluoride levels in human and cow milk and commer-

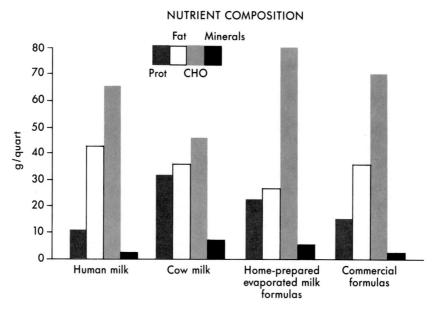

FIG. 15-1 Nutrient composition comparison of human milk/commercial formulas and cow milk/home-prepared milk formulas. (Modified from Dallman PR: Nutritional anemia of infancy. In Tsang RC, Nichols BL, editors: *Nutrition during infancy,* Philadelphia, 1988, Hanley & Belfus.)

cial formulas prepared without fluoridated water are low. This mineral is involved in tooth development, which is very active during early infancy. A reduction in dental caries is seen in children who receive adequate fluoride from birth. Thus a supplement is recommended for infants not receiving fluoridated water or those fed formula reconstituted with unfluoridated water.

Vitamin K levels in human milk are much lower than in cow milk or formulas. This vitamin, which is required for blood coagulation, can be produced by intestinal bacteria. However, the gut is sterile at birth, and time is required for intestinal flora to become established and produce vitamin K. Hemorrhagic disease of the newborn results from low vitamin K levels; therefore vitamin K injections are given at birth. Excessive bruising, petechiae, prolonged bleeding from blood-sampling sites or circumcisions, and intracranial hemorrhage may occur in affected infants.

Cow milk is low in vitamins C and E, but human milk and commercial formulas provide sufficient amounts. See Fig. 15-1 for a graphic comparison of the nutrient composition of human milk and other infant feedings.

LACTATION

Lactation is under the control of numerous endocrine glands, particularly the pituitary hormones prolactin and oxytocin. It is influenced by the suckling process and by maternal emotions. The establishment and maintenance of lactation in the human are determined by at least four factors: (1) the anatomic structure of the mammary gland and the development of alveoli, ducts, and nipples; (2) the initiation and maintenance of **milk secretion;** (3) **milk ejection,** or propulsion of milk from the alveoli to the nipple; and (4) the efficient and regular removal of milk from the breasts.

Breast Development

The female breast, a large exocrine gland, is quiescent during most of the woman's life span. It is composed of about 18 segments embedded in fat and connective tissues and lavishly supplied with blood vessels, lymphatic vessels, and nerves. The size of the breast is related to the amount of fat present and gives no indication of functional capacity. The principal feature of mammary growth in pregnancy is a great increase in ducts and alveoli under the influence of many hormones. Fig. 15-2 shows glandular (alveolar) tissue of each lobule leading into the duct system, which enlarges into lactiferous ducts and sinuses (ampullae). The lactiferous sinuses are under the areola and converge at the nipple pores. Late in pregnancy there is maximum development of the lobuloalveolar system and presumably a sensitization of glandular tissue for action by prolactin. Colostrum is present in the breasts from the fourth month of pregnancy.

Lactation Process

Breastfeeding depends on the interplay of hormones, reflexes, and learned behavior of the mother and newborn, and consists of the following factors:

- Lactogenesis. **Lactogenesis** (initiation of milk production) begins during the later part of pregnancy. Colostrum is secreted as a result of stimulation of the mammary alveolar cells by placental lactogen, a prolactin-like substance. Milk production continues after birth as an automatic process as long as milk is removed from the breast.

- Milk production. The continuing secretion of milk is mainly related to (1) sufficient production of the anterior pituitary hormone prolactin and (2) efficient removal of milk. Maternal nutrition and fluid intake are contributing factors to the quantity and quality of milk.

- Milk ejection. Movement of milk from the alveoli (where it is secreted by a process of extrusion from the cells) to the mouth of the infant is an active process within the breast. This process depends on the **let-down,** or **milk ejection, reflex.** The let-down reflex is primarily a response to an infant's sucking. The sucking stimulates the posterior pituitary gland to secrete oxytocin. Under the influence of oxytocin, the cells surrounding the alveoli contract, propelling the milk through the ductal system into the infant's mouth.

- Colostrum. Thick yellow **colostrum** is uniquely suited to the needs of the newborn. It provides vital antibodies and concentrated nutrition in the small volume typical of most early feedings. Early efficient breastfeedings correlate with decreased blood levels of bilirubin. The high protein level of colostrum facilitates binding of bilirubin and the laxative action of colostrum promotes early passage of meconium. Colostrum gradually changes to breast milk between the third and fifth postpartum day.

- Breast milk. At the beginning of each feeding, the foremilk contains less fat and flows at a faster rate than at the end of feeding. Toward the end of the feeding the hindmilk is whiter and contains more fat. The higher fat content at the end of the feeding satisfies the infant. Feeding long enough to thor-

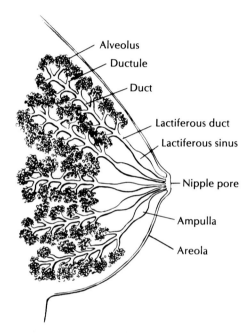

FIG. 15-2   Detailed structural features of human mammary gland. (From Worthington-Roberts B, Williams SR: *Nutrition in pregnancy and lactation,* ed 5, St. Louis, 1993, Mosby.)

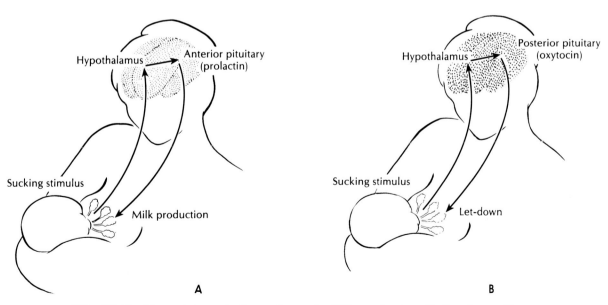

FIG. 15-3   Maternal breastfeeding reflexes. **A,** Milk production. **B,** Let-down. (From Worthington-Roberts B, Williams SR: *Nutrition in pregnancy and lactation,* ed 5, St. Louis, 1993, Mosby.)

oughly soften at least one breast at each feeding provides the calories needed for good weight gain, allows more time between feedings, and decreases gas and fussiness because the higher fat feedings are digested more slowly (Woolridge, Fisher, 1988).

The full-term, healthy newborn baby possesses three reflexes needed for successful breastfeeding: the rooting, sucking, and swallowing reflexes. However, to breastfeed efficiently, some infants may need practice to coordinate sucking, swallowing, and breathing.

Maternal Breastfeeding Reflexes

Three major maternal reflexes involved in breastfeeding are secretion of prolactin, nipple erection, and the letdown reflex (Fig. 15-3).

Prolactin is the key lactogenic hormone in initiating and maintaining milk secretion. The sucking stimulus provided by the baby sends a message to the hypothalamus, which stimulates the anterior pituitary to release prolactin, the hormone that promotes milk production by the alveolar cells of the mammary gland. The amount of prolactin secreted, and hence the milk produced, is related to the amount of sucking stimulus, that is, the frequency, intensity, and duration with which the baby breastfeeds (Garza, Hopkinson, 1988; Lawrence, 1994; Worthington-Roberts, 1993).

Stimulation of the nipple by the infant's mouth leads to erection. The **nipple erection reflex** assists in the propulsion of milk through the lactiferous sinuses to the nipple pores.

The ejection of milk from the alveoli and milk ducts occurs because of the let-down reflex. As a result of the sucking stimulus, the hypothalamus releases oxytocin from the posterior pituitary. Oxytocin stimulates contraction of the myoepithelial cells around the alveoli in the mammary glands. Contraction of these musclelike cells causes milk to be propelled through the duct system and into the lactiferous sinuses, where it becomes available to the nursing infant (Lawrence, 1994).

The let-down reflex may be felt as a tingling sensation or there may be no sensation perceived by the mother. Other signs of let-down are milk dripping from the breasts before the baby starts to suckle, milk leaking from the breast opposite to the one being used, uterine cramping during feeding caused by the action of oxytocin on the uterus, and increased vaginal bleeding during or just after feeding. Many women experience the letdown reflex when simply thinking about their baby or hearing another baby cry. Let-down may occur during sexual activity, since oxytocin is released during orgasm. Most mothers feel very relaxed or drowsy as they breastfeed. Increased thirst is also a sign that breastfeeding is going well.

Although the attitude of the mother toward breastfeeding may be a powerful factor in achieving successful lactation, the remarkable survival of the human race with mothers breastfeeding under extremely stressful conditions suggests that lactation does not require an idyllic setting.

Cultural Aspects of Lactation

To promote lactation and provide proper assistance to a new mother, nurses should consider cultural beliefs. For instance, in the Philippines, if the mother's milk does not flow regularly, a meal of chicken and green papaya boiled in coconut milk is suggested (Hart, 1965). A Filipina mother may be advised to eat a soup of boiled clams and ginger. Some Filipina mothers use hot applications of special medicinal preparations to stimulate lactation. Furthermore, some Filipina mothers believe that raising an arm over the head while lying down will decrease, if not actually stop, lactation. Hart also reported the belief of some Filipina women that heavy work makes their milk "hot." Korean mothers eat seaweed soup with rice to increase milk production (Park, Peterson, 1991). Currier (1978) reported that Hispanic Americans believe that exposing mothers to cold diminishes the flow of milk.

Other differences can be observed in Finland, where no infant formula is manufactured. All women breastfeed (Carr, 1989). Countries such as Colombia, Brazil, Thailand, and New Guinea have reversed the recent decline in breastfeeding through breastfeeding promotion.

Filipinas, Mexican-Americans, Vietnamese, and some Nigerians typically do not give colostrum to their infants. These mothers begin breastfeeding after their milk has come in. Some Korean women do not begin breastfeeding until 3 days after birth, whereas others begin breastfeeding immediately and offer the breast every time the infant cries (Choi, 1986). Morse et al (1990) found that 50 out of 120 cultures studied withheld colostrum at least 2 days. Mexican-Americans tend to overfeed their babies because they believe that a fat baby is a healthy baby (Alexander, Blank, 1988).

In Kenya, mothers feed preterm neonates only by breast. They also begin breastfeeding preterm infants earlier than is the practice in most other countries. Kenyans

CULTURAL CONSIDERATIONS

SOME CULTURAL BELIEFS ABOUT BREASTFEEDING

Cultures in which breastfeeding is common but infants are not given colostrum, because colostrum is believed to be bad or unclean, include the following: Japanese, Laotian, Cambodian, Vietnamese, Korean, Mexican, Filipino, and Haitian.

Cultures in which breastfeeding is common include the following: Swedish, Finnish, Chinese, Indian, Saudi Arabian Muslim, and South African.

never use gavage tubes. They feed preterm infants from small cups until they can suck (Armstrong, 1987) (see Cultural Considerations).

Care Management

The nurse can be an important contributor to the health care team. Nurses can assess the progress of the mother and the baby in learning how to breastfeed successfully. They can provide education, support, and counseling in the breastfeeding process.

✤ ASSESSMENT

Feeding an infant involves the infant and the parents. Therefore both need to be assessed.

Assessment of the Infant

The infant is assessed for developmental readiness for feeding, nutritional needs, and success of the feeding program (Shrago, Bocar, 1990). Infant factors affecting readiness for feeding are assessed shortly after birth for the breastfed and bottle-fed infant. These factors include age, condition at birth, maturity, and energy level. The suck is evaluated by placing a gloved finger in the baby's mouth, with the finger pad touching and stroking the palate. The examiner should be able to feel the tongue cushioning the joint of the finger and stroking the finger.

If there are no complications, the infant can be put to breast immediately after birth. The initial feeding allows the nurse to assess the newborn for any signs of tracheoesophageal fistula or atresia. It used to be the practice in many nurseries to offer the newborn plain sterile water 1 to 4 hours after birth. This is not necessary. Colostrum is not irritating if aspirated; it is readily absorbed by the respiratory system. With encouragement and by taking advantage of the normal period of alertness following birth, the newborn can breastfeed from the start. Early and prolonged contact (i.e., rooming-in) promotes continuation of breastfeeding (Lindenberg et al, 1990).

The success of the breastfeeding program can be assessed by direct observation of the baby at the breast. The baby who sucks well on a finger may not be able to coordinate sucking, breathing, and swallowing milk. Signs that breastfeeding is going well must be elicited from both the mother and the newborn.

As the infant grows and matures, nutritional needs change. The infant who is obtaining the necessary nutrients and fluid exhibits a steady increase in weight, good skin turgor and muscle tone, vigorous feeding behavior, and satisfaction. The satisfied newborn sleeps, cries in moderation, and is interested in socializing.

Assessment of the Parents

The couple is assessed as follows:

1. Physical ability and psychologic readiness for feeding the newborn
2. Knowledge of breastfeeding and formula-feeding so that an informed choice of method can be made
3. Knowledge of the infant's nutrition needs and capabilities
4. Knowledge and skill in feeding methods
5. Knowledge of an adequate and safe diet during lactation

The techniques used to assess these areas include interviews, discussion, and observation of skill in feeding.

The nurse must be alert for signs that the parents need information about the newborn's reflexes (rooting, sucking, gagging, extrusion), cues indicating readiness to feed, and feeding techniques (either breast or bottle). Lack of knowledge can lead to parent and child frustration and loss of self-esteem and can negatively affect the parent-child relationship. Mother-related problems and nursing actions are described in Table 15-1. The infant is assessed for readiness to feed, feeding skill, frequency and character of passage of urine and stool, weight, and general behavior. Factors that cause *failure to thrive* must be identified promptly (Fig. 15-4). Gestational age and birth weight and developmental and acquired disorders influence infant nutrition and feeding.

✤ NURSING DIAGNOSES

When observations have been made, data collected and analyzed, nursing diagnoses relative to the infant's nutrition status can be made. Examples include the following:

High risk for ineffective breastfeeding related to
- Maternal anxiety or ambivalence
- Nonsupportive partner/family

High risk for situational low self-esteem related to
- Difficulties encountered in breastfeeding secondary to knowledge deficit

Effective family coping, potential for growth related to
- Knowledge of infant readiness to feed
- Skill in implementing chosen feeding method

A nursing plan of care on p. 431 presents examples of nursing diagnoses based on assessment findings.

✤ PLANNING

While planning care, the nurse needs to consider many factors. These factors include the infant's and parent's readiness for feeding, the chosen feeding method, and relevant cultural influences. Community resources such as breastfeeding support groups can be helpful, as can teaching aids such as videotapes available in the hospital or clinic.

TABLE 15-1 Mother-Related Problems in Breastfeeding

PROBLEM	NURSING ACTION
ENGORGED BREASTS	
Engorgement is a response of the breasts to the hormones of lactation and the presence of milk. The breasts swell and pinch the ducts shut so the baby cannot breastfeed. The tenderness extends into the axilla. The breasts usually feel firm, tense, and warm as a result of the increased blood supply, and the skin may appear shiny and taut. The unyielding areolae make it difficult for the infant to grasp the nipple. Breastfeeding can be uncomfortable to the mother and frustrating for both mother and infant. Engorgement must be treated aggressively. Breast milk contains prolactin inhibiting factor. Any time the breasts stay full, the milk glands get the message to make less milk.	1. Apply ice to the breasts. Ice will reduce the swelling so enough of the milk can be removed to soften the areola for the baby to latch on. 2. After 15 minutes of ice, the mother should use the electric pump; then nurse, ice, pump, and nurse until her breasts are softened. 3. Heat or cold? If a mother realizes that she is getting engorged and a warm shower makes her milk flow, application of warm, moist heat may help lessen the engorgement. However, most mothers' breasts are so swollen that heat only brings more blood to an already congested area. For these mothers, ice and pumping are the best treatment.
SORE NIPPLES	
The nipples may become sore during the early days of breastfeeding. **Sore nipples** may be prevented or limited by using a correct position and avoiding undue breast engorgement. Pain is a clear sign that intervention is necessary. Is the baby sucking properly while feeding? Could the mother have a monilial infection on her nipples?	1. Assess position of infant at breast. 2. Evaluate baby's sucking during a feeding. 3. Expose the nipples to air. 4. Use a heat lamp to dry the nipples after the feeding (40-W bulb in a desk lamp, positioned 45 cm [18 in] from the breast). 5. If soreness occurs, feed from less sore side first when sucking is more vigorous.
PLUGGED DUCTS	
Occasionally a milk duct will become plugged, creating a tender spot on the breast, which may appear lumpy and hot. **Plugged ducts** might result from inadequate emptying of the breasts, wearing a bra that is too tight, incorrect positioning for feeding, or always using the same position.	1. Offer the sore breast first so that it will be emptied more completely. 2. Nurse longer and more often; if the breast gets too full, the plugged duct becomes worse and infection may develop. 3. Change positions at every feeding so that the pressure of the feeding will be applied to different places on the breast. 4. Apply warm compresses to the breasts between feedings to increase milk flow.
AFTERPAINS	
The breastfeeding mother may experience afterpains. Afterpains are more common in multiparous women than in primiparas. The afterpains may be intense enough that the mother is uncomfortable and her tension interferes with feeding the infant. The mother may note an increase in lochial flow due to the uterine contractions that cause the afterpains.	1. Offer a mild analgesic for pain 40 minutes before the feeding period. The mother may be reassured that this discomfort is transitory and will be gone in about 2 days. 2. Explain to the parents that the uterine contractions are a sign that the hormones needed for breastfeeding are functioning.

TABLE 15-1 Mother-Related Problems in Breastfeeding—cont'd

PROBLEM	NURSING ACTION
PERCEPTION OF INADEQUATE AMOUNT OF MILK Insufficient milk supply rarely is a problem (see Clinical Application of Research, p. 422). Because sucking stimulates the flow of milk, feeding on demand for adequate duration should supply ample amounts of milk.	1. Increase frequency of feedings to increase supply. 2. Note frequency of infant urination and bowel movements; six to eight voidings and one stool every 24 hours are adequate. 3. Weight gain of ¾ to 1 oz/day indicates adequate intake. 4. Reassure mother if infant seems satisfied and is gaining weight.
BREAST PUMPING For a number of reasons, mothers may wish to remove milk from their breasts and save it for a later feeding or take to their hospitalized newborn. Milk can be expressed by hand satisfactorily. For many women, however, a manual or electric breast pump provides a better stimulus for milk flow and is a more efficient mode of milk collection.	Instruct the mother in the use of a breast pump (see Fig. 15-12).
MATERNAL INFECTION If breast tenderness is accompanied by fever and a general flulike feeling, a breast infection is probably present.	Instruct the mother to notify her primary health care provider.
SEXUAL SENSATIONS For some women the rhythmic uterine contractions occurring while breastfeeding are similar to those experienced during orgasm. These sensual feelings while nursing an infant may disturb the mother.	Reassure the mother that such feelings are normal.
RELACTATION AND LACTATION AFTER ADOPTING Occasionally a mother starts breastfeeding late or discontinues it but decides at a much later date that she would like to begin again. After adopting an infant, a small number of women decide to attempt lactation. Some have never done so before; others have breastfed a baby of their own. With much sucking stimulus, lactation can be induced. It requires great perseverance. Because the mammary glands complete their development for lactation during the first 6 months of pregnancy, a woman who has never been pregnant or never carried a pregnancy beyond the first trimester is a poor candidate for successful induction of lactation.	Instruct the mother to attempt relactation or induced lactation by providing the infant substantial opportunities to suck at the breast. With much sucking stimulus over several days' time, many patient and persistent women can initiate the lactation process or restore it. Their volume of milk production may be less than the infant demands, in which case a supplemental feeding after breastfeeding may be necessary. Alternatively, some women use the Lact-Aid Nursing Trainer or the Medela S.N.S. to complement their own milk production (Fig. 15-5) (Edgehouse and Radzyminski, 1990). While sucking at the breast, the baby also obtains milk via suction through a small tube leading to a container of fresh formula that is clipped to the mother's bra. As the infant sucks, the mother's milk supply is built up and the infant receives adequate nutrition through the feeding device.

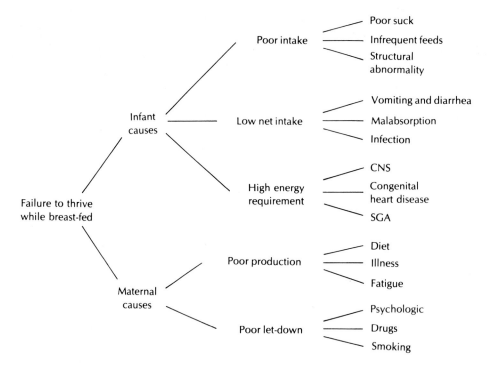

FIG. 15-4 Diagnostic flow chart for failure to thrive. (From Lawrence RA: *Breastfeeding: a guide for the medical profession,* ed 4, St. Louis, 1994, Mosby.)

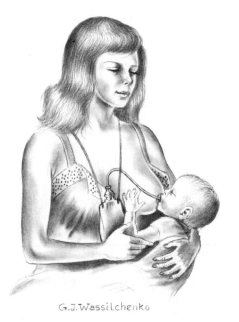

G.J.Wassilchenko

FIG. 15-5 Lact-Aid Nursing Trainer in use.

❖ EXPECTED OUTCOMES

The expected outcomes for the infant include the following:

1. The infant will receive the necessary nutrients to grow well.

2. The infant will have minimal physiologic stress associated with digestion, metabolism, and excretion of nutrients.

The expected outcomes for the parents include the following:

1. The parents will verbalize understanding of sound feeding practices.

2. The parents will demonstrate skill and confidence in feeding and caring for their infant.

3. The parents will enjoy feeding their infant.

❖ COLLABORATIVE CARE

General Considerations

Prenatal Period

An expectant couple is encouraged to select a method of infant feeding before the birth. Information should be provided so that the couple can make a knowledgeable choice.

Counseling about infant feeding should begin during the first trimester of pregnancy when the parents are unrushed and have time to consider their choices. Parents are encouraged to express their opinions and feelings so that they can be discussed and any misinformation can be corrected. Classes should teach what breastfeeding is like and focus on how to utilize the baby's reflexes.

Fathers and partners are encouraged to participate in counseling sessions because their encouragement and emotional support contribute to successful lactation. Many parents have never seen a woman breastfeeding an infant; they therefore find it especially helpful to have a couple who are successfully breastfeeding an infant available to answer questions and to provide reinforcement.

Over the past 10 years there has been an increase in the number of women who choose to breastfeed. This increase is more likely to be seen among middle class and educated couples. Reports indicate that low-income women participate in Special Supplement Food Programs for Women, Infants, and Children (WIC) and tend to bottle-feed instead of breastfeed (Barber-Madden, 1990). However, WIC has initiated successful programs to encourage mothers to breastfeed their babies.

Postnatal Period

Feeding is an emotionally charged area of infant care. The size and growth of an infant are often equated with excellence and evidence of mothering or parenting ability. The infant who is a fussy eater can raise parental anxiety levels. The anxious parent appears to compound the problem, and a vicious cycle can develop. Getting help from a knowledgeable source for a feeding or two will break the cycle. Parents need positive feedback to develop a feeling of confidence in their own abilities. Often just listening and praising are the most effective interventions. The first few days the parents are home with the baby often are filled with excitement and anxiety about infant care activities. Entertaining company and other family commitments may have to be restricted. Many parents need considerable assistance with infant feeding. Both group and individual teaching may be necessary.

Breastfeeding

Breast milk is the food of choice for infants. Breastfeeding offers many advantages: nutritional, immunologic, and psychologic. According to Worthington-Roberts (1993), breastfeeding offers the following advantages:

1. Breastfed infants receive immunoglobulins to protect against many diseases and infections.
2. Breastfed babies have fewer ear and upper respiratory tract infections.
3. Breastfed infants have less diarrhea and fewer gastrointestinal problems.
4. Breastfed infants' risk of developing juvenile-onset diabetes is diminished.
5. Breastfed babies are less likely to develop certain types of lymphoma.
6. The type of protein ingested is less likely to cause allergic reactions.
7. Breastfed infants have fewer problems with overfeeding because the need to "empty the bottle" is eliminated.
8. Breastfed infants have a decreased incidence of obesity and hypertension in adulthood.

9. Bottle washing, preparation of formula, and refrigeration are unnecessary.
10. Maternal organs return more quickly to their nonpregnant condition.
11. Breastfeeding promotes close mother-child contact.

Women who have had no contact with mothers who breastfeed and who have had little or no contact with newborns may require assistance to become proficient in breastfeeding (Lawrence, 1994). Attending meetings of a community breastfeeding support group before the baby's birth can meet this need (see the Home Care box on p. 418).

Immunologic Benefits

Evidence shows that the newborn infant acquires important elements of host resistance from breast milk while maturation of the infant's own immune system is taking place. Human milk contains high levels of immunoglobulin A (IgA) and affords protection against several bacterial and viral diseases, especially those of the respiratory and gastrointestinal systems (Whaley, Wong, 1995).

Immunoglobulins are believed to function directly in the infant's gastointestinal tract by diminishing antigen contact with intestinal mucosa until the infant's own antibody responses are developed. **Lactoferrin,** which is secreted in human milk, is believed to play a role in controlling bacterial growth in the gastrointestinal tract. It works by competing with microorganisms that require iron for replication. The presence of these factors is believed to explain the reduced incidence of illness in breastfed babies that has been reported not only in developing countries but also in the United States.

IgA protects against development of many allergies. In addition, human milk contains numerous other host defense factors, such as macrophages, granulocytes and T- and B-lymphocytes (Lawrence, 1994).

Jaundice

Some researchers suggest that insufficient feeding and hyperbilirubinemia are related. Early and unlimited breastfeeding stimulates milk production and encourages elimination of meconium through stimulation of the gastrocolic reflex and the laxative effects of colostrum (de Steuben, 1992).

Care of the Breasts

Daily washing of the breasts with water is sufficient for cleanliness. It is helpful to air-dry the nipples after each feeding. Expressed breast milk may be massaged gently around the nipple. No breast creams, lotions, or ointments should be applied because they block the secretion of a natural bacteriostatic oil by the Montgomery glands. Some infants object to either the taste or the smell of creams and refuse to suckle until the breast has been washed.

HOME CARE

BREASTFEEDING

Here are some things to know before you start.

ABOUT YOURSELF

You can assume any comfortable position (Figs. 15-8). Let the breast fall forward without tension. Leave one hand free to guide the nipple into the child's mouth.

The nipple can be made more prominent by gently rolling it between your fingers. Some of the areola will be put in the baby's mouth with the nipple. This prevents bruising the nipple.

Colostrum is the yellow fluid you can express from your breasts now. It is good for the baby. It contains some fat and protein and helps the baby resist infections.

Milk may be expected to appear 48 to 96 hours after birth. Before the milk comes in, the breasts feel soft to the touch. After the milk comes in, the breasts may feel full and hard.

THE BREASTFEEDING TECHNIQUE

Hold the baby so that the infant's cheek touches the breasts. The pressure against the lower lip begins the rooting reflex. The baby will turn toward the nipple. The baby can smell the colostrum and milk, which also will cause turning toward the nipple.

Put the baby to breast by guiding the nipple and areolar tissue into the infant's mouth and over the tongue. Compress the breast with thumb above and fingers below the areola to permit the infant to latch on effectively.

EXPECTED INFANT RESPONSES AND MATERNAL SENSATIONS

At first the baby sucks in short bursts of three to five sucks followed by single swallows. In 1 to 2 days a sucking pattern evolves. This consists of 10 to 30 sucks followed by swallowing. The infant's lips exert pressure on the areola, and the tongue "cradles" the nipple so that the tip is not retracted. The pressure, combined with negative intraoral pressure, brings milk into the mouth (Fig. 15-6).

When the baby is sucking properly, there is no "clicking" noise. This clicking noise means the infant is sucking on her or his own tongue in the back of the throat,

past the nipple. You should hear the rhythmic suck-swallow breathing pattern that indicates milk is flowing. Some mothers can sense if the infant has drawn the areolar tissue into the mouth along with the nipple.

BREASTFEEDING THE BABY

Get the baby ready to put to breast by first making sure the infant is awake. If necessary, waken the baby by stroking the cheek, rubbing the feet, and talking to her or him. The nurse may help you position the baby so that the head is directly facing the breast and the nipple is not pulled to one side.

Now put the infant to breast by bringing the baby to the breast, not the breast to the baby. The baby's face, chest, abdomen, and knees should all be facing your body. Touch the infant's upper lip with your nipple, and watch how the baby will turn toward you with an open mouth (Fig. 15-7, *A, B*). Pull the baby as close to you as you can.

Feel how the baby's jaws fit behind the nipple and the nipple is deep in the infant's mouth (Fig. 15-7, *C*).

If infant needs more breathing space, lift the baby's hips to enlarge the breathing space. Do *not* make a "dimple" in your breast for breathing space; it may dislodge the nipple.

You may need to hold your breast throughout the entire feeding for a few weeks.

It is a good idea to use both breasts at each feeding. You need to empty both breasts because an empty breast signals the woman's body to produce more milk. You can tell which breast to start with next time by feeling the weight. The heaviest one has the most milk, so start with that one.

To remove the baby from the breast, place a finger in the corner of the baby's mouth and keep it there until the breast has been comfortably removed (Fig. 15-7, *D*).

Before putting the baby to the other breast, burp the infant (Fig. 15-9). Some babies never burp; others do so frequently, Gently rub or pat the baby's back.

After feeding, place the baby on the right side. This allows air in the stomach to come up and not bring the milk with it (see Fig. 14-3).

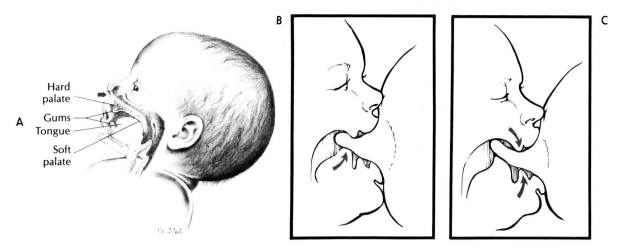

FIG. 15-6 Suckling process: **A,** Infant breathes through nose *(arrow)*. Tongue and palate meet, closing esophagus. **B,** Tongue thrusts up and forward to grasp nipple. **C,** Gums compress areola and tongue moves backward, creating negative pressure for suction. (**B** and **C** from Riordan J: *A practical guide to breastfeeding,* St. Louis, 1987, Mosby.)

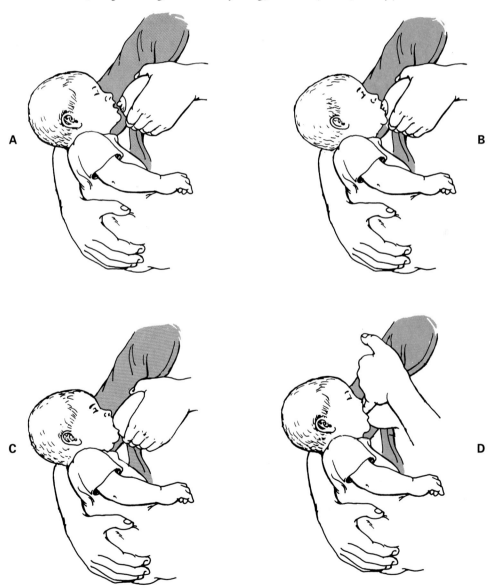

FIG. 15-7 Cradle hold. **A,** Mother touches the infant's lower lip to elicit rooting reflex; infant responds by turning to breast and opening mouth. **B,** Infant begins to latch on. **C,** Infant latched on correctly. **D,** Mother uses finger to release suction at end of feeding.

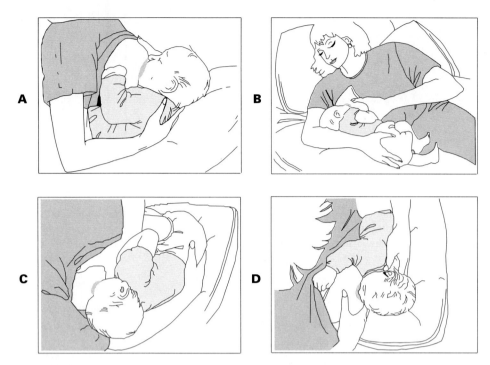

FIG. 15-8 Common positions for breastfeeding. **A,** Football hold (right breast). **B,** Side-lying. **C,** Cradling. **D,** Across lap. (Copyright 1991 Lactation Consultants of North Carolina.)

If a mother needs a bra, she will be uncomfortable without one. If she wishes to wear a bra, it needs to be well fitted, with comfortable shoulder straps and with flaps over the breasts large enough to release the breast without discomfort. Milk leaking from the breasts, particularly just before the feeding (milk ejection reflex), can be uncomfortable and embarrassing. The bra can be padded with folded squares of soft cotton cloth, a perineal pad cut in two, or commercially designed pads. Lining the cup with plastic material is not recommended because trapped moisture tends to cause sore nipples.

A tingling sensation in the nipple usually precedes leaking of milk. Pressure with the heel of the hands over the nipples often will prevent leaking.

Diet and Fluids

During lactation there is increased need for maternal energy, protein, minerals, and vitamins. This increase restores what the mother loses in producing milk, it provides adequate nutrients for the nourishment of the infant, and it protects the mother's own stores. A well-balanced diet containing an extra 500 calories per day (per baby) is usually necessary for both mother and infant. Because this amount of calories is inadequate to compensate completely for the energy costs of producing milk, the mother will experience a gradual weight loss as fat stores deposited during pregnancy are expended.

Although the breastfeeding mother requires adequate fluids, drinking to satisfy thirst is sufficient. Glasses of wa-

ter, fruit juices, decaffeinated tea, and milk can be alternated. The mother can keep a pitcher of water close by when breastfeeding because she often becomes thirsty. The use of beer or wine while breastfeeding is not recommended (Blume et al, 1987).

Breastfeeding Positions and Techniques

There are several positions for nursing a baby. The mother should find a position that is comfortable for her (Fig. 15-7 and 15-8). The baby should be in a comfortable position to facilitate feeding and should not have to turn the head or strain the neck to reach the nipple. When the mother lightly touches the baby's lips with her nipple, the baby will respond with a natural rooting reflex and turn toward the nipple and open his or her mouth. The nipple and as much of the areola as possible should be in the baby's mouth. If the baby's nose seems to be blocked by the breast, the mother can elevate the baby's hips, which will provide more breathing space. Depressing the breast usually pulls the nipple out of position for proper latch-on. When the mother is ready to give the baby a chance to burp, she should gently insert her finger into the corner of the baby's mouth between the gums to break the suction (Fig. 15-7, *D*). Pulling the baby away without breaking suction can be painful and lead to sore nipples. There are several positions for burping (bubbling) the baby (Fig. 15-9). After burping the baby, the mother should check to see that the first breast was thoroughly softened. If it is still full, the baby

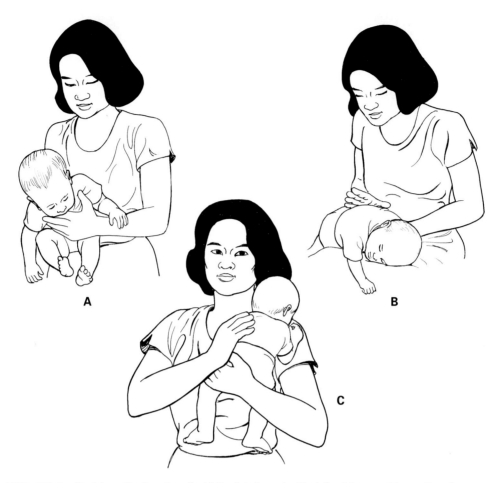

FIG. 15-9 Positions for burping (bubbling) infant. **A,** Upright. Note position of hand on jaw supporting head. **B,** Across lap. **C,** Over shoulder.

needs to be put back on the same breast. After the first breast is soft, the mother should offer the second one.

At the next breastfeeding the mother should offer the breast from which the infant last nursed. An easy way to know which breast to offer is for the mother to lift both to determine which is heavier.

Breastfeeding is more successful when the baby is awake and eager to eat. When the infant must be awakened to eat, parents can talk to, massage, wash the face with a warm washcloth, pat, and unwrap the baby. It may take several minutes to awaken the infant, but newborns need to be fed every 2 to 3 hours for a total of 8 to 12 times each 24 hours for at least 1 month.

Limiting time at the breast does not prevent sore nipples. When the baby is nursing correctly, there will not be pain or tissue damage. Getting the baby on and off the breast carefully, positioned correctly, and sucking properly may require practice for both the mother and the baby. Pain is usually a sign that the baby is not positioned correctly. For example, the mother may need to learn to hold the baby closer, support the weight of her

breast more, get the baby's mouth open wider, or hold the baby's chin down to help stick out the tongue. Often pain occurs only at the beginning of a feeding. When the milk lets down and lubricates the nipple, the soreness abates. Expressing a few drops of milk to wet the nipple facilitates latching-on. The mother may need to try a different position to adjust the infant's sucking (Fig. 15-8). This often decreases discomfort (Storr, 1988).

Infant Responses
When breastfed babies are feeding efficiently, they do *not* feed more often than formula-fed babies. Gavage-fed babies in intensive care nurseries are fed the same volumes and frequency whether given breast milk or formula. The problem has been that health care professionals have not known how to facilitate efficient feedings.

Breastfed babies consume what they need and no more. Breastfeeding whenever the baby is hungry is easy to do because the milk is always ready. Some babies may be hungry as frequently as every hour or two on some days, on other days only every 4 hours. The more often

CLINICAL APPLICATION OF RESEARCH

INSUFFICIENT MILK SUPPLY SYNDROME

Mothers often stop breastfeeding because they think they do not have enough milk. Whether the milk produced is insufficient or whether mothers perceive that it is insufficient is unknown. This study was conducted to determine what factors are associated with an inadequate supply of breast milk. The sample included 384 mothers with infants between 8 and 14 weeks of age; 190 mothers participated in the Women, Infants, and Children (WIC) supplemental food program and 194 did not. Data were collected using an author-developed breastfeeding questionnaire that addressed factors such as maternal time constraints, maternal comfort factors, breastfeeding behaviors, maternal psychologic and physiologic factors, sociocultural factors, infant factors, and possible insufficient milk syndrome (IMS) factors. Of the mothers, 100 (26%) reported they did not have enough milk to satisfy their baby during the first 8 postpartum weeks.

Mothers who had IMS knew less about breastfeeding, did not intend to breastfeed as long, and were less confident about breastfeeding. Lack of support from the mother-in-law was associated with IMS. Mothers with IMS reported more illness and poorer health while breastfeeding. Larger babies breastfed longer. Introducing solid food was associated with IMS.

Since some of the factors associated with IMS are identifiable during pregnancy, nurses can address these factors in childbirth preparation classes and reinforce the teaching in breastfeeding classes after childbirth. Education about breastfeeding and support from significant others are necessary for successful breastfeeding. Nurses can play an important role in breastfeeding success.

Reference: Hill PD, Aldag J: Potential indicators of insufficient milk supply syndrome, *Res Nurs Health* 14:11, 1991.

---

the baby breastfeeds, the more milk the breasts produce. Thus, when a baby needs to increase the mother's supply of breast milk during a growth spurt, she or he should breastfeed more often. Some babies breastfeed on only one side at a feeding and gain weight well.

Crying does not always mean that the baby is hungry. The baby may be physically uncomfortable or just want to be held, burped, or changed. The mother can be reassured that she is producing sufficient milk if the infant has at least 6 to 8 voidings of pale, straw-colored urine and 1 bowel movement in 24 hours (see Clinical Application of Research box above). In warm weather the baby may be thirsty and will increase the number of breastfeedings.

The stools of breastfed babies are loose. Some infants have a bowel movement at each feeding. Older breastfed babies may go a week without having a bowel movement, but a newborn should have at least one per day. The change from black, sticky meconium to yellow, soft stools reassures parents that the baby is digesting breast milk. Babies who are fed only breast milk do not become constipated, although they may strain considerably in passing the stool. The stool does not have a foul smell and is not irritating to the skin.

Breastfeeding Twins

Many families find it easier to breastfeed twins than to bottle feed because giving a bottle requires both hands, whereas breastfeeding leaves one hand free. Also, some mothers breastfeed twins simultaneously (Fig. 15-10). Parents do not have to shop for and prepare formula, wash bottles, nipples and caps, get up at night to warm bottles, and carry bottles when going out.

Many mothers of twins use a modified **demand feeding** schedule. They feed the first baby who wakes up and then awaken the second baby to feed.

A record of the feeding times, which breast was used by which baby, and which side was used first may be helpful during the early weeks. If one twin feeds more readily than the other, an effort should be made to have that twin feed on alternate breasts to equalize stimulation. If feeding the babies simultaneously, the mother should experiment with positions. Both babies may be cradled. One baby may be held in the football hold and the other in the cradle hold. If both babies are in football holds, it may be difficult for the mother to remove them without help. Obviously the mother with twins will need extra assistance from her family, extra nourishment (500 calories a day for each baby), and extra rest.

Breastfeeding Preterm Infants

When a mother wishes to feed a preterm infant, she is taught to use a breast pump every 3 to 4 hours to stimulate milk production and then to maintain a supply of milk. The milk can be collected in a bottle, frozen, and taken to the nursery for gavage or bottle feedings of her infant. When the baby's condition permits, the baby will be put to breast.

Expressing and Storing Breast Milk

During the early days of breastfeeding, engorgement may make the mother very uncomfortable. Expressing breast milk will provide her some relief and soften the breast so the baby can nurse.

If a mother returns to work, it may be necessary for her to pump her breasts while away from the baby. Breast

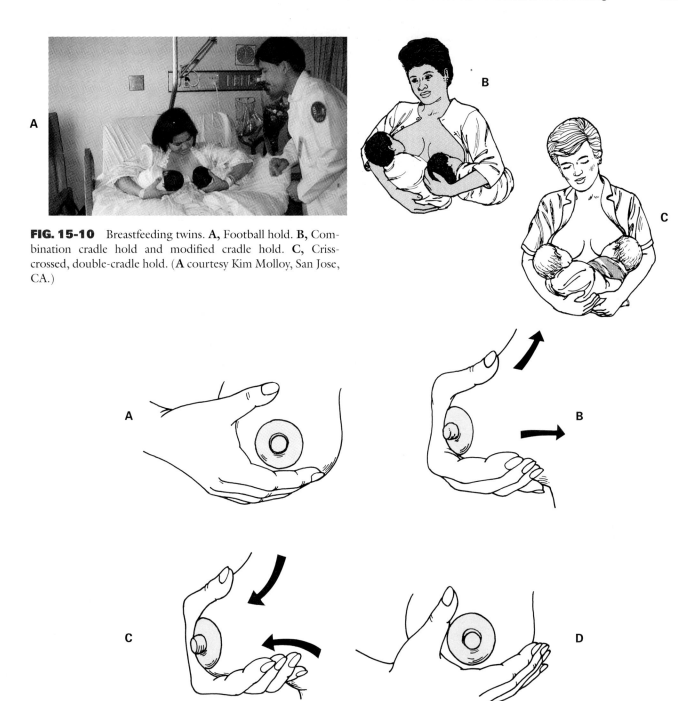

FIG. 15-10   Breastfeeding twins. **A,** Football hold. **B,** Combination cradle hold and modified cradle hold. **C,** Crisscrossed, double-cradle hold. (**A** courtesy Kim Molloy, San Jose, CA.)

FIG. 15-11   Manual expression of human milk. **A,** Start with thumb above areola and other fingers below. **B,** Press in toward chest. **C,** Squeeze milk from lactiferous sinuses by compressing breast as thumb and fingers slide forward. **D,** Rotate hand one-fourth turn around breast, and repeat steps in a rhythmic motion until milk begins to flow. Fingers should not slip across areola to nipple.

milk can be expressed by hand **(manual expression of milk)** (Fig. 15-11) or with the aid of a breast pump. The process is facilitated if the mother is relaxed. The mother may want to drink liquids before expressing milk.

Several types of breast pumps are available on the market today (Fig. 15-12). Some are easier to use than others, and they vary greatly in price. Hand-held pumps are not as efficient as the electric pumps. Electric pumps can be purchased or rented from home health agencies or breastfeeding support groups.

After the mother has selected a pump, she should

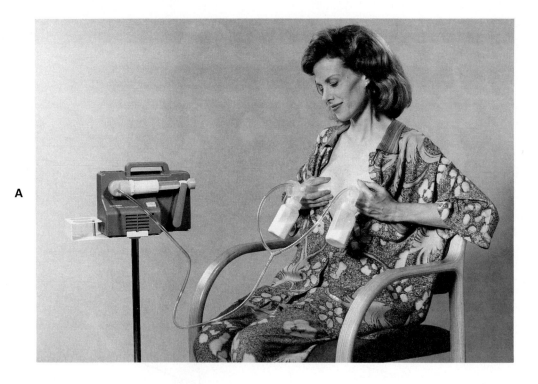

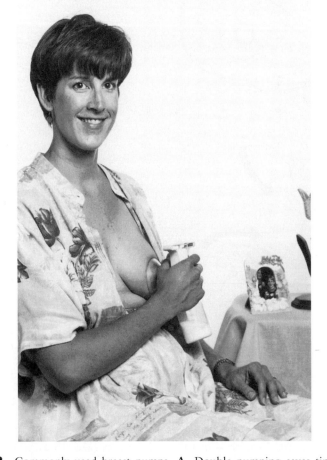

FIG. 15-12 Commonly used breast pumps. **A,** Double pumping saves time and energy when a mother must provide milk for a baby from whom she is separated. **B,** Ameda-Egnell One-hand pump; each pumping action requires only one motion of energy per pump. (**A,** Courtesy Medela Breast Pump Company, McHenry, IL. **B,** From Ameda-Egnell, courtesy Brett Thomas Photography, Woodstock, IL.)

moisten the inside of the breast cup with warm water. This forms a better seal. The mother should be instructed to lean over slightly and place the nipple and areola in the cup. The cup is gently pressed toward the chest, and the pump is turned on. When the flow of milk decreases, the pump should be moved to the other breast. When the milk flow decreases in the second breast, the woman returns to the first breast.

The expressed milk may be fed to the baby in a bottle, or the milk can be stored and frozen. If breast milk is to be transported, it should be kept cold. Breast milk can be safely stored in a refrigerator 24 to 48 hours. If it is not to be used within 48 hours, it should be frozen immediately after being expressed. Breast milk may be frozen for 6 months. To thaw, the container should be placed in lukewarm tap water. Thawed breast milk should be used right away. It should not be refrozen, and a microwave oven should not be used to thaw or heat breast milk (Worthington-Roberts, 1993). Microwaving causes hot spots, which can cause thermal burns in the infant's mouth and throat.

Breastfeeding by Diabetic Women

Breastfeeding by diabetic women is encouraged not only for its psychologic benefits and its advantages for the infant but also for its antidiabetogenic effect. Breastfeeding decreases the insulin requirements for insulin-dependent women. The insulin dosage must be readjusted at the time of weaning.

Contaminants in Maternal Milk

Nonnutrients enter human milk from the bloodstream of the lactating mother. Such compounds include environmental pollutants, nicotine, methadone, marijuana, caffeine, and alcohol. The distribution of a compound across the membrane between plasma and milk is influenced by (1) its solubility in fat, (2) its degree of ionization, (3) its degree of protein binding, and (4) active vs. passive transport.

Substance abuse creates significant difficulties for the nursing infant. Regular use of *alcohol* is common in our society. However, during both pregnancy and lactation, even moderate drinking can cause problems (Little et al, 1989). *Smoking* by the lactating woman can cause a decrease in her milk supply. Another reason not to smoke tobacco is the secondhand smoke in the baby's atmosphere. This smoke can aggravate or even trigger asthma symptoms, and babies of parents who smoke have a higher incidence of lung disease. *Caffeine* should be taken in moderation by the breastfeeding mother. Although only 1% of the mother's ingested caffeine passes to the milk, the baby's immature system cannot excrete the caffeine as effectively as an adult can. Some babies are sensitive to even a small amount of caffeine. Caffeine is found in coffee, tea, chocolate, and some soft drinks. It is best to limit these drinks to no more than a total of

24 oz per day. If laxatives are taken, they may cause loose stools in the infant.

Since the human immunodeficiency virus (HIV) passes into breast milk, mothers who are HIV positive should not breastfeed. Exceptions are made in countries where lack of sanitation places a bottle-fed infant at greater risk (Goldfarb, 1993).

Drugs in Breast Milk

Mothers should be cautioned about taking any but essential medications, since virtually all drugs ingested by a mother pass into her breast milk (Kacew, 1993). The majority of drugs do not cause significant problems in infants and in most instances breastfeeding can continue. When medications are necessary, mothers should consult with their health care providers about the effects of prescribed medications to determine the safety of continuing breastfeeding (see Appendix G).

Effect of Menstruation

If menstruation occurs, the mother can continue to breastfeed. Although some babies may act fussy on the first day, the quality and quantity of the milk are not affected (Lawrence, 1994).

Maternal Commitments

On occasions when the mother needs to be away from the infant at feeding time, a bottle of breast milk can be substituted. If the mother returns to the workplace, she can continue to breastfeed (Morse, Bottorff, 1989). Some mothers pump while at work; others simply breastfeed when at home. The length of time a woman breastfeeds her infant will depend on her own feelings and situation. Milk will continue to be produced as long as it taken from the breast.

Concerns

The inexperienced breastfeeding mother is likely to encounter major or minor problems in the course of adjusting to breastfeeding. Success or failure at breastfeeding may depend largely on the availability of help in the early weeks and the support of her partner and a clinician or friend who provides useful tips.

Dealing with Early Feeding Difficulties

In the beginning the infant may make frantic rooting, mouthing motions but will not grasp the nipple and eventually begins to cry and stiffen his or her body. The mother should stop trying to feed for a few minutes. After she comforts the infant and takes time to relax herself, she may begin again.

If the infant does not open his or her mouth wide enough to grasp the nipple, the mother can stroke the baby's lower lip and put her finger in the baby's mouth to tickle the tongue. Several minutes of playing with the baby's mouth and tongue will usually get a baby to open wider. She should not try to depress the infant's lower jaw with one finger as she guides the nipple into the mouth because the baby will root toward her finger. Sometimes the infant may latch on properly but will not suck. If this occurs, the mother can stimulating sucking motions by pressing upward under the baby's chin. Expression of colostrum results, and the infant is stimulated by the taste and begins sucking.

Usually an infant will suck vigorously at first and then may begin taking short, rapid sucks with frequent rest periods. This behavior indicates a slowing of the flow of milk. If the mother massages the breast toward the nipple, the flow of milk will resume. As soon as sucking resumes, the massage should be discontinued so that the infant will not be overwhelmed and choked by the milk flowing too rapidly.

The infant may suck for a few minutes and then fall asleep. Stimulation to awaken the baby may include unwrapping the baby, holding the baby upright, talking to the baby, or gently rubbing the back and the soles of the feet. A sleepy infant will not nurse satisfactorily. If it is impossible to awaken the baby, it is better to postpone the feeding for 20 to 30 minutes and then try again to awaken the baby.

Individual counseling by a skilled clinician or lactation consultant can greatly simplify the process of learning to cope with breastfeeding problems. Table 15-1 presents mother-related problems in breastfeeding.

Breastfeeding and Birth Control

Breastfeeding is not considered an effective method of birth control, although it has been found to delay the return of ovulation after childbirth. To be effective, the infant must breastfeed every 2 to 3 hours around the clock to keep prolactin levels high enough to prevent ovulation. Predicting the return of ovulation is difficult because it may occur before menses resumes. Basal body temperature, presence of cervical mucus, and the cervical position may be used to predict the onset of ovulation. Depoprovera and Norplant contraceptive use should not be started before 6 weeks postpartum. If these agents or oral contraceptives are taken sooner than 6 weeks after birth, the amount of milk a woman produces may be diminished. Other forms of contraception are preferable while breastfeeding.

Support Systems/Referrals

New parents may need some advice or encouragement when they begin breastfeeding (such as being shown how to position the baby correctly to help prevent sore nipples). Childbirth educators, lactation consultants, perinatal nurses, and local support groups for breastfeeding mothers can provide valuable information and suggestions for breastfeeding. The mother's commitment to breastfeeding and the support from partner, family, and friends greatly increase the chances of success. The fa-

ther will find he has a very definite role in helping his child wake for feedings and calm down when fussy, answering cries for help, diapering, bathing, and walking and playing with the baby.

Formula-Feeding

Formula-feeding is a successful alternative to breastfeeding in certain instances, including the following:
1. The family decides against breastfeeding or the mother is unable to breastfeed because of disease or anomalies.
2. The mother's schedule does not permit her to breastfeed.
3. Special formula is required because of infant allergies or special dietary needs.
4. It provides supplementation for infants of mothers who occasionally choose to omit breastfeeding.
5. It complements human milk if the mother's milk production is inadequate (Tsang, Nichols, 1988.)
6. The infant is adopted.

Formula-feeding should be the choice if the mother has an active infection such as tuberculosis, syphilitic breast lesions, or acquired immunodeficiency syndrome (AIDS). Other medical reasons need to be evaluated.

Formulas are recommended on the basis of the infant's nutrition needs, the parent's preferences, cost, need for refrigeration, convenience, and the parents' ability to prepare the formula accurately and safely.

Feeding Process and Care of the Mother and Infant

Inexperienced mothers who are formula-feeding their infants need teaching, counseling, and support. They need assistance with the feeding process and with problems they experience. Some parents who elect formula-feeding express concern that the baby will suffer as a result of their decision. They need assurance that knowledge of their infant's nutrition needs and skill in use of formula-feeding can be an acceptable alternative to breastfeeding. Emphasis on the beneficial use of the feeding time for close contact with their infant can help relieve their tensions (see guidelines for teaching of self-care to parents in the Home Care box on p. 427).

Feeding Skills

Formula-feeding parents need teaching regarding feeding skills. During feedings, they should be encouraged to assume an *en face* position with the infant (looking into each other's eyes) and to hold the infant closely and securely. Feedings provide a good time to talk, sing, or read to the infant or simply enjoy a time of peaceful relaxation with the baby.

A *bottle should never be propped* with a pillow or other inanimate object and left with the infant. This practice may result in choking, and it deprives the infant of important interaction during feeding. Moreover, propping the bottle has been implicated in causing **nursing bottle caries,** or decay of the first teeth resulting from continuous bathing of the teeth with carbohydrate-containing fluid as the infant sucks sporadically on the nipple.

The bottle should be held so that fluid fills the nipple and none of the air in the bottle is allowed to enter the nipple (Fig. 15-13). After the newborn period the infant who falls asleep, turns aside the head, or ceases to suck usually is signaling that enough formula has been taken. Parents should be taught to look for these cues and avoid overfeeding, which could contribute to obesity.

Care of Breasts

The breasts should be washed daily with clear water or mild soap. A well-fitting brassiere provides needed support. During the early postpartum period a tight binder, ice pack, and mild analgesic may be necessary to relieve discomfort caused by pressure if the milk comes in. Nipple and breast stimulation should be avoided. When showering, women should stand so that the shower sprays their back and not their breasts. Medication to suppress lactation may be prescribed. *Note:* as of August 1994, bromocriptine (Parlodel) was voluntarily withdrawn by the manufacturer as an indication for lactation suppression due to reports of serious adverse effects.

HOME CARE

FORMULA-FEEDING

Baby needs to be wide awake.

The hospital bottles of formula can be stored at room temperature. You may use this brand or the one your pediatrician recommends. They contain 4 oz of formula (120 ml) Your baby will probably drink 2 to 3 oz (60 to 90 ml) at a feeding for a few days and then increase. If you do not use all the formula, throw the remainder away because it spoils once opened.

You can keep track of how many ounces the baby drinks in 1 day by writing it down. When you take the baby for a checkup, your physician or nurse will ask you the amount of intake.

Your baby will probably be hungry every 3 to 5 hours. If your baby fusses or cries in between feedings, check the diaper or the infant's need to be picked up and cuddled. As the baby gets older, thirst may occur. Check with the pediatrician concerning water supplementation.

Test the temperature of the formula by letting a few drops fall on the inside of your wrist. If the formula feels comfortably warm to you, it is the correct temperature. If the formula is refrigerated, warm it by placing the bottle in a pan of hot water. Check it often for correct temperature.

Test the size of the nipple hole by holding the bottle and nipple upside down. The formula should drip from the nipple. If it runs in a stream, the hole is too big. If it has to be shaken for the formula to come out, the hole is too small. To correct this, you can try a softer nipple or enlarge the hole in the nipple or both. To enlarge the hole, heat a needle stuck into a cork (used as a handle) and insert the hot needle into the nipple. New nipples may be softened by boiling for 5 minutes before using. If the nipple collapses, unscrew the bottle lid to let air in.

Most newborns need burping. They tend to swallow air when sucking. Burp the baby who has been crying before feeding, then after every ounce of formula. As the

infant gets older and you get more experienced, you will know when to burp the baby.

To feed the baby, place the nipple in the infant's mouth over the tongue. It should rest against the roof of the mouth. This stimulates the sucking reflex.

Hold the bottle like a pencil. Keep nipple filled with milk so that the infant does not suck in air.

Start out with the baby held away from you until the nipple is in the mouth. The baby who is too close will turn toward you and not the nipple; this is the rooting reflex.

After the baby starts feeding, you can hold the infant close.

Some newborns take longer to feed than others. Slow patient feeding, keeping the baby awake and encouraging the infant to take more may be necessary.

The stools of a formula-fed newborn are soft but formed. They will be yellow with a characteristic odor. The baby probably will defecate either during the feeding or after. Change the diaper immediately because the composition of the stool is irritating to the skin.

SAFETY TIPS

Do not prop the bottle. The nipple may fall against the throat and block the air, or the baby could drown in the formula or aspirate any that was regurgitated.

Infants should never be left alone while feeding until they are old enough to remove the bottle from their mouth.

Bottles taken to bed can lead to early dental problems in young children (nursing bottle caries, or baby bottle syndrome).

Practice how to hold the newborn, and learn to use the bulb syringe in case the baby should choke.

After the baby is finished eating, place the infant in the crib on the right side so air can come up easily.

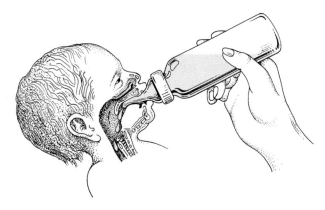

FIG. 15-13 Bottle-feeding. Bottle is held in hand like a pencil. Note milk covers nipple area so infant will not suck in air.

Diet and Fluids

A formula-feeding mother needs a well-balanced diet to restore maternal energy, provide protein for healing, and provide minerals and vitamins. An adequate fluid intake is important to maintain renal function and bowel regularity.

Infant Responses

Because cow milk formula forms a larger curd, stomach emptying time is slower than with breast milk. Formula-fed babies eat every 3 to 5 hours. The primary health care provider gives instructions as to the amounts of formula to be fed the infant over 24 hours and when to increase the amounts to ensure that the growing infant's nutrition needs are met. Formula may be fed at room temperature or warmed until the milk feels warm when tested on the caregiver's inner arm. The infant may need extra fluids in warm weather.

Infants swallow air when fed from a bottle and should be burped after every ½ to 1 oz of formula. Unused formula should be discarded after a feeding. Bottles, nipples, water, and formula need not be sterilized unless the water is not safe.

The stools of formula-fed babies are firmer than those of breast-fed babies and have a characteristic odor. Infants may have one or two stools per day. The diaper should be changed and the skin cleaned thoroughly to prevent irritation.

Infant Feeding Formulas

Commercial Formulas. Commercial formulas are available in three forms: ready-to-feed, concentrate, and powder. All forms are equivalent in nutritional content, but there may be a considerable difference in price. Parents should be helped to weigh the considerations of convenience and cost carefully and to choose the form that best suits their needs. Powdered formulas are especially well suited to the needs of families who travel or who are away from home frequently at feeding time, because they are lightweight, not bulky, and require no re-

frigeration. Ready-to-feed and condensed formulas usually come in multiserving cans that must be refrigerated after opening. Some ready-to-feed formula is sold in disposable bottles, but ordinarily this is the most costly type of formula. Families should be counseled to comparison shop since prices may vary among brands and among stores.

Cow milk is used as the basis of most formulas, although soy-based formulas and other specialized formulas are available for the infant who does not tolerate milk-based formulas. A comparison of human milk with commercial formulas is given in Fig. 15-1. The following list summarizes the modifications used in preparing milk-based commercial formulas:

1. Butterfat is removed and vegetable oils are added to ensure adequate fat absorption and to provide essential fatty acids.
2. Protein is heated to produce a softer, more flocculent curd that is more easily digested by the infant.
3. Protein and mineral concentrations are decreased to more nearly resemble those in human milk. Carbohydrate is then added to provide sufficient calories.

Evaporated Milk Formulas. Some families may wish to make their own formula at home using evaporated milk to reduce the expense of formula feeding. However, it is impossible for these formulas to resemble human milk as closely as do commercial products (Fig. 15-1). Because human milk is uniquely designed to meet the needs of the human infant, it is commonly used as the standard for judging all infant feedings. Thus mothers who do not breastfeed should be encouraged to use commercial formulas whenever possible. For eligible families, the WIC program will provide iron-fortified infant formula.

Caution: Honey sometimes is used as a sweetener for home-prepared infant foods or formula, and occasionally it is recommended for use on pacifiers to promote sucking in hypotonic babies. Use of honey for any of these purposes, however, is contraindicated because some sources contain spores of *Clostridium botulinum* (Whaley, Wong, 1995). These spores are extremely resistant to heat and are not destroyed in the processing of honey. If ingested by an infant, spores may germinate and lethal toxin may be released into the lumen of the bowel. Infant botulism may ultimately develop, and in some cases it is fatal.

Formula Preparation. Recent recommendations for labeling commercial infant formulas require that the directions for preparation and use of the formula include pictures and symbols for nonreading individuals. In addition, manufacturers are translating the directions into a variety of languages, such as Spanish and Vietnamese, to prevent misunderstanding and errors in formula preparation. It is important to impress upon families that the proportions *must not be altered*—neither diluted to extend the amount of formula nor concentrated to provide more calories.

Although manufacturers of commercial formula include directions for preparing and administering their products, the nurse should review **formula preparation** with the mother. It is especially important that formula be diluted properly. The newborn's kidneys are immature, and overly concentrated formula may provide protein and minerals that exceed the kidneys' excretory ability. However, if formula is too dilute (a practice sometimes followed to conserve formula and save money), the infant may be unable to consume a sufficient volume to ensure growth.

Sterilization of formula rarely is recommended now where families have access to a safe public water supply. Instead, formula is prepared with scrupulous cleanliness. Where water comes from a private well or a public supply of questionable safety, parents should be advised to boil for 15 minutes all water that is to be fed to the infant or used for formula preparation.

If sanitary conditions within the home appear unsafe, it may be necessary to teach the mother to sterilize the formula. The two traditional methods for sterilization are terminal heating and the aseptic method. In the terminal heating method the prepared formula is placed in the bottles, which are topped with the nipples and caps, and they are boiled together in a water bath for 25 minutes. In the aseptic method the bottles, nipples, and any other necessary equipment such as a funnel are boiled separately, after which the formula is poured into the bottles. (The Teaching Approaches box below summarizes steps in formula preparation)

Unmodified Cow Milk. Unmodified cow milk is unsuited to meet the nutritional needs of the infant (Fig. 15-1). Specific concerns include its excessive amounts of calcium, phosphorus, and other minerals, imbalance of

calcium and phosphorus, excessive protein content, poorly absorbed fat, and low iron concentration. In addition, for reasons that are not completely understood its use is apt to cause gastrointestinal blood loss in the infant (Zeigler et al, 1990). This blood loss, as well as the low levels of iron in the milk, increases the likelihood of iron-deficiency anemia. Anemia in the infant may have serious and long-lasting consequences; some evidence suggests that anemic infants (corrected with iron therapy) have learning delays that may persist throughout the preschool years (Oski, 1990). Unmodified cow milk should not be used before the end of the first year of life.

Some infants have an allergic reaction to the formula and may be switched to a soy milk formula (Tsang, Nichols, 1988). The soy protein used in infant formulas appears to equal and, in some cases, exceed the amount of protein in cow milk formula. Some infants benefit from a change from one brand of formula to another.

Discharge Planning

If the mother elects early discharge, anticipatory guidance can be given before the mother leaves the hospital, at the well-baby checkups, or during a home visit. The following information is helpful to the parents.

Frequency of Feeding

During the daytime, the mother feeds the infant so that the baby is not sleeping more than 3-4 hours at a time. At night, the infant is allowed to sleep and is fed only upon awakening. Night feedings should be business-like so that the baby learns that nights are not play time.

Ideally for the newborn, feeding schedules are determined by the infant's hunger. Feeding infants when they signal readiness is called *demand feeding. Scheduled feedings* are arranged at predetermined intervals to meet family routines. The newborn will breastfeed every 1½ to 3 hours during the daytime and usually every 3 to 5 hours at night. Breast-fed infants need to feed at least every 3 hours during the daytime. "Good" babies who rarely cry, who sleep, and who awaken only to nurse every 4 to 6 hours usually do not have an adequate weight gain, and the mother may not maintain an adequate milk supply. Most babies will average 10 feedings during a 24 hours period. The following guide illustrates the average intake by formula-fed infants:

Age	Quantity/feeding	Number of feedings 24 hours
Birth to 3 wk	2 to 3 oz (60 to 90 ml)	6 to 10
3 wk to 2 mo	5 oz (150 ml)	5 to 8
2 to 3 mo	5 to 7 oz (150 to 210 ml)	5 to 6

Mothers will notice spurts in the infant's appetite between 10 days and 2 weeks; 6 weeks and 9 weeks; and 3 months and 6 months. These appetite spurts correspond to growth spurts. The infant wants to breastfeed more

TEACHING APPROACHES

FORMULA PREPARATION

- Clean all necessary equipment (bottle, nipple, can opener), and wash hands carefully before preparing formula.
- Read formula label and dilute formula exactly as recommended by the manufacturer.
- Use tap water for preparation of concentrated or powdered formula, unless directed otherwise by physician or nurse.
- Opened cans of ready-to-feed or concentrated formula should be discarded after 24 hours.

frequently and for longer periods. For the breastfeeding baby, increasing the feedings results in a greater production of milk. The satisfied infant then tapers off her or his demands. For the formula-fed baby, the amount of formula offered can be increased by 2 to 4 oz (60 to 120 ml).

Supplemental Feedings for Breastfed Babies

Supplemental feedings should *not* be offered to breastfed infants in the nursery because, if satiated, they will not suck vigorously at the breast. Lactation depends on emptying the breast at each feeding. If milk is allowed to accumulate in the ducts, breast engorgement and ischemia result, suppressing the activity of the acini (milk-secreting cells). Consequently milk production is reduced. In addition, the process of sucking from a bottle is different from breast-nipple compression. The relatively inflexible rubber nipple prevents the tongue from its usually rhythmic action. Infants learn to put the tongue against the nipple holes to slow down the more rapid flow of fluid. When infants use these same tongue movements during breastfeeding, they may push the human nipple out of the mouth and may not grasp the areola properly (Lawrence, 1994).

Usually by 3 to 4 weeks after birth, lactation is well established and a feeding schedule has been formed. Larger infants are able to retain increased amounts because of greater stomach capacity; as a result they generally sleep through the night sooner than do smaller infants. After the milk supply is established, an occasional bottle will not affect lactation and breastfeeding.

Mineral and Vitamin Supplementation

Shortly after birth vitamin K is administered intramuscularly to prevent hemorrhagic disease of the newborn. Normally vitamin K is synthesized by the intestinal flora. However, because the infant's intestine is sterile at birth and breast milk contains low levels of vitamin K, the supply is inadequate for at least the first 3 to 4 days.

The normal infant receiving breast milk from a well-nourished mother needs no specific vitamin and mineral supplements, with the exceptions of fluoride in a dosage of 0.25 mg daily and iron by 6 months of age (when fetal iron stores are depleted). Supplements of 5 to 7.5 mg of vitamin D daily are indicated if the infant does not have adequate ultraviolet light because of pigmented skin color or little exposure to light (Bronner and Paige, 1992).

Milk from strict vegetarian mothers (those who include no animal products in their diet) may be too low in vitamin B_{12} to meet the infant's needs. These infants (and mothers) require a supplement (Specker et al, 1988). Like human milk, commercial iron-fortified formula supplies all the nutrients needed by the infant for the first 6 months. The only supplementation required

HOME CARE

FLUORIDE SUPPLEMENTATION

- Administer fluoride drops daily as prescribed by your health care provider.
- Leave supplement in childproof container, and store it where children cannot reach it. (The drops have a pleasant taste. Long-term overdose causes mottling of teeth, and acute poisoning can cause symptoms ranging from vomiting and other gastrointestinal disturbances to death.)
- If infant begins to consume 240 ml or more of fluoridated water per day (either alone or in other feedings such as juices), consult your health care provider regarding discontinuing the supplement.

is 0.25 mg of fluoride if the local water supply is not fluoridated or if the infant is given ready-to-feed formula, which eliminates the use of fluoridated tap water (Bronner, Paige, 1992) (see Home Care box above).

Weaning

Weaning the baby from the breast can be a smooth process if it is done gradually. Gradual elimination of feedings over a period of several weeks creates less discomfort for both mother and infant and gradually decreases the amount of milk being produced.

One breastfeeding a day can be substituted with formula if the infant is younger than 1 year of age. Many mothers wean directly from the breast to a cup. The feeding eliminated is a matter of personal choice. Frequently the feeding before bedtime is the last feeding eliminated. The weaning process should continue until all breastfeeding is eliminated.

Sometimes situations require the mother to stop breastfeeding suddenly. If this happens, the mother may have engorgement. This discomfort can be diminished by wearing a snug brassiere and avoiding stimulation of the breast. Ice packs and a mild analgesic may help.

Introducing Solid Foods

The infant receives the right balance of nutrients from breast milk or formula during the first 4 to 6 months (Bronner, Paige, 1992). It is not true that the feeding of solids will help the baby sleep through the night. Introduction of solid foods before the infant is 4 to 6 months of age may result in overfeeding and decreased intake of breast milk or formula. The infant cannot communicate feeling full as can an older child, who is able to turn the head away. The proper balance of carbohydrate, protein, and fat for an infant to grow properly is in the breast milk or formula.

PLAN OF CARE

Maternal Self-Esteem, Breastfeeding, and Infant Nutrition

Case History
Mindy Jonus, a 32-year-old first-time mother, called for a nurse to help her with breastfeeding. Jason (7 lb 10 oz) is 1 day old and is making frantic rooting and mouthing motions but appears unable to latch on. When you enter the room, the baby is crying lustily and is very stiff. Mindy is trying to push Jason's cheek to turn his head to face the breast. Mindy is near tears and equally frustrated. She cries out, "I just do not know what to do! I can't remember everything the nurse did for me last night. I feel like such a failure."

EXPECTED OUTCOMES	IMPLEMENTATION	RATIONALE	EVALUATION
Nursing Diagnosis: Situational low self-esteem related to lack of experience with breastfeeding			
Mindy's anxiety will be relieved.	Suggest that she wrap Jason snugly, pick him up, "bubble," cuddle, and talk or sing to him to relax him.	A frantic, frustrated newborn is unable to initiate feeding; he may have a bubble causing abdominal discomfort.	Jason relaxes and stops frantic rooting, mouthing, and crying.
Mindy's self-esteem will be maintained as she understands that she and Jason both need to learn to breastfeed.	Comment on her success in relaxing Jason.	Focuses mother on her accomplishment of a parental skill.	Mindy states her pleasure from seeing Jason respond to her.
	Touch her neck and shoulders to teach her to relax specific tense muscle groups (as she had learned to do in parent education classes for childbirth).	Reinforces self-care method to reduce muscle tension.	Mindy's posture and facial expression indicate relaxed muscles in neck and shoulders.
Mindy's self-esteem will be enhanced as she learns and implements methods to console Jason.	Remark that this is the first time for both her and Jason to breastfeed, and each needs time to learn.	Reaffirms that breastfeeding is a learned behavior for both and learning takes time.	Mindy states she had never grasped the fact that breastfeeding needs to be learned by both of them.
Mindy will feel supported.	State that you will remain with her as *she* initiates the feeding.	Offers supportive presence while Mindy *learns by doing*.	Mindy states she "would feel better having someone nearby" as she starts the feeding.
Nursing Diagnosis: High risk for ineffective breastfeeding related to insufficient knowledge regarding newborn reflexes and breastfeeding techniques			
Mindy will verbalize understanding of newborn reflexes, such as rooting.	Describe and demonstrate rooting reflex.	Provides knowledge so newborn reflexes can be used effectively.	Mindy states she understands content taught and demonstrated.
Mindy will demonstrate breastfeeding techniques.	Ask Mindy to assume a comfortable position and let the breast fall forward without tension.	Provides support as Mindy learns by doing.	Mindy completes breastfeeding at this time. Mindy is able to breastfeed successfully at the next feeding. Mindy states pleasure with her accomplishment and with breastfeeding.
	Assist Mindy to position Jason so that his face, chest, and knees face her body.		

Continued.

PLAN OF CARE—CONT'D

Maternal Self-Esteem, Breastfeeding, and Infant Nutrition

EXPECTED OUTCOMES	IMPLEMENTATION	RATIONALE	EVALUATION
	Coach Mindy to bring Jason to the breast, compress her breast with thumb above and fingers below areola, touch his cheek and outer angle of his lip, and guide her nipple and areolar tissue into his mouth and over his tongue. Describe, demonstrate, and watch Mindy do the following: • Make a breathing space by lifting Jason's hips • Remove baby from breast • Bubble him • Try alternate positions • Care for breasts • Lay Jason on his right side after feeding		

Nursing Diagnosis: Potential for altered nutrition related to parent's lack of knowledge of infant's behaviors, elimination patterns, and growth (weight)

Mindy will verbalize understanding of infant's behaviors and elimination patterns. Jason will sleep after feedings. Jason will void pale, straw-colored urine 6-10 times/day	Discuss infant's: • Behavior indicating satiety (enough food), such as sleeping 3 hours • Stooling pattern • Voiding pattern • Immediate weight loss less than 10% of birth weight • Regaining birth weight within 10 days	Anticipatory guidance provides reassurance and serves as a basis for decision making. Knowledge helps to allay anxiety regarding the unknown and thereby assists in maintaining parent's self-confidence.	Mindy states she understands content. Jason loses less than 10% of his birth weight and has normal elmination patterns.
Jason will not lose more than 10% of his birth weight and will regain his birth weight within 10 days.	Discuss need to empty each breast at each feeding. While Mindy is changing Jason's diaper, encourage questions regarding Jason's elimination pattern. Encourage questions regarding Jason's behaviors, characteristics, and parameters of normal growth and development.	Emptying the breasts is the stimulus for lactation. Readiness for learning enhances retention of content. Reassures Mindy that all questions are legitimate and that answers are available for the asking.	At his next visit to the physician, nurse practitioner, or home health care nurse, Jason's growth is within normal parameters; he shows no signs of failure to thrive. Mindy indicates satisfaction with her mothering.

The infant's individual growth pattern should help determine the right time to start solids (Bronner, Paige, 1992). The primary health care provider will advise when to introduce solid foods. The schedule for introducing solid foods and the type of foods to serve will be discussed during well-baby supervision visits with the pediatrician or pediatric nurse practitioner.

Referrals

Referral procedures provide an opportunity for individuals and groups to take advantage of services available from other sources. A properly coordinated health service delivery for infants and children that includes a registered dietitian can contribute to a sense of continuity and to consistency of care and advice. The mother is encouraged to contact the local association that assists with breastfeeding (see Appendix H).

✤ EVALUATION

Parental knowledge and infant well-being and the findings that represent normal response form the basis for selecting appropriate nursing actions and evaluating their effectiveness. The nurse can be reasonably assured that care was effective to the degree that the following expected outcomes for care have been met:

- The infant received the level and type of nutrients to support body composition, activity, and growth.
- The infant experienced minimal physiologic stress associated with digestion, metabolism, and excretion of nutrients.
- The infant received sufficient fluids to maintain adequate body water balance.

The following expected outcomes apply to the mother/parents.

- They verbalized understanding of sound nutritional selection and feeding practices.
- They demonstrated skill and confidence in the feeding method of choice.
- They developed closeness and pleasure with the child during feeding.

KEY POINTS

- Healthy term babies are developmentally ready for feeding.
- Teaching and counseling about the feeding of infants are important aspects of the daily care plan for maternity patients.
- Parents are provided with information about breastfeeding and formula-feeding so that an informed choice about method of feeding can be made.
- The attitude of the parents toward breastfeeding is a powerful factor in achieving successful lactation.

- The size of the breast is not related to its functional capacity.
- Limiting breastfeeding time does not prevent nipple soreness.
- The composition and characteristics of commercial formulas are based on those of mature human milk.
- Use of honey in formula or on pacifiers can cause botulism and be fatal.
- Neither skim nor low-fat milk is suitable for infant feeding.

CRITICAL THINKING EXERCISES

1. A new mother calls you to assist her with breastfeeding. She is crying as she hands you the baby, saying, "I just can't do this."
    a. What additional information do you need?
    b. Based on assessment data, formulate nursing diagnoses. Plan and prioritize patient-centered goals for the diagnosis that takes priority. Choose interventions, giving rationale and expected outcomes. Justify your decisions and actions.

2. You overhear two mothers talking. One says she plans to start feeding her infant cereal as soon as possible so that the baby will sleep all night. The other mother states she wants to feed her baby only natural foods and that she plans to use honey as a natural sweetener. Role-play how you would approach this situation, what you plan to say, and how you will say it while showing respect for each woman. Justify your decisions and actions.

REFERENCES

Alexander MA, Blank JJ: Factors related to obesity in Mexican-American preschool children, *Image* 20(2):79, 1988.

Armstrong H: Breastfeeding and low birth weight babies: advances in Kenya, *J Hum Lact* 3:34, 1987.

Barber-Madden R: Design and implementation of a citywide breastfeeding promotion program: the New York City approach, *Fam Community Health* 12:71, 1990.

Blume S et al: Beer and breastfeeding mom, *JAMA* 258:2126, 1987.

Bronner YL, Paige DM: Current concepts in infant nutrition, *J Nurse-Midwifery* 37:43S, 1992.

Carr C: A four-week observation of maternity care in Finland, *JOGNN* 18:100, 1989.

Choi EC: Unique aspects of Korean-American mothers, *JOGNN* 15:394, 1986.

Currier RL: The hot-cold syndrome and symbolic balance in Mexican and Spanish-American folk medicine. In Martinez RA, editor: *Hispanic culture and health care: fact, fiction, folklore,* St Louis, 1978, Mosby.

de Steuben C: Breast-feeding and jaundice: a review, *J Nurse-Midwifery* 37:59S, 1992.

Garza C, Hopkinson J: Physiology of lactation. In Tsang RC, Nichols BL, editors: *Nutrition during infancy,* Philadelphia, 1988, Hanley & Belfus.

Goldfarb J: Breastfeeding: AIDS and other infectious diseases, *Clin Perinatol* 20:225, 1993.

Hart DV: From pregnancy through birth in a Bisayan Filipino village. In Hart DV, Rajadhon PA, Coughlin RJ, editors: *Southeast Asian birth customs: three studies in reproduction,* New Haven, CT, 1965, Human Relations Area Files.

Hoekelman RA et al, editors: *Primary pediatric care,* ed 2, St Louis, 1992, Mosby.

Kacew S: Adverse effects of drugs and chemicals in breast milk on the nursing infant, *J Clin Pharmacol* 33:213, 1993.

Lawrence RA: *Breastfeeding: a guide for the medical professional,* ed 4, St Louis, 1994, Mosby.

Lindenberg CS, Artola RC, Jimenez V: The effect of early postpartum mother-infant contact and breast-feeding promotion on the incidence and continuation of breast-feeding, *Int J Nurs Stud* 27:179, 1990.

Little RE et al: Maternal alcohol use during breastfeeding and infant mental and motor development at one year, *N Engl J Med* 321:425, 1989.

Morse JM, Bottorff JL: Intending to breastfeed and work, *JOGNN* 18:493, 1989.

Morse JM, Jehle C, Gamble D: Initiating breastfeeding: a world survey of the timing of postpartum breastfeeding, *Int J Nurs Stud* 27:303, 1990.

Oski FA: Whole cow milk feeding between 6 and 12 months of age? Go back to 1976, *Pediatr Rev* 12:187, 1990.

Park K-JY, Peterson LM: Beliefs, practices, and experiences of Korean women in relation to childbirth, *Health Care Women Internat* 12:261, 1991.

Riordan J, Auerbach KG: *Breastfeeding and human lactation,* Boston, 1993.

Shrago L, Bocar D: The infant's contribution to breastfeeding, *JOGNN* 19:209, 1990.

Specker BL et al: Increased urinary methylmalonic acid excretion in breast-fed infants of vegetarian mothers and identification of an acceptable dietary source of vitmain B_{12}, *Am J Clin Nutr* 47:89, 1988.

Storr GB: Prevention of nipple tenderness and breast engorgement in the post-partal period, *JOGNN* 17:203, 1988.

Tsang RC, Nichols BL, editors: *Nutrition during infancy,* Philadelphia, 1988, Hanley & Belfus.

Whaley LE, Wong DL: *Nursing care of infants and children,* ed 4, St Louis, 1995, Mosby.

Witherly SA: Soy formulas are not hypoallergenic, *Am J Clin Nutr* 51:705, 1990.

Woolridge M, Fisher O: Colic, "overfeeding," and symptoms of lactose malabsorption in the breastfed baby: a possible artifact of feed management? *Lancet* 1:382, 1988.

Worthington-Roberts B: Lactation and human milk: nutritional considerations. In Worthington-Roberts B, Williams SR, editors: *Nutrition in pregnancy and lactation,* ed 5, St Louis, 1993, Mosby.

Zeigler EE et al: Cow milk feeding in infancy: further observations on blood loss from the gastrointestinal tract, *J Pediatr* 116:11, 1990.

BIBLIOGRAPHY

Anderson E, Geden E: Nurses' knowledge of breastfeeding, *JOGNN* 20:58, 1991.

Gamble D, Morse JM: Fathers and breastfed infants: postponing and types of involvement, *JOGNN* 22:358, 1992.

Hill PD, Aldag J: Potential indicators of insufficient milk supply syndrome, *Res Nurs Health* 14:11, 1991.

Maecagno-Smith R, Young M: Breastfeeding the sleepy infant, *Can Nurse* 89:20, 1993.

Matthews MK: Mother's satisfaction with their neonates' breastfeeding behaviors, *JOGNN* 20:49, 1991.

Medoff-Cooper B: Changes in nutritive sucking patterns with increasing gestational age, *Nurs Res* 40:245, 1991.

Raisler J: Promoting breastfeeding among vulnerable women, *J Nurs-Midwifery* 38(1):1, 1993.

Serdula MK et al: Correlates of breast-feeding in a low-income population of whites, blacks, and Southeast Asians, *J Am Diet Assoc* 91:41, 1991.

Ziemer M, Pigeon J: Skin changes and pain in the nipple during the first week of gestation, *JOGNN* 22(3):247, 1993.

Five

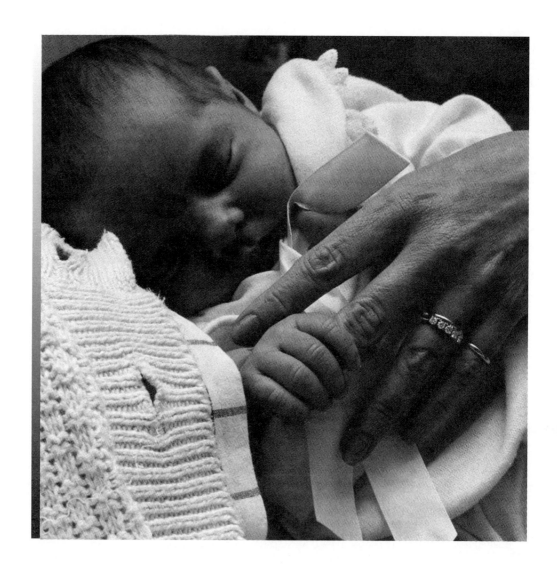

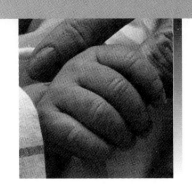

Postpartum Period

16 **Maternal Physiology during the Postpartum Period**

17 **Family Dynamics after Childbirth**

18 **Nursing Care during the Postpartum Period**

19 **Home Care**

CHAPTER 16

Maternal Physiology during the Postpartum Period

KITTY CASHION

LEARNING OBJECTIVES

Define the key terms listed.

Describe the anatomic and physiologic changes that occur during the postpartum period.

Identify characteristics and measurement of uterine involution and lochial flow.

Recognize expected values for vital signs and blood pressure, deviations from normal findings, and probable causes of the deviations.

KEY TERMS

autolysis
colostrum
diaphoresis
diastasis recti abdominis
diuresis
engorgement (breast)
fourth trimester of pregnancy
hemorrhoids
involution
lochia alba
lochia rubra
lochia serosa
pelvic relaxation
puerperium
subinvolution
thromboembolism

RELATED TOPICS

Autoimmune disorders *(Chap. 22)* • Breastfeeding *(Chap. 15)* • Dependent edema *(Chap. 7)* • Diastasis recti abdominis *(Chap. 5)* • Hemorrhagic shock *(Chap. 21)* • Physiologic anemia of pregnancy *(Chap. 5)* • Pregnancy-induced hypertension *(Chap. 21)* • Uterine atony *(Chap. 18)* • Postpartum infection *(Chap. 21)* • Pelvic relaxation (uterine prolapse, rectoceles, cystoceles) *(Chap. 30)* • Menstrual cycle *(Chap. 3)*

The postpartum period is the 6-week interval between the birth of the newborn and the return of the reproductive organs to their normal nonpregnant state. This period is sometimes referred to as the **puerperium,** or **fourth trimester of pregnancy.** The physiologic changes that occur are distinctive, although considered normal, as the processes of pregnancy are reversed. Many factors, including energy level, degree of comfort, health of the newborn, and care and encouragement given by the health professionals, contribute to the mother's response to her infant during this time. To provide care beneficial to the mother, her infant, and her family, the nurse must synthesize knowledge from maternal anatomy and physiology of the recovery period, the newborn's physical and behavioral characteristics, infant care activities, and family response to the birth of the child. This chapter focuses on anatomic and physiologic changes of the woman after childbirth.

439

REPRODUCTIVE SYSTEM AND ASSOCIATED STRUCTURES

Uterus

Involution Process

The return of the uterus to a nonpregnant state following birth is called **involution.** This process begins immediately after expulsion of the placenta with contraction of the uterine smooth muscle.

At the end of the third stage of labor the uterus is in the midline, about 2 cm *below* the level of the umbilicus with the fundus resting on the sacral promontory. At this time uterine size approximates the size at 16 weeks of gestation (about the size of a grapefruit), and weighs about 1000 g (2 lb).

Within 12 hours the fundus may be approximately 1 cm *above* the umbilicus (Fig. 16-1). Involution progresses rapidly during the next few days. The fundus descends about 1 to 2 cm every 24 hours. By the sixth postpartum day the fundus normally will be half the distance from the symphysis pubis to the umbilicus. The uterus should not be palpable abdominally after the ninth postpartum day.

The uterus, which at full term weighs about 11 times its prepregnant weight, involutes to about 500 g (1 lb) 1 week after birth and 350 g (11 to 12 oz) 2 weeks after birth. A week after birth the uterus lies in the true pelvis once again. At 6 weeks it weighs 50 to 60 g.

Increased estrogen and progesterone levels are responsible for the massive growth of the uterus during

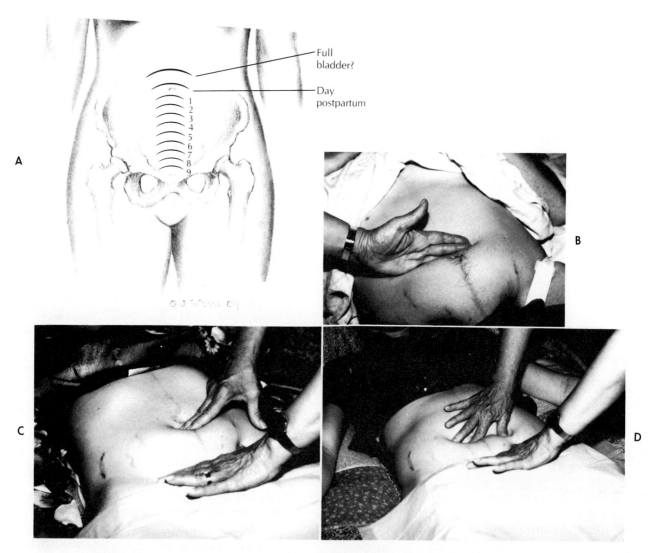

FIG. 16-1 Assessment of involution of uterus after childbirth. **A,** Normal progress, days 1 through 9. **B,** Size and position of uterus 2 hours after childbirth. **C,** Two days after childbirth. **D,** Four days after childbirth. (**B, C,** and **D** courtesy Marjorie Pyle, RNC, *Lifecircle,* Costa Mesa, CA.)

pregnancy. Prenatal uterine growth is due both to *hyperplasia,* an increase in the number of muscle cells, and to *hypertrophy,* enlargement of the existing cells. Postpartally the decrease in these hormones causes *autolysis,* a self-destruction of excess hypertrophied tissue. The additional cells laid down during pregnancy remain, however, and account for the fact that uterine size increases slightly after each pregnancy.

Subinvolution is the failure of the uterus to return to a nonpregnant state. The most common causes of subinvolution are retained placental fragments and infection.

Contractions

The intensity of uterine contractions increases significantly immediately after birth, presumably in response to the greatly diminished intrauterine volume. Postpartum hemostasis is achieved primarily by compression of intramyometrial blood vessels, rather than platelet aggregation and clot formation. The hormone oxytocin, released from the pituitary gland, strengthens and coordinates uterine contractions, compressing blood vessels and aiding in hemostasis. During the first 1 to 2 postpartum hours uterine contractions may decrease in intensity and become uncoordinated. Because it is vital that the uterus remain firm and well contracted, exogenous oxytocin (Pitocin) is usually administered intravenously or intramuscularly immediately after expulsion of the placenta. Mothers who plan to breastfeed may be encouraged to put the baby to breast immediately after birth as well, since suckling stimulates oxytocin release.

Afterpains

In primiparas the tone of the uterus is increased so that the fundus generally remains firm. Periodic relaxation and contraction are more common for multiparas and may cause uncomfortable afterpains that persist throughout the early puerperium. Afterpains are more noticeable after births where the uterus was overdistended (e.g., large baby, twins). Breastfeeding and exogenous oxytocic medication usually intensify these afterpains, since both stimulate uterine contractions.

Placental Site

Immediately after the placenta and membranes are expelled, vascular constriction and thromboses reduce the placental site to an irregular nodular and elevated area. Upward growth of the endometrium causes sloughing of necrotic tissue and prevents the scar formation that is characteristic of normal wound healing. This unique healing process enables the endometrium to resume its usual cycle of changes and to permit implantation and placentation in future pregnancies. Endometrial regeneration is completed by the end of the third postpartum week except at the placental site. Regeneration at the placental site usually is not complete until 6 weeks after birth.

Lochia

Postchildbirth uterine discharge, commonly called lochia, is initially bright red, changing later to a dark red or reddish brown. It may contain small clots. For the first 2 hours after birth the amount of uterine discharge should be about that of a heavy menstrual period. After that time, the lochia flow should steadily decrease.

Lochia rubra consists mainly of blood and decidual and trophoblastic debris. The flow pales, becoming pink or brown after 3 to 4 days (lochia serosa). **Lochia serosa** consists of old blood, serum, leukocytes, and tissue debris. About 10 days after childbirth the drainage becomes yellow to white (lochia alba). **Lochia alba** consists of leukocytes, decidua, epithelial cells, mucus, serum, and bacteria. Lochia alba may continue 2 to 6 weeks after childbirth.

Judging the amount of lochial flow based on observation of perineal pads is difficult. Jacobson (1985) suggested one method for subjectively estimating postpartal blood loss based on the amount of staining on a perineal pad (see Fig. 12-29). Weighing perineal pads before and after use provides a more objective measurement of lochial flow. Each gram of weight increase is roughly equivalent to 1 ml of blood loss. Any estimation of lochial flow is inaccurate and incomplete without consideration of the time factor involved. The woman who saturates a peripad in 1 hour or less is bleeding much more than the woman who saturates one peripad over the course of an 8-hour shift.

If the woman receives an oxytocic medication, regardless of the route of administration, the flow of lochia is usually scant until the effects of the medication wear off. Also, the amount of lochia is usually less after cesarean

TABLE 16-1   Lochial and Nonlochial Bleeding

LOCHIA	NONLOCHIAL BLEEDING
Lochia usually trickles from the vaginal opening. The steady flow is greater as the uterus contracts.	If the bloody discharge spurts from the vagina, there may be cervical or vaginal tears in addition to the normal lochia.
A gush of lochia may result as the uterus is massaged. If it is dark in color, it has been pooled in the relaxed vagina, and the amount soon lessens to a trickle of bright red lochia (in the early puerperium).	If the amount of bleeding continues to be excessive and bright red, a tear may be the source.

births. Flow of lochia usually increases with ambulation and breastfeeding. After lying in bed for a prolonged period, the woman may experience a gush of blood upon standing, which is not to be confused with hemorrhage.

Persistence of lochia rubra early in the postpartum period suggests continued bleeding as a result of retained fragments of the placenta or membranes. Recurrence of bleeding about 10 days after birth indicates bleeding from the placental site, which is healing. However, after 3 to 4 weeks, bleeding may be caused by infection or subinvolution. Continued lochia serosa or lochia alba may indicate endometritis, particularly if fever, pain, or abdominal tenderness is associated with the discharge. Lochia should smell like normal menstrual flow; an offensive odor usually indicates infection.

It is important to remember that all postpartal vaginal bleeding is not necessarily lochia. Another common source of vaginal bleeding after birth is unrepaired vaginal or cervical lacerations. Table 16-1 distinguishes between lochial and nonlochial bleeding.

Cervix

Immediately after birth the cervix is soft. By 18 hours postpartum, however, it has shortened, developed a firm consistency, and regained its form. The cervix up to the lower uterine segment remains edematous, thin, and fragile for several days after birth. The ectocervix (portion of the cervix that protrudes into the vagina) appears bruised and has some small lacerations—optimal conditions for the development of infection. The cervical os, dilated to 10 cm during labor, closes gradually. Two fingers may still be introduced into the cervical os for the first 4 to 6 days postpartum; however, only the smallest curette may be introduced by the end of 2 weeks. The external cervical os never regains its prepregnant appearance; it is no longer shaped like a circle but appears as a jagged slit, often described as a fish mouth (see Fig. 3-9). Lactation delays production of cervical and other estrogen-influenced mucus and mucosal characteristics.

Vagina and Perineum

Postpartum estrogen deprivation is responsible for the thinness of the vaginal mucosa and the absence of rugae. The greatly distended, smooth-walled vagina gradually returns to its nonpregnant size by 6 to 8 weeks after childbirth. Rugae reappear by about the fourth week, although they are never as prominent as they are in the nulliparous woman. Most rugae may be permanently flattened. The mucosa remains atrophic in the lactating woman at least until menstruation begins again. Thickening of the vaginal mucosa occurs with the return of ovarian function. Estrogen deficiency is responsible for a decreased amount of vaginal lubrication and thinner vaginal mucosa. Localized dryness and coital discomfort (dyspareunia) may persist until ovarian function returns and menstruation resumes. Use of a water-soluble lubri-

cant during intercourse is usually recommended, since it is helpful in reducing discomfort.

Initially the *introitus* is erythematous and edematous, especially in the area of the episiotomy or laceration repair. Careful repair, prevention, or early treatment of hematomas and good hygiene during the first 2 weeks after birth usually result in an introitus barely distinguishable from that of a nulliparous woman.

Most *episiotomies* are visible only if the woman is lying on her side with her buttock raised or placed in lithotomy position. A good light source is essential for visualization of some episiotomies. The healing process of an episiotomy is the same as for any surgical incision. Signs of infection (pain, redness, warmth, swelling, or discharge) or loss of approximation (separation) of the incision edges may occur. Healing should occur within 2 to 3 weeks.

Hemorrhoids (anal varicosities) are commonly seen (see Fig. 7-11, *B*). Women often experience associated symptoms such as itching, discomfort, and bright red bleeding with defecation. These hemorrhoids usually decrease in size within weeks of childbirth.

Pelvic Muscular Support

The supporting structure of the uterus and vagina may be injured during childbirth and may contribute to gynecologic problems later. Supportive tissues of the pelvic floor, torn or stretched during childbirth, may require up to 6 months to regain tone. The term **pelvic relaxation** refers to the lengthening and weakening of the fascial supports of pelvic structures. These structures include the uterus, upper posterior vaginal wall, urethra, bladder, and rectum. Although relaxation can occur in any woman, it is usually a direct but delayed complication of childbirth (see Clinical Application of Research).

ENDOCRINE SYSTEM
Placental Hormones

Great hormonal changes occur during the postpartal period. Expulsion of the placenta results in dramatic decreases of the hormones produced by that organ. Decreases in human placental lactogen (hPL), estrogens, and cortisol, and in the placental enzyme insulinase reverse the diabetogenic effects of pregnancy, resulting in significantly lower blood sugar levels in the immediate puerperium. Diabetic mothers will likely require much less insulin for several days. Because these normal hormonal changes make the puerperium a transitional period for carbohydrate metabolism, interpretation of glucose tolerance tests is more difficult at this time.

Estrogen and progesterone levels drop markedly following expulsion of the placenta, reaching their lowest levels 1 week postpartum. Decreased estrogen levels are associated with breast engorgement and with the diure-

INCONTINENCE FOLLOWING RUPTURE OF THE ANAL SPHINCTER DURING BIRTH

Midline episiotomy is liberally used in the United States. Third-degree and fourth-degree lacerations occur in 17% to 25% of midline episiotomies. This study was undertaken to determine whether differences exist in the symptoms reported by women with these lacerations and those reported by women without injury to the sphincter. Data were collected by chart review and by telephone interview. Participants were 70 primiparous women, half of whom had anal sphincter rupture while giving birth and half who did not. The interviews occurred 9 to 12 months after they gave birth. The women were asked about perineal pain, painful intercourse, and incontinence of gas and liquid or formed stool. More women with rupture (17%) reported incontinence of gas than those women without rupture (3%). The groups were similar in incidence of incontinence of stool, painful intercourse, and perineal pain. In prenatal classes, childbirth educators can describe episiotomy and possible sequelae. Pregnant couples can be encouraged to discuss the relative merits of mediolateral vs. midline episiotomies, especially when the fetus is large and shoulder dystocia may occur, or when forceps are needed. Although not addressed in this study, perineal exercises (e.g., Kegel exercises) should be encouraged.

Crawford LA et al: Incontinence following rupture of the anal sphincter during delivery, *Obstet Gynecol* 82:527, 1993.

sis of excess extracellular fluid accumulated during pregnancy. In nonlactating women estrogen levels begin to rise by 2 weeks after birth and are higher than in women who breastfeed by postpartum day 17 (Bowes, 1991).

Pituitary Hormones and Ovarian Function

Lactating and nonlactating women differ considerably in the time of appearance of the first ovulation and the reestablishment of menstruation. The persistence of elevated serum prolactin levels in breastfeeding women appears to be responsible for suppressing ovulation. Because levels of follicle-stimulating hormone (FSH) have been shown to be identical in lactating and nonlactating women, it is thought that the ovary does not respond to FSH stimulation when increased prolactin levels are present (Bowes, 1991).

Prolactin levels in blood rise progressively throughout pregnancy. In women who breastfeed, prolactin levels remain elevated into the sixth week after birth (Bowes, 1991). Serum prolactin levels are influenced by the frequency of breastfeeding, the duration of each feeding, and the degree to which supplementary feedings are used. The individual differences in the strength of the infant's sucking stimulus probably also affect prolactin levels. This emphasizes the fact that breastfeeding is not a reliable form of birth control. After birth, in nonlactating women, prolactin levels decline, reaching the prepregnant range within 2 weeks.

Ovulation occurs as early as 27 days after birth in nonlactating women, with a mean time of about 70 to 75 days. In women who breastfeed, the mean time to ovulation is about 190 days (Bowes, 1991). Among lactating women 15% have resumed menstruation by 6 weeks and 45% by 12 weeks. Among nonlactating women 40% menstruate by 6 weeks, 65% by 12 weeks, and 90% by 24 weeks. For lactating women 80% of first menstrual cycles are anovulatory; for nonlactating women 50% of first cycles are anovulatory (Scott et al, 1990).

The first menstrual flow after childbirth is usually heavier than normal. Within three to four cycles the amount of menstrual flow has returned to the woman's prepregnant volume.

ABDOMEN

When the woman stands up during the first days after birth, the abdomen protrudes and gives the woman a still-pregnant appearance. During the first 2 weeks after birth the abdominal wall is relaxed. About 6 weeks are required before the abdominal wall returns to its nonpregnant state. The skin regains most of its previous elasticity, but some striae persist. The return of muscle tone depends on previous tone, proper exercise, and the amount of adipose tissue. On occasion, with or without overdistention because of a large fetus or multiple fetuses, the abdominal wall muscles separate, a condition termed **diastasis recti abdominis** (see Fig. 5-11). Persistence of this defect may be disturbing to the woman, but surgical correction is rarely necessary. With time, the defect becomes less apparent.

URINARY SYSTEM

The hormonal changes of pregnancy (high steroid levels) contribute to the increase in renal function, whereas the diminishing steroid levels after birth may partly explain the reduced renal function during the puerperium. Kidney function returns to normal within a month after birth. About 2 to 8 weeks are required for the pregnancy-induced hypotonia and dilatation of the ureters and renal pelves to return to the prepregnant state (Cunningham et al, 1993). In a small percentage of women dilatation of the urinary tract may persist for 3 months.

Urine Components

The renal glycosuria induced by pregnancy disappears. Lactosuria may be expected in lactating women. The blood urea nitrogen (BUN) increases during the puerperium as **autolysis** of the involuting uterus is accomplished. This breakdown of excess protein in the uterine muscle cells also results in a mild (+1) proteinuria for 1 to 2 days after childbirth in about 50% of women. Acetonuria may occur in women with an uncomplicated birth or after a prolonged labor with dehydration.

Postpartal Diuresis

Within 12 hours of birth women begin to lose excess tissue fluid accumulated during pregnancy. One mechanism that reduces these retained fluids of pregnancy is the profuse **diaphoresis** that often occurs, especially at night, for the first 2 or 3 days after childbirth. Postpartal **diuresis,** caused by decreased estrogen levels, removal of increased venous pressure in the lower extremities, and loss of the remaining pregnancy-induced increase in blood volume, is another mechanism by which the body rids itself of excess fluid. Fluid loss through perspiration and increased urinary output accounts for a weight loss of approximately 5 lb during the puerperium. This elimination of excess fluid accumulated during pregnancy is sometimes referred to as *reversal of the water metabolism of pregnancy.*

Urethra and Bladder

Trauma may occur to the urethra and bladder during the birth process as the infant passes through the birth canal. The bladder wall may be hyperemic and edematous, often with small areas of hemorrhage. Clean-catch or catheterized urine specimens after birth often reveal hematuria from bladder trauma. The urethra and urinary meatus may also be edematous.

Birth-induced trauma, increased bladder capacity following childbirth, and the effects of conduction anesthesia combine to cause a decreased urge to void. In addition, pelvic soreness caused by the forces of labor, vaginal lacerations, or the episiotomy reduces or alters the voiding reflex. Decreased voiding, along with postpartal diuresis, may result in bladder distention. Immediately after birth a distended bladder can lead to excessive bleeding, since it prevents the uterus from firmly contracting. Later in the puerperium overdistention can make the bladder more susceptible to infection as well as impede the resumption of normal voiding (Cunningham et al, 1993). If prolonged bladder overdistention occurs, further damage to the bladder wall (atony) may result. With adequate emptying of the bladder, bladder tone is usually restored 5 to 7 days after childbirth.

GASTROINTESTINAL SYSTEM
Appetite

The mother is usually hungry shortly after giving birth and can tolerate a light diet. After full recovery from analgesia, anesthesia, and fatigue, most new mothers are ravenously hungry. Requests for double portions of food and frequent snacks are not uncommon.

Motility

Typically, decreased muscle tone and motility of the gastrointestinal tract persist for only a short time after childbirth. Excess analgesia and anesthesia may delay a return to normal tonicity and motility.

Bowel Evacuation

A spontaneous bowel evacuation may be delayed until 2 to 3 days after childbirth. This can be explained by decreased muscle tone in the intestines during labor and the immediate puerperium, prelabor diarrhea or a prebirth enema, lack of food, or dehydration. The mother often anticipates discomfort during the bowel movement because of perineal tenderness as a result of episiotomy, lacerations, or hemorrhoids. Regular bowel habits need to be reestablished when bowel tone returns.

BREASTS

The concentrations of hormones that stimulated breast development during pregnancy (estrogen, progesterone, human chorionic gonadotropin, prolactin, cortisol, and insulin) decrease promptly after childbirth. The time it takes for the return of these hormones to prepregnancy levels is determined in part by whether the mother breastfeeds her infant.

Nonbreastfeeding Mothers

The breasts feel generally nodular (in nonpregnant women they feel granular). The nodularity is bilateral and diffuse.

If the woman chooses not to breastfeed and no antilactogenic medication is taken, prolactin levels drop rapidly. **Colostrum** secretion and excretion persist for the first few days after birth. Palpation of the breast on the second or third day, as milk production begins, may reveal tissue tenderness in some women. On the third or fourth postpartum day **engorgement** may occur. The breasts are distended (swollen), firm, tender, and warm to the touch (vasocongestion makes them feel warm). Breast distention is primarily caused by temporary congestion of veins and lymphatics rather than from an accumulation of milk. Milk can be expressed from the nipples. Axillary breast tissue (the tail of Spence) and any accessory breast or nipple tissue along the milk line may be involved. Engorgement resolves spontaneously, and discomfort decreases usually within 24 to 36 hours. If suckling is never begun (or is discontinued), lactation ceases within a few days to a week.

Breastfeeding Mothers

As lactation is established, a mass (lump) may be felt; however, a filled milk sac will shift position from day to day. Before lactation begins, the breasts feel soft and a yellowish fluid, colostrum, can be expressed from the nipples. After lactation begins, the breasts feel warm to the touch and firm. Tenderness persists for about 48 hours. Bluish white milk (skim-milk appearance) can be expressed from the nipples. The nipples are examined for erectility as opposed to inversion and for cracks or fissures.

CARDIOVASCULAR SYSTEM

Blood Volume

Changes in blood volume depend on several factors, for example, blood loss during childbirth and mobilization and subsequent excretion of extravascular water (physiologic edema). Blood loss results in immediate but limited decrease in total blood volume. Thereafter normal shifts in body water cause a slow decline in blood volume. By the third to fourth week after the birth the blood volume usually has regressed to nonpregnant values.

Pregnancy-induced hypervolemia (increase of at least 40% over nonpregnant values near term) allows most women to tolerate a considerable blood loss during childbirth. Many women lose 300 to 400 ml of blood during vaginal birth of a single fetus and about twice this amount during cesarean birth.

Readjustments in the maternal vasculature after childbirth are dramatic and rapid. The woman's response to blood loss during the early puerperium differs from that in a nonpregnant woman. Three postpartum physiologic changes protect the woman: (1) elimination of uteroplacental circulation reduces the size of the maternal vascular bed by 10% to 15%, (2) loss of placental endocrine function removes the stimulus for vasodilation, and (3) mobilization of extravascular water stored during pregnancy occurs. Thus hypovolemic shock usually does not occur with normal blood loss.

Cardiac Output

Pulse rate, stroke volume, and cardiac output increase throughout pregnancy. Immediately after the birth these remain elevated or rise even higher for 30 to 60 minutes, as the blood that was shunted through the uteroplacental circuit suddenly returns to the general circulation. These values increase regardless of type of birth or use of conduction anesthesia (Bowes, 1991). Data regarding the exact return of cardiac hemodynamic levels to nor-

mal are not available, but normal cardiac output values are found when measurements are taken 8 to 10 weeks after childbirth (Bowes, 1991).

Vital Signs

Few alterations in vital signs are seen under normal circumstances. There may be a small, transient rise in both systolic and diastolic blood pressure lasting about four days after the birth (Bowes, 1991) (Table 16-2). Respiratory function returns to nonpregnant levels by 6 months after birth. After the uterus is emptied, the diaphragm descends, the normal cardiac axis is restored, and the point of maximum impulse (PMI) and the electrocardiogram (ECG) are normalized.

Blood Components

Hematocrit and Hemoglobin

During the first 72 hours after childbirth there is a greater loss in plasma volume than in blood cells. The decrease in plasma volume plus the increase in red blood cell (RBC) mass of pregnancy is associated with a rise in hematocrit by the third to seventh day postpartum. There is no RBC destruction during the puerperium, but any gain will disappear gradually in accordance with the life span of the RBC. The exact time at which RBC volume returns to prepregnancy values is not known but is within normal limits when measured 8 weeks after childbirth (Bowes, 1991).

White Blood Cell Count

Normal leukocytosis of pregnancy averages about 12,000/mm^3. During the first 10 to 12 days after childbirth values between 20,000 and 25,000/mm^3 are common. Neutrophils are the most numerous white blood cells (WBCs). Leukocytosis coupled with the normal increase in erythrocyte sedimentation rate may confuse the diagnosis of acute infections at this time.

Coagulation Factors

Clotting factors and fibrinogen are normally increased during pregnancy and remain elevated in the immediate puerperium. This hypercoagulable state, when combined with vessel damage and immobility, causes an increased risk of **thromboembolism,** especially after cesarean birth. Fibrinolytic activity also increases during the first few days after childbirth (Bowes, 1991). Factors I, II, VIII, IX, and X decrease within a few days to prepregnant levels. Fibrin split products, probably released from the placental site, can also be found in maternal blood.

Varicosities

Varicosities of the legs and around the anus (hemorrhoids) are common during pregnancy. Varices, even the less common vulvar varices, empty rapidly immediately after childbirth. Surgical correction of varicosities is not

TABLE 16-2 Vital Signs After Childbirth

NORMAL FINDINGS	DEVIATIONS FROM NORMAL FINDINGS AND PROBABLE CAUSES
TEMPERATURE During first 24 hours may rise to 38° C (100.4° F) as a result of dehydrating effects of labor. After 24 hours the woman should be afebrile.	A diagnosis of puerperal sepsis is suggested if a rise in maternal temperature to 38° C (100.4° F) is noted after the first 24 hours after childbirth and recurs or persists for 2 days. Other possibilities are mastitis, endometritis, urinary tract infections, and other systemic infections.
PULSE Pulse, along with stroke volume and cardiac output, remains elevated for the first hour or so after childbirth. It then begins to decrease at an unknown rate. By 8 to 10 weeks after childbirth the pulse has returned to a nonpregnant rate.	A rapid pulse rate or one that is increasing may indicate hypovolemia as a result of hemorrhage.
RESPIRATIONS Respirations should fall to within the woman's normal prebirth range.	Hypoventilation may follow an unusually high subarachnoid (spinal) block.
BLOOD PRESSURE Blood pressure is altered *slightly* if at all. Orthostatic hypotension, as indicated by feelings of faintness or dizziness immediately after standing up, can develop in the first 48 hours as a result of the splanchnic engorgement that may occur after birth.	A low or falling blood pressure may reflect hypovolemia secondary to hemorrhage. However, it is a late sign, and other symptoms of hemorrhage usually alert the staff. An increased reading may result from excessive use of vasopressor or oxytocic medications. Since pregnancy-induced hypertension (PIH) can persist into or occur first in the postpartum period, routine evaluation of blood pressure is needed. If a woman complains of headache, hypertension must be ruled out as a cause before analgesics are administered. If the blood pressure is elevated, the woman is confined to bed and the health care provider notified.

considered during pregnancy. Total or the nearly total regression is anticipated after childbirth.

NEUROLOGIC SYSTEM

Neurologic changes during the puerperium are those resulting from a reversal of maternal adaptations to pregnancy and those resulting from trauma during labor and birth.

Pregnancy-induced neurologic discomforts abate after birth. Elimination of physiologic edema through the diuresis that follows childbirth relieves carpal tunnel syndrome by easing the compression of the median nerve. The periodic numbness and tingling of fingers that afflict 5% of pregnant women usually disappear after childbirth unless lifting and carrying the baby aggravates the condition. Headache requires careful assessment. Postpartum headaches may be caused by various conditions,

including pregnancy-induced hypertension (PIH), stress, and leakage of cerebrospinal fluid into the extradural space during placement of the needle for epidural or spinal anesthesia. Duration of the headaches varies from 1 to 3 days to several weeks, depending on the cause and effectiveness of the treatment.

MUSCULOSKELETAL SYSTEM

Adaptations in the mother's musculoskeletal system that occurred during pregnancy are reversed in the puerperium. The adaptations include those that contribute to relaxation and subsequent hypermobility of the joints and a change in the mother's center of gravity because of the enlarging uterus. Stabilization of joints is complete by 6 to 8 weeks after birth. However, although all other joints return to their normal prepregnant position before restabilization, those in the parous woman's feet do not.

The new mother may notice a permanent increase in shoe size.

INTEGUMENTARY SYSTEM

Chloasma of pregnancy usually disappears at the termination of pregnancy. Hyperpigmentation of the areolae and linea nigra may not regress completely after childbirth. Some women will have permanent darker pigmentation of those areas. Stretch marks on breasts, abdomen, hips, and thighs may fade but usually do not disappear.

Vascular abnormalities such as spider angiomas (nevi), palmar erythema, and epulis generally regress in response to the rapid decline in estrogens after the end of pregnancy. For some women spider nevi persist indefinitely.

The abundance of fine hair seen during pregnancy usually disappears after giving birth; however, any coarse or bristly hair that appears during pregnancy usually remains. Fingernails return to their nonpregnancy characteristics of consistency and strength.

Diaphoresis is the most noticeable change in the integumentary system (see p. 444).

IMMUNE SYSTEM

The mother's need for rubella vaccination or for prevention of Rh isoimmunization is determined.

KEY POINTS

- The uterus involutes rapidly after birth, returning to the true pelvis within 1 week.
- The rapid drop in estrogen and progesterone following expulsion of the placenta is responsible for many of the anatomic and physiologic changes in the puerperium.
- Assessment of lochia and fundal height is essential to monitoring the progress of normal involution and identifying potential problems.
- Breastfeeding is a *not* a reliable form of birth control.
- Few alterations in vital signs are seen under normal circumstances after childbirth.
- Activation of blood clotting factors, immobility, and sepsis predispose the woman to thromboembolism.
- Marked diuresis, decreased bladder sensitivity, and overdistention of the bladder can lead to problems with urinary elimination.
- Postpartum physiologic changes allow the woman to tolerate considerable blood loss at birth.

CRITICAL THINKING EXERCISES

1. Prepare a teaching plan for the new mother that will cover all aspects of postpartum anatomic and physiologic changes.
   a. Correlate these changes with prenatal adaptations.
   b. Describe the differences and similarities in multiparous women and primiparous women.
   c. Examine myths and common misunderstandings about changes that can affect postpartum recovery.
2. Conduct an assessment of the ability to estimate blood loss.
   a. Pour measured amounts of a red fluid (e.g., 25 ml, 50 ml, 75 ml, 100 ml, 250 ml) on perineal pads and on plastic-backed underpads.
   b. Ask students, faculty, staff nurses, medical students, nurse midwives and physicians to make independent assessments of the volume and record their assessments.
   c. Collect the records of the assessments. Calculate percentage of correct responses among the total group and within each category of observer.
   d. Were estimates of volume closer on perineal pads or on underpads? Were the errors in judgment large enough to cause concern about estimates of actual blood loss? How might you improve your ability to estimate blood loss?

REFERENCES

Bowes WA: Postpartum care. In Gabbe SG, Niebyl JR, Simpson JL, editors: *Obstetrics: normal and problem pregnancies,* ed 2, New York, 1991, Churchill Livingstone.

Cunningham FG et al: *Williams obstetrics,* ed 19, Norwalk, CT, 1993, Appleton & Lange.

Jacobson H: A standard for assessing lochia volume, *MCN* 10(3):174, 1985.

Scott JR et al: *Danforth's obstetrics and gynecology,* ed 6, Philadelphia, 1990, JB Lippincott.

BIBLIOGRAPHY

Brewer MM et al: Postpartum change in maternal weight and body fat deposits in lactating vs. non-lactating women, *Am J Clin Nutr* 49(2):259, 1989.

Butters L et al: The influence of breast and bottlefeeding on blood pressure, *Midwifery* 4(3):130, 1988.

Greene GW et al: Postpartum weight change: how much of the weight gained in pregnancy will be lost after delivery? *Obstet Gynecol* 71(51):701, 1988.

Luegenbiehl DL et al: Standardized assessment of blood loss, *MCN* 15(4):241, 1990.

17

Family Dynamics after Childbirth

RHEA P. WILLIAMS

LEARNING OBJECTIVES

Define the key terms listed.

Describe the two components of the parenting process.

Discuss five preconditions that influence attachment.

List the sensual responses that strengthen attachment.

Differentiate the three periods in parental role change following childbirth.

List six parental tasks and responsibilities.

Identify infant behaviors that facilitate and inhibit parental attachment.

Identify behaviors of the three phases of maternal adjustment.

Discuss maternal age over 35 as a factor influencing parental response.

Explain paternal adjustment.

List three ways to facilitate parent-infant adjustment.

Describe sibling adaptation.

Describe grandparent adjustment.

KEY TERMS

attachment

biorhythmicity

claiming process

cognitive-affective skills

cognitive-motor skills

en face

engrossment

entrainment

executive behaviors

fingertip exploration

habituation

infant-parent interaction

   rhythm

   behavioral repertoires

   responsivity

maternal adjustment

   dependent phase

   dependent-independent phase

   interdependent phase

mothering function

mutuality

positive feedback

postpartum depression ("baby blues")

sibling rivalry

signaling behaviors

taking-hold phase

taking-in phase

RELATED TOPICS

Affective disorders *(Chap. 23)* · Body image *(Chap. 6)* · Developmental tasks *(Chap. 6)* · Emotional lability *(Chap. 6)* · Sexuality *(Chap. 6)* · Adolescent pregnancy *(Chap. 25)* · Infant behavioral states *(Chap. 13 and 14)*

The birth of a child poses a fundamental challenge to the existing interactional structure of the family. Becoming a parent creates a period of instability that requires behaviors that promote the transition to parenthood. Parents must explore their relationship with the infant as well as redefine the relationship between themselves. If there are other children, parents must adjust their own life space to include another child, and the older children must adjust to the infant's claim on parental time and love (Walz, Rich, 1983). The nurse

449

who understands the parenting process, including adjustments of parents, siblings, and grandparents is well prepared to assist family members with the transition to parenthood.

PARENTING PROCESS

During the prenatal period the mother is the primary agent in providing an environment in which the fetus may develop and grow. This close symbiotic union of mother and child ends with birth. Others may then assume partial or complete involvement in the infant's care. Whoever—whether biologic or substitute parent(s), woman or man—assumes the parental role enters into a crucial relationship with a child that will persist throughout the life of each. Women and men, of course, may exist without a child; thus, in essence, parenthood is optional. Parenthood may serve as a maturation factor in the life of a woman and man regardless of whether it is biologically based. For children, parenting is all important; their continued existence depends on receiving adequate care.

The tasks, responsibilities, and attitudes that make up parenting care have been designated by Steele and Pollack (1968) as the **mothering function.** It is a process in which an adult (a mature, caring, capable, self-sufficient person) assumes the care of an infant (an immature, helpless, dependent person). Either parent may exhibit motherliness. Motherliness is now recognized to be a non–gender-related ability. The ability to show gentleness, love, and understanding and to place another's welfare above one's own is not limited to women—it is a human characteristic.

Steele and Pollack (1968) describe parenting as one process with two components. The first component, being practical or mechanical in nature, involves cognitive and motor skills; the second component, emotional in nature, involves cognitive and affective skills. Both components are essential to the infant's well-being and future development.

Cognitive-Motor Skills

The first component in the process of parenting includes childcare activities such as "feeding, holding, clothing, and cleaning the infant, protecting it from harm, and providing mobility for it" (Steele, Pollack, 1968). These task-oriented activities, or **cognitive-motor skills,** do not appear automatically as efficient caregiving behaviors at the birth of one's child. The parents' abilities in these respects are influenced by their own cultural and personal experiences. Many parents have to learn how to do these tasks, and this learning process can be difficult for them. However, almost all parents with the desire to learn and with the support of others become adept in caregiving activities.

Cognitive-Affective Skills

The psychologic component in parenting, motherliness or fatherliness, appears to stem from the *parents'* earliest experiences with a loving, accepting mother figure. In this sense parents may be said to inherit the ability to show concern and tenderness and to pass on this ability to the next generation by repeating the kind of parent-child relationship they experienced. The **cognitive-affective skills** of parenting include an attitude of tenderness, awareness, and concern for the child's needs and desires. This component of parenting has a profound effect on the manner in which the practical aspects of child care are performed and on the emotional response of the child to the care. A positive parent-child relationship is mutually rewarding. This relationship is fundamental to a person's development of confidence in the expectations that others will be willing to help and that the person is worth helping.

Erikson's concept (1959, 1964) of basic trust is similar. He claims that development of a sense of trust determines the infant's responses to others throughout life. Persons who experienced a positive parent-child relationship tend to be social or outgoing and to be able to seek and accept assistance from others. In contrast, those deficient in a sense of trust tend to be alienated and isolated. They are most likely to have crises because of their inability to make use of situational supports in times of stress.

PARENTAL ACQUAINTANCE, BONDING, AND ATTACHMENT

Although much research has been directed toward unraveling the process by which a parent comes to love and accept a child and a child comes to love and accept a parent, researchers still do not know what motivates and commits parents and their children to decades of supportive and nurturing care of each other. This process often is referred to as attachment or bonding, terms that often are used interchangeably even though definitions differ somewhat. *Bonding,* as defined by Brazelton (1978), describes the initial mutual attraction between people, such as between parent and child at first meeting. **Attachment** occurs at critical periods, such as birth or adoption. It describes a feeling of affection or loyalty that binds one person to another; it is unique, specific, and enduring (Klaus, Kennell, 1982). The attachment process has been described as linear, beginning during pregnancy, intensifying during the early postpartum period, and being constant and consistent once established. It is critical to mental and physical health across the life span (Parkes, Stevenson-Hinde, 1982).

Mercer (1982) lists *five preconditions that influence attachment:*

1. A parent's emotional health (including the ability to trust another person)
2. A social support system encompassing mate, friends, and family
3. A competent level of communication and caregiving skills
4. Parental proximity to the infant
5. Parent-infant fit (including infant state, temperament, and sex)

If any of these preconditions is not present or is distorted, skilled intervention is necessary to ensure the attachment process.

According to Stainton (1983), attachment is a mutual exchange of feelings predicated by attractiveness, responsiveness, and satisfaction and is subject to changes in intensity as circumstances change over time. Attachment is developed and maintained by proximity and interaction. As with any developmental process, it is characterized by periods of progress and regression, and temporary or permanent withdrawal from attachment figures can occur.

Mercer (1982) notes that attachment is facilitated by **positive feedback:** "Positive feedback includes the social, verbal and nonverbal responses, either real or perceived, that indicate acceptance of one partner by the other." She goes on to say that attachment occurs through a "mutually satisfying experience." The newborn infant grasps a finger or a strand of hair, becoming attached to the parent (Fig. 17-1).

Bowlby (1958) and others (Ainsworth, 1969, 1970; Ainsworth, Bell, 1970; Brazelton, 1963, 1973) have extended the concept of attachment to include **mutuality;** that is, the infant's behaviors and characteristics call forth a corresponding set of maternal behaviors and characteristics. The infant displays **signaling behaviors** such as crying, smiling, and cooing that initiate the contact and

bring the mother near the child. These behaviors are followed by **executive behaviors** such as rooting, grasping, and postural adjustments that maintain the contact. The caregiver is more attracted to an alert, responsive, cuddly infant than to one who is irritable and apparently disinterested. Attachment occurs more readily with the infant whose temperament, social capabilities, appearance, and sex fit the parent's expectations. If the child does not meet these expectations, resolution of disappointment can delay the attachment process.

An important part of attachment is acquaintance (Klaus, Kennell, 1982). Parents use eye contact, touching, talking, and exploring as they become acquainted during the immediate postpartum period. Adoptive parents undergo the same process when they first meet their new child. During this period families engage in identification of the new baby through the **claiming process.** The child is first identified in terms of "likeness" to other family members, then in terms of "differences," and finally in terms of "uniqueness." The unique newcomer is thus *incorporated* into the family. Mothers and fathers scrutinize an infant carefully. They point out characteristics that the child shares with other family members and indicate recognition of a relationship between them. Mothers may make comments such as the following that reveal the claiming process: "Russ held him close and said, 'He's the image of his father,' but I found one part like me—his toes are shaped like mine. Look, he's smiling; he likes his mother's jokes."

Parental responses have direct implications for nursing. Nurses can establish an environment that enhances frequent and positive parent-child contacts. They can encourage parental awareness of infant responses and ability to communicate, provide support and encouragement as parents attempt to become competent and loving in their role, and enhance the attachment process.

Communication Between Parent and Child

Attachment is strengthened through the use of sensual responses or abilities by both partners in the parent-child interaction. The sensual responses and abilities used in communication between parent and child include the following. The nurse should keep in mind, however, that there may be cultural variations in the described behaviors.

Touch

Touch, or the tactile sense, is used extensively by parents and other caregivers as a means of becoming acquainted with the newborn. Many mothers reach out for their infants as soon as they are born and the cord is cut. They lift them to their breasts, enfold them in their arms, and cradle them. Once the child is close to them they

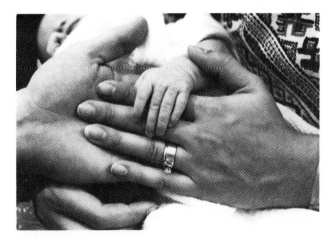
FIG. 17-1 Hands. (Courtesy St. Luke's Hospital, Kansas City, MO.)

begin the exploration process with their fingertips, one of the most touch-sensitive areas of the body. For some other mothers and other caregivers (fathers, nursing and medical students) studies have depicted a predictable pattern of touch behavior (Rubin, 1963; Klaus, Kennell, 1982; Tulman, 1985). The caregiver begins with a **fingertip exploration** of the infant's head and extremities. Within a short time the caregiver uses the palm to caress the baby's trunk and eventually enfolds the infant in her or his arms (Fig. 17-2). Gentle stroking motions are used to soothe and quiet the infant. Mothers pat or gently rub their infant's back after feedings. Infants pat the mother's breast as they nurse. Mothers and fathers want to touch, pick up, and hold their infant. Parents and infant seem to enjoy sharing each other's body warmth. Mothers will say, "I love her warm little body against mine." Variations in touching behaviors may be noted in mothers from some cultural groups. For example, minimal touching and cuddling is a traditional Southeast Asian practice. These practices are thought to protect the child from evil spirits (Galanti, 1991).

Eye-to-Eye Contact

Interest in having eye contact is demonstrated again and again. Some mothers remark that once their babies have looked at them, they feel much closer to them (Klaus, Kennell, 1982). Parents spend much time getting their babies to open their eyes and look at them.

As newborns become functionally able to sustain eye contact, parents and infant spend much time gazing at one another (Fig. 17-3), often in the *en face* position. **En face** (face to face) is a position in which two faces are approximately 8 inches apart and on the same plane. We need to implement medical and nursing practices that encourage this exchange. Newborns can be held close enough to see the parent's face. Instillation of protective eye ointment can be withheld until the infant and parents have some time together. Lights can be dimmed so that the child's eyes will open.

Voice

The shared response of parents and infant to one another's voice is also remarkable. Parents wait tensely for the first cry. Once the sound has reassured them of the baby's life and health, they begin comforting behaviors. As the parents talk in high-pitched voices, the infant is calmed and alert and turns toward them.

Odor

Another behavior shared by parents and infant is responsiveness to each other's odor. Mothers comment on the smell of their babies when first born and have noted that each child has a unique odor (Porter, Cernoch, Perry, 1983). Infants learn rapidly to distinguish the odor of their own mother's breast milk (Stainton, 1985).

Entrainment

Newborns have been found to move in time with the structure of adult speech (Condon, Sander, 1974). They wave their arms, lift their heads, kick their legs, seemingly dancing in tune to their parent's voice. This means that the infant has developed *culturally determined rhythms* of speech long before using the spoken language in communicating. A *carryover* (**entrainment**) occurs once the child begins to talk. This shared rhythm also acts to give the parent positive feedback and to establish a positive setting for effective communication.

Biorhythmicity

The unborn child can be said to be in tune with the mother's natural rhythms, such as heartbeats. After birth a crying infant may be soothed by being held in a posi-

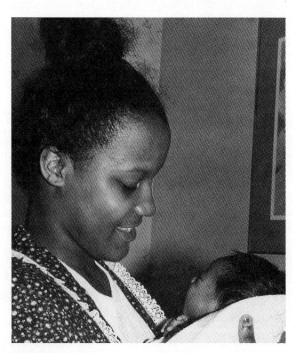

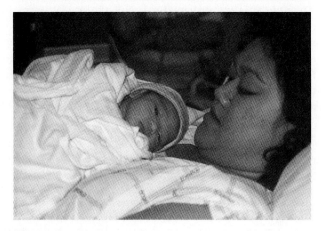

FIG. 17-2 Mother interacts with newborn. (Courtesy Marjorie Pyle, RNC, *Lifecircle*, Costa Mesa, CA.)

FIG. 17-3 Mother and new baby make eye contact in *en face* position. (Courtesy Caroline E. Brown, Hershey, PA.)

tion in the mother's arms where her heartbeat can be heard or by hearing a recording of a heartbeat. One of the newborn's tasks is to establish a personal rhythm (**biorhythmicity**). Parents can help in this process by giving consistent loving care and by using their infant's alert state to develop responsive behavior and thereby increase social interactions and opportunities for learning. The more quickly parents become competent in childcare activities, the more quickly their psychologic energy can be directed toward observing the communication cues the infant gives them.

More research with mothers and infants from culturally diverse groups is needed to help nurses understand the pattern of communication between parent and child so that culturally sensitive assessments and interventions are made to support the attachment process.

Early Contact

Research with mammals other than humans indicates that early contact between mother and offspring is important in developing future relationships. To date, *no* scientific evidence has demonstrated that *immediate contact* after birth is essential for the human parent-child relationship. According to Siegel (1982), findings from carefully controlled replicated investigations appear to document that:

> Early contact, irrespective of its supplementation by extended contact, favorably affects maternal affectional behavior during the first postpartum days. The results are consistent across low and middle socioeconomic status mother-infant pairs as well as in developed and less developed countries.

He also notes that early contact has a positive effect on the duration of breastfeeding.

The physiologic benefits of early contact between mother and infant have been documented (Klaus, Kennell, 1982). For the mother, levels of oxytocin and prolactin rise; for the infant, sucking reflexes are employed early. The process of developing active immunity begins as the infant ingests flora from the mother's skin.

The first hours or days after birth may be a sensitive time for parent-infant interaction. Early close contact may *facilitate* the attachment process between parent and child. This is not to say a delay will inhibit this process (humans are too resilient for that), but additional psychologic energy may be needed to accomplish the same effect. Parents who can not expend this energy, the delay may affect the infant's future well-being.

Research in the area of child abuse documents the greater percentage of neglect, abuse, and failure to thrive among infants separated from parents for relatively long periods because of illness or preterm birth (Klaus, Kennell, 1982).

Parents who desire but are unable to have early contact with their newborn infant can be reassured that such contact is not essential for optimum parent-child inter-

actions. Otherwise, adopted infants would not form the usual affectional ties with their parents. Nor does the mode of infant-mother contact after birth (skin-to-skin vs. wrapped) appear to have any important effect. Nurses need to counsel mothers to allay fears that their emotional bond to their infant is not necessarily weaker because they missed early contact or because the contact was not skin-to-skin (Curry, 1979). Indeed, in some cultures a mother's contact with her newborn may be limited to the baby's feeding. In some East Indian families, for example, a family member takes over all baby care except the feeding. Mothers from this culture may refuse to hold their baby at other times (Galanti, 1991).

Extended Contact

Since the early 1970s consumers have worked toward childbirth practices that establish the family as the focus of care. The alternatives of home birth, birthing centers, and family-centered maternity care units reflect this desire by parents to share in the birth process and to have extended, uninterrupted contact with their infants.

One method of family-centered care is the provision of rooming-in facilities for the mother and her baby. The infant is transferred to the area from the transitional nursery (if the facility uses one) after showing satisfactory extrauterine adjustment. The father is encouraged to visit and to participate in the infant's care. Siblings and grandparents are also encouraged to visit and become acquainted with the infant. Many hospitals have established family birth units. The mother is accompanied by the father during the birth of the infant, and all three may remain together until discharged. Medical and nursing personnel are available for any care necessary for the mother and child. Other hospitals arrange for the discharge of mother and infant any time from 2 to 24 hours after birth if the condition of the mother and that of the infant warrants it. Follow-up care with nursing personnel from a health agency is usually part of this plan.

Mother-baby care is another form of family-centered care. Care for the mother and baby is provided by a primary nurse, fostering family unity (Fig. 17-4). Parents are more likely to be more self-confident in care and maternal attachment and maternal role attainment is promoted (NAACOG, 1989).

Extended contact with the infant should be available for all parents, but especially for those assessed to be at risk for parenting inadequacies. Any activity that optimizes family-centered care is worthy of serious consideration by postpartum nurses.

PARENTAL ROLE AFTER CHILDBIRTH

For the biologic parent the parental role begun during pregnancy enlarges and intensifies at birth. Care and nurturing of the child is initiated before birth when the

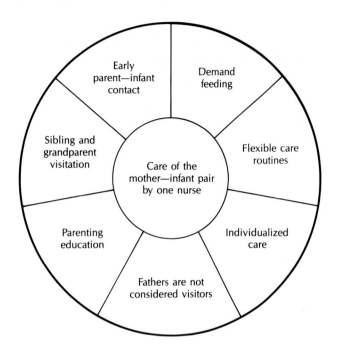

FIG. 17-4 The wheel of family-centered postpartum and newborn care. (Adapted From Watters NE: Combined mother-infant nursing care, *JOGNN* 14:480, 1985.)

mother carried out the dictates of health (e.g., diet, rest, exercise) for the "good of her baby" and the father who nurtured his mate and took an interest in his unborn child were already functioning in the parental role.

During the postpartum period new tasks and responsibilities arise and old behaviors need to be modified or new ones added. Mothers' and fathers' responses to the parental role change over time and tend to follow a predictable course.

During the early period parents have to recognize their relationship with their infant. The infant's needs for shelter, nourishment, protection, and socializing continue. What was accomplished through the biologic process of pregnancy now requires an array of caregiving activities. This period is characterized by intense learning and need for nurturing. The family structure and functioning as a system has been forever altered. The duration of this period varies but generally lasts about 4 weeks.

The next period represents a time of drawing together and uniting the family unit. This consolidation period involves negotiating roles (wife-husband/partners, mother-father, parent-child, sibling-sibling). It involves a stabilizing of tasks, a coming to terms with commitments. Parents demonstrate growing competence in infant care activities and become sensitive to the meaning of their infant's behavior. This period lasts approximately 2 months and in conjunction with the early period forms what is now termed the *fourth trimester.*

Parents and children grow in their roles until separated by death. The most outstanding feature of the life-

long process of parent-child interaction is change, consistent evolution over time. The individuals involved deal not only with the present but also with the future. They need support and care in the here and now and anticipatory guidance for coming changes.

Parental Tasks and Responsibilities

Parents need to reconcile the actual child with the fantasy and dream child. This means coming to terms with the infant's physical appearance, sex, innate temperament, and physical status. If the real child differs greatly from the fantasy child, parents may delay acceptance for a period.

Some parents are startled by the appearance of the infant—size, color, molding of the head, or bowed appearance of the legs. Many fathers have commented that they thought the odd shape of the child's head (molding) meant the child would be mentally retarded.

Disappointment over the sex of the infant can take time to resolve. Some parents may actually grieve over "loss" of sex of the child before they can accept that child. The mother or father may be able to give adequate physical mothering but may find it difficult to be sincerely involved with the infant until these feelings have been resolved.

Parents need to establish the newborn as a person separate from themselves, that is, as someone having many dependency needs and requiring much nurturing.

Parents need to become adept in the care of the infant. This includes caregiving activities, noting the communication cues given by the infant to indicate needs, and responding appropriately to them.

Parents need to establish reasonable evaluative criteria to use in assessing the success or failure of the care given the infant. Parents are surprisingly sensitive to infant responses. One father told of his first attempt to give his child a kiss. At that moment the child turned her head. The father felt hurt, although he understood that the baby was totally unaware of her own movements. How the infant responds to parental care and attention is interpreted by the parent as a comment on the quality of the care being given. These responses may include crying, weight gain or loss, or sleeping at a designated time. Continued responses deemed negative by the parent can result in alienation of parent and child to the infant's detriment (Table 17-1).

Self-esteem grows with competence. Mothers of preterm infants have noted that the adept handling of their infants by nurses made their own efforts to sustain their child appear inadequate. Nurses therefore have the opportunity to instruct the new mother and enhance her self-esteem. Mothers who have supplied breast milk for their infant comment that this makes them feel they are contributing in a unique way to the welfare of their child.

TABLE 17-1 Infant Behaviors Affecting Parental Attachment

FACILITATING BEHAVIORS	INHIBITING BEHAVIORS
Visually alert; eye-to-eye contact; tracking or following of parent's face	Sleepy; eyes closed most of the time; gaze aversion
Appealing facial appearance; randomness of body movements reflecting helplessness	Resemblance to person parent dislikes; hyperirritability or jerky body movements when touched
Smiles	Bland facial expression; infrequent smiles
Vocalization; crying only when hungry or wet	Crying for hours on end; colicky
Grasp reflex	Exaggerated motor reflex
Anticipatory approach behaviors for feedings; sucks well; feeds easily	Feeds poorly; regurgitates; vomits often
Enjoys being cuddled, held	Resists holding and cuddling by crying, stiffening body
Easily consolable	Inconsolable; unresponsive to parenting, caretaking tasks
Activity and regularity somewhat predictable	Unpredictable feeding and sleeping schedule
Attention span sufficient to focus on parents	Inability to attend to parent's face or offered stimulation
Differential crying, smiling, and vocalizing; recognizes and prefers parents	Shows no preference for parents over others
Approaches through locomotion	Unresponsive to parent's approaches
Clings to parent; puts arms around parent's neck	Seeks attention from any adult in room
Lifts arms to parents in greeting	Ignores parents

From Gerson E: *Infant behavior in the first year of life*, New York, 1973, Raven Press. Copyright 1973. With permission.

Criticism, real or imagined, of new parents' ability to provide adequate physical care, nutrition, or social stimulation for their infant can prove devastating. Assistance, including advice by husbands, wives, mothers, mothers-in-law, and other relatives and professional workers, can be seen as supportive. Conversely, it can be seen as an indication of how inept these individuals have judged the new parent to be.

Parents must establish a place for the newborn within the family group. Whether the infant is the first born or last born, all family members must adjust their roles to accommodate the newcomer. An only child needs support to accept a rival to parental affections. An older child needs support when she loses her place as the family baby. The parents are expected to negotiate these changes.

Parents need to establish the primacy of their adult relationships to maintain the family as a group. Since this includes reorganizing many roles, for example, sex roles, child-care roles, career roles, and community roles, time and energy must be provided for this vital task.

Maternal Adjustment

Three phases are discernible as the mother adjusts to her version of the parental role. These phases of **maternal adjustment** are characterized by dependent behavior, dependent-independent behavior, and interdependent behavior.

Dependent Phase

During the first 1 to 2 days after birth the mother's dependency needs predominate. To the extent that these needs are met by others, the mother is able to divert her psychologic energy to her child rather than to herself. She needs "mothering" to "mother." Rubin (1961) has aptly described these few days as the **taking-in phase,** a time when nurturing and protective care are required by the new mother. In Rubin's classic description the taking-in phase lasted 2 to 3 days. A more recent study (Ament, 1990) supported Rubin's work, except women were now found to move more quickly through the taking-in. A strong taking-in phase was noted only in the first 24 hours after birth.

For a few hours or days following birth, mature and healthy women appear to suspend involvement in everyday responsibilities. They rely on others to respond to their needs for comfort, rest, and nourishment.

The **dependent phase** is a time of great excitement, and most parents are extremely talkative. They need to verbalize their experience of pregnancy and birth. Focusing on, analyzing, and accepting these experiences help the parents move on to the next phase. Some parents are able to use the staff or other mothers as an audience. Others are more comfortable verbalizing these feelings to family or friends.

Anxiety and preoccupation with her new role often narrow a mother's perceptual field; therefore information given during this time may have to be repeated.

Dependent-Independent Phase

If the mother has received adequate nurturing in the first few hours or days, by the second or third day her desire for independent action reasserts itself. In the **dependent-independent phase** the mother alternates between a need for extensive nurturing and acceptance by others and the desire to take charge once again. She responds enthusiastically to opportunities to learn and practice the care of the baby or, if she is an accomplished mother, to carry out or direct this care. Rubin (1961) describes this as the **taking-hold phase,** noting that it lasts approximately 10 days.

In the period of 6 to 8 weeks after birth the mastery of the tasks of parenthood is crucial. Realistic expectations facilitate the subsequent functioning of the family as a unit.

Some women adjust with considerable difficulty to the isolation of infant care and resent the endless coping with home and child-care responsibilities. The mothers who appear to need additional support include:

1. Primiparas inexperienced in child care
2. Women whose careers had provided outside stimulation
3. Women who lack friends or family members with whom to share delights and concerns
4. Adolescent mothers
5. Women without partners

Depressive states are not uncommon during this phase. Feelings of extreme vulnerability may arise from a number of factors. Psychologically the mother may be overwhelmed by the actuality of parental responsibilities. She may feel deprived of the supportive care she received from family members and friends during pregnancy. Some mothers regret the loss of the mother–unborn child relationship and mourn its passing. Still others experience a letdown feeling when labor and birth are complete.

Fatigue following birth is compounded by around-the-clock demands of the new baby and can accentuate the feelings of depression. It has been suggested that a lowered level of circulating glucocorticoids or a condition of subclinical hypothyroidism may exist during the puerperium. This physiologic state could explain some minor degrees of **postpartum depression ("baby blues").** Depressive reactions are not necessarily expressed verbally. A depressive state signified by typical behaviors (withdrawal, loss of interest in surroundings, and crying) can be manifested. Once immediate tasks and adjustments have been undertaken and brought under control, a plateau is reached. At this time the lifelong effects of the parents' new responsibility come into focus.

It is hoped that toward the end of the dependent-independent phase the tasks and adjustments of daily routine will begin to follow a pattern. The baby begins to take an established position in the family. Many of the feeding problems, whether related to breastfeeding or bottle-feeding, have been largely resolved. The mother's physical energy and strength return. By the fifth week the infant has been examined by the health care provider and the mother also has been examined or has made arrangements for a checkup. It is time to move on to the next phase of adjustment.

Interdependent Phase

In this phase interdependent behavior reasserts itself, and the mother and her family move forward as a system with interacting members. The relationship between partners, although altered by the introduction of a child, resumes many of its former characteristics. A primary need is to establish a lifestyle that includes, but in some respects excludes, the child. The couple must share interests and activities that are adult in scope.

Most couples resume sexual intercourse by the third or fourth week after the child is born; some begin earlier, as soon as it can be accomplished without discomfort for the woman. Sexual intimacy increases the man-woman aspect of the family, and the adult pair shares a closeness denied to other family members. Many new fathers speak of the alienation experienced when they observe the intimate mother-child relationship, and some are frank in expressing feelings of jealousy toward the infant. The resumption of the marital relationship seems to bring the parents' relationship back into focus.

The **interdependent phase** *(letting-go)* is stressful for the parental pair. Interests and needs often diverge during this time. Men and women must resolve the effects of their individual roles on childrearing, homemaking, and career on their relationship. A special effort must be undertaken to strengthen the adult-adult relationship as a basis for the family unit.

Paternal Adjustment

It is now recognized that the mother-child relationship exists not in a vacuum but within the context of the family system. Parents' attitudes toward and expectations of one another's parental behavior affect the behavior of each dyad. In American culture the newborn has been found to have a powerful impact on the father. Fathers have demonstrated intense involvement with their babies. Greenberg and Morris (1976) named the father's absorption, preoccupation, and interest in the infant **engrossment.** These researchers delineate a number of characteristics of engrossment. Some of the sensual responses relating to touch and eye-to-eye contact are the same as discussed earlier. The father's keen awareness of features both unique and similar to himself is another characteristic related to the father's need to claim the infant. An outstanding response is one of *strong attraction* to the newborn. Much time is spent communicating with the infant and taking delight in the infant's response to the father. Fathers feel a sense of increased self-esteem, a sense of being "proud, bigger, more mature, and older" after seeing their baby for the first time.

Research focusing on paternal relationships gives the nurse some insight about paternal adjustment. For example, a study by Henderson and Brouse (1991) on the experiences of new fathers during the first 3 weeks of life suggests that new fathers go through a predictable three-stage process during the transition to fatherhood. *Stage 1* involves coming to the experience with preconceptions

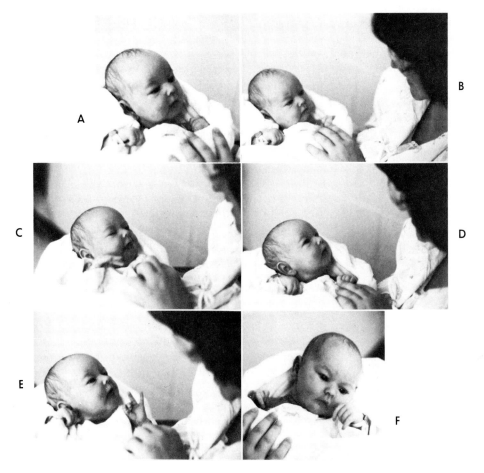

FIG. 17-5   Holding newborn in *en face* position, mother works to alert her daughter, 6 hours old. **A,** Infant is quiet and alert. **B,** Mother begins talking to daughter. Note frown of concentration. **C,** Infant responds, opens mouth like her mother. **D,** Infant gazes at her mother. **E,** Infant waves hand, opens mouth. **F,** Infant glances away, resting. Hand relaxes. (Courtesy Colleen Stainton.)

about what it will be like when they take the baby home. *Stage 2* is the uncomfortable reality of being a new father. Some fathers begin to realize that their expectations are not based on fact. Feelings of sadness and ambivalence often accompany reality. *Stage 3* involves a conscious decision to take control and become more actively involved in their infant's life.

Much has still to be learned about the relationships between fathers and their offspring. Research should be expanded to include fathers from diverse cultural backgrounds and those in nontraditional family forms to more fully explain this phenomenon. Based on current knowledge, however, nurses can assist fathers in the transition to fatherhood. Interventions that increase feelings of competence, confidence, and comfort will assist fathers during this difficult transition (Henderson, Brouse, 1991). Such assistance includes helping fathers explore their expectations of fatherhood, providing realistic and consistent information about infant behavior, and including interested fathers in infant care instructions. New fathers should also be encouraged to share their feelings about this new experience with their partners.

Infant-Parent Adjustment

Newborn babies are active participants in shaping their parents' reaction to them (Brazelton, Cramer, 1990). The **infant-parent interaction** is characterized by a "set of rhythms, behavioral repertoires, and responsivity or response styles" (Field, 1978) (Fig. 17-5). These traits are unique to each partner. Interactions can be facilitated in any of three ways: (1) modulation of **rhythm,** (2) modification of **behavioral repertoires,** and (3) mutual **responsivity.**

Rhythm

To regulate the rhythm, both parent and infant must be able to interact. Therefore the infant must be in the alert state, one of the most difficult of the sleep-wake states to maintain (Fig. 17-6). The alert state occurs most often during a feeding or in face-to-face play. The parent must work hard to help the infant maintain the alert state long enough and often enough for interactions to take place (see Fig. 17-5, *A*). The *en face* position is usually assumed. Multiparous mothers show particular sensitivity and responsiveness to their infant's feeding rhythms.

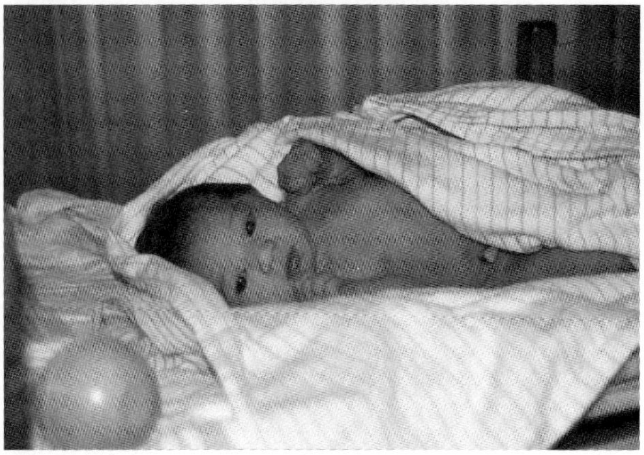

FIG. 17-6 Infant in alert state. (Courtesy Marjorie Pyle, RNC, *Lifecircle,* Costa Mesa, CA.)

The mother who is sensitive to feeding rhythms reserves stimulation for pauses in sucking activity. For example, the mother learns not to talk or smile excessively while the infant is sucking because the infant will stop feeding to interact with her (Field, 1978). With maturity the infant can sustain longer interactions by adjusting activity rhythms, that is, limb movement, sucking, gaze alteration, and **habituation** (see Fig. 17-5, *F*). "In the interim, the adult learns to attend to these rhythms, modulate her or his own rhythms, and thereby facilitate a rhythmical turn-taking interaction" (Field, 1978).

Repertoires

Both contributors to the infant-parent interaction have a repertoire of behaviors they can use to facilitate interactions. Fathers and mothers engage in these behaviors depending on the amount of contact and caregiving of the infant.

The *infant's repertoire* includes gaze behaviors, vocalizing, and facial expressions. The infant is able to focus and follow the human face from birth. The infant is also able to use gaze alternation. These abilities are under voluntary control. "The infant appears to look away from the mother's face when under- or over-aroused to modulate his or her arousal level and process the stimulation he or she is receiving" (Field, 1978) (Fig. 17-5, *F*). Brazelton et al (1974) suggest that one of the key responses for the parents to learn is awareness of *the infant's capacity for attention and inattention.* Developing this awareness is especially important in interacting with premature infants (Sammons, Lewis, 1985).

Body gestures form a part of the infant's early language. Babies greet parents with waving hands (Fig. 17-5, *E*) or with a reaching out of hands. They can raise an eyebrow or soften their expression to elicit loving attention. They can be stimulated to smile or laugh with game playing. To end an interaction they use pouting or crying, arching of the back, and general squirming.

The parents' repertoire includes various behaviors for interacting with their infant. One of these behaviors is constantly looking at the infant and noting the infant's behavior. Adults also infantilize their speech to help the infant listen. They do this by slowing the tempo, speaking loudly and rhythmically, and by emphasizing key words. They repeat phrases frequently. Infantilizing is not the same as "baby talk," which involves distortion of sounds.

Parents also use facial expressions as a means of interaction. They may slow and exaggerate expressions such as surprise, happiness, and confusion to communicate them to the infant. Playing games, such as "peek-a-boo," is another means of interaction. Parents can also be observed imitating the infant's behaviors. If the baby smiles, the parent will also smile. If the baby frowns, the parent responds in kind.

Responsivity

Contingent responses are those that occur within a specific time and are similar in form to a stimulus behavior. They elicit a feeling in the person originating the behavior of having an influence on the interaction. In other words, they act as positive feedback. Adults view infant behaviors such as smiling, cooing, and sustained eye contact, usually in *en face* position, as contingent responses. The adults are encouraged to continue the same game when the infant responds in such a way. These responses act as rewards to the initiator. When the adult imitates the infant, the infant appears to enjoy the responses. The infant in turn imitates behaviors of adults soon after birth. The parent shows progression in presenting behaviors for the baby to imitate; for example, in early interactions the parent will grimace rather than laugh, which is in keeping with the infant's developmental level. Such turnabout behaviors sustain interactions and promote harmony in the relationship.

Factors Influencing Parental Responses

How the parents respond to the birth of their child is influenced by various factors, including age, social networks, culture, socioeconomic conditions, and personal aspirations for the future.

Maternal Age Over 35

Maternal age has a definite effect on pregnancy outcome. The mother and fetus are generally thought to be at highest risk when the mother is an adolescent or over 35 years old. Adolescent pregnancy is a significant issue in North America and is addressed in Chapter 25.

Issues and concerns related to the over-35 age group have become increasingly more prominent in the last decade. Studies have identified certain factors that can influence parental responses in this older group. *Fatigue and the need for more rest* seem to be the major concerns of older parents with newborns (Queenan, 1987; Winslow, 1987).

Measures designed to assist the mother in regaining strength and muscle tone (e.g., prenatal and postpartum exercises) are emphasized. Some older mothers may find that the care of the newborn infant exhausts their physical capabilities. Many women might benefit from referral to supportive resources in the community (Scott, Meredith, Angwin, 1986).

Social Networks

Primiparas and multiparas may have different needs. Multiparas may be more realistic in anticipating their physical limitations and can adjust to changes in roles and relationships more easily. Primiparas may need more supportive care and follow-up for parenting, including referral to community resources. The families and friends of the parents and their newborn child form an important dimension of the parent's social network, much of which may be culturally determined. Social networks provide a support system on which parents can rely for assistance (Crawford, 1985; Cronenwett, 1985a, b). Positive emotional and affectional relationships appear critical to the enhancement of parenting skills and nurturance of children (Gottlieb, 1980; Schornkoff, 1984). Social networks promote the growth potential of children and the prevention of their maltreatment. Mercer (1982) and Crawford (1985) found that social networks provided support but were also a source of conflict. Grandparents or in-laws who assisted with household responsibilities and who did not intrude into the parents' privacy or critically judge them were most appreciated. Sometimes a large network caused problems in that it generated conflicting advice to the new parents. In some cultural networks, however, a large network may be an important element of support.

Culture

Cultural beliefs and practices are important determinants of parenting behaviors. They influence the interactions with the baby as well as the parent or family's caregiving style. (See Chapter 2 for discussion about culture and childbearing. Table 2-2 gives examples of some traditional cultural beliefs that may be important to parents from African-American, Asian-American, and Mexican-American cultures.)

Knowledge of these cultural beliefs can help the nurse make more accurate assessments and diagnosis of observed parenting behaviors. For example, nurses may become concerned when they observe cultural practices that appear to reflect poor bonding (Galanti, 1991). The nurse may observe a Vietnamese woman who gives minimal care to her infant but refuses to cuddle and further interact with the child. This apparent lack of interest in the newborn is this cultural group's attempt to "ward off evil spirits." This belief demonstrates an intense love and concern for the child (Galanti, 1991).

Since all members of a cultural group do not necessarily adhere to traditional practices, it is important to validate which cultural practices are important to individual parents.

Socioeconomic Conditions

Socioeconomic conditions often determine access to available resources. Families who can afford the added expenses of a newborn may experience minimal financial stress. In families where the birth of a newborn is seen as a financial burden, increased levels of stress may be evident. This stress may interfere with parenting behaviors, making the transition to parenthood more difficult.

Nursing measures designed to help persons experiencing stress due to economic circumstances involve referrals to social and economic community agencies as well as health agencies.

Personal Aspirations

For some women parenthood interferes with or curtails their plans for personal freedom or advancement in their career. Resentment concerning their loss may not have been resolved during the prenatal period. If this resentment is not resolved, it will spill over into caregiving activities and may result in indifference and neglect. Or, conversely, it may result in oversolicitousness and the setting of impossibly high standards by the mother for her behavior or the child's performance (Shainess, 1970).

Nursing intervention includes providing opportunities for parents to vent their feelings freely to an objective listener; to discuss measures to permit personal growth of the parent, for example, by part-time employment, volunteer work, and use of agencies that provide babysitting care or mother substitutes during parents' vacations; and to learn about the care of the child.

SIBLING ADAPTATION

Introduction of the infant into a family with one or more children may pose problems for the parents. They are faced with the task of caring for a new child while not neglecting the others. Parents need to distribute their attention in a manner that they consider fair.

Older children have to assume new positions within the family hierarchy. The older child's goal is to maintain a leading position. The child who is next in birth order to the infant has to gain a superior position over the newcomer (Kreppner et al, 1982). As the infant develops and begins to assert herself or himself, the older child works toward dominance.

Regression to an infantile level of behavior may be seen in some children. They may revert to bed-wetting, whining, or refusing to feed themselves. Because the baby absorbs time and attention of the important person in the other children's lives, jealous reactions are to be expected once the initial excitement of having a new baby in the home is over.

Parents, especially mothers, spend much time and energy promoting sibling acceptance of a new baby. Older children are involved actively in preparation for the infant, and involvement intensifies after the birth of the child. Mother and father face a number of tasks related to **sibling rivalry** and adjustment. The tasks include the following:

1. Making the older child feel loved and wanted
2. Managing guilt arising from feelings that older children are being deprived of parental time and attention
3. Developing feelings of confidence in their ability to nurture more than one child
4. Adjusting time and space to accommodate the new baby
5. Monitoring behavior of older children toward the more vulnerable infant and diverting aggressive behavior

Sibling preparation classes have been shown to be one effective way to help decrease sibling rivalry when a second child joins the family (Fortier et al, 1991).

Acquaintance behaviors of siblings with the newborn have been described by Marecki et al (1985) and Anderberg (1988). The acquaintance process depends on the information given to the child before the baby is born and on the cognitive developmental level of the child. The initial behaviors of siblings with the newborn include looking at the infant and touching the head (Fig. 17-7).

The initial adjustment of older children to a newborn takes time. Children should be allowed to interact at their own pace rather than being forced. To expect a young child to accept and love a rival for the parents' affection assumes a too-mature response. Sibling love grows as does other love, that is, by being with another person and sharing experiences.

GRANDPARENT ADAPTATION

The amount of grandparent involvement in the newborn's care depends on many factors, for example, willingness of the grandparents to become involved, proximity of the grandparents, and ethnic and cultural expectations of the role grandparents play (Grosso et al, 1981).

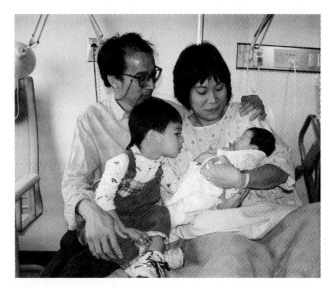

FIG. 17-7 Parents introducing infant daughter to "big" brother. (Courtesy Kim Molloy, San Jose, CA.)

The woman's mother is an important model for child-rearing practices (Rubin, 1975). She acts as a source of knowledge and as a support person. Grandchildren are tangible evidence of continuity, of immortality. Often grandparents comment that the presence of grandchildren helps relieve loneliness and boredom.

New parents can be encouraged to include grandparents; this inclusion will enrich their lives and those of their children. As parents are assisted in working through differing opinions and unresolved conflicts (e.g., dependency, control) between themselves and their parents, they can move toward mastery of the developmental tasks of adulthood. Grandparental support can be a stabilizing influence for families undergoing developmental crises such as childbearing and new parenthood (Newell, 1984). Grandparents can foster the learning of parental skills and preserve cultural tradition.

One way to help grandparents bridge the generation gap and help them understand parenting concepts that their adult children are using is to offer classes (Maloni, McIndue, Rubenstein, 1987). Included in these classes is information about up-to-date childbearing practices, especially family-centered care; infant care, feeding, and safety (car seats); and exploration of roles grandparents play in the family unit. This can foster open discussion between the generations about feelings and needs of parents and grandparents.

KEY POINTS

- The birth of a child poses a fundamental challenge to the existing interactional structure of a family.
- Either parent may exhibit "motherliness."
- Attachment is the process by which parent and child come to love and accept each other.
- Attachment is strengthened through the use of sensual responses or abilities by both partners in the parent-child interaction.
- Early contact with the newborn is not essential for optimum parent-child interactions.
- For the biologic parent, the parental role does not begin at birth, but rather enlarges and intensifies.
- In adjusting to the parental role, the mother moves from a dependent state to an interdependent state.
- Mothers may be overwhelmed by the actuality of parenting responsibilities and may exhibit signs of postpartum depression ("baby blues").

- A primary need of parents is to establish a lifestyle that includes, but in some respects excludes, the child.
- In Western culture the newborn has been found to have a powerful impact on the father.
- Modulation of rhythm, modification of behavioral repertoires, and mutual responsivity facilitate infant-parent adjustment.
- Many factors influence parental responses (for example, their age, culture, socioeconomic level, and their expectations of what their child will be like).
- Parents face a number of tasks related to sibling adjustment that require creative parental interventions.
- Grandparental support can be a stabilizing influence during developmental crises such as childbearing.

CRITICAL THINKING EXERCISES

1. You are asked to participate in a group discussion on parenthood. Consider the following.
   a. Examine your feelings regarding parenthood and how these might affect your perceptions of parenting.
   b. Identify how experiences with your own parents might affect your parenting style.
   c. Discuss your feelings with the group and compare experiences.
   d. Identify possible interventions to facilitate parenting in the postpartum period.

2. You are providing postpartum care for a woman and her newborn. The woman's 2-year-old daughter comes for a visit and states that she "hates the baby."
   a. What are possible reasons for this reaction?
   b. How can you check them out? What assessments are needed to determine if sibling rivalry is a problem?
   c. Formulate a plan of care to counteract the problem and justify choices.

REFERENCES

Anderberg GJ: Initial acquaintance and attachment behavior of siblings with the newborn, *JOGN Nurs* 17(1):49, 1988.

Ainsworth MD, Bell SM: Attachment, exploration and separation: illustrated by the behavior of one-year-olds in a strange situation, *Child Dev* 41:49, 1970.

Ainsworth MD: Object relations, dependency, and attachment: a theoretical review of the infant-mother relationship, *Child Dev* 40:969, 1969.

Ainsworth MD: The development of infant-mother attachment. In Caldwell BM, Reccurti HN, editors: *Review of child development research,* vol 3, New York, 1970, Russell Sage Foundation.

Ament LA: Maternal tasks of the puerperium reidentified, *JOGNN* 19(4):330, 1990.

Bowlby J: The nature of the child's tie to his mother, *Int J Psychoanal* 39:350, 1958.

Brazelton TB, Cramer BG: *The earliest relationship,* Reading, MA, 1990, Addison-Wesley.

Brazelton TB: Effect of maternal expectations on early infant behavior, *Early Child Dev Care* 2:259, 1973.

Brazelton TB et al: The origins of reciprocity: the early mother-infant interaction. In Lewis M, Rosenblum LA, editors: *The effect of the infant on its caregiver,* New York, 1974, John Wiley & Sons.

Brazelton TB: The early mother-infant adjustment, *Pediatrics* 32:931, 1963.

Brazelton TB: The remarkable talents of the newborn, *Birth Fam J* 5:187, 1978.

Condon W, Sander L: Neonate movement is synchronized with adult speech: interactional participation and language acquisition, *Science* 183:99, 1974.

Crawford J: A theoretical model of support network conflict experienced by new mothers, *Nurs Res* 34:100, 1985.

Cronenwett LR: Network structure, social support, and psychological outcomes of pregnancy, *Nurs Res* 34:93, 1985a.

Cronenwett LR: Parental network structured and perceived support after birth of first child, *Nurs Res* 34:347, 1985b.

Curry MS: Contact during first hour with the wrapped or naked newborn: effect on maternal attachment behaviors at 36 hours and three months, *Birth Fam J* 6:4, 1979.

Erikson EH: *Childhood and society,* New York, 1964, WW Norton.

Erikson EH: Identity and the life cycle: selected papers. In *Psychological issues,* vol 1, no 1, New York, 1959, International Universities Press.

Field T: The three Rs of infant-adult interactions: rhythms, repertoires, and responsibility, *J Pediatr Psychol* 3:131, 1978.

Fortier JC et al: Adjustment to a newborn: sibling preparation makes a difference, *JOGNN* 20(1):73, 1991.

Galanti GA: *Caring for patients from different cultures,* Philadelphia, 1991, University of Pennsylvania Press.

Gerson E: *Infant behavior in the first year of life,* New York, 1973, Raven Press.

Gottlieb BH: The role of individual and social support in preventing child maltreatment. In Garbarino J, Stocking S, editors: *Protecting children from abuse/neglect,* San Francisco, 1980, Jossey-Bass.

Greenberg M, Morris N: Engrossment: the newborn's impact on the father, *Nurs Digest* 4:19, 1976.

Grosso C et al: Bridging cultures. The Vietnamese American family . . . and grandma makes three, *MCN* 6:177, 1981.

Henderson AD, Brouse AJ: The experiences of new fathers in the first 3 weeks of life, *J Adv Nurs* 16:293, 1991.

Klaus MH, Kennell, JH: Parent-infant bonding, ed 2, St Louis, 1982, Mosby.

Kreppner K et al: Infant and family development from triads to tetrads, *Hum Dev* 25:373, 1982.

Maloni JA, McIndue JE, Rubenstein G: Expectant grandparents classes, *JOGNN* 16(1):26, 1987.

Marecki M et al: Early sibling attachment, *JOGNN* 14(5):418, 1985.

Mercer RT: Parent-infant attachment. In Sonstegard LJ et al, editors: *Women's health, vol 2: Childbearing,* New York, 1982, Grune & Stratton.

NAACOG Committee on Practice: *Mother-baby care,* NAACOG OGN Nursing Practice Resource, Washington, DC, 1989, NAACOG.

Newell NJ: Grandparents, the overlooked support system for new parents during the fourth trimester, *NAACOG Update Series 1* (lesson 21), 1984.

Parkes CM, Stevenson-Hinde J: *The place of attachment in human behavior,* New York, 1982, Basic Books.

Porter RH, Cernoch JM, Perry S: The importance of odors in mother-infant interactions, *Matern Child Nurs J* 2:147, 1983.

Queenan JT, moderator: Managing pregnancy in patients over 35, *Contemp OB/GYN* 29(5):180, 1987.

Rubin R: Maternal behavior, *Nurs Outlook* 9:682, 1961.

Rubin R: Maternal tasks in pregnancy, *Matern Child Nurs J* 4:143, 1975.

Rubin R: Maternal touch at first contact with the newborn infant, *Nurs Outlook* 11:828, 1963.

Sammons WA Lewis JM: *Premature babies: a different beginning,* St. Louis, 1985, Mosby.

Schornkoff JP: Social support and the development of vulnerable children, *Am J Public Health* 74:310, 1984.

Scott L, Meredith A, Angwin, J: *Time out for motherhood: a guide for today's working woman to the financial, emotional and career aspects of having a baby,* Los Angeles, 1986, Jeremy P Tarcher.

Shainess N: Abortion is no man's business, *Psychology Today,* p. 18, March, 1970.

Siegel E: A critical examination of studies of parent-infant bonding. In Klaus M, Robertson M, editors: *Birth, interaction and attachment,* Evansville, IL, 1982, Johnson & Johnson.

Stainton MC: Origins of attachment: culture and cue sensitivity, *Dissertation Abstracts International,* 46, 3786-B. (University Microfilms No. 8600606), 1985.

Steele B, Pollock C: A psychiatric study of parents who abuse infants and small children. In Helfer RE, Kempe C, editors: *The battered child,* Chicago, 1968, University of Chicago Press.

Tulman L: Mothers and unrelated persons' initial handling of newborn infants, *Nurs Res* 34:205, 1985.

Walz B, Rich O: Maternal tasks of taking on a second child in the postpartum period, *Matern Child Nurs J* 12:3, 1983.

Winslow W: First pregnancy after 35: what is the experience? *MCN* 12(2):92, 1987.

BIBLIOGRAPHY

Coffman S: Parent and infant attachment: review of nursing research 1981-1990, *Pediatric Nursing* 18(4):421, 1992.

Denehy JA: Interventions related to parent-infant attachment, *Nurs Clin North Am* 27:425, 1992.

Donaldson NE: A review of nursing intervention research on maternal adaptation in the first 8 weeks postpartum, *J Perinat Neonat Nurs* 4(4):1, 1991.

Hassan SA: Maternal behaviors and initial maternal-infant interaction of vaginally and cesarean delivered mothers, *Matern Child Nurs J* 19(2):177, 1990.

Kemp VH, Sibley DE, Pond EF: A comparison of adolescent and adult mothers on factors affecting maternal role attainment, *Matern Child Nurs J* 19(1):63, 1990.

Makey M, Miller H: Women's views of postpartum sibling visitation, *Matern Child Nurs J* 20(1):40, 1992.

Mercer RT, Ferketich SL: Predictors of parental attachment during early parenthood, *J Adv Nurs* 15(3):268, 1990.

Palkovitz R: Changes in father-infant bonding beliefs across couples' first transition to parenthood, *Matern Child Nurs J* 20(3-4):141, 1992.

Tomlinson PS, Rothenberg MA, Carver LD: Behavioral interaction of fathers with infants oand mothers in the immediate postpartum period, *J Nurse Midwifery* 36(4):232, 1991.

Tomlinson PS: Verbal behavior associated with indicators of maternal atachment with the neonate, *JOGNN* 19(1): 76, 1990.

18 Nursing Care during the Postpartum Period

KITTY CASHION
CAROL LEE A. JOHNSTON

LEARNING OBJECTIVES

Define the key terms.

List the components of a complete postpartum physical and psychosocial assessment.

List signs of physical and psychosocial complications during the postpartum period.

Give examples of nursing diagnoses for physical and psychosocial care.

Identify goals for postpartum physical and psychosocial care.

Summarize nursing interventions to prevent infection and excessive bleeding.

Summarize nursing interventions to promote normal bowel and bladder patterns, care of the breasts of women who are breastfeeding or bottle-feeding, and the health of future pregnancies and children.

Summarize nursing interventions to support women and their families in developing parenting skills and in adjusting to the birth of a new baby.

Describe a variety of methods of family planning.

State the advantages and disadvantages of commonly used methods of family planning.

Explain the common nursing interventions that facilitate the use of family planning.

Recognize ethical and legal considerations of control of fertility.

Explain the influence of cultural expectations on postpartum adjustment.

Discuss the nurse's responsibilities related to discharge teaching and preparation for home care.

KEY TERMS

adaptive behavior
afterbirth pains
basal body temperature (BBT)
calendar method
cervical mucus method
condom
contraception
couplet care
diaphragm
engorgement
fertile period
fourth stage of labor
Homans' sign
intrauterine device (IUD)
Kegel exercises
Kleihauer-Betke test
lactation suppression
oral hormonal contraceptives
oxytocic medications
periodic abstinence
postpartum blues
Rh immune globulin
rubella vaccine
safe period
sibling rivalry
sitz bath
spermicide
spinnbarkheit
thromboembolism
thrombus
uterine atony

RELATED TOPICS

Breastfeeding *(Chap. 15)* • Engorgement *(Chap. 15 and 16)* • Episiotomy *(Chap. 12)* • Family dynamics after childbirth *(Chap. 17)* • Hemorrhagic disorders *(Chap. 21)* • Infection *(Chap. 21)* • Menstrual cycle *(Chap. 3)* • Neurobehavior of the newborn *(Chap. 13 and 14)* • Nutrition *(Chap. 8)* • Postpartum depression *(Chap. 23)* • Postpartum psychosis *(Chap. 23)* • Taking in, taking hold phases *(Chap. 17)* • Toxic shock syndrome *(Chap. 21)* • Uterine involution *(Chap. 16)*

The goal of nursing care in the immediate postpartum period is to assist women and their partners during their initial transition to parenting. The approach to the care of women after birth has changed from one modeled on sick care to one that is wellness oriented. Consequently, in the United States most women remain hospitalized no more than 1 or 2 days after giving birth. Because there is so much important information to be shared with these women in a very short time, it is vital that their care be thoughtfully planned and provided. The nurse provides care that focuses on the woman's physiologic recovery, her psychologic well-being, and her ability to care for herself and her new baby. In addition, the nurse considers the needs of other family members and includes strategies in the plan of care to assist the family in adjusting to the new baby.

To provide quality care, the nurse must be knowledgeable about physical changes in the mother (see Chapter 16) and psychosocial and emotional changes in the entire family (see Chapter 17). This chapter focuses on using the nursing process to meet both the mother's and the family's needs during this crucial time.

Care Management—Physical Needs

✧ ASSESSMENT

After completion of the initial 1-hour to 2-hour recovery period following childbirth, a time often referred to as the **fourth stage of labor,** mothers are usually transferred by wheelchair or gurney from the labor and birth unit to a postpartum unit. At this time the nurse who was present for the birth may continue to provide care, or a postpartum nurse may assume this responsibility. In hospitals using the labor, delivery, recovery, postpartum (LDRP) concept, however, the woman remains in the same room where she labored and gave birth.

A complete physical assessment, including measurement of vital signs, is performed upon admission to the postpartum unit. Another essential piece of assessment data that must be obtained on admission to the postpartum unit is a comprehensive report of intrapartal events (see Table 12-7). Other components of the initial assessment include the mother's emotional status, energy level, degree of physical discomfort, hunger, and thirst. To some degree, her knowledge level concerning self-care and infant care can also be determined at this time.

Vital Signs

Assessment of the patient's blood pressure, pulse, and respirations is usually performed every 15 minutes during the first hour after childbirth (see Procedure 12-3 on p. 307). If the woman's condition remains stable, these assessments are made less frequently after completion of the initial recovery period, for example, every 30 minutes for 2 hours and then hourly for another 2 hours. The mother's temperature is assessed upon admission to the recovery area and again 1 hour later. If the woman's vital signs remain within normal limits, they will likely be assessed every 4 to 8 hours for the remainder of her hospitalization.

Ongoing Physical Assessment

The postpartum woman should be thoroughly evaluated each shift throughout hospitalization. Physical assessments include evaluation of the breasts, uterine fundus, lochia, perineum, bladder and bowel function, vital signs, and legs. An example of a critical care path for progression of postpartum physical changes over the first 3 days appears on p. 465. Signs of potential problems that may be identified during the assessment process are listed in the Signs of Potential Complications box on page 465.

Routine Laboratory Tests

Several laboratory tests may be performed in the immediate postpartum period. Hemoglobin and hematocrit values are often requested on the first postpartum day to assess blood loss during childbirth. In some hospitals a clean-catch or catheterized urine specimen may be obtained and sent for routine urinalysis or culture and sensitivity, especially if an indwelling urinary catheter was inserted during the intrapartum period. In addition, the woman's prenatal record should be reviewed to determine her rubella and Rh status and the need for possible treatment.

✧ NURSING DIAGNOSES

Although all women experience similar physiologic changes during the postpartum period, certain factors act to make each woman's experience unique. From a physiologic standpoint the length and difficulty of the labor, type of birth (vaginal or cesarean), presence of episiotomy and/or lacerations, and whether she plans to breastfeed or bottle-feed are factors to be investigated with each woman. After analyzing the data obtained during the assessment process, the nurse establishes nursing diagnoses that will provide a guide for planning care. Examples of nursing diagnoses frequently established for the postpartum patient include the following:

High risk for infection related to
- Childbirth trauma to tissues

Constipation or urinary retention related to
- Postchildbirth discomfort
- Childbirth trauma to tissues

Sleep pattern disturbance related to
- Discomforts of postpartum period
- Long labor process
- Infant care and hospital routine

Pain related to
- Involution of uterus

CAREPATH

Care Path Postpartum Changes (Days 1 through 3)

Assessment	2 to 24 Hours (Day 1)	25 to 48 Hours (Day 2)	49 to 72 Hours (Day 3)
TEMPERATURE	97.1° F (36.2° C) 100.4° F (38° C)	Within normal range	Within normal range
PULSE	Bradycardia: 50 to 70 beats/min	Bradycardia may persist or rate may return to normal range	Bradycardia may persist or rate may return to normal range
BLOOD PRESSURE	Within normal range	Within normal range	Within normal range
ENERGY LEVEL	Euphoric, happy, excited, or fatigued; may show need for sleep	Often tired, slow moving	Anxious to go home; level returning to normal
UTERUS	At umbilicus or just below; firm	1 cm or more below umbilicus; firm	2 cm or more below umbilicus; firm
LOCHIA	Rubra; moderate; few clots, if any; fleshy odor of normal menstrual flow	Rubra to serosa; moderate to scant; odor continues to be fleshy or absent	Rubra to serosa; scant; odor continues to be fleshy or absent
PERINEUM	Edematous; clean, healing, intact; episiotomy edges approximated	Edema lessening; clean, healing	Edema lessening or absent; clean, healing
LEGS	Pretibial or pedal edema; Homans' sign negative	Edema lessening; Homans' sign negative	Edema minimal or absent; Homans' sign negative
BREASTS	Remain soft to palpation; colostrum can be expressed	Begin to feel firmer; occasionally feel lumpy	Increase in vascularity and initiation of swelling; feel firmer and warmer to touch; milk expected within 2 to 4 days after birth
APPETITE	Excellent; may ask for double helpings, snacks	Usually remains excellent	Varies; appetite may have returned to normal or may lessen (especially if patient is constipated)
ELIMINATION Voiding Defecation	Up to 3000 ml None expected; stool softener	Large amounts None expected; stool softener	Amount/24 hours is lessening Usually defecates
DISCOMFORT	Generalized aching; perineal area; episiotomy, hemorrhoids, afterbirth pains	Muscle aches; perineal area: episiotomy, hemorrhoids	Possible tension headache, perineal area: usually lessening; breasts, nipples

SIGNS OF POTENTIAL COMPLICATIONS

PHYSIOLOGIC PROBLEMS

Temperature	More than 100.4° F (38° C) after the first 24 hours
Pulse	Tachycardia, marked bradycardia
Blood pressure	Hypotension or hypertension
Energy level	Lethargy, extreme fatigue
Uterus	Deviated from the midline, boggy, remains above the umbilicus after 24 hours
Lochia	Heavy, foul odor; bright red bleeding that is not lochia
Perineum	Pronounced edema, not intact, signs of infection, marked discomfort
Legs	Homans' sign positive; painful, reddened area; warmth on posterior aspect of calf
Breasts	Redness, heat, pain, cracked and fissured nipples, inverted nipples, palpable mass
Appetite	Lack of appetite
Elimination	*Urine:* inability to void, urgency, frequency, dysuria; *bowel:* constipation, diarrhea
Rest	Inability to rest or sleep

- Trauma to perineum
- Episiotomy
- Hemorrhoids
- Engorged breasts

High risk for injury related to

- Postpartum hemorrhage
- Effects of anesthesia

Knowledge deficit related to

- Importance of voiding as deterrent to hemorrhage

Ineffective breastfeeding related to

- Maternal discomfort
- Infant positioning
- Normal physiologic response

✤ EXPECTED OUTCOMES

The nursing plan of care includes both the postpartum woman and her infant, even if the nursery nurse retains primary responsibility for the infant. In many hospitals, **couplet care** (also called mother and baby care or single room maternity care) is practiced. In this approach the nurse has been educated in both mother and infant care and functions as the primary nurse for both mother and infant, even if the infant is kept in the nursery. This approach is a variation of rooming-in, in which the mother and child room together and mother and nurse share the care of the infant. The organization of the mother's care must take the newborn into consideration. The day actually revolves around the baby's feeding and care times. In couplet care, responsibility and accountability for infant care and patient education rest with the primary nurse.

Once the nursing diagnoses are formulated, the nurse plans with the patient what nursing measures will be appropriate and which are to be given priority. During her hospital stay the mother is encouraged to assume increasing responsibility for her self-care and her infant's care. As the patient and her partner provide more care for herself and the baby, the nurse's role changes from one of providing direct care to one primarily of teaching, encouragement, and support.

The nursing plan of care will include assessments to detect deviations from normal physical changes, measures to relieve discomfort or pain, and safety measures to prevent injury or infection. The plan of care will also include teaching and counseling measures designed to promote the patient's feelings of competence in self-care and baby care. Family members are included in the teaching. The nurse evaluates continuously and is ready to change the plan if indicated. Almost all hospitals use standardized care plans as a base. The nurse's ability to adapt the standardized plan to specific medical and nursing diagnoses results in individualized patient care. Caution is advised against total reliance on a standardized plan; by doing so the uniqueness of the individual may be overlooked.

Expected outcomes for the postpartum period are based on the nursing diagnoses identified for the individual patient. Examples of common expected outcomes for physiologic needs are that the woman will:

1. Remain free from infection
2. Demonstrate normal involution and lochial characteristics
3. Remain comfortable and injury free
4. Demonstrate normal bowel and bladder patterns
5. Demonstrate knowledge of breast care for breastfeeding and nonbreastfeeding, as appropriate
6. Protect the health of future pregnancies and children
7. Integrate the newborn into the family

✤ COLLABORATIVE CARE

Nurses play many roles while implementing the nursing plan of care. They provide direct physical care, teach mother and baby care, and provide anticipatory guidance and counseling. Perhaps most important of all they nurture the patient by providing encouragement and support as the woman begins to assume the many tasks of motherhood. Nurses who take the time to "mother the mother" do much to increase feelings of self-confidence in new mothers.

The first step in providing individualized care is to confirm the patient's identity by checking her wrist band. At the same time the infant's identification number is matched with the corresponding band on the mother's wrist. The nurse demonstrates caring and respect by determining how the mother wishes to be addressed and then notes her preference in her record and in her nursing plan of care.

The woman and her family are oriented to their surroundings. Familiarity with the unit, routines, resources, and personnel reduces one potential source of anxiety—the unknown. The mother is reassured through knowing whom and how she can call for assistance and what she can expect in the way of supplies and services. If the woman's usual daily routine before admission differs from the facility's routine, the nurse works with the woman to develop a mutually acceptable and workable routine.

Implementation of the nursing care plan involves putting into practice specific activities that should result in achieving the expected outcomes planned for each individual patient.

Prevention of Infection

One important means of preventing infection is maintenance of a clean environment. Bed linens should be changed daily, and disposable pads and draw sheets may need to be changed even more frequently. Patients should avoid walking about barefoot to avoid contaminating bed linens when they return to bed. Supervision of use of facilities to prevent cross-contamination is also necessary. For example, a common sitz bath or heat lamp must be scrubbed after each woman's use. Staff members are another important part of the hospital environment. Personnel must be conscientious about their hand-washing techniques to prevent cross infection. Universal precautions must be practiced. Staff members with colds, coughs, or skin infections (for example, a cold sore on the lips [herpes simplex virus, type 1]) must follow hospital protocol when in contact with postpartum patients.

Proper care of the episiotomy site and any perineal lacerations prevents infection in the genitourinary area and aids the healing process. Educating the woman to wipe from front to back (urethra to anus) after voiding or defecating is a simple but extremely effective first step. In many hospitals a squeeze bottle filled with warm water

---

BOX 18-1

Interventions for Episiotomy, Lacerations, and Hemorrhoids

Explain both procedure and rationale before implementation

CLEANSING

Wash perineum with mild soap and warm water at least once daily.

Cleanse from symphysis pubis to anal area.

Apply peripad from front to back, protecting inner surface of pad from contamination.

Wrap soiled pad and place in covered waste container.

Remind to change pad every time she voids or defecates or at least 4 times per day.

Wash hands before and after changing pads.

Assess amount and character of lochia with each pad change.

ICE PACK

Apply a covered ice pack to perineum from front to back.
1. During first 2 hours to decrease edema formation and increase comfort
2. After the first 2 hours following the birth to provide anesthetic effect

SQUEEZE BOTTLE

Demonstrate for and assist woman: explain rationale.

Fill bottle with tap water warmed to approximately 100° F (38° C) (comfortably warm on the wrist).

Instruct woman to position nozzle between her legs so that squirts of water reach perineum as she sits on toilet seat. Explain that it will take whole bottle of water over perineum.

Remind her to blot dry with toilet paper or clean wipes.

Remind her to avoid contamination from anal area.

Apply new clean pad.

SITZ BATH

Built-in type (Fig. 18-1):

Prepare bath by thoroughly scrubbing with cleaning agent and rinsing.

Pad with towel before filling.

Fill one-half to one-third full with water of correct temperature: 100.4° F to 105° F (38° to 40.6° C).*

Encourage woman to use at least twice a day for 20 minutes.

Place call bell within easy reach.

Teach woman to enter bath by tightening gluteal muscles and keeping them tightened and then relaxing them after she is in the bath.

Place dry towels within reach.

Ensure privacy.

Check woman in 15 minutes; assess pulse as needed.

Disposable type:

Clamp tubing and fill bag with warm water.

Raise toilet seat, place bath in bowl with overflow opening directed toward back of toilet.

Place container above toilet bowl.

Attach tube into groove at front of bath.

Loosen tube clamp to regulate rate of flow: fill bath to about one-half full; continue as above for built-in sitz bath.

SURGI-GATOR

Assemble Surgi-Gator (Fig. 18-2).

Instruct woman regarding use and rationale.

Follow package directions.

Instruct woman to sit on toilet with legs apart and to put nozzle so tip is just past the perineum, adjusting placement as needed.

Remind her to return her applicator to her bedside stand.

DRY HEAT

Inspect lamp for defects.

Cover lamp with towels.

Position lamp 50 cm (20 in) from perineum: use 3 times a day for 20-minute periods.

Teach regarding use of 40-W bulb at home.

Provide draping over woman.

If same lamp is being used by several women, clean it carefully between uses.

TOPICAL APPLICATIONS

Apply anesthetic cream or spray: use sparingly 3 to 4 times per day.

Offer witch hazel pads (Tucks) after voiding or defecating; woman pats perineum dry from front to back, then applies witch hazel pads.

---

*Some authors propose cool sitz bath (Ramler, Roberts, 1986).

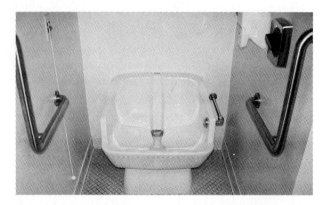

FIG. 18-1 Sitz bath. (Courtesy Kim Molloy, San Jose, CA.)

or a betadine solution is used after each voiding to cleanse the perineal area (Box 18-1). The patient should also be taught to change her perineal pad from front to back, each time she voids or defecates, and to wash her hands thoroughly before and after doing so.

Prevention of Excessive Bleeding

The most common cause of excessive bleeding following childbirth is **uterine atony,** failure of the uterine muscle to contract firmly. The uterus feels soft and limp to palpation. The two most important interventions for preventing excessive bleeding, therefore, are maintaining good uterine tone and preventing bladder distention.

Maintenance of Uterine Tone

A major intervention to maintain good tone is stimulation by gently massaging the uterine fundus until firm. Fundal massage may cause a temporary increase in the amount of vaginal bleeding seen as pooled blood leaves the uterus. Clots may also be expelled. Patient education is extremely important in maintaining uterine tone. Fundal massage can be a very uncomfortable procedure. Understanding the causes and dangers of uterine atony and the purpose of fundal massage can help the woman to be more cooperative. Teaching her to do self-fundal massage enables the patient to maintain some control and decreases her anxiety. The uterus may remain boggy even after massage and expulsion of clots. If this occurs, it is important that the nurse remain with the patient and summon help. The primary health care provider should be notified immediately. Additional interventions likely to be employed are administration of intravenous fluids and **oxytocic medications** (drugs that stimulate contraction of the uterine smooth muscle). Table 18-1 contains information about common oxytocic medications.

Prevention of Bladder Distention

A full bladder causes the uterus to be displaced above the umbilicus and well to one side of midline in the abdomen. It also prevents the uterus from contracting normally. Nursing interventions focus on helping the

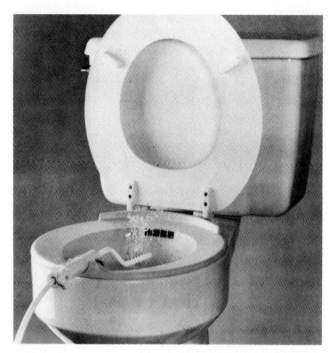

FIG. 18-2 Hygienic sitz bath (SurgiGator) for perineal care. (Courtesy Andermac, Inc., Yuba City, CA.)

woman spontaneously empty her bladder as soon as possible. The first priority is to assist the woman to the bathroom or onto a bedpan if she is unable to ambulate. Having the woman listen to running water, placing her hands in warm water, or pouring water from a squeeze bottle over her perineum may stimulate voiding. Other techniques include assisting the woman into the shower or sitz bath and encouraging her to void or placing oil of peppermint in a bedpan under the woman. The vapors may relax the urinary meatus and trigger spontaneous voiding.

If these measures are unsuccessful, a sterile catheter may be inserted to drain the urine. In the past, nurses were taught that suddenly emptying a distended bladder could result in hemorrhage, syncope, sepsis, and shock. Nursing textbooks usually recommended that no more than 750 to 1000 ml of urine be removed at one time. Little scientific evidence exists to support this practice, however. Complete bladder emptying is surely more comfortable, and probably at least as safe, as serial drainage (Bristoll et al, 1989).

LEGAL TIP: **Patient Abandonment**

 In an emergency situation the nurse must remain with the patient and call for help. Leaving the patient can lead to a charge of patient abandonment.

Evaluation of the woman's responses to intervention is an ongoing part of the nursing process. All responses to interventions should be carefully recorded. If the expected outcomes are not met or new needs emerge, the plan of care is modified accordingly. For example, if the

TABLE 18-1 Pharmacologic Measures to Stimulate Uterine Tone

INTERVENTION	ACTION, USES DURING PUERPERIUM	ONSET OF EFFECT, DURATION, USUAL DOSE	CONTRAINDICATIONS, PRECAUTIONS	COMMENTS
Oxytocin injection, USP (10 U/ml) (Pitocin, Syntocinon, Uteracon); oxytocic, synthetic posterior pituitary hormone	Stimulates phasic uterine muscle contraction; promotes milk ejection (let-down) reflex, facilitates flow of milk during engorgement	IV injection, 10 U; onset in 1 min IV infusion, 10 to 40 U/1000 ml 5% dextrose or physiologic electrolyte solution IM injection, 3 to 10 U; onset in 3 to 7 min; duration 30 to 60 min	Hypersensitivity; return of atony when effect wears off; may cause severe hypertension if patient is also receiving ephedrine, methoxamine, or other vasopressors	Alert: Assess for return of atony; store in cool place
Ergonovine, USP, NF (Ergotrate maleate); oxytocic, ergot alkaloid	Stimulates prolonged, nonphasic uterine contractions	Oral: 0.2 to 0.4 mg every 6 to 12 hours for 48 hours; onset in 6 to 15 min IM injection: 0.2 mg (1 ml) if nausea precludes oral preparation, onset in a few minutes Initial response: firm, tetanic contraction Subsequent response: alternating minor relaxations/contractions for 1½ hour; strong rhythmic contractions for 3 to 4 hours after injection	Severe hypertensive episodes may occur if given to hypertensive patients or those receiving vasoconstrictors; hypersensitivity; nausea, vomiting; sudden change in blood pressure or pulse; rare cases of myocardial infarction have been associated with postpartum use	Alert: Assess for changes in blood pressure, pulse; store in cool place in a light-resistant container
Methylergonovine, NF (Methergine); oxytocic, ergot alkaloid and congener of lysergic acid (LSD)	Stimulates rapid, sustained tetanic uterine contractions; used in treatment of subinvolution; has only minimum vasoconstrictive effect	Oral: 0.2 mg tab every 6 to 8 hours for maximum of 1 week; onset in 5 to 10 min IM injection 0.2 mg (1 ml) every 2 to 4 hours; onset in 2 to 5 min IV infusion (*emergency only*): 0.2 mg (1 ml) *slowly over 60 sec;* onset immediate	Nausea, vomiting; transient hypertension; dizziness, headache; tinnitus; diaphoresis; palpitations; temporary chest pains	Alert: Do not administer with Percodan—may result in hallucinations; assess blood pressure; store in cold place, away from light
Carboprost (Prostin/M15); oxytocic, prostaglandin	Stimulates rapid, sustained uterine contractions; used for treatment of uterine atony and uterine inversion	IM injection 1 ampule (250 μg), onset within minutes; intramyometrial injection (by primary care provider only), ½ to 2 ampules (125 to 500 μg) diluted with 10 ml saline (injected transabdominally into anterior wall of uterus); onset within minutes	Severe hypertension (systolic >170 mm Hg or diastolic >100 mm Hg) and with severe symptomatic asthma Diarrhea seen with dosage above 1 ampule; systolic and diastolic blood pressure usually rises; bronchoconstriction and wheezing are concerns	Alert: Monitor blood pressure and for adverse reactions; store in refrigerator

uterus is firm and the bladder empty, something other than uterine atony is causing the excessive bleeding. Immediately following childbirth other causes of excessive bleeding include unrepaired vaginal or cervical lacerations and disseminated intravascular coagulation (DIC). Later in the postpartum period subinvolution of the placental site, retained placental fragments, and infection can cause excessive uterine bleeding. Further assessment is necessary to determine the cause and correct the problem.

Promotion of Comfort, Rest, Ambulation, and Exercise

Comfort

Most women experience some degree of discomfort during the immediate postpartum period. Common causes of discomfort include afterbirth pains, episiotomy or perineal lacerations, hemorrhoids, and breast engorgement. The woman's description of the type and severity of her pain is the nurse's best guide in choosing an appropriate intervention. To confirm the location and extent of discomfort, the nurse inspects and palpates areas of pain as appropriate for redness, swelling, discharge, and heat, and observes for body tension, guarded movements, and facial tension. Blood pressure, pulse, and respirations may be elevated in response to acute pain. Diaphoresis may accompany severe pain. A lack of objective symptoms does not necessarily mean there is no pain, since there may also be a cultural component to the expression of pain. Nursing interventions are intended to eliminate the pain sensation entirely or reduce it to a tolerable level that allows the woman to care for herself and her baby. Nurses may employ both nonpharmacologic and pharmacologic interventions to promote comfort. As a rule, nonpharmacologic measures should be employed first, either alone or in combination with pharmacologic interventions. Pain relief is enhanced by using more than one method or route.

Nonpharmacologic Interventions. **Afterbirth pains** are the menstrual-like cramps experienced by many women as the uterus contracts following childbirth. Warmth, distraction, imagery, therapeutic touch, relaxation, and interaction with the infant may decrease the discomfort associated with these uterine contractions.

Simple interventions that can decrease the discomfort associated with an episiotomy or perineal lacerations are to encourage the woman to lie on her side whenever possible and to use a pillow when sitting. Other interventions include application of an ice pack, topical applications (if ordered), dry heat, cleansing with a squeeze bottle or Surgi-Gator, and a cleansing shower, tub bath, or sitz bath. Many of these interventions are also effective for hemorrhoids, especially ice packs,

sitz baths, and topical applications (such as witch hazel pads). Box 18-1 gives more specific information about these interventions.

The discomfort associated with engorged breasts may be lessened by applying either ice or heat to the breasts and wearing a well-fitted support bra. Decisions about specific interventions for engorgement are based on whether the woman chooses breastfeeding or bottle-feeding (see Chapter 15).

Pharmacologic Interventions. Most health care providers routinely order a variety of analgesics to be administered as needed, including both narcotic and non-narcotic choices, with their dosage and time frequency ranges. Patient-controlled analgesia (PCA) pumps and continuous epidural analgesia infusions are two newer technologies now frequently used to provide postpartum pain relief. Many women want to participate in decisions about analgesia. Severe pain, however, may interfere with active participation in choosing pain relief measures. If an analgesic is to be given, the nurse must make a clinical judgment of the type, dosage, and frequency from the medications ordered. The woman is informed of the prescribed analgesic and its common side effects.

Breastfeeding mothers often have concerns about the effects on the infant of taking an analgesic. Often the timing of medications can be adjusted to minimize infant exposure. A mother may be given pain medication immediately after breastfeeding, for example, so that the interval between medication administration and the next nursing period is as long as possible. Although nearly all drugs present in maternal circulation are also found in breast milk, many analgesics commonly used during the postpartum period are considered relatively safe for breastfeeding mothers (see Appendix G). The decision to administer medications of any kind to a breastfeeding mother must always be made by carefully weighing the woman's need for the drug against actual or potential risks to the infant (Briggs et al, 1990; Anderson, 1991).

Pain is a frightening, lonely experience, and a woman should feel confident that her need for pain relief will be attended to. Therefore the nurse evaluates the effectiveness of the pain relief measures employed until acceptable pain relief is achieved. When acceptable analgesia has been achieved, the nurse evaluates with the woman what pain relief measures were helpful and modifies the plan of care if necessary.

If acceptable pain relief has not been obtained in 1 hour and there has been no change in the initial assessment, the nurse may need to contact the primary care provider for additional pain relief orders or further directions. Unrelieved pain results in fatigue, anxiety, and a worsening perception of the pain. It might also indicate the presence of a previously unknown or untreated problem. Further assessment and treatment will likely be necessary to determine the cause of the pain and correct it.

Rest, Ambulation, and Exercise

Rest. The excitement and exhilaration experienced after the birth of the infant may make rest difficult. The new mother, who is often anxious about her ability to care for her infant or is uncomfortable, may also have difficulty sleeping. In the days that follow, the demands of the infant, along with the influence of the hospital environment and routines, contribute to alterations in her sleep pattern.

Interventions must be planned to meet the woman's individual needs for sleep and rest. Backrubs, other comfort measures, and medication for sleep for the first few nights may be necessary. Hospital and nursing routines also may be adjusted to meet individual needs. In addition, the nurse can help the family limit visitors and provide a comfortable chair or bed for the partner.

Ambulation. Early ambulation is successful in reducing the incidence of thromboembolism and in promoting women's more rapid recovery of strength. Confinement to bed is not required for women who had general anesthesia, who had epidural or spinal anesthesia, or who had local anesthesia such as pudendal block. Free movement is permitted once the anesthetic wears off unless an analgesic has been administered. After the first vital rest period is over, the mother is encouraged to ambulate frequently.

Prevention of **thrombus** (clot formation) is part of the nursing care plan. If a woman remains in bed longer than 8 hours (e.g., after cesarean birth), exercise to promote circulation in the legs is indicated using the following routine:

1. Alternate flexion and extension of feet.
2. Rotate ankle in circular motion.
3. Alternate flexion and extension of legs.
4. Press back of knee to bed surface; relax.

If the woman is susceptible to **thromboembolism,** the use of estrogens to inhibit or suppress lactation should be avoided. Women with varicosities are encouraged to wear support hose. The woman is encouraged to walk about actively for true ambulation and discouraged from sitting immobile in a chair. If a thrombus is suspected, as evidenced by a positive **Homans' sign** (complaint of pain in calf muscles when dorsiflexion of foot is forced), warmth, redness, or tenderness in the suspected leg, the primary health care provider should be notified immediately; meanwhile the woman should be confined to bed, with the affected limb elevated on pillows.

Exercise. Most women who have just given birth are extremely interested in regaining their nonpregnant figure. Postpartum exercise can begin soon after birth, although the woman should be encouraged to start with simple exercises and gradually progress to more strenuous ones. Fig. 18-3 illustrates a number of exercises appropriate for the new mother. Kegel pelvic exercises to strengthen muscle tone are extremely important, particularly after vaginal birth. To perform them, the woman alternately contracts and relaxes the muscles in her vagina, rectum, and buttocks. **Kegel exercises** help women to regain the muscles tone that is often lost as pelvic tissues are torn and stretched during pregnancy and birth (p. 137). Women who maintain muscle strength may benefit years later by experiencing less stress urinary incontinence (Sampselle, 1990).

Promotion of Normal Bowel and Bladder Patterns

Bladder

After giving birth the mother should void spontaneously within 6 to 8 hours. The first several voidings should be measured to document adequate emptying of the bladder. A volume of at least 150 ml is expected for each voiding. Some women experience difficulty in emptying the bladder, possibly a result of diminished bladder tone, edema from trauma, or fear of discomfort. Nursing interventions for inability to void and bladder distention are discussed on p. 468.

Bowel

Nursing interventions to promote normal bowel elimination include educating the woman about measures to avoid constipation. These include ensuring adequate roughage and fluid intake and promoting exercise. Alerting the woman to side effects of medications such as narcotic analgesics (i.e., decreased gastrointestinal tract motility) may encourage her to implement measures to reduce the risk of constipation. Stool softeners are often routinely ordered, and laxatives may be necessary during the early postpartum period. With early discharge a new mother may be home before having a bowel movement.

Breastfeeding Promotion and Lactation Suppression

Breastfeeding Promotion

The first 2 hours after birth are an excellent time to encourage the mother to breastfeed. The infant is in an alert state and ready to breastfeed, which will aid in the contraction of the uterus and prevention of maternal hemorrhage. This is a wonderful opportunity for the nurse to instruct the mother in breastfeeding and to assess the physical appearance of the breasts. (See Chapter 15 for further information on assisting the breastfeeding woman.)

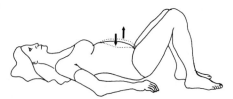

Abdominal Breathing. Lie on back with knees bent. Inhale deeply through nose. Keep ribs stationary and allow abdomen to expand upwards. Exhale slowly but forcefully while contracting the abdominal muscles; hold for 3 to 5 seconds while exhaling. Relax.

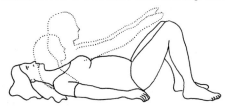

Reach for the Knees. Lie on back with knees bent. While inhaling deeply lower chin onto chest. While exhaling, raise head and shoulders slowly and smoothly and reach for knees with arms outstretched. The body should only rise as far as the back will naturally bend while waist remains on floor or bed (about 6 to 8 inches). Slowly and smoothly lower head and shoulders back to starting position. Relax.

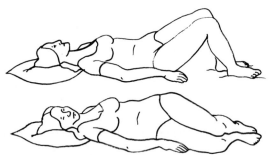

Double Knee Roll. Lie on back with knees bent. Keeping shoulders flat and feet stationary, slowly and smoothly roll knees over to the left to touch floor or bed. Maintaining a smooth motion, roll knees back over to the right until they touch floor or bed. Return to starting position and relax.

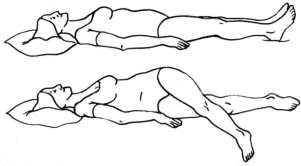

Leg Roll. Lie on back with legs straight. Keeping shoulders flat and legs straight, slowly and smoothly lift left leg and roll it over to touch the right side of floor or bed and return to starting position. Repeat, rolling right leg over to touch left side of floor or bed. Relax.

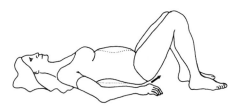

Combined Abdominal Breathing and Supine Pelvic Tilt (Pelvic Rock). Lie on back with knees bent. While inhaling deeply, roll pelvis back by flattening lower back on floor or bed. Exhale slowly but forcefully while contracting abdominal muscles and tightening buttocks. Hold for 3 to 5 seconds while exhaling. Relax.

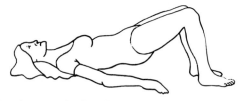

Buttocks Lift. Lie on back with arms at sides, knees bent and feet flat. Slowly raise buttocks and arch back. Return slowly to starting position.

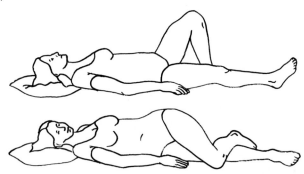

Single Knee Roll. Lie on back with with right leg straight and left leg bent at the knee. Keeping shoulders flat, slowly and smoothly roll left knee over to the right to touch floor or bed and then back to starting position. Reverse position of legs. Roll right knee over to the left to touch floor or bed and return to starting position. Relax.

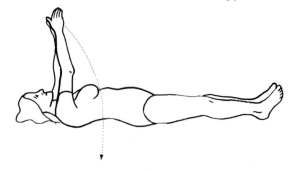

Arm Raises. Lie on back with arms extended at 90° angle from body. Raise arms so they are perpendicular and hands touch. Lower slowly.

FIG. 18-3 Postpartum exercise should begin as soon as possible. The woman should start with simple exercises and gradually progress to more strenuous ones.

Lactation Suppression

Suppression of lactation is necessary when the woman has decided not to breastfeed or in the case of neonatal death. One very important nonpharmacologic intervention is wearing a well-fitted support bra or breast binder continuously for at least the first 72 hours after giving birth. Women should also avoid any breast stimulation, including running warm water over the breasts, newborn suckling, or pumping of the breasts. Few nonbreastfeeding mothers experience severe breast **engorgement** (swelling of breast tissue caused by increased blood and lymph supply to the breasts preceding lactation). If breast engorgement occurs, it can usually be managed satisfactorily with these nonpharmacologic interventions.

In the past an estrogen (Tace), a combination of estrogen and testosterone (Deladumone), or bromocriptine (Parlodel) was often prescribed for lactation suppression. Recently there has been a shift away from the use of these drugs. Lactation suppression is no longer considered an indication for the use of Tace, Deladumone, or Parlodel. Parlodel inhibits prolactin secretion, thus preventing milk production and possible subsequent breast engorgement. Recently seizures, strokes, and myocardial infarctions have been reported in postpartum women taking Parlodel for lactation suppression. The exact relationship between Parlodel use and these adverse reactions has not been established. The drug should definitely be used with caution. Women who develop severe or progressive headaches unresponsive to usual treatment while taking Parlodel should contact their health care providers immediately (Drug Facts and Comparisons, 1993; United States Pharmacopeial Convention, 1993).

Health Promotion of Future Pregnancies and Children

If the assessment data indicate the need, rubella vaccination and Rh immune globulin (RhoGam) are administered during the puerperium. Failure to administer these products to women at risk of contracting rubella or developing Rh isoimmunization can seriously jeopardize the health of any future pregnancies and children.

Rubella Vaccination

For women who have not had rubella (10% to 20% of all women) or women who are serologically negative (i.e., titer of 1:8 or less), a subcutaneous injection of **rubella vaccine** is recommended in the immediate postbirth period to prevent fetal anomalies in future pregnancies. Seroconversion occurs in approximately 90% of women vaccinated after birth. The live attenuated rubella virus is not communicable; therefore breastfeeding mothers can be vaccinated. However, the live attenuated rubella vaccine is made from duck eggs, so women who have allergies to these eggs may develop a hypersensitivity reaction to the vaccine, for which they will need

adrenalin. A transient arthralgia or rash is common in vaccinated women but is benign. The vaccine may be teratogenic, the patient should be informed about the vaccine (see Legal Tip).

LEGAL TIP: Rubella Vaccination

Informed consent for Rubella vaccination in the postpartum period includes information about the possible side effects and the risk of teratogenic effects. Women must understand that they must practice contraception to avoid pregnancy for 2 to 3 months after being vaccinated.

Prevention of Rh Isoimmunization

Injection of **Rh immune globulin** (a solution of gamma globulin that contains Rh antibodies) within 72 hours after birth prevents sensitization in the Rh-negative woman who has had a fetomaternal transfusion of Rh-positive red blood cells (RBCs). The Rh immune globulin promotes lysis of the fetal Rh-positive blood cells before the mother forms her own antibodies against them. Rh immune globulin is administered prenatally at 28 to 30 weeks' gestation to all Rh-negative, antibody (Coombs')-negative women as well as earlier in gestation should invasive procedures, such as amniocentesis, be performed. Postpartally Rh immune globulin is administered to all Rh-negative, antibody (Coombs')-negative women who give birth to Rh-positive infants. Also, it is extremely important that Rh immune globulin be administered after all known abortions occurring at or after 8 weeks' gestation.

The administration of 300 µg (1 vial) of Rh immune globulin is usually sufficient to prevent maternal sensitization. If a large fetomaternal transfusion is suspected, however, the dosage needed should be determined by performing a **Kleihauer-Betke test,** which detects fetal blood in the maternal circulation. If more than 15 ml fetal blood is present in maternal circulation, the dosage of Rh immune globulin must be increased.

A 1:1000 dilution of Rh immune globulin is crossmatched to the mother's RBCs to ensure compatibility. Since Rh immune globulin is a blood product, precautions similar to those used for transfusing blood are necessary when it is given.* The identification number on the patient's hospital wristband should correspond to the identification number found on the laboratory slip. The nurse must also check to see that the lot number on the laboratory slip corresponds to the lot number on the vial. Finally, the expiration date on the vial should be checked to ensure a usable product. Rh immune globulin is ad-

---

*There is some disagreement about whether Rh immune globulin should be considered a blood product. Health care providers need to discuss the most current information about this issue with women whose religious beliefs conflict with having blood products administered to them.

PLAN OF CARE

Spontaneous Vaginal Birth

Case History

Mary Williams, a 24-year-old first-time mother experienced a spontaneous vaginal birth with a midline episiotomy after 15 hours of labor and epidural analgesia. She plans to breastfeed her healthy daughter, who weighs 9 pounds 2 ounces. She is admitted to the postpartum unit after 2 hours in the recovery room.

Mary had a period of heavy vaginal bleeding after the birth; however, her fundus is now firm, and the lochia is moderate rubra. Her vital signs are temperature 99° F (37.2° C, BP 110/70 mm Hg, pulse 80 beats/min, respirations 18/min. An IV infusion of 5% dextrose and ½ normal saline with Pitocin is infusing at 20 drops per minute. Although fatigued and hungry, Mary and her husband, who was with her throughout the labor and birth, verbalize their excitement about the birth of their daughter.

Two hours later, Mary's postpartum assessment reveals that her fundus is 3 cm above the umbilicus, to the right side, and is boggy. Mary has saturated one peripad in the last 2 hours and has passed a few small clots. She is also complaining of pain at the episiotomy site.

EXPECTED OUTCOMES	IMPLEMENTATION	RATIONALE	EVALUATION
Nursing Diagnosis: High risk for fluid volume deficit related to uterine atony			
Mary's fundus will remain firm, lochia moderate without evidence of hemorrhage.	Assess tone and response to gentle massage.	Massage promotes contraction of uterus. Continued assessment determines need for further interventions.	Mary's fundus is firm at midline, and lochia rubra is moderate in amount.
	Check IV flow of oxytocin (Pitocin).	Pitocin stimulates uterine contraction; adequate infusion maintains level of oxytocin.	
	Express clots.	Empties uterus and promotes contractions.	
	Assess bladder for fullness and encourage voiding.	Full bladder interferes with uterine contraction.	
	Assess amount and character of lochia.	Indicates amount of blood loss.	
	Assess vital signs.	Further indication of amount of blood loss.	Mary's vital signs are normal and stable.
	Teach Mary how to assess and massage fundus.	Involvement in self-care maintains sense of control.	Mary demonstrates ability to assess and massage uterus.
Nursing Diagnosis: Perineal pain related to episiotomy and hemorrhoids			
Mary will state decreasing level of pain in the perineal area.	Explain and demonstrate: Use of hot or cold procedures to perineal area	Knowledge promotes self-care. Decreases pain: heat increases circulation; cold decreases edema.	Mary states stitches feel more comfortable.
Mary will state and demonstrate understanding of proper perineal self-care techniques.	Perineal hygiene: proper wiping, proper changing, and placement of peripad	Prevents contamination and infection that could cause pain.	Mary performs self-perineal care using proper technique at appropriate times.
	Side-lying position and sitting technique through tensing of gluteal muscles	Decreases pressure on area.	
	Use of analgesics	Reduces pain perception.	

PLAN OF CARE—cont'd

Spontaneous Vaginal Birth

EXPECTED OUTCOMES	IMPLEMENTATION	RATIONALE	EVALUATION
Nursing Diagnosis: Sleep pattern disturbances related to excitement, interrupted sleep, and discomfort			
Mary will state ability to sleep restfully and to feel rested while awake.	Individualize nursing routine to fit Mary's schedule.	Promotes individual sleep pattern.	Mary states, "I slept well during night and at nap time."
	Keep noise level in hall and at nursing station to minimum; close Mary's door while resting.	Reduces distracting external stimuli.	
	Arrange uninterrupted nap while baby sleeps.		Mary states, "I feel rested and refreshed."
	Advise Mary to limit visitors and telephone calls.		
	Discuss with Mary techniques used by her in the past to promote rest, for example, warm drink, reading, TV at bedtime.	Provides feeling of control. Promotes relaxation.	
	Provide specific comfort measures if experiencing pain: back rub, analgesics.	Reduces pain and tension. Promotes relaxation and rest.	

ministered to the mother intramuscularly. It should never be given to an infant. Rh immune globulin suppresses the immune response. Therefore the woman who receives both Rh immune globulin and rubella vaccine must be tested at 3 months to see if she has developed rubella immunity. If not, the woman will need another dose of rubella vaccine.

✦ EVALUATION

Evaluation of nursing care is ongoing and begins when the patient is admitted to the unit and ends only after discharge. If progress toward meeting the expected outcomes of care is not evident, interventions may need to be modified. As the patient's condition changes during her hospitalization, expected outcomes may need to be added or deleted. The nurse can be reasonably assured that care was effective when the expected outcomes of care have been achieved (see Plan of Care).

Care Management— Psychosocial Needs

Meeting the psychosocial needs of new mothers involves planning care that considers the composition and functioning of the entire family. Nurses assess the parents' reactions to the birth experience, feelings about them-

selves, and interactions with the new baby and other family members. Specific interventions are then planned to increase the parents' knowledge and self-confidence as they assume the care and responsibility of the new baby and integrate a new member into their existing family structure in a way that meets their cultural expectations.

✦ ASSESSMENT OF ADAPTATION TO PARENTHOOD

Impact of the Birth Experience

Many women indicate a need to examine the birth process itself and look at their own intrapartal behavior in retrospect (Konrad, 1987). Their partners may express similar desires. During pregnancy the woman and her partner may have developed a specific birth plan that includes a vaginal birth and very little medical intervention. If their birth experience was quite different (e.g., induction, epidural anesthesia, cesarean birth), both partners may need to mourn the loss of their expectations before they can adjust to the reality of their birth experience. Inviting them to review the events and describe how they feel helps the nurse assess how well they understand what happened and how well they have been able to put their childbirth experience into perspective. Feelings about giving birth can certainly affect both partners' adaptation to parenting.

Maternal Self-Image

An important assessment concerns the woman's self-concept, body image, and sexuality. How this new mother feels about herself and her body during the puerperium may affect her behavior and adaptation to parenting. The woman's self-concept and body image may also affect her sexuality.

Feelings related to sexual adjustment after childbirth are often a cause of concern for new parents. Women who have recently given birth may be reluctant to resume sexual intercourse for fear of pain or may worry that coitus could damage healing perineal tissue. Because many new parents are anxious for information but reluctant to bring up the subject, postpartum nurses should matter-of-factly include the topic of postpartum sexuality during their routine physical assessment. While examining the episiotomy site, for example, the nurse can say, "I know you're sore right now, but it probably won't be long until you (or you and your partner) are ready to make love again. Have you thought about what that might be like? Would you like to ask me questions?" This approach assures the woman and her partner that resuming sexual activity is a legitimate concern for new parents, and indicates the nurse's willingness to answer questions and share information.

Parent-Infant Interactions

A thorough postpartum psychosocial assessment includes evaluation of the parents' interactions with the new baby. Parental responses to the birth of a child include behaviors that are either adaptive or maladaptive. Both mother and father exhibit these behaviors, although to date most research has centered on the mother.

Many new parents experience parenting difficulties until their skills become established. Once they feel confidence in their skills, the increase in self-esteem promotes a positive affective response to the child. However, some parents exhibit parenting disorders (a matter of degree) that place the child in jeopardy and at risk. Protocols for the physical screening of high-risk pregnant women and fetuses have been developed and confirmed. However, tools predicting high-risk parenting behaviors require more replication over larger population samples before they can be used with the same precision.

The quality of motherliness or fatherliness in a parent's behavior prompts nurturing and protection as opposed to neglect or abuse of the child. Cues indicating the presence or absence of this quality appear early in the postbirth period as parents react to the newborn infant and continue the process of establishing a relationship (Table 18-2).

Adaptive Behavior

Adaptive behaviors stem from the parents' realistic perception and acceptance of their newborn's needs and her or his limited abilities, immature social responses, and helplessness. Parents exhibit adaptive behaviors when they find pleasure in their infant and in the tasks done for and with him or her; when they understand their infant's emotional states and provide comfort; and when they read the infant's cues for new experience and can sense the infant's fatigue level.

Maladaptive Behavior

Maladaptive behaviors are exhibited when parents respond inappropriately to the needs of their infant. They expect responses from the infant far in excess of the infant's ability to perform. They interpret inadequate responses as defiance or as negative judgment of parental capabilities. They obtain no pleasure from physical contact with their child. Such infants tend to be handled roughly. They are held in a manner that allows the head to dangle without support, and are not cuddled. The parents see the child as unattractive. The child-caring tasks of bathing and changing are viewed with disgust or annoyance. There is a lack of discrimination in responding to the infant's signals relative to hunger, fatigue, need for soothing or stimulating speech, and need for comforting body or eye contact. The parents of these infants often show excessive concern over the health of their child and cannot distinguish between the expected minor illnesses of childhood and serious disabilities. It appears difficult for them to accept their child as healthy and happy.

Interpretation of Infant Behavior

The parents' view of and response to their infant is profoundly affected by their interpretation of his or her behavior. Mothers and fathers often make value judgments about their infant's behavior and respond as though the baby had either praised or criticized them. They may see their infant as good and themselves as good parents if their infant sleeps and eats well, cries very little, and is easily consoled. On the other hand, parents of babies who cry excessively, are difficult to feed, exhibit an apathetic affect, or stiffen when held may feel that the baby is bad and see themselves as failures. If parents can be helped to see newborn behavior not as bad or good, but as their baby's unique way of communicating personality, needs, and desires, they will be well on the way to developing a healthy parent-child relationship.

Family Structure and Functioning

Another important component of the psychosocial assessment is looking at the family composition and functioning. A woman's adjustment to her role as mother is affected greatly by her relationships with her partner, her mother and other relatives, and any other children. Nurses can help to ease the new mother's return home by assessing for conflicts likely to occur among family members and helping the woman to plan strategies for dealing with those problems before discharge. For ex-

TABLE 18-2   Mothering Behaviors*

ADAPTIVE BEHAVIORS	MALADAPTIVE BEHAVIORS
FEEDING	
Offers appropriate amount and type of food to infant	Provides inadequate type or amount of food for infant
Holds infant in comfortable position during feeding	Does not hold infant, or holds in uncomfortable position during feeding
Burps baby during and after feeding	Does not burp infant
Prepares food appropriately	Prepares food inappropriately
Offers food at comfortable pace for infant	Offers food at pace too rapid or slow for infant's comfort
INFANT STIMULATION	
Provides appropriate verbal stimulation for infant during visit	Provides no, or only aggressive, verbal stimulation for infant during visit
Provides tactile stimulation for infant at times other than during feeding or moving infant away from danger	Does not provide tactile stimulation or only that of aggressive handling of infant
Provides age-appropriate toys	No evidence of age-appropriate toys
Interacts with infant in a way that provides for infant's satisfaction	Frustrates infant during interactions
INFANT REST	
Provides quiet or relaxed environment for infant's rest, including scheduled rest periods	Does not provide quiet environment or consistent schedule for rest periods
Ensures that infant's needs for food, warmth, and dryness are met before sleep	Does not attend to infant's needs for food, warmth, and dryness before sleep
PERCEPTION	
Demonstrates realistic perception of infant's condition in accordance with medical and nursing diagnoses	Shows unrealistic perception of infant's condition
Has realistic expectations for infant	Demonstrates unrealistic expectations of infant
Recognizes infant's unfolding skills or behavior	Has no awareness of infant's development
Shows realistic perception of own mothering behavior	Shows unrealistic perception of own mothering behavior
INITIATIVE	
Shows initiative in attempts to manage infant's problems, including actively seeking information about infants	Shows no initiative in attempts to meet infant's needs or to manage problems; does not follow through with plans
RECREATION	
Provides positive outlets for own recreation or relaxation	Does not provide positive outlets for own recreation or relaxation
INTERACTION WITH OTHER CHILDREN	
Demonstrates positive interaction with other children in home	Demonstrates hostile-aggressive interaction with other children in home
MOTHERING ROLE	
Expresses satisfaction with mothering	Expresses dissatisfaction with mothering

Reprinted by permission from Mercer RT: In Sonstegard LJ et al, editors: *Women's health: childbearing,* vol 2, New York, 1982, Grune & Stratton.
*These describe paternal as well as maternal behaviors.

SIGNS OF POTENTIAL COMPLICATIONS

PSYCHOSOCIAL NEEDS

Inability or refusal to discuss labor and birth experience

Refusal to interact with or care for baby (e.g., does not name baby, does not want to hold or feed baby)

Refusal to attend infant care (including breastfeeding) classes

Refusal to discuss contraception

Refers to self as ugly and useless

Excessive preoccupation with self (body image)

Marked depression

Lack of support system

ample, couples may have very different ideas about parenting. Dealing with the stresses of sibling rivalry and unsolicited grandparent advice can also affect the woman's transition to motherhood. Only by asking about other nuclear and extended family members can the nurse discover potential problems in family relationships and help to plan workable solutions for them. The Signs of Potential Complications box lists some signs that indicate a need for further assessment.

Impact of Cultural Diversity

The final component of a complete psychosocial assessment is the patient's cultural beliefs and values. Much of a woman's behavior during the postpartum period is strongly influenced by her cultural background. In today's world, where travel is commonplace, nurses are likely to come in contact with women from many different countries and cultures. The nurse must remember that all cultures have developed safe and satisfying methods of caring for new mothers and babies. Only by understanding and respecting the values and beliefs of each woman can the nurse design a plan of care to meet her individual needs.

Following is an example of one "clash of cultures." The nurse in this case was able to take this information and modify her plan of care to make it culturally congruent, and therefore more satisfying, for the patient.

▪ A Vietnamese woman who had been in the United States for 4 years requested rooming-in facilities following childbirth. Instead of participating in the care of her infant, she refused to do so, remained in bed, wore a woolen cap, and appeared distressed and angry. The staff were puzzled and upset by her behavior. One nurse decided to put newly learned concepts concerning cross-cultural nursing into effect. She began by praising the woman's ability to speak English and, after eliciting a smile, remarked, "Every country has developed good ways to look after mothers and babies. Would you tell me about the care in Vietnam?" There was

an immediate response. The woman explained that in her country women remained in bed for 10 days after birth and the biggest danger to their health was getting a cold. The baby was kept in the room with his mother, but either a grandmother or nurse took complete charge of the care.

✦ NURSING DIAGNOSES

After analyzing the data obtained during the assessment process, the nurse establishes nursing diagnoses to provide a guide for planning care. Examples of nursing diagnoses related to psychosocial issues that are frequently established for the postpartum patient include the following:

Altered family processes related to
- Unexpected birth of twins

Impaired verbal communication related to
- Patient's deafness
- Patient's language not the same as nurse's

Altered parenting related to
- Long, difficult labor
- Unmet expectations of labor and the birth

Knowledge/skill deficit related to
- Meaning of infant behavioral cues
- Holding, cuddling, interacting with infant

Anxiety related to
- Newness of parenting role, sibling rivalry, or response of grandparent

High risk for situational low self-esteem related to
- Lack of knowledge of infant characteristics or of caregiving skills
- Grandparent responses

Anxiety related to
- Insufficient knowledge of contraception and resumption of sexual activity

✦ EXPECTED OUTCOMES

The psychosocial plan of care for the postpartum woman includes all family members. The postnatal period is a crucial one for the family, since it contains the potential for crisis in family adjustment. Developing a plan of care that recognizes family strengths and provides support for family weaknesses does much to help family members take on new tasks and responsibilities.

Cultural issues must also be considered when planning care. It is important that nurses do not use their own cultural beliefs as a framework for care. Though the beliefs and behaviors of other cultures may seem strange, they should be encouraged so long as the mother wants to conform to them and she and the baby suffer no ill effects. On the other hand, the nurse should never assume that a mother wishes to participate in the behaviors practiced by a particular cultural group simply because she is a member of that culture. Many young women who are first-generation or second-generation

BOX 18-2

Some Cultural Beliefs about the Postpartum Period and Conception

POSTPARTUM CARE

Chinese, Mexican, Korean, and Southeast Asian women may wish to eat only warm foods and drink hot drinks to replace blood loss and to restore the balance of hot and cold in their bodies. These women may also wish to stay warm and avoid bathing, exercises, and hair washing for 7 to 30 days after childbirth. Self care may not be a priority; care by family members is preferred. These women may wear abdominal binders. They may prefer not to give their babies colostrum.

Haitian women may request to take the placenta home to bury or burn.

CONTRACEPTION

Birth control is government mandated in *China*. Most Chinese women will have an IUD inserted after the birth of their first child.

Saudi Arabian women will usually not practice birth control.

Mexican women will likely choose the rhythm method because most are Catholic.

(East) Indian men are encouraged to have a voluntary sterilization by vasectomy.

Americans follow their cultural traditions only when older family members are present.

Nonwestern cultures hold two general beliefs about the postpartum period. The first is that new mothers have a body imbalance between heat and cold. The Chinese, for example, believe that a postpartum woman's blood is weak (cold) and thickened (Ludman et al, 1989). Specific foods should be eaten and certain practices followed to restore the balance (Coughlin, 1965; Campbell, Chang, 1975; Hahn, Muecke, 1987; Lee et al, 1988; Lee, 1989; Horn, 1990; Ahumada, 1991; Park, Peterson, 1991; D'Avanzo, 1992; Geissler, 1994).

The second general belief is that mother and baby remain in an unclean state for a period of several weeks following birth. During this time mothers are to remain secluded, with limited activity. This period often ends with a ritual cleansing ceremony that restores purity (Stern et al, 1980; Horn, 1990; Geissler, 1994). Women who have immigrated to the United States or other Western nations may not have much help at home, making it extremely difficult for them to observe these activity restrictions (Park; Peterson, 1991). Box 18-2 lists some common cultural beliefs about the postpartum period.

As in planning care to meet physiologic needs, standardized care plans must be adapted to meet the specific needs of individual families. The nurse evaluates continuously and is ready to change the plan if necessary.

Expected psychosocial outcomes during the postpartum period are based on the nursing diagnoses identified for the individual patient and her family. Examples of common expected outcomes are listed below. The patient (family) will:

1. Demonstrate self-confidence in providing essential newborn care
2. Identify measures that promote a healthy personal adjustment in the postpartum period
3. Maintain healthy family functioning based on cultural norms and personal expectations

❖ COLLABORATIVE CARE

The nurse functions in the roles of teacher, encourager, and supporter, rather than doer, while implementing the psychosocial plan of care for a postpartum patient. Implementation of the psychosocial care plan involves carrying out specific activities to achieve the expected outcomes of care planned for each individual patient.

Promotion of Parenting Skills

New parents may well feel overwhelmed at the prospect of caring for a helpless, demanding newborn. Because today's families are smaller than in the past, many women and men grow up with little chance to gain knowledge and experience in infant care. In our mobile society extended family members such as aunts and grandparents often live too far away to provide much support and assistance. Many parents hesitate to seek help from professionals, friends, or family members or feel that they have no one to call upon, should they want to do so. Therefore one of the main concepts to be stressed repeatedly is that parenthood is a learned role. As with any other learned role, it takes time to master, improves with experience, and evolves gradually and continually as the needs of the parents and child change. Parents first begin to get acquainted with their new baby as the nurse performs a physical examination and describes any normal variations present. At this time the nurse can also discuss the baby's behavior, pointing out normal characteristics such as activity states and reflexes. Demonstrations and discussions of basic infant care skills, such as feeding, bathing, and diaper changing, are also included in nursing care. Through the loving and attentive manner nurses exhibit while providing physical care, they act as role models. As one nurse described it:

> ▪ I found the mother crying and distraught as she wrapped and unwrapped her baby. She said, "I don't seem to be able to do anything right." I took the baby from her and talked to him. "What are you doing to your mother? You've got her all upset!" The baby alerted to my voice and looked at me. Then I said to the mother, "Now, you talk to him." She said, "You're a big lovely boy, don't cry so much." The baby, hearing her voice, promptly turned his head from me to look at her. I said, "You see, he knows his mother's voice and pre-

fers it to mine." The mother was surprised and seemed very pleased and excited. We then reviewed how to wrap a baby snugly.

Parents should be given the opportunity to practice the infant care skills demonstrated by the nurse. Recognition and praise of their successes increase the parents' feelings of competence and confidence in their caretaking skills.

Because many mothers are discharged within 24 to 48 hours after giving birth, teaching often takes place during a period when the mother may have difficulty absorbing a great deal of information. Ament (1990) suggested that the presentation of only vital highlights may be more practical during the early puerperium. Telephone hotlines to hospital, clinic, or physician's office, home visits, books, pamphlets, and videotapes are all excellent resources that can be most helpful to parents after hospital discharge. Several well-done, inexpensive videotapes on baby and child care are listed in the bibliography at the end of this chapter.

Coping Strategies for New Parents
Healthy Personal Adjustment

Since hospital stays are usually short, parents leave the protective environment of the hospital in the "honeymoon" period of parenthood. The realities of recovery and the parenting role become evident quickly, especially for those without assistance in the home. Women may misjudge the actual amount of physical and emotional energy they possess and that care of an infant requires. They may expect to resume tasks too soon and then feel discouraged when they are unable to do so.

Tulman and Fawcett (1991) interviewed 96 mothers of healthy, full-term infants about their recovery from childbirth when the babies were 6 months of age. Al-most half the women had found the first 6 months after childbirth to be more difficult than they had expected. Perhaps providing pregnant women with more information on lifestyle changes after giving birth would help to ease their transition to motherhood.

Many women experience **postpartum blues,** feelings of sadness and depression, sometimes called the baby blues, in the immediate postpartum period. Symptoms begin 2 or 3 days after childbirth and usually disappear within a week or two. The woman experiences a letdown feeling accompanied by irritability. She may cry easily, lose her appetite, have trouble sleeping, and feel anxious. Mothers of preterm infants have been found to initially experience higher levels of anxiety and depression (Gennaro, 1988). Severe depressive psychosis occurs rarely.

The nurse can best assist the woman and family by assuring them that this depression is both normal and temporary. Recognizing the state, helping the woman verbalize her feelings, and providing support and understanding are important nursing actions. The nurse can explain to the woman and family that the depression may be caused by hormonal changes, emotional reaction to the role transition, discomfort, or fatigue. Setting up tasks the woman can accomplish easily and successfully are interventions that can help counteract the feelings of depression. It is also important to encourage adequate rest and nutrition. Since the woman will likely continue to experience symptoms after discharge, the nurse should always include the woman's partner in all interventions to support the woman and express concerns (see the Clinical Application of Research box).

Adjusting to a New Family Member

The birth of a baby causes enormous, permanent changes in family relationships. In addition to being a romantic

---

 CLINICAL APPLICATION OF RESEARCH

MATERNITY BLUES AND POSTPARTUM DEPRESSION

Research has documented that mothers who experience maternity blues are at increased risk for postpartum depression. Beck, Reynolds, and Rutowski (1992) investigated whether early discharge (first or second day postpartum) as compared to the customary discharge (3 days postpartum) was a risk factor in developing either the blues or postpartum depression. The researchers found that equal numbers of women in both groups (early discharge or customary discharge) experienced the blues and depression. They also found that women who experienced the blues were more likely to experience postpartum depression. For those women affected, the peak experience of the blues occurred 5 days postpartum and depression was present at each of the times it was mea-sured: 1 week, 6 weeks, and 12 weeks.

The researchers concluded that early discharge did not contribute to these conditions. Nurses providing care in the postpartum unit should discuss maternity blues and postpartum depression with women before discharge. Women should be counseled to call the health care provider if feelings of depression persist beyond the fifth day postpartum. Telephone follow-up or home visits could be scheduled for the fourth or fifth day so that an assessment of the level of depression can be made.

References: Beck CT, Reynolds MA, Rutowski P: Maternity blues and postpartum depression, *JOGNN* 21(4):287, 1992.

twosome, the couple have become, and will always be, parents. Couples often come from very different families of origin and have conflicting expectations regarding family roles. Working through these differences in beliefs and values occurs over time as the family grows and matures.

Most couples have fantasized during pregnancy about how their new baby would behave. New parents can find it disconcerting to discover that their baby's behavior is not at all what they expected. Some babies cry more than expected or do not seem satisfied with their feedings. Many babies have fussy periods, often late in the after-noon or around dinner time, when they are nearly impossible to console.

Box 18-3 presents practical suggestions for families adjusting to life with a new baby.

Grandparents/Extended Family

Grandparents and other extended family members often provide much needed emotional support for new families. In addition, they can assist with housework, meals, babysitting with older children, and eventually the new baby. Being able to verbalize experiences with others who are interested and experienced also tends to reassure the

---

BOX 18-3

Coping Mechanisms for New Families

- *Set priorities for tasks.* Many tasks can be left for a later period or done by others. Be firm about not taking on extra tasks for family, friends, or community. Try not to schedule a move to a new location soon after giving birth.
- *Do not become overly concerned with appearances.* Tidiness in the home is not as important as time spent with the family. Taking up the role of super housekeeper can be postponed until other adjustments are made.

  Sometimes new mothers become overburdened with visits from relatives eager "to take over the baby." Husbands or partners can help redirect these well-meaning people toward helping with the housework and cooking. This leaves the parent free to interact with the child.
- *Get plenty of rest and sleep.* Rearrange schedules if necessary. Because naps may not be possible if there are other children in the family, going to bed early is recommended; let friends know when to visit.
- *Do not undertake the care of another incapacitated relative at this point.* Such responsibilities should be undertaken by other family members.
- *Arrange for some time away from the baby.* Enlist the help of friends, family, or others for baby-sitting. Relaxation for parents is necessary. Baby-sitting, if at all possible, must be planned and a regular schedule developed. This includes time off during the day so that you can get away from the home and its responsibilities. In some localities churches or other agencies have developed programs attuned to the needs of mothers. The young children are cared for while the mothers take part in activities with other mothers. This helps them establish relationships with others who also are involved in the care of young children. A mutual sharing of successes and failures in this regard helps a new mother maintain a feeling of equilibrium.

  At the very least you need to plan to get out of the house at least once each day. Access to a car and being able to drive are assets. Taking the baby out for a walk or shopping helps break up the daily routine.
- *Make plans regarding fertility management* before intercourse is resumed and the possibility of pregnancy arises.
- *Be open in your communication with others.* Share incidents of delight or of worry with others. Be open in your requests for support. Discussions with other mothers are helpful.
- *Learn what health facilities are available,* for example, well-baby centers, immunization clinics, mother-infant classes (e.g., exercise, massage) and how to get in touch with the health care provider. If you have questions, remember that the hospital is open all day and night and you can call the emergency or maternity department at any time.
- *Prepare for returning to work.* Most women are physically able to return to work by the end of the sixth week. If plans for child care were not in place before the birth, adjustments for child care must be made. Ideally a substitute parent would be one who could come to the home and provide love, as well as care, for the child. Some parents are fortunate enough to have grandparents or other relatives willing and able to fill such a role. Others must take the child to another person's home or a day-care center early in the morning and pick the child up at night. The care provided by day-care centers is needed by some children whose mothers must work to help support them or who are the sole support of the child. For families who require this type of service, assistance in locating such help can be obtained from the local health department and parent referrals. Unfortunately there are not enough quality places available for all children requiring day-care.
- *Include the father/partner in caregiving activities.* Research shows that most fathers/partners participate in infant care to the extent that the mother allows (Stainton, 1985).

new mother. A mother, in discussing visits by the family to see the new baby commented as follows:

- I want the family to come. You people praise him so and think he is the most wonderful baby. All my friends have their own babies and are too busy trying to get compliments for them to give us any. All babies need aunties and grandmothers!

Grandparents, especially, often feel the need to advise new parents on caring for the new baby. Many communities now offer grandparent classes, where grandparents can be updated on contemporary thinking. Examples of contemporary child-rearing theories with which grandparents may be unfamiliar are that one cannot spoil a newborn, that breastfeeding is superior to bottle-feeding, and that bright colors are better than pastels for the baby's room because they are more stimulating. Safer infant car seats and disposable diapers are advances that most grandparents readily appreciate.

Siblings

Sibling rivalry (competition between brothers and sisters) may require much parental time and attention

---

HOME CARE

SUGGESTIONS FOR DECREASING SIBLING RIVALRY

- Make changes in sleeping arrangements early enough before the birth so that the child doesn't feel the new baby is taking over his or her bed.
- Make arrangements for the child's care well before the birth and discuss with the child where he/she will stay and who will keep him/her.
- Talk about the care that new babies require. Explain that it is okay to sometimes be angry with the baby, but never okay to hurt the baby.
- Spend special time with the older child. For example, Dad or another relative might take the child on an outing to the park. Mom might be able to read a story or play a game while the new baby is sleeping or feeding.
- Expect babyish behavior for a while. The older child needs extra love and attention, not punishment.
- Don't let relatives and friends ignore the older child. For example, they might bring a small gift for the older child when giving a present to the new baby.
- Let the older child help care for the new baby: sing or talk to the baby, bring Mom a diaper, help pick the clothes the baby wears home from the hospital, help select the baby's name, and help dress, feed, burp, and hold the new baby with assistance.

---

to be handled successfully. Jealousy is usually present to some extent, even when brothers and sisters have been prepared for the new baby's coming. Older siblings may wonder, "Why would Mommy and Daddy be getting a new baby unless the old one (me!) wasn't good enough?" Acting-out behavior, especially in preschool siblings, is common. Examples of common acting-out behaviors include whining, wetting pants or bed, asking for bottle or breast, acting silly, having temper tantrums, asking if babies die, and suggesting that the baby be returned to the hospital or put in the garbage. The Home Care box below at left contains suggestions for decreasing sibling rivalry.

✤ EVALUATION

Evaluating nursing care in relation to psychosocial concerns can be difficult in the early postpartum period. Parental, infant, and family relationships are still undergoing rapid changes at the time most mothers are discharged home. Healthy family adjustments to the birth of a child will continue in the weeks ahead. However, the nurse can be reasonably assured that care was effective if expected outcomes for care have been met, at least to some extent. Families should demonstrate competency in providing essential newborn care, exhibit healthy personal adjustment, and have developed plans for maintaining healthy family functioning that are congruent with their cultural norms and their personal expectations.

DISCHARGE FROM HOSPITAL

Bridging the gap between hospital and home care requires sensitive and knowledgeable nursing care. Discharge planning begins at the time of admission to the unit and should be reflected in the plan of care developed for each individual patient. For example, a great deal of time during the hospital stay is usually spent in teaching about maternal and newborn care, since all women must be capable of providing basic care for themselves and their infants at the time of discharge. It is also crucial that every woman be taught to recognize physical signs and symptoms that might indicate problems and how to obtain advice and assistance quickly if these signs appear. The Signs of Potential Complications box on p. 465 lists several common indications of maternal physical problems in the postpartum period. Before discharge women also need basic instruction regarding the resumption of intercourse, prescribed medications, routine mother-baby checkups, and contraception.

Just before the time of discharge the nurse reviews the woman's chart (audits the chart) to see that laboratory reports, medications, signatures, and so on are in order. Some hospitals have a checklist to follow before the woman's discharge. The nurse verifies that medications, if ordered, have arrived on the unit, that any valuables kept secured during the woman's stay have been returned to her and that she has signed a receipt for them, and that the infant is ready to be discharged.

The nurse is careful not to administer any medication that would make the mother sleepy if she is the one who will be holding the baby on the way out of the hospital. In most instances the woman is seated in a wheelchair and usually is given the baby to hold. Some families leave unescorted and ambulatory, depending on hospital protocol. The woman's possessions are gathered and taken out with her and her family; usually they are placed on some type of cart or carried by family members. *The woman's and the baby's identification bands are carefully checked.* As the woman and the baby are assisted into the car, the nurse should make sure that there is a car seat in which to secure the baby (see Legal Tip).

LEGAL TIP: **Early Discharge**

Whether or not the woman and her family have chosen early discharge, the nurse and the primary care provider are held responsible if the woman is discharged before her condition has stabilized within normal limits. If complications occur, the medical and nursing staff could be sued for abandonment.

Sexual Activity

Many couples resume sexual activity before the traditional postpartum checkup 6 weeks after childbirth. They may be anxious about the topic but uncomfortable and unwilling to bring it up. Since health care providers often fail to mention the subject, it is important that the nurse discuss the physical and psychologic effects that giving birth can have on lovemaking. The Home Care box at right contains helpful information about the resumption of sexual intercourse.

Prescribed Medications

Most patients have at least one medication prescribed for their use after discharge. Many health care providers routinely have women continue to take their prenatal vitamins and iron during the postpartum period. It is especially important that women who are breastfeeding or who are discharged with a lower than normal hematocrit take these medications as ordered. Women with extensive episiotomies (third or fourth degree) or vaginal lacerations are usually given stool softeners to take at home. The nurse should make certain that the patient knows the route, dosage, and frequency of all ordered medications, as well as common side effects.

Routine Mother and Baby Checkups

Women who have experienced uncomplicated vaginal births are still commonly scheduled for the traditional

HOME CARE

RESUMPTION OF SEXUAL INTERCOURSE

You can safely resume sexual intercourse by the third or fourth postbirth week if bleeding has stopped and the episiotomy has healed. For the first 6 weeks to 6 months the vagina does not lubricate well because steroid depletion inhibits the vasocongestive response to sexual tension.

Your physiologic reactions to sexual stimulation for the first 3 postbirth months are marked by a reduction in both rapidity and intensity of response. Vasocongestion of the labia major and minora is delayed well into the plateau phase. The walls of the vagina are thin and pink, a condition similar to senile vaginitis. This results from the hormonal starvation of the involutional period. Finally, the size of the orgasmic platform and strength of the orgasmic contractions are reduced.

A water-soluble gel, cocoa butter, or a contraceptive cream or jelly might be recommended for lubrication. If some vaginal tenderness is present, your partner can be instructed to insert one or more clean, lubricated fingers into the vagina and rotate them within the vagina to help relax it and to identify possible areas of discomfort. A coital position in which the woman has control of the depth of the penile penetration also is useful. The side-by-side or female-superior position often is recommended.

The presence of the baby influences postbirth lovemaking. Parents hear every sound made by the baby; conversely you may be concerned that the baby hears every sound you make. In either case any phase of the sexual response cycle may be interrupted by hearing the baby cry or move, leaving both of you frustrated and unsatisfied. The amount of psychologic energy expended by you in child care activities may lead to fatigue. Newborns require a great deal of attention and time, not to mention what is necessary to take care of twins or triplets, and older children as well.

Some women have reported sexual stimulation to plateau and orgasmic levels when nursing their babies. Although nursing mothers have a longer delay in ovarian steroid production, they often are interested in returning to sexual activity before nonnursing mothers. Nursing mothers also report higher levels of postbirth eroticism.

You should be instructed to perform the Kegel exercises to strengthen your pubococcygeal muscle. This muscle is the major sphincter of the pelvis. It is associated with bowel and bladder function and with vaginal perception and response during intercourse.

6-week postpartum examination. Patients who have had a cesarean birth are often seen in the health care provider's office or clinic 2 weeks after hospital discharge. The time for the follow-up appointment should be included in the discharge orders. If an appointment for a specific date and time was not made for the patient prior to leaving the hospital, she should be encouraged to call the health care provider's office or clinic immediately and schedule an appointment herself .

Parents who have not already done so need to make plans for well child care at the time of discharge. Most offices and clinics like to see newborns for an initial examination at 2 weeks of age. Again, if an appointment for a specific date and time was not made for the infant before leaving the hospital, the parents should be encouraged to call the office or clinic right away.

Care Management—Contraception

Contraceptive options should also be discussed with couples before discharge so that they can make informed decisions about fertility management prior to resuming sexual activity. Waiting to discuss contraception at the 6-week checkup may be too late. It is possible, particularly in women who bottle-feed, for ovulation to occur as soon as 1 month after giving birth. A woman who engages in unprotected sex risks the possibility of becoming pregnant much sooner than she planned. **Contraception** is the voluntary prevention of pregnancy, having both individual and social implications. Today, couples choosing contraception must be informed about prevention of unintended pregnancy as well as protection against sexually transmitted diseases (STDs). Nurses can be instrumental in the decision-making process.

✤ ASSESSMENT

The woman's knowledge about contraception and her sexual partner's commitment to any particular method are determined. Data are required about the frequency of coitus (once every so often or several times per week), whether the woman has one sexual partner or several, the level of involvement the woman wishes to assume, and her (their) objections to any methods. The woman's level of comfort and willingness to touch her genitals and cervical mucus are assessed. Myths are identified and religious and cultural factors are determined. The woman's verbal and nonverbal responses to hearing about the various available methods are carefully noted. An individual's reproductive-life plan needs to be considered.*

---

*When contraception is begun other than immediately postpartum, a history, physical examination, and laboratory tests precede its initiation for some forms. A complete gynecologic examination is done. Menstrual, contraceptive, and obstetric histories are taken.

Informed consent is a vital component in the education of the patient concerning contraception or sterilization. The nurse has the responsibility of documenting information provided and the understanding of that information by the patient. The acronym BRAIDED (NAACOG, 1991a) may be useful to ensure that all elements of an informed consent are covered (see Legal Tip).

LEGAL TIP: **Informed Consent**
B— Benefits: information about advantages and success rates
R— Risks: information about disadvantages and failure rates
A—Alternatives: information on other methods available
I—Inquiries: opportunity to ask questions
D—Decisions: opportunity to decide or change mind
E—Explanations: information about method and how it is used
D—Documentation: information given and patient's understanding

✤ NURSING DIAGNOSES

Nursing diagnoses reflect analysis of the assessment findings. Following are examples of nursing diagnoses that may emerge:

High risk for decisional conflict related to
• Contraceptive alternatives
Fear related to
• Contraceptive method side effects
High risk for infection related to
• Being sexually active
• Use of contraceptive method
High risk for altered sexuality patterns related to
• Fear of pregnancy
High risk for infection related to
• Broken skin or mucous membrane secondary to surgery, IUD insertion, hormonal implant
Pain related to
• Postoperative recovery after sterilization
Spiritual distress related to
• Discrepancy between religious or cultural beliefs and choice of contraception

✤ EXPECTED OUTCOMES

Planning is a collaborative effort among the woman, her sexual partner (when appropriate), the primary health care provider, and the nurse. The expected outcomes are determined and stated in patient-centered terms, and may include the following:
1. The woman will verbalize understanding about contraceptive methods.

2. The woman will state that she is comfortable and satisfied with the chosen method.
3. If further childbearing is desired, the woman or couple will achieve pregnancy when planned.
4. The woman or couple will experience no adverse sequelae as a result of the chosen method of contraception.
5. The woman will receive and understand all information necessary to give informed consent.

❖ COLLABORATIVE CARE

Unbiased patient teaching is fundamental to initiating and maintaining any form of contraception. A care provider relationship based on trust is an important facet in patient compliance. The nurse counters myths with facts, clarifies misinformation, and fills in gaps of knowledge. There are various contraceptive techniques used in North America. The ideal contraceptive should be safe, easily available, economical, acceptable, simple to use, and promptly reversible. Although no means or method may ever achieve all these objectives, impressive progress has been made recently.

Contraception failure rate refers to the percentage of contraceptive users expected to experience an accidental pregnancy during the first year, even when they use a method consistently and correctly. Contraceptive effectiveness or failure varies from couple to couple (see Box 18-5). Nurses have an obligation to provide unbiased information about failure rates and method effectiveness.

Safety of a method depends on the patient's medical history, tobacco use, and age. Barrier methods offer some protection from STDs, and oral contraceptives may lower the incidence of ovarian and endometrial cancer. "While there are risks associated with contraceptive use, the risk of death from a full-term pregnancy exceeds the risk of death from the use of any method of contraception, with the exception of the woman over age 35 who smokes and takes oral contraceptives" (NAACOG, 1991a).

Methods of Contraception

The following discussion of contraceptive methods provides the nurse with information needed for patient teaching. After implementing the appropriate teaching for contraceptive use, the nurse supervises return demonstrations and practice to assess patient understanding. The woman is given written instructions and phone numbers for questions. If the woman has difficulty understanding written instructions, she (couple) is offered graphic material and a phone number to call as necessary or an offer to return for further instruction.

Nonprescription Methods

Several nonprescription methods for control of fertility (contraception) are practiced. Prescription and supervi-

---

BOX 18-5

Factors Affecting Method Effectiveness

Frequency of intercourse
Motivation to prevent pregnancy
Understanding use of the method
Compliance with method
Provision of short-term or long-term protection
Likelihood of pregnancy for the individual woman

---

sion are unnecessary for barrier methods, that is, condom, foam, spermicide, and vaginal sponges, as well as for periodic abstinence.

Two methods practiced but not recommended are douching and coitus interruptus. *Coitus interruptus,* a method practiced for centuries, requires the man to withdraw before ejaculation. Extreme self-discipline is needed, and the sexual relationship may be strained. The danger of pregnancy from sperm in the preejaculatory drops is ever present. No advantages are given for this method, which has the lowest rate of effectiveness, comparable to the use of no contraceptive method (Lethbridge, 1991).

Periodic Abstinence. Although **periodic abstinence,** or natural family planning (NFP), is not a method of contraception, it does provide contraception by using methods that rely on avoidance of intercourse during fertile periods. *Fertility awareness* is the combination of charting signs and symptoms with the use of abstinence or other contraceptive methods during fertile periods (Davis, 1992).

Knowledge of the menstrual cycle is basic to the practice of NFP. To review, the human ovum can be fertilized no later than 16 to 24 hours after ovulation. Motile sperm have been recovered from the uterus and the oviducts as long as 60 hours after coitus. However, their ability to fertilize the ovum probably lasts no longer than 24 to 48 hours. Pregnancy is unlikely to occur if a couple abstains from intercourse for 4 days before and for 3 or 4 days after ovulation (**fertile period**). Unprotected intercourse on the other days of the cycle (**safe period**) should not result in pregnancy. However, there are two principal problems with this method: the exact time of ovulation cannot be predicted accurately, and couples may find it difficult to exercise restraint for several days before and after ovulation. Women with irregular menstrual periods have the greatest risk of failure with this form of contraception (Medical Letter, 1988). The typical failure rate is 20% during the first year of use (Hatcher et al, 1994).

Ovulation usually occurs about 14 days before the onset of menstruation. Therefore variations in the length of menstrual cycles are usually a result of differences in the length of the preovulatory phases. The fertile period can be anticipated by the following:

1. Calculating the time at which ovulation is likely to occur based on the lengths of previous menstrual cycles (*calendar method*)
2. Recording the rise in basal body temperature (BBT), a result of the thermogenic effect of progesterone (*temperature method*)
3. Recognizing the changes in cervical mucus at different phases of the menstrual cycle (*ovulation or Billings method*)
4. Using a predictor test for ovulation
5. Utilizing a combination of several methods

Calendar Method. Practice of the **calendar method,** (also known as the *rhythm method* or menstrual cycle charting), is based on a count of the number of days in each cycle counting from the first day of menses (Labbok, Queenan, 1989). With the calendar method the fertile period is determined after accurately recording the lengths of menstrual cycles for 1 year. The first unsafe day (beginning of the fertile period) can be determined by subtracting 18 days from the length of the shortest cycle. The last unsafe day (beginning of postovulatory safe period) can be calculated by subtracting 11 days from the length of the longest cycle. If the shortest cycle is 24 days and the longest is 30 days, application of the formula is as follows:

Shortest Cycle	Longest Cycle
24	30
− 18	− 11
6th day	19th day

To avoid conception the couple would abstain during the fertile period—days 6 through 19.

If the woman has very regular cycles of 28 days each, the formula indicates the fertile days to be:

Shortest Cycle	Longest Cycle
28	28
− 18	− 11
10th day	17th day

To avoid pregnancy, the couple abstains from day 10 through 17 because ovulation occurs on day 14 ±2 days. A major drawback of the calendar method is that one is trying to predict future events with past data. The unpredictability of the menstrual cycle is also not taken into consideration.

The method is most useful as an adjunct to the BBT or cervical mucus method. It is *not* useful in the postpartum period, during lactation, or at extremes of reproductive age when cycles are most variable (Labbok, Queenan, 1989).

Basal Body Temperature. The **basal body temperature (BBT)** is the lowest body temperature of a healthy

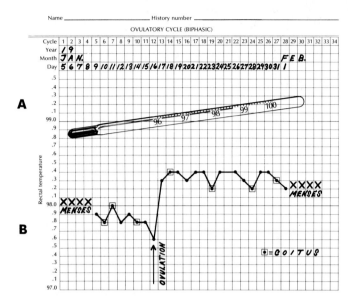

FIG. 18-4 **A,** Special thermometer for recording BBT, marked in tenths to enable person to read more easily. **B,** Basal temperature record shows drop and sharp rise at time of ovulation. Biphasic curve indicates ovulatory cycle.

person that is taken immediately after waking and before getting out of bed. The BBT usually varies from 97.2° to 97.4° F (36.2° to 36.3° C) during menses and for about 5 to 7 days afterward (Fig. 18-4).

If ovulation fails to occur, this pattern of lower body temperature continues throughout the cycle. Infection, fatigue, less than 3 hours of sleep per night, awakening late, and anxiety may cause temperature fluctuations, altering the expected pattern. If a new BBT thermometer is purchased, this fact is noted on the chart because the readings may vary slightly. Jet lag, alcohol taken the evening before, or sleeping in a heated waterbed must also be noted on the chart because each affects the BBT.

About the time of ovulation a slight drop in temperature [about 0.1° F (0.05° C)] may be seen; after ovulation, in concert with the increasing progesterone levels of the early luteal phase of the cycle, the BBT rises slightly [about (0.3° to 0.7°F, 0.2° to 0.4° C)] (Labbok, Queenan, 1989). The temperature remains on an elevated plateau until 2 to 4 days before menstruation. Then it drops to the low levels recorded during the previous cycle unless pregnancy has occurred and temperature remains elevated.

The drop and subsequent rise in temperature are referred to as the *thermal shift.* When the entire month's temperatures are recorded on a graph, the pattern described is more apparent. It is more difficult to perceive day-to-day variations without the entire picture (see Fig. 18-4). Therefore the BBT alone is not a reliable method to predict ovulation (Labbok, Queenan, 1989). To determine if a rise in temperature is indeed the thermal shift, the woman must be aware of other signs approach-

TEACHING APPROACHES

BASAL BODY TEMPERATURE

Discuss BBT with the woman.

Show woman a diagram depicting the phases of the menstrual cycle.

Discuss the different hormones in the woman's body that are responsible for her menstrual cycle and ovulation. Leave time for questions.

Show the woman a sample BBT graph (see Fig. 18-4) and the biphasic line seen in ovulatory cycles.

Show the woman the BBT thermometer and how it is calibrated.

Provide a demonstration.

Encourage woman to demonstrate taking and reading the thermometer and how she will graph the temperature while the nurse watches.

Encourage the woman to start a log at the same time that keeps track of any other activity that might interfere with her true BBT.

TEACHING APPROACHES

CERVICAL MUCUS CHARACTERISTICS

SETTING THE STAGE

Show charts of menstrual cycle along with changes in the cervical mucus.

Have woman practice with raw egg white.

Supply her with a BBT log and graph if she doesn't already have one.

Explain that assessment of cervical mucus characteristics is best when mucus is not mixed with semen, contraceptive jellies or foams, or discharge from infections.

CONTENT RELATED TO CERVICAL MUCUS

Explain to woman (couple) how cervical mucus changes throughout the menstrual cycle.

Right before ovulation, the watery, thin, clear mucus becomes more abundant and thick. It feels like a lubricant and can be stretched 5+ cm between the thumb and forefinger; this is called **spinnbarkheit.** This indicates the period of maximum fertility. Sperm deposited in this type of mucus can survive until ovulation occurs.

ASSESSMENT TECHNIQUE

Stress that good hand-washing is imperative to begin and end all self-assessment.

Start observation from last day of menstrual flow.

Assess cervical mucus several times a day for several cycles. Mucus can be obtained from vaginal introitus; no need to reach into vagina to cervix.

Record findings on the same record on which her BBT is entered. Record any other events also.

ing ovulation while she continues to assess the BBT (see later discussion of symptothermal method for other indicators of ovulation).

Most counselors advise the couple who wish to prevent conception to avoid unprotected intercourse from the day of the drop in the BBT and for 3 days of elevated temperature (Labbok, Queenan, 1989). Others require the woman to abstain for the entire preovulatory period, starting with day 1 of menses until the third consecutive day of elevated BBT (Mishell, 1989) (see the Teaching Approaches box above).

Cervical Mucus Method. The **cervical mucus method** (also called the *Billings method* and the *Creighton model ovulation method*) requires that the woman recognize and interpret the characteristic cyclic changes in the amount and consistency of cervical mucus (see the Teaching Approaches box above right). Each woman has her own unique pattern of mucus changes. The cervical mucus that accompanies ovulation is necessary for viability and motility of sperm. Without adequate cervical mucus, coitus does not result in conception. To ensure an accurate assessment of changes, the cervical mucus should be free from semen, contraceptive gels or foams, and blood or discharge from vaginal infections for at least one full cycle. Other factors that create difficulty in identifying mucus changes include douches and vaginal deodorants, being in the sexually aroused state (which thins the mucus), and taking medications such as antihistamines, which dry up the mucus.

Some women may find this method unacceptable if they find touching their genitals uncomfortable. Whether or not the individual wants to use this method

for contraception, it is to the woman's advantage to learn to recognize mucus characteristics at ovulation. Self-evaluation of cervical mucus can be highly accurate (Fehring et al, 1994) and can be useful diagnostically for any of the following purposes:

1. To alert the couple to the reestablishment of ovulation while breastfeeding and after discontinuation of oral contraception
2. To note anovulatory cycles at any time and at the commencement of menopause
3. To assist couples in planning a pregnancy

Symptothermal Method. The symptothermal method combines the BBT and cervical mucus methods with awareness of secondary, cycle phase-related symptoms (see Table 3-1). Both partners take responsibility for assessments, recordings, and evaluation of their findings. Together they determine the days for abstinence. Couples who use the symptothermal method commonly report an improvement in their sexual relationship.

The couple gains fertility awareness as they learn the

woman's individual psychologic and physiologic symptoms that mark the phases of her cycle. Secondary symptoms include increased libido, midcycle spotting, mittelschmerz, pelvic fullness or tenderness, and vulvar fullness. The couple, perhaps using a speculum, looks at the cervix to assess for changes indicating ovulation: that is, the os dilates slightly, the cervix softens and rises in the vagina, and cervical mucus is copious and slippery. To complete their records, the couple notes days on which coitus, changes in routine, illness, and so on have occurred (Fig. 18-5). Calendar calculations and cervical mucus changes are used to estimate the onset of the fertile period; changes in cervical mucus or the BBT are used to estimate its end.

Effectiveness of the symptothermal method with abstinence during the fertile period ranges between 73% and 97%.

Predictor Test for Ovulation. All of the preceding discussion is about assessments that are indicative of but do not prove the occurrence and exact timing of ovulation. The *predictor test* for ovulation is a major addition

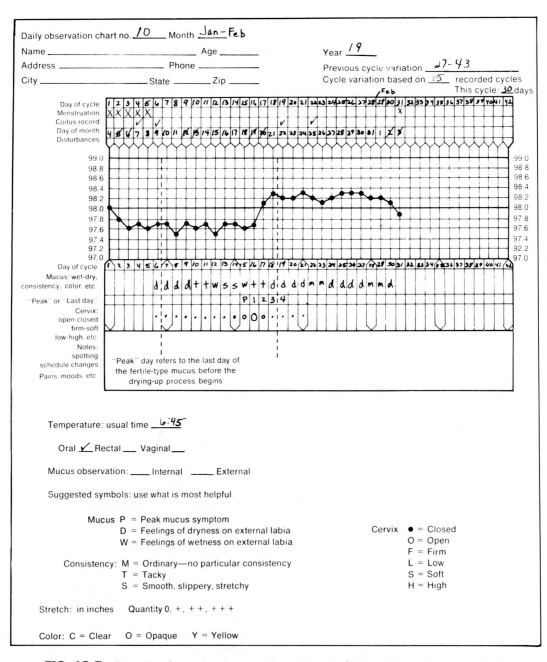

FIG. 18-5 Example of completed symptothermal method chart. (From Fogel C, Woods NF: *Health care of women,* St Louis. 1981, Mosby.)

to the periodic abstinence methods to help women who want to plan the time of their pregnancies and those who are trying to conceive. The *predictor test* for ovulation detects the sudden surge of luteinizing hormone (LH) that occurs approximately 12 to 24 hours *before* ovulation (Fehring, 1990). Unlike BBT, the test is not affected by illness, emotional upset, or physical activity. Available for home use, a test kit contains sufficient material for several days' testing during each cycle. A positive response indicative of an LH surge is noted by color change that is easy to read. Directions for use of this home test kit vary with the manufacturer.

Chemical and Mechanical Contraceptive Barriers. Barrier contraceptives are currently receiving great attention and increased use (Connell, 1989). This method has an additional distinct advantage of reducing the spread of STDs (Mishell, 1989).

Spermicides. A vaginal **spermicide** is a physical barrier to sperm penetration that also has a chemical action on sperm. *Nonoxynol 9* (N-9) and octoxynol 9 are the most commonly used spermicidal chemicals. Intravaginal spermicides are marketed as aerosol foams, foaming tablets, suppositories, creams, films, and gels (Fig. 18-6). Preloaded, single-dose applicators small enough to be carried in a small purse are available (Grimes, 1986). *Vaginal sponges* are also over-the-counter spermicides. Water is needed to activate the spermicide (nonoxynol 9) and facilitate insertion. Spermicide is released continuously for 24 hours. A woven loop is used for retrieval from the vagina. Box 18-6 provides patient teaching information about spermicide use.

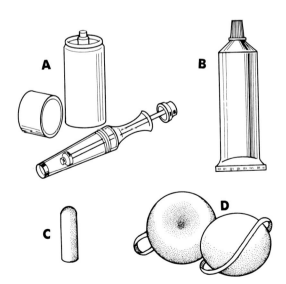

FIG. 18-6   Vaginal spermicides. **A,** Foam with applicator. **B,** Cream, **C,** Suppository. **D,** Sponge.

BOX 18-6

Spermicides

MODE OF ACTION

Provides a physical and chemical barrier that prevents viable sperm from entering the cervix. Effect is local within the vagina. The spermicide is placed deep in the vagina in contact with the cervix before each incidence of coitus.

FAILURE RATE

Typical failure: 21%. With vaginal sponges, parous women are more likely to become pregnant than nulliparous women.

ADVANTAGES

- Easy to apply.
- Safe.
- Low cost.
- Available without a prescription or previous medical examination.
- Delicate vaginal mucosa is not harmed unless the woman is allergic to a particular preparation.
- Aid in lubrication of the vagina.
- Vaginal sponges are less messy than other spermicides.
- Alternative for nursing mothers (does not interfere with lactation).
- Alternative for the premenopausal woman (to prevent masking symptoms of onset of the climacterium).
- Backup when the woman forgets her oral contraceptive.
- Increase the effectiveness of condoms and other forms of contraception.

STD PROTECTION

- The barrier method containing Nonoxynol 9 provides some protection against STDs through bacteriostatic action. Needs to be used with condoms if protection from STDs is needed.

DISADVANTAGES

- Maximum spermicidal effectiveness lasts usually no longer than 1 hour.
- If intercourse is to be repeated, reapplication of additional spermicide must precede it.
- Some users complain it is messy and has an unpleasant fizz and taste.
- Allergic response or irritation of vaginal or penile tissue may occur.
- Possible decreased tactile sensation.
- Vaginal sponges may be difficult to remove.

NURSING CONSIDERATIONS/PATIENT TEACHING

- Can must be shaken to distribute foam spermicide before use.
- Tablets and suppositories take from 10 to 30 minutes to dissolve.

Continued.

BOX 18-6

Spermicides—cont'd

- Douching must be avoided for at least 6 hours after coitus.
- Encourage open communication between sexual partners to discuss intravaginal contraception.
- Provide opportunity to see and handle a variety of samples.
- Provide anatomical model to practice insertion into the vagina.
- Vaginal sponges should never be reused, need to be left in place for 6 hours after coitus, and should *not* be used during menses or within 6 weeks of childbirth to prevent toxic shock syndrome (Connell, 1989).
- Nurse needs to feel comfortable teaching both male and female partners.

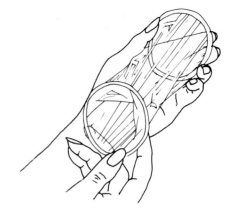

FIG. 18-7 WPC-333 soft polymer vaginal sheath.

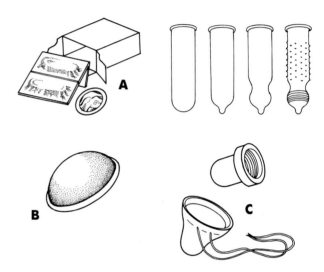

FIG. 18-8 Mechanical barriers. **A,** Types of condoms. **B,** Diaphragm. **C,** Cervical caps.

Vaginal Sheath (Female Condom). The vaginal sheath of natural latex rubber has flexible rings at both ends (Connell, 1989) (Fig. 18-7). Basically this device is a combination of a diaphragm and a condom. The closed end of the pouch is inserted into the vagina and is anchored around the cervix: the open ring covers the labia. It can be applied well in advance of intercourse so that spontaneity is unaffected. Before intercourse, a spermicide is added. Since it is a relatively loose sheath, it tends to heighten sensation for the man. Both women and men report that intercourse with the sheath is generally about as satisfying as intercourse without the sheath. Application of this disposable barrier requires no special training. It comes in one size and is available over the counter (Greydanus, Lonchamp, 1990). This device may provide more protection against STDs than do condoms.

Condom. The **condom** is a thin, stretchable sheath to cover the penis (Fig. 18-8, *A*). In addition to three available sizes, four basic features differ among condoms marketed in the United States. These features are material, shape, lubricants, and spermicides. Ninety-nine percent are made of latex rubber. A functional difference in condom shape is the presence or absence of a sperm reservoir tip. To enhance vaginal stimulation, some condoms are contoured and rippled or have ribbed or roughened surfaces. Thinner construction increases heat transmission and sensitivity; a variety of colors increases their acceptability and attractiveness (Connell, 1989). A wet jelly or dry powder lubricates some condoms. Since 1982 spermicide (0.5 g of nonoxynol 9) has been added to the interior or exterior surfaces of some condoms. The addition of nonoxynol 9 to latex condoms not only increases contraceptive effectiveness, it also increases pro-

tection against transmission of STDs, including HIV (Hatcher et al, 1994).

For years, health care providers assumed that everyone knew how to use condoms, so proper instruction was not provided. To prevent unintended pregnancy and the spread of STDs, it is essential that condoms be used correctly. Instructions, such as those listed in Box 18-7, can be used for patient teaching.

Methods Requiring Prescription

Several methods for the control of fertility require prescription and supervision. Interview, physical examination, and occasionally laboratory tests are prerequisites for some forms of contraception. These methods of contraception include hormonal therapy, use of diaphragms or cervical caps, and IUDs.

Hormonal Contraception. Over 30 different oral contraceptive formulations are available in the United

Condoms

MECHANISM OF ACTION

Sheath is applied over the erect penis before insertion or loss of preejaculatory drops of semen. Used correctly, condoms prevent sperm from entering the cervix. Spermicide-coated condom cause ejaculated sperm to be immobilized rapidly, thus increasing contraceptive effectiveness.

FAILURE RATE

- Typical users, 12%.
- Correct and consistent users, 2%.

ADVANTAGES

- Safe.
- No side effects.
- Readily available.
- Premalignant changes in cervix can be prevented or ameliorated in women whose partners use condoms.
- Method of male nonsurgical contraception.

DISADVANTAGES

- Must interrupt lovemaking to apply sheath.
- Sensation may be altered.
- If used improperly, spillage of sperm can result in pregnancy.
- Occasionally condoms may tear during intercourse.

STD PROTECTION

- If a condom is used throughout the act of intercourse and there is no unprotected contact with female genitals, a latex rubber condom, which is impermeable to viruses, can act as a protective measure against STDs.

NURSING CONSIDERATIONS

- Use a new condom (check expiration date) for each act of sexual intercourse or other acts between partners that involve contact with the penis.
- Place condom after penis is ercet and before intimate contact
- Place condom on head of penis (Fig. A) and unroll it all the way to the base (Fig B).
- Leave an empty space at the tip (Fig A); remove any air remaining in the tip by gently pressing air out towards the base of the penis.
- If a lubricant is desired, use water-base products such as K-Y Jelly.
- After ejaculation, carefully withdraw still erect penis, holding onto condom rim; discard.
- Store unused condoms in cool, dry place.
- Do not use condoms that are sticky, brittle, or obviously damaged.

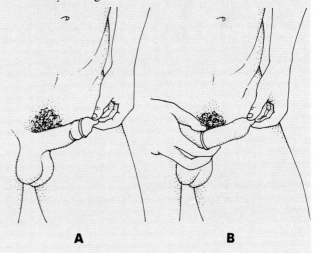

A   B

States today. General classes are described in Table 18-3. Because of the wide variety of preparations available, the woman and nurse need to read the package insert for information about specific products prescribed. Formulations include combined estrogen-progestin steroidal medications, progestational agents, and an estrogenic agent. The formulations are administered orally, subdermally, or by implantation. Combined estrogen-progestin steroidal medications are discussed first.

Combined Estrogen-Progestin Oral Contraceptives

Mode of action. The normal menstrual cycle is maintained by a feedback mechanism. Follicle-stimulating hormone (FSH) and luteinizing hormone (LH) are secreted in response to *fluctuating* levels of ovarian estro-gen and progesterone. Regular ingestion of combined estrogen-progestin steroidal medication suppresses the action of the hypothalamus and anterior pituitary leading to inappropriate secretion of FSH and LH. Therefore follicles do not mature; ovulation is inhibited.

Other contraceptive effects are induced by the combined steroids. Maturation of the endometrium is altered, making it a less favorable site for implantation should ovulation and conception occur. It also has a direct effect on the endometrium, so that from 1 to 4 days after the last steroid tablet is taken, the endometrium sloughs and bleeds as a result of hormone withdrawal. The withdrawal bleeding usually is less profuse than that of normal menstruation and may last only 2 to 3 days. Some women have no bleeding at all.

The cervical mucus remains thick as a result of the ef-

TABLE 18-3 Hormonal Contraception

COMPOSITION	ROUTE OF ADMINISTRATION	DURATION OF EFFECT
Combination of an estrogen and a progestin	Oral	24 hours
Minipill: progestin (norethindrone, 0.35 mg) only	Oral	24 hours
Morning-after pill: estrogen (diethylstilbestrol [DES]) in very high doses—25 mg	Oral	Taken within 72 hours of unprotected coitus during fertile period: because of DES effect on fetus, abortion advised if method fails
Depo-Provera: progestin only (medroxyprogesterone acetate), 150 mg	Intramuscular injection	From 3 to 6 months
Norplant system: progestin (Levonorgestrel) in Silastic containers	Implant, subdermal	Up to 5 years

fect of the progestin. Cervical mucus under the effect of progesterone does not provide as suitable an environment for sperm penetration as does the thin, watery mucus at ovulation (Willson, Carrington, 1991).

The possible effect, if any, of altered tubal and uterine motility induced by the steroidal hormones is not clear. Nevertheless, **oral hormonal contraceptives,** if taken daily for 3 weeks of every 4, provide virtually absolute protection against conception (Cunningham et al, 1993).

Phasic pills (e.g., triphasic oral contraceptives) are those which alter the amount of progestin and sometimes the amount of estrogen within each cycle. These preparations reduce the total dosage of steroid hormones in a single cycle without sacrificing contraceptive efficacy or cycle control (Cunningham et al, 1993).

Advantages. For motivated women it is easy to take an oral contraceptive at about the same time each day. Taking the pill does not relate directly to the sexual act; this fact increases its acceptability to some women. Commonly there is an improvement in sexual response once the possibility of pregnancy is not an issue. For some it is convenient to know when to expect the next "menstrual" flow.

Oral contraceptives are considered to be a safe option for older, nonsmoking women until menopause. Perimenopausal women can benefit from regular bleeding cycles, a regular hormonal pattern, and the noncontraceptive health benefits of oral contraceptives (Contraception, 1992).

The noncontraceptive health benefits of oral contraceptives include decreased menstrual blood loss and decreased iron-deficiency anemia, regulation of menorrhagia and irregular cycles, lowered incidence of dysmenorrhea (menstrual cramps) and premenstrual syndrome (PMS). Oral contraceptives also offer protection against endometrial adenocarcinoma and possibly ovarian cancer, reduced incidence of benign breast disease, protec-

tion against the development of functional ovarian cysts, and some types of pelvic inflammatory disease (PID), and decreased risk of ectopic pregnancy (NAACOG, 1991a).

Women taking steroidal contraceptives are examined before the medication is prescribed and yearly thereafter. The examination includes medical and family history, weight, blood pressure, general physical and pelvic examination, screening cervical cytologic analysis (Pap smear), and hemoglobin determination. Consistent monitoring by the health care provider is valuable in the detection of noncontraception-related disorders as well, so that timely treatment can be initiated.

Use of oral hormonal contraceptives is initiated on one of the first 7 days of the menstrual cycle (day 1 of the cycle is the first day of menses). Other women start their use after childbirth or abortion. If contraceptives are to be started at any time other than during normal menses, or within 3 weeks after birth or abortion, another method of contraception should be used throughout the first week to avoid the risk of pregnancy (Cunningham et al, 1993). The combined estrogen-progestin pill taken daily 3 weeks out of every 4 is the most effective reversible form of contraception available (Cunningham et al, 1993). Taken exactly as directed, oral contraceptives prevent ovulation and pregnancy cannot occur; the overall effectiveness rate is almost 100%. Almost all failures (i.e., pregnancy occurs) are caused by omission of one or more pills during the regimen. The typical failure rate due to omission is 3%.

Disadvantages and side effects. Since hormonal contraceptives have come into use, the amount of estrogen and progestational agent contained in each tablet has been reduced considerably (Cunningham et al, 1993). This is important because adverse effects are, to a degree, dose related.

Women must be screened for conditions that present

absolute or relative contraindications to oral contraceptive use. *Absolute contraindications* include a history of thromboembolic disorders, cerebrovascular or coronary artery disease, breast cancer, estrogenic-dependent tumors, pregnancy, impaired liver function, liver tumor, and previous cholestasis. Strong *relative contraindications* include migraine headaches, hypertension, acute mononucleosis, surgery requiring immobilization for 4 weeks, long-leg cast or major lower leg injury, age of 40 years or older accompanied by a second cardiovascular risk factor, age of 35 years or older and heavy smoking (more than 15 cigarettes per day), and abnormal genital bleeding (Hatcher et al, 1994). The main causes of hospitalization and death are cardiovascular problems (e.g., myocardial infarction [heart attack], cerebrovascular accident [stroke], and thromboembolism) (Grimes, 1986).

Certain side effects of anovulatory drugs are attributable to estrogen and progestin or both. Side effects of *estrogen excess* include nausea and vomiting, dizziness, edema, leg cramps, increase in breast size, chloasma (mask of pregnancy), visual changes, hypertension, and vascular headache. Side effects of *estrogen deficiency* include early spotting (days 1 to 14), hypomenorrhea, nervousness, and atrophic vaginitis leading to painful intercourse (dyspareunia). Side effects of *progestin excess* include increased appetite, tiredness, depression, breast tenderness, vaginal yeast infection, oily skin and scalp, hirsutism, and postpill amenorrhea. Side effects of *progestin deficiency* include late spotting and breakthrough bleeding (days 15 to 21), heavy flow with clots, and decreased breast size. One of the most common side effects is bleeding irregularities (Hillard, 1989).

In the presence of side effects, especially those which are bothersome to the woman, a different product, a different drug content, or another method of contraception may be required. The "right" product for a woman contains the lowest dose of sex steroid hormones that prevents ovulation and that has the fewest and least harmful side effects. There is no way to predict the right dosage for any particular woman; trial and error is the main method for prescribing oral contraceptives, starting with the lowest possible estrogen dose.

The *changes in glucose tolerance* that occur in some women taking oral contraceptives are similar to those changes that occur during pregnancy. The dosage, type, and potency of progestin (not estrogen) produce some deterioration of glucose tolerance in normal women, as well as in those with a history of gestational diabetes (Mishell, 1989).

The effectiveness of oral contraceptives is decreased when the following drugs are taken at the same time:

- Barbiturates (for sedation)
- Phenytoin sodium (for seizure disorders)
- Antibiotics

Also, the use of oral contraceptives can decrease the effectiveness of several drugs (e.g., insulin and oral anticoagulants) (Orshan, 1988).

Research on use of oral contraceptives and risk of breast cancer has been inconsistent (NAACOG, 1991 a,b); investigation continues on this important concern.

Women who discontinue oral contraception for a planned pregnancy commonly ask whether they should wait before attempting to conceive. Although data are controversial, studies indicate that these infants have no greater chance of being born with any type of birth defect than do infants born to women in the general population, even if conception occurred in the first month after the medication was discontinued (Mishell, 1989).

After discontinuing oral contraception there is usually a delay before ovulation and menstrual cycles recur, similar to that experienced by a new mother. However, *postpill amenorrhea* exceeding 6 months should be investigated.

Nursing considerations. There are many different preparations of oral hormonal contraceptives. The nurse reviews the prescribing information in the package insert with the woman. Because of the wide variations, each woman must be clear about the unique dosage regimen for the preparation prescribed for her. Directions for care after missing one or two tablets also vary. Recent findings indicate that if one or two tablets are missed, another form of contraception needs to be used until the required regimen is reestablished (see the Home Care box below).

HOME CARE

ADMINISTRATION OF ORAL CONTRACEPTIVE PILLS

- A pill should be taken at the same time every day for 21 (or 28) days.
- If one pill is missed, take it as soon as you remember it, and take the next one at the usual time.
- If you miss two or more pills in a row in the first 2 weeks of the cycle, take two for 2 days and use a backup method of contraception for the next 7 days.
- If you miss two or more pills in the third week, or three or more pills anytime: *Sunday starters* keep on taking pills until the next Sunday. Start a new pack on that day. Use a backup method of contraception for the next 7 days. *Day 1 starters* throw out the rest of the pack and start a new pack that day. Use a backup method of contraception for the next 7 days.
- *28-day pill pack:* If you miss any of the seven pills that do not have any hormones, throw out the pills you missed and keep taking one pill a day until the pack is empty. You do not need a backup method of contraception.

Modified from: Family Health International: *An example of OC use instructions for PPIs,* Research Triangle Park, NC, 1990.

Withdrawal bleeding ("periods") tends to be short and scanty when some combination pills are taken. A woman may see no fresh blood at all. Some women may have only a drop of blood or a brown smudge on their tampon or underwear. This counts as a period. This fact may explain why some women have difficulty remembering the first day of their last period.

No more than 50% to 70% of women who start taking oral contraceptives are still taking them after 1 year. It is therefore important that nurses recommend that all women choosing to use oral contraceptives also be provided with a second method of birth control and that women be instructed and comfortable with this backup method. Most women stop taking oral contraceptives for nonmedical reasons; that is, they *choose* to stop, not because they develop a complication or a serious side effect.

The nurse also reviews the signs of potential complications associated with the use of oral contraceptives (see the Signs of Potential Complications box at right).

Oral contraceptives do not protect a woman against STDs. A barrier method such as condoms and spermicide should be used as well if protection is desired (NAACOG, 1991a).

Progestin-Only Contraception

Oral progestins (Minipill). The minipill of 0.5 mg or less of a progestational agent daily presumably impairs fertility. Ovulation may occur. Progestational impact on cervical mucus decreases sperm penetration and alters endometrial maturation to discourage implantation should conception occur. Users report a higher incidence of irregular bleeding.

Injectable progestins. The advantages of medroxyprogesterone (DMPA, Depo-Provera) include a contraceptive effectiveness comparable to combined oral contraceptives, long-lasting effects, the requirement of injections only 2 to 4 times a year, and lactation not likely to be impaired (Cunningham et al, 1993). The modes of action include inhibition of ovulation and alteration in endometrial maturation and cervical mucus. Disadvantages are prolonged amenorrhea or uterine bleeding, increased risk of venous thrombosis and thromboembolism, and no protection against STDs.

Implantable progestin (Norplant). The Norplant system consists of six flexible, nonbiodegradable Silastic capsules. They contain progestin providing up to 5 years of contraception. Insertion and removal of the capsules are minor surgical procedures involving a local anesthetic, a small incision, and no sutures. The capsules are placed subdermally in the inner aspect of the upper arm (Fig. 18-9). The progestin prevents some, but not all, ovulatory cycles and thickens cervical mucus. The effectiveness is greater than 99% over 5 years. Other advantages include long-term continuous contraception, not coitus related, and reversibility (see the Ethical Consid-

SIGNS OF POTENTIAL COMPLICATIONS

ORAL CONTRACEPTIVES

Before oral contraceptives are prescribed and periodically throughout hormone therapy the woman is alerted to stop taking the pill and to report any of the following symptoms to the health care provider immediately. The word *aches* helps in retention of this list:

A—Abdominal pain: may indicate a problem with the liver or gallbladder
C—Chest pain or shortness of breath: may indicate possible clot problem within lungs or heart
H—Headaches (sudden or persistent): may be caused by cardiovascular accident or hypertension
E—Eye problems: may indicate vascular accident or hypertension
S—Severe leg pain: may indicate a thromboembolic process

ETHICAL CONSIDERATIONS

ENFORCED CONTRACEPTION

The nurse may be confronted with an ethical dilemma concerning enforced contraception for a patient. There have been some judicial rulings for a woman convicted of child abuse to either obtain a Norplant device or face a jail term. Other women receiving public assistance for children may be told to get the implant or be faced with decreased or even no payments.

Some nurses may consider this punitive approach to be effective in preventing the birth of more children to unsuitable mothers; however, some individuals strongly believe that forcing women to have such procedures is interfering with her constitutional rights.

erations box). Irregular menstrual bleeding is the most common side effect (Darney et al, 1990). Other side effects, including headaches, nervousness, nausea, skin changes, and vertigo, are less common. Changes in glucose and insulin values have occurred after 6 months, especially in women who are diabetic (Konje et al, 1992). No STD protection is provided with the Norplant method, so condoms should be used if protection is desired.

Diaphragm With Spermicide. The vaginal **diaphragm** is a shallow, dome-shaped rubber device with a flexible wire rim that covers the cervix (see Fig. 18-8, *B*). There are three main styles of diaphragms available in a wide range of diameters (50 to 95 mm). Diaphragms differ in the inner construction of the circular rim. The

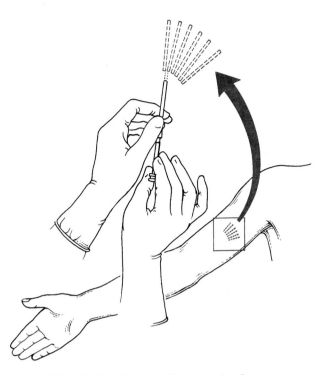

FIG. 18-9 Norplant Contraceptive System.

three types of rims are flat spring, coil spring, and arch-ing spring.

The diaphragm should feel comfortable. It should be the largest size the woman can wear without her being aware of its presence. The use of a contraceptive gel or cream with the diaphragm offers both mechanical and chemical barriers to pregnancy.

The diaphragm is a mechanical barrier preventing the meeting of the sperm with the ovum. The diaphragm holds the spermicide in place against the cervix for the 6 hours it takes to destroy the sperm. The *effectiveness* of this combined method is approximately 83% to 90%. Highly motivated women may achieve rates of 99%.

Nursing Considerations. The woman is informed that she needs an annual gynecologic examination. The device may need to be refitted after 2 years, the loss or gain of 9 kg (20 lb) or more, term birth, or second tri-mester abortion (Kugel, Verson, 1986; Connell, 1989). Since there are various types of diaphragms on the mar-ket, the nurse uses the package insert for teaching the woman how to use and care for the diaphragm (see the Teaching Approaches box p. 496).

Except for occasional allergic responses to the dia-phragm or spermicide, there are no side effects from a well-fitted device. The diaphragm can be inserted as long as 6 hours before intercourse to increase spontaneity, but spermicide must be added each time intercourse is re-peated (Medical Letter, 1988). It must be left in place for at least 6 hours after the last intercourse. The woman

who engages in intercourse infrequently may choose this barrier method. The spermicide does offer additional lu-brication if it is needed. A decreased incidence of vagini-tis, cervicitis (including cervicitis caused by *Chlamydia trachomatis* and *Neisseria gonorrhoeae*), PID, and cervi-cal intraepithelial neoplasia is noted among women who use contraceptive creams, foams, and gels with the dia-phragm.

This method is contraindicated for the woman with relaxation of her pelvic support (uterine prolapse) or a large cystocele.

Disadvantages include the reluctance of some women to insert and remove the diaphragm. A cold diaphragm and a cold gel temporarily reduce vaginal response to sexual stimulation if insertion of the diaphragm occurs immediately before intercourse. Some women or couples object to the messiness of the spermicide. These annoy-ances of diaphragm use, along with failure to insert the device once foreplay has begun, are the most common reasons for failures of this method. Side effects may in-clude irritation of tissues related to contact with spermi-cides. Urethritis and recurrent cystitis (Strom, 1987) caused by upward pressure of the diaphragm rim against the urethra may be increased by the use of the contra-ceptive diaphragm.

Toxic shock syndrome (TSS), although reported in very small numbers, can occur in association with the use of the contraceptive diaphragm (Connell, 1989). The nurse should instruct the woman about ways to reduce her risk for TSS. These measures include prompt removal 6 to 8 hours after intercourse, not using the diaphragm during menses, and learning and watching for danger signs of TSS. These danger signs include temperature of 101° F (38.4° C), diarrhea, vomiting, muscle aches, and sunburnlike rash.

Cervical Cap. The cervical cap has a 1¼-inch to 1½-inch soft natural rubber dome with a firm but pliable rim (see Fig. 18-8, *C*). It fits snugly around the base of the cervix close to the junction of the cervix and vaginal for-nices (Hatcher et al, 1994). The device is available in four sizes. It is recommended that the cap remain in place no less than 8 hours and not more than 48 hours at a time (Secor, 1992). It is left in place 6 to 8 hours after the last act of intercourse. The seal provides a physical bar-rier to sperm: spermicide inside the cap adds a chemical barrier.

The extended period of wear is an added convenience for women who previously used the diaphragm. Instruc-tions for the actual insertion and use of the cervical cap closely resemble the instructions for use of the contra-ceptive diaphragm. Some of the differences are that the cervical cap can be inserted hours before sexual inter-course without a need for additional spermicide later, no additional spermicide is required for repeated acts of in-tercourse when the cap is used, and the cervical cap re-

USE AND CARE OF THE DIAPHRAGM

POSITIONS FOR INSERTION OF DIAPHRAGM

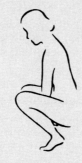

Squatting

This is the most commonly used position, and most women find this position satisfactory.

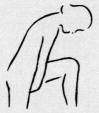

Leg Up Method

Another position is to raise the left foot (if right hand is used for insertion) on a low stool, and in a bending position the diaphragm is inserted.

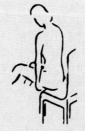

Chair Method

Another practical method for diaphragm insertion is for you to sit far forward on the edge of a chair.

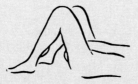

Reclining

You may prefer to insert the diaphragm while in a semi-reclining position in bed.

INSPECTION OF DIAPHRAGM

Your diaphragm must be inspected carefully before each use. The best way to do this is:

Hold the diaphragm up to a light source. Carefully stretch the diaphragm at the area of the rim, on all sides, to make sure there are no holes. Remember, it is possible to puncture the diaphragm with sharp fingernails.

Another way to check for pinholes is to carefully fill the diaphragm with water. If there is any problem, it will be seen immediately.

If your diaphragm is puckered, especially near the rim, this could mean thin spots.

The diaphragm should not be used if you see any of the above; consult your health care provider.

PREPARATION OF DIAPHRAGM

Rinse off cornstarch. Your diaphragm must always be used with a spermicidal lubricant to be effective. Pregnancy cannot be prevented effectively by the diaphragm alone.

Always empty your bladder before inserting the diaphragm. Place about 2 teaspoonful of contraceptive jelly or contraceptive cream on the side of the diaphragm that will rest against the cervix (or whichever way you have been instructed). Spread it around to coat the surface and the rim. This aids in insertion and offers a more complete seal. Many women also spread some jelly or cream on the other side of the diaphragm (see Fig. A).

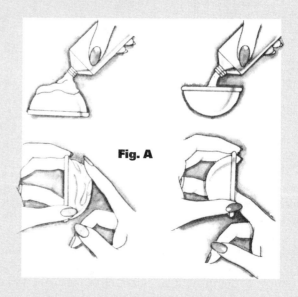

Fig. A

INSERTION OF DIAPHRAGM

The diaphragm can be inserted as much as 6 hours before intercourse. Hold the diaphragm between your thumb and fingers. The dome can either be up or down, as directed by your health care provider. Place your index finger on the outer rim of the compressed diaphragm (see Fig. B). Use the fingers of the other hand to spread the labia (lips of the vagina). This will assist in guiding the diaphragm into place.

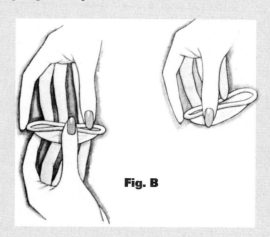

Fig. B

USE AND CARE OF THE DIAPHRAGM—cont'd

INSERTION OF DIAPHRAGM

Insert the diaphragm into the vagina. Direct it inward and downward as far as it will go to space behind and below the cervix (see Fig. C).

Fig. C

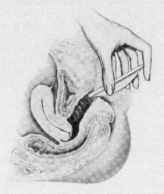

Tuck the front of the rim of the diaphragm behind the pelvic bone so that the rubber hugs the front wall of the vagina (see Fig. D).

Fig. D

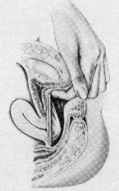

Feel for your cervix through the diaphragm to be certain it is properly placed and securely covered by the rubber dome (see Fig. E).

Fig. E

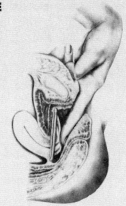

To clean the introducer (if one is used), wash with mild soap and warm water, rinse and dry thoroughly.

Fig. F

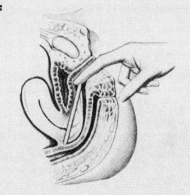

GENERAL INFORMATION

Regardless of the time of the month, this method of contraception must be used each and every time intercourse takes place. Your diaphragm must be left in place for at least 6 hours after the last intercourse. If you remove your diaphragm before the 6-hour period, your chance of becoming pregnant could be greatly increased.

REMOVAL OF DIAPHRAGM

The only proper way to remove the diaphragm is to insert your forefinger up and over the top side of the diaphragm, and slightly to the side.

Next, turn the palm of your hand downward and backward hooking the forefinger firmly on top of the inside of the upper rim of the diaphragm, *breaking the suction.*

Pull the diaphragm down and out. This avoids the possibility of tearing the diaphragm with the fingernails. The diaphragm *should not* be removed by trying to catch the rim from *below* the dome (see Fig. F).

CARE OF DIAPHRAGM

When using a vaginal diaphragm, avoid using products that may contain petroleum, such as certain body lubricants, vaginal lubricants, or vaginitis preparations. These products can weaken the rubber.

A little care means longer wear for your diaphragm. After each use the diaphragm should be washed in warm water and mild soap. Do not use detergent soaps, cold cream soaps, deodorant soaps, and soaps containing petroleum, since they can weaken the rubber.

After washing, the diaphragm should be dried thoroughly. All water and moisture should be removed with your towel. The diaphragm should then be dusted with *cornstarch.* Scented talc, body powder, baby powder, and the like should not be used because they can weaken the rubber.

The diaphragm should then be placed back in the plastic case for storage. It should not be stored near a radiator or heat source or exposed to light for an extended period.

quires less spermicide than the diaphragm when initially inserted (Secor, 1992). If the cap is left in place more than 48 hours, it will produce an odor.

Some women are not good candidates for wearing the cervical cap. They include women with abnormal Pap test results, women who cannot be fitted properly with the existing cap sizes, women who find the insertion and removal of the device too difficult, women with a history of TSS, women with vaginal or cervical infections (NAACOG, 1988), and women who experience allergic responses to the cap or spermicide.

Nursing Considerations. The angle of the uterus, the vaginal muscle tone, and the shape of the cervix may interfere with the cervical cap's ease of fitting and use. Correct fitting requires time, effort, and skill from both the woman and the clinician (Secor, 1992). The woman must check the cap's position before and after each act of intercourse.

After 3 months of use cervical cap users had a higher rate of conversion from class I (no abnormal cells present) to class III (suspicious abnormal cells present) Pap tests when compared with diaphragm users (NAACOG, 1988; Mishell, 1989). These conversions may be manifestations of the human papillomavirus (HPV). Women using the cap should have a Pap test at least every year.

Whereas no link has been discovered between TSS and the use of the cervical cap, such an association remains possible (Secor, 1992). The package insert recommends that another form of birth control be used during menstrual bleeding and up to at least 6 weeks postpartum.

The cap should be refitted after any gynecologic surgery or birth and after major weight losses or gains. Otherwise, the size should be checked at least once a year (Secor, 1992).

Strong patient motivation is the most important criterion for successful cap use. First-year failure rates range from 8 to 27 pregnancies per 100 women who initiate the use of this method (Mishell, 1989; Women's Health, 1989; Hatcher et al, 1994). That failure rating is similar to the one given the diaphragm.

The woman must be given the information available for this product as presented above. The nurse needs to assess the woman's understanding and skill in the use of the cervical cap (see Teaching Approaches box).

Intrauterine Devices. An **intrauterine device (IUD)** is a small, T-shaped device inserted into the uterine cavity. Medicated IUDs are loaded with either copper or a progestational agent (Fig. 18-10). These chemically active substances are released continuously, for example, copper-bearing devices for 4 to 8 years (at present) and progesterone devices for 1 year (*Contraception Report,* 1992). IUDs are impregnated with barium sulfate for radiopacity.

TEACHING APPROACHES

USE AND CARE OF THE CERVICAL CAP

Push cap up into vagina until it covers cervix.

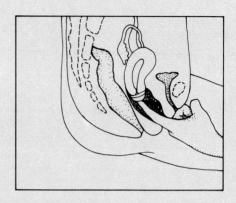

Press rim against cervix to create a seal.

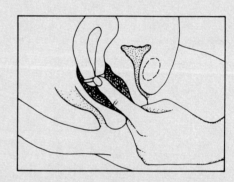

To remove: Push rim toward right or left hip to loosen from cervix and then remove.

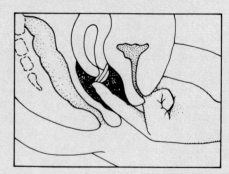

The woman can assume a number of positions to insert the cervical cap. See the four positions shown for inserting the diaphragm, p. 496.

Recent evidence strongly supports a true contraceptive effect in preventing fertilization (*Contraception Report,* 1992). The copper-bearing IUD damages sperm in transit to the uterine tubes and "interferes with the reproductive process anatomically and temporally before

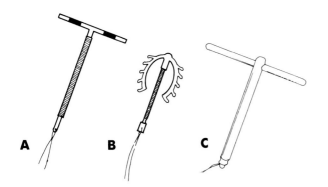

FIG. 18-10 Intrauterine devices. **A,** Copper-T 380A; 380 signifies total of 380 mm² of copper (mounted on polyethylene) exposed to endometrium; *A* refers to copper on the arms (approved by FDA). **B,** Multiload devices come in different sizes and are prepared with different loads of copper. Not yet available in United States, they are widely available outside of United States. **C,** Progestasert.

SIGNS OF POTENTIAL COMPLICATIONS

IUDs

Signs of potential complications related to IUDs can be remembered in this manner (Hatcher et al, 1994):
P—Period late, abnormal spotting or bleeding
A—Abdominal pain, pain with coitus
I—Infection exposure, abnormal vaginal discharge
N—Not feeling well, fever, or chills
S—String missing

ova reach the uterus" (WHO, 1987; Ortiz, Croxatto, 1987; Grimes, 1989) (Fig. 18-10, *A* and *B*). The progesterone-bearing IUD causes progestin-related effects on cervical mucus and endometrial maturation (Fig. 18-10, *C*). Because the effect is local, there is no disruption of the woman's ovulatory pattern. Copper-bearing IUDs have a lower failure rate than the progesterone-releasing IUDs (NAACOG, 1991a). The typical failure rate is 3%.

The IUD offers constant contraception without the need to remember to take pills each day or engage in other manipulation before or between coital acts. If pregnancy can be excluded, an IUD may be placed at any time during the menstrual cycle. An IUD may be inserted immediately after abortion (Liskin, Fox, 1982).

The absence of interference with hormonal regulation of menstrual cycles makes the IUD more appropriate than hormonal contraception for heavy smokers, women over 35, women who have hypertension, or those with a history of vascular disease or familial diabetes. Contraceptive effects are reversible. When pregnancy is desired, the IUD may be removed by the health care provider.

The Progestasert offers two important noncontraceptive progesterone-related advantages: less blood loss during menstruation and decreased primary dysmenorrhea. The mean blood loss is increased for the copper IUD. This blood loss may be clinically significant in undernourished populations.

The use of an IUD is contraindicated for women with a history of PID, known or suspected pregnancy, undiagnosed genital bleeding, suspected genital malignancy, or a distorted intrauterine cavity.

Disadvantages of IUD use include risk of PID, especially within 3 months of insertion, and risk of bacterial vaginosis, uterine perforation, and infection at time of in-

sertion. The IUD offers no protection against STDs. The IUD is not recommended for teenagers, but primarily for women who have had at least one child and who are involved in stable monogamous relationships (NAACOG, 1991b).

Nursing Considerations. The woman should be taught to check for the presence of the IUD thread after menstruation and at the time of ovulation as well as before coitus to rule out expulsion of the device. If pregnancy occurs with the IUD in place, the IUD should be removed immediately, if possible (Grimes, 1986). Retention of the IUD during pregnancy increases the risk of septic spontaneous abortion (Liskin, Fox, 1982). Some women allergic to copper develop a rash, necessitating the removal of the copper-bearing IUD. Signs of Potential Complications to be taught to the woman are listed in the box above.

Sterilization

Sterilization refers to surgical procedures intended to render the person infertile. Most procedures involve the occlusion of the passageways for the ova and sperm (Fig. 18-11). For the female the oviducts (uterine tubes) are occluded; for the male the sperm ducts (vas deferens) are occluded. Only surgical removal of the ovaries (oophorectomy) or uterus (hysterectomy) or both will result in absolute sterility for the woman. All other operations have a small but definite failure rate; that is, pregnancy may result. In the United States voluntary sterilization is the most common choice of contraception for couples who are 30 years of age or older.

Laws and Regulations. All states have strict regulations for informed consent. Many states in the United States permit voluntary sterilization of any mature, rational woman without reference to her marital or pregnancy status. Although the partner's consent is not required by law, the patient is encouraged to discuss the situation with the partner, and health care providers may request the partner's consent.

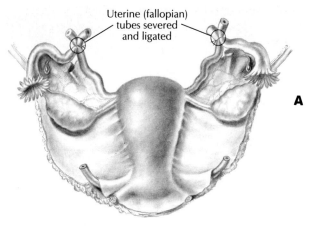

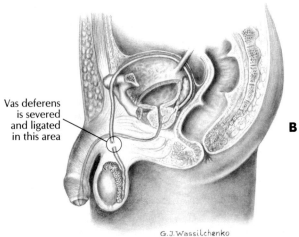

G.J.Wassilchenko

FIG. 18-11 Sterilization. **A,** Oviduct ligated and severed (tubal ligation). **B,** Sperm duct ligated and severed (vasectomy).

Sterilization of minors or mentally incompetent females is restricted by most states. The operation often requires the approval of a board of eugenicists or other court-appointed individuals (see Legal Tip).

LEGAL TIP: **Female Sterilization**

- If Federal funds are used for sterilization, the person must be at least 21 years old.
- Informed consent must include an explanation of the risks, benefits, and alternatives; a statement that describes sterilization as a permanent, irreversible method of birth control; and a statement that mandates a 30-day waiting period between giving consent and the sterilization.
- Informed consent must be in the person's native language or an interpreter must be provided.

Nursing Considerations. *Assessment* data include the history, physical examination, and laboratory data.

The nurse assesses motivation for sterilization, and alternatives are discussed. Motivation for elective sterilization includes personal preference; obstetric reasons such as multiparity, medical reasons such as hypertensive, cardiovascular, or renal disease in the woman or recurrent acute epididymitis in the man, and diagnosis of inheritable disease.

The patient's knowledge of the sterilization methods and of the chosen method is assessed. Gaps in knowledge and misinformation are noted. The record is reviewed for the signed informed consent.

Information must be given about what is entailed in various procedures, how much discomfort or pain can be expected, and what type of care is needed. Many individuals fear sterilization procedures because of the imagined effect on their sexual life. They need reassurance concerning the hormonal and psychologic basis for sexual function and the fact that uterine tube occlusion or vasectomy has no biologic sequelae in terms of sexual adequacy (Shain et al, 1991).

Preoperative care includes health assessment, which includes a psychologic assessment, physical examination, and laboratory tests. The nurse assists with the health assessment, answers questions, and confirms the patient's understanding of printed instructions (e.g., nothing by mouth [NPO] after midnight). Ambivalence and extreme fear of the procedure are reported to the health care provider.

Postoperative care depends on the procedure performed, for example, laparoscopy, laparotomy for tubal occlusion, or vasectomy. General care includes recovery after anesthesia, vital signs, fluid and electrolyte balance (intake and output, laboratory values), prevention of or early identification and treatment for infection or hemorrhage, control of discomfort, and assessment of emotional response to the procedure and recovery.

Discharge planning depends on the type of procedure performed. In general, the patient is given written instructions about observing for and reporting symptoms and signs of complications, the type of recovery to be expected, and the date and time for a follow-up appointment.

Female Sterilization. Female sterilization may be done immediately after birth (within 24 to 48 hours), concomitantly with abortion, or as an interval procedure (during any phase of the menstrual cycle). Most sterilization procedures are performed immediately after a pregnancy, probably because of heightened motivation or increased practicality. Out-of-hospital sterilization is also safe and effective (Nisanian, 1990).

Tubal Occlusion. The operation used commonly is the laparoscopic tubal fulguration (destruction of tissue by means of an electric current [electrocoagulation]) See Fig 30-4 for laparoscopy examination, a procedure of en-

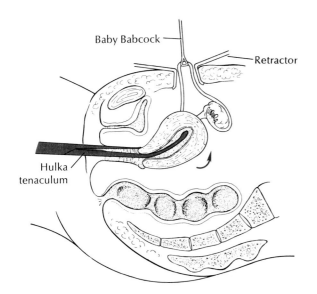

FIG. 18-12 Use of minilaparotomy to gain access to oviducts for tubal occlusion procedures. Tenaculum is used to lift uterus upward *(arrow)* toward incision.

TEACHING APPROACHES

WHAT TO EXPECT AFTER TUBAL LIGATION

You should expect no change in hormones and their influence.

Your menstrual period will be about the same as before the sterilization.

You may feel pain at ovulation.

The ovum disintegrates within the abdominal cavity.

It is highly unlikely that you will get pregnant.

You should not experience a change in sexual functioning; in fact, you may enjoy sexual relations more since you won't be concerned about getting pregnant.

Sterilization offers no protection against STDs; therefore you may need to use condoms.

tering the abdomen for access to the uterine tubes. A minilaparotomy may be used for tubal ligation (Fig. 18-12) or for the application of bands or clips. Bands (e.g., Falope ring) and clips (e.g., Hulka-Clemens) are placed around the tubes to block them (Cunningham et al, 1993). Fulguration and ligation are considered to be permanent methods. Use of the bands or clips has the theoretic advantage of possible removal and return of tubal patency. Transcervical approaches to inject occlusive material into the tubes are being investigated (NAACOG, 1991a).

For the minilaparotomy approach the woman is admitted the morning of surgery, having received nothing by mouth (NPO) since midnight. Preoperative sedation is given. The procedure may be carried out with a local anesthetic, but a regional or general anesthetic may also be used. A small vertical incision is made in the abdominal wall below the umbilicus. The woman may experience sensations of tugging but no pain, and the operation is completed within 20 minutes. She may be discharged several hours later if she has recovered from anesthesia. Any abdominal discomfort usually can be controlled with a mild analgesic (e.g., acetaminophen). Within 10 days the scar is almost invisible (see the Teaching Approaches box). As occurs with any surgery, there is always a possibility of complications of anesthesia, infection, hemorrhage, and trauma to other organs. Failures, although less than 0.5%, can occur (NAACOG, 1991a).

Tubal Reconstruction. Restoration of tubal continuity (reanastomosis) and function is technically feasible except after laparoscopic tubal fulguration. Sterilization reversal, however, is costly, difficult (requiring microsur-

gery), and uncertain (Cunningham et al, 1993). The success rate varies with the extent of tubal destruction and removal. The incidence of successful pregnancy after reanastomosis is only about 15%. The loss of a segment of tube necessary for sperm capacitation and fertilization is the probable reason for low pregnancy rates.

Male Sterilization. Vasectomy is the easiest and most commonly employed operation for male sterilization. In the United States 500,000 men undergo vasectomy each year (Cunningham et al, 1993). Vasectomy can be carried out with local anesthesia and on an out-of-hospital basis.

In vasectomy small right and left incisions are made into the anterior aspect of the scrotum above and lateral to each testis over the spermatic cord (Fig. 18-11, *B*). Each vas deferens is identified and doubly ligated with fine, nonabsorbable sutures. Then each vas deferens is severed between the ligatures. Occasionally the surgeon cauterizes the cut stumps of the sperm ducts. Many surgeons bury the cut ends into scrotal fascia to lessen the chance of reunion. Then the skin incisions are closed. Usually one nonabsorbable suture is used for closure of each skin incision. A dressing is applied.

The man is instructed in self-care to promote a safe return to routine activities. To reduce swelling and relieve discomfort, ice packs are applied to the scrotum intermittently for a few hours postoperatively. A scrotal support may be applied to decrease discomfort. Moderate inactivity for about 2 days is advisable because of local scrotal tenderness. The skin suture can be removed 5 to 7 days postoperatively. Sexual intercourse may be resumed as desired.

Sterility is not immediate. Some sperm will remain in

the proximal portions of the sperm ducts after vasectomy. One week to several months are required to clear the ducts of sperm (i.e., after approximately 15 ejaculations). Therefore some form of contraception is needed until the sperm count in the ejaculate on two consecutive tests is down to zero (Cunningham et al, 1993).

Vasectomy has no effect on potency (ability to achieve and maintain an erection) or volume of ejaculate. Endocrine production of testosterone continues so that secondary sex characteristics are not affected. Sperm production continues. Men occasionally may develop a hematoma, infection, or epididymitis (Hatcher et al, 1994). Less common are painful granulomas from accumulation of sperm. Sperm unable to leave the epididymis are lysed by the immune system.

Complications after bilateral vasectomy are uncommon and usually not serious (Giovannucci, 1992). They include bleeding (usually external), suture reaction, and reaction to anesthetic agent. Sterilization failures are rare, occurring in about 2 per 1000 men.

Tubal Reconstruction. Microsurgery to reanastomose (restoration of tubal continuity) the sperm ducts can be accomplished successfully in 90% of cases (i.e., sperm in the ejaculate) (Jarow, 1987). However, the fertility (pregnancies) rate is much lower (40% to 60%). The rate of success decreases as the time since the procedure increases. The vasectomy may result in permanent changes in the testes that leave men unable to father children. The changes are those ordinarily seen only in the elderly (e.g., interstitial fibrosis [scar tissue between the seminiferous tubules]). Some men develop antibodies against their own sperm (autoimmunization). The role of antisperm antibodies in fertility after vasectomy reversal has not been completely determined.

Future Trends

Contraceptive options are more limited in the United States and Canada than some other industrialized countries. Lack of funding for research, governmental regulations, conflicting values about contraception, and high costs of liability coverage for contraception have been cited as blocks to new and improved methods.

Methods that are currently being investigated include a contraceptive vaccine, vaginal rings, transdermal patches, biodegradable implants, and sublingual tablets for delivering hormonal contraception, more reliable ovulation predictors, and reversible sterilization methods using silicone blocks and other materials (Hatcher et al, 1994).

PLAN OF CARE

Sexually Active 22-Year-Old Woman

Case History

Jayne is a 22-year-old woman who has just become sexually active. She and her partner are high school graduates with 1 year of education at a community college.

The interview reveals that Jayne has not previously used any method of contraception. She and her partner want to choose a reliable method before they have coitus again. She expresses concern about the ease of use and possible side effects of the different methods. The nurse-practitioner found the physical examination to be within normal limits. The Pap smear and STD tests are negative.

EXPECTED OUTCOMES	IMPLEMENTATION	RATIONALE	EVALUATION
Nursing Diagnosis: Fear related to contraceptive method side effects			
Jayne and George will state they are less fearful.	The nurse discusses potential side effects for the chosen methods.	Knowledge of information reduces fear of the unknown. Knowledge strengthens one's ability to cope.	Jayne and George verbalize reasonable comfort with the knowledge.
Nursing Diagnosis: High risk for infection related to being sexually active			
Jayne and George's risk for STDs will be reduced.	The nurse discusses safer sex practices and barrier methods.	Couples in monogomous relationships are at least risk for STDs. Certain barrier methods can reduce the risk of STD transmission.	Jayne and George choose to use foam and condom. They exhibit no signs and symptoms of STDs at this time and at subsequent visits.

✤ EVALUATION

The nurse can be reasonably assured that care was effective if the goals of care have been achieved: the woman (couple) learns about the various methods of contraception; the couple achieves pregnancy only when it has been planned; and they experience no adverse sequelae as a result of the chosen method of contraception (see Plan of Care).

KEY POINTS

- Postpartum care is modeled on the concept of health.
- Cultural beliefs and practices affect the patient's response to the puerperium.
- The nursing plan of care includes assessments to detect deviations from normal, comfort measures to relieve discomfort or pain, and safety measures to prevent injury or infection.
- The nurse provides teaching and counseling measures designed to promote the patient's feelings of competence in self-care and baby care.
- The nurse must exhibit both clinical and decision-making skills to provide safe and effective physical care. Common nursing interventions include evaluating and treating the boggy uterus and the full urinary bladder, providing for pharmacologic and nonpharmacologic relief of pain and discomfort associated with the episiotomy or lacerations, and instituting measures to promote or suppress lactation.
- Nurses can help to promote the health of the patient's future pregnancies and children by administering rubella vaccine and Rh immune globulin if indicated.
- Meeting the psychosocial needs of new mothers involves planning care, which considers the composition and functioning of the entire family.

- Parenthood is a learned role. It requires time to master, improves with experience, and evolves gradually and continually as the needs of the parents and child change.
- Mothers (and fathers) often misjudge the actual amount of physical and emotional energy required for the role transition to parenthood.
- The nurse provides anticipatory guidance that helps new mothers and their families plan ways to achieve healthy adjustments to a new family member, deal with sibling responses, and interact positively with grandparents and other extended family members.
- There are a variety of contraceptive methods and various effectiveness ratings, advantages, and disadvantages of these methods.
- Nurses need to provide accurate information to couples to enable them to choose the contraceptive method(s) best suited to them.
- Proper concurrent use of spermicides and latex condoms provides protection against HIV and other STDs.
- Tubal ligations and vasectomies are sterilization methods used by increasing numbers of women and men.

CRITICAL THINKING EXERCISES

1. You are assigned to care for a Korean mother on the postpartum unit. She does not want to get out of bed, and you think it is related to her cultural practices. Nursing staff members tell you to make her follow the physician's order for activity, that is, to get out of bed as needed and to perform self-care activities.
   a. Identify the issues that are in conflict in this situation.
   b. Analyze arguments pro and con for integrating the woman's cultural practices into a plan of care.
   c. Formulate a plan of care based on your analysis.
2. During clinical experience with newborns, select a baby that you "really like" and the one that you "can't stand."
   a. Identify those characteristics of the newborn that influence your response to the babies.
   b. Reflect on what you would do if *your* baby had the characteristics of the one you "can't stand."
   c. Devise strategies for intervention for the mother (or father) whose baby does not meet her (or his) expectations.
3. You are working in a family planning clinic. A 17-year-old single woman and a 35-year-old married mother of two children are requesting birth control information.
   a. Examine your beliefs about who should have access to birth control and which methods are perceived by you to be acceptable. How might these beliefs affect your ability to provide birth control information?
   b. What patient information is needed as you assist these two women in making a decision about a birth control method?
   c. What information is needed by the women for them to make an informed decision about a method of contraception?
   d. Select one method for each of the above women; justify your choices.
   e. Write a teaching plan to provide specific instructions for each method.

REFERENCES

Ahumada LS: Multicultural perinatal health care, *Matern Child Health Educ Resources* vol 6, 1991.

Ament LA: Maternal tasks of the puerperium reidentified, *JOGNN* 19(4):330, 1990.

Anderson PO: Therapy review: drug use during breast-feeding, *Clin Pharmacy* 10:594, 1991.

Briggs GG et al: *Drugs in pregnancy and lactation: a reference guide to fetal and neonatal risk,* ed 3, Baltimore, 1990, Williams & Wilkins.

Bristoll SL et al: The mythical danger of rapid urinary drainage, *Am J Nurs* 89(3):344, 1989.

Campbell T, Chang B: Health care of the Chinese in America. In Spradley BW, editor: *Contemporary community nursing,* Boston, 1975, Little & Brown.

Connell EB: Barrier contraceptives, *Clin Obstet Gynecol* 32(2):377, 1989.

Contraception choices for women over age 35: focus on benefits and risks, *The contraception report* 3(2):4, 1992.

Coughlin R: Pregnancy and birth in Vietnam. In Hart D, Rajadhon PA, Coughlin RJ, editors: *Southeast Asian birth customs: three studies in human reproduction,* New Haven, CT, 1965, Human Relations Area Files.

Cunningham FG et al: *Williams obstetrics,* ed 19, Norwalk, CT, 1993, Appleton & Lange.

Darney PD et al: Acceptance and perceptions of Norplant among users in San Francisco, *Stud Fam Plann* 21(3):152, 1990.

D'Avanzo CE: Bridging the cultural gap with Southeast Asians, *MCN* 17(4):204, 1992.

Davis MS: Natural family planning, *NAACOG Clin Issues Perinat Women Health Nurs* 3(2):280, 1992.

Drug facts and comparisons, ed 47, St Louis, 1993, Facts and Comparisons Wolters Kluewer Co.

Family Health International: *An example of OC use instructions for PPIs,* Research Triangle Park, NC, 1990.

Fehring RJ et al: Use effectiveness of the Creighton model ovulation method of natural family planning, *JOGNN* 23(4):303, 1994.

Geissler E: *Pocket guide to cultural assessment,* St Louis, 1994, Mosby.

Gennaro S: Postpartal anxiety and depression in mothers of term and preterm infants, *Nurs Res* 37(2):82, 1988.

Giovannucci E et al: Vasectomy and its effects on lifespan, *N Engl J Med* 326:1392, 1992.

Greydanus DE, Lonchamp D: Contraception in the adolescent: preparation for the 1990s, *Med Clin North Am* 74(5):1205, 1990.

Grimes DA: Reversible contraception for the 1980s, *JAMA* 255(1):69, 1986.

Grimes DA: Whither the uterine device? *Clin Obstet Gynecol* 32(2):369, 1989.

Hahn RA, Muecke MA: The anthropology of birth in five U.S. ethnic populations: implications for obstetrical practice, *Curr Probl Obstet Gynecol Fertil* vol 138, 1987.

Hatcher RA et al: *Contraceptive technology: 1994-1996,* ed 16, New York, 1994, Irvington Publishers.

Hillard PA: The patient's reaction to side effects of oral contraceptives, *Am J Obstet Gynecol* 161(5)1412, 1989.

Horn B: Cultural concepts and postpartal care, *J Transcultural Nurs,* 2(1):48, 1990.

Jarow JP: Vasectomy: autoimmunity and reversal, *JAMA* 257(15):2087, 1987.

Konje J, Otolorin E, Ladipo O: The effect of continuous subdermal levonorgestrol (Norplant) on carbohydrate metabolism, *Am J Obstet Gynecol* 166:15, 1992.

Konrad CJ: Helping mothers integrate the birth experience, *MCN* 12(4):268, 1987.

Kugel C, Verson H: Relationship between weight change and diaphragm size change, *JOGNN* 15:123, 1986.

Labbok M, Queenan JT: The use of periodic abstinence for family planning, *Clin Obstet Gynecol* 32(2):387, 1989.

Lee RV: Understanding Southeast Asian mothers-to-be, *Childbirth Educ* 8(3):32, 1989.

Lee RV et al: Southeast Asian folklore about pregnancy and parturition, *Obstet Gynecol* 71:643, 1988.

Lethbridge DJ: Coitus interruptus—considerations as a method of birth control, *JOGNN* 20(1):80, 1991.

Liskin LS, Fox G: IUDs: an appropriate contraceptive for many women, *Popul Rep* (B), no 4, 1982.

Ludman EK et al: Blood-building foods in contemporary Chinese populations, *Perspect Pract* 89(8):1122, 1989.

Medical Letter: Choice of contraceptives, *Med Lett* 30(779), whole issue, Nov 18, 1988.

Mercer RT: Parent infant interaction. In Sonstegard LJ et al, editors: *Women's health: childbearing* vol 2, New York, 1982, Grune & Stratton.

Mishell DR: Contraception, *N Engl J Med* 320(12):777, 1989.

NAACOG: Cervical cap enters North American market, *NAACOG Newsletter* 15(9):1, 1988.

NAACOG: *Contraceptive options* (OGN Practice Resource), Washington, DC, 1991a, NAACOG.

NAACOG: *Contraception for special populations: teenagers and women over thirty-five*, Palo Alto, 1991b, Syntex.

Nisanian A: Outpatient minilaparotomy sterilization with local anesthesia, *J Reprod Med* 35(4):380, 1990.

Orshan SA: The pill, the patient, and you, *RN* 51(7):49, 1988.

Ortiz MF, Croxatto HB: The mode of action of IUDs, *Contraception* 36:37, 1987.

Park KJY, Peterson LM: Beliefs, practices, and experiences of Korean women in relation to childbirth, *Health Care Women Internat* 12:261, 1991.

Ramler D, Roberts J: A comparison of cold and warm sitz baths for relief of postpartum perineal pain, *JOGNN* 15:471, 1986.

Sampselle CM: Changes in pelvic muscle strength and stress urinary incontinence associated with childbirth, *JOGNN* 19(5):371, 1990.

Secor RMC: The cervical cap. *NAACOG Clin Issues Perinat Women Health Nurs* 3(2):236, 1992.

Shain RN et al: Impact of tubal sterilization and vasectomy on female marital sexuality: results of a controlled longitudinal study, *Am J Obstet Gynecol* 164(3):763, 1991.

Stainton MC: *Maternal newborn attachment origins and processes III. Interactional synchrony: the prelude to attachment.* Doctoral dissertation, San Francisco, 1985, University of California.

Stern PN et al: Culturally induced stress during childbearing: the Filipino-American experience, *Issues Health Care Women* 2(3-4):67, 1980.

Strom BL et al: Diaphragms, *Ann Intern Med* 107:816, 1987.

Tulman L, Fawcett, J: Recovery from childbirth: looking back 6 months after delivery, *Health Care Women Internat* 12:341, 1991.

United States Pharmacopeial Convention, Inc: *Drug information for the health care professional*, ed 13, Taunton, MA, 1993, Rand McNally.

Williams LR, Cooper MK: Nurse-managed postpartum home care, *JOGNN* 22(1):25, 1993.

Willson JR, Carrington ER: *Obstetrics and gynecology*, ed 9, St Louis, 1991, Mosby.

Women's Health: Cervical cap approved for marketing, *Am J Nurs* 89(2):165, 1989.

World Health Organization: Mechanism of action, safety, and efficacy of intrauterine devices, *Technical Report Series 753*, Geneva, 1987, World Health Organization.

BIBLIOGRAPHY

Aderhold KJ, Perry L: Jet hydrotherapy for labor and postpartum pain relief, *MCN* 16(2):97, 1991.

Beck CT, Reynolds MA, Rutowski P: Maternity blues and postpartum depression, *JOGNN* 21(4):287, 1992.

Berchtold N, Burrough M: Reaching out: depression after delivery support group network, *NAACOG Clin Issues Perinat Women Health Nurs* 1(3):385, 1990.

Boyer KB: Prediction of postpartum depression, *NAACOG Clin Issues Perinat Women Health Nurs* 1(3):359, 1990.

Flagler S: Relationships between stated feelings and measures of maternal adjustment, *JOGNN* 19(5):411, 1990.

Fortier JC et al: Adjustment to a newborn: sibling preparation makes a difference, *JOGNN* 20(1):73, 1991.

Gardner DL, Campbell B: Assessing postpartum fatigue, *MCN* 16(5):264, 1991.

Hinkle LT: Counseling for the Norplant user, *JOGNN* 23(5):387, 1994.

Kaunitz A: Oral contraceptives and gynecologic cancer: an update for the 1990s, *Am J Obstet Gynecol* 167(4, Part 2):1171, 1992.

King J: Helping patients choose an appropriate method of birth control, *MCN* 17(2):91, 1992.

Lamp JM: Humor in postpartum education: depicting a new mother's worst nightmare, *MCN* 17(2):82, 1992.

Lommel LL et al: Adolescent use of contraceptives, *NAACOG Clin Issues Perinat Women Health Nurs* 3(2):199, 1992.

Martell LK: Postpartum depression as a family problem, *MCN* 15(2):90, 1990.

Rempusheski VF: Role of the extended family in parenting: a focus on grandparents of preterm infants, *J Perinat Neonat Nurs* 4(2):43, 1990.

Spadt SK, Martin KR, Thomas AM: Experiential classes for siblings-to-be, *MCN* 15(3):184, 1990.

Sweezy SR: Contraception for the postpartum woman, *NAACOG Clin Issues Perinat Women Health Nurs* 3(2):209, 1992.

Videotapes For Parents

All are available from Childbirth Graphics Ltd, Rochester, NY.

Baby Basics (VHS, 110 minutes)

Excellent and entertaining resource on infant care in the first few months. Topics include the newborn at birth, parents caring for themselves postpartum, the first few days at home, daily care, feeding, health and safety, crying and sleeping, growth and development.

Baby Talk (VHS, 60 minutes)

Excellent new video on early parenting concerns and baby care. Topics include newborn appearance, sleep and awake patterns, crying and colic, illness and doctor visits, bottle feeding, and the importance of parents taking care of themselves.

Hey, What About Me? (VHS, 25 minutes)

Video on sibling adjustment. Contains songs about feelings, games and lullabies, bouncing rhymes to do with the new baby, and suggestions on what the siblings can do when they feel angry or lonely.

19 Home Care

DEITRA LEONARD LOWDERMILK

LEARNING OBJECTIVES

Define the key terms.
Identify common selection criteria for safe early postpartum discharge.
List the potential advantages and disadvantages of early postpartum discharge, including those justified by research findings.
Summarize the nurse's role in these postpartum follow-up strategies: early discharge preparatory classes, home visits, telephone follow-up, warm lines, and support groups.

KEY TERMS

care path case management
early postpartum discharge
postpartum support group
warm lines

RELATED TOPICS

Home care for newborns *(Chap. 14)* • Parenting skills *(Chap. 18)* • Postpartum assessment *(Chap. 18)* • Newborn assessment *(Chap. 14)* • Family relationships *(Chap. 17)*

Early postpartum discharge is a trend affecting increasing numbers of maternity clients and the nurses who provide their care. Early postpartum discharge refers to a postbirth hospital stay of 48 hours or less and is generally based on criteria that indicate low-risk status (Box 19-1). In 1994 a woman who has experienced an uncomplicated vaginal birth is often discharged after 24 hours.

The nurse in contemporary maternity practice is well advised to examine the circumstances contributing to early postpartum discharge and the implications of shorter stays for the well-being of patients and families and for maternity practice. The first issue is best addressed by examining the role of the current health care environment in early discharge.

THE HEALTH CARE ENVIRONMENT THAT SUPPORTS EARLY DISCHARGE

Escalation of health care costs has contributed to cost containment efforts on the part of both care providers and agencies that fund care. One such measure, prospective payment, enables the fee structures to be determined in advance of treatment, rather than retrospectively. Prospective payment systems impose cost containment measures and provide incentives to providers who decrease costs. A prospective payment system, the diagnosis related group (DRG), was initiated by the federal government in 1983 to enable containment of Medicare costs so that the system might remain solvent. The DRG fee structure specifies that providers may recover only the preset (prospective) fee associated with a particular diagnosis, regardless of the actual cost incurred in delivering such care. Hospitals that contain costs are allowed to keep the overage in payment. In the event that actual costs incurred are greater than those allowable by diagnosis, hospitals absorb the loss.

Success of prospective payment systems, including the DRG model for cost containment, have encouraged other health care financiers (private insurers, the health maintenance organization [HMO]), and the preferred provider organization [PPO] to enact similar measures. Prospective payment systems have resulted in other major changes in health care: fewer unnecessary hospital-

BOX 19-1

Criteria for Early Discharge

MOTHER

Uncomplicated pregnancy, labor, birth, and postpartum course
No evidence of premature rupture of membranes
Stable blood pressure; temperature < 100.4° F (38° C)
Ability to ambulate
Ability to void without difficulty
Intact perineum without third- or fourth-degree perineal laceration
Hemoglobin > 10 g
No significant vaginal bleeding

INFANT

Term infant (38 to 41 weeks) with birth weight of 2500 to 4500 g*
Normal findings on physical assessment performed by health care provider*
Normal laboratory data, including negative Coombs' test result and hematocrit 40% to 65%*
Stable vital signs*
Temperature stability*
Successful feeding (normal sucking and swallowing)*
Apgar score > 7 at 1 and 5 minutes
Normal voiding and stooling
PKU and thyroid screening tests completed, repeat of PKU test scheduled for 2 weeks*

GENERAL

Attendance at classes that include maternal and infant care, with an emphasis on problems of the first week at home*
Presence of a support person in the home to assist with care*
Presence of a strategy for follow-up*
Uncomplicated pregnancy, labor, birth, and postpartum course for mother and baby*
Demonstration of skill by mother in feeding, providing skin and cord care, measuring temperature with a thermometer, assessing infant well-being and signs of illness, and providing emergency care*

PKU, Phenylketonuria.
*Recommendations of American Academy of Pediatrics: Criteria for early infant discharge and follow-up evaluation, *Pediatrics* 65:651, 1980.

izations, more diagnostic tests and minor procedures performed in out-of-hospital settings, increasing acuity of in-hospital health problems, and early discharge.

An appreciation of the potential effects of those changes, especially early discharge, and the existence of an intensely competitive health care market have led to the development of innovative services to bridge hospi-

tal and home. The maternity nurse can play a vital role in developing and implementing home care options. To do so effectively involves first recognizing the advantages and disadvantages of early discharge, including those with research support.

Potential Advantages of Short-Stay Maternity Care

Proponents of early postpartum discharge cite the following advantages of the practice:
- Reinforce the concept of childbirth as a normal physiologic event.
- Allow shorter separations between mothers and other children.
- Extend a couple's sense of control and participation beyond the birth itself.
- Capitalize on the security of the home environment during the stressors of early parenting.
- Decrease unnecessary exposure to the pathogens in the hospital environment (Harrison, 1990).
- Allow beds on the maternity service to be used more effectively (i.e., quick turnover in patients or for someone with a complication).
- Take advantage of increasing numbers of nonmedicated births.
- Allow more time for mother/father/partner/infant and other family members to bond (Fig. 19-1).
- Create less disruption in the daily life of the family.

Potential Disadvantages of Short-Stay Maternity Care

The day that a couple brings the newborn home for the first time is generally joyous and memorable. It also can be profoundly unsettling. Although some new parents anticipate early discharge eagerly, others feel unprepared for the reality they face. The woman with another child or children, feeling unrested, may be concerned about going home to their demands. Not uncommonly, the first-time mother will report astonishment at her level of discomfort. As one young mother explained, "I thought when labor was over, there would be no more pain. Why didn't someone warn me about stitches and sore nipples?" Another, while packing to go home, shared these feelings, "Almost from the minute I was brought from the delivery room, I have been bombarded with facts about baby care. There's so much to learn, everything is jumbled in my brain. What if I don't remember something or do it backwards and hurt my baby? The ink isn't dry on the birth records and I'm about to be wheeled out the door."

During the immediate days and weeks of the fourth trimester, the parents will be experiencing a major life transition: recovering from the events surrounding birth, adjusting to the demands of a newborn, parenting, applying the knowledge and skill from their postdischarge instructions, shifting priorities, and realigning some roles while assuming new ones. When there are other children, an additional challenge occurs: helping them to adjust to sharing home and parents with the newborn. The stress inherent in such profound transitions contributes tremendous crisis potential to the early postpartum experience.

Opponents of early postpartum discharge cite these predominant concerns: the risk of undetected complications and the vulnerability and crisis potential that exists for both the patients and families. Goer (1990) cites recommendations of the American College of Obstetrics and Gynecologists (ACOG) for a 96-hour recovery time after a cesarean birth and a 48-hour recovery time after vaginal birth: "ACOG also recommends 96 hours following uncomplicated abdominal hysterectomy—and hysterectomy [patients] won't be taking home a new baby."

The protest against early discharge becomes magnified in the conventional health care arena, in which there is a 4- to 6-week interval between discharge and the first scheduled visit to a health care provider for follow-up. To some extent, without some innovative approach, families are on their own, attempting a major life transition without benefit of health care resources. Postpartum nurses have been expected to be responsive to the changes in practice dictated by cost containment. In a small pilot survey, Lukacs (1991) found postpartum nurses frustrated, feeling harried, and occasionally ineffective in meeting the needs of the short-stay patient. Continued attention must be given to the ways in which

nurses and nursing are affected by this short-stay model of practice.

The Future of Early Postpartum Discharge

As evaluative studies and research continue to show favorable patient and economic outcomes of early postpartum discharge, the approach will likely become more common. Caseloads will tend to be increased as selection criteria are relaxed, so that those at minor risk will experience shorter postpartum hospitalization. In addition, common problems such as maternal infection and infant hyperbilirubinemia, identified after discharge, may be treated in the home (Norr, Nacion, 1986).

Existing home care follow-up programs are likely to extend their services to greater numbers of patients, including those from lower socioeconomic groups and those who stay longer than 24 hours in the hospital setting (Evans, 1991). Programs will offer increased outreach services, allowing those at greater geographic distances to take advantage of the short-stay option. As more maternity nurses extend their practice into homes, the subspecialty of postpartum home care will emerge.

NURSING CARE AND EARLY POSTPARTUM DISCHARGE: BRIDGING HOSPITAL AND HOME

The hospital-based maternity nurse assumes an invaluable role as caregiver, teacher, and patient/family advo-

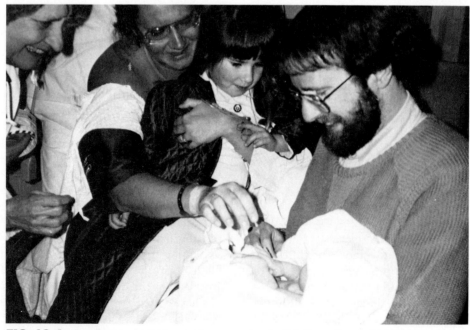

FIG. 19-1 Bonding and attachment begun early after birth are fostered in postpartum period. Grandmother, parents, and older sibling meet newborn. (Courtesy Nancy Mason, MD.)

cate in settings with early postpartum discharge options. In collaboration with other health care providers, the nurse is instrumental in determining the readiness of mother and infant for early discharge. On the basis of careful assessment, the nurse plans an approach for meeting the needs of mother and infant during the brief hospitalization and provides anticipatory guidance, teaching, and referral to help to ensure continued well-being at home.

Care Path

One innovation to achieve these ends during the shortened hospital stay is the use of **care path case management** for delivery of nursing care. The care path clearly delineates what teaching/discharge planning should occur within specified times. Nurses have an average of only 24 hours to prepare the postpartum mother for discharge. Therefore each nurse on each shift is expected to complete the prescribed interventions.

For example, the mother-baby care path standard after vaginal birth may include the following schedule—as long as maternal or newborn recovery continues (see Care Path). Starting with admission to the postpartum unit or 2 hours after birth if the woman remains in an LDRP setting until the end of the first 8 hours, the woman is assisted with ambulation; is taught about perineal self-care (including medication), hand washing, involution, and bleeding (lochia); and is given booklets and introduced to available videotapes. When the baby is with her, she learns about supporting the infant's head and extremities and proper positioning for feeding and burping. If she is breastfeeding, she also learns about rooting, latching on, and release of the nipple. She is taught about safety: use of the suction bulb, baby positioning, need for a car seat, and the need for the baby to be attended at all times.

By the end of the second 8 hours the woman is taught about diet, activity and rest, elimination, and medication. When her baby is with her, she is taught about bonding and attachment, usual parent concerns, normal newborn characteristics, diaper changes, cord care, frequency and timing of feedings, use of water feedings, pacifiers, and suckling patterns.

By the end of the third 8 hours the woman needs a review of warning signs for which to call her health care provider. If she needs a consultation—for example, with a lactation specialist—this call is made before discharge. Sibling rivalry is discussed. Teaching is reinforced, and questions are answered. The mother is asked whether she needs repeat demonstrations or explanations, for example, newborn characteristics, including crying, sneezing, diaper changes, feeding, circumcision care, and recognition of jaundice. As the woman is preparing to go home, she is reminded again of the person to call should a question arise and of the follow-up appointments.

The care path provides clear direction to coordinat-ing care, teaching essentials of information, preparing the postpartum woman for discharge, and supporting the parent toward independence (Gillerman, Beckham, 1991).

The care plan needs to be adapted to a woman's special needs (e.g., English as a second language or inability to read, impaired mental capacity such as retardation, substance abuse, very young chronologic age, or physical problems such as extreme fatigue, infection, or anemia). The care plan is a standard. Any deviation is noticed quickly and must be acted on. Therefore the care path can enhance and secure quality care. It is one appropriate vehicle for high-technology nursing and developing professional independence. It provides one method to effect the transition from hospital to home care.

Postpartum Follow-Up Services

For women discharged early, there is an obvious need for bridging hospital and home, especially early in the course of the fourth trimester when rapid physiologic and psychosocial transitions are occurring. Maternity nurses, wishing to offer continuity of care, have extended their practice arena outside the hospital, offering a variety of postpartum follow-up services:

- Early-discharge preparatory classes
- Telephone follow-up
- Home visit follow-up
- Warm lines/help lincs
- Parent support groups

Although home care packages for postpartum follow-up may be offered by hospitals, maternity centers, public health agencies, private physicians, or independent entrepreneurs, it is the nurse who is a constant presence in each of these approaches.

Care Management

✦ ASSESSMENT

Systematic nursing assessment of the postpartum woman and her newborn assumes special significance when anticipating early discharge. Nurses may use assessment data to help establish that criteria have been met for early discharge, thereby safe-guarding mother and infant. A careful assessment enables the nurse to note normality of findings and to recognize and promptly report any complications. Furthermore, these assessment findings represent baseline data for continued assessment in the home.

The postpartum assessment focuses on the mother's physiologic and psychologic status, her level of comfort, any relevant knowledge deficit and readiness to learn, the bonding behaviors evident, and adjustment to the transitions required for mothering. The focus of the newborn assessment is physiologic adjustment to an extrauterine environment, normality of physical and behavioral findings, and ability of the parents to meet the infant's needs.

CARE PATH

Mother-Baby Vaginal Birth Without Complications: Expected Length of Stay—24 Hours

	4th Stage Labor	By 4 Hours after Birth	1st Baby Visit	By 8 Hours after Birth
ASSESSMENTS		PP admission assessment and care plan completed		
VITAL SIGNS	every 15 min times 1 hour WNL	every 1 hour times 3 WNL		every 8 hours WNL
POSTPARTUM ASSESSMENT	every 15 min times I hour WNL	every 1 hour times 3 WNL		every 8 hours WNL
VOIDING	Empty bladder or fundus firm and not displaced	Empty bladder or fundus firm and not displaced		Empty bladder each void
SENSORY	Fully alert; moving all extremities	Ambulating with help		Ambulating without help
BONDING	Evidence of parent/ infant bonding at first breastfeeding		Parent/infant bonding continues	
LABS		Intrapartal CBC results on chart/computer; determine Rh status and need for anti-Rh globulin;check for Rubella immunity		
INTERVENTIONS IV	IV	May be discontinued		
PERINEAL	Ice pack to perineum; pericare by nurse	Self perineal care		
ACTIVITY	Up to BR with help	Ambulates with help	Assisted to comfortable position for holding and feeding baby	Ambulates without help
MEDICATIONS	Pitocin added to IV; analgesics PRN	Pitocin discontinued		Stool softener; PNV
TEACHING/ DISCHARGE PLAN	Breastfeeding positioning; call for help with first ambulation	Verbalizes understanding/ unit routines and how to achieve rest, pericare, involution, pain control	Handwashing, infant safety, positioning for breastfeeding, and-burping; if breastfeeding, positioning baby, latching on, timing, removing from breast	Comfort measures and care related to bowel and bladder function, nutrition, lactation promotion or suppression
REFERRAL/ CONSULT				

PP, Postpartum; *WNL*, within normal limits; *CBC*, complete blood count; *HCT*, hematocrit; *BR*, bathroom; *PRN*, as needed; *PNV*, prenatal vitamin; *Rx*, prescription.

CARE PATH

Mother-Baby Vaginal Birth Without Complications: Expected Length of Stay—24 Hours

2nd Baby Visit	By 16 Hours After Birth	3rd Baby Visit	By 24 Hours After Birth	Discharge Shift
Parent/infant bonding progressing	PP HCT if ordered; give anti-Rh globulin if indicated			PP HCT WNL; give Rubella vaccine if indicated
	Sitz bath if ordered			Rx filled or given to take home
Bonding, parent concerns, feeding	Use of sitz bath	Infant bath, cord care, need for car seat, newborn characteristics, circumcision care if needed; answer questions; return demonstration for diaper change and feeding	Home care: signs of complications (infection, bleeding), normal psychologic adjustments, resumption of normal activities of daily living; resumption of sexual activities, contraception; identification of support system at home	Return demonstration infant care; reinforce use of booklets for infant and self-care; inform whom to call if problems; review need for follow-up appt; provide information about community resources; discuss immunization needs; provide copy of home care instructions
	Assess need for referral/consults, i.e., social work, lactation consultant		Referral as needed before discharge	Refer to community agency as needed

✤ NURSING DIAGNOSIS

As each woman and family anticipate postpartum discharge, they will have unique responses. After a careful analysis of data obtained from the assessment, the nurse establishes data-based nursing diagnoses that will guide nursing actions. The following nursing diagnoses may be relevant for a woman or family experiencing early postpartum discharge:

Altered health maintenance related to
- Insufficient knowledge of signs of complications

Anxiety related to
- Perceived lack of readiness for early discharge

Ineffective breastfeeding related to
- Inadequate knowledge or insufficient support

Ineffective family coping related to
- Disorganization and role changes of early discharge and parenting

Fatigue related to
- Lack of opportunities to rest during brief hospitalization

High risk for altered parenting related to
- Lack of knowledge/skill and unrealistic expectations

✤ EXPECTED OUTCOMES

A plan of care is formulated that relates specifically to the needs of the woman and her family. To the extent possible, the nurse involves them all in the planning and incorporates their priorities and preferences for any actions planned. *Expected outcomes* are set in patient-centered terms and prioritized in collaboration with the woman and family. Expected outcomes appropriate for women/families experiencing early postpartum discharge include the following:

1. The postpartum woman will experience uncomplicated physiologic recovery.
2. The woman will experience uncomplicated psychologic adjustment to parenting.
3. The postpartum woman will verbalize an accurate knowledge base and/or demonstrate appropriate care of self and infant.
4. The woman will list available resources for home care and support and the manner in which these may be accessed.
5. The new parents will demonstrate positive interactions with each other, the newborn, and other family members.
6. The postpartum woman will attend preparatory classes for early discharge and will be scheduled for follow-up at home.

✤ COLLABORATIVE CARE

Nurses assume both caregiving and teaching roles in preparing the woman and her family for early discharge.

They know what home care follow-up alternatives are available to their postpartum patients and make appropriate referrals. Nurses who are providers of postpartum home care extend continuity of care to the postdischarge setting in a variety of ways: supportive counseling, teaching, and referral, which are based on continued additions to the data base.

✤ EVALUATION

Evaluation of outcomes is a continuous process. To be effective, evaluation is based on patient-centered expected outcomes identified during the planning stage of nursing care. The nurse can be reasonably assured that care was effective if the following outcomes have been achieved:

- The postpartum woman has experienced uncomplicated physiologic recovery and psychologic adjustment to parenting.
- She verbalizes an accurate knowledge base and/or demonstrates appropriate self-care and infant care.
- She lists available resources for home care and support and the manner in which these may be obtained.
- The new parents demonstrate positive interactions with each other, the newborn, and other family members.
- The postpartum woman has attended preparatory classes for early discharge and has scheduled a follow-up visit.

If the nurse determines that expected outcomes are being achieved, implementation of the nursing actions continues as planned. When evaluation data suggest that expected outcomes have not been attained, the plan is revised.

EARLY DISCHARGE PREPARATORY INSTRUCTION

To ensure the woman's safety and well-being, a basic criterion for patient selection in short-stay maternity programs is educational preparation before discharge. Either formal classes or one-on-one instruction, both supplemented with written material, may be provided at various times throughout the pregnancy. The necessary instructions may be given initially or expanded during the short hospital stay. Attempting to provide essential teaching only within the time constraints of a short-stay setting presents a special challenge for nurses who are trying to teach more in less time, often with fewer staff members. In addition, the nurse who is doing the teaching may be carrying a caseload that also includes women with complications. Postpartum teaching is further complicated because the learner is tired and uncomfortable from the demands of labor and distracted by visitors and her desire to spend time with the baby and her family:

"The attention span of short-stay mothers may be affected by sensory overload, postdelivery fatigue, and sleep deprivation" (Martell et al, 1989).

The nurse recognizes that the adult's *readiness to learn* is associated with an acknowledgment that a problem exists or with recognition of a gap or deficit in knowledge or skill. The postpartum woman may not identify knowledge deficit as a priority concern (Blackburn et al, 1988; Tribotti et al, 1988). The inexperienced mother may not realize her limitations or know what questions to ask until she is at home with the dependent newborn. The multiparous woman, not yet appreciating how unique each child is, may not realize that her existing knowledge base is insufficient. (Pridham et al, 1991). For example, one mother of an especially fussy newborn son reported that she had not learned quieting behaviors when caring for her first baby, a quiet, easily comforted daughter.

A *teaching plan* is essential to avoid duplication of content and to ensure that all essential information is given. A teaching plan also offers consistency of the information being provided. Few things are more frustrating than hearing conflicting information, especially when the learner is pressed for time or is feeling stressed. Written and audiovisual materials can be used effectively to reinforce the verbal instructions.

Teaching plans should be based on systematic assessment of the woman's learning needs, rather than on the nurse's perceptions of what constitutes essential information. Blackburn et al (1988) and Tribotti et al (1988) indicate that differences often exist between what nurses believe patients should know and what patients want to know. However, focusing on the informational needs common to new mothers can assist the nurse in collaborating with the woman in planning instruction. Mothers in short-stay perinatal programs have identified as priorities health threats to themselves and their babies, feeding, and infant care (Davis et al, 1988; Martell et al, 1989). Of concern to multiparous women are family relationships (Hiser, 1987).

Once home, the postpartum woman is likely to turn to the infant's father or another support person as a source of information. For that reason it is imperative to include the woman's partner or support person in the instruction whenever possible. Grandparents also may be invited because they frequently are caregivers for the new family during early days at home (Fig. 19-2).

When postpartum follow-up is planned, especially home visits, not all the essential teaching must be provided during the hospital stay. Some information, even if considered somewhat essential, can be temporarily delayed to the next nurse-patient contact. The nurse can help the family to anticipate what their most pressing information needs will be between discharge and the initial follow-up contact. Together, nurse and patients can plan to meet those prioritized needs. For example, the mother and nurse may reach a mutual decision to delay the total bath demonstration until the first home visit,

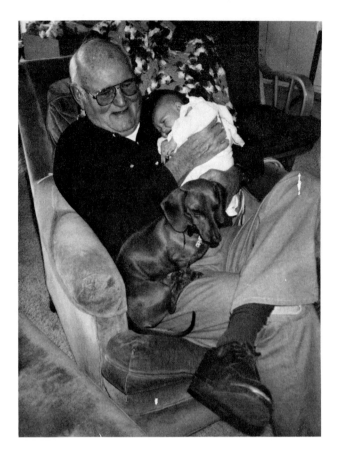

FIG. 19-2 Grandfather tends to newborn while assisting family dog with "sibling" rivalry. (Courtesy Nancy Mason, MD.)

focusing in-hospital teaching on cleaning the diaper area. Subsequently, the mother will learn to bathe her infant in the home, where she can work with the items she will use on a daily basis. Learning is facilitated because she is not forced to adapt to agency routine, supplies, or equipment; instead, she works within the security of her home with items familiar to her (Evans, 1991).

The nurse is, of course, compelled to provide emergency information and to help women gain knowledge or skills they will need between discharge and the initial postdischarge contact (see Signs of Potential Complications). All couples need to be helped to anticipate the reality of homecoming with a new infant and the stressors of the first hours and days of transition. Table 19-1 shows a checklist devoted to self-assessment of learning needs of women anticipating early postpartum discharge. Other topics include breastfeeding, formula-feeding, and infant care.

Instructions for the First Hours or Days at Home

New parents often romanticize homecoming with their newborn to the extent that they are inadequately prepared for the reality. One new mother explains, "By the time we drove an hour through traffic, my stitches were hurting and all I wanted was a warm sitz bath and some private time with Bill and the baby, in that order. Instead, a carload of visitors pulled into the driveway as we were unbuckling the baby from his car seat. I thought I would surely cry."

All couples, especially those anticipating early discharge, must be helped to anticipate what the transition from hospital to home will be like so that reality shock will not negate their joy or cause undue stress. Anticipatory guidance should focus on the immediacy of home-coming: the trip itself, providing essential infant care, ensuring rest and comfort for the mother, dealing with visitors, and enlisting help. Sometimes the most simple nursing strategies provide enormous support.

The Trip Home

With guidance from the nurse, the couple anticipates the actual journey home. The nurse reinforces the use of an infant car seat that meets appropriate safety standards and helps the parents consider how they will respond if the baby becomes fussy during the trip. Some new mothers prefer to ride home sitting in the back seat beside the infant in the car seat. A fluffy pillow on the seat can provide comfort for a painful perineum, especially during a long trip. Before discharge the nurse may wish to administer whatever mild analgesic has been ordered for postpartum pain relief. The nurse first determines that the mother has had at least one previous dose of the medication without untoward effect.

Before the discharge a family member may wish to take all unnecessary items and any flowers or gifts home and to have any prescriptions filled. This minimizes the time necessary for unloading the car or shopping, thereby increasing the availability of that person as a support after the trip home.

Dealing with Activities of Daily Life

Even the small details of daily life may become stressful, given the demands of a newborn or the discomfort or

---

SIGNS OF POTENTIAL COMPLICATIONS

WARNING SIGNS—POSTPARTUM (PHYSICAL)

1. Fever, with or without chills
2. Foul-smelling or irritating vaginal discharge
3. Excessive lochia or vaginal discharge
4. Recurrence of bright red vaginal bleeding after the lochia has changed to rust color
5. A swollen area on the leg that is painful, red, or hot to the touch
6. Localized swelling or a painful, hot area on the breast
7. A burning sensation during urination or an inability to urinate
8. Pelvic or perineal pain

TABLE 19-1 Self-Assessment of Learning Needs: Early Postpartum Discharge Unit

As a patient anticipating early postpartum discharge, your time in the hospital will be limited. To help the nursing staff make sound use of that time to meet your learning needs, please complete this checklist by placing a check (✔) in the column that best describes your priority for learning the information listed. Use the following key:
CR, Critical to know before discharge
HV, Prefer to learn during home visit
PI, Printed sheet or brochure will be adequate
OK, Knowledge in area is adequate or not desired

TOPIC	LEARNING PRIORITY				DOCUMENTATION OF TEACHING/DATE/NURSE	PATIENT OUTCOME
	CR	HV	PI	OK		
Self-care of vaginal flow						
Care of stitches						
Afterpains						
Diet						
Postbirth exercises						
Warning signs						
Resuming sex/birth control						

fatigue associated with birth and a busy homecoming day, or both. The nurse may intervene by suggesting that even if the plan is to use cloth diapers, the parents may wish to purchase one box of disposables for those first hours at home. The nurse, offering preparatory instructions during the pregnancy, may encourage the woman to freeze extra casseroles or leftovers to be ready for use for the first few meals at home. Even a take-out meal can be planned if necessary to decrease one additional parental responsibility or concern during the initial hours at home.

Planning for discharge soon after an infant feeding ensures that the couple will have adequate time to get home and relatively settled before the next feeding (Fig. 19-3). Offering a sample carton of premixed bottles for the formula-fed infant prevents an immediate need for rushed preparation of formula. *Offering the samples to nursing mothers is inappropriate because it may be confused as discouragement of breastfeeding.*

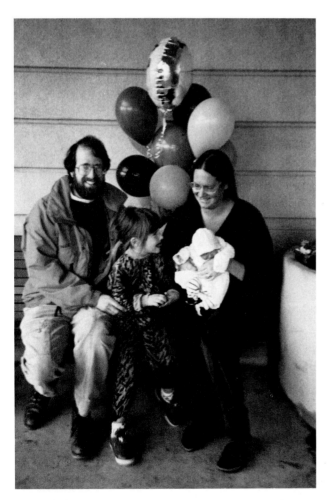

FIG. 19-3 Happy homecoming requires some planning. (Courtesy Nancy Mason, MD.)

Dealing with Visitors

A newborn in the family or neighborhood often seems to draw visitors like a magnet. Although the new parents may be unsettled by the trip home, they may serve as unwilling hosts to avoid strained relationships with friends and family. The nurse can help the parents in advance to explore ways in which they can assert their needs in such situations. They also may want to work out some signal for alerting the partner that the new mother is becoming tired or uncomfortable and needs to have a partner invite the visitors into another part of the house.

POSTPARTUM CARE
Home Visits

Many early discharge programs are using postpartum home visits as an additional measure for postpartum follow-up. Home visits may be a service of the hospital, the private physician, a public health department, or a private agency providing home care to maternity patients (Mitchell et al, 1993). Regardless of their source, home visits are planned collaboratively with the family and are scheduled on the basis of identified need. A visit may occur as early as 24 hours after discharge; rarely would an initial visit be delayed beyond the third day at home. Additional visits are planned throughout the course of the first week, as needed. A decision to extend the contract for home visits beyond that time will be made on the basis of the family's needs.

Assessment

During the home visit the nurse conducts a systematic assessment of mother and newborn to determine physiologic adjustment and to identify any existing complications. The assessment also focuses on the mother's emotional adjustment, including the presence of balancing factors (perception, coping, and support) that prevent crisis, and her knowledge of self-care and infant-care. Ideally, the father is present during a home visit so that the couple's adjustment to parenting can be considered. If not, the mother's perception of their adjustment can be noted. The visit also affords the nurse an opportunity to observe interaction among those family members present within the familiarity and security of their home setting where they are in control. Observing new parents, the newborn, and other family members in this natural setting enables the nurse to elicit data about their life circumstances not accessible in any other way (Clemen-Stone et al, 1991). The Home Care box on p. 516 indicates criteria for evaluating the visit's outcome.

Interventions

Although the primary nursing interventions during a home visit involve supportive counseling, anticipatory guidance, teaching, or referral, on occasion physical care

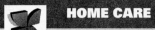

OUTCOME CRITERIA—PHYSIOLOGIC RECOVERY, INVOLUTION, AND HEALING IN MOTHER

- Lists signs of problems that should be reported to primary care provider immediately
- Verbalizes understanding of normal findings
- Confirms decreasing discomfort, controlled by prescribed comfort measures
- Confirms patterns reflecting adequate rest

Breasts

- Supported by well-fitted brassiere
- Nontender; no signs of inflammation
- Intact nipples without cracks, fissures, or undue soreness
  If breastfeeding:
- Describes or demonstrates technique for placing baby on and removing baby from breast, positioning to decrease stress of nipple area
  If not breastfeeding:
- No engorgement
- Taking lactation suppressants correctly (if prescribed) and knows warning signs to report
- Discusses importance of not stimulating breasts

Uterus

- Fundus firm, descending below umbilicus ~1 cm/day

Bowels/bladder

- Resumption of usual pattern of bowel elimination
- Hemorrhoids (if present) decreasing in size; not causing undue discomfort
- Resumption of usual pattern of urinary elimination; no burning or difficulty in initiating stream

Lochia

- Reveals normally progressing involution—rubra, serosa, alba in decreasing amounts—normal fleshy odor, no clots

Incision: perineal or abdominal

- Episiotomy (if present) well approximated without undue redness, edema, ecchymosis, discharge, or tenderness
- Cesarean incision (if present) clean, dry, well approximated; skin staples, sutures, or Steri-strips intact (if still present); evidence of normal healing process

Legs

- Nontender, with negative Homans' sign bilaterally

PHYSIOLOGIC ADAPTATION OF INFANT

Temperature

- 97.6° to 99° F (36.5° to 37.2° C) axillary route

Heart rate

- 120 to 160 beats/min, strong, regular, normal variations with activity

Respiration

- 30 to 60 breaths/min, normal breath sounds, irregular rhythm; no retractions, or grunting; normal variations with activity

Skin

- Warm, good turgor; no rashes

Head

- Symmetric, with flat fontanels; molding or caput decreasing; no hematoma

Abdomen

- Soft, nondistended; audible bowel sounds

Color

- Consistent with racial background; no jaundice

Activity

- Alert with good muscle tone; moving all extremities normally

Umbilical cord

- Normal atrophy noted, dry base without redness; not malodorous

Circumcision

- Bell in place (if appropriate); clean and healing; no evidence of oozing; urinary stream normal

Elimination

- Wetting a minimum of 6 to 10 diapers/day; stools consistent with feeding method in color, number, and consistency

Sleep pattern

- Sleeps well

Feeding

- Sucking well without excessive spitting
- Burping well
- Length of breastfeeding (if done) consistent with recommendations
- Amount of formula per feeding (if done) consistent with recommendations

EFFECTIVE ADJUSTMENT TO PARENTING

- Parents interact with newborn in a loving and nurturing way.
- Parenting behaviors reflect appreciation of sensory and behavioral capacities of infant.
- Parents respond to cues provided by infant.
- Parents verbalize increasing confidence and competence in physical care of infant feeding, diapering, dressing, hygiene, sensory stimulation.
- Parents identify deviations from normal in the infant that should be brought to the immediate attention of the primary caregiver.
- Parents relate not only stressful or challenging factors in lifestyle change but also positive or joyous ones.
- Parents describe or demonstrate emergency procedures and verbalize ways for accessing emergency help.
- Parents interact in a supportive manner.
- Parents collaborate effectively with each other in caring for newborn and other children.
- Parents relate effectively to newborn's relatives.

might be given. For example, on order from the health care provider, the nurse may remove sutures or staples from the mother's abdominal incision, change a dressing, or initiate home phototherapy for the infant (Fig. 19-4). On occasion it may be necessary for the nurse to collect blood or urine specimens for laboratory study. For example, a clean-catch urine specimen might be needed for a mother with suspected urinary tract infection; infant blood might be collected to follow up hyperbilirubinemia in the newborn. Throughout procedures of this kind, careful techniques are used to prevent the spread of pathogens.

Documentation

It is imperative that nurses keep careful records documenting their assessment findings and all interventions, including counseling and teaching. Not only does such documentation serve as a legal record of the visit; it also justifies appropriate reimbursement. Fig. 19-5 shows an example of a document for recording a postpartum home visit.

Previsit Plans

Although a nurse's purpose in visiting is different from that of a guest in the home, visiting nurses extend the same courtesy they would show to friends they might visit. For example, the nurse will call ahead to verify that the time scheduled for the visit is still convenient. (Not only is this common courtesy; it occasionally saves an unnecessary, sometimes costly trip.) Nurses will show respect for the privacy and personal property of family members. For example, the woman is given the choice of where the interview and physical examination will be conducted to best safeguard her privacy. The nurse will seek permission before using the family's hand washing facilities, placing equipment in a particular place, or using the family telephone to call the health care provider.

A home visit progresses more effectively if it is planned and well organized. The nurse reviews the hospital's discharge summary, teaching plan, and any other records, including orders of the health care provider that will serve to structure the interview and physical assessment and that will provide a sense of continuity in care. After

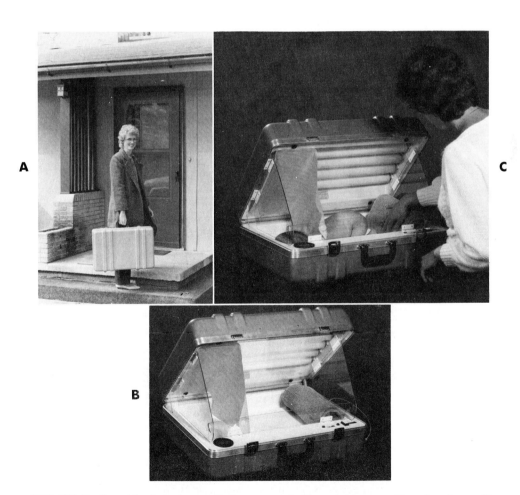

FIG. 19-4   Portable phototherapy for home use. **A,** Nurse brings portable unit to home. **B,** Assembled unit. **C,** Infant under phototherapy with face shielded from light. (Courtesy PEP Inc., Park Rapids, MN.)

MATERNAL ASSESSMENT

HEALTH PERCEPTION – HEALTH MANAGEMENT
_____ Reports overall health status as positive.
_____ Free from signs/symptoms of infection.
_____ Lochia is scant; reddish-brown or serosanguineous; no clots or foul odor.
_____ Exhibits behaviors compliant with plan of care.
_____ Verbalizes plan for medical follow-up.
Comments:

NUTRITION – METABOLIC
_____ Usual food intake is adequate for healing/lactation.
_____ Usual fluid intake is adequate for healing/lactation.
Comments:

ELIMINATION
_____ Reports an acceptable, regular pattern of bowel movements.
_____ Reports a normal pattern of urinary elimination.
Comments:

ACTIVITY – EXERCISE
_____ Activity level and exercise activities are appropriate.
Comments:

COGNITIVE – PERCEPTUAL
_____ Communicates effectively.
_____ Verbalizes relief from or a minimal amount of pain.
_____ No behavioral characteristics/physical responses to pain are observed.
_____ Verbalizes comfort with current knowledge level related to self and newborn care.
_____ Expresses correct knowledge related to self and newborn care.
_____ Demonstrates cognitive ability to problem solve and/or to make appropriate decisions for self and newborn.
Comments:

SLEEP – REST
_____ Recognizes need for sleep and/or rest.
_____ Reports napping and/or retiring early.
_____ Reports feeling rested.
_____ No behavioral characteristics related to fatigue are observed.
Comments:

SELF-PERCEPTION – SELF-CONCEPT
_____ Experiencing a low to normal level of anxiety.
_____ Exhibits a positive self-image, body image, and sense of personal identity.
Comments:

ROLE – RELATIONSHIP
_____ Verbalizes and/or demonstrates signs of newborn attachment.
_____ Mother/father/siblings show signs of adaptation to new roles.
+/– If relevant, exhibits appropriate grief response.
Comments:

SEXUALITY – REPRODUCTIVE
_____ Verbalizes a positive adaptation to restrictions and/or changes in sexual relations.
Comments:

COPING – STRESS TOLERANCE
_____ Verbalizes experiencing an appropriate amount of stress and a smooth transition to changes.
_____ Verbalizes use of positive coping mechanisms.
_____ Verbalizes assistance and/or support from another person.
_____ Verbalizes family (or family verbalizes) experiencing an appropriate amount of stress and a smooth transition to changes.
_____ Verbalizes family (or family verbalizes) use of positive coping mechanisms.
Comments:

VALUE – BELIEF
+/– If relevant, shows signs of spiritual well-being.
Comments:

NEWBORN ASSESSMENT

HEALTH PERCEPTION – HEALTH MANAGEMENT
_____ Overall health status reported as positive.
_____ Free from all signs/symptoms of infection.
_____ Free from signs/symptoms of increasing jaundice.
_____ Free from presence of rash or skin irritation.
_____ Environment free from obvious threats to newborn's safety.
_____ Caregiver exhibits behaviors compliant with plan of care for newborn.
_____ Caregiver verbalizes plan for medical follow-up of newborn.
Comments:

NUTRITIONAL – METABOLIC
_____ Weight gain is appropriate   (Weight: _____ Date: _____).
_____ Observable signs of adequate infant intake.
_____ Caregiver verbalizes satisfaction with feeding process.
Comments:

ELIMINATION
_____ Stool is yellow-brown, soft and passed easily.
_____ Voids at least six times in 24 hours.
Comments:

SWEDISH HOSPITAL MEDICAL CENTER
MATERNAL-NEWBORN HOME SERVICES
SEATTLE, WASHINGTON 98104

© 1991 SWEDISH HOSPITAL MEDICAL CENTER

NB-1207   Rev. 6/91   FC/SHMC   SN-5846

FIG. 19-5   Document for recording postpartum home visit, and example of standard of care. (Copyright jointly held by Swedish Hospital Medical Center and Cynthia J. Evans, RN, MN, Coordinator, Maternal-Newborn Home Services, Seattle, WA.)

CONTACT RECORD

	TELEPHONE / HOME VISIT			CALLS RECEIVED		
DATE / TIME	NURSING NOTES	STANDARDS OF CARE	SIGNATURE	DATE / TIME	STANDARDS OF CARE	SIGNATURE
	No answer – 1st attempt					
	No answer – 2nd attempt					
	No answer – 3rd attempt					
	No answer – 4th attempt					
	Message left to call MNHS					
	Message left to call MNHS					
	Telephone Assessment Protocol completed					
	Home Visit Assessment Protocol completed					

STANDARDS OF CARE INDEX

A = Anxiety	F = Coping, Family	I = Infection	K = Knowledge Deficit	X = Sexuality
B = Breastfeeding, Ineffective	O = Coping, Individual	i = Infection, Newborn	N = Nutrition	t = Skin Integrity
b = Breastfeeding, Interruption	D = Diarrhea	V = Involution	n = Nutrition, Newborn	S = Sleep
C = Constipation	d = Diarrhea, Newborn	Y = Injury	P = Pain	U = Urinary
c = Constipation, Newborn	G = Grieving	j = Jaundice	R = Parenting	u = Urinary, Newborn

NURSING NOTES

DATE / TIME	

FIG. 19-5, cont'd For legend see opposite page.

SLEEP PATTERN DISTURBANCE — STANDARD OF CARE

INITIATED: DATE / TIME _____

RN _____

RESOLVED: DATE / TIME _____

RN _____

RELATED TO:
1. Frequent night feedings.
2. Infant waking periods at night.
3. Inability to take naps/rest due to:
   a. other children.
   b. outside responsibility.
   c. limited help.
   d. difficulty sleeping.
4. Knowledge deficit of need for rest.
5. Pain/discomfort.
6. Anxiety/emotional state.
7. Inactivity.
8. Pregnancy.
9. Other:

CHARACTERIZED BY:
1. Verbal complaints of not feeling rested.
2. Verbal complaints of interrupted sleep.
3. Verbal complaints of difficulty falling asleep.
4. Observation of physical characteristics related to fatigue.
5. Other:

OUTCOME STANDARDS

DATE / RN

_____ 1. Recognizes need for sleep/rest.
_____ 2. Reports feeling rested.
_____ 3. Verbalizes retiring early and/or naps during the day.
_____ 4. Nurse does not observe any of the behavioral characteristics related to fatigue.

INTERVENTIONS

DATE / RN

_____ 1. Stress importance of rest.
_____ 2. Recommend resting if unable to sleep.
_____ 3. Provide positive reinforcement for any attempts at resting/sleeping.
_____ 4. Teach relaxation techniques.
_____ 5. Recommend restricting or lessening outside activities.
_____ 6. Remind of importance of vitamin/iron and balanced diet.
_____ 7. Teach techniques to minimize night time interruptions.
_____ 8. Encourage having someone else attend to household chores.
_____ 9. Recommend priority setting; do only highest priority items or basic tasks.
_____ 10. Recommend napping during infant's longest nap period.
_____ 11. Recommend lying down when infant first goes down.
_____ 12. Recommend unplugging telephone when napping.
_____ 13. If bottle feeding, suggest having someone else feed infant at night.
_____ 14. Encourage separating daytime rest from night time sleep.
_____ 15. Provide comfort measures and aids.
_____ 16. Other:

EVALUATION

DATE / RN

_____ 1. Receptive to interventions.
_____ 2. Other:

ADDRESSOGRAPH

SWEDISH HOSPITAL MEDICAL CENTER
MATERNAL-NEWBORN HOME SERVICES
Seattle, Washington 98104

© 1991 Swedish Hospital Medical Center

NB-1323   6/91   FC/SHMC

FIG. 19-5, cont'd   For legend see p. 518.

the visit is planned, the nurse collects necessary equipment, supplies, and instructional materials and ensures that they are clean and in working order before placing them securely in the bag. In addition to a name tag, the nurse who is not known to the family places other identification in the bag for use in securing access to the home.

Before the visit, the nurse obtains directions to the family's home and secures a map, if necessary. If public transportation will be used, it is necessary to become familiar with the route and to obtain the necessary fare or tokens. Before using a personal or agency automobile, the nurse ensures that it has been adequately serviced and fueled for the trip. In case of emergency, the agency should always have a copy of the nurse's daily itinerary and the nurse should have emergency telephone numbers and appropriate coins for toll calls and emergency transportation. Box 19-2 summarizes the protocol for a postpartum home visit.

Safety Concerns

The visiting nurse will need to enter unsafe areas on occasion. Taking necessary safety precautions and avoiding dangerous visits is imperative. A confident, nonvulnerable manner is appropriate. For visits in particularly dangerous settings, nurses may wish to visit in pairs. Nurses also may wish to report to the agency by telephone at specified intervals. The same precautions and common sense that guide a lone person's behavior in any potentially hazardous setting should be used on home visits. For example, the nurse should park near the home or in a well-lighted public area with an unobstructed route to the home's entrance. Automobile keys spread between the fingers with sharp ends outward not only allow quick access to an automobile but also can be used as a weapon if necessary. The automobile should always be locked and any valuables stored out of sight. The nurse should not accept rides with strangers, enter vacant buildings, walk near groups of strangers in doorways or alleys, enter a yard with an unrestrained dog, or carry valuables. Neither should unfamiliar shortcuts be used. If nurses are concerned about entering a home or other building, they are best advised not to enter without an escort (Humphrey, 1986). If the nurse has an intuitive feeling that the house is unsafe, it is wise to leave immediately.

Advantages and Limitations

A home visit has the obvious advantage of allowing the visitor to observe and interact with family members in their most natural and secure environment. Because they are at home, they are no longer anticipating how an infant will affect their lives; they are experiencing it. For that reason family members may have questions or concerns about areas that had not been anticipated before discharge. The use of open-ended questions by the nurse

may serve to elicit those kinds of issues. For example, "What is it like being home?" "What has happened that you least expected?" "What has been your greatest joy in bringing the baby home?" "Now that you are at home, what needs do you have?"

The nurse is able to assess the adequacy of resources in the home, as well as evidence of safety in both the home and immediate surroundings. Both kinds of data are helpful in planning health teaching. Teaching that was not possible during the short hospital stay can be continued on a priority basis. For example, nurse and mother may explore what must be learned to get through the hours until the next visit. Learning about infant care is facilitated because the exact items to be used on a daily basis are available for demonstration and return demonstration; the mother is not required to adapt what she has learned to her own setting.

Although telephone follow-up must, of necessity, address the mother's perceptions of her status and that of the newborn and family, home visit allows direct assessment. It is therefore more likely to facilitate identification of complicated physical or psychologic adjustment.

There are several limitations in home visits as a postpartum follow-up strategy: (1) the cost of visiting families separated by great geographic distances, (2) the availability of the number of nurses with expertise in caring for maternity patients and newborns in the home, and (3) concerns about safety in accessing families in certain areas.

Telephone Follow-Up

As part of their early discharge package, many providers are implementing one or more postpartum telephone follow-up calls to their patients for assessment, provision of health teaching, identification of complications to effect timely intervention, and referrals. Telephone follow-up may be part of the services offered by the hospital, private physician, or a private agency and may be used separately or in combination with other strategies for extending postpartum care.

The nature of the telephone follow-up calls should be explained to the family before discharge from the hospital. A mutually agreeable time is scheduled for the initial call. The ideal time for a telephone call varies according to family needs and provider philosophy and protocol. In some cases the initial call might be placed within the first few hours after early discharge to ascertain that the homecoming has not been a problem. Donaldson (1977), in her classic work on postpartum telephone follow-up suggests that an ideal time for the follow-up call is 3 to 7 days after discharge, and she provides a scientific rationale in support of that schedule. By that time the reality of the transition home has been realized and couples have begun to explore their concerns and options. Calls made earlier than 3 days may not allow ad-

BOX 19-2

Protocol for Postpartum Home Visit

PREVISIT INTERVENTIONS

1. Contact family to arrange details for home visit:
   a. Identify self, credentials, and agency role.
   b. Review purpose of home visit follow-up.
   c. Schedule convenient time for visit.
   d. Confirm address and route to family home.
2. Review and clarify appropriate data.
   a. All available assessment data for mother and infant (i.e., referral forms, hospital discharge summaries, family identified learning needs).
   b. Review records of any previous nursing contacts.
   c. Contact other professional caregivers as necessary to clarify data (i.e. obstetrician, nurse-midwife, pediatrician, referring nurse).
3. Identify community resources and teaching materials appropriate to meet needs already identified.
4. Plan the visit, and prepare bag with equipment, supplies, and materials necessary for assessments of mother and infant, actual care anticipated for mother and infant, and teaching.

IN-HOME INTERVENTIONS: ESTABLISHING A RELATIONSHIP

1. Reintroduce self and establish purpose of postpartum follow-up visit for mother, infant, and family; offer family opportunity to clarify their expectations of contact.
2. Spend brief time socially interacting with family to become acquainted and establish trusting relationship.

IN-HOME INTERVENTIONS: WORKING WITH FAMILY

1. Conduct systematic assessment of mother and newborn to determine physiologic adjustment and any existing complications.
2. Throughout visit, collect data to assess the emotional adjustment of individual family members to newborn and lifestyle changes. Note evidence of family-newborn bonding and sibling rivalry; note relationships among mother, father, children, and grandparents.
3. Determine adequacy of support system.
   a. To what extent does someone help with cooking, cleaning, and other home management tasks?
   b. To what extent is help being provided in caring for the newborn and any other children?
   c. Are support persons encouraging the new mother to care for herself and get adequate rest?
   d. Who is providing helpful information? Emotional support?
4. Throughout the visit, observe home environment for adequacy of resources:
   a. Space: privacy, safe play of children, sleeping.
   b. Overall cleanliness and state of repair.
   c. Number of steps new mother must climb.
   d. Adequacy of cooking arrangements.
   e. Adequacy of refrigeration and other food storage areas.
   f. Adequacy of bathing, toileting, and laundry facilities.

g. Arrangements in home for newborn: sleeping, bathing, formula preparation (if needed), layette items and diapers.
5. Throughout the visit, observe home environment for overall state of repair and existence of safety hazards:
   a. Storage of medications, household cleaners, and other substances hazardous to children.
   b. Presence of peeling paint on furniture, walls, or pipes.
   c. Factors that contribute to falls, such as dim lighting, broken steps, scatter rugs.
   d. Presence of vermin.
   e. Use of crib or playpen that fails to meet safety guidelines.
   f. Existence of emergency plan in case of fire; fire alarm or extinguisher.
6. Provide care to mother and/or newborn as prescribed by their respective primary care provider or in accord with agency protocol.
7. Provide teaching on basis of previously identified needs.
8. Refer family to appropriate community agencies or resources, such as warm lines and support groups.
9. Ascertain that woman knows potential problems to watch for and whom to call if they occur.
10. Ensure that used disposable items have been handled appropriately and that reusable items are cleaned and repacked appropriately in the nurse's bag.

IN-HOME INTERVENTIONS: ENDING THE VISIT*

1. Summarize the activities and main points of the visit.
2. Clarify future expectations, including schedule of next visit.
3. Review teaching plan, and provide major points in writing.
4. Provide information about reaching the nurse or agency if needed before the next scheduled visit.

POSTVISIT INTERVENTIONS

1. Document the visit thoroughly, using the necessary agency forms to serve as a legal record of the visit and to allow third-party reimbursement, as possible.
2. Initiate the plan of care on which the next encounter with the patient/family will be based.
3. Communicate appropriately (by telephone, letter, progress notes, or referral form) with primary care provider, other health professionals, or referral agencies on behalf of patient/family.

---

*If this is the nurse's final planned encounter with the woman/family, it is important to recognize that both the women and nurse may have feelings evoked by ending a meaningful relationship and by saying goodbye. Such feelings as anger, denial, and sadness are normal in this situation. Freely expressing these feelings at the end of the relationship is encouraged. Often patients are encouraged to do so if the nurse shares such feelings first.

equate time for the "honeymoon" phase of homecoming to disappear, therefore the woman's perception of the situation may not be realistic.

The number of calls and the time intervals between calls also vary and may be based on the family's assessed need and the other strategies being provided.

All therapeutic dialogue between nurse and patient, including that by telephone, is purposive and goal directed. This is not a social call even though there may be limited small talk in reestablishing rapport between nurse and patient. During the telephone follow-up the nurse will ask questions with the following goals:

- To determine evidence of the mother's physiologic recovery, comfort, and rest
- To determine evidence of psychologic well-being in the mother, including the presence of crisis-preventing balancing factors
- To determine selected evidence of physiologic adaptation in the newborn
- To establish the perceived level of parental adjustment to parenthood and the stresses inherent in the early fourth trimester

- To identify learning needs of the family
- To determine the extent to which a relationship is being formed between the newborn, siblings, parents, and grandparents (Fig. 19-6)
- To explore the areas creating special concerns or challenges, as well as placing unsettling demands on family members

In opening the conversation, the nurse should provide reintroduction to family members and reinforce the reason for the telephone call. The nurse should ascertain if the call has been made at a convenient time; otherwise, the effectiveness of the call is questionable. For example, a mother who has just settled a fussy baby and is attempting to relax herself will not be well served by a follow-up call at this time. Furthermore, common courtesy dictates that nurses determine if the call will create an unwelcome interruption for whatever reason. If so, a more suitable time should be mutually set.

The particulars of a follow-up call are planned on the basis of the discharge summary or records from the postpartum hospital stay. The use of discharge notes to guide the assessment ensures that an area of particular concern

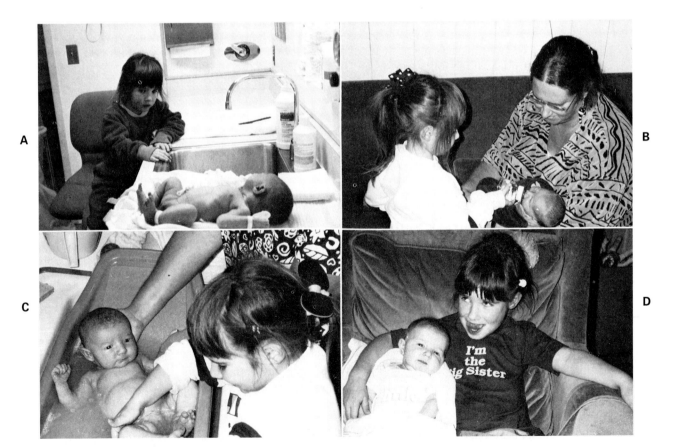

FIG. 19-6 Progress in sibling bonding and attachment. **A,** Watching during her new sister's first bath before discharge. **B,** Sibling feeds new sister under mother's watchful eye. **C,** Sibling gives her 2-week-old sister a bath; both seem to be enjoying this time together. **D,** Sibling bonding and attachment between big sister and 1-month-old little sister. (Courtesy Nancy Mason, MD.)

will not be overlooked. It also prompts the nurse to follow up on the basis of the woman's history. An additional advantage is in the personalization and sense of warmth and regard it communicates. For example, rather than asking how other children are reacting to the new baby, the nurse can ask specifically, "How is Leslie responding to his new brother?" or "Is your Mom still with you, or has she gone back to South Carolina?" The latter question shows more interest than "Who is helping you at home?"

The nurse allows the conversation to develop as naturally as possible so that the woman will not feel rushed or interrupted as rapport is established. This will be particularly important if the telephoner is not the nurse who cared for the family in the health care facility. A natural progression has the additional advantage of providing cues, such as the topic the mother chooses to address first, which often indicates her area of greatest concern. Open-ended questions facilitate the telephone interaction most effectively, for example: "How are things going since you left the hospital?" "You mentioned frequent headaches since you got home. Tell me more about those." Or "How are you and Peter collaborating on the baby's care?" Because specific assessment data about the mother, infant, and family are necessary, the nurse eventually will guide the assessment to these areas so that the aforementioned goals for the call can be met.

An effective postpartum telephone follow-up should assess the well-being of mother and infant and the transitions each family member is making to the new lifestyle and changes in the family constellation. To determine the crisis potential in the family, the nurse is careful to address each of the balancing factors. Consider, for example, the nurse making a return call to check on the status of a new mother who has been experiencing sore nipples. At an earlier call, the nurse had reinforced teaching about varying the infant's position on the breast to minimize stress to the nipple and had referred the mother to La Leche League. Today the nurse moves quickly to an assessment of the balancing factors, starting with "How have things been going since we spoke last?" Depending on the answer, the nurse may address a second factor by asking, "What have you been able to try?" After hearing the answer, the nurse might follow up by asking, "And how is that working?" The nurse would determine if the mother has called La Leche and how productive this intervention has been. Additional teaching or referral, possibly to the primary caregiver, may be necessary at this time.

The primary interventions available to providers extending care by telephone include patient advocacy, provision of teaching, reassurance/positive feedback, corrective feedback, supportive counseling, anticipatory guidance, and referral. Interventions are selected on the basis of a careful assessment and are provided in collaboration with the family.

Both the assessment data elicited and interventions employed during the postpartum follow-up call are recorded. Documentation serves both legal and reimbursement purposes (see Plan of Care.)

Advantages and Limitations

Telephone follow-up affords contact with the postpartum family during the vulnerable time interval in which support and intervention may be particularly effective. Most patients can be reached by telephone; according to Donaldson's research (1988), 92% of homes are accessible by telephone. Calls are more cost-effective than are home visits but are limited by the indirect nature of the assessment. If the mother's perception of her well-being (or that of the newborn or family) is inaccurate or falsely reported, problems may be missed and intervention will not be supported by relevant data. This disadvantage can be overcome by combining both strategies: telephone calls and home visits.

An average call lasts 19 minutes (Rhode, Groejes-Finke, 1980). Planning and documentation time can easily expand the time commitment to 30 minutes per call. Consequently, there is a potential limit to the number of calls that can be handled each day. The effectiveness of telephone calls to postpartum women also is limited by the telephone skills and listening ability of the caller and by the comfort the mother experiences in providing personal data to the faceless caller.

Warm Lines/Help Lines

The **warm line** represents another type of telephone link between the new family and concerned caregivers or experienced parent volunteers. Warm line services sometimes are best understood in contrast to hot lines, which may be more familiar to new parents. For example, they might have seen advertisements of hot lines in their area that provide emergency help to prevent suicide or child abuse.

In contrast, *a warm line is a helpline,* or consultation service, not a crisis line. The warm line is appropriately used for less extreme concerns that may seem urgent at the time the call is placed but are not actual emergencies. Calls to warm lines commonly relate to infant feeding, prolonged crying, or sibling rivalry. One new mother called because she noticed a drop of blood on her daughter's diaper. With an explanation of the reason for the blood and that its presence was normal, she was appropriately reassured. Another mother called to talk about how it felt when her 4-year-old son screamed out, "I hate you and I hate that baby." Warm line services may extend beyond the fourth trimester. Even parents with adolescent children may profit from the helping relationship of a warm line.

Individuals who answer warm line calls need to be good listeners who are empathic and able to use techniques such as open-ended questions, restating, and re-

Telephone Follow-Up after Early Postpartum Discharge

Case History

Ann Klaric is a 27-year-old postpartum patient who was discharged from a short-stay unit 48 hours after the birth of her first child, a son named Jason. At midnight on her day of discharge, Ann called the warm line with medically related questions. She was referred to a hospital-based maternity clinical nurse specialist.

The telephone interview revealed that Ann expelled "a large blood clot" when she last voided 10 minutes earlier. This is the first blood clot she has experienced since the birth, and even though she is now bleeding much less, Ann has obviously been alarmed by the experience. She says, "I'm so keyed up that I don't think I can relax enough to rest. Plus, I'm afraid to go to sleep—what if I start to hemorrhage and don't wake up?"

Prompted by the nurse's assessment, Ann describes the expelled clot as golf-ball size, dark red, and smooth; she did not notice any tissue fragments. The mild cramping she experienced earlier has ceased. In response to the nurse's specific inquiries, Ann describes her physical activity since leaving the hospital at 7 PM as follows. She unpacked, breastfed and provided other care for the baby, prepared a snack for her and her husband, and washed a load of clothes.

Later, after resolution of her more urgent problems, Ann says, "While I have you on the line, let me ask you another question. I've noticed that my bra is becoming tighter. Can that affect my breasts and cause me not to have enough milk for the baby? I wish I knew more about breastfeeding."

EXPECTED OUTCOMES	IMPLEMENTATION	RATIONALE	EVALUATION
Nursing Diagnosis: Fluid volume deficit related to postpartum bleeding secondary to overactivity during first hours at home			
Ann will decrease her activity level, and bleeding will have decreased when she calls the nurse in 2 hours.	Assess amount of blood loss on basis of perineal pad count, Ann's description of blood clot expelled, and history of bleeding since discharge from hospital.	Accurate assessment of actual/potential hemorrhage and contributing factors enables planning appropriate interventions.	
	Identify Ann's activity level since discharge as a possible contributing factor in increased bleeding.	Decreasing activity level and avoiding heavy lifting generally is associated with decreased uterine bleeding.	After 2 hours in bed, Ann reports that bleeding has decreased in amount.
	Instruct Ann to feel her fundus to make sure it is firm. If it is not firm, Ann should massage it until it becomes firm.	The uterus should be firm. If it is boggy, hemorrhage could occur.	Ann reports that her fundus feels firm.
	Encourage decreased activity (bed rest) for next 2 hours followed by reassessment. Suggest that applying a clean perineal pad before bed rest will facilitate more accurate data about the effects of decreased activity.		
	Review telephone number of nurse, and encourage Ann to call back in 2 hours to report on condition. Advise Ann to call earlier if heavy bleeding recurs (>1 pad/hr).	Offering the woman an opportunity to provide self-care to the extent possible increases self-confidence in decision making and in ability to cope with future emergency.	

Continued.

EXPECTED OUTCOMES	IMPLEMENTATION	RATIONALE	EVALUATION
Nursing Diagnosis: Anxiety related to concerns about possibility of postpartum hemorrhage			
Ann will report diminished anxiety, and her concerns about excessive bleeding will be resolved.	Listen carefully with an attitude of warm regard and empathy to establish a trusting relationship. Assist Ann to acknowledge and express her feelings and concerns. Clarify misconceptions, and provide accurate information about uterine bleeding and overactivity. Suggest that Ann lie down for 2 hours and use familiar Lamaze techniques. Provide positive reinforcement for Ann's decision making/coping as demonstrated by her calling for help. Assure Ann that nurse is immediately accessible by telephone, if needed, and that her call in 2 hours with a status report is welcomed and anticipated.	An atmosphere of trust is basic to sharing private feelings, anxiety, and concerns not only with this care provider but also in future health care encounters. Relaxation techniques and knowledge that a concerned caregiver is immediately available will decrease anxiety and enhance the woman's feelings of emotional comfort.	By the end of the telephone call, Ann reports that she is more relaxed and reassured about her condition.
Nursing Diagnosis: Altered health maintenance related to knowledge deficit regarding breastfeeding			
Ann will verbalize understanding of the process of production of breast milk and will evaluate her nursing bra according to criteria provided by nurse.	Assess learning needs. Prioritize learning needs to plan timely teaching that capitalizes on readiness to learn. Answer Ann's questions first. Provide opportunity for follow-up to meet other learning needs at more opportune time. Provide telephone number of contact person to answer questions and validate information or arrange home visit.	Prioritizing instructions in such a way that the woman's most urgent need for information is met early reduces anxiety and enhances learning.* Ensuring readiness to learn, eliminating environmental barriers, and being responsive to patient's needs and preferences are essential components in providing instruction for health maintenance.	Ann acknowledges understanding of the concept of supply and demand in breastmilk production and determines that her nursing bra is providing nonconstrictive support according to the following criteria: • Nonbinding • No underwires • Seams stitched toward underarm (to prevent obstruction of milk ducts) • 1 to 2 cup sizes larger than prepregnancy • Nonelastic straps • Comfortable and easy to fasten • Support to place nipples at midline Ann requests a home visit to learn more about breastfeeding.
Ann will identify her preference for follow-up to enable additional learning, as needed.			

*Only Ann's most pressing concern and request for information was addressed during this telephone encounter because of the late hour (midnight) and her need to rest. Follow-up to meet Ann's other learning needs is essential.

flecting to encourage the caller to communicate. The caller is given an unhurried opportunity to share feelings or concerns. It is her story, and she is allowed to tell it in her own way. Questions often are used to clarify what the caller is saying.

The caller is assessed for evidence of impending crisis: What is the situation or concern? What has already been tried in order to cope? What resources are available? Advice is not given; rather callers are helped to explore options available to them. Referrals may be made to support groups or to community agencies. When medical problems are identified, referrals are made to the appropriate physician.

Rauen (1985), who refers to the "telephone as stethoscope," maintains that communication can be blocked when the caregiver "talks too much, makes judgmental remarks, conveys differences, takes sides, dwells on personal experiences or assumes that the first problem mentioned is the real problem." Warm line calls always end with the caregiver summarizing the call—what concerns were identified and what resolutions have been explored. Also, the caller is invited to call again if the need arises.

Advantages and Limitations

The primary advantage of the warm line is quick access to a good listener, whether nurse or trained volunteer, 24 hours a day, 365 days a year. Because it is an advertised helpline, couples may feel more comfortable and less intimidated about making the call.

Inasmuch as the warm line offers round-the-clock service, there are potential difficulties in staffing, when a limited staff necessitates an answering recorder or message service, the resource is less effective. Having to leave a message negates the advantage of immediate access. Although some individuals welcome the anonymity of a faceless listener, they may be less willing to record a message.

The cost of the warm line is minimal if volunteers are used; the only costs are the telephone service itself and advertisement. The financial commitment obviously increases when any of the staff members are salaried.

For some nurses the inability to evaluate the effectiveness of their interventions is frustrating. There are generally no provisions for follow up with the caller to determine the extent to which the problem has been resolved, if at all.

Support Groups

Humans are inherently social beings, involved on a daily basis in some kind of group—groups of family members, classmates, co-workers, and friends. Often education, work, worship, and leisure time take place in groups. Thus it seems reasonable that at times of difficult transitions, people might turn to groups for support. Nurses are generally familiar with the benefits of support groups for such diverse groups as the newly divorced or widowed, those with recently diagnosed acquired immuno-

deficiency syndrome (AIDS) or cancer, and those undergoing mastectomy, colostomy, or heart attack.

A special group experience is sometimes sought by the woman adjusting to motherhood. On occasion, postpartum women who have met earlier in prenatal clinics or on the hospital unit may begin to associate for mutual support. Members of Lamaze classes who attend a postpartum reunion may decide to extend their relationship during the fourth trimester. Realizing the value of group support, nurses may wish to make postpartum support groups available as a strategy for bridging hospital and home.

A **postpartum support group** is a collection of individuals living the postpartum experience who are (1) striving to satisfy a personal need by belonging to a group, (2) interacting with respect to mutual goals, common interests or concerns, and (3) experiencing the reward of an interdependent relationship. They perceive themselves to be members of a group; others recognize them as a group. Group behavior is governed by rules and norms that are collectively chosen; for example, "We will protect each other's confidences" and "Husbands are invited to group meetings only when members agree unanimously to invite them."

Recognizing the universality of their feelings—that others feel the same way and that they are not alone or unique by virtue of their feelings or concerns—decreases anxiety and reassures members of their normality. It is comforting and offers a sense of catharsis to feel free to share feelings with others. For many women, it is a welcome relief to unburden deeply held emotions such as guilt, anger, or grief in a supportive setting where others, because of their shared emotions, are likely to be nonjudgmental.

Often in a postpartum support group, an experienced mother can impart concrete information that can be valuable to other group members. For example, one new mother shared her nurse-midwife's advice about placing warm, newly brewed tea bags on sore nipples for the comfort and healing value of warmth and the tannic acid. Another shared the use she had made of her husband's socks with the foot cut out. Sliding the sock over her left arm provided enough traction to keep the wet, soapy baby from slipping off the supporting arm while she gave the infant his bath. An inexperienced mother may find herself imitating the behavior of someone in the group whom she perceives as particularly capable. She may imitate someone's way of positioning a baby or find herself folding her daughter's diapers differently after watching someone else's technique.

Finally, sharing oneself in a group, whether in expressing feelings or expertise, has the therapeutic value of altruism. When the woman believes that she has helped someone else, it increases her sense of esteem and self-worth. In addition to its therapeutic benefit, this factor, as well as those discussed, encourage ongoing group membership.

KEY POINTS

- The trend for early postpartum discharge will continue as a result of cost containment measures, increasing technologic advances, and consumer demand.
- The short-stay option in perinatal care is safer when selection criteria are used and when home care follow-up is available.

- Early discharge classes, postpartum telephone follow-up, home visits, warm lines, and support groups used individually or in combination are effective means of preventing crisis and facilitating physiologic and psychologic adjustments in the postpartum period.

CRITICAL THINKING EXERCISES

1. You are making a home visit to a new mother on her third postpartum day. She has two other children, ages 2 and 4. Assessment reveals the following findings:
   - Skin problems show that the infant is not being bathed properly.
   - Interactions of siblings with the newborn show that they have not accepted the necessity for correct hand washing and negative attitudes toward the newborn.
   - The mother shows a lack of knowledge concerning the newborn's jaundice.
   - The mother quotes family members regarding proper care of the umbilicus; the infant is wearing a flannel belly band that overlaps the diaper.

   For each of the identified problems:
   a. Formulate a nursing diagnosis.
   b. Prioritize nursing diagnoses.
   c. Plan and prioritize patient-centered goals and expected outcomes.
   d. Choose interventions and indicate rationale.
   e. Indicate how you would know your interventions were effective.
   f. Verify and justify your claims, beliefs, conclusions, decisions, and actions.

References

Blackburn S et al: Patients' and nurses' perception of patient problems during the immediate postpartum period, *Appl Nurs Res* 1:141, March 1988.

Clemen-Stone S, Eigsti DG, McGuire SL: *Comprehensive family and community health nursing*, ed 3, St Louis, 1991, Mosby.

Davis JH et al: A study of mothers' postpartum teaching priorities, *Matern Child Nurs J* 17:41, 1988.

Donaldson NE: Effect of telephone postpartum follow-up: a clinical trial, *Diss Abstr Int* 49:2567B (University Microfilms No. DA8809495), 1988.

Donaldson NE: Fourth trimester follow-up, *Am J Nurs* 77:1176, 1977.

Edwards M: The crisis of the fourth trimester, *Birth Fam J* 1:19, 1974.

Evans CL: Description of a home follow-up program for childbearing families, *JOGNN* 20:113, 1991.

Gillerman H, Beckham MH: The postpartum early discharge dilemma: an innovative solution, *J Perinat Neonatal Nurs* 5:9, 1991.

Goer H: The incredible shrinking postpartum stay, *Bay Area Baby*, vol 25, 1990.

Harrison LL: Patient education in early postpartum discharge programs, *MCN* 15:39, 1990.

Hiser PL: Concerns of multiparas during the second postpartum week, *JOGNN* 16:195, 1987.

Humphrey CJ: *Home care nursing handbook*, Norwalk, CT, 1986, Appleton-Century-Crofts.

Lukacs A: Issues surrounding early postpartum discharge: effects on the caregiver, *J Perinat Neonatal Nurs* 5:33, 1991.

Martell LK et al: Information priorities of new mothers in a short-stay program, *West J Nurs Res* 11:320, 1989.

Mitchell A et al: Comparison of liason and staff nurses in discharge referrals of postpartum patients for public health nursing follow-up. *Nurs Res* 42:245, 1993.

Norr KF, Nacion KW: Early postpartum discharge, *NAACOG Nursing Update Series* 4:2, 1986.

Pridham KF et al: Early postpartum transition: progress in maternal identity and role attainment, *Res Nurs Health* 14:21, 1991.

Rauen KC: The telephone as stethoscope, *MCN* 10:122, 1985.

Rhode MA, Groenjes-Finke JM: Evaluation of nurse initiated telephone calls to postpartum women, *Issues Health Care Women* 2:23, 1980.

Tribotti S et al: Nursing diagnoses for the postpartum woman, *JOGNN* 17:410, 1988.

Bibliography

Ament LA: Maternal tasks of the puerperium reidentified, *JOGNN* 19:330, 1990.

Arnold LS, Blakewell-Sacho S: Models of perinatal home follow-up, *J Perinat Neonatal Nurs* 5:18, 1991.

Auerbach KS, Jacobi AM: Postpartum depression in the breast-feeding mother, *NAACOG's Clin Issues Perinat Womens Health Nurs* 12:375, 1990.

Donaldson NE: A review of nursing intervention research on maternal adaptation in the first 8 weeks postpartum, *J Perinat Neonatal Nurs* 4(4):1, 1991.

Gillerman H, Beckham MH: The postpartum early discharge dilemma: an innovative solution, *J Perinat Neonatal Nurs* 5:9, 1991.

Gjerdingen DK, Froberg DG, Fontaine P: A causal model describing the relationship of women's postpartum health to social support, length of leave, and complications of childbirth, *Women Health* 16:71, 1990.

Martell LK: Postpartum depression as a family problem, *MCN* 15:90, 1990.

NAACOG: Physical assessment of the neonate, *OGN Nursing Practice Resource*, Washington, DC, 1991, NAACOG.

NAACOG: Postpartum nursing care: vaginal delivery, *OGN Nursing Practice Resource*, Washington, DC, 1991, NAACOG.

Stern TE: An early discharge program: an entrepreneurial nursing practice becomes a hospital-affiliated agency, *J Perinat Neonatal Nurs* 5:1, 1991.

Six

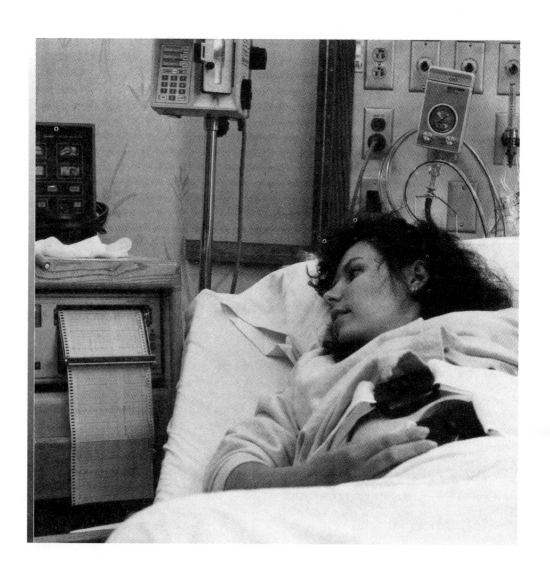

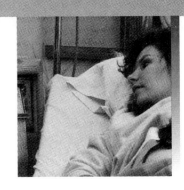

Complications of Childbearing

20 Assessment for Risk Factors

21 Hypertension, Hemorrhage, and Maternal Infections

22 Endocrine, Cardiovascular, and Medical-Surgical Problems during Pregnancy

23 Psychosocial Problems

24 Labor and Birth at Risk

25 Adolescent Sexuality, Pregnancy, and Parenthood

CHAPTER 20

Assessment for Risk Factors

SUSAN MATTSON

LEARNING OBJECTIVES

Define the key terms.

Explore the scope of high-risk pregnancy.

List risk factors identified through history, physical examination, and diagnostic techniques.

Understand various diagnostic modalities and implications of findings.

Explain diagnostic techniques to women and their families.

KEY TERMS

alpha-fetoprotein (AFP)
amniocentesis
biophysical profile (BPP)
chorionic villus sampling (CVS)
contraction stress test (CST or OCT)
daily fetal movement count (DFMC)
Doppler ultrasound
intrauterine growth retardation (IUGR)
lecithin/sphingomyelin (L/S) ratio
magnetic resonance imaging (MRI)
nonstress test (NST)
percutaneous umbilical blood sampling
    (PUBS) or cordocentesis
ultrasonography
uteroplacental insufficiency

RELATED TOPICS

Fetal monitoring *(Chap. 11)* • Hypertensive complications *(Chap. 21)* • Anemia *(Chap. 21)* • Hemorrhage complications *(Chap. 21)* • Infections *(Chap. 21)* • Diabetes mellitus *(Chap. 22)* • Cardiovascular complications *(Chap. 22)* • Substance abuse *(Chap. 23)* • Dystocia *(Chap. 24)* • Preterm labor and birth *(Chap. 24)* • Oxytocin stimulation of labor *(Chap. 24)* • Low-birth-weight infants *(Chap. 27)*

Of the approximately 6 million births that occur in the United States each year, 500,000 will be categorized as high risk because of maternal or fetal complications. The united efforts of all members of the obstetric team and close collaboration with other medical personnel are required to adequately care for the high-risk woman. In this chapter the high-risk woman and the factors associated with diagnosis of high risk are identified. Techniques of biophysical monitoring of fetal health are emphasized.

SCOPE OF THE PROBLEM

A high-risk pregnancy is one in which the life or health of the mother or fetus is jeopardized by a disorder coincidental with or unique to pregnancy. For the mother the high-risk status extends (arbitrarily) through the puerperium, that is, until 29 days after birth. Postbirth maternal complications are usually resolved within a month of birth, but perinatal morbidity may continue for months or years.

533

A better understanding of human reproduction has greatly reduced maternal morbidity and mortality. Knowledge of the fetus and neonatal disorders has increased dramatically in the last 10 to 15 years. This has led to a gratifying drop in perinatal morbidity and mortality during this period. Since 1969, when the perinatal death rate dropped below 30 per 1000 live births for the first time, the rate has steadily declined. In 1991, the death rate was estimated to be 8.5 per 1000 live births, a record low (National Center for Health Statistics, 1994).

Each year about 3.5 million pregnancies reach viability (22 to 24 weeks' gestation), but of these at least 30,000 fetuses fail to survive. About the same number of newborns die during the first month of life. High-risk pregnancy thus presents one of the most critical problems of modern medical and nursing care. Emphasis is on the safe birth of normal infants who can develop to their maximum potential. Advances along many scientific fronts have provided the technology to achieve a level of perinatal health care far beyond that previously available.

Although pregnancy is often referred to as a maturational crisis, the diagnosis of high risk also imposes a situational crisis (e.g., the pregnancy terminates before the anticipated date, the woman develops gestational diabetes mellitus with its potential complications, a neonate is born who does not meet cultural, societal, or familial norms and expectations). Understanding of the high-risk patient allows the nurse to provide individualized therapeutic care.

Maternal Health Problems

Although different parts of the world have different leading causes of maternal death attributable to pregnancy, in general, three major disorders have persisted for the last 35 years: hypertensive disorders, infection, and hemorrhage. The number of maternal deaths overall is small; however, maternal mortality remains a significant problem because a high proportion of deaths are preventable, mainly through improving the access to and utilization of prenatal care services. Nurses can be instrumental in educating the public about the importance of obtaining early and regular care during pregnancy.

Fetal and Neonatal Health Problems

Fetal death (demise) is defined as the death in utero before complete expulsion of the product of human conception. It does not result from therapeutic or elective abortion. Fetal death is also called intrauterine death and results in stillbirth.

Neonatal death is the death of a liveborn neonate at 20 weeks' gestation or more. A liveborn neonate is one who shows any evidence of life after birth, even if only momentary (respiration, heartbeat, voluntary muscle movement, or pulsation within the umbilical cord), and who dies within 28 days.

Perinatal death rate is defined as the sum of fetal and neonatal death rates. This statistic is considered the most sensitive indicator of the effectiveness of perinatal care.

The incidence of *infant mortality* is expressed as the number of deaths per 1000 live births.

Infant mortality includes the neonatal death rate. As Table 20-1 demonstrates, the majority of the 10 leading causes of death during infancy continue to occur during the perinatal period. Although a number of perinatal problems have benefited from improved treatment, congenital anomalies continue to be the leading cause of infant mortality. The incidence of most birth defects has

TABLE 20-1 Deaths Under 1 Year and Infant Mortality Rates for the 10 Leading Causes of Infant Death: United States, 1989*

RANK ORDER	CAUSE OF DEATH (NINTH REVISION INTERNATIONAL CLASSIFICATION OF DISEASES, 1975)	NUMBER	RATE
	All causes	39,655	981.3
1	Congenital anomalies	8,120	200.9
2	Sudden infant death syndrome	5,634	139.4
3	Disorders relating to short gestation and unspecified low birth weight	3,931	97.3
4	Respiratory distress syndrome	3,631	89.9
5	Newborn affected by maternal complications of pregnancy	1,534	38.0
6	Accidents and adverse effects	996	24.6
7	Newborn affected by complications of placenta, cord, and membranes	984	24.4
8	Infections specific to the perinatal period	892	22.1
9	Intrauterine hypoxia and birth asphyxia	725	17.9
10	Pneumonia and influenza	636	15.7
	All other causes	12,572	311.1

Modified from National Center for Health Statistics: Advanced report of final mortality statistics, 1989, *Monthly Vital Statistics Report* 40(8):2, 1992.
*Rates per 100,000 live births; beginning in 1989, race for live births is tabulated according to race of mother.

neither substantially decreased nor increased. Problems related to low birth weight and preterm birth are chiefly responsible for deaths during the first 4 weeks of life.

The leading causes of death in the neonatal period are congenital anomalies, disorders relating to short gestation and low birth weight, respiratory distress syndrome, and the effects of maternal complications. The four leading causes of death after the neonatal period are sudden infant death syndrome (SIDS), congenital anomalies, injuries and infections (National Center for Health Statistics, 1992). African-American women are twice as likely as whites to experience prematurity, low birth weight, and infant and fetal death (Kessel et al, 1988).

HIGH-RISK FACTORS

The idea that certain prenatal and intrapartal events can have an adverse effect on the infant in later life is not a new one. Serious biologic handicaps, health problems, obstetric disorders, and social deprivation may compromise the mother and the infant in subtle or more obvious ways. Identification of the high-risk patient is critical to minimize maternal and neonatal mortality and morbidity. There is ample evidence that known risk factors can be used to identify high-risk patients early in the prenatal course as well as intrapartally. Approximately 20% of pregnant women can be identified prenatally to be at risk, accounting for 55% of poor pregnancy outcomes (ACOG, 1988). Commonly it is the alert nurse, familiar with deviations from normal, who notes and re-

ports potential or real high-risk factors. Many factors from within the woman and from her surrounding environment influence the outcome of her pregnancy (Fig. 20-1).

Several factors place the pregnancy at high risk: poverty, inadequate nutrition, infection, sexually transmitted diseases (STDs), medical conditions, and use of substances such as tobacco, alcohol, cocaine, and other drugs jeopardize the entire childbearing experience for the mother, fetus/neonate, and family.

Early in pregnancy abnormalities in the mother's reproductive or endocrine systems may lead to spontaneous abortion (miscarriage). Problems of implantation or genetic defects often result in spontaneous abortion. During the *second trimester* maternal and fetal conditions may lead to late abortion or preterm labor. Uterine abnormalities or an incompetent cervical os, cyanotic heart disease, Rh incompatibility, and hypertension are among maternal conditions that may complicate pregnancy and its outcome. Gross abnormality of the fetus and multifetal gestation are two fetal risk factors. Additional risk factors may occur during the *third trimester.* Fetal malformations or malpresentations, umbilical cord complications, placenta previa, abruptio placentae, preterm rupture of membranes, preterm labor, postterm labor, hydramnios, or oligohydramnios may jeopardize maternal and fetal/neonatal well-being (Box 20-1).

Hemorrhage, infection, abnormal vital signs, traumatic labor or birth, and some psychosocial events are specific factors that place the new mother at risk during the *early puerperium.*

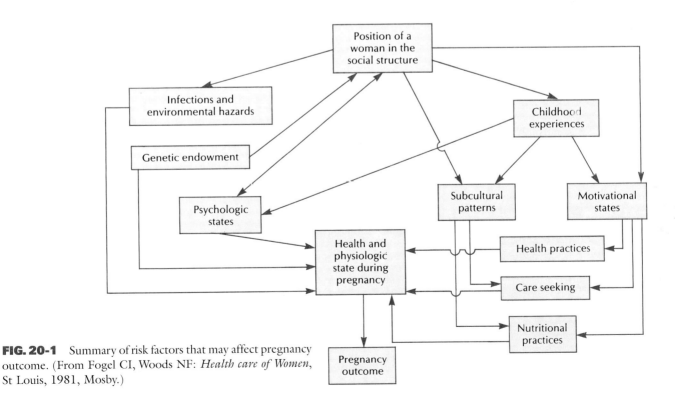

FIG. 20-1   Summary of risk factors that may affect pregnancy outcome. (From Fogel CI, Woods NF: *Health care of Women,* St Louis, 1981, Mosby.)

BOX 20-1

Categories of High-Risk Pregnancy

MATERNAL AGE AND PARITY FACTORS

1. Age 16 years or under
2. Nullipara 35 years or over
3. Multipara 40 years or over
4. Interval of 8 years or more since last pregnancy
5. High parity (5 or more)
6. Pregnancy occurring 3 months or less after last birth

NONMARITAL PREGNANCY

PREGNANCY-INDUCED HYPERTENSION (PIH), HYPERTENSION, KIDNEY DISEASE

1. Preeclampsia with hospitalization before labor
2. Eclampsia
3. Kidney disease—pyelonephritis, nephritis, nephrosis, etc.
4. Chronic hypertension, severe (160/100 mm Hg or over)
5. Blood pressure 140/90 mm Hg or above on 2 readings 30 minutes apart

ANEMIA AND HEMORRHAGE

1. Hematocrit 30% or below in pregnancy
2. Hemorrhage (previous pregnancy)—severe, requiring transfusion
3. Hemorrhage (present pregnancy)
4. Anemia (hemoglobin below 10 g) for which treatment other than oral iron preparations is required (hemolytic, macrocytic anemias, etc.)
5. Sickle cell trait or disease
6. History of bleeding or clotting disorder at any time

FETAL FACTORS

1. Two or more previous preterm births (twins = one birth)
2. Two or more consecutive spontaneous abortions (miscarriages)
3. One or more stillbirths at term gestation
4. One or more gross anomalies
5. Rh incompatibility or ABO isoimmunization problems
6. History of previous birth defects—cerebral palsy, brain damage, mental retardation, metabolic disorders such as phenylketonuria (PKU)
7. History of large infants (over 4032 g [9 lb])

PATERNAL AGE AND OTHER FACTORS

DYSTOCIA (HISTORY OF OR ANTICIPATED)

1. Contracted pelvis or cephalopelvic disproportion (CPD)

2. Multifetal pregnancy in current pregnancy
3. Two or more breech births
4. Previous operative births (e.g., cesarean or midforceps birth)
5. History of prolonged labor (more than 18 hours for nullipara; more than 12 hours for multipara)
6. Previously diagnosed genital tract anomalies (incompetent cervix, cervical or uterine malformation, solitary ovary or tube) or problem (ovarian mass, endometriosis)
7. Short stature (1.5 m [60 in] or less)

HISTORY OF OR CONCURRENT CONDITIONS

1. Diabetes mellitus; gestational diabetes
2. Hyperemesis gravidarum
3. Thyroid disease (hypothyroidism or hyperthyroidism)
4. Malnutrition or extreme obesity (20% over ideal weight for height; 15% under ideal weight for height)
5. Organic heart disease
6. Syphilis and TORCH infections: toxoplasmosis, rubella in first 10 weeks of *this* pregnancy, cytomegalovirus (CMV), and herpes simplex; HIV positive status, or acquired immunodeficiency syndrome (AIDS); *Chlamydia;* human papillomavirus (HPV)
7. Tuberculosis or other serious pulmonary pathologic condition (e.g., emphysema, asthma)
8. Malignant or premalignant tumors (including hydatidiform mole)
9. Alcoholism, substance dependency
10. Psychiatric disease or epilepsy (documented)
11. Mental retardation

THOSE WITH PREVIOUS HISTORY OF

1. Late registration, or poor clinic attendance
2. Family violence including battery, rape, incest
3. Home situation making clinic attendance and hospitalization difficult
4. Mothers, including minors, without family resources (including desertions, adoptions, injuries, separations, family withdrawals, sole support)

Modified from Fogel CI, Woods NF: *Health care of women: a nursing perspective*, St Louis, 1981, Mosby.

DIAGNOSTIC TECHNIQUES

The major goal of antepartum fetal surveillance is the detection of potential fetal compromise. Ideally, the technique used will identify the compromise before intrauterine asphyxia of the fetus so that the health care provider can take measures to prevent or minimize adverse perinatal outcomes (see Ethical Considerations). The results of any such tests must be interpreted in light of the complete clinical picture. The remainder of this chapter describes the diagnostic techniques available, their use in detecting fetuses at risk, and the nurse's role in assisting patients during these procedures.

Each diagnostic procedure involves some degree of risk. In addition, the cost of the procedures varies, with some tests being quite costly. These factors must be weighed and discussed with the woman and family to determine whether the advantages of the test outweigh the potential risks and additional expense. Since these tests have limitations in terms of diagnostic accuracy and applicability, no one test should be used as the basis for determining health status or planning care.

Biophysical Assessment
Ultrasonography

Sound is a waveform of energy that causes small particles in a medium to oscillate. The frequency of sound refers to the number of peaks or waves that traverse a given point per unit of time, and is expressed in hertz (Hz). Sound with a frequency of one peak per second would have a frequency of one Hz. When directional beams of sound strike an object, an echo is returned. The time delay between the emission of the sound and the return of the echo is noted, as well as the direction from which the echo comes. From these data the object's distance and location can be calculated.

Ultrasound is sound having a frequency higher than that of normal human hearing, that is, greater than 20,000 Hz. First introduced in the 1960s, diagnostic ultrasound has developed rapidly to enjoy a principal position in antepartum fetal surveillance. Diagnostic ultrasound instruments operate in a range of frequency varying from 2 to 10 million Hz (or 2 to 10 megahertz [mHz]), still well below that used by sonar and radar.

Operational Modes

Table 20-2 presents a summary of modalities, imaging, and principal uses of diagnostic ultrasound. Static image scanners are useful for gynecologic as well as obstetric diagnoses. Dynamic image scanners provide direct visualization of indicators of fetal viability—fetal cardiac and body movement.

ETHICAL CONSIDERATIONS

FETAL RIGHTS

Amniocentesis, percutaneous umbilical blood sampling, and chorionic villus sampling are prenatal tests used for diagnosing fetal defects in early pregnancy. All are invasive and carry risks to the mother and fetus. They may also involve issues of abortion because there is no treatment for genetically affected fetuses. Thus the issue of fetal rights is a key ethical concern in prenatal testing for fetal defects.

TABLE 20-2 Diagnostic Ultrasound: Operational Modes*

MODALITY	PRODUCT	PRINCIPAL USE
PULSED WAVE		
A Mode	Static image	Diagnostic evaluation of brain
B Mode (gray scale)*	Static image	Images of abdominal and pelvic structures
M Mode	Dynamic imaging	Monitoring of heart and measuring of heart wall displacement
Real time*	Static image and dynamic imaging	Provides dynamic imaging and static images
CONTINUOUS WAVE		
Doppler mode*	Ranging mode	Fetal heart monitoring

Pulsed wave, Sound emitted at intervals; *continuous wave,* sound emitted continuously; *A mode,* one-dimensional image that appears as spikes on a horizontal base; distance between spikes can be measured (e.g., biparietal diameter [BPD]); *B mode (gray scale),* rough, two-dimensional image of various tissue densities for visualizing tissue texture and contour; *M mode,* time-related tracings showing straight lines for motionless structures and wiggly lines for structural motion (e.g., atrial septal defects and patent ductus arteriosus); *static,* stationary; *dynamic,* moving; *real time,* dynamic imaging (limb and respiratory movements), as well as static images (BPD, placental location); *Doppler mode,* detection of change in frequency (wavelength) of structures rather than in amplitude motion (e.g., blood flow in umbilical cord and placenta, closure of fetal cardiac valves).
*Used extensively in obstetrics and gynecology.

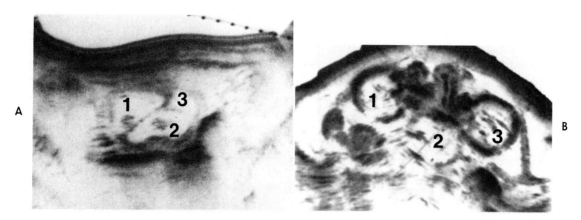

FIG. 20-2 **A,** Transverse static image scan demonstrates three well-formed gestational sacs. **B,** Subsequent static image scan demonstrates three well-defined fetal heads in woman carrying triplets. (From Athey PA, Hadlock FP: *Ultrasound in obstetrics and gynecology,* ed 2, St Louis, 1985, Mosby.)

BOX 20-2

Major Indications for Obstetric Sonography

FIRST TRIMESTER

Confirm pregnancy
Confirm viability
Rule out ectopic pregnancy
Confirm gestational age*
  Birth control use
  Irregular menses
  No dates
  Postpartum pregnancy
Previous complicated pregnancy
  Cesarean birth
  Rh incompatibility
  Diabetes mellitus
  Fetal growth retardation
    Clarify dates/size discrepancy
Large for dates—rule out:
  Leiomyomata
  Bicornuate uterus
  Adnexal mass
  Multifetal gestation
  Poor dates
  Molar pregnancy*†‡
Small for dates—rule out:
  Poor dates
  Missed abortion
  Blighted ovum

SECOND TRIMESTER

Establish or confirm dates†
If no fetal heart tones:
  Clarify dates/size discrepancy
Large for dates—rule out:
  Poor estimate of dates
  Molar pregnancy
  Multifetal gestation
  Leiomyomata
  Polyhydramnios
  Congenital anomalies

SECOND TRIMESTER—cont'd

Small for dates—rule out:
  Poor estimate of dates
  Fetal growth retardation
  Congenital anomalies
  Oligohydramnios
If history of bleeding—rule out total placenta previa
If Rh incompatibility—rule out fetal hydrops

THIRD TRIMESTER

If no fetal heart tones:
  Clarify dates/size discrepancy
Large for dates—rule out:
  Macrosomia (diabetes mellitus)
  Multifetal gestation
  Polyhydramnios
  Congenital anomalies
  Poor estimate of dates§
Small for dates—rule out:
  Fetal growth retardation
  Oligohydramnios
  Congenital anomalies
  Poor estimate of dates§
Determine fetal position—rule out:
  Breech
  Transverse lie
If history of bleeding—rule out:
  Placenta previa
  Abruptio placentae
  Determine fetal lung maturity
  Amniocentesis for lecithin/sphingomyelin ratio
  Placental maturity (grade 0-3)
If Rh incompatibility—rule out fetal hydrops

Modified from Athey PA, Hadlock FP: *Ultrasound in obstetrics and gynecology,* ed 2, St Louis, 1985, Mosby.
*Accuracy ± 3 days.
†Accuracy ± 1 to 1½ weeks.
‡Hydatidiform mole.
§Accuracy only ± 3 weeks.

Applications in Pregnancy

When carefully performed and accurately interpreted, ultrasonography can supply vital information. During the *first trimester* ultrasound examination is performed to obtain the following information: (1) number, size, and location of gestational sacs (Fig. 20-2), (2) presence or absence of fetal cardiac and body movement, (3) presence or absence of uterine abnormalities (e.g., bicornuate uterus, fibroids) or adnexal masses (e.g., ovarian cysts, ectopic pregnancy), (4) pregnancy dating (e.g., *biparietal diameter [BPD],* crown-rump length), and (5) coexistence and location of an intrauterine device (IUD).

During the *second and third trimesters* the following information is sought: (1) fetal viability, number, position, gestational age, growth pattern, and anomalies such as conjoined (Siamese) twins, (2) amniotic fluid volume, (3) placental location, maturity, or anomalous development, (4) uterine fibroids and anomalies, and (5) adnexal masses. Major indications for obstetric ultrasonography are found in Table 20-2 on p. 537. In general, the use of ultrasound has hastened diagnoses so that appropriate therapy can be instituted early in the pregnancy. Early therapy may decrease the severity and duration of morbidity, both physical and emotional, of the mother (family). Early diagnosis of fetal anomaly, for instance, makes possible choices such as intrauterine surgery or other therapy for the fetus, discontinuation of the pregnancy, and preparation of the family for the care of a child with a disorder or planning for placement of child after birth.

Findings

Fetal Viability. Fetal heart activity can be demonstrated as early as 6 to 7 weeks by real time echo scanners and at 10 to 12 weeks by Doppler mode. Confirmation of fetal death can be detected by lack of heart motion, the presence of fetal scalp edema (maceration), and overlap of the cranial bones. By 9 to 10 weeks, molar pregnancy (hydatidiform mole) can be diagnosed (Fig. 20-3).

Gestational Age. Several indicators have been established for gestational dating: (1) uncertain dates for the last normal menstrual period, (2) recent discontinuation of oral contraceptives, (3) bleeding episode during the first trimester, (4) uterine size that does not agree with dates, and (5) other high-risk conditions.

When performed during the first 18 weeks of gestation, ultrasound permits an extremely accurate assessment of gestational age by measurement of a single parameter. During this time most normal fetuses grow at the same rate. However, they do not continue to do so as the gestation advances, and accuracy of fetal age diagnosis decreases as the fetal age increases. With advanced fetal age, ensuring the accuracy of gestational age estimates by ultrasound depends on the additional measurement of more variables (Manning, 1989).

Four methods of estimation of fetal age are used: (1) determination of gestational sac dimensions (obtainable at about 8 weeks); (2) measurement of crown-rump length (obtainable between 7 and 14 weeks); (3) measurement of the BPD (obtainable at about 12 weeks); and (4) measurement of femur length (after 12 weeks).

Fetal BPD at 36 weeks should be approximately 8.7 cm. Term pregnancy and fetal maturity can be diagnosed with some confidence if the biparietal cephalometry by ultrasonography is greater than 9.8 cm (Fig. 20-4), especially when combined with appropriate femur length measurement. An estimate of fetal weight is based on BPD. With a BPD of 9.8 cm, fetal weight is estimated at over 3180 g (7 lb).

Fetal Growth and Anatomy. Fetal growth may be jeopardized under certain conditions. Some of the con-

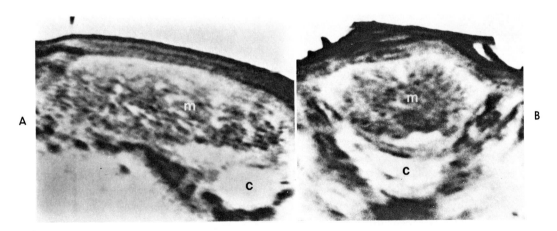

FIG. 20-3 Longitudinal (**A**) and transverse (**B**) scans of molar pregnancy. (**M**). Note typical vesicular (grape-like) pattern. Also shown are lutein cysts (C) (From Athey PA and Hadlock FP: *Ultrasound in obstetrics and gynecology,* ed 2, St Louis, 1985, Mosby.

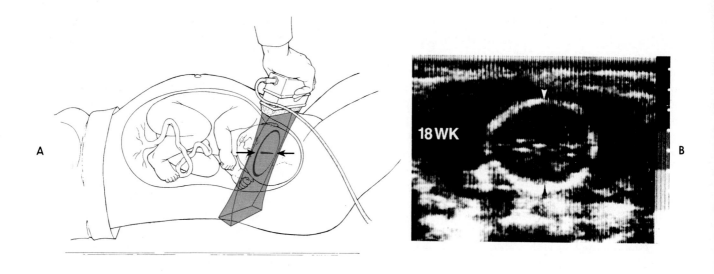

FIG. 20-4 **A,** Biparietal cephalometry by ultrasound. **B,** Linear array, real-time image demonstrates fetal biparietal diameter (BPD) at 18 weeks. (From Athey PA, Hadlock FP: *Ultrasound in obstetrics and gynecology*, ed 2, St Louis, 1985, Mosby.)

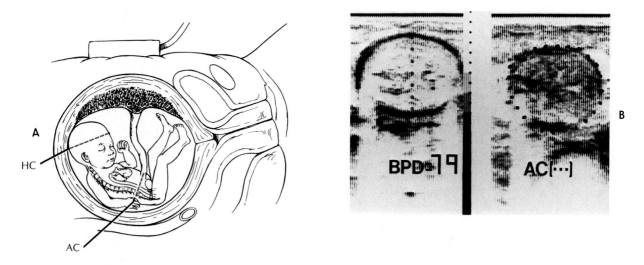

FIG. 20-5 **A,** Schematic presentation of appropriate planes of sections for head circumference HC and abdominal circumference AC. **B,** Real-time ultrasound image demonstrates typical head and body images that correspond to planes in **A.** (From Athey PA, Hadlock FP: *Ultrasound in obstetrics and gynecology*, ed 2, St Louis, 1985, Mosby.)

ditions that serve as indicators for ultrasound assessment of fetal growth include the following: poor maternal weight gain or pattern of weight gain; previous **intrauterine growth retardation (IUGR);** chronic infections; ingestion of certain legal and illegal drugs; diabetes mellitus; pregnancy-induced or other hypertension; multifetal pregnancy; other medical or surgical complications; and little or no prenatal care. Serial evaluations of BPD and limb length can differentiate between wrong dates and true IUGR. IUGR may be symmetric (the fetus is small in all parameters) or asymmetric (head and body growth vary). Symmetric IUGR may be caused by low genetic growth potential, intrauterine infection, maternal undernutrition or heavy smoking, or chromosomal

aberration. Asymmetric IUGR may reflect placental insufficiency secondary to hypertension, renal disease, or cardiovascular disease.

Reduced fetal growth is still among the most frequent complications associated with stillbirth (Morrison, Olsen, 1985). Macrosomic infants (those weighing over 4000 g) are at increased risk for birth trauma; macrosomic fetuses associated with maternal glucose intolerance are at increased risk of intrauterine death as well (Manning, 1989).

The BPD, head circumference, abdominal circumference, and estimated fetal weight for a normal 32-week fetus are illustrated in Fig. 20-5.

Depending on the gestational age, the following

structures may be identified: head (including ventricles and blood vessels), neck, spine, heart, stomach, small bowel, liver, kidneys, bladder, and limbs. Ultrasonography permits the confirmation of normal anatomy and the detection of major fetal malformations. The recognition of an anomaly may influence the location and method of birth so that neonatal outcomes may be optimal.

Beyond 36 weeks of gestation, more than 85% of all major anomalies can be detected by ultrasound. As a general rule, the earlier in gestation a lesion is detected, the worse the prognostic significance (Manning, 1989).

The number of fetuses and their presentation may also be assessed. This knowledge will often govern therapy and mode of birth.

Adjunct to Amniocentesis. The safety of amniocentesis is increased when the physician knows the exact position of the fetus, placenta, and pockets of amniotic fluid. Ultrasonography has greatly reduced previous risks associated with amniocentesis such as a fetal-maternal hemorrhage from a pierced placenta.

Placental Position and Function. The pattern of uterine and placental growth and the fullness of the bladder influence the apparent location of the placenta. By the middle of the second trimester the placenta can be clearly defined, but if it is seen to be low lying, its relationship to the internal cervical os can sometimes be altered by changing the degree of fullness of the maternal bladder. Additionally, scans done during this time report a placenta overlying the os in 15% to 20% of pregnancies; at term the incidence of placenta previa is only 0.5%. This error may be due to the subsequent elongation of the lower uterine segment as pregnancy progresses or distortion of the uterine cavity by the maternal bladder. The diagnosis of *placenta previa* can seldom be confirmed until the third trimester.

Fetal Well-being. Among the many physiologic measurements that can be accomplished with ultrasound are the following: heart motion, *fetal breathing movements (FBMs)*, fetal urine production (following serial measurements of bladder volume), fetal limb and head movements, and analysis of vascular waveforms from the fetal circulation (McCallum, 1984). It has been noted that FBMs are decreased with maternal smoking and alcohol ingestion and increased with hyperglycemia. Fetal limb and head movements serve as an index of neurologic development.

Amniotic Fluid Volume. Abnormalities of amniotic fluid volume, whether excessive or diminished, are frequently associated with fetal disorders. The total volume can be evaluated by a method developed by Rutherford et al (1987) whereby the depths (in centimeters) of amniotic fluid in all four quadrants surrounding the maternal umbilicus are totaled, resulting in an *amniotic fluid*

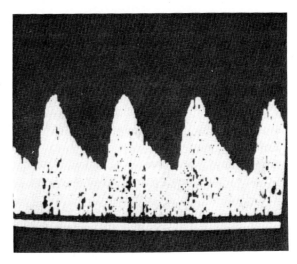

FIG. 20-6 Normal umbilical artery velocity waveforms and measurements from systole and end diastole. (From Schulman H: Doppler ultrasound. In Eden R, Boehm R, editors: *Assessment and care of the fetus: physiological, clinical, and medicological principles.* Norwalk, CT, 1990, Appleton and Lange.)

index (AFI). An AFI of less than 5 cm is considered to be indicative of oligohydramnios (decreased fluid), 5 to 8 cm is thought to be normal, and a measurement greater than 8 cm reflects polyhydramnios (increased fluid). Oligohydramnios has been associated with congenital anomalies (such as renal agenesis), growth retardation, and fetal distress in labor. Polyhydramnios has been found with neural tube defects, obstruction of the fetal GI tract, multifetal pregnancies, and fetal hydrops (Gabbe, 1986).

Doppler Blood Flow Measurements. Doppler ultrasound is used to study blood flow noninvasively in the fetus and placenta in pregnancies at risk due to hypertension, IUGR, diabetes mellitus, preterm labor, and multifetal gestations.

When a sound wave is reflected from a moving target, there is a change in frequency of the reflected wave relative to the transmitted wave. This is called the Doppler effect. An ultrasound beam scattered by a group of red blood cells (RBCs) is an example of this effect. The velocity of the RBCs can be determined by measuring the change in the frequency of the sound wave reflected off them (Trudinger, 1989).

Velocity waveforms from umbilical and uterine arteries, reported in systolic/diastolic (S/D) ratios, can first be detected at 15 weeks of pregnancy. Because of progressive decline in resistance in both the umbilical and uterine artery circulation, decreasing measurement values occur as pregnancy advances. Most fetuses will achieve an S/D ratio of 3 or less by 30 weeks. Persistent elevation of S/D ratios after 30 weeks is associated with IUGR (Fig. 20-6).

Biophysical Profile. The advent of real time ultrasound now permits detailed assessment of the physical and physiologic characteristics of the developing fetus to such an extent that it is possible to examine the fetus in detail and to catalogue normal and abnormal biophysical responses to stimuli. The **biophysical profile (BPP)** is a noninvasive dynamic assessment of a fetus and its environment, employing ultrasonography and external fetal monitoring.

Fetal BPP scoring is a method of fetal risk surveillance. The procedure may be viewed as undertaking a physical examination of the fetus, including determination of vital signs. The fetus responds to central hypoxia by alterations in movement, muscle tone, breathing, and heart rate patterns. The presence of normal fetal biophysical activities shows that the central nervous system is fully functional and therefore not hypoxemic (Manning,

Harman, 1990). Attention is paid to the presence or absence of three discrete biophysical variables (Table 20-3) for scoring, interpretation, and management:

1. Fetal breathing movements (FBMs): Defined by initial inward movement of the thorax with descent of the diaphragm and abdominal contents, followed by a return to the original position.
2. Fetal movements (FMs): Defined as single or clusters of activity of the limbs and fetal body; isolated hand and arm movements represent normality.
3. Fetal tone (FT): The definition has been refined to at least one episode of opening of the hand with finger and thumb extension with a return to closed fist formation. In the absence of any hand movement, tone is still recorded as normal if the hand remains in the fist formation for the entire 30-minute observation.

TABLE 20-3 Biophysical Profile

VARIABLES	NORMAL (SCORE = 2)	ABNORMAL (SCORE = 0)
Fetal breathing movements	One or more episodes in 30 min, each lasting ≥30 sec	Episodes absent or no episode of ≥30 sec in 30 min
Gross body movements	Three or more discrete body/limb movements in 30 min (episodes of active continuous movement considered as a single movement)	Less than three episodes of body/limb movements in 30 min
Fetal tone	One or more episodes of active extension with return to flexion of fetal limb(s) or trunk; opening and closing of hand considered normal tone	Slow extension with return to flexion; movement of limb in full extension, or fetal movement absent
Reactive fetal heart rate	Two or more episodes of acceleration (≥15 beats/min) in 20 min, each lasting ≥15 sec and associated with fetal movement	Less than two episodes of acceleration or acceleration of <15 beats/min in 20 min
Qualitative amniotic fluid volume	One or more pockets of fluid measuring ≥1 cm in two perpendicular planes	Pockets absent or pocket <1 cm in two perpendicular planes

SCORE	INTERPRETATION	RECOMMENDED MANAGEMENT
10	Normal infant, low risk for chronic asphyxia	Repeat testing at weekly intervals; repeat twice weekly in diabetic women and women ≥42 weeks
8	Normal infant, low risk for chronic asphyxia	Repeat testing at weekly intervals; repeat twice weekly in diabetic women and women ≥42 weeks; oligohydramnios is indication for delivery
6	Suspected chronic asphyxia	Repeat testing within 24 hr; oligohydramnios or repeat score ≤6 is indication for delivery
4	Suspected chronic asphyxia	Indications for delivery are ≥36 weeks and favorable cervix; if <36 weeks and lecithin/sphingomyelin ratio <2.0, repeat test in 24 hr; repeat score ≤6 or oligohydramnios is indication for delivery
2	Strong suspicion of chronic asphyxia	Extend testing time to 120 min; persistent score ≤4, regardless of gestational age, is indication for delivery

Reprinted with permission from Manning FA et al: Fetal assessment based on fetal biophysical profile scoring: experience in 12,620 referred high risk pregnancies, *Am J Obstet Gynecol* 151:345, 1985.

Scoring also includes:

- Qualitative amniotic fluid volume: Normal is a finding of at least one pocket that measures at least 1 cm in two perpendicular planes.
- Nonstress test: Often performed before the BPP as a screening procedure.
- Placental grading: Included by some (Vintzileos et al, 1985); the placenta is given 2 points for grades I or II and 0 points for a grade III.

The BPP provides an accurate estimate of the risk of fetal death in the 24 to 48 hours following the test. Additionally, when an abnormal score and oligohydramnios are encountered, labor induction is warranted (Manning, Harman, 1990). The BPP has also proven effective as an early predictor of fetal infection in women whose membranes rupture prematurely (at less than 37 weeks' gestation). The change in biophysical activities, similar to those seen when a fetus is hypoxic, precedes the clinical signs of infection and indicates the necessity for immediate birth (Gaffney, Salinger, Vintzileos, 1990). When risk is low, as with a normal score, intervention is indicated only for obstetric or maternal factors.

Nursing Role

Although an increased number of nurses with additional training do perform ultrasound and biophysical profiles in certain centers, the majority of nurses will find themselves counseling and educating women about the procedure (see Legal Tip). Accurate information regarding the procedure is imperative to allay anxiety. Although ultrasound has become a widely used diagnostic tool, recommendations for the procedure are based on expectations of a fetal problem. Therefore the procedure may provoke anxiety in the woman. The nurse should give her ample opportunity to have her questions answered, and be reassured as to the safety of ultrasound.

LEGAL TIP: **Performance of Limited Ultrasound Examinations**

Nurses who have the training and competence may perform limited ultrasound examinations if it is within the scope of practice in their state or area, and if it is consistent with regulations of the agencies in which they practice. Limited ultrasound examinations include identification of fetal number, fetal presentation, fetal cardiac activity location of the placenta, and biophysical profile including amniotic fluid volume assessment. Patients should be informed about the limited information provided by these examinations. They are not meant to evaluate or identify fetal anomalies, assess fe-

tal age, or estimate fetal weight. The obstetric health care provider is responsible for obtaining a basic or targeted examination when complete patient assessment is necessary (AWHONN, 1993).

Early in pregnancy the woman is usually directed to come for the examination with a full bladder, since it supports the uterus in position for the imaging. She is then positioned comfortably in a supine position with small pillows under her head and knees. It is most important that the uterus be displaced to one side by a wedge under the right hip, or by tilting the woman to one side to avoid supine hypotension and vena cava syndrome. The display panel should be positioned so that the woman can observe the images on the screen of the machine if she so desires; some women may not want to watch.

The transvaginal approach is also used to evaluate the fetus by ultrasound. This can be very effective because of the nearness of the fetal parts to be evaluated, and not needing to traverse the abdominal wall. Some women do not wish this method to be employed, however, due to modesty or discomfort, so the patient's wishes should be accommodated if possible. The transvaginal mode is not very useful if the presenting part is very low in the pelvis, particularly near term; the presenting part will be the only structure viewed.

There is no conclusive evidence that humans have been harmed by diagnostic ultrasound during the 25 years it has been used (Athey, Hadlock, 1985; Cunningham, MacDonald, Gant, 1993). No detrimental effects have been observed to date on the fetus or mother either histologically, functionally, or embryologically in experimental work; however, there is a hypothetical risk that cannot be ignored or overlooked. Benefit must be weighed against hypothetical risk. Pregnant women should be informed of the clinical indication for ultrasound, specific benefit, potential risk, and alternatives.

Magnetic Resonance Imaging

Magnetic resonance imaging (MRI) is a noninvasive tool that can be used for obstetric and gynecologic diagnosis. MRI can evaluate (1) fetal structure—CNS, thorax, abdomen, genitourinary tract, musculoskeletal system, and overall growth; (2) placenta—position, density, and evaluation of gestational trophoblastic disease; (3) amniotic fluid quantity; (4) maternal structures—uterus, cervix, adnexa, and pelvimetry; (5) biochemical status (pH, ATP content) of tissues and organs; and (6) soft tissue, metabolic, or functional malformations. Although the procedure appears to have many advantages, its complete safety has not been accurately determined. Thus broad usage should not be encouraged until further studies are made (Mattison, Angtuaco, 1988). Currently it is not used widely in all centers.

Biochemical Assessment
Amniocentesis

An **amniocentesis** is performed to obtain amniotic fluid, which contains fetal cells. Under direct ultrasound visualization, a needle is inserted transabdominally into the uterus. Amniotic fluid is withdrawn into a syringe, and various analyses are performed. Amniocentesis is possible after the fourteenth week of pregnancy, when the uterus becomes an abdominal organ and when there is sufficient amniotic fluid for this procedure (Fig. 20-7).

Overall complications are less than 1% for both mother and fetus and include the following:

Maternal: hemorrhage, fetal-maternal hemorrhage with possible maternal Rh isoimmunization, infection, labor, abruptio placentae, inadvertent damage to the intestines or bladder, amniotic fluid embolism.

Fetal: death, hemorrhage, infection (amnionitis), direct injury from the needle, abortion or premature labor, leakage of amniotic fluid.

Many of the complications have been minimized or eliminated by performing the procedure under ultrasound and by adequate monitoring of the woman and fetus afterward. Nursing actions at that time include (1) continuous electronic monitoring of fetus (for nonreassuring heart rate patterns) and uterus (for contractions),

(2) administration of RhoGam (immune globulin) to Rh-negative women, and (3) instructions for daily fetal movement counts.

Indications for the procedure include prenatal diagnosis of genetic disorders, assessment of pulmonary maturity, and diagnosis of fetal hemolytic disease. Amniotic fluid may be analyzed for the following conditions.

Genetic Problems

Prenatal assessment of genetic disorders is indicated in women of advanced age, those with a previous child with a chromosome abnormality, or a family history of chromosome anomalies. Inherited errors of metabolism may also be detected (such as Tay-Sachs disease, hemophilia, and thalassemia) and other disorders for which marker genes are known.

Cells are cultured for *karyotyping* of chromosomes. Fetal cells are also assessed for *sex chromatin;* sex determination is important if a sex-linked disorder such as hemophilia (occurring almost always in a male fetus) is suspected.

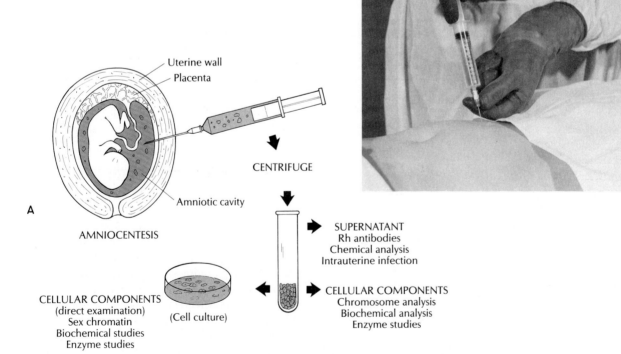

FIG. 20-7 **A,** Amniocentesis and laboratory utilization of amniotic fluid aspirant. **(B),** Transabdominal amniocentesis. (**A** From Whaley LF: Understanding inherited disorders, St. Louis, 1974, Mosby. **B** Courtesy March of Dimes.)

Alpha-Fetoprotein (AFP)

The normal source of **alpha-fetoprotein (AFP)** in amniotic fluid is fetal urine. Some of the protein crosses fetal membranes into maternal circulation. Correct interpretation of concentration of AFP requires precise knowledge of gestational age. AFP levels may be elevated in the presence of a variety of conditions in which fetal integument is not intact and the protein leaks from the capillaries into the amniotic fluid. Elevated levels are associated with neural tube defects, such as spina bifida and anencephaly (Table 20-4). AFP may also be elevated with severe fetal hemolytic disease, esophageal atresia, congenital nephrosis, omphalocele, fetal hemorrhage into amniotic fluid, oligohydramnios, low birth weight, and fetal death. Levels may also be elevated in a normal multifetal pregnancy. Low levels may be associated with chromosomal trisomies (e.g., Down syndrome), gestational trophoblastic disease, fetal death, increased maternal weight, and overestimation of gestational age (Cunningham, MacDonald, Gant, 1993). *It must be remembered that this screening test is not perfect. There will be false positives as well as false negatives.*

Fetal Lung Maturity

Greater accuracy in estimating fetal maturity is now possible through use of amniotic fluid or its exfoliated cellular content. Term pregnancy and fetal maturity can be demonstrated by the following laboratory studies.

A **lecithin/sphingomyelin (L/S) ratio** greater than 2:1 indicates adequate lung maturity for extrauterine life (see Chapter 4 and Table 20-4). This is generally achieved by 36 weeks' gestational age. A quick means of determining the L/S ratio is the rapid surfactant test, also known as the *shake test* or foam stabilization test. Equal parts of fresh amniotic fluid and normal saline solution are added to two parts 95% ethyl alcohol. The mixture is shaken vigorously for 30 seconds. If bubbles are still present at the meniscus 15 minutes after shaking, the fetal lung is judged to be mature.

An L/S ratio of 2 does not necessarily mean that the neonate will not develop respiratory distress syndrome (RDS). This is especially true with certain pregnancy complications. The conditions in which an L/S ratio of 2 is not reassuring include the following: maternal diabetes mellitus (Quirk, Bleasdale, 1986), erythroblastosis fetalis, and fetal/neonatal sepsis (Cunningham, MacDonald, Gant, 1993).

The presence of *phosphotidiglycerol* (PG), another phospholipid, also reflects fetal lung maturity. In the presence of PG the incidence of RDS is virtually 0%. The turbidity of the specimen itself is believed to be dependent on the total amniotic fluid phospholipid concentration. Delta optical density (ΔOD) 650 nm > 0.15 correlates extremely well with the absence of RDS (Sonek, Reiss, Gabbe, 1990).

When the *bilirubin* level or ΔOD (of bilirubinoid pigments is 450 nm < 0.015,) the gestational age is greater than 36 weeks.

When the *creatinine* (estimate of renal maturity) value is greater than 2.0 mg/dl, the gestational age is greater

---

TABLE 20-4   Summary of Biochemical Monitoring Techniques

TEST	POSSIBLE FINDINGS	CLINICAL SIGNIFICANCE
MATERNAL BLOOD		
Coombs' test	Titer of 1:8 and rising	Significant Rh incompatibility
Alpha-fetoprotein	See below	
AMNIOTIC FLUID ANALYSIS		
Color	Meconium	Possible hypoxia or asphyxia
Lung profile		Fetal lung maturity
Lecithin/sphingomyelin (L/S) ratio	>2	
Phosphatidylglycerol (PG)	Present	
Creatinine	>2 mg/dl	Gestational age >36 weeks
Bilirubin (ΔOD 450/nm)	<0.015	Gestational age >36 weeks, normal pregnancy
	High levels	Fetal hemolytic disease in Rh isoimmunized pregnancies
Lipid cells	>10%	Gestational age >35 weeks
Alpha-fetoprotein	High levels after 15-week gestation	Open neural tube or other defect
Osmolality	Decline after 20-week gestation	Advancing nonspecific gestational age
Genetic disorders	Dependent on cultured cells for karyotype and enzymatic activity	Counseling may be required
Sex-linked		
Chromosomal		
Metabolic		

than 36 weeks in the absence of maternal renal disease and dehydration or of fetal anomaly.

After *fetal lipid-containing exfoliated cells* are stained with Nile blue sulfate, a finding of more than 20% orange-staining cells indicates a gestational age of greater than 35 weeks; the fetus probably weighs 2500 g.

Fetal Hemolytic Disease

Identification and follow-up of fetal hemolytic disease in isoimmunized pregnancies is another indication for amniocentesis. The first ΔOD analysis for amount of bilirubin in amniotic fluid is postponed until the second trimester. Therapy by intrauterine transfusion of packed, Rh-negative, type O red blood cells is not possible before that time.

Apt Test

This test is used to differentiate maternal and fetal blood when there is vaginal bleeding during pregnancy or labor. To perform the test quickly, add 0.5 ml bloody fluid to 4.5 ml distilled water and shake. Then add 1 ml 0.25 normal sodium hydroxide. Fetal and cord blood will remain pink for 1 to 2 minutes. Maternal blood becomes brown in 30 seconds. For further confirmation, a Kleihauer-Betke examination for fetal red blood cells can be done in the laboratory (see p. 473).

Meconium in Amniotic Fluid

There are three possible reasons for the passage of meconium during the intrapartum period: (1) it is a normal physiologic function that occurs with maturity (meconium passage is infrequent before weeks 32 to 34, with an increased incidence after 38 weeks), (2) it is the result of hypoxia-induced peristalsis and sphincter relaxation, and (3) it may be a sequela to umbilical cord compression–induced vagal stimulation in mature fetuses.

The appearance of meconium-stained fluid is an indication for careful evaluation. Meconium is usually described as occurring from a trace amount through a rating of 4+, with respective pigmentation of a slightly green tinge up to a dark brown. The following criteria are proposed for evaluating meconium passage during the intrapartum period (Scott et al, 1990):

1. Consistency: old and thin vs. new and thick. A new and thick consistency is more likely to be the result of fetal stress.
2. Timing: thick, fresh meconium passed for the first time in late labor, associated with nonremediable severe variable or late FHR decelerations, is an omninous sign. However, *the presence of meconium alone is not necessarily a sign of fetal distress.*
3. Presence of other indicators: meconium passage and nonremediable severe variable or late decelerations (especially with poor baseline variability) with or without acidosis confirmed by scalp blood sampling are ominous signs.

In the presence of meconium, the birthing team should anticipate the need for careful suctioning of the nasopharynx at time of birth, ideally before the first breath is taken. Suctioning at this time is effective in reducing the incidence and severity of meconium aspiration in the neonate (Brady, Goldman, 1986).

Percutaneous Umbilical Blood Sampling (PUBS) or Cordocentesis

Direct access to the fetal circulation during the second and third trimesters is now possible through **percutaneous umbilical blood sampling (PUBS)** or *cordocentesis*. It is the most widely used method for fetal blood sampling and transfusion (Nicolaides, Thorpe-Beeston,

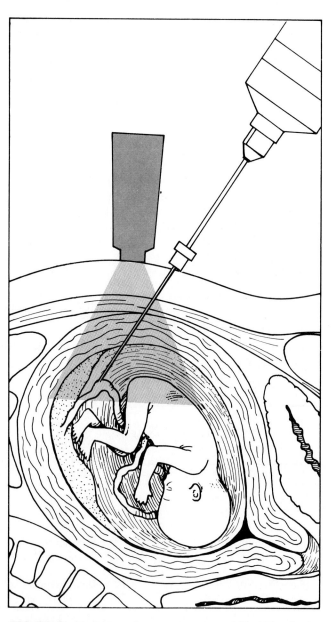

FIG. 20-8 Technique for percutaneous umbilical blood sampling guided by ultrasound.

Noble, 1990). PUBS involves the insertion of a needle directly into a fetal umbilical vessel under ultrasound guidance. Ideally, the umbilical cord is punctured 1 to 2 cm from its placental insertion. At this point the cord is well anchored and will not move, and the risk of maternal blood contamination (from the placenta) is slight (Ludomirski, Weiner, 1988). Generally, 1 to 4 ml of blood is removed during the puncture and immediately tested by Kleihauer-Betke method to ensure it is fetal blood (Fig. 20-8).

The three main complications reported are blood leakage from the puncture site, fetal bradycardia, and chorioamnionitis; none of the procedures was followed by premature rupture of the membranes (Ludomirski, Weiner, 1988).

Indications for use include prenatal diagnosis of inherited blood disorders or karyotyping of malformed fetuses, detection of fetal infection, determination of the acid-base status of IUGR fetuses, and assessment and treatment of isoimmunized and thrombocytopenic pregnancies.

Since a fetal blood specimen will yield a karyotype in 2 or 3 days, PUBS may be the procedure of choice when time limitations do not permit amniotic fluid cultures to be used.

In fetuses at risk for isoimmune hemolytic anemia, PUBS now permits identification of fetal blood type and count precisely and may avoid further interventions. If the fetus is antigen positive for maternal antibodies, a direct Coombs' test can be done to confirm the degree of anemia through hemolysis. PUBS is now the route of choice for intrauterine transfusion for severely anemic fe-

tuses; it can be started as early as 19 weeks' gestation, 4 to 5 weeks earlier than through the intraperitoneal route (Ludomirski, Weiner, 1988).

Follow-up includes continuous fetal heart rate monitoring for several minutes up to 1 hour and a repeat ultrasound 1 hour later to ensure that there was no further bleeding or hematoma formation.

Chorionic Villus Sampling

Chorionic villus sampling (CVS) could partially replace amniocentesis for genetic diagnosis. Although there are risks to the fetus, the greatest advantage in this new technique (Fig. 20-9) is that genetic diagnosis can be moved ahead from the second to the first trimester—as early as the eighth week—and can produce results rapidly. This increases the potential for improving fetal treatment by allowing earlier intervention (Golbus, 1987). Earlier diagnosis also reduces a couple's waiting period, imposes less social and psychologic stress, permits the couple privacy because the pregnancy is not obvious as yet, and allows for an earlier and safer abortion if the couple so chooses.

This procedure is done between weeks 8 and 14 (see Fig. 20-9) and involves the removal of a small tissue specimen from the fetal portion of the placenta. Since chorionic villi originate in the zygote, that tissue reflects the genetic makeup of the fetus. The specimen is removed either from the chorion frondosum or the chorion laeve.

Real time ultrasound is used to guide the procedure. The aspiration cannula and obturator must negotiate the cervical canal, must be placed at a suitable site, and must avoid rupturing the amniotic sac.

Two other techniques used in CVS are direct vision biopsy using a hysteroscope and transabdominal aspiration guided by ultrasound. The magnitude of the procedure-related risk in CVS is around 2% (Jackson, 1988), and includes possible complications such as spontaneous abortion, infection, hematoma, intrauterine

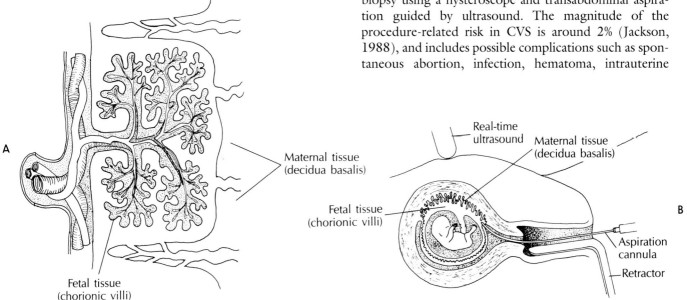

FIG. 20-9 Chorionic villus sampling. **(A),** Chorionic villi at time of sampling (between 8 and 14 weeks). **(B),** Taking sample by transcervical method.

death, growth retardation, Rh isoimmunization, trauma, and birth defects. At present, if the risk of a fetal genetic disorder (e.g., hemoglobinopathies) is 25% or more, CVS is one possible diagnostic alternative.

Maternal Blood Assessments

Coombs' Test

Coombs' test for Rh incompatibility is discussed at length in Chapter 27. If Coombs' titer is greater than 1:8 to 1:16, amniocentesis for ΔOD is indicated to determine a need for intrauterine transfusion (see Table 20-4).

Alpha-Fetoprotein (AFP)

The most exciting development in recent years has been the emergence of maternal serum alpha-fetoprotein (MSAFP) as a screening tool for neural tube defects in pregnancy. Through this technique approximately 80% to 85% of all open neural tube defects (NTDs) can be detected early in pregnancy.

The cause of NTDs is not well understood, but it is important to note that 95% of all affected infants are born to women with no previous family history of similar anomalies. There are 1 to 2 per 1000 births in most parts of the United States. The risk of recurrence is 2% to 3% (10 to 15 times) the general population after one affected child. After two affected children the risk rises to 6% to 8% (Burton, 1988).

AFP is produced by the fetal liver and is detectable in increasing quantities in the serum of pregnant women from 14 to 34 weeks. One must keep in mind that, although amniotic fluid AFP is diagnostic, MSAFP is a screening tool only and identifies candidates for the more definitive procedures of amniocentesis and ultrasound examination. MSAFP screening can be done with reasonable reliability any time between 15 and 21 weeks' gestation (17 weeks is ideal).

Once the woman's level is determined, it is compared with normal values established within each laboratory for each week of gestation. Most use a value 2 to 2.5 times the normal median as abnormal (reported as multiples of the mean, or MOM). An abnormal test should be repeated in 1 week; if two sequential MSAFPs are elevated, the woman should be counseled regarding the significance of the findings, the nature of NTDs, and options for further testing.

The next step is ultrasound, since besides NTD, the most common reasons for elevated AFPs are underestimated gestational age, multiple pregnancy, unrecognized fetal demise, and severe oligohydramnios. If the fetus appears normal and of correct gestational age, an amniocentesis should be done for AFP (Burton, 1988). See the previous discussion of amniotic fluid AFP p. 545.

There is a convincing body of evidence that Down syndrome and probably other autosomal trisomies are as-

sociated with lower than normal MSAFP and amniotic fluid AFP (Burton, 1988).

Electronic Monitoring

Whereas first and second trimester antenatal assessment is directed primarily at the diagnosis of fetal anomalies, the goal of third trimester testing is to determine whether the intrauterine environment continues to be supportive to the fetus (Halle, 1993). The testing is often used to determine the timing of birth for women at risk for **uteroplacental insufficiency** (the gradual decline in the delivery of needed substances by the placenta to the fetus). It has been suggested that a gradual loss of placental function occurs in which nutritive function is lost first, leading to IUGR. Subsequently, respiratory function is compromised, resulting in fetal hypoxia (Freeman, Lagrew, 1990).

The two most frequently used third trimester tests are the **nonstress test (NST)** or fetal activity test (FAT) and the **contraction stress test (CST)** or oxytocin challenge test (OCT).

The NST monitors the fetus for acceleration of the FHR in response to movement, indicative of a healthy fetus. The CST, a more specific test, identifies the fetus who is stable at rest but shows evidence of compromise when stressed. This fetus demonstrates late decelerations when contractions are induced, which stress the fetus through decreased uterine blood flow and placental perfusion.

The desired goals of antepartum monitoring are to prevent intrauterine fetal death and avoid unnecessary premature intervention.

Indications for both the NST and the CST include the following:

Maternal diabetes mellitus
Chronic hypertension
Hypertensive disorders in pregnancy
IUGR
Sickle cell disease
Maternal cyanotic heart disease
Suspected postmaturity
History of previous stillbirth
Rh sensitization (isoimmunization)
Meconium-stained amniotic fluid (at amniocentesis)
Hyperthyroidism
Collagen diseases
Older pregnant women
≥40 weeks' gestation
Chronic renal disease

There are no contraindications for the NST. Absolute contraindications for the CST are rupture of membranes, previous classic cesarean birth, preterm labor, placenta previa or abruptio placentae. The following are considered relative contraindications for the CST: multifetal pregnancy, previous preterm labor, hydramnios less than

36 weeks' gestation, and incompetent cervix (Freeman, Lagrew, 1990). As a rule, reactive patterns with the NST or negative results with the CST are associated with favorable outcomes. In general, biophysical assessment is considered reliable, but false negatives and false positives do occur (Haesslein, 1987; Scott et al, 1990).

Nonstress Test

The basis for the NST, is that the normal fetus will produce characteristic heart rate patterns. Acceleration of FHR in response to fetal movement is the desired outcome of the NST. This then allows most high-risk pregnancies to continue, with the test being repeated twice a week. A *reactive pattern* suggests fetal well-being with an associated good perinatal outcome.

In the healthy fetus with an intact central nervous system, 90% of gross fetal body movements are associated with fetal heart rate accelerations. This response can be blunted by hypoxia or acidosis, drugs (analgesics, barbiturates, and beta-blockers), fetal sleep, and some congenital anomalies (Sonek, Reiss, Gabbe, 1990).

Advantages include the fact that it is easy to perform in an outpatient setting, since it is noninvasive. It is also relatively inexpensive and has no known contraindications.

Disadvantages center around the high false positive rate for nonreactive findings secondary to fetal sleep cycles, medications, and fetal immaturity. There is slightly lower sensitivity to fetal compromise than with CST or biophysical profile.

Procedure

The woman is seated in a reclining chair (or in semi-Fowler's position) to avoid supine hypotension. The FHR is recorded by Doppler transducer, and a toco-transducer is applied to detect uterine contractions or fetal movements (FMs). The nurse observes the strip chart for signs of *fetal activity* and a concurrent acceleration of FHR. If evidence of fetal movement is not apparent on the strip, the woman may be asked to depress a button on a hand-held event marker that is connected to the monitor when she feels fetal movement. The movement is then noted on the strip. Since almost all accelerations are accompanied by FM, it need not be recorded with accelerations for the test to be considered reactive (Gabbe, 1986). The test usually takes 20 to 30 minutes but may take longer if the fetus needs to be awakened because of a sleep state.

Interpretation

Generally accepted criteria for a reactive tracing are two or more accelerations of 15 beats/min lasting for 15 seconds over a 20-minute period, normal baseline rate, and long-term variability amplitude of 10 or more beats/min. If the test does not meet the criteria after 40 minutes, it is considered nonreactive, and a CST should be performed (Fig. 20-10).

Fetal Acoustic Stimulation (FAS)

The acoustic stimulation test is another method of testing antepartum FHR response. The test takes approximately 10 minutes to complete, with the fetus monitored for 5 minutes before stimulation to obtain a baseline FHR. The sound source (usually a laryngeal stimulator) is then applied briefly to the maternal abdomen over the fetal head. Monitoring continues for another 5 minutes and the chart is assessed. A reactive test is achieved if there is FHR acceleration of at least 15 beats/min for at least 120 seconds, or two accelerations of at least 15 beats/min for at least 15 seconds within 5 minutes of stimulus. FAS may also be applied during an NST if the fetus appears to be in a sleep state.

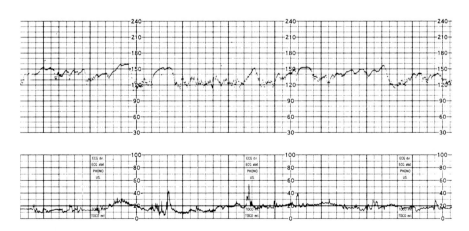

FIG. 20-10 Reactive nonstress test. (FHR accelerations with fetal movement.) (From Tucker SM: *Pocket Guide to Fetal Monitoring*, St Louis, 1992, Mosby.)

Contraction Stress Tests

The basis for the CST is that a healthy fetus can withstand a decreased oxygen supply during the physiologic stress of an oxytocin-stimulated contraction, whereas a compromised fetus will demonstrate late decelerations that are nonreassuring and indicative of uteroplacental insufficiency. **A negative test suggests fetal well-being.**

Contraindications include the following: threatened preterm labor, placenta previa, hydramnios, multifetal pregnancy, rupture of membranes, previous preterm labor, and previous classic cesarean birth (Cunningham, MacDonald, Gant, 1993).

Advantages of the CST are that it provides an earlier warning of fetal compromise than the NST, and there are fewer false positive tests. *Disadvantages* include the contraindications described earlier, as well as the fact that it is more time consuming and expensive than an NST; it is an invasive procedure if exogenous oxytocin is required.

Procedure

The woman is placed in semi-Fowler's position or sits in a reclining chair. She is monitored externally, and the nurse observes the strip for 10 minutes for baseline rate, long-term variability, and the possible occurrence of spontaneous contractions.

Nipple-stimulated Contraction Stress Test

If the woman has three or more spontaneous contractions within a 10-minute period, the nipple-stimulated contractions need not be initiated. If less than three spontaneous contractions occur within the period, and if late decelerations do not occur with intermittent spontaneous contractions, nipple stimulation can be initiated. The nurse explains the procedure to the woman and then proceeds by applying warm, moist washcloths to both breasts for several minutes. The woman is instructed to massage or roll the nipple of one breast for four cycles of 2 minutes on and 2 minutes off. If unsuccessful,

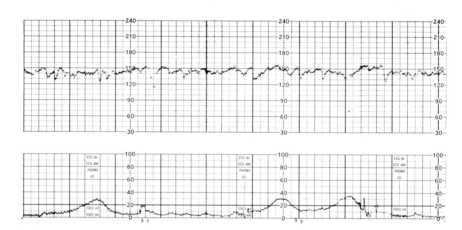

FIG. 20-11 Negative CST. (From Tucker SM: *Pocket Guide to Fetal Monitoring*, St Louis, 1992, Mosby.)

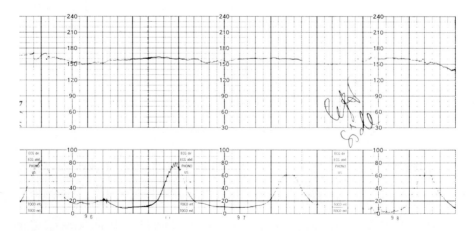

FIG. 20-12 Positive CST, compromised fetus. (From Tucker SM: *Pocket Guide to Fetal Monitoring*, St Louis, 192, Mosby.)

stimulate the breast for 10 minutes, stopping when a contraction begins and starting when it stops. If uterine contractions do not occur, both nipples should be stimulated for 10 minutes. The nipples should be restimulated intermittently as needed to maintain uterine contractions. If nipple stimulation does not produce the desired uterine activity, an oxytocin-stimulated CST is indicated.

Oxytocin-Stimulated Contraction Stress Test

The health care provider orders the dosage, which usually starts at 0.5 mU/min. The oxytocin is always diluted in an IV solution and piggybacked into the tubing of the main IV. The infusion is usually delivered by an infusion pump or controller to ensure accurate dosage. The oxytocin infusion is usually increased by 0.5 mU/min at 15-minute to 20-minute intervals until three uterine contractions of good quality are observed within a 10-minute period. The FHR pattern is then interpreted. The oxytocin infusion is discontinued and the maintenance IV solution infused until such time as uterine activity has returned to the preoxytocin infusion level. The IV is then removed, and the fetal monitor is discontinued. The woman can be sent home on the health care provider's orders.

Interpretation of Results

A guide for the interpretation of the CST follows:

Result	Interpretation
Negative	No late decelerations with a minimum of three uterine contractions lasting 40 to 60 seconds within a 10-minute period (Fig. 20-11)
Positive	Persistent and consistent late decelerations occurring with more than half the contractions (Fig. 20-12)
Suspicious	Late decelerations occurring with less than half the uterine contractions once an adequate contraction pattern has been established
Hyperstimulation	Late decelerations occurring with excessive uterine activity (contractions more often than every 2 minutes or lasting longer than 90 seconds) or a persistent increase in uterine tone
Unsatisfactory	Inadequate uterine contraction pattern or tracing too poor to interpret

The clinical significance of the CST is as follows:

Result	Interpretation
Negative	Reassurance that the fetus is likely to survive labor, should it occur within 1 week; more frequent testing may be indicated by the clinical situation
Positive	Management lies between use of other tools of fetal assessment and termination of pregnancy; a positive test indicates that the fetus is at increased risk for perinatal morbidity and mortality; the health care provider may perform an expeditious vaginal birth following a successful induction or may proceed directly to cesarean birth
Suspicious, hyperstimulation, or unsatisfactory	NST and CST should be repeated within 24 hours; if interpretable data cannot be achieved, other methods of fetal assessment must be used

Daily Fetal Movement Count (DFMC) or Kick Counts

Maternal assessment of fetal activity is a simple yet valuable method for monitoring the fetal condition. It can be done at home, is noninvasive, is simple to understand, and does not interfere with most daily routines. In general, the presence of fetal movements is a reassuring sign of fetal health. It has been well documented in the literature that decreased or absent fetal movements was noted by a majority of women who experienced stillbirth (Calhoun, 1990).

Maternal awareness of fetal movements is reported to be at least 90% accurate as demonstrated by simultaneous observation of the fetus by real time ultrasound. It is also important to note that no mothers reported *more* movements than were documented.

Several protocols for counting are in existence and vary with the practitioner. Thus no one method is described here. Except for very low daily fetal movements, or where there is a trend toward decreased motion, the clinical value of the absolute number of fetal movements has not been established. The only exception is when fetal movements cease entirely for 12 hours (the fetal alarm signal), at which time the woman should seek immediate medical attention. Generally, less than three FMs within 1 hour warrant further evaluation through NST, CST, BPP, or a combination (Freda et al, 1993).

KEY POINTS

■ A high-risk pregnancy is one in which the life or well-being of the mother or infant is jeopardized by a biophysical or psychosocial disorder coincidental with or unique to pregnancy.

■ Factors that place the pregnancy and fetus-neonate at risk include anatomic, physiologic, therapeutic, environmental, and idiopathic events.

■ Psychosocial perinatal warning indicators include

characteristics of the parents, the child, their support systems, and family circumstances.

- Maternal and perinatal mortality for whites is considerably lower than for other races in the United States.
- There is excellent evidence that mortality decreases when high risk is identified early and intensive care applied.
- Diagnostic techniques include ultrasonography, MRI, PUBS, CVS, and EFM. CVS could partially replace amniocentesis for genetic diagnosis.

- Biochemical monitoring techniques involve assessment of maternal urine and blood, and of amniotic fluid and its components.
- Electronic monitoring that results in a *reactive* NST and a *negative* CST suggest fetal well-being.
- The biophysical profile uses ultrasonography and external fetal monitoring to assess the fetus and its environment.

CRITICAL THINKING EXERCISES

1. Review several patients' charts. Identify risk factors and give rationale for each choice.

2. Assist with a CST or NST. Evaluate the fetal monitor strip and determine if it is an example of a reactive nonstress test, a nonreactive nonstress test, a positive contraction stress test, or a negative contraction stress test.

References

American College of Obstetricians and Gynecologists: *Guidelines for perinatal care,* ed 2, Elk Grove Village, IL, 1988, American Academy of Pediatrics and ACOG.

Athey P, Hadlock F: *Ultrasound in obstetrics and gynecology,* ed 2, St Louis, 1985, Mosby.

Association of Women's Health, Obstetric, and Neonatal Nurses: *Nursing practice competencies and educational guidelines for limited ultrasound examinations in obstetric and gynecologic/infertility settings,* Washington, DC, AWHONN, 1993.

Brady J, Goldman S: Management of meconium aspiration syndrome. In Thibeault D, Gregory G, editors: *Neonatal pulmonary care,* Norwalk, CT, 1986, Appleton-Century-Crofts.

Burton B: Elevated maternal serum alpha-fetoprotein (MSAFP): interpretation and follow up, *Clin Obstet Gynecol* 31(2):293, 1988.

Calhoun S: "Ask the experts": daily fetal movement counts, *NAACOG Newsletter* 17(8):6, 1990.

Cunningham F, MacDonald P, Gant N: *Williams obstetrics,* ed 19, Norwalk, CT, 1993, Appleton & Lange.

Freda et al: Fetal movement counting: which method? *MCN* 18:314, 1993.

Freeman R, Lagrew D, Jr: The contraction stress test. In Eden R, Boehm F, editors: *Assessment and care of the fetus: physiological, clinical and medicolegal principles,* Norwalk, CT, 1990, Appleton & Lange.

Gabbe S: Antepartum fetal evaluation. In Gabbe S, Niebyl J, Simpson J, editors: *Obstetrics: normal and problem pregnancies,* New York, 1986, Churchill Livingstone.

Gaffney S, Salinger L, Vintzileos A: The biophysical profile for fetal surveillance, *MCN* 15:356, 1990.

Golbus M, Appleman Z: Chorionic villus sampling. In Eden R, Boehm F, editors: *Assessment and care of the fetus: physiological, clinical and medicolegal principles,* Norwalk, CT, 1990, Appleton & Lange.

Haesslein H: Antepartum fetal assessment. Paper presented at UCSF antepartum and intrapartum management conference, San Francisco, June 1987.

Halle J: Diagnostic evaluation of pregnancy. In Mattson S, Smith J, editors: *Core curriculum for maternal newborn nursing,* Philadelphia, 1993, WB Saunders.

Jackson L: *CVS Newsletter,* No. 24, Feb. 14, 1988.

Kessel S et al: Racial differences in pregnancy outcomes, *Clin Perinatol* 14:745, 1988.

Ludomirski A, Weiner S: Percutaneous fetal umbilical blood sampling, *Clin Obstet Gynecol* 3(1):19, 1988.

Manning F: General principles and application of ultrasound. In Creasy R, Resnik R, editors: *Maternal-fetal medicine: principles and practices,* Philadelphia, 1989, WB Saunders.

Manning F, Harman C: The fetal biophysical profile. In Eden R, Boehm F, editors: *Assessment and care of the fetus: physiological, clinical and medicolegal principles,* Norwalk, CT, 1990, Appleton & Lange.

Manning F, Platt L, Supos L: Antepartum fetal evaluation: development of a fetal biophysical profile, *Am J Obstet Gynecol* 136:787, 1980.

Mattison D, Angtuaco T: Magnetic resonance imaging in prenatal diagnosis, *Clin Obstet Gynecol* 31(2):353, 1988.

McCallum W: Ultrasound applications in pregnancy, Midcoastal California Perinatal Outreach Program, Jan 1984.

Morrison I, Olsen J: Weight-specific stillbirth and associated causes of death: an analysis of 765 stillbirths, *Am J Obstet Gynecol* 152:975, 1985.

National Center for Health Statistics: Advance report of final mortality statistics, 1989, *Monthly Vital Statistics Report* 40(8S), 1992.

National Center for Health Statistics: Births, marriages, divorces, and deaths, 1993, *Monthly Vital Statistics Report,* 42:19, 1994.

Nicolaides K, Thorpe-Beeston J, Noble P: Cordocentesis. In Eden R, Boehm F, editors: *Assessment and care of the fetus: physiological, clinical and medicolegal principles,* Norwalk, CT, 1990, Appleton & Lange.

Quirk J, Bleasdale J: Fetal lung maturation in the pregnancy complicated by diabetes melitus. In DiRenzo G, Hawkins P, editors: *Perinatal medicine: updates and controversies,* New York, 1986, Cortina Learning International, Inc.

Rutherford S et al: The four-quadrant assessment of amniotic fluid volume: an adjunct to antepartum fetal heart rate testing. Part 1. *Obstet Gynecol,* 70(3):353, 1987.

Scott J et al: *Danforth's obstetrics and gynecology,* ed 6, Philadelphia, 1990, JB Lippincott.

Sonek J, Reiss R, Gabbe S: Antenatal fetal assessment. In Iams J, Zuspan F, Quilligan E, editors: *Zuspan and Quilligan's manual of obstetrics and gynecology,* St. Louis, 1990, Mosby.

Trudinger B: Doppler ultrasound assessment of blood flow. In Creasy R, Resnik R, editors: *Maternal fetal medicine: principles and practices,* ed 2, Philadelphia, 1989, WB Saunders.

Vintzileos A et al: The fetal biophysical profile in patients with premature rupture of the membranes: an early predictor of fetal infection, *Am J Obstet Gynecol* 152(5):510, 1985.

Bibliography

Affonso D, Mayberry L: Common stressors reported by a group of childbearing American women. *Health Care Women Internat* 11(3):331, 1990.

Chez B et al: Interpretations of nonstress tests by obstetric nurses, *JOGNN* 19(3), 227, 1990.

Copel J et al: The antenatal diagnosis of congenital heart disease using fetal echocardiography: is color flow mapping necessary? *Obstet Gynecol* 78(1):1, 1991.

Gilbert E, Harmon J: *High-risk pregnancy and delivery,* ed 2, St Louis, 1993, Mosby.

Heaman M: Psychosocial aspects of antepartum hospitalization, *NAACOG's Clinical Issues in Perinatal and Women's Health Nursing* 1(3):333, 1990.

Madel A et al: Absence of need for amniocentesis in patients with elevated levels of maternal serum alpha-fetoprotein and normal ultrasonographic examinations, *N Engl J Med* 323(9):557, 1990.

Maloni J et al: Physical and psychosocial side effects of antepartum bedrest, *Nurs Res* 42(4):28, 1993.

Mandeville LK, Troiano NM, editors: *High risk intrapartum nursing,* Philadelphia, 1992, JB Lippincott.

NAACOG: *Standards for the nursing care of women and newborns,* ed 4, Washington, DC, 1991, NAACOG.

21

Hypertension, Hemorrhage, and Maternal Infections

JUDITH H. POOLE

LEARNING OBJECTIVES

Define the key terms.

Describe the assessment techniques and formulate a nursing plan of care for the woman with preeclampsia.

Describe the HELLP syndrome and list appropriate nursing actions.

Compare abruptio placentae and placenta previa.

Discuss clotting disorders in pregnancy with emphasis on disseminated intravascular coagulation (DIC).

Identify postpartum hemorrhage causes, signs and symptoms, possible complications, and management.

Describe hemorrhagic shock including management and hazards of therapy.

Summarize assessment and care of women with HIV, STDs, and postpartum infections.

Review infection control protocols to minimize nosocomial infections to patients and occupational risk for infection to the health care provider.

KEY TERMS

abortion
abruptio placentae
bacteremic shock
cerclage
clonus (ankle)
deep tendon reflexes (DTRs)
disseminated intravascular coagulation (DIC)
eclampsia
ectopic pregnancy
HELLP syndrome
hemorrhagic shock
hydatidiform mole
incompetent cervix
placenta previa
preeclampsia
pregnancy-induced hypertension (PIH)
puerperal infection
sexually transmitted diseases (STDs)
trophoblastic disease
uterine atony

RELATED TOPICS

Adult respiratory distress syndrome (ARDS) *(Chap. 22)* · Blood pressure assessment *(Chap. 5)* · Fetal assessment tests *(Chap. 20)* · Fetal and uterine monitoring at home *(Chap. 24)* · Immunology *(Chap. 3)* · Infertility *(Chap. 30)* · Intrauterine growth retardation (IUGR) *(Chap. 27)* · Mean arterial pressure (MAP) *(Chap. 5)* · Therapeutic abortion *(Chap. 30)* · Tocolysis *(Chap. 24)* · TORCH infections in the neonate *(Chap. 27)*

Providing safe and effective care for the high-risk patient requires a joint effort from all members of the health care team, with each member contributing unique skills and talents to provide optimum outcomes for mother and infant. This chapter focuses on the three major maternal conditions that can affect the health of the woman, fetus, or newborn: hypertensive states, hemorrhage, and maternal infections.

HYPERTENSION IN PREGNANCY
Significance and Incidence

Hypertensive disorders of pregnancy greatly contribute to maternal and perinatal morbidity and mortality. It is estimated that hypertension complicates approximately 7% to 10% of all pregnancies. Of the women with hypertension during pregnancy, between one half and two thirds are diagnosed with preeclampsia or eclampsia (Brown, 1991). The prevalence is increased to as many as 20% to 40% of pregnancies in women with chronic renal disease or vascular disorders such as essential hypertension, diabetes mellitus, and lupus erythematosus (Scott et al, 1990; Fairlie, Sibai, 1993).

Morbidity and Mortality

Hypertension complicating pregnancy is a leading cause of maternal and infant morbidity and mortality. Preeclampsia-eclampsia may predispose the woman to potentially lethal complications such as abruptio placentae, disseminated intravascular coagulation (DIC), cerebral hemorrhage, cerebral vascular accident, hepatic failure, and acute renal failure (Consensus Report, 1990).

Preeclampsia contributes to intrauterine fetal death and perinatal mortality. The main causes of neonatal death from preeclampsia are placental insufficiency and abruptio placentae. Also, intrauterine growth retardation (IUGR) is common in infants of preeclamptic women (Roberts, 1990; Sibai, 1990a).

Eclampsia (seizures) from profound cerebral effects of preeclampsia-eclampsia is the major maternal hazard. As a rule maternal and perinatal morbidity and mortality are highest in cases where eclampsia presents early in gestation (before 28 weeks), maternal age is over 25 years, the woman is a multigravida, and chronic hypertension or renal disease is present. Outcomes are also more complicated in women who receive little or no prenatal care or who are transported from other health care facilities (Fairlie, Sibai, 1993). The fetus of the eclamptic woman is at increased risk from abruptio placentae, preterm birth, intrauterine growth retardation (IUGR), and acute hypoxia (Sibai et al, 1983).

Classification

The hypertensive disorders of pregnancy refer to a variety of conditions in which there is an elevation of maternal blood pressure with a corresponding risk to maternal and fetal well-being. Originally the hypertensive disorders of pregnancy were termed *toxemia;* however, this is inappropriate, in that no toxic agent or toxins have been identified. Confusion over classification continues today, causing difficulties in establishing a clinical diagnosis of the specific hypertensive disorder (ACOG, 1986; Sibai, Anderson, 1991). The following classification is the one most commonly used today (Consensus Report, 1990):

Preeclampsia-eclampsia
  Mild
  Severe
Chronic hypertension (precedes pregnancy)
Chronic hypertension with superimposed preeclampsia-eclampsia
Transient hypertension

Preeclampsia, eclampsia, and transient hypertension are gestational hypertensive disorders, often referred to as **pregnancy-induced hypertension (PIH)**. Chronic hypertensive states are related to preexisting conditions.

Preeclampsia

Preeclampsia is a pregnancy-specific condition in which hypertension develops after 20 weeks of gestation in a previously normotensive woman. **Preeclampsia** is a multisystem, vasospastic disease process characterized by hemoconcentration, hypertension, and proteinuria. The diagnosis of preeclampsia has traditionally been based on the presence of hypertension with proteinuria and/or edema. However, the most significant finding is hypertension in that 20% of eclamptic patients have no significant proteinuria before their first seizure (Willis, Blanco, 1990).

Hypertension is defined as an elevation of systolic and diastolic pressures equal to or exceeding 140/90 mm Hg. When first trimester blood pressures are known, they serve as the woman's baseline values. Using this information, an alternative definition for hypertension is a rise in systolic pressure of 30 mm Hg or a rise in diastolic pressure of 15 mm Hg above the woman's baseline values. This latter definition is useful because blood pressure varies with age, race, physiologic state, dietary habits, and heredity. The Committee on Terminology of the American College of Obstetricians and Gynecologists (ACOG) has also defined hypertension as an increase in mean arterial pressure (MAP) of 20 mm Hg; or if prior blood pressures are unknown, a MAP of 105 mm Hg is definitive for hypertension.

The blood pressure elevation must be present on at least two occasions 4 to 6 hours apart (Fairlie, Sibai, 1993). Techniques of measurement must be standardized.

Proteinuria is defined as a concentration of 0.1 g/L (> 2+ on the dipstick) or more in at least two random urine specimens collected at least 6 hours apart. In a 24-

hour specimen proteinuria is defined as a concentration of 0.3 g per 24 hours.

Edema is no longer necessary for the diagnosis of preeclampsia (Sibai, Rodriguez, 1992). If present, edema is a generalized accumulation of interstitial fluid after 12 hours of bed rest or a weight gain of more than 2 kg (4½ to 5 lb) per week. In the presence of hypertension and/or proteinuria edema should be evaluated as a reflection of end-organ edema and possible organ hypoxia.

Eclampsia

Eclampsia is the development of convulsions or coma in patients with signs and symptoms of preeclampsia. The convulsion or coma can be attributed to no preexisting neurologic disorder.

Chronic hypertension

Chronic hypertension is defined as hypertension present before the pregnancy or diagnosed before the twentieth week of gestation. Hypertension that persists longer than 6 weeks postpartum is also classified as chronic hypertension.

Chronic Hypertension with Superimposed Preeclampsia-Eclampsia

Women with chronic hypertension may develop preeclampsia or eclampsia. The development of preeclampsia or eclampsia in the woman with chronic hypertension increases maternal and perinatal morbidity and mortality. ACOG recommends that the diagnosis of superimposed preeclampsia be made on the basis of an increase of blood pressure together with the presence of proteinuria or generalized edema (Consensus Report, 1990).

Transient Hypertension

Transient hypertension is the development of hypertension during pregnancy or the first 24 hours postpartum without other signs of preeclampsia or preexisting hypertension. The presence of transient hypertension may be predictive of the eventual development of essential hypertension.

Etiology of Preeclampsia

Preeclampsia is a condition unique to human pregnancy; signs and symptoms develop only during pregnancy and disappear quickly after birth of the fetus and placenta. There is no one patient profile that identifies the woman who will develop preeclampsia. However, there are certain high-risk factors that are associated with developing the disease: primigravidity, grand multigravidity, large fetus, multifetal pregnancy, morbid obesity. Approximately 85% of preeclampsia is seen during the first pregnancy. It occurs in 14% to 20% of multifetal pregnancies and 30% of patients with major uterine anomalies. In women

with chronic hypertension or renal disease the incidence may be as high as 25% (Zuspan, 1991). Preeclampsia is a disease that progresses along a continuum from mild disease to severe preeclampsia, HELLP syndrome, or eclampsia.

Pathophysiology of Preeclampsia

The pathophysiology of preeclampsia-eclampsia is somehow related to the physiologic changes of pregnancy. Normal physiologic adaptations to pregnancy include an increase in blood plasma volume, vasodilatation, decreased systemic vascular resistance (SVR), elevated cardiac output (CO), and a decreased colloid osmotic pressure (COP) (Box 21-1). In preeclampsia there is a decrease in circulating plasma volume resulting in hemoconcentration and an increase in maternal hematocrit. These changes lead to a decrease in maternal organ perfusion, including the uteroplacental-fetal unit. Cyclic vasospasms further decrease organ perfusion by destroying red blood cells, thereby decreasing maternal oxygen-carrying capacity.

BOX 21-1

Normal Physiologic Adaptations to Pregnancy

CARDIOVASCULAR

↑ Blood volume; plasma volume expansion increases red cell mass expansion, leading to a physiologic anemia of pregnancy

↓ Total peripheral resistance; will see decreases in blood pressure readings

↑ Cardiac output; results from increased blood volume; slight increase in heart rate to compensate for peripheral relaxation

↑ Oxygen consumption

Physiologic edema related to ↓ plasma colloid osmotic pressure and ↑ venous capillary hydrostatic pressure

HEMATOLOGIC

↑ Clotting factors; predisposes to DIC and clotting

↓ Serum albumin results in decreases in colloid osmotic pressure; predisposes to pulmonary edema

RENAL

↑ Renal plasma flow and glomerular filtration rate

ENDOCRINE

↑ Estrogen production results in ↑ renin-angiotensin II–aldosterone secretion

↑ Progesterone production blocks aldosterone effect (slight ↓ Na)

↑ Vasodilator prostaglandins result in resistance to angiotensin II (slight ↓ BP)

In part *vasospasms* are the underlying mechanism for the signs and symptoms present with preeclampsia. Vasospasms result from an increased sensitivity to circulating pressors, such as angiotensin II, and possibly an imbalance between the prostaglandins prostacyclin and thromboxane A$_2$ (Consensus Report, 1990).

Investigators have tested the ability of aspirin (a prostaglandin inhibitor) to alter the pathophysiology of preeclampsia by interfering with the production of thromboxane (Schiff et al, 1989; Walsh, 1990). Investigation of the use of aspirin as a prophylactic treatment in the prevention of preeclampsia and its risk-benefit ratio for the mother and fetus/neonate is continuing. Other investigators are studying the use of calcium supplementation to prevent hypertension in pregnancy.

In addition to endothelial damage (Fig. 21-1), arterial vasospasm may contribute to an increased capillary permeability. This increases edema and further decreases intravascular volume, predisposing the patient with preeclampsia to pulmonary edema (Dildy et al, 1991).

Easterling and Benedetti (1989) propose that preeclampsia is a hyperdynamic condition in which the characteristic findings of hypertension and proteinuria result from renal hyperperfusion. To control the large volume of blood perfusing the kidney, renal vasospasm is initiated as a protective mechanism; but it eventually produces the proteinuria and hypertension characteristic of preeclampsia.

The relationship of the immune system to preeclampsia suggests that immunologic factors play an important role in the development of preeclampsia (Sibai, 1991a). The presence of foreign protein, the placenta, or the fetus may trigger an adverse immunologic response. This theory is supported by the increased incidence of preeclampsia-eclampsia in first-time mothers (first exposure to fetal tissue) and in women pregnant by a new partner (different genetic material) (Fig 21-2).

Genetic predisposition may be another immunologic factor (Chesley, 1984). Sibai (1991a) found a greater frequency of preeclampsia and eclampsia in daughters and granddaughters of women with a history of eclampsia, which suggests an autosomal recessive gene controlling the maternal immune response. Paternal factors also are being examined (Klonoff-Cohen et al, 1989).

Mild vs. Severe Preeclampsia

As preeclampsia worsens, regardless of etiology, a multiorgan system involvement is evidenced from the disease process. Renal involvement is demonstrated by changes in urinary output and serum chemistries. Renal blood flow and glomerular filtration are decreased resulting in oliguria, decreased urine creatinine clearance, and increases in blood urea nitrogen, serum creatinine, and serum uric acid (Dildy et al, 1991).

The pathophysiology of preeclampsia affects the central nervous system (CNS) by inducing cerebral edema and increased cerebral resistance (Dildy et al, 1991). Complications include headaches, seizures, and cerebral vascular accidents. As CNS involvement advances, the woman complains of headaches and visual disturbances (scotoma) or exhibits changes in mentation and level of consciousness. A life-threatening complication is the development of eclampsia, or the onset of seizures.

Impaired placental perfusion leads to early degenerative aging of the placenta and possible IUGR of the fetus. Decreased perfusion of the liver leads to impaired function. Hepatic edema and subcapsular hemorrhage, experienced by the woman as *epigastric* or *right upper quadrant pain,* is one sign of impending eclampsia. Liver enzyme levels rise in response to liver damage. Rupture of the liver is a rare but catastrophic complication (Cunningham et al, 1993).

Debate continues whether preeclampsia contributes to or is the result of disseminated intravascular coagulation (DIC) or whether DIC occurs with preeclampsia (Perry, Martin, 1992; Poole, 1993, Weiner, 1991). The most common coagulation abnormality seen in preeclampsia is platelet consumption resulting in thrombocytopenia (Sibai, 1990d).

The HELLP Syndrome

HELLP syndrome, a multisystem condition, is a form of severe preeclampsia-eclampsia in which the woman presents with a variety of complaints and exhibits common laboratory markers for a syndrome of hemolysis *(H)* of red blood cells, elevated liver enzymes *(EL),* and low platelets *LP).* The complaints range from malaise, epigastric pain, nausea and vomiting, to nonspecific viral syndrome–like symptoms. On presentation these women are generally in the second or early third trimester and initially may show few signs of preeclampsia. These women often receive a nonobstetric diagnosis that delays treatment and increases maternal and perinatal morbidity and mortality (Martin et al, 1991a).

HELLP syndrome affects approximately 2% to 12% of the severe preeclamptic population, with a mortality rate of 2% to 24% (Sibai et al, 1986). The incidence is high-

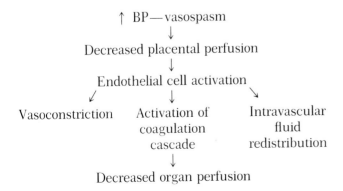

FIG. 21-1 Endothelial cell dysfunction and preeclampsia.

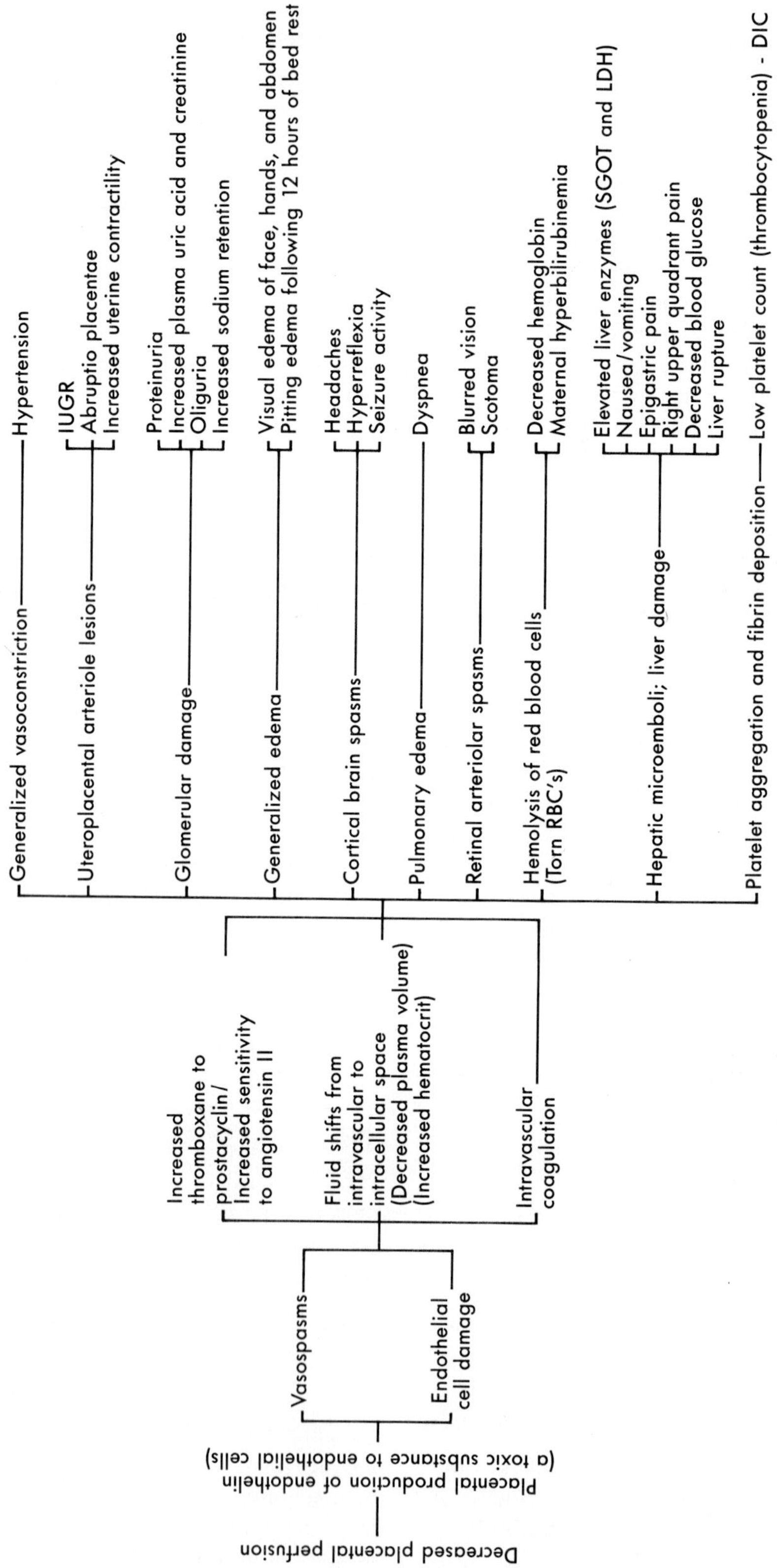

Decreased placental perfusion

Placental production of endothelin (a toxic substance to endothelial cells)

Vasospasms

Endothelial cell damage

Increased thromboxane to prostacyclin/ Increased sensitivity to angiotensin II

Fluid shifts from intravascular to intracellular space (Decreased plasma volume) (Increased hematocrit)

Intravascular coagulation

Generalized vasoconstriction —— Hypertension

Uteroplacental arteriole lesions —— IUGR
                                      Abruptio placentae
                                      Increased uterine contractility

Glomerular damage —— Proteinuria
                        Increased plasma uric acid and creatinine
                        Oliguria
                        Increased sodium retention

Generalized edema —— Visual edema of face, hands, and abdomen
                        Pitting edema following 12 hours of bed rest

Cortical brain spasms —— Headaches
                            Hyperreflexia
                            Seizure activity

Pulmonary edema —— Dyspnea

Retinal arteriolar spasms —— Blurred vision
                                Scotoma

Hemolysis of red blood cells (Torn RBC's) —— Decreased hemoglobin
                                                Maternal hyperbilirubinemia

Hepatic microemboli; liver damage —— Elevated liver enzymes (SGOT and LDH)
                                        Nausea/vomiting
                                        Epigastric pain
                                        Right upper quadrant pain
                                        Decreased blood glucose
                                        Liver rupture

Platelet aggregation and fibrin deposition —— Low platelet count (thrombocytopenia) - DIC

FIG. 21-2 Pathophysiology of preeclampsia-eclampsia.

TABLE 21-1   Common Laboratory Changes in Preeclampsia

	NORMAL	PIH	HELLP
Hemoglobin/hematocrit	12 to 16/37 to 47	May ↑	↓
Platelets	Unchanged	Unchanged	$<100,000$ mm^3
PT/PTT	Unchanged	Unchanged	Unchanged
Fibrinogen	150 to 400	300 to 600	↓
Fibrin split products (FSP)	Absent	Absent	Present
Blood urea nitrogen (BUN)	9 to 20	<10	↑
Creatinine	0.5 to 1.3	<1.0	↑
Lactate dehydrogenase (LDH)	84 to 220	Unchanged	↑
Aspartate aminotransferase (AST) (formerly SGOT)	4 to 20	Unchanged	↑
Alanine aminotransferase (ALT) (formerly SGPT)	3 to 21	Unchanged	↑
24° Protein	0 to 100	0 to 300	↑
Creatinine clearance	97 to 137	130 to 180	↓
Burr cells/schistocytes	Absent	Absent	Present

est among older, white, and multiparous women.

Although the exact mechanism is unknown, HELLP syndrome is thought to occur secondary to changes occurring with preeclampsia (see Fig. 21-2). Arterial vasospasm, endothelial damage, and platelet aggregation with resultant tissue hypoxia are the underlying mechanisms for the pathophysiology of HELLP syndrome (Poole, 1988, 1993).

The coagulopathy seen in HELLP syndrome is similar to that in DIC, except that coagulation factor assays, prothrombin time (PT), partial thromboplastin time (PTT), and bleeding time usually remain normal (Guyton, 1992; Leduc et al, 1992; Perry, 1992) (Table 21-1). In evaluating the degree of coagulopathy present in HELLP syndrome, it must be kept in mind that thrombocytopenia is a common finding (Perry, 1992).

CARE MANAGEMENT

✦ ASSESSMENT

Hypertensive disorders of pregnancy can occur without warning or with the gradual development of symptoms. A key goal is early identification of pregnant women at risk for the development of preeclampsia (Box 21-2). Therefore each woman is assessed for etiologic factors during the first prenatal visit. During each subsequent visit the woman is assessed for symptoms that suggest the onset or presence of preeclampsia.

Factors such as parity, age, and geographic location need to be taken into consideration. First-time mothers, or women with a new partner, have been found to be six to eight times more susceptible than multiparous women are to the development of preeclampsia (Consensus Report, 1990). Daughters and sisters of preeclamptic women have a higher tendency to develop preeclampsia than do unrelated women (O'Brien, 1992). Women younger than 18 or older than 35 years of age,

BOX 21-2

Risk Factors for Preeclampsia-Eclampsia

Primigravida or older multipara
Age: <18 or >35
Weight: <100 pounds or obesity
Presence of chronic disease process: diabetes mellitus, hypertension, renal disease, vascular disease, collagen vascular disease (systemic lupus erythematosus)
Hydatidiform mole
Pregnancy complications: multiple gestation, large fetus, fetal hydrops, polyhydramnios
Preeclampsia in previous pregnancy
New genetic material

unmarried, and residing in the southern and western regions of the United States have a significantly higher incidence of preeclampsia. Race alone was not found to be a significant factor for either preeclampsia or eclampsia (Saftlas et al, 1990).

Obstetric conditions associated with increased placental mass such as multifetal gestation and hydatidiform moles, as well as chronic medical disorders such as hypertension, collagen vascular disease, renal disease, and diabetes mellitus, lead to a greater risk for preeclampsia (Roberts, 1990).

Interview

The nurse reviews the woman's admission form and prenatal record. When the nurse and pregnant woman are comfortable, the nurse begins with the interview to clarify, expand, or complete the form. Medical history is reviewed, especially the presence of diabetes mellitus, renal disease, and hypertension. Family history is explored for occurrence of preeclamptic or hypertensive conditions, diabetes mellitus, and other chronic conditions.

The social and experiential history provides information about the woman's marital status, nutritional status, cultural beliefs, activity level, and health habits such as smoking, drug use, and alcohol consumption.

A review of systems adds to the data base for detecting blood pressure changes from baseline, abnormal weight gain and pattern of weight gain, increased signs of edema, and presence of proteinuria. It is also important to note whether the woman is having unusual, frequent, or severe headaches, visual disturbances, or epigastric pain.

Physical Examination

Lack of specific reliable diagnostic tests currently hinder early detection and treatment of preeclampsia. Women with a MAP greater than 85 mm Hg during the second trimester are at greater risk for developing hypertension during the third trimester (O'Brien, 1992).

Accurate and consistent *blood pressure assessment* is important for establishing a baseline and monitoring subtle changes throughout the pregnancy. Many variables can influence blood pressure measurements, such as position, cuff size, arm used, and emotional state. Personnel caring for pregnant women need to be consistent in taking and recording blood pressure measurements in a standardized manner (Box 21-3). If electronic blood pressure devices are used, there should be a manual reading to validate the electronic device reading. Electronic blood pressure devices show a widening of the pulse pressure compared to manual readings; however, the MAP is unchanged (Marx et al, 1993).

Observation of *edema* plus hypertension warrants additional investigation. Edema is assessed by distribution, degree, and pitting. If periorbital or facial edema is not obvious, the pregnant woman is asked if it was present when she awoke. Edema may be described as dependent or pitting.

Dependent edema is edema of the lower or most dependent parts of the body, where hydrostatic pressure is greatest. If a person is ambulatory, this edema may first be evident in the feet and ankles. If the person is confined to bed, the edema is more likely to occur in the sacral region.

Pitting edema leaves a small depression or pit after finger pressure is applied to the swollen area. The pit is caused by movement of fluid to adjacent tissue, away from the point of pressure. Within 10 to 30 seconds the pit normally disappears. Although the amount of edema is difficult to quantitate, the method described in Fig. 21-3 may be used to record relative degrees of edema formation.

Symptoms reflecting CNS and visual system involvement usually accompany facial edema. Although it is not a routine assessment during the prenatal period, evaluation of the fundus of the eye yields valuable data. An initial baseline finding of normal eyegrounds assists in differentiating preexisting from new disease processes. The woman may be unable to relate other symptoms such as epigastric pain or oliguria.

Deep tendon reflexes (DTRs) are evaluated if preeclampsia is suspected. The biceps and patellar reflexes and ankle clonus are assessed and the findings recorded (Fig. 21-4; Table 21-2). *The evaluation of DTRs is especially important if the woman is being treated with magnesium*

BOX 21-3

Blood Pressure Measurement Protocol

1. Attempt to have woman relaxed before taking blood pressure; then measure the blood pressure with the woman in a sitting position and use the same arm for each measurement.
2. Have the arm resting on a table at heart level.
3. Use the proper cuff size.
4. Assess for approximate systolic blood pressure level using the palpation method before taking measurement.
5. Maintain a slow, steady deflation rate.
6. Take the average of two readings, at least 6 hours apart, to minimize recorded blood pressure variations across time.
7. Use accurate equipment.

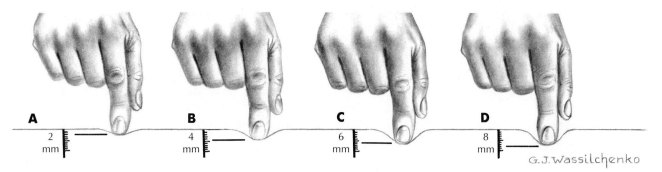

FIG. 21-3 Assessment of pitting edema. **A,** 1+; **B,** 2+; **C,** 3+; **D,** 4+.

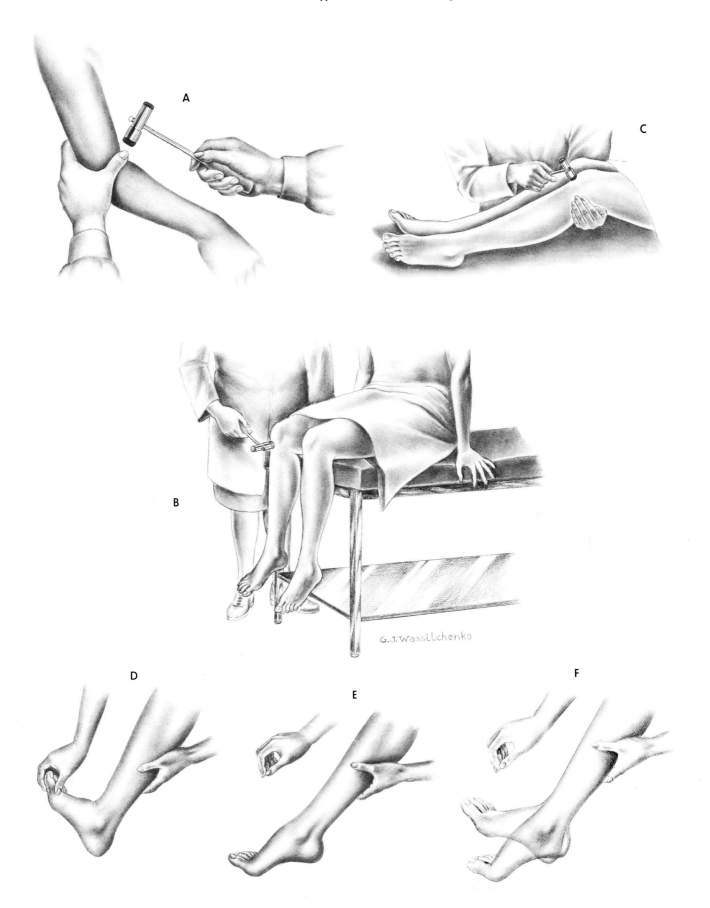

FIG. 21-4   Deep tendon reflexes. **A,** Biceps reflex. **B,** Patellar reflex with woman's legs hanging freely over end of examining table. **C,** With woman in supine position. **D,** Hyperactive reflexes (clonus) at ankle joint. **E,** Normal (negative clonus) response. **F,** Abnormal (positive clonus) response.

TABLE 21-2 Assessing Deep Tendon Reflexes	
DEGREE	**GRADING**
Brisk with sustained clonus	5+
Hyperactive response (brisk with transient clonus)	4+
More than normal (brisk)	3+
Normal, active	2+
Low response (sluggish or dull)	1+
No response	0

sulfate; absence of DTRs is an early indication of impending magnesium toxicity. The *patellar reflex* is elicited with the woman's legs hanging freely over the end of the examination table, or with the woman lying on her side with the knee slightly flexed, or both legs supported by the examiner. A blow with a percussion hammer is dealt directly to the patellar tendon, inferior to the patella. *Normal response is the extension or kicking out of the leg.* To assess for hyperactive reflexes (**clonus**) at the ankle joint, the leg should be supported with the knee flexed. With one hand the foot is sharply dorsiflexed and the position maintained for a moment. The foot is then released. *Normal (negative clonus)* response is elicited when no rhythmic oscillations (jerking) are felt while the foot is held in dorsiflexion. When the foot is released, no oscillations are seen as the foot drops to the plantar flexed position. *Abnormal (positive clonus)* response is recognized by rhythmic oscillations of one or more beats felt when the foot is in dorsiflexion and seen as the foot drops to the plantar flexed position.

An important assessment is determination of fetal status. Uteroplacental perfusion is decreased in women with preeclampsia, thereby placing the fetus in jeopardy. The fetal heart rate (FHR) should be assessed for baseline rate, variability, periodic changes, and nonperiodic changes. Abnormal baseline rate, decreased or absent variability, or late decelerations are indications of fetal intolerance to its intrauterine environment. Biophysical or biochemical monitoring for fetal well-being may be ordered: fetal movement counts, nonstress testing (NST), contraction stress testing (CST), biophysical profile (BPP), and serial ultrasonography.

Considered experimental, Doppler flow velocimetry studies are now being used for evaluating maternal-fetal well-being (see p. 541). A systolic/diastolic ratio over 3 after 26 weeks is considered abnormal, and ratios of 3.8 have been associated with preeclampsia (Fairlie, 1991, Farmakides et al, 1992).

Uterine tonicity is evaluated for signs of labor and abruptio placentae. If labor is suspected, a vaginal examination for cervical changes is indicated.

During the physical examination the pregnant woman is examined for signs of deterioration of mild preeclampsia to severe preeclampsia or eclampsia. Signs of worsening liver involvement, renal failure, worsening hypertension, cerebral involvement, and developing coagulopathies must be assessed and documented. Respirations are assessed for rales (crackles) or diminished breath sounds, which may indicate pulmonary edema. Warning signs of preeclampsia and the differentiation of mild from severe preeclampsia are summarized in Table 21-3. Noninvasive assessment parameters include level of consciousness, blood pressure, hemoglobin oxygen saturation (pulse oximetry), electrocardiographic (ECG) findings, and urine output. Invasive hemodynamic monitoring may be indicated in selected patients (ACOG, 1992).

Laboratory Tests

The nurse assists in obtaining a number of blood and urine specimens to aid in the diagnosis of preeclampsia, HELLP syndrome, or chronic hypertension. At present no known laboratory tests are available to detect the development of preeclampsia. However, baseline laboratory test information is useful in the early diagnosis of preeclampsia and for comparison with results obtained to evaluate progression and severity of disease. An initial blood specimen is obtained for the following tests to assess the disease process and its effect on renal and hepatic functioning:

- Complete blood cell count (including a platelet count)
- Clotting studies (including bleeding time, PT, PTT, and fibrinogen)
- Liver enzymes (lactate dehydrogenase [LDH], aspartate aminotransferase [AST] [SGOT], alanine aminotransferase [ALT] [SGPT])
- Chemistry panel (blood urea nitrogen [BUN], creatinine, glucose, uric acid)
- Type and screen, possible crossmatch

The hematocrit, hemoglobin, and platelets are monitored closely for changes indicating a worsening of patient status. Since hepatic involvement is a possible complication, serum glucose levels are monitored if liver function tests indicate elevated liver enzymes (Egley et al, 1985). Once platelets drop below 100,000, the patient warrants coagulation profiles to identify developing DIC (Leduc et al, 1992).

Proteinuria is determined from dipstick testing of a clean-catch or catheter urine specimen. A reading greater than +1 on two or more occasions, at least 4 hours apart, should be followed by a 24-hour urine collection (Gilbert, Harmon, 1993). A 24-hour collection for protein and creatinine clearance are more reflective of true renal status. Proteinuria usually is a late sign in the course of preeclampsia (Consensus Report, 1990). Protein readings are designated as follows:

TABLE 21-3 Differentiation of Mild and Severe Preeclampsia

	MILD PREECLAMPSIA	SEVERE PREECLAMPSIA
MATERNAL EFFECTS		
Blood pressure	Rise in systolic blood pressure of 30 mm Hg or more; a rise in diastolic blood pressure of ≥15 mm Hg or a reading of 140/90 mm Hg × 2, 6 hr apart	Rise to ≥160/110 mm Hg on two separate occasions 6 hr apart with pregnant woman on bed rest
MAP	140/90 = 107	160/110 = 127
Weight gain	Weight gain of more than 0.5 kg (1 lb)/wk during the second and third trimesters, or a sudden weight gain of 2 kg (4 to 4½ lb)/wk at any time	Same as mild preeclampsia
Proteinuria Qualitative dipstick Quantitative 24-hr analysis	Proteinuria of 300 mg/L in a 24-hr specimen or >1 g/L in a random daytime specimen on two or more occasions 6 hr apart because protein loss is variable; with dipstick, values vary from trace to 1+	Proteinuria of 5-10 g/L in 24 hr or ≥2+ protein on dipstick
Edema	Dependent edema, some puffiness of eyes, face, fingers; pulmonary rales absent	Generalized edema, noticeable puffiness of eyes, face, fingers; pulmonary rales may be present
Reflexes	Hyperreflexia 3+; no ankle clonus	Hyperreflexia 3+ or more; ankle clonus
Urine output	Output matches intake; ≥30 ml/hr	Oliguria: <30 ml/hr or 120 ml/4 hr output
Headache	Transient	Severe
Visual problems	Absent	Blurred, photophobia, blind spots on funduscopy
Irritability/affect	Transient	Severe
Epigastric pain	Absent	Present
Serum creatinine	Normal	Elevated
Thrombocytopenia	Absent	Present
AST elevation	Minimal	Marked
Hematocrit	Increased	Increased
FETAL EFFECTS		
Placental perfusion	Reduced	Decreased perfusion expressed as IUGR in fetus; FHR: late decelerations
Premature placental aging	Not apparent	At birth placenta appears smaller than normal for duration of pregnancy; premature aging is apparent with numerous areas of broken syncytia; ischemic necroses (white infarcts) are numerous, and intervillous fibrin deposition (red infarcts) may be recorded

0

Trace

+1 30 mg/dl (equivalent to 300 mg/L)

+2 100 mg/dl

+3 300 mg/dl

+4 Over 1000 mg (1 g)/dl

Urine output is assessed for volume of at least 30 ml per hour or 120 ml in 4 hours.

✤ NURSING DIAGNOSES

Nursing diagnoses are derived by carefully analyzing the assessment findings. Common nursing diagnoses for patients with hypertensive disorders in pregnancy include the following:

Anxiety related to
- Preeclampsia and its effect on mother and infant

Knowledge deficit regarding
- Management (diet, bed rest)

Ineffective individual/family coping related to
- The mother's restricted activity and concern over a complicated pregnancy or the mother's inability to work outside the home

Powerlessness related to
- Inability to prevent control condition outcomes

Alteration in tissue/organ perfusion, decreased, related to
- Hypertension
- Cyclic vasospasms
- Cerebral edema
- Hemorrhage

High risk for pulmonary edema related to
- Decreased colloid osmotic pressure
- Increased systemic vascular resistance
- Pulmonary vascular endothelial damage

High risk for impaired gas exchange related to
- Magnesium sulfate therapy
- Pulmonary edema

High risk for alteration in cardiac output, decreased, related to
- Excessive antihypertensive therapy
- Cardiac involvement of the disease process

High risk for infection related to
- Hospital environment and compromised host

High risk for abruptio placentae related to
- Systemic vasospasms
- Hypertension
- Decreased uteroplacental perfusion

High risk for injury to fetus related to
- Uteroplacental insufficiency
- Preterm birth
- Abruptio placentae

High risk for injury to mother related to
- CNS irritability secondary to cerebral edema, vasospasm, decreased renal perfusion
- Magnesium sulfate and antihypertensive therapies

✤ EXPECTED OUTCOMES

Planning care follows medical diagnosis, choice of home or hospital management, and the woman's and family's resources. A plan is developed mutually with the woman, if possible, and should be individualized and related specifically to the needs of the patient and her family. Expected outcomes for care of patients with hypertensive disorders of pregnancy include the following:

1. The woman will recognize and immediately report abnormal signs and symptoms to prevent worsening of condition.
2. The woman will adhere to the medical regimen to minimize risk to herself and her fetus.
3. Significant other(s) will become involved and supportive in the woman's care and management of the disease to optimize emotional and physical outcomes.
4. The woman will verbalize her fears and concerns to cope with the condition and situation.
5. The woman and fetus will not suffer adverse sequelae from preeclampsia or its management.
6. The woman will not experience eclampsia and the severity of its complications.
7. The fetus will not experience distress; the newborn will be born in optimal condition with no adverse sequelae to the maternal condition and its management.
8. The woman will give birth in optimal condition with no sequelae to her condition and its management.
9. The family will be able to cope effectively with the mother's high-risk condition, its management, and outcomes.

✤ COLLABORATIVE CARE

Preeclampsia

Nursing actions are derived from medical management, health care provider directives, and nursing diagnoses.

The most effective therapy is *prevention*. Early prenatal care, identification of the at-risk woman during pregnancy, and recognition and reporting of physical warning signs are essential components for optimizing maternal and perinatal outcomes. The nurse's skills in assessing the woman for factors and symptoms of preeclampsia cannot be overestimated.

Nurses can do much in the advocacy role. Measurements should be taken to improve public education and access to antenatal care. Counseling, referral to community resources, mobilization of support systems, nutrition counseling, and information about normal adaptation to pregnancy are essential preventive components of care. The nurse's role as educator is important in informing the woman about her condition and responsibilities in preeclampsia management, whether in the home or hospital.

Emotional and psychologic support is essential to help the woman and her family cope. Their perception of the disease process, the reasons for it, and the care received will affect their compliance with and participation in therapy. The family will need to use coping mechanisms and support systems to help them through this crisis. A plan of care for the woman suffering from preeclampsia is superimposed on the nursing care all women need during labor and the birth process.

Home Care

Interventions for preeclampsia such as bed rest and diet are considered palliative (Consensus Report, 1990). The most effective therapy for preeclampsia is preventing progression of the condition and enabling the pregnancy to continue (see Home Care box on p. 566).

LEGAL TIP: **Standard of Care for the Preeclamptic Patient at Home**
Home care of the preeclamptic patient requires the same level of nursing expertise as the intrapartum setting. The standard of care for the preeclamptic patient at home is that the nurse should be prepared to assess the condition, provide care, identify deviations from normal, intervene accordingly, and refer when appropriate.

Management at home can be satisfactory if preeclampsia is mild and fetal growth retardation is not a problem. For home care to be effective, the nurse needs to assess the home environment and the woman's ability to assume responsibility. In addition, the effects of illness, language, age, culture, beliefs, and support system need to be considered. The woman's support systems need to be mobilized and involved in planning and implementing her care. A knowledge of the subjective symptoms and objective signs that indicate deterioration of the condition is vital. If these symptoms occur, the woman must call her health care provider immediately (see the Home Care box above at right).

Bed rest in the lateral recumbent position is a standard therapy for preeclampsia and maximizes uteroplacental blood flow. It has been shown to be beneficial in decreasing blood pressure and promoting diuresis. Since women with mild preeclampsia feel reasonably well, boredom from being restricted is common. Diversionary activities provide a means of coping with the restricted lifestyle changes (see the Home Care box at right).

Learning relaxation can help to reduce stresses associated with the high-risk condition and to prepare the woman for labor and the birth. Progressive relaxation studies also have shown relaxation effective in lowering blood pressures of persons with chronic hypertension as well.

The woman is instructed in how to take her own

HOME CARE

ASSESSING AND REPORTING CLINICAL SIGNS OF PREECLAMPSIA

- Report immediately any increase in your blood pressure, protein in urine, weight gain greater than 1 pound/week, or edema.
- Take your blood pressure on the same arm in a sitting position each time for consistent and accurate readings. Support arm on a table in a horizontal position at heart level.
- Use the same scale, wearing the same clothes, at the same time each day, after voiding, before breakfast, for reliable daily weights.
- Dipstick your clean-catch urine sample for assessing proteinuria; report frequency or burning on voiding.
- Report to your health care provider if proteinuria is +2 or more or if you have a decrease in urine output.
- Daily assess your baby's activity. Decreased activity (three or fewer movements per hour) may indicate fetal distress.
- It is important to keep your scheduled prenatal appointments so that any changes in your or the baby's condition can be detected immediately.
- Keep a daily log/diary of your assessments for your home health care nurse, or bring it with you to your next prenatal visit.

HOME CARE

COPING WITH BED REST

- In bed, lie on your left side (and alternate to right side as needed). This allows more blood to get to your uterus (womb) and baby.
- Increase your fluid intake to 8 glasses/day, and add roughage (e.g., bran, fruits, leafy vegetables) to your diet to decrease constipation.
- Include diversional activities such as puzzles, reading, and crafts to reduce boredom.
- Do gentle exercises such as circling your hands and feet or gently tensing and relaxing arm and leg muscles. This improves muscle tone, circulation, and sense of well-being.
- Encourage family participation in your care.
- Have significant others assist you with care of the house, children, etc.
- Use relaxation to help you cope with stress. Relax your body one muscle at a time or imagine some pleasant scene, word, or image. Soothing music can also help you to relax.

HOME CARE

LEARNING ABOUT PREECLAMPSIA CONDITION

- The cause of pregnancy-induced hypertension is not known; symptoms are believed to occur from changes in body organ functioning.
- Decreased perfusion to organs can result in symptoms of preeclampsia.
- An increase in blood pressure, edema, weight, and proteinuria indicates disease process is worsening.
- Decreased fetal movement may indicate fetal hypoxia.

BOX 21-4

Nutrition

- There is no sodium restriction; however, avoid salty foods (e.g., canned foods, sodas, pretzels, potato chips, pickles, sauerkraut).
- Eat a nutritious, balanced diet. Collaborate with registered dietitian for diet best suited for individual woman (for discussion of nutrition, see Chapter 8).
- Avoid alcohol, smoking.
- Drink 8 to 10 8-ounce glasses of water per day.
- Eat foods with roughage, e.g., whole grains, raw fruits, and vegetables.

blood pressure and keep a record of the measurements. Women should have formal instruction in using correct, standardized techniques for obtaining accurate blood pressure measurements. Electronic devices have been found to be as accurate as mechanical aneroid units for hypertensive pregnant women. They are easy to apply and read without need for a stethoscope or another person (Smith et al, 1990). This is particularly advantageous for women having their blood pressure monitored on an outpatient basis.

The woman is taught to weigh daily and check for proteinuria. The initial appearance of proteinuria usually indicates progressive severity of preeclampsia. An increase in weight is associated with edema formation.

Because the disease has potential adverse effects on uterine blood flow, the fetus must be regularly evaluated for hypoxia. The woman is instructed about the importance of keeping appointments for fetal monitoring tests. Explanation of the purpose of the tests and what the woman may experience during the procedures is also necessary. For home management the woman may be instructed in how to do daily fetal movement counts (see Chapter 20).

Diet and fluid recommendations are much the same as for typical pregnant women. Diets high in protein and low in salt have been suggested to prevent preeclampsia; however, the efficacy of this has not been proven (Fairlie and Sibai, 1993). Pregnant women with hypertension have less plasma volume; thus sodium restriction is not recommended. Salt is needed for maintenance of blood volume and placental perfusion. Adequate fluid intake helps to maintain optimal fluid volume and aids in renal perfusion and filtration. The nurse uses assessment data about the woman's diet and counsels her in areas of deficiency, if needed (Box 21-4 and Plan of Care on p. 571).

Severe Preeclampsia/HELLP Syndrome

The woman diagnosed with severe preeclampsia/HELLP syndrome is critically ill and warrants appropri-

ate management, usually in a tertiary care center. Management protocols are controversial among the medical authorities; recommendations range from immediate birth to conservative management of the pregnancy (Dildy et al, 1991; Harvey, Burke, 1992; Sibai, 1991b). Recognition of the clinical and laboratory findings of severe preeclampsia/HELLP syndrome is important if early, aggressive therapy is to be initiated to prevent maternal and perinatal mortality. An unfavorable (uneffaced and undilated) cervix due to the gestational age and the aggressive nature of this disorder support cesarean birth. Prolonged induction of labor could increase maternal morbidity.

Regardless of the treatment modality initiated, birth is the only definitive treatment for severe preeclampsia and the HELLP syndrome. Important components of management include the administration of magnesium sulfate ($MgSO_4$) as a seizure prophylaxis and the administration of an antihypertensive agent if diastolic blood pressure is higher than 110 mm Hg. Hypoglycemia may be present in the woman with the HELLP syndrome; blood sugar less than 40 mg/dl is associated with an increased maternal mortality (Egley et al, 1985).

Hospital Care

The woman with severe preeclampsia/HELLP syndrome has multiple problems and is a tremendous challenge for the health care team. Nurses caring for this woman need a strong knowledge of the disease process, treatment regimen, and possible complications to the mother and fetus (see Table 21-3). Nursing care must focus on both the mother and fetus.

Severe preeclampsia is diagnosed when one of the following is present (Fairlie, Sibai, 1993):

1. Blood pressure ≥ 160 mm Hg systolic or ≥ 110 mm Hg diastolic on two occasions at least 6 hours apart with the woman on bed rest
2. Proteinuria ≥ 5 g in a 24-hour urine collection or ≥3+ on dipstick in at least two random clean-catch samples at least 4 hours apart

3. Oliguria ≤ 400 ml in 24 hours
4. Cerebral or visual disturbances
5. Epigastric pain
6. Pulmonary edema or cyanosis
7. HELLP syndrome

Antepartum care focuses on stabilization and preparation for birth. Maternal and fetal surveillance, patient education regarding the disease process, and supportive measures directed toward the patient and her family are initiated. Assessments include a review of the cardiovascular, pulmonary, renal, hematologic, and central nervous systems. Fetal assessments for well-being (e.g., NST, biophysical profile, Doppler velocimetry) are important due to the potential for hypoxia related to uteroplacental insufficiency. Baseline laboratory assessments include metabolic package for liver enzyme determination, complete blood count with platelets, coagulation profile to assess for DIC, and electrolyte package to establish renal functioning (Farmarkides et al, 1990).

The extensiveness of health assessment on admission is governed by the severity of the woman's condition. Weight is taken on admittance and every day thereafter. An indwelling urinary catheter facilitates monitoring of renal function and effectiveness of therapy. If appropriate, vaginal examination reveals the status of the cervix. Abdominal palpation establishes uterine tonicity and fetal size, activity, and position. Electronic fetal monitoring is initiated to determine fetal status. The nurse's skill in implementing the techniques described can be reassuring to the woman and her family. The patient's room must be close to staff and emergency drugs, supplies, and equipment. Noise and external stimuli must be minimized. *Seizure precautions* are taken (Box 21-5).

Commonly, bed rest is ordered. The nurse's ingenuity may be called on to help the woman cope physically and psychologically with the side effects of immobility and an environment limited in stimuli and support. Thromboembolic events, which are a risk factor during normal pregnancy, pose an even greater risk with preeclampsia.

Intrapartum nursing care of the woman with severe preeclampsia or the HELLP syndrome involves maternal and fetal assessments as labor progresses. The assessment and prevention of tissue hypoxia and hemorrhage, both of which can lead to permanent compromise of vital organs, continue throughout the intrapartum and postpartum periods (Harvey, Burke, 1992).

Magnesium Sulfate

One of the important goals of care for the woman with severe preeclampsia/HELLP syndrome is preventing or controlling convulsions. An infusion of magnesium sulfate is started to decrease the incidence of seizures. This is the drug of choice in the treatment of preeclampsia-eclampsia; however, seizures may develop during magnesium sulfate therapy if the dosage is not correctly titrated according to the individual patient's clinical re-

---

BOX 21-5

Hospital Precautionary Measures

Environment
  Quiet
  Nonstimulating
  Lighting subdued
Seizure precautions
  Padded side rails
  Suction equipment tested and ready to use
  Oxygen administration equipment tested and
    ready to use
Call button within easy reach
Emergency medication tray immediately accessible
  Hydralazine and magnesium sulfate in or adjacent
    to woman's room
  Calcium gluconate immediately available in a
    well-labeled syringe
Emergency birth pack accessible

---

sponse (Sibai, 1990b, c; 1991b). Benefits of magnesium sulfate therapy include an increase in uterine blood flow to protect the fetus and an increase in prostacyclin to prevent uterine vasoconstriction (Iams, Zuspan, Quilligan, 1990).

Magnesium sulfate is administered as a secondary infusion by volumetric infusion pump. An initial or loading dose of 4 to 6 g is given over 15 to 30 minutes, followed by a maintenance infusion of 2 to 4 g per hour. A therapeutic serum level between 4.8 and 9.6 mg/dl is maintained by a constant infusion (Fairlie, Sibai, 1993). Following the loading dose, there may be a transient lowering of the arterial blood pressure secondary to relaxation of smooth muscle. However, within an hour of initiating therapy arterial blood pressures will return to pretherapy levels; *magnesium sulfate is not a hypotensive drug. It is an anticonvulsant drug.*

Intramuscular (IM) magnesium sulfate rarely is used because the drug absorption rate cannot be controlled, injections are painful, and tissue necrosis can occur. The IM dose is 4 to 5 g given in each buttock by deep Z-track method (1% procaine may be ordered added to the solution to reduce injection pain) and can be followed at 4-hour intervals with IM doses of 4 to 5 g. When magnesium sulfate is given IM, levels are adequate during the first 1 to 2 hours of administration but inadequate for the next 3 to 4 hours (Sibai, 1988).

Magnesium sulfate interferes with the release of acetylcholine at the synapses, decreasing neuromuscular irritability, depressing cardiac conduction, and decreasing CNS irritability (Dildy et al, 1991). Since magnesium circulates free and unbound to protein and is excreted in the urine, accurate recordings of maternal urine output must be obtained. Because magnesium sulfate is a CNS depressant, the nurse assesses for signs and symptoms of magnesium toxicity, including loss of knee-jerk reflexes, respiratory depression, oliguria, respiratory arrest, and cardiac arrest (see the Emergency box below). The woman's blood pressure, pulse, and respiratory status are monitored every 15 minutes. Administration of magnesium sulfate is continued for at least the first 12 to 24 hours postpartum to prevent the occurrence of seizures.

Strict monitoring of intravenous fluid, oral intake, and urinary output is important to avoid fluid overload. Magnesium sulfate increases sodium retention and is excreted by the kidneys. Magnesium toxicity can develop very quickly and easily in women with renal involvement. Hourly urinary output must be measured when magnesium sulfate is administered. The most accurate measure of urinary output is with a retention catheter. *The woman's urinary output must total at least 120 ml every 4 hours. Also be aware of serum creatinine levels: as serum levels approach 1 mg/dl, the kidney does not excrete magnesium.* If output is less than 30 ml per hour, or less than 120 ml every 4 hours or if serum creatinine levels are elevated, the health care provider is notified. In the presence of oliguria or renal involvement the infusion of magnesium sulfate may be reduced or discontinued.

Diuresis within 24 to 48 hours is an excellent prognostic sign. It is considered evidence that perfusion of the kidney has improved as a result of relaxation of arteriolar spasm. With improved perfusion, fluid moves from the interstitial spaces to the intravascular bed, and edema is reduced. Diuresis results in weight loss. In the presence of a large urinary output (>200 ml/hr), the dosage of magnesium sulfate may need to be increased.

Uterine activity and sensitivity to oxytocin are in-

creased. *Therefore increased sensitivity to the effects of oxytocin must be taken into account when the drug is used for induction or augmentation of labor.*

Serum levels are obtained 4 to 6 hours after the initial loading dose. Additional serum magnesium levels are then obtained based on the woman's response and if any signs of toxicity are present.

Magnesium sulfate does not seem to affect fetal heart rate variability in a healthy term fetus and rarely is toxic in the healthy term newborn whose weight is within normal range for gestational age. Neonatal serum magnesium levels approximate the mother's hypermagnesemia and result in depressed respirations and hyporeflexia (Sibai, 1988). Neonatal hypermagnesemia may require assisted mechanical ventilation until serum levels normalize.

Calcium gluconate, the antidote for magnesium sulfate, should be kept at the bedside. If toxicity occurs, 1 g of 10% calcium gluconate is administered by slow intravenous push (over at least 3 minutes) and repeated every hour until the respiratory, urinary, and neurologic depression has been alleviated.

If the woman develops eclampsia, magnesium sulfate may be administered by slow intravenous push in 1-g or 2-g boluses (see Emergency box on p. 569). For seizures unresponsive to magnesium sulfate, amobarbital sodium, 250 mg, can be administered by slow intravenous push over 3 minutes (Sibai, 1990b, c). In patients who have seizures unresponsive to therapy, a neurologic assessment of the brain is indicated.

Control of Blood Pressure

For the severely hypertensive preeclamptic/HELLP syndrome woman antihypertensive medications are ordered to lower the diastolic blood pressure. Initiation of antihypertensive therapy reduces maternal morbidity and mortality associated with left ventricular failure and cerebral hemorrhage (Harvey, Burke, 1992). Because a degree of maternal hypertension is necessary to maintain uteroplacental perfusion, antihypertensive therapy must not decrease the arterial pressure too low or too rapidly. Therefore the target range for the diastolic pressure is 90 to 100 mm Hg (Harvey, Burke, 1992).

Intravenous labetalol hydrochloride, an antihypertensive agent, is commonly administered. Other antihypertensive agents such as those described in Box 21-6 may be employed (Harvey, Burke, 1992). The choice of agent depends on patient response and health care provider preference.

Eclampsia

The reported incidence of eclampsia is from 0.5% to 2% of all pregnancies. A wide range of signs and symptoms besides convulsions are associated with eclampsia: extreme hypertension, hyperreflexia, 4+ proteinuria, generalized edema to mild hypertension without edema. The woman reports headaches with or without visual distur-

EMERGENCY

MAGNESIUM SULFATE TOXICITY

SIGNS/SYMPTOMS

Respirations <12/min
Hyporeflexia, absence of reflexes
Urinary output <30 ml/hr
Toxic serum levels >9.6 mg/dl
Signs of fetal distress (e.g., sudden drop in FHR)
Significant drop in maternal pulse or blood pressure

INTERVENTION

Discontinue MgSO₄ immediately, and change to maintenance solution.
Call for assistance and notify health care provider for immediate care.
Administer calcium gluconate or calcium chloride as ordered (e.g., 1 g for IV injection given over 3-min period).
Provide frequent to continuous monitoring of DTRs, respiration rate, urine output.
Monitor MgSO₄ level as indicated by patient response.

bances for 1 to 4 days before the onset of convulsions; proteinuria is absent in 20% of the women (Villar, Sibai, 1988). Laboratory findings also vary. Hemoconcentration is evidenced by an increased hematocrit. Serum uric acid, creatinine, liver function tests, and urine creatinine

clearance are elevated. DIC may be present if treatment is delayed or abruptio placentae occurs.

Immediate Care

The immediate care during a convulsion is to ensure a patent airway (see Emergency box). Once this has been attained, adequate oxygenation must be maintained by use of supplemental oxygen. When convulsions occur, the woman is turned to her side to prevent aspiration of vomitus and the supine hypotension syndrome. After the convulsion ceases, food and fluid are suctioned from the glottis or trachea. Magnesium sulfate (and amobarbital sodium for recurrent convulsions) is given as ordered (Sibai, 1990a). If an IV infusion is not in place, it is begun with a large-bore needle. Time, duration, and description of convulsions are recorded, and any urinary or fecal incontinence noted. The fetus is monitored for adverse effects. A transient bradycardia and decreased fetal heart rate variability are common.

Aspiration is a leading cause of maternal morbidity and mortality following an eclamptic seizure. After ini-

---

BOX 21-6

Pharmacologic Control of Hypertension in Pregnancy

Hydralazine (Apresoline, Neopresol)
  Action: Arteriolar vasodilator
  Target tissue: Peripheral arterioles—decreases muscle tone, thereby decreasing peripheral resistance; hypothalamus and medullary vasomotor center—minor decrease in sympathetic tone
  Maternal effects: Headache, flushing, palpitation, tachycardia, some decrease in uteroplacental blood flow, increase in HR and cardiac output, increases oxygen consumption
  Fetal effects: Tachycardia: late decelerations and bradycardia if maternal diastolic pressure below 90 mm Hg
  Nursing actions: Assess for effects of medications; alert mother (family) to expected effects of medications; assess BP because precipitous drop can lead to shock and perhaps to abruptio placentae; assess urinary output; maintain bed rest in a lateral position with side rails up
Labetalol hydrochloride (Normodyne)
  Action: Beta-blocking agent causing vasodilatation without significant change in cardiac output
  Target tissue: Peripheral arterioles (see Hydralazine)
  Maternal and fetal effects: Minimum
  Nursing actions: See Hydralazine
Methyldopa (Aldomet)
  Action: Used if maintenance therapy is needed: 250 to 500 mg orally every 8 hours (alpha$_2$-receptor agonist)
  Target tissue: Postganglionic nerve endings—interferes with chemical neurotransmission to reduce peripheral vascular resistance; CNS—sedation
  Maternal effects: Sleepiness, postural hypotension, constipation; rare: drug-induced fever in 1% of women and positive Coombs' test in 20%
  Fetal effects: After 4 months of maternal therapy, positive Coombs' test in infant
  Nursing actions: See Hydralazine
Nitroglycerin
  Action: Potent vasodilator
  Target tissue: Venous system
  Maternal effects: Decreases BP by decreasing cardiac output; antihypertensive effect related to maternal intravascular volume status
  Fetal effects: Stress may be noted with MAP <106 mm Hg, decreased FHR variability
  Nursing actions: Requires special IV setup, see Hydralazine; to monitor BP electronically

---

EMERGENCY

ECLAMPSIA

TONIC-CLONIC CONVULSION SIGNS
Stage of invasion: 2 to 3 sec; eyes fixed; twitching of facial muscles.
Stage of contraction: 15 to 20 sec; eyes protrude and are bloodshot; all body muscles in tonic contraction.
Stage of convulsion: Muscles relax and contract alternately (clonic). Respirations are halted and then begin again with long, deep, stertorous inhalation. Coma ensues.

INTERVENTION
Keep airway patent, turn head to one side; place pillow under one shoulder or back, if possible.
Call for assistance.
Protect with side rails up and padded.
Observe and record convulsion activity.

AFTER CONVULSION/SEIZURE
Observe for postconvulsion coma, incontinence.
Use suction as needed.
Administer oxygen via face mask at 10 L/min.
Start IV fluids and monitor for potential fluid overload.
Give MgSO$_4$ or anticonvulsant drug as ordered.
Insert indwelling catheter.
Monitor blood pressure.
Monitor fetal and uterine status.
Expedite laboratory work as ordered to monitor kidney function, liver function, coagulation system, and drug levels.
Provide hygiene and a quiet environment.
Support and keep woman and family informed.
Be prepared for birth when woman is stable.

tial stabilization and airway management, the nurse should anticipate orders for a chest x-ray and possibly arterial blood gases (ABGs) to rule out the possibility of aspiration.

A rapid assessment of uterine activity, cervical status, and fetal status is performed. During the convulsion, membranes may rupture and the cervix may dilate because the uterus becomes hypercontractile and hypertonic; birth may be imminent. If not, *once the woman's seizure tendency and blood pressure are controlled, a decision should be made as to whether the birth should take place*. The more serious the condition of the woman, the greater the need to proceed to the birth, which is the definitive cure for the disease. The route of birth—induction of labor vs. cesarean birth—depends on the maternal and fetal condition. All medications and therapy are merely temporary measures (Iams et al, 1990). If fetal lungs are not mature and the birth can be delayed for 48 hours, steroids such as betamethasone may be given.

Determination of pulmonary artery wedge pressure (PAWP) (Swan-Ganz catheter) may be required for accurate fluid monitoring in the presence of pulmonary edema or acute renal failure (ACOG, 1992). An indwelling catheter is required for accurate measurement of hourly urinary output. Blood sugar is evaluated by bedside fingerstick or venous draw every 1 to 8 hours as ordered. Glucose solutions are administered as ordered. To correct hypovolemia, crystalloids (0.9% saline or Ringer's lactated solution) are infused intravenously at a rate that maintains a urine output of at least 30 ml per hour, and the maternal response is recorded.

Medications (e.g., magnesium sulfate, antihypertensive agents) are given as directed. The woman's response is monitored and recorded and all drugs, dosages, and times recorded.

Laboratory tests are ordered to assess for the HELLP syndrome and to have blood typed and crossmatched. Other tests include determination of electrolytes, liver function battery, and complete hemogram and clotting profile.

The woman may have been incontinent of urine and stool or the membranes may have ruptured during the convulsion; she will need assistance with hygiene and a change of gown. Oral care with a soft toothbrush may be of comfort to her.

The health care provider explains procedures briefly and quietly. *The woman is never left alone*. The family is also kept informed of management, rationale, and the woman's progress.

Postpartum Nursing Care

Following birth the symptoms of preeclampsia-eclampsia resolve quickly, usually within 48 hours. The hematopoietic and hepatic complications of HELLP syndrome may persist longer. It is not uncommon for these patients to show an abrupt decrease in platelets with a concomitant increase in LDH and AST after a trend toward normalization of values has begun. Generally, the laboratory abnormalities seen with HELLP syndrome resolve in 72 to 96 hours.

The nursing care of the woman with hypertensive disease differs from that required in a normal postpartum period in a number of respects. The following variations in the nursing process are emphasized.

Careful assessment of the woman with a hypertensive disorder continues throughout the postpartum period. Blood pressure is measured at least every 4 hours for 48 hours or more frequently as the woman's condition warrants. Even if no convulsions occurred before the birth, they may occur within this period. Magnesium sulfate infusion is continued up to 48 hours after the birth. The same assessments continue until the drug is discontinued. The woman is at risk for a boggy uterus and a large lochia flow as a result of the magnesium sulfate therapy; therefore assessments of the uterine tone are necessary. The preeclamptic woman is hemoconcentrated and unable to tolerate excessive postpartum blood loss. Oxytocin or prostaglandin products are used to control bleeding. Ergot products (e.g., Ergotrate, Methergine) are contraindicated because they increase blood pressure. The woman is asked to report symptoms such as headaches and blurred vision. The nurse assesses affect, level of consciousness, blood pressure, pulse, and respiratory status before an analgesic is given for headache. It must be remembered that magnesium sulfate potentiates the action of narcotics, CNS depressants, and calcium channel blockers; these drugs need to be administered with caution. The woman may need to continue medication if her diastolic blood pressure exceeds 100 mm Hg at the time of discharge.

The woman's and family's responses to labor, the birth, and the newborn are monitored. Interactions and involvement in the care of the newborn are encouraged as much as the woman and her family desire. In addition, the woman and her family need opportunities to discuss their emotional response to complications. The nurse also provides information concerning the prognosis. Preeclampsia and eclampsia do not necessarily recur in subsequent pregnancies, but careful prenatal care is essential (recurrence rate is about 30%).

✦ EVALUATION

Evaluation is a continuous process. To be effective, it needs to be based on measurable criteria that reflect the expected outcomes of nursing care. Thus for severe preeclampsia and/or the HELLP syndrome, the following conditions should be met:

- The woman and fetus will not suffer adverse sequelae from preeclampsia or its management.

PLAN OF CARE

Preeclampsia: Home Care

Case History

Olga is a 38-year-old gravida 3, para 0-1-1-0, at 32 weeks' gestation. She noticed feeling "puffy" and found it difficult to get into her shoes.

During her prenatal visit nursing assessment reveals +2 pedal edema, BP 140/90 (MAP = 107), +2 DTRs, no clonus, and +1 proteinuria. Olga is very concerned about her condition and that of her baby. She expresses concern about constipation and anticipates becoming very bored on prolonged bed rest at home.

EXPECTED OUTCOME	IMPLEMENTATION	RATIONALE	EVALUATION
Nursing Diagnosis: High risk for injury, mother and fetus, related to not identifying a worsening of the preeclamptic condition			
Olga will be able to monitor and assess herself and her fetus and immediately report any changes to her health care provider.	Discuss warning signs/symptoms, and instruct Olga to notify health care provider immediately of any changes.	Knowledge enables Olga to become a partner in her own care; knowledge provides the basis for decision making.	Olga correctly verbalized signs/symptoms of worsening preeclampsia; written diary/log demonstrated understanding.
	Instruct Olga how to assess and record BP, fetal activity, urine for protein, edema, and daily weight in daily log; observe return demonstration.	Observing and practicing new skills increases self-confidence and provides reassurance.	Olga correctly demonstrates assessment and recording BP, fetal activity, urine testing, edema, and daily weight. Olga recorded: BP 130/76, fetal activity ≥3/hr, voiding large amounts of urine negative for protein, weight loss of 4 lb.
Nursing Diagnosis: Constipation related to decreased physical activity, decreased motility, and iron supplementation			
Olga will experience bowel regularity.	Counsel concerning diet high in fiber and fluid intake (8 to 10 8-oz glasses per day) and setting a routine time for bowel movements.	A side effect of iron supplementation is constipation; roughage/fluids and regularity stimulate bowel movement.	Olga reports regular daily bowel movements without discomfort.
	Instruct/demonstrate how to do gentle exercise; observe return demonstration.	Exercise facilitates bowel regularity.	Olga reports that her friend exercises with her every morning and her husband every evening.
	Explain reasons for tendency toward constipation during pregnancy.	Hormones relax smooth muscles of bowel; increase stomach-emptying time and decrease bowel motility.	Olga states she understands reasons.

Continued.

PLAN OF CARE—cont'd

Preeclampsia: Home Care

EXPECTED OUTCOMES	IMPLEMENTATION	RATIONALE	EVALUATION
Nursing Diagnosis: Diversional activity deficit related to imposed bed rest			
Olga will report minimal or no boredom.	Refer to home health care nurse.	Home visit provides information regarding setting potential.	Home health nurse visit is scheduled.
	Give Olga telephone numbers of other women on bed rest and suggest she network with them.	Provides mutual support through ventilation of feelings, ideas for activity, socializing.	Olga states she looks forward to talking with others who are "in the same boat."
	Explore Olga's interests: quilt making, other handwork, crafts, reading, TV, videotapes, visits with family/friends.	Enables Olga to look at alternatives and make decisions that will best meet her needs.	Olga begins to make telephone calls as soon as she gets home.
	Discuss home management and mobilization of help from significant others and community resources.	Enables Olga to start thinking about and problem solving regarding home management.	Olga reports that her mother had offered to come whenever needed; states she has many friends.
	Teach/demonstrate/ask for return demonstration of relaxation techniques.	Provides another means of coping; empowers her in self-care.	At next visit, Olga states she is not bored. Friends/husband relax with her; have set up visiting/helping schedules.

- The woman will not experience eclampsia or the severity of its complications.
- The fetus will not experience distress.
- The newborn will be born in optimal condition with no adverse sequelae resulting from the maternal condition and its management.
- The woman will give birth in optimal condition with no sequelae to her condition and its management.
- The family will be able to cope effectively with the mother's high-risk condition, its management, and outcomes.

If the outcome for the mother or baby is unfavorable, the family is assisted in coping with loss and grief (see Plan of Care on p. 571).

MATERNAL HEMORRHAGIC DISORDERS

Hemorrhagic disorders in pregnancy are medical emergencies. Maternal mortality has decreased significantly in recent years; however, hemorrhage remains a major cause of maternal death (Suresh, Kinch, 1991). Prompt, expert teamwork on the part of the health care providers is needed to save the life of the mother and infant.

Early Pregnancy Bleeding

Bleeding during early pregnancy is alarming to the woman and of concern to the health care provider. The common bleeding disorders of early pregnancy include abortion, incompetent cervix, ectopic pregnancy, and hydatidiform mole.

Spontaneous Abortion

Abortion is the termination of pregnancy before viability of the fetus. Viability is reached about 22 to 24 weeks' gestation—a fetal weight over 500 g, or a crown-rump length of 18 cm—when the fetus is able to survive in an extrauterine environment. With today's technology for newborn care, such an infant has at least a chance for survival. There are three types of abortions: *spontaneous* abortions result from natural causes; with *therapeutic* abortions the pregnancy is interrupted deliberately for medical reasons; and *elective* abortions are performed for personal reasons. This discussion includes only spontaneous abortions; for therapeutic and elective abortions see Chapter 30.

An early spontaneous abortion, or miscarriage, is one that occurs before 12 weeks' gestation; a late abortion is one occurring between 12 and 20 weeks of gestation. The rate of spontaneous abortion is difficult to deter-

PLAN OF CARE

Preeclampsia: Hospital Care

Case History

At 35 weeks, Olga comes for her scheduled prenatal appointment. The interview reveals that she has not been eating well because she feels nauseated and has had a dull headache for 2 days. Findings of physical examination include BP 150/98 (MAP = 115); DTRs 3+; Ø clonus; digital and facial edema; weight gain, 3 kg (6.6 lb). Urinalysis revealed proteinuria +2. Olga was admitted to the hospital, and IV $MgSO_4$ was started.

EXPECTED OUTCOMES	IMPLEMENTATION	RATIONALE	EVALUATION
Nursing Diagnosis: High risk for injury to mother and fetus related to CNS irritability			
Olga will experience decreased CNS irritability to normal levels.	Establish baseline data (e.g., DTRs, clonus). Monitor IV $MgSO_4$ and serum levels of $MgSO_4$. Assess for $MgSO_4$ toxicity.	Baseline needed to monitor effect of therapy. $MgSO_4$ is an anticonvulsant that acts on the myoneural junction. An overdose can decrease muscle activity, resulting in severe respiratory depression.	Olga's DTRs were at 2+ with no clonus. Olga's $MgSO_4$ serum levels remained within normal range. No $MgSO_4$ toxicity was noted.
Olga will not convulse.	Maintain a quiet, non-stimulating, dark environment.	Strong stimuli such as bright light and loud noises can precipitate a seizure (convulsion).	Olga experienced no seizure activity.
Nursing Diagnosis: Altered tissue perfusion related to preeclampsia secondary to arteriole vasospasm			
Olga will experience vasodilatation as evidenced by diuresis and decreased edema and weight loss.	Monitor oral intake and IV $MgSO_4$ infusion. Monitor urinary output. Monitor visible edema and daily weight loss. Maintain on complete bed rest in side-lying position.	$MgSO_4$, acting on the myoneural junction, relaxes the vasospasm. This relaxation often results in increased perfusion of the kidneys, mobilization of extravascular fluid (edema), and diuresis. Bed rest maximizes uteroplacental blood flow, which often reduces BP and promotes diuresis.	Olga's periorbital tissues, fingers, and sacral edema is decreasing; she experiences diureses. Olga experiences a weight loss.
Nursing Diagnosis: Fear related to threat of injury to Olga and couple's unborn baby			
The couple will state a decrease in fear.	Keep couple informed about the management of Olga's condition, as well as baby's status (e.g., FHR). Remain close by, listen to their fears, clarify information. Involve them in decisions about their care (e.g., comfort measures preferred, selection of oral fluid [if allowed], mouth care).	Knowledge reduces the fear of the unknown. Validation that one's feelings are legitimate increases one's ability to cope and relieves stress.	Couple state they do not feel as alone and different as they did before. Couple expresses relief that they can do something for themselves, that they have a say in matters—they don't feel so helpless.

TABLE 21-4 Assessing Abortion

TYPE OF ABORTION	AMOUNT OF BLEEDING	UTERINE CRAMPING	PASSAGE OF TISSUE	TISSUE IN VAGINA	INTERNAL CERVICAL OS	SIZE OF UTERUS
Threatened	Slight	Mild	No	No	Closed	Agrees with length of pregnancy
Inevitable	Moderate	Moderate	No	No	Open	Agrees with length of pregnancy
Incomplete	Heavy	Severe	Yes	Possible	Open with tissue in cervix	Smaller than expected for length of pregnancy
Complete	Slight	Mild	Yes	Possible	Closed	Smaller than expected for length of pregnancy
Missed	Slight	No	No	No	Closed	Smaller than expected for length of pregnancy
Septic	Varies; usually malodorous; fever present	Varies; fever present	Varies; fever present	Varies; fever present	Usually open; fever present	Any of the above with tenderness

From Gordon RT: Emergencies in obstetrics and gynecology. In Warner CG, editor: *Emergency care: assessment and intervention,* ed 3, St Louis, 1983, Mosby.

mine; approximately 15% of all clinically apparent pregnancies end in spontaneous abortion (Glass, Golbus, 1989; Simpson, 1990). More than half of all early spontaneous abortions are caused by abnormal embryonic development, chromosomal defects, and inherited disorders (McBride, 1991; Simpson, 1990). Late spontaneous abortions result from maternal causes such as advancing maternal age and parity, chronic infections, chronic debilitating diseases, poor nutrition, and recreational drug use; the reasons for the remainder are speculative (Cunningham et al, 1993; McBride, 1991). The diagnosis of the type of abortion a woman is experiencing is based on the signs and symptoms present (Table 21-4; Fig. 21-5).

Causes

Recurrent, early (habitual) spontaneous abortion is the loss of three or more previable pregnancies. The causes of recurrent early abortion may include (1) endocrine imbalance—women with a luteal phase defect (Carp et al, 1990) or insulin-dependent diabetics with both an elevated blood glucose and hemoglobin A$_{1C}$ in the first trimester have a significantly increased risk of spontaneous abortion (Mills et al, 1988); (2) infections—systemic and endometrial infections caused by rubella, cytomegalovirus, active genital herpes, toxoplasmosis, *Treponema, Listeria, Chlamydia,* and *Mycoplasma* (Arias, 1993; Gilbert & Harmon, 1993; McBride, 1991); (3)

systemic disorders (e.g., lupus erythematosus); (4) genetic factors; and (5) cocaine use (Cunningham et al, 1993; Rosenak et al, 1990).

Anomalies of the reproductive tract cause second or third trimester pregnancy loss. Little can be done to avoid genetic causes of pregnancy loss, but prepregnancy correction of maternal disorders, immunization against infectious diseases, adequate early prenatal care, and treatment of pregnancy complications will do much to prevent abortion.

Types

The types of spontaneous abortion include threatened, inevitable, incomplete, complete, septic, and missed (see Fig. 21-5). Symptoms of a *threatened abortion* (Fig. 21-5, *A*) include spotting of blood and a closed cervical os. Management includes bed rest and avoidance of stress and orgasm. Follow-up treatment is individualized.

Inevitable (Fig. 21-5, *B*) and *incomplete* (Fig. 21-5, *C*) abortions involve a moderate to heavy amount of bleeding with an open cervical os. Tissue may also be present with the bleeding. Prompt termination of the pregnancy, usually by curettage, is the suggested treatment.

In a *complete abortion* (Fig. 21-5, *D*) all of the fetal tissue is passed, the cervix is closed, and there may be slight bleeding. Usually no further treatment is required.

Presenting symptoms of a *septic,* or infected, abortion

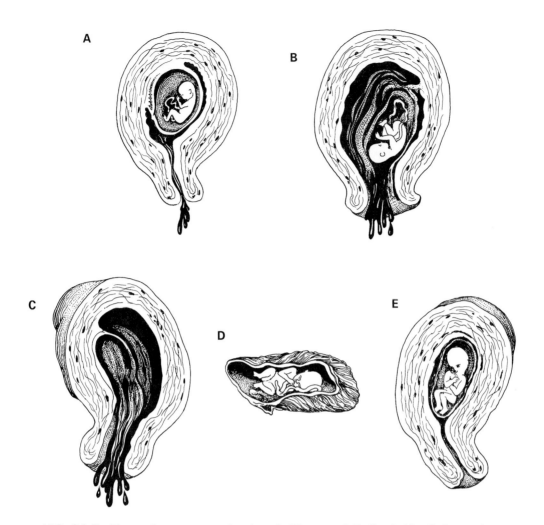

FIG. 21-5   Types of spontaneous abortion. **A,** Threatened. **B,** Inevitable. **C,** Incomplete. **D,** Complete. **E,** Missed.

include fever and abdominal tenderness. Vaginal bleeding, which may be slight to heavy, is usually malodorous. Termination of the pregnancy, antibiotic therapy, and treatment of septic shock are initiated.

A *missed abortion* (Fig. 21-5, *E*) refers to a pregnancy in which the fetus has died but spontaneous abortion does not occur. It may be diagnosed when the uterus is smaller than expected for the duration of the pregnancy. There may be no bleeding or cramping and the cervical os is closed. Treatment may include waiting up to 1 month for spontaneous abortion to occur with frequent monitoring of the woman's clotting factors. If spontaneous abortion does not occur, the health care provider will terminate the pregnancy to prevent DIC and/or sepsis in the woman.

Signs and Symptoms

Signs and symptoms of spontaneous abortion depend on the duration of pregnancy. The woman may feel she is experiencing a heavy menstrual flow if abortion occurs before the sixth week of pregnancy. Abortion that occurs between the sixth and twelfth weeks of pregnancy

will cause moderate discomfort and blood loss. After the twelfth week, abortion is typified by severe pain, similar to that of labor, because the fetus must be expelled.

Medical management (Table 21-5) depends on the classification of spontaneous abortion. Therefore, an early accurate diagnosis of spontaneous abortion is vital.

Incompetent Cervix

An **incompetent cervix** is characterized by painless dilatation of the cervical os without labor or contractions of the uterus in the second trimester or early in the third trimester of pregnancy. Miscarriage or preterm birth may result. The incidence of cervical incompetence is 20% or more of all second trimester losses (Iams, Zuspan, Quilligan, 1990).

Causes

Etiologic factors include a history of traumatic birth, forceful dilatation and curettage (D&C), or ingestion of diethylstilbestrol (DES) by the woman's mother while pregnant with the woman. Other instances may result from a congenitally short cervix or uterine anomalies.

TABLE 21-5 Types of Spontaneous Abortion and Usual Management

TYPE OF ABORTION	MANAGEMENT
Threatened	Bed rest, sedation, and avoidance of stress and orgasm are recommended. Further treatment will depend on woman's response to treatment.
Inevitable and incomplete	Prompt termination of pregnancy is accomplished, usually by dilatation and curettage (D & C).*
Complete	No further intervention may be needed if uterine contractions are adequate to prevent hemorrhage and if there is no infection.
Missed	If spontaneous evacuation of the uterus does not occur within 1 month, pregnancy is terminated by method appropriate to duration of pregnancy.* Blood clotting factors are monitored until uterus is empty. DIC and incoagulability of blood with uncontrolled hemorrhage may develop in cases of fetal death after the twelfth week if products of conception are retained for longer than 5 weeks (see p. 591 for discussion of DIC).
Septic	Immediate termination of pregnancy by method appropriate to duration of pregnancy.* Cervical culture and sensitivity (C & S) studies are done, and broad-spectrum antibiotic therapy (e.g., ampicillin) is started. Treatment for septic shock is initiated if necessary.

*See Chapter 30 for discussion of these procedures.

The diagnosis of cervical incompetence is difficult and is based upon clinical history. A presumptive diagnosis can usually be made if a woman experiences appreciable cervical dilatation and prolapse of the membranes through the cervix without labor. In a woman with a history of repeated second trimester terminations, cervical incompetence should be suspected.

Medical Management

The woman with an incompetent cervix may be managed conservatively with bed rest, hydration, and tocolysis (inhibition of uterine contractions) or actively by performing a cervical cerclage. Correction of the weakened cervix is possible by wedge trachelorrhaphy (removal of a wedge from the anterior segment of the cervix with closure) in the nonpregnant woman. During pregnancy a *McDonald cerclage,* band of homologous fascia, or nonabsorbable ribbon (Mersilene) may be placed around the cervix beneath the mucosa to constrict the internal os (Fig. 21-6). Successful continuation of the pregnancy to viability or beyond occurs in approximately 40% of women, provided the membranes remain intact and that the cervix is not more than 3 cm dilated or more than 50% effaced at the time of correction. The suture is left in place until close to term, when it is removed and labor is allowed to begin spontaneously. This procedure must be repeated with each pregnancy.

A second method involves placement of a pursestring ligature to maintain a closed cervix. This procedure, the *Shirodkar,* allows for the suture to remain in place permanently for the woman that anticipates future pregnancies. Births are accomplished by cesarean.

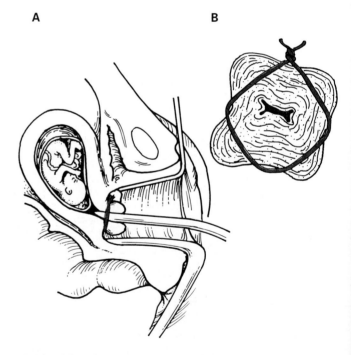

A   B

FIG. 21-6 **A,** Cerclage correction of incompetent cervical os. **B,** Cross-section of closed internal os.

Ectopic Pregnancy

Ectopic pregnancy is one in which the fetus is implanted outside the uterine cavity (Fig. 21-7). Most extrauterine pregnancies result from abnormalities that impede or prevent the passage of the fertilized ovum through the fallopian tube (e.g., peritubal adhesions following pelvic inflammatory disease). Approximately one of every 100 pregnancies in the United States is ectopic, and at least

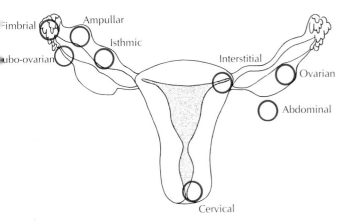

FIG. 21-7   Sites of implantation of ectopic pregnancies. Order of frequency of occurrence is ampulla, isthmus, interstitium, fimbria, tuboovarian ligament, ovary, abdominal cavity, and cervix (external os).

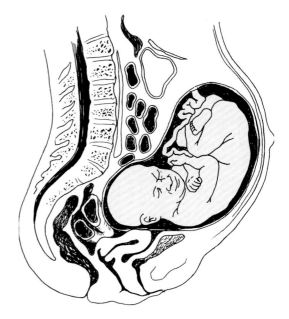

FIG. 21-8   Ectopic pregnancy, abdominal.

three fourths of these become symptomatic and are diagnosed during the first trimester. Ectopic pregnancy is a significant cause of maternal morbidity and mortality with mortality increased 10 times more than for a vaginal birth and 50 times for an induced abortion (Cunningham et al, 1993).

Ectopic pregnancy is classified according to the site of implantation (e.g., tubal, ovarian). The uterus is the only organ capable of containing and sustaining a term pregnancy. However, the rare abdominal pregnancy, with birth by laparotomy, may result in a living infant (Fig. 21-8).

Signs and Symptoms

There are no signs or symptoms diagnostic of early ectopic pregnancy. A missed period, adnexal fullness, and tenderness may suggest an unruptured tubal pregnancy. In contrast, the following triad is associated with early ruptured extrauterine pregnancy in almost 50% of cases: amenorrhea or an abnormal menstrual period followed by slight uterine bleeding, adnexal or cul-de-sac mass, and unilateral pelvic pain over the mass. Decidua but no placental villi may be found on curettage. Additional findings of *acute rupture* may include shock out of proportion to visible blood loss, or referred shoulder pain.

In *chronic ruptured* tubal pregnancy, which represents slightly more than half the total of ectopic pregnancies, internal bleeding usually has been slow and the symptoms atypical or inconclusive. In addition to slight, dark vaginal bleeding, a sense of pelvic pressure or fullness, lower abdominal tenderness, flatulence, a tense, tender, semicystic, perhaps crepitant, cul-de-sac mass may be felt. Slight fever, leukocytosis, and a falling hematocrit or hemoglobin level may be noted. An ecchymotic blueness of the umbilicus *(Cullen's sign),* which is indicative of hematoperitoneum, may develop in a neglected, ruptured intraabdominal ectopic pregnancy.

Medical Management

The use of ultrasound as an aid in the management of an ectopic pregnancy has allowed improved accuracy in the preoperative diagnosis. The differential diagnosis of ectopic pregnancy involves a consideration of numerous disorders that share many, perhaps all, of the same signs and symptoms (Table 21-6).

The major management problem in ectopic pregnancy is hemorrhage; bleeding must be quickly and effectively controlled. Blood transfusions must be available. Laparotomy is performed immediately after the diagnosis of ectopic pregnancy is made. Blood and clots are evacuated, and bleeding vessels are controlled.

Advanced ectopic abdominal pregnancy requires laparotomy as soon as the woman is fit for surgery. If the placenta of a second or third trimester abdominal pregnancy is attached to a vital organ, such as the liver, no attempt at separation and removal should be made. The cord should be cut flush with the placenta. Degeneration and absorption of the placenta usually occur without complication.

The diagnosis and management of ectopic pregnancy are rapidly changing as technology improves. The use of methotrexate therapy is being explored for patients with ectopic pregnancy (Stoval, Ling, and Buster, 1990). Current evidence demonstrates that laparoscopic management of ectopic pregnancies is equally safe, equally effective, and less traumatic than laparotomy and may replace laparotomy as treatment for most ectopic pregnancies (Nager, Murphy, 1991).

Prognosis varies. The success of a subsequent pregnancy is dependent on specifics of the woman's reproductive history. Ectopic pregnancy recurs in approximately 10% of women, but more than 50% of women who have had an ectopic pregnancy achieve at least one normal pregnancy thereafter.

Hydatidiform Mole

Hydatidiform mole is one of three types of gestational trophoblastic neoplasms (ACOG, 1993). There are two distinct types: complete, or classic, mole and partial mole, which may or may not be part of the accepted continuum of **trophoblastic disease** (DePetrillo et al, 1987).

Hydatidiform mole occurs in 1 of every 1200 pregnancies in the United States, but a much higher inci-

dence is seen in Asia and tropical areas (Berman, DiSaia, 1989). It is most often seen in women who have had ovulation stimulation with clomiphene (Clomid), in women of lower socioeconomic groups, and in women at both ends of the reproductive spectrum (early teens or perimenopausal). The risk of developing a second mole is four to five times higher than the risk of the first.

Types

The complete or classic mole results from fertilization of an egg whose nucleus has been lost or inactivated (Fig.

TABLE 21-6 Differential Diagnosis of Ectopic Pregnancy

	ECTOPIC PREGNANCY	APPENDICITIS	SALPINGITIS	RUPTURED CORPUS LUTEUM CYST	UTERINE ABORTION
Pain	Unilateral cramps and tenderness before rupture	Epigastric, peri-umbilical, then right lower quadrant pain; tenderness localizing at McBurney's point; rebound tenderness	Usually in both lower quadrants with or without rebound	Unilateral, becoming general with progressive bleeding	Midline cramps
Nausea and vomiting	Occasionally before, frequently after rupture	Usual; precedes shift of pain to right lower quadrant	Infrequent	Rare	Almost never
Menstruation	Some aberration; missed period, spotting	Unrelated to menses	Hypermenorrhea or metorrhagia or both	Period delayed, then bleeding, often with pain	Amenorrhea, then spotting, then brisk bleeding
Temperature and pulse	37.2°-37.8° C (99°-100° F); pulse variable; normal before, rapid after rupture	37.2°-37.8° C (99°-100° F): pulse rapid: 99-100	37.2°-40° C (99°-104° F): pulse elevated in proportion to fever	Not over 37.2° C (99° F): pulse normal unless blood loss marked, then rapid	To 37.2° C (99° F) if spontaneous: to 40° C (104° F) if induced (infected)
Pelvic examination	Unilateral tenderness, especially on movement of cervix; crepitant mass on one side or in cul-de-sac	No masses; rectal tenderness high on right side	Bilateral tenderness on movement of cervix: masses only when pyosalpinx or hydrosalpinx present	Tenderness over affected ovary: no masses	Cervix slightly patulous: uterus slightly enlarged, irregularly softened: tender with infection
Laboratory findings	WBC to 15,000/mm³; RBC strikingly low if blood loss large; sedimentation rate slightly elevated	WBC: 10,000-18,000/mm³ (rarely normal); RBC normal: sedimentation rate slightly elevated	WBC: 15,000-30,000/mm³; RBC normal: sedimentation rate markedly elevated	WBC normal to 10,000/mm³: RBC normal: sedimentation rate normal	WBC: 15,000/mm³ if spontaneous: to 30,000/mm³ if induced (infection); RBC normal: sedimentation rate slightly to moderately elevated

From Benson RC, editor: *Current obstetric and gynecologic diagnosis and treatment*, ed 5, 1984 Lange Medical Publications

21-9). The mole resembles a bunch of white grapes. The hydropic (fluid-filled) vesicles grow rapidly, causing the uterus to be larger than expected for the duration of the pregnancy. Usually the mole contains no fetus, placenta, amniotic membranes or fluid. Maternal blood has no placenta to receive it; therefore hemorrhage into the uterine cavity and vaginal bleeding occur. In about 3% of these hydatidiform moles a progression toward choriocarcinoma (a rapid-growing malignant neoplasm) occurs. The potential for malignant transformation of partial moles is much less than that associated with the complete mole (Scott et al, 1990).

Signs and Symptoms

In the early stages the signs and symptoms of hydatidiform mole cannot be distinguished from normal pregnancy. Later, vaginal bleeding occurs in almost every case. The vaginal discharge may be dark brown (resembling prune juice) or bright red, either scant or profuse. It may continue for only a few days or intermittently for weeks. Early in pregnancy about half the women have a uterus significantly larger than expected from the menstrual dates.

Anemia from blood loss, excessive nausea and vomiting (hyperemesis gravidarum), and abdominal cramps caused by uterine distention are relatively common findings. Anemia results from intrauterine bleeding. Preeclampsia occurs in about 15% of cases, usually between 9 and 12 gestational weeks.

Medical Management

Many moles abort spontaneously. When hydropic vesicles are passed vaginally and the woman saves the specimen, the diagnosis can be established with certainty. The sonographic pattern of a molar pregnancy is character-ized by a diffuse snowstorm pattern (Kulb, 1990). Any uncertainty in diagnosis is usually clarified by clinical history, human chorionic gonadotropin (hCG) titer (although not considered diagnostic), and if necessary a repeat sonogram in 2 weeks.

Suction curettage offers a safe, rapid, and effective method of evacuation of hydatidiform mole in almost all women (Scott et al, 1990). Follow-up management includes frequent physical and pelvic examinations along with measurement of serum hCG levels for at least 1 year. A rising titer and an enlarging uterus may indicate choriocarcinoma. Therefore, to avoid confusion with signs of pregnancy, pregnancy should be avoided for 1 year. Oral contraceptives are usually prescribed. Cure of the malignant condition is defined as a complete absence of all clinical and hormonal evidence of disease for 5 years.

Care Management—Early Pregnancy Bleeding

Upon admission of the woman to the hospital, the nurse obtains a history of the woman's chief complaint, pain, bleeding, and last menstrual period (LMP) to determine the approximate length of gestation. The initial data base includes vital signs, previous pregnancies, previous pregnancy outcomes, type and location of pain, quantity and nature of bleeding (Box 21-7), allergies, and emotional status. It is not uncommon for the woman to be anxious and fearful of what may happen to herself or her pregnancy.

If an incompetent cervix is suspected, the assessment includes exploring the woman's feelings about her preg-

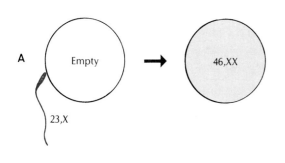

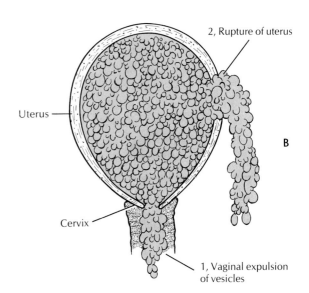

FIG. 21-9   A, Chromosomal origin of complete mole. Single sperm *(color)* fertilizes an "empty" ovum. Reduplication of the sperm's 23, X set gives a completely homozygous diploid 46, XX. A similar process follows fertilization of an empty ovum by two sperm with two independently drawn sets of 23, X or 23, Y; therefore both karyotypes of 46, XX and 46, XY can result. **B,** Uterine rupture with hydatidiform mole. *1,* Evacuation of mole through cervix. *2,* Rupture of uterus and spillage of mole into peritoneal cavity (rare).

BOX 21-7

Assessment of Bleeding in Pregnancy

INITIAL DATA BASE
Chief complaint
Vital signs
Gravidity, parity
LMP/EDB
Pregnancy history (previous and current)
Allergies
Nausea and vomiting
Pain (onset, quality, precipitating event)
Bleeding or coagulation problems
LOC
Emotional status

EARLY PREGNANCY
Confirmation of pregnancy

Bleeding (bright or dark, intermittent or continuous)
Pain (type, intensity, persistence)
Vaginal discharge

LATE PREGNANCY
EDB
Bleeding (quantity, associated pain)
Vaginal discharge
Amniotic membrane status
Uterine activity
Abdominal pain
Fetal status/viability

EDB, Estimated date of birth; *LMP*, last menstrual period; *LOC*, level of consciousness.

---

nancy and her understanding about an incompetent cervix. It is also important to evaluate the woman's support systems. Since the diagnosis of an incompetent cervix usually is not made until the woman has lost one or more previous pregnancies, she may feel guilty or to blame for this impending loss.

The nurse should suspect the possibility of an ectopic pregnancy in a woman who has missed a menstrual period, has spotting and pelvic pain, and who has a history of pelvic infection, IUD use, or tubal surgery. If the woman has internal bleeding, assessment will reveal the presence of vertigo, shoulder pain, hypotension, and tachycardia. Any patient suspected of having an ectopic pregnancy should be immediately referred to a primary care provider for a confirmative diagnosis and medical intervention.

Physical examination with an ectopic pregnancy reveals unilateral pain over the tube and ovary, and an adnexal mass is often palpated. Laboratory testing reveals a low hCG level. An ultrasound examination for the woman at risk allows earlier diagnosis and a resultant reduction in the mortality and morbidity resulting from the condition (de Crespigny, 1987).

A negative or weakly positive urine pregnancy test is characteristic of abortion. With considerable or persistent blood loss, anemia is likely. If sepsis is present, temperature is greater than 38° C (100.4° F) and white blood cell count (WBC) is greater than 12,000/mm^3. Endocrine studies show that hCG, estrogen, and progesterone titers are minimal or absent in established abortions.

After assessing the patient, immediate nursing care focuses on stabilization of the woman. Psychosocial aspects of care focus on what this pregnancy loss means to the woman and her family. Care is patient and family cen-

tered. Careful explanations are provided as to the nature of the complication, expected procedures, and possible future implications.

The woman should be told that spontaneous abortions occur frequently and are not usually related to behavior. If the woman has a history of cigarette, alcohol, or drug use she should be told of the increased risk of early pregnancy loss in relation to these behaviors (Deutchman, 1989; Glass, Golbus, 1989).

The nurse reinforces explanations given by the primary care provider and carries out appropriate orders. An intravenous line is started, laboratory work obtained, and possibly an ultrasound test performed. Laboratory tests include a complete blood count (CBC), blood typing for group, Rh factor, and crossmatching, and urinalysis. Chest x-ray films and ECG evaluation are obtained if necessary. Blood, fluid, and electrolyte imbalances are corrected as soon as possible.

If a D&C is scheduled, the nurse reinforces explanations, answers any questions or concerns, and prepares the patient for surgery. *Dilatation and curettage* is a surgical procedure in which the cervix is dilated and a curette is inserted to scrape the uterine walls and remove uterine contents. General preoperative and postoperative care is appropriate for the woman requiring surgical intervention for spontaneous abortion.

Analgesics and/or anesthetic appropriate to the procedure are used. IV administration of oxytocin, 10 U in 500 ml of infusate, may be needed to induce or augment abortion. After evacuation of the uterus, 10 to 20 U of oxytocin in 1000 ml of infusate may be given to prevent hemorrhage.

Ergot products such as ergonovine, which contract the uterus and cervix, are contraindicated until the uterus is emptied to avoid retention of fragments or tissue. Retained fragments of fetal or placental tissue predispose to uterine relaxation and puerperal infection. Three or four doses of ergonovine, 0.2 mg orally or intramuscularly every 4 hours, may be given if the woman is normotensive. Antibiotics are given as necessary. Transfusion may be required for shock or anemia. If the woman is Rh negative and has not developed isoimmunization, she is given an intramuscular injection of $Rh_o(D)$ immune globulin within 72 hours of the abortion. The usual dose of $Rh_o(D)$ immune globulin at less than 12 weeks' gestation is 50 µg; if greater than 12 weeks, 300 µg. (See Box 21-8 for patient teaching following an abortion.)

For the woman with an incompetent cervix, implementation of the nursing plan of care is determined by medical management. If conservative management is the treatment of choice, the woman must understand the importance of bed rest at home and the need for close observation and supervision. Instructions include the rationale for bed rest, restricting activity, and warning signs to report. Tocolytics may be given prophylactically to prevent uterine contractions and further dilatation of the cervix. The woman must be instructed on the importance of taking oral tocolytic medication as prescribed, the expected response, and possible side effects. If home-monitoring is implemented, she is taught how to apply a contraction monitor and transmit the monitor tracing by telephone to the monitoring center (see Fig. 24-13). Nurses at the monitoring center assess the tracing for contractions, answer questions, provide emotional support and education, and report information to the woman's primary care provider (Robichaux et al, 1990).

If management of early pregnancy bleeding is unsuccessful and the fetus is born before viability, appropriate grief support should be provided. If the neonate is born prematurely, appropriate anticipatory guidance and sup-

BOX 21-8

Discharge Teaching for the Woman after Spontaneous Abortion

- Refer to appropriate support groups, clergy, or professional counseling.
- Advise woman to report any heavy, profuse, or bright red bleeding to health care provider.
- Reassure woman that a scant, dark discharge may persist for 1 to 2 weeks.
- To reduce the risk of infection, remind woman not introduce anything into the vagina until bleeding has stopped.
- Acknowledge that she has experienced a loss and that time is required for recovery. She may experience mood swings and depression.

port are necessary. Follow-up care should assess the woman's physical and emotional recovery. Referrals to local support groups or counseling are provided as needed.

Late Pregnancy Bleeding
Placenta Previa

In **placenta previa** the placenta is implanted in the lower uterine segment. The degree to which the internal cervical os is covered by the placenta determines how the placenta previa is classified. Placenta previa often is described as *complete, total,* or *central* if the internal os is entirely covered by the placenta, when the cervix is fully dilated (Fig. 21-10). *Partial placenta previa* implies incomplete coverage. *Marginal placenta previa* indicates that only an edge of the placenta approaches the internal os. The term *low-lying (low) implantation* is used

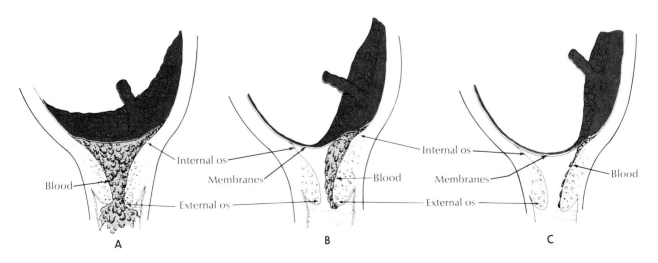

FIG. 21-10 Types of placenta previa after onset of labor. **A,** Complete, or total. **B,** Incomplete, or partial. **C,** Marginal, or low lying.

when the placenta is situated in the lower uterine segment but away from the os. By term, the incidence of placenta previa is 0.5% to 1% (Kulb, 1990; Lavery, 1990).

Painless uterine bleeding, especially during the third trimester, characterizes placenta previa (Table 21-7). The first significant bleeding episode usually occurs between 29 and 30 weeks' gestation. Rarely is the first episode life threatening or a cause of hypovolemic shock. The *bright red bleeding* may be intermittent, may occur in gushes, or, more rarely, may be continuous.

Diagnosis

Currently the standard for the diagnosis of placenta previa is transabdominal ultrasound. If ultrasound reveals a normally implanted placenta, a speculum examination is performed to rule out local causes of bleeding (e.g., cervicitis, polyps, or carcinoma of the cervix), and a coagulation profile is obtained to rule out other causes of bleeding.

Medical Management

Conservative management (e.g., bed rest to extend the period of gestation) is usually possible when the fetus is not mature because the initial spontaneous bleed with a placenta previa is rarely life threatening to the mother or fetus. When fetal lung maturity is achieved and survival is likely, the birth is accomplished.

After the diagnosis of placenta previa has been made, the woman usually remains in the hospital under close supervision. The duration of pregnancy should be confirmed and, except in an emergency, birth postponed until after the thirty-sixth week. A cesarean birth is usually performed for women with placenta previa (Cunningham et al, 1993).

Abruptio Placentae

Abruptio placentae, or *premature separation of the placenta,* is the detachment of part or all of the placenta from its implantation site (Fig. 21-11). Separation oc-

TABLE 21-7 Summary of Findings: Abruptio Placentae and Placenta Previa

	ABRUPTIO PLACENTAE			
	MARGINAL SEPARATION	**MODERATE SEPARATION**	**SEVERE SEPARATION* (MORE THAN 66%)**	**PLACENTA PREVIA**
Bleeding: external, vaginal	Minimal	Absent or moderate	Absent to moderate	Minimal to severe and life threatening
Color of blood	Dark red	Dark red	Dark red	Bright red
Shock	Absent	Common	Very common: often sudden	Occasional
Coagulopathy	Rare	Occasional	Common	Rare
Uterine tonicity	Normal	Increased—may be localized to one region or diffuse over uterus: uterus fails to relax between contractions	Tetanic, persistent uterine contraction: boardlike uterus	Normal
Tenderness (pain)	Usually absent; if present, is localized	Increased—usually diffuse over uterus	Agonizing, unremitting uterine pain	Absent
Ultrasonographic findings:				
Location of placenta	Normal—upper uterine segment	Normal—upper uterine segment	Normal—upper uterine segment	Abnormal—lower uterine segment
Station of presenting part	Variable to engaged	Variable to engaged	Variable to engaged	High—not engaged
Fetal position	Usual distribution†	Usual distribution	Usual distribution	Commonly transverse, breech, or oblique
Concurrent hypertensive state	Usual distribution	Commonly present	Commonly present	Usual distribution

*Onset is usually abrupt; fetus usually dies.
†Usual distribution refers to the usual variations or incidence seen when there is no concurrent problem.

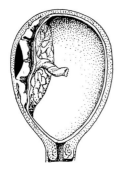 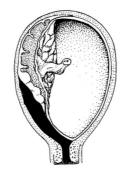 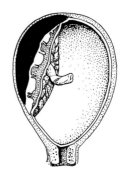

FIG. 21-11 Abruptio placentae. Premature separation of normally implanted placenta.

curs in the area of the decidua basalis after the twentieth week of pregnancy, before the birth of the baby.

Premature separation of the placenta is a serious event and accounts for about 15% of all perinatal deaths. More than 50% of these deaths are the result of preterm birth; many others die from intrauterine hypoxia.

There are two classification systems for identifying placental abruption based on type and severity. The first classification system grades an abruption based on the degree of placental separation (Green, 1989). The second system classifies abruption based on signs and symptoms.

The separation may be partial or complete, or only the margin of the placenta may be involved. Bleeding from the placental site may dissect (separate) the membranes from the decidua basalis and flow out through the vagina; it may remain concealed (retroplacental hemorrhage); or it may do both (see Fig. 21-11). Clinical symptoms vary with the degree of separation (see Table 21-7).

Diagnosis

The diagnosis of placental abruption is based on the woman's history, physical examination, and laboratory studies. Abruptio placentae is suspected in the woman presenting with sudden onset, intense, usually localized uterine pain, with or without vaginal bleeding. Sonography is utilized to rule out placenta previa; however, it is not diagnostic for an abruption (Cunningham et al, 1993; Lowe, Cunningham, 1990).

Medical Management

Treatment is dependent on maternal and fetal status. In the presence of fetal distress, severe hemorrhage, coagulopathy, poor labor progress, or increasing uterine resting tone, a cesarean birth is performed. If the mother is hemodynamically stable, a vaginal birth may be attempted when the fetus is alive and in no acute distress, or if the fetus is dead. Fluid replacement must be aggressive in the presence of hemorrhage. Whole blood and Ringer's lactate are infused in quantities necessary to maintain a urine output of 30 to 60 ml per hour and a hematocrit of approximately 30% (Lowe, Cunningham, 1990).

Care Management—Placenta Previa and Abruptio Placentae

With the woman's admission to the hospital, the nurse begins with an assessment of the bleeding. Abdominal assessment reveals a soft, relaxed, nontender uterus of normal tone for placenta previa; uterine tenderness and increased tone are present with abruptio. Laboratory studies include a CBC, blood type and Rh, possible type and crossmatch for packed red blood cells, and a coagulation profile.

Nursing interventions depend on whether the woman is managed conservatively or actively. Information is given to the woman and her family about placenta previa or abruptio placentae, including causes, treatment, and expected outcomes. Vital signs and noninvasive assessments of cardiac output (Box 21-9) are obtained frequently to observe for signs of declining hemodynamic status. Fetal status is continuously monitored if the fetus has survived the initial insult. If placental abruption is suspected, the uterus is palpated to assess for tenderness and uterine activity. If appropriate, an intrauterine pressure catheter is placed to evaluated uterine tone; normal uterine resting tone is less than 20 mm Hg. For the

---

BOX 21-9

Noninvasive Assessments of Cardiac Output

Palpation of pulses
  Arterial
  Blood pressure
Auscultation
  Heart sounds/murmurs
  Breath sounds
Inspection
  Skin color, temperature, turgor
  Level of consciousness (LOC)
  Capillary refill
  Urinary output
  Neck veins
  Pulse oximetry
  Mucous membranes

PLAN OF CARE

Placenta Previa

Case History

Joyce, a 25-year-old healthy primigravida at 33 weeks' gestation, comes to the labor and birth unit with her husband. The admission diagnosis is probable placenta previa. After an ultrasound examination the diagnosis was changed to bleeding secondary to central previa.

The admission interview revealed that Joyce awoke this evening and found she was bleeding. She states that the bleeding was painless and bright red and that when she got out of bed, the blood ran down her legs. Joyce keeps asking, "What did I do to cause this?" and "Is my baby going to be OK?" Joyce states she has no history of bleeding disorders and no significant medical or obstetric history. During the physical examination the nurse notes the following vital signs: temperature 97.6° F, pulse 110 beats/min, respirations 28/min, BP 100/68 mm Hg, fetal heart rate 156 beats/min. The uterus is soft and nontender, with no contractions palpated. Fundal height is 34 cm. On admission the peripad Joyce had worn to the hospital was noted to be two thirds saturated with bright red blood. There was no active bleeding at present. The following laboratory tests were ordered: CBC, DIC profile, bleeding time, blood type and Rh. An IV infusion was started with a 16-gauge angiocatheter to infuse at 125 ml/hr. A review of laboratory findings revealed hemoglobin 9.3 g/dl, hematocrit 27%, platelets 145,000 mm^3 with normal coagulation studies.

EXPECTED OUTCOMES	IMPLEMENTATION	RATIONALE	EVALUATION
Nursing Diagnosis: Decreased cardiac output related to excessive bleeding secondary to placenta previa			
Joyce's intravascular blood volume and cardiac output will be restored as evidenced by normal pulse, blood pressure, hemodynamic values and laboratory values.	Assess and record vital signs, blood pressure, LOC, CVP/PAWP, peripheral perfusion, intake and output, and amount of bleeding. Assist health care provider, or initiate IV fluid therapy and/or blood replacement therapy as ordered; administer medications per health care provider's orders.	Accurate assessment of hemodynamic status provides a basis for planning and evaluating interventions. Restoration of vascular volume requires IV therapy and pharmacologic interventions. Lost blood volume must be restored to prevent further complications such as infections, fetal compromise, and compromise to maternal vital organ systems.	Joyce's bleeding stops, and hemodynamic profile is restored. Her laboratory values return to normal.
Nursing Diagnosis: Potential for infection related to anemia and bleeding secondary to placenta previa			
Joyce will remain physiologically safe as evidenced by absence of infection and restoration of normal laboratory values.	Assess and document vital signs, blood pressure, uterine tenderness, malodorous vaginal discharge. Monitor laboratory results for shifting of differential or rising WBC. Assess fetus for signs of intrauterine infection such as fetal tachycardia and decreasing biophysical profile scores.	Accurate assessment of subtle changes in Joyce's status can detect early signs of infection. In placenta previa, placental tissue is exposed, increasing the risk of infection.	Joyce remains afebrile, free of any signs of infection for the next 6 weeks, and gives birth to a viable mature fetus.

PLAN OF CARE—cont'd

Placenta Previa

EXPECTED OUTCOMES	IMPLEMENTATION	RATIONALE	EVALUATION

Nursing Diagnosis: Potential for injury (fetal) related to decreased uterine/placental perfusion secondary to bleeding

The fetus will remain physiologically safe as evidenced by reactive nonstress test, normal biophysical profile scores, absence of late decelerations during labor, and uncompromised birth.	Monitor fetus at least daily for signs of tachycardia, decreased movement, loss of reactivity on nonstress test, and presence of late decelerations with fetal monitoring. Obtain biophysical profiles as ordered to assess for signs of intrauterine infection. Obtain ultrasonographic examination as ordered to evaluate fetal growth and amniotic fluid volume.	This fetus is at increased risk for intrauterine compromise; careful and consistent assessments will identify changes in fetal status early so that interventions can be implemented.	The fetus reached maturity (39 weeks' gestation) without compromise. At birth the infant had normal Apgar scores (9/9), cord pH (7.32), and required no resuscitation. He weighed 3345 g and went home with his family on the third postbirth day.

woman diagnosed with an abruptio placentae, preparations are made for birth, remembering that an emergency cesarean birth is always a possibility.

If conservative management is utilized in the management of a placenta previa, nursing care focuses on accurate assessments and appropriate referrals. The woman is instructed on the importance of bed rest and the need to report any further spotting or bleeding. Maternal vital signs are assessed as indicated based on her condition. Serial laboratory values are evaluated for the presence of falling hemoglobin/hematocrit and changes in coagulation studies. Fetal well-being is evaluated by the use of nonstress testing, biophysical profiles, and ultrasonography. Any indication of fetal compromise is reported immediately to the health care provider.

If active management is undertaken for placenta previa, the nurse continuously assesses maternal and fetal status while preparing the woman for surgery. Maternal vital signs are assessed frequently for decreasing blood pressure, rising pulse rate, changes in LOC, and oliguria. Fetal assessment is maintained by continuous electronic fetal monitoring to assess for signs of hypoxia.

Emotional support for the woman and her family is extremely important. If actively bleeding, the woman is concerned not only for her own well-being but for the well-being of her fetus. All procedures should be explained and a support person should be present.

If the woman is discharged home after stabilization to be managed conservatively following diagnosis of placenta previa, discharge teaching focuses on the prevention of further complications. The woman will know to notify her health care provider of any further spotting or

bleeding episodes and to be prepared to return to the hospital immediately. She must understand the importance of maintaining bedrest and the need for close follow-up.

Expected outcomes to be evaluated after birth are that the woman's laboratory values will return to normal, that she will be hemodynamically stable, and that she will be discharged without signs of complications.

If the fetus survived the initial insult, the expected outcome for the baby is to be discharged with the woman with no significant compromise. If the fetus died, the woman is referred as appropriate for follow-up care (see Plan of Care on p. 584).

Cord Insertion and Placental Variations

A *velamentous* insertion of the cord is a rare placental anomaly in which the cord vessels begin to branch at the membranes and then course onto the placenta (Fig. 21-12, *A*). Rupture of the membranes or traction on the cord may tear one or more of the fetal vessels. As a result the fetus may quickly bleed to death. *Battledore* (marginal) insertion of the cord (Fig. 21-12, *B*) increases the risk of fetal hemorrhage, especially following marginal separation of the placenta.

Rarely the placenta may be divided into two or more separate lobes, resulting in *succenturiate* placenta (Fig. 21-12, *C*). Blood vessels joining the lobes may be supported only by the fetal membranes and are therefore in danger of tearing during labor or during the birth of the baby or of the placenta. During expulsion of the pla-

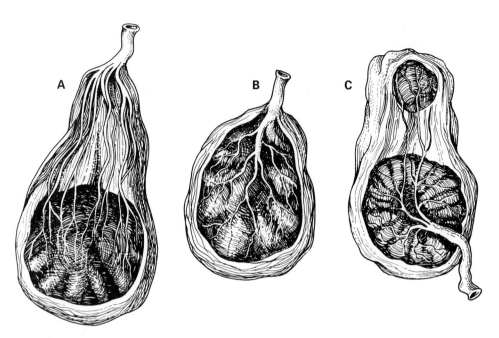

FIG. 21-12 Cord insertion and placental variations. **A,** Velamentous insertion of cord. **B,** Battledore placenta. **C,** Placenta succenturiate.

centa, one or more of the separate lobes may remain attached to the decidua basalis, preventing uterine contraction, and increasing the risk of postpartum hemorrhage.

Postpartum Hemorrhage

Postpartum hemorrhage, traditionally the loss of 500 ml of blood or more after vaginal birth, is the most common and most serious type of excessive obstetric blood loss. A more meaningful definition of postpartum hemorrhage is the loss of 1% or more of body weight, since 1 ml of blood weighs 1 g. Postpartum hemorrhage is a leading cause of maternal morbidity and mortality, accounting for approximately 10% of nonabortive maternal deaths. Approximately 8% of all births are complicated by postpartum hemorrhage (Murahata, 1991).

Postpartum hemorrhage may be sudden and even exsanguinating. Moderate but persistent bleeding may continue for days or weeks. Postpartum hemorrhage may be early, within the first 24 hours after birth, or late, from 24 hours after birth until the twenty-eighth postpartum day.

Control of bleeding from the placental site is accomplished by prolonged contraction and retraction of interlacing strands of myometrium, the living ligature. A firm or contracted uterus does not normally bleed after birth unless placenta previa had existed. Therefore careful assessment of uterine tone and the maintenance of uterine contractions through manual massage or oxytocic stimulation, as needed, are important parts of postpartum care.

Early postpartum hemorrhage almost invariably is caused by uterine atony, lacerations of the birth canal, or DIC. *Late postpartum hemorrhage* most commonly is

the result of subinvolution of the placental site, retained placental tissue, or infection.

It is helpful to consider the problem of excessive bleeding with reference to the stages of labor. From birth of the fetus until separation of the placenta the character and quantity of blood passed may suggest excessive bleeding. For example, *dark blood* is probably of venous origin, perhaps from varices or superficial lacerations of the birth canal. *Bright blood* is arterial and indicates, for example, deep lacerations of the cervix. *Spurts of blood* with clots may indicate partial placental separation. *Failure of blood to clot* or remain clotted is indicative of coagulopathy.

The period from the separation of the placenta to its expulsion may be when excessive bleeding occurs. This is the result of incomplete placental separation. After the placenta has been expelled, persistent or excessive blood loss usually is the result of atony of the uterus (i.e., its failure to contract well or maintain its contraction) or prolapse of the uterus into the pelvis.

Complications of postpartum hemorrhage are either immediate or delayed. Hemorrhagic (hypovolemic) shock and death may occur from sudden, exsanguinating hemorrhage. Delayed complications provoked by postpartum hemorrhage include anemia, puerperal infection, and thromboembolism.

Uterine Atony

Uterine atony is marked hypotonia of the uterus. Uterine atony occurs in at least 5% of births, particularly when the woman is a grand multipara. It also can occur with hydramnios, when the fetus is large, or after the births of a multifetal gestation. In such conditions the uterus is overstretched and contracts poorly. Other causes of atony include traumatic birth, use of halogenated anesthesia, magnesium sulfate, rapid or prolonged labor, chorioamnionitis, and use of oxytocin for labor induction or augmentation. Uterine atony is the principal cause of postpartum hemorrhage.

Lacerations of the Birth Canal

Lacerations of the birth canal are the second major cause of postpartum hemorrhage. Continued bleeding despite efficient postpartum uterine contractions demands inspection or reinspection of the birth passage. Continuous bleeding from so-called minor sources may be just as dangerous as a sudden loss of a large amount of blood, although often it is ignored until shock develops. Birth canal lacerations may include injuries to the labia, perineum, vagina, and cervix.

Factors that influence the causes and incidence of obstetric lacerations of the lower genital tract include operative birth; uncontrolled spontaneous birth; congenital abnormalities of the maternal soft parts; contracted pelvis; size, abnormal presentation, and position of the fetus; relative size of the presenting part and the birth canal; prior scarring from infection, injury, or surgery; vulvar, perineal, and vaginal varices; and abnormalities of uterine action, for example, precipitate birth.

Medical Management

The first step in the treatment of uterine bleeding is to elevate the uterus to determine if it is firmly contracted. The health care provider orders oxytocin, 20 to 40 units to 1 L of crystalloid to infuse at 10 to 15 ml per minute (Zahn, Yeomans, 1990); this infusion should be continued for at least 3 or 4 hours. If the uterus fails to respond to oxytocin, 0.2 mg of IM methylergonovine produces tetanic uterine contraction and is effective in treating hemorrhage from uterine atony. However, its use is contraindicated in the presence of hypertension. If methylergonovine fails or is contraindicated, 15-methyl PGF_{2a} becomes the oxytocic of choice. Most hemorrhage can be controlled after one or two injections of 0.25 mg IM; the majority of failures occur in women with chorioamnionitis (Baskett, Writer, 1991; Zahn, Yeomans, 1990). Blood transfusion for the treatment of shock may be urgently needed.

Retained Placenta

Nonadherent Retained Placenta

With no significant bleeding and with proper management the normally implanted placenta separates within 15 minutes of birth in about 90% of women; within 30 minutes 95% of women will have a separated placenta. If the placenta has not been recovered within 30 minutes of birth, most health care providers attempt to remove it manually. No supplementary anesthesia is needed for

parturients who have had regional anesthesia for birth. For other women, administration of light nitrous oxide and oxygen inhalation anesthesia or IV thiopental (Pentothal) facilitates intrauterine exploration, placental separation, and recovery of the placenta. If preterm birth occurs, placental retention is common.

Adherent Retained Placenta

Abnormal adherence of the placenta occurs for unknown reasons, but it is thought to be the result of zygote implantation in a zone of defective endometrium. There is no zone of separation between the placenta and the decidua. Abnormal adherence of the placenta is diagnosed in only about 1 of every 12,000 births. The mother with an abnormally attached placenta is at increased risk for postpartum hemorrhage leading to hypovolemic shock.

Unusual placental adherence may be partial or complete. The following degrees of attachment are recognized:

- *Placenta accreta (vera):* slight penetration of myometrium by placental trophoblast (unusual)
- *Placenta increta:* deep penetration by placenta (rare)
- *Placenta percreta (destruens):* perforation of uterus by placenta (exceptional)

At least 15% of cases of abnormally adherent placenta (all types) are associated with placenta previa (Zahn, Yeomans, 1990). The diagnosis of an abnormally adherent placenta generally is made when manual separation of a retained placenta is attempted. If the placenta does not separate readily (even a portion), immediate abdominal hysterectomy may be indicated.

Inversion of the Uterus

Inversion of the uterus (turning inside out) after birth is a potentially life-threatening complication. The incidence of uterine inversion is approximately 1 in 2500 births (Zahn, Yeomans, 1990). The inversion may be partial or complete. Fundal pressure and traction applied to the cord may result in inversion. Although proper management of the third stage of labor prevents the majority of uterine inversions, some are unavoidable. Regardless of the precipitating factor, once an inversion occurs prompt recognition and correction are necessary to reduce maternal morbidity and mortality.

Prevention—always the easiest, cheapest, and most effective therapy—is especially appropriate in the avoidance of puerperal uterine inversion. *One must not pull on the umbilical cord until the placenta has definitely separated.* Uterine inversion may occasionally recur in a subsequent birth.

Medical Management

Medical management of this condition involves all of the following interventions (Zahn, Yeomans, 1990):

1. Treatment of shock, which invariably is out of proportion to the blood loss. Oxytocic agents are

withheld until the uterus has been repositioned.
2. Replacement of the uterus, after the woman has received tocolysis or is under deep anesthesia. Oxytocics are ordered.
3. Abdominal or vaginal surgery may be necessary to reposition the uterus if manual replacement is unsuccessful.
4. Blood replacement therapy as indicated.

Also initiated are broad-spectrum antibiotic therapy and a nasogastric tube to minimize paralytic ileus.

Care Management—Postpartum Hemorrhage

Postpartum hemorrhage can progress rapidly to shock; therefore the nurse must assess the woman carefully and thoroughly. The woman's history should be reviewed for factors that would predispose to postpartum hemorrhage (Box 21-10). The bleeding should be assessed as to color, amount, and, if possible, source. Vital signs may not be reliable indicators of shock in the immediate postpartum period due to the increased blood volume of this period. Assessments include an evaluation for bladder distention because a distended bladder prevents uterine contraction.

Immediate care of the woman experiencing a postpartum hemorrhage includes assessment of vital signs and uterine consistency along with administration of oxytocin. Explanations are given to the patient regarding rationale for procedures and the need to act quickly.

The care of the woman who has suffered lacerations of the perineum is similar to that advocated for episiotomies, that is, analgesia as needed for pain, and heat or cold applications as necessary. *To avoid injury to the suture line, a woman with third- or fourth-degree lacerations is not given routine postpartum rectal suppositories or enemas.* Attention to diet and intake of fluids is emphasized, as well as oral stool softeners to assist her in reestablishing bowel habits.

The care of the woman experiencing an inversion of the uterus focuses on immediate stabilization of hemodynamic status. If the uterus has been replaced manually, care must be taken after birth to avoid aggressive fundal massage.

Hemorrhagic Shock

Hemorrhage is a major threat to the mother during the childbearing cycle. **Hemorrhagic shock** is an emergency situation in which the perfusion of body organs becomes severely compromised, and death may ensue. Aggressive treatment is necessary to prevent adverse sequelae (e.g., cellular death, fluid overload, shock lung, and oxygen toxicity).

Physiologic compensatory mechanisms are activated in response to hemorrhage. The adrenals release catecholamines, causing arterioles and venules in the skin, lungs, gastrointestinal tract, liver, and kidneys to constrict. The available blood flow is diverted to the brain and heart and away from other organs, including the uterus. If shock is prolonged, the continued reduction in cellular oxygenation results in an accumulation of lactic acid and acidosis. Acidosis (lowered serum pH) causes arteriole vasodilatation; venule vasoconstriction persists. A circular pattern is established: decreased perfusion, increased tissue anoxia and acidosis, edema formation, and pooling of blood further decrease the perfusion. Cellular death occurs.

Care Management—Hemorrhagic Shock

Hemorrhagic shock often occurs rapidly. During pregnancy however, the increased blood volume can mask early signs of shock. An early sign of shock in the pregnant woman is a mild tachycardia. As the shock state worsens, heart rate continues to increase with a corresponding decrease in blood pressure. If the woman is still pregnant, there is a shunting of blood from the placenta; nonreassuring fetal heart rate patterns may be the earliest sign of shock. As soon as a woman exhibits the signs and symptoms of shock (Table 21-8) the nurse summons assistance and equipment. The nurse should have standing orders to start IV fluids and know the type of infusion to use and laboratory tests to order. While waiting for the primary care provider, the nurse ensures a patent airway, which may include airway insertion, and facilitates oxygen administration. The nurse can elevate one of the patient's hips to avoid supine hypotensive syndrome. Trendelenburg's position (with head down and feet elevated) is not advised, since this position may interfere with cardiopulmonary function.

BOX 21-10

Risk Factors for Postpartum Hemorrhage

Cesarean birth
Birth of a large infant
Birth assisted by forceps or vacuum extractor
Overdistended uterus from hydramnios, multifetal gestations, large fetus
Intrauterine manipulation/manual removal of the placenta
Lacerations of the birth canal
Magnesium sulfate administration during labor or postpartum
Multiparity
Previous postbirth hemorrhage
Placental abruption, retained placental fragments
Pitocin-induced/augmented labor
Uterine atony
Uterine inversion
Uterine subinvolution

When the primary care provider arrives, the nurse helps with instituting and monitoring measures to increase tissue perfusion. To maintain circulating volume it is necessary to administer large volumes of fluid; a second intravenous line is started with a large-bore needle. The nurse should be prepared to assist with placement of a central venous or Swan-Ganz catheter if needed. Large amounts of crystalloids (lactated Ringer's or normal saline) expand plasma volume; however, they decrease the colloid oncotic pressure (COP). As COP decreases, the risk for pulmonary edema increases. To compensate for this, colloid solutions (albumin) should be used to balance the effect of volume and COP (Dorman, 1989). The nurse continues to monitor, assess, and record respirations, pulse, blood pressure, skin condition, urinary output, level of consciousness (LOC), and hemodynamic parameters (CVP or Swan-Ganz) to evaluate effectiveness of management (see Figs. 21-13 and 21-14).

Effective respiratory status is essential in that the body rids itself of excess acids by increasing the respiratory rate. Ventilatory assistance with oxygen and/or mechanical ventilation may be needed.

The pulse rate increases and becomes irregular as shock progresses in severity. In early stages of shock during pregnancy systolic blood pressure increases, whereas in later stages of shock the systolic blood pressure decreases. *In pregnancy, blood pressure is not a sensitive indicator of impending shock.* Because of the increased blood volume during pregnancy, up to a 30% blood loss can occur before signs of shock appear (Dorman, 1989). Nonreassuring fetal heart rate patterns usually occur before changes are seen in maternal vital signs.

Perfusion of the skin is sacrificed in the body's attempt to maintain blood flow to the heart and brain. Therefore the condition of the skin is a valuable index to the severity of shock. The nurse assesses the degree of ischemia or cyanosis of the nail beds, eyelids, and skin inside the mouth (buccal mucosa, gums, tongue). The nurse notes the degree of coolness and clamminess of the skin to palpation.

The nurse measures hourly urine output. Poor urinary output (less than 30 ml per hour) may indicate worsening of shock or inadequate fluid therapy; an increased output indicates improvement in the woman's condition.

The adequacy of cerebral perfusion may be estimated by an evaluation of the woman's level of consciousness. In early stages of decreased cerebral blood flow the woman may complain of "seeing stars," feeling dizzy, or feeling nauseated. She may become restless and orthopneic. As cerebral hypoxia increases, she may become confused and react slowly or not at all to stimuli. An improved sensorium is an indicator of improvement.

CVP readings measure the function (e.g., blood pressure) of the right side of the heart (Fig. 21-13). Normal values range between 1 and 7 cm H_2O (Clark et al, 1989). A low or falling value indicates inadequate blood volume or hypovolemia. A high or rising value indicates impaired contractility of the heart. A more precise method for evaluating hemodynamic status and heart function is by using a *Swan-Ganz (PA) catheter,* a multiple-lumen pulmonary artery (PA) catheter that measures both right- and left-side heart functions (Fig. 21-14). By inflating the balloon at the catheter tip one can measure the pulmonary artery wedge pressure

TABLE 21-8   Symptoms of Shock

	MILD	MODERATE	SEVERE	IRREVERSIBLE
Respirations	Rapid, deep	Rapid, becoming shallow	Rapid, shallow, may be irregular	Irregular, or barely perceptible
Pulse	Rapid, tone normal	Rapid, tone may be normal but is becoming weaker	Very rapid, easily collapsible, may be irregular	Irregular apical pulse
Blood pressure	Normal or hypertensive	60 to 90 mm Hg systolic	Below 60 mm Hg systolic	None palpable
Skin	Cool and pale	Cool, pale, moist, knees cyanotic	Cold, clammy, cyanosis of lips and fingernails	Cold, clammy, cyanotic
Urinary output	No change	Decreasing to 10 to 22 ml/hr (adult)	Oliguric (less than 10 ml) to anuric	Anuric
Level of consciousness	Alert, oriented, diffuse anxiety	Oriented, mental cloudiness or increasing restlessness	Lethargic, reacts to noxious stimuli, comatose	Does not respond to noxious stimuli
CVP	May be normal (1 to 7 cm H_2O)	3 cm H_2O	0 to 3 cm H_2O	

Modified from Royce JA: *Nurs Clin North Am* 8:377, 1973; Wagner MM, Clinical Nursing Specialist, University of Iowa Hospitals and Clinics.

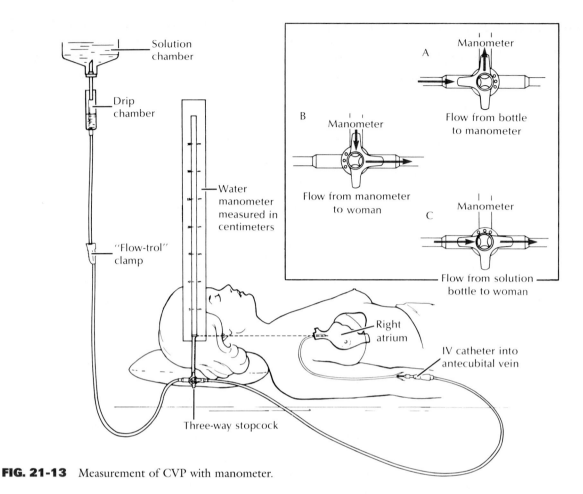

FIG. 21-13 Measurement of CVP with manometer.

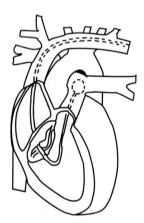

FIG. 21-14 Swan-Ganz pulmonary artery (PA) catheter.

(PAWP), an indicator of left-side heart function. In the hemodynamically compromised patient the ability to evaluate left-side heart function is important; left-sided failure precedes right-side heart failure by up to 12 hours. Normal values range between 6 and 10 mm Hg during pregnancy (Clark et al, 1989). Because pulmonary edema can occur at lower wedge pressures during preg-

nancy, the use of a PA catheter yields more useful information than only CVP readings.

Anxiety is contagious. The nurse's calm, confident manner, coupled with brief, simple explanations, is an important aspect of care.

Blood replacement therapy is not uncommon in the management of hemorrhage (Table 21-9). Common clinical symptoms of inadequate intravascular volume (hypovolemia) that necessitates blood replacement include the following:

1. Evidence of hemorrhage (loss of a large amount of blood externally or internally in a short time)
2. Evidence of hypovolemic shock (increasing pulse, cool clammy skin, rapid breathing, restlessness, reduced urine output)
3. Decrease in hemoglobin and hematocrit below acceptable level for trimester of pregnancy or the nonpregnant state

Aggressive fluid and blood replacement is not without risk.

The 24 hours after the shock period are critical. The nurse observes for fluid overload, shock lung, and oxygen toxicity (Table 21-10).

Transfusion reactions may follow administration of

TABLE 21-9   Replacement Clotting Factors

INFUSATE AND FACTORS	NEED	RISK	EXPECTED OUTCOME
Fresh-frozen plasma: clotting factors	Depleted clotting factors	Hepatitis B, HIV	Increase fibrinogen to 10 mg/dl per unit infused
Cryoprecipitate: I, V, VII, XIII	Fibrinogen concentration <50 mg/dl; a level of 50,000/mm^3 should be sought	Hepatitis, HIV	Increase fibrinogen 2 to 5 mg/dl to 10 mg/dl per unit infused
Platelet concentrate; platelets	<20,000/mm^3	Rhesus isoimmunization in Rh-negative women	Increase platelet count 7500 mm^3 per unit infused

blood or blood components. Even in an emergency, each must be checked per hospital protocol (see Legal Tip). Complications include hemolytic reactions, febrile reactions, allergic reactions, circulatory overload, and air embolism. Rapid transfusion with ice-cold blood can chill the heart and cause arrhythmia or arrest. It must be remembered that banked blood is calcium deficient, increasing the risk for arrhythmias and further bleeding.

LEGAL TIP: **Standard of Care for Seizures and Bleeding Emergencies**

The standard of care for obstetric emergency situations is that provision should be made for implementing independent nursing actions. Policies, procedures, and protocols for managing emergencies may include those relating to (1) seizures, (2) hemorrhage and shock, and (3) abruptio placentae.

Infection is another complication of hemorrhage. Causes may include surgical procedures, multiple pelvic examinations, anemia, and loss of the WBC component of the blood.

Clotting Disorders in Pregnancy
Normal Clotting

Normally there is a delicate balance (homeostasis) maintained between two opposing systems, the hemostatic system and the fibrinolytic system. The *hemostatic system* is involved in the life-saving process by stopping the flow of blood from injured vessels, in part through the formation of insoluble fibrin that acts as a hemostatic platelet plug. The phases of the coagulation process involve an interaction of the coagulation factors in which each factor sequentially activates the factor next in line in the so-called cascade effect sequence. The *fibrinolytic system* refers to the process by which the fibrin is split into fibrin degradation products (FDPs) and circulation is restored.

A history of abnormal bleeding, inheritance of unusual bleeding tendencies, and a report of significant ab-

TABLE 21-10   Hazards of Shock Therapy

HAZARD	NURSING ACTION
Fluid overload: moist respirations, stridor, or dyspnea	Alert health care provider, decrease the drip rate
Shock lung: tachypnea, dyspnea, anxiety, a rise in blood pressure, cyanosis, and harsh loud breaths	Alert health care provider, maintain ventilator between 50 and 70 mm Hg
Oxygen toxicity: muscular twitching about the face, followed by convulsions resembling grand mal seizures	Alert health care provider; take convulsion precautions

errations of laboratory findings indicate a bleeding or clotting problem. Table 21-11 describes the tests that are used to determine mechanisms for the control of bleeding, that is, the function of platelets and the necessary clotting factors.

Disseminated Intravascular Coagulation

Disseminated intravascular coagulation (DIC, defibrination syndrome, defibrination coagulopathy, consumptive coagulopathy) is a pathologic form of clotting that is diffuse and consumes large amounts of clotting factors, causing widespread external and/or internal bleeding. Simply, DIC is an overzealous consumption of clotting factors (Dorman, 1989).

Physical examination reveals unusual bleeding. Spontaneous bleeding from the woman's gums or nose may be noted. Petechiae may appear around the blood pressure cuff on her arm. Excessive bleeding may occur from the site of trauma (e.g., venipuncture sites, injection sites,

TABLE 21-11 Coagulation Tests

TEST	COMMENTS
Activated partial thromboplastin time (PTT: measures intrinsic system): 25 to 36 sec	Screening test of choice; very sensitive, relatively easy to perform, inexpensive; all coagulation factors except proconvertin are measured
One-stage prothrombin time (PT: Quick's test: measures extrinsic system): 9.5 to 11.3 sec	Test for proconvertin (VII), proaccelerin (V), Stuart-Prower factor (X), prothrombin (II), and fibrinogen deficiencies; unfortunately, it does not measure factors necessary for earlier stages of coagulation
Thrombin time (plasma): 10 to 15 sec	Test measures conversion of fibrinogen to fibrin and depends on concentration of fibrinogen or inhibitors such as fibrin split-products, antithrombins, and heparin
Platelet count: 150,000 to 300,000/ mm^3	*Most reliable index for DIC*
Specific factor assays (e.g., plasma fibrinogen): 195 to 365 mg/dl	Each coagulation factor can be assessed by indirect clotting method using natural or synthetic factor-deficient substrates and compared with activity of normal plasma (100%); however, fibrinogen is only factor that can be measured directly by chemical method
Bleeding time Template: 2 to 8 min Ivy: 1 to 7 min Duke: 1 to 3 min	Finger or earlobe puncture 5 mm deep and 2 mm wide (Bard-Parker blade No. 11) is made after antiseptic preparation of skin; note time of puncture: touch bleeding point gently with sterile filter paper to absorb blood every 30 sec until bleeding stops

nicks from shaving of perineum or abdomen, injury from insertion of urinary catheter). Maternal symptoms may include tachycardia and diaphoresis. Laboratory tests reveal decreased platelets, fibrinogen, and prothrombin (the factors consumed during coagulation). Fibrinolysis is first increased but later is severely depressed. Breakdown of fibrin increases the accumulation of fibrin degradation (fibrin split) products in the blood. Fibrin degradation products have anticoagulant properties and thus prolong PT. Bleeding time is normal; coagulation time shows no clot; clot retraction time shows no clot; and PTT is increased.

The primary management of all cases of DIC involves correction of the underlying cause, for example, removal of the dead fetus, treatment of existing infection or preeclampsia-eclampsia, or removal of a placental abruption. Packed RBCs may be transfused to correct anemia. Deficiencies secondary to DIC primarily involve platelets, factors V and VIII, fibrinogen, and prothrombin. Administration of fresh frozen plasma (FFP) in combination with platelet concentrates is effective in all these conditions when replacement therapy is warranted (Dorman, 1989).

Renal failure is one consequence of DIC; therefore urinary output is monitored. Output must be maintained at more than 30 ml per hour, and supportive measures are initiated. Oxygen is administered by a tight-fitting rebreathing mask at 10 to 12 L per minute.

The emotional needs of the family are recognized and supported. Anxiety, grief, and altered self-concept can result from fetal or maternal loss.

Maternal and fetal prognosis depends on the degree and extent of the underlying disorder as well as the response of the woman to prompt and proper treatment. Maternal risk is further increased if the fetus dies in utero.

Other Clotting Disorders

Autoimmune thrombocytopenic purpura (ATP) is an autoimmune disorder in which antiplatelet antibodies decrease the life span of the platelets. Thrombocytopenia, capillary fragility, and increased bleeding time are diagnostic.

ATP may result in severe hemorrhage after cesarean birth or from cervical or vaginal lacerations. The incidence of postpartum uterine bleeding or vaginal hematomas is also increased in ATP.

Platelet transfusions are given to maintain the platelet count at 100,000/mm^3. Corticosteroids are given if the diagnosis is made before or during pregnancy. Splenectomy, if needed, is deferred until after the puerperium. Neonatal thrombocytopenia, a result of the maternal disease process, occurs in about 50% of the cases and is associated with a high mortality.

von Willebrand's disease, a type of hemophilia, is probably the most common of all hereditary bleeding disorders (Cunningham et al, 1993). It results from a factor VIII deficiency and platelet dysfunction. It is transmitted as an incomplete autosomal dominant trait to both sexes. Although von Willebrand's disease is rare, it is one of the most common congenital clotting defects in American women of childbearing age. Since factor VIII increases during pregnancy, this increase may be sufficient to offset danger from hemorrhage during childbirth. However, the woman should be observed for at least 1 week postpartum. Treatment of von Willebrand's disease consists of replacement of factor VIII through administration of cryoprecipitate or fresh frozen plasma.

MATERNAL INFECTIONS

Infections in pregnancy are responsible for significant morbidity and mortality. The direct financial costs of disease can be substantial. Indirect costs can be as startling and are much more difficult to measure. Some consequences of maternal infection last a lifetime, such as infertility and sterility. Psychosocial sequelae may include altered interpersonal relationships and lowered self-esteem. Other conditions, such as a congenitally acquired infection, often affect a child's length and quality of life.

Pregnancy generally is regarded as an immunosuppressed condition. Altered immune responses in pregnancy may decrease maternal ability to fight infection. In addition, genital tract changes also may affect susceptibility. These intravaginal changes, accompanied by decreasing vaginal pH, may contribute to increased susceptibility (Brunham et al, 1990).

Education and counseling are important aspects of care for the prevention of maternal infections. Adolescent mothers are at high risk because of earlier onset of intercourse and increased likelihood of multiple partners. The recent trend of exchanging sex for drugs is contributing to a rise in infection rates, especially among urban, poor, and minority women (Aral, Holmes, 1990). The prevention of disease and the reduction of maternal and neonatal effects continue to be monumental challenges.

Sexually Transmitted Disease

The term **sexually transmitted disease (STD)** reflects the definition as any microbe that is passed from one person to another through close, intimate contact (Spense, 1989) (Box 21-11).

Chlamydial Infections

Chlamydial infections are epidemic in the United States. *Chlamydia trachomatis,* the most common sexually transmitted bacterial pathogen, is responsible for substantial morbidity, personal suffering, and heavy economic burden. Estimated cost exceeds $1.5 billion per year (Schachter, 1989). An estimated 3 to 5 million adults are infected each year; however, infection with *C. trachomatis* is not a reportable STD. Difficulty in diagnosis, limited screening resources, and inadequate follow-up affect disease reporting.

C. trachomatis can exist only within living cells, and transmission occurs by direct sexual contact or exposure at birth. Fifteen known immunotypes of *C. trachomatis* are responsible for adult and neonatal infections (Bourcier, Seidler, 1987; Marvin, Slevin, 1987).

BOX 21-11

Sexually Transmitted Diseases

BACTERIAL
Chlamydia
Gonorrhea
Syphilis
Chancroid
Lymphogranuloma venereum
Gardnerella
Shigellosis
Salmonellosis
Genital mycoplasmas
Group B streptococci

VIRAL
Human immunodeficiency virus
Herpes simplex virus, types 1 and 2
Cytomegalovirus
Viral hepatitis, A and B
Human papillomavirus

PROTOZOAL
Trichomoniasis
Giardiasis
Amebiasis

PARASITIC
Pediculosis
Scabies

FUNGAL
Candidiasis

Definitive laboratory diagnosis is possible with tissue culture (McGregor, 1989). However, it is expensive, requires skill to perform, and requires 4 to 7 days for results. There are two antigen detection methods: (1) a direct immunofluorescent test (e.g., MicroTrak), which requires a fluorescent microscope and takes 30 minutes, and (2) an enzyme-linked immunosorbent assay (ELISA) test (e.g., Chlamydiazyme), which gives a color signal in 4 hours. The 30-minute test is more appropriate for screening low-risk populations, whereas the ELISA test is used for high-risk populations.

Populations at risk have been identified (Centers for Disease Control [CDC], 1993; Marvin, Slevin, 1987). The sexually active female under 20 years of age is two to three times more likely to become infected than are women between 20 and 29. Women over 30 have the lowest rate. Women and men with multiple sexual partners are at highest risk. People who do not use barrier methods of birth control (condom, spermicide, diaphragm) have a high incidence.

The CDC guidelines recommend screening the populations at risk, treating all those who are presumably infected, and educating the medical profession and public. Combination antibiotic therapy is recommended for heterosexual men and women infected with gonorrhea because 20% to 50% harbor *C. trachomatis.* Priority groups for screening are high-risk pregnant women, adolescents, and women with multiple sexual partners (CDC, 1993).

Infections often are asymptomatic, although women usually have a history of mucopurulent discharge and bleeding resulting from inflammation and erosion of cervical columnar epithelium. Dysuria and other urinary tract discomfort, as well as dyspareunia may occur.

The role of *C. trachomatis* in spontaneous abortion, preterm birth, low birth weight, and postpartum endometritis needs further investigation (Brunham, Holmes, and Embree 1990). Fetal or neonatal effects are common. Stillbirth and neonatal death are 10 times more common than in noninfected women (Schachter, 1989). Aftereffects of the infection include salpingitis, ectopic pregnancy, pelvic inflammatory disease (PID), infertility, and sterility.

Preferred antimicrobial treatment of urethral, cervical, and rectal chlamydial infections is with doxycycline or azithromycin. If the woman is pregnant, erythromycin is used, and all sexual partners should be tested and treated (CDC, 1993).

Gonorrhea

Gonorrhea is caused by *Neisseria gonorrhoeae,* a type of diplococcus bacteria. Although gonorrhea is an STD, it also is spread by direct contact with infected lesions and indirectly by transfer from inanimate objects, or *fomites.* Self-inoculation with contaminated hands is common.

Gonorrhea often produces only mild symptoms in women, or may persist unsuspected in the lower genital tract. The incubation period is 2 to 5 days. Symptoms of lower urogenital tract infection include dysuria and frequency, heavy green-yellow purulent discharge at the cervical os, cervical tenderness, vulvovaginitis, bartholinitis, dyspareunia, and postcoital bleeding. Swollen and painful Bartholin's glands and tender lymph nodes in the groin usually accompany infection. Lower abdominal pain, cervical tenderness, fever, nausea, and vomiting are accompanying symptoms. Anorectal infection is diagnosed by local inflammation, burning, and pruritus. Oropharyngeal infection may be asymptomatic or result in inflammation and sore throat. Systemic infection results in gonococcemia, skin rashes, arthritis, pericarditis, and meningitis.

Increasing evidence suggests that antepartum gonococcal infection may be related to preterm birth, premature or prolonged rupture of membranes, and chorioamnionitis (Brunham, Holmes, and Embree, 1990). Postnatal maternal complications of untreated gonorrhea include gonococcal endometritis, acute salpingitis, dermatitis, and arthritis.

Ceftriaxone in a single dose is recommended for treatment. Spectinomycin is the preferred alternative therapy. Among high-risk women, especially those with multiple partners, numerous STDs are common. Therefore prac-

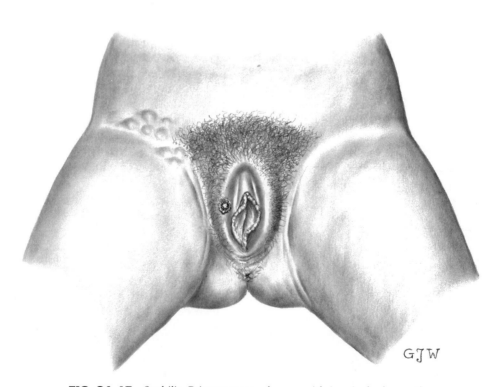

FIG. 21-15 Syphilis. Primary stage: chancre with inguinal adenopathy.

titioners suggest testing for and treating chlamydial infection and syphilis if maternal history warrants. All sexual partners should be treated and condom use encouraged for oral and genital intercourse.

Syphilis

Syphilis is caused by the spirochete *Treponema pallidum* after an incubating period of several weeks. The incidence of syphilis in the United States is increasing and has serious sequelae during pregnancy.

Several methods of clinical assessment of syphilis are available. Any test for antibodies may not be reactive in the presence of active infection because it takes time for the body's immune system to develop antibodies to any antigen.

Nonspecific serologic tests used for screening purposes are of two types: complement fixation (Kolmer, Wasserman) and flocculation (Kahn, RPR [rapid plasma reagin], Venereal Disease Research Laboratories [VDRL]). VDRL test results are not positive until 10 to 90 days after infection. Therefore infection may exist in the presence of a negative result from the VDRL test. If the antibodies in the newborn have been acquired from the mother, titers should drop to zero by 3 months. False positive results may occur if the newborn has an acute infection of any kind or a collagen disease. Even in the presence of a syphilitic infection a false negative result may occur, for example, if the mother became infected late in pregnancy. A false positive result may occur in the presence of heroin dependence.

Specific tests for treponemal antigen are more expensive and are used for differential diagnosis. These tests include *T. pallidum* immobilization (TPI), fluorescent treponemal antibody absorption (FTA-ABS), and fluorescent treponemal antibody absorption, immunoglobulin M (FTA-ABS IgM). The FTA-ABS IgM is most specific for neonatal syphilis; a positive result is especially valuable in diagnosis of the condition in the symptom-free child.

Pregnancy does not alter the progression of syphilis (Fig. 21-15). Primary and secondary stages of untreated syphilis lead to stillbirth. Latent and tertiary stages of untreated syphilis lead to secondary syphilis (congenital syphilis) in the newborn.

Penicillin is preferred for the treatment of syphilis. In penicillin-allergic persons, alternate choices include tetracycline or doxycycline, erythromycin, and ceftriaxone. Tetracycline is contraindicated in pregnancy because of its effects on liver function in the mother and tooth discoloration and decreased bone growth in the fetus.

Human Immunodeficiency Virus/Acquired Immunodeficiency Syndrome

Transmission of *human immunodeficiency virus (HIV)*, a retrovirus, occurs primarily through the exchange of body fluids (e.g., blood, semen, perinatal events) (Friedland, Klein, 1987; Hecht, 1987; Landesman et al, 1987). Severe depression of the cellular immune system characterizes *acquired immunodeficiency syndrome (AIDS)*. Although the populations at high risk have been well documented, all women should be assessed for the possibility of HIV exposure. HIV infection in women commonly is reported at a later stage in the disease, and they usually enter the hospital for initiation of treatment when the illness is more severe. The delay may be due in part to the occurrence of symptoms different from those of men (Bendell, Efantis-Potter, 1992). Chronic vaginitis and candidiasis are common presenting problems.

Once HIV enters the body, seroconversion to HIV positivity occurs within the first 10 weeks of exposure. Although seroconversion may be totally asymptomatic, it usually is accompanied by a viremic, influenza-type response to initial HIV infection. Symptoms include fever, malaise, myalgias, nausea, diarrhea, sore throat, and rash and may persist for 2 to 3 weeks.

Laboratory studies may reveal leukopenia, thrombocytopenia, anemia, and an elevated erythrocyte sedimentation rate. In addition, HIV has a strong affinity for surface-marker proteins on T-lymphocytes. This affinity of HIV for T-lymphocytes leads to significant T-cell destruction. T helper cell titers of less than 400 cells/mm^3 are associated with a more rapid progression to AIDS.

Delay in diagnosis must be avoided when the woman is pregnant. Pregnancy is not encouraged with positive HIV status; preconception counseling is recommended. Exposure to the virus has a significant impact on the woman's pregnancy and newborn feeding method and on the newborn's health status. It is hypothesized that HIV from infected women is transmitted to the fetus and newborn in three ways: (1) to the fetus as early as the first trimester via maternal circulation; (2) to the infant during labor and birth by inoculation or ingestion of maternal blood and other infected fluids; (3) to the infant through breast milk (ACOG, 1992a; Bendell, Efantis-Potter, 1992). Infants born to seropositive mothers seem to be at greater risk for an HIV infection and AIDS than are infants born to seronegative mothers who later show seroconversion.

Prenatal Period

The incidence of HIV in pregnant women is expected to increase (ACOG, 1992a). The health history, physical examination, and laboratory testing must reflect this expectation if women and their newborns are to receive appropriate care. Those who fall into the high-risk category for HIV infection include (1) women and partners from geographic areas where HIV is prevalent; (2) women and partners who use intravenous drugs; (3) women with persistent and recurrent STDs; (4) women who received blood transfusions between 1978 and 1985; (5) any woman who believes she may have been exposed to HIV. Information about HIV and the availability of HIV testing should be offered to high-risk women at their initial entry into prenatal care. Testing is voluntary and requires informed consent. A negative result on the first prenatal HIV test is not a guarantee for continued negative titers (see Ethical Considerations).

Prenatal testing also can reveal gonorrhea, syphilis, prolonged and persistent episodes of herpes, *C. trachomatis,* hepatitis B, *Mycobacterium tuberculosis,* candidiasis (oropharyngeal or chronic vaginal infection), cytomegalovirus (CMV), and toxoplasmosis. About half of AIDS sufferers have elevated CMV titers.

History of vaccinations and immune status is documented. The titers for chickenpox and rubella are determined, and tuberculosis skin testing (purified protein derivative [PPD]) is done. Previous vaccination with Recombivax HB vaccine is noted because the vaccine once contained human blood products.

The woman may be a candidate for receiving $Rh_o(D)$ immune globulin. Transmission of HIV has not been traced to the Rh vaccine (Francis, Chin, 1987).

Some prenatal discomforts (e.g., fatigue, anorexia, and weight loss) mimic signs and symptoms of HIV infection. Differential diagnosis of all pregnancy-induced complaints and symptoms of infections is warranted. Major signs of worsening HIV infection include a weight loss of greater than 10% of prepregnancy body weight, chronic diarrhea for longer than 1 month, and fever (intermittent or constant) for longer than 1 month.

To support any pregnant woman's immune system, appropriate counseling is provided for optimum nutrition, sleep, rest, exercise, and stress reduction. If HIV infection is diagnosed, the woman is advised of the possible consequences for her infant. If she chooses to continue the pregnancy, she is counseled regarding safer sex techniques (Box 21-12). Use of condoms and nonoxynol 9 spermicide is encouraged to minimize further exposure to HIV if her partner is the source. Orogenital sex is discouraged. As necessary, the woman is referred for drug rehabilitation to discontinue substance abuse. Abuse of alcohol or other drugs compromises the body's immune system and increases the risk for AIDS and associated conditions: (1) HIV may require the presence of an already damaged immune system before it can cause disease; (2) alcohol and drugs interfere with many medical and alternative therapies for AIDS; (3) alcohol and drugs affect the judgment of the user, who may become more prone to engage in activities that place persons at high risk for AIDS or increase exposure to HIV; and (4) alcohol and drug abuse causes stress, including sleep problems, which harms the functioning of the immune system.

Pharmacologic treatment for HIV infection has progressed rapidly since the discovery of the virus. The primary drug approved for treatment of HIV infection is 3′ azido-3′-deoxythymidine (zidovudine, AZT [Retrovir]). Although this medication shows promise for treatment of HIV infection, its use in pregnancy has been limited because of the potentially toxic or mutagenic effects on the fetus. Azidothymidine is being tested in some controlled studies with pregnant women who have T-helper cell counts of less than 400 cells/mm³ and has been found to significantly reduce the risk of HIV transmission from an infected woman to her fetus (Boyer et al, 1994). Unfortunately funding sources to make the drug available to HIV positive pregnant women is a problem. Other opportunistic infections that persist concurrently with HIV infection are treated with medications specific to the infection.

Intrapartum Period

Care of the woman in labor is not substantially altered by asymptomatic infection with HIV. The mode of birth is based only on obstetric considerations because the virus crosses the placenta early in pregnancy.

The primary focus is the prevention of *nosocomial* spread of HIV and the protection of care providers. The risk of transmission of HIV is considered to be low during vaginal birth despite the exposure to the infected woman's blood, amniotic fluid, and vaginal secretions.

External electronic fetal monitoring (EFM) is preferred if monitoring is needed. There is a possibility of

 ETHICAL CONSIDERATIONS

CONFIDENTIALITY

Although confidentiality in the nurse-patient relationship is a basic ethical belief, sometimes the nurse is faced with a decision of whether to notify the sexual or IV needle partner who is placed at risk by the HIV-positive woman. This is an ethical dilemma involving personal and professional values regarding the issue of the patient's rights to privacy and requires careful values clarification and discussion.

BOX 21-12

"Safer" Sex

- "Safer" sex is possible only if there is no oral or genital exchange of body fluids.
- Correct use of condoms, while greatly reducing risk, is not exclusively protective.
- Use of spermicides containing nonoxynol 9 may offer additional protection.
- Select sexual partners with extreme care.
- Ask partner about history of STDs.

inoculation of the virus into the neonate if fetal scalp blood sampling is done or if a fetal scalp electrode is applied. In addition, the one who performs either of these procedures is placed at risk by accidental sticks to the finger.

Postpartum Period

Little is known of the clinical course during the postpartum period for the woman infected with HIV. Although the immediate postpartum period has not been noted to be significant, longer follow-up has revealed a high frequency of clinical illness in mothers whose children develop disease (Minkoff et al, 1987a, b; Scott et al, 1985). Counseling may be required regarding placement of children if the parents are no longer able to care for themselves (Bendell, Efantis-Potter, 1992).

Regardless of whether infection is diagnosed, the nursing process is implemented in a culturally sensitive and humane manner. "HIV infection is a biologic event, not a moral comment. It is vital to remember, to model,

and to teach that [personal] reactions to particular lifestyles, practices, or behaviors must not influence [the nurse's] ability to provide objective, compassionate, and effective health care to all" (Keeling, 1987).

The newborn can be with the mother, however, breastfeeding is usually contraindicated. Universal precautions should be implemented for both the mother and newborn, as they are with all patients. The woman and her infant are referred to primary care providers who are experienced in the treatment of AIDS and associated conditions.

TORCH Infections

*T*oxoplasmosis, *o*ther infections (e.g., hepatitis), *r*ubella virus, *c*ytomegalovirus, and *h*erpes simplex viruses, known collectively as *TORCH infections,* comprise a group of organisms capable of crossing the placenta and adversely affecting the development of the fetus. TORCH infections and their maternal and fetal effects are outlined in Table 21-12.

TABLE 21-12   Maternal Infection: TORCH

INFECTION	MATERNAL EFFECTS	FETAL OR NEONATAL EFFECTS	COUNSELING PREVENTION, IDENTIFICATION, AND MANAGEMENT
Toxoplasmosis (protozoa)	Acute infection: similar to influenza; lymphadenopathy	With maternal acute infection: parasitemia Less likely to occur with maternal chronic infection Abortion likely with acute infection early in pregnancy	Avoid eating raw meat and exposure to litter used by infected cats; if cats in house, have toxoplasma titer checked If titer is rising during early pregnancy, abortion may be considered an option
Other: Hepatitis A (infectious hepatitis) (virus)	Abortion—cause of liver failure during pregnancy Fever, malaise, nausea, and abdominal discomfort	Exposure during first trimester: fetal anomalies; fetal or neonatal hepatitis; preterm birth; intrauterine fetal death	Usually spread by droplet or hand contact especially by culinary workers; gamma-globulin can be given as prophylaxis for hepatitis A
Hepatitis B (serum hepatitis) (virus)	May be transmitted sexually. Symptoms variable: fever, rash, arthralgia, depressed appetite, dyspepsia, abdominal pain, generalized aching, malaise, weakness, jaundice, tender and enlarged liver	Infection occurs during birth Maternal vaccination during pregnancy should present no risk for fetus; however, data are not available	Generally passed by contaminated needles, syringes, or blood transfusions; also can be transmitted orally or by coitus, but incubation period is longer; hepatitis B immune globulin can be given prophylactically after exposure Hepatitis B vaccine recommended for populations at risk; vaccine consists of series of 3 IM doses.

Continued.

TABLE 21-12   Maternal Infection: TORCH—cont'd

INFECTION	MATERNAL EFFECTS	FETAL OR NEONATAL EFFECTS	COUNSELING PREVENTION, IDENTIFICATION, AND MANAGEMENT
Hepatitis B (serum hepatitis) (virus)			Populations at risk: women from Asia, Pacific islands, Haiti, sub-Africa, Alaska (women of Eskimo descent); other women at risk include health care providers, intravenous drug users, those sexually active with multiple partners and single partner having multiple risks
Rubella (3-day German measles, virus)	Rash, fever, mild symptoms; suboccipital lymph nodes may be swollen; some photophobia Occasionally arthritis or encephalitis Spontaneous abortion	Incidence of congenital anomalies: first month, 50%; second month, 25%, third month, 10%, fourth month, 4% Exposure during first 2 months: malformations of heart, eyes, ears, or brain, abnormal dermatoglyphics Exposure after fourth month: systemic infection, hepatosplenomegaly, intrauterine growth retardation, rash At 15 to 20 years of age, the affected child may experience deterioration of intellect and development or may develop epilepsy	Vaccination of pregnant women contraindicated; pregnancy should be prevented for 3 months after vaccination; pregnant women nonreactive to hemagglutinin-inhibition antigen can be safely vaccinated after the birth
Cytomegalovirus (CMV) (a herpes virus)	Respiratory or sexually transmitted asymptomatic illness or mononucleosis-like syndrome: may have cervical discharge	Fetal or neonatal death or severe, generalized disease—hemolytic anemia and jaundice: hydrocephaly or microcephaly; pneumonitis; hepatosplenomegaly	Virus may be reactivated and cause disease in utero or during birth in subsequent pregnancies: fetal infection may occur during passage through infected birth canal; disease is commonly progressive through infancy and childhood
Herpes genitalis (herpes simplex virus, type 2 [HSV-2])	See discussion that follows cytomegalovirus		

Toxoplasmosis

Toxoplasmosis is a protozoan infection associated with the consumption of raw meat or poor hand washing after handling raw meat or infected cat litter. Pregnant women with HIV antibodies are at risk because toxoplasmosis is one of the common accompanying opportunistic infections. The presence of toxoplasmosis can be determined with blood studies, and women in at-risk groups should have toxoplasmosis titers evaluated. Acute infection in pregnancy produces influenza-like symptoms and lymphadenopathy. The pharmaceutic treatment of choice for toxoplasmosis is spiramycin; sulfa (and clindamycin in sulfa-allergic women) is also used (ACOG, 1993).

Other Infections

The primary infection included in this category is hepatitis. *Hepatitis A,* or *infectious* hepatitis, is a virus spread by droplets and is associated with poor hand washing after defecation. Pregnancy effects include spontaneous abortion and influenza-like symptoms. If exposure to the fetus occurs in the first trimester and is untreated, possible effects include fetal anomalies, preterm birth, fetal or neonatal hepatitis, and intrauterine fetal death. Gamma globulin vaccination is given to mothers and newborns for prophylaxis.

Hepatitis B, or *serum hepatitis,* is a virus transmitted in a manner similar to that of HIV. Routes of transmission include contaminated needles, syringes or blood products, sexual intercourse, and body fluid exchange. When maternal infection occurs in the first trimester, up to 10% of neonates will be seropositive for the hepatitis B surface antigen (HBsAg). If the woman is acutely infected in the third trimester, 80% to 90% of the neonates will be infected (ACOG, 1992d).

The CDC and ACOG recommend hepatitis B virus screening for all pregnant women at an early prenatal visit. Women at risk should be given the hepatitis B vaccine. If she is exposed to the hepatitis B virus before she is able to be vaccinated, she should initially receive passive immunization with hepatitis B immune globulin (HBIG) and then undergo the vaccination series. Pregnancy is not a contraindication to vaccination (ACOG, 1992d).

Rubella

Rubella, also known as German measles, is a viral infection transmitted by droplets. Fever, rash, and mild lymphedema usually are seen in an infected mother. Consequences for the fetus are much more serious and include spontaneous abortion, congenital anomalies (referred to as congenital rubella syndrome), and death. Preventing maternal rubella infection and its subsequent fetal effects is the major focus of rubella immunization programs (ACOG, 1992c). Vaccination of pregnant women is contraindicated because a rubella infection may develop after the vaccine is administered. As part of preconception counseling or during the postpartum stay, rubella vaccine is given to women who are not rubella immune, and they are counseled to use contraception for at least 3 months after vaccination.

Cytomegalovirus

Cytomegalovirus (CMV) is the primary cause of congenital viral infection in the fetus and neonate and is the most common infectious cause of mental retardation. Infectious viral sources include saliva, urine, semen, breast milk, blood, and cervical/vaginal secretion. CMV also has been isolated from placental tissue. Most primary CMV infections are asymptomatic, and most women who show CMV infection in pregnancy (by positive titers) have a chronic or recurrent infection (Brunham, Holmes, and Embree, 1990). No effective pharmacologic treatment exists for CMV; therapies focus on treatment of symptoms.

Herpes Simplex Virus

Herpes simplex virus type 1 (HSV-1) infections predominate during childhood. The virus is transmitted primarily by contact with oral secretions and causes cold sores and fever blisters. HSV-2 infections usually occur after puberty as sexual activity increases. HSV-2 is transmitted primarily by contact with genital secretions. Public health experts believe that within the United States 10 to 40 million people carry the HSV-2. Many genital infections show a mixture of HSV-1 and HSV-2.

HSV interacts with epithelial or neuroepithelial cells and neurons. The incubation period is between 2 and 4 weeks. During the initial infection, HSV migrates to one or more sensory nerve ganglia, where it remains latent and dormant indefinitely (Fig. 21-16, *A*). An intact immune system cures the infection at the place of entry. The *primary* infection involves mucocutaneous cells; recurrent infection involves stratified epithelial cells. Stressor stimuli trigger recurrent infection (Fig. 21-16, *B*). Fever, another infection, emotions, menstruation, intercourse, and ultraviolet light are some common stressors. Infections seem to be more severe in the woman during pregnancy.

HSV infections may involve external genitals, the vagina, and cervix. Symptoms are more pronounced with first infections of HSV. Painful blisters form (Fig. 21-17), rupture, and then drain, leaving shallow ulcers that crust over and disappear after 2 to 6 weeks. A vaginal discharge is seen if the cervix or vaginal mucosa is involved. The woman may have fever, malaise, anorexia, painful inguinal lymphadenopathy, dysuria, and dyspareunia. Recurrences sometimes are preceded by itching, a burning sensation in the genital area, tingling in the legs, or a slight increase in vaginal discharge.

The pregnancy effects of primary genital herpes infection include spontaneous abortion, preterm labor, and IUGR. The likelihood of a poor outcome increases with advancing gestational age. The frequency and severity of recurrent infection also appear to increase with gestation (Brown, Baker, 1989).

The route of HSV transmission from mother to newborn is via an infected birth canal during birth. The risk of maternal-infant transmission is greater during a primary HSV-2 infection than during a recurrent episode (Corey, 1990). Cesarean birth is no longer recommended for all mothers with HSV because transplacental infection can occur. Only those mothers with clinical evidence of *active lesions* should give birth abdominally (Corey, 1990).

Acyclovir has been used since 1977 to treat life-threatening HSV infections in adults and newborns. When used for primary infections, it decreases the duration of viral shedding, pain, new lesion formation, and

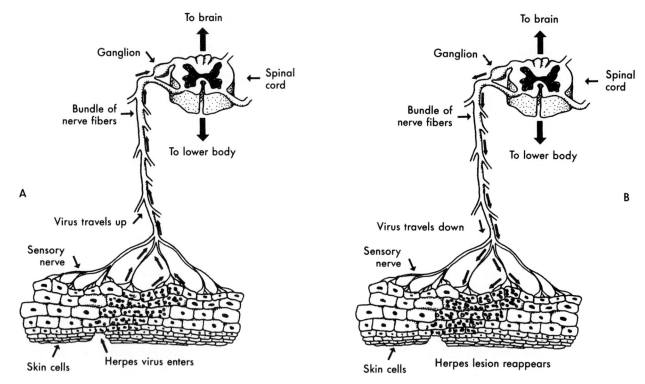

FIG. 21-16 **A,** Initial herpes infection takes place when virus *(color dots)* enters cells of mucous membranes, eyes, or skin. They reproduce and travel up *(colored arrows)* sensory nerves until they reach ganglion (cluster of nerve cell bodies). There they are protected by body's immune system, which overcomes infection at place of entry. **B,** Though entry wound soon heals, when conditions allow, virus may later travel back down nerve pathway to reinfect skin cells again.

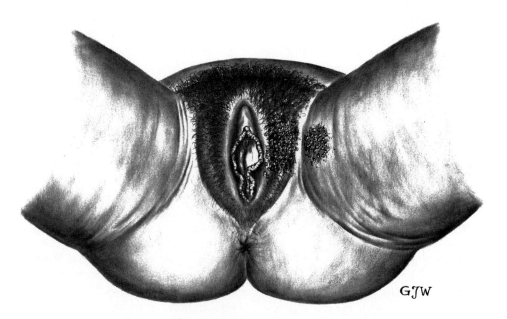

FIG. 21-17 Herpes genitalis.

time to complete healing; it is effective in suppressing recurrences with long-term use. Data are not clear regarding safety or efficacy in pregnancy (Brown, Baker, 1989).

Infection control measures are an important part of treatment. Thorough hand washing should be practiced by health care providers as well as by family members. Gloves should be worn during contact with lesions or secretions. Family members with oral lesions should be discouraged from kissing the newborn. Instruction on genital hygiene and prevention of infection also should be given (Box 21-13).

Health care providers with HSV infections also should take precautions. Anyone with oral HSV lesions should wear a mask if in close contact with newborns, and anyone with skin lesions (herpetic whitlow) should not give direct care until lesions are dried and crusted.

Human Papillomavirus

Condylomata acuminata infection, sexually transmitted lesions caused by *human papillomavirus (HPV),* is the most common viral sexually transmitted infection—three times greater than genital herpes (Oriel, 1990). More than 50 HPVs infect skin and mucosal surfaces, with HPV-6, HPV-11, and HPV-16 most commonly infecting the genital tract (Oriel, 1990; Shah, 1990).

Disease occurs at the entry site of the virus after an incubation period of 2 to 3 months. *HPV is disseminated by skin-to-skin contact, not through body fluid exchange.* Exposure to the virus is by sexual contact with an infected partner; multiple partners increase the likelihood of HPV infection. Others at risk include smokers and oral contraceptive users. HPV is clinically significant because various types are associated with congenitally derived respiratory papillomatosis in children and with cervical carcinoma.

Condyloma acuminatum infection causes dry, wartlike growths on the vulva, vagina, cervix, or rectum (Fig. 21-18). These growths may be small or large, single or multiple, or have a cauliflower appearance. Chronic vaginal discharge, pruritus, or dyspareunia can occur. Diagnosis is by colposcopy and direct visualization of the growths, by biopsy, or by Papanicolaou smears.

In many persons the condition is difficult to treat. Available therapy is primarily cytotoxic or destructive. Cytotoxic agents are podophyllin and 5-fluorouracil (5-FU). Podophyllin, 20% to 30% in tincture of benzoin, is used for lesions 2 cm or less in diameter, but not in the vagina or on the cervix. Petrolatum is used to protect surrounding skin because podophyllin is caustic and cy-

---

BOX 21-13

Genital Hygiene

- Wash hands before and after genital contact.
- After urination or defecation, wipe and cleanse with a single front-to-back motion and discard tissue.
- Change sanitary napkins (pads) and tampons frequently as directed and after every use of bathroom.
- Scrub and rinse tub before and after bathing.

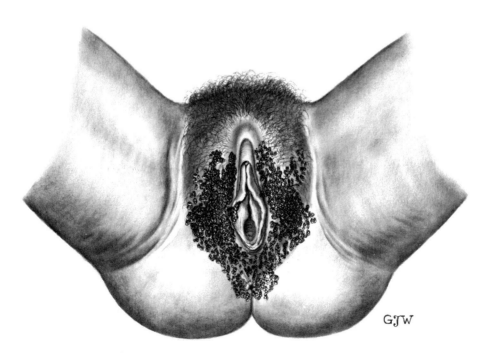

FIG. 21-18 Human papillomavirus infection (condylomata acuminata).

totoxic. The woman must wash the medication off after 4 hours or sooner if burning occurs. She is treated for 6 weeks. Therapy may not produce a cure; recurrence rate is 70%. *Podophyllin is not to be used during pregnancy;* its use is associated with fetal death and preterm labor. The more effective cytotoxic agent is 5-FU in 5% cream. This highly toxic agent is used for resistant condyloma and has a cure rate that approaches 90%. Local pain and epithelial erosion are side effects of local application. Treatment with 5-FU is most effective when used in conjunction with laser therapy.

The most effective destructive method is a carbon dioxide laser used with local anesthesia. It is precise and sterile and is accompanied by minimum bleeding and trauma. The treated area does not regain its normal pigmentation for several years. Post-laser therapy instructions are as follows:

1. Keep area clean by irrigating with warm water twice a day.
2. Dry with electric hair dryer.
3. Apply antibacterial cream twice a day.
4. Use gauze dressing to prevent rubbing against clothing.
5. Use lidocaine ointment 5% for discomfort.
6. Return to clinic as instructed.
7. Use latex condoms until disease is cured in the woman. Today condoms are dense enough to prevent passage of viruses.

Trichloroacetic acid, 50% solution, is a destructive therapy that is somewhat safer to use than podophyllin. It can be self-applied with a cotton swab and does not need to be washed off. Cryotherapy with liquid nitrogen also is used with some success for external condyloma.

Some pregnant women harbor HPV in the genital tract. Pregnancy effects of HPV infection include proliferation and increased friability of lesions. Many experts recommend removal of large, outward-growing lesions during pregnancy; carbon dioxide laser treatments have been used between 30 and 32 weeks' gestation. Treatment usually is followed by vaginal birth without complications (Ferenczy, 1984). Cesarean birth is indicated when the pelvic outlet is obstructed or when vaginal birth would result in excessive blood loss.

Genital Tract Infections
Vaginal Infections

The three most common vaginal infections are bacterial vaginosis, candidiasis, and trichomoniasis. Vaginal infections may be sexually transmitted.

Infections must be distinguished from normal vaginal discharge, *leukorrhea*, a whitish discharge. It consists of mucus and exfoliated vaginal epithelial cells as a result of hyperplasia of the vaginal mucosa such as occurs during pregnancy, at the time of ovulation, and before menstruation. If it is copious, it can cause discomfort.

Altered vaginal physiology during pregnancy may precipitate *vaginitis* (inflammation of the vagina). Vaginal secretions are increased, and the vagina is less acidic during pregnancy. These conditions provide an environment that promotes microbial growth.

The most common cause of vaginal symptoms among childbearing women is *bacterial vaginosis,* also referred to as nonspecific vaginosis. By-products of bacterial metabolism affect vaginal pH, thus altering the flora of the vagina. The predominant microorganism is *Gardnerella vaginalis*. The homogeneous vaginal discharge has an amine (fishy) odor when mixed with 10% potassium hydroxide. "Clue cells" are seen on microscopic examination of vaginal discharge.

The maternal effect of this bacterial infection is usually a mild illness. Signs and symptoms may include a milklike discharge and itching, burning, and pain in the vagina and around the introitus. Obstetric complications include amniotic fluid infection, premature rupture of membranes (PROM), preterm labor and birth, and postpartum endometritis. Bacterial vaginosis also may be a risk factor for PID.

Treatment of bacterial vaginosis is most effective with oral metronidazole. However, because of its potential teratogenic effects, metronidazole should be given only in the second and third trimester. Topical preparations of metronidazole and clindamycin also have been used to successfully treat the condition. Although sexual partners usually are treated, disagreement exists as to its actual effectiveness.

Vulvovaginal Candidiasis

Vulvovaginal candidiasis, or candidal vaginitis, occurs throughout the world. Most trends suggest that the disease is increasing, in part as a result of the widespread use of antimicrobial agents. Similarly, the number of healthy, symptom-free women who harbor *Candida* organisms also is increasing.

Most yeastlike organisms isolated from the vagina are *Candida albicans,* a fungus normally found in the intestines. Dysuria and dyspareunia are common complaints. Speculum examination usually reveals thick, white, cheeselike patches adhering to the pale, dry, and sometimes cyanotic vaginal mucosa.

Maternal effects of vaginal candidiasis usually are not health threatening, but affected mothers may be extremely uncomfortable from the pain, itching, and vaginal discharge. Pregnancy predisposes women not only to an increased rate of infection but also to increased recurrences and increased treatment failures. Recurrent candidal vaginitis in the antepartum period necessitates screening for gestational diabetes and HIV infection, if appropriate. Treatment goals include measures to relieve symptoms and topical or vaginal antifungal agents such as clotrimazole.

Trichomoniasis

Trichomonas vaginalis is a hearty protozoan that thrives in an alkaline milieu. The role of sexual contact in the transmission of *T. vaginalis* is well documented; trichomoniasis is prevalent in approximately 30% of sexually active women (Rein, Müller, 1990).

In symptom-free persons the infection may be identified during a routine examination or with a Papanicolaou smear. *T. vaginalis* has an affinity for mucous membranes, and 75% of infected women report a profuse, frothy vaginal discharge that may be malodorous, usually gray or yellow-green, and may stream from the vagina when a speculum is inserted.

Trichomoniasis seems to have few maternal effects other than symptomatic discomfort. However, perinatal infection by *T. vaginalis* is the most frequent form of nonvenereal transmission of disease. Fetal and neonatal effects include fever and irritability. The preferred treatment, administration of metronidazole, should be administered to pregnant women only in the second and third trimesters. Partners should also be treated.

Group B Streptococcus

Group B streptococcal (GBS) bacterial infections have been recognized as the leading cause of life-threatening perinatal infections in the United States (ACOG, 1992b). The transmission rate of infection from mother to infant near the time of birth ranges between 50% and 75% (Hill, 1990). Women with preterm labor or PROM are at increased risk for maternal infection as well as neonatal infection. Maternal effects include miscarriage, stillbirth, preterm birth, fever, septicemia, and puerperal infection.

Treatment of GBS infections is accomplished with penicillin, ampicillin, cephalothin, or erythromycin. Intrapartum antibiotic chemoprophylaxis for women who are GBS carriers reduces the frequency of GBS disease (ACOG, 1992b).

Urinary Tract Infections

Urinary tract infections (UTIs) affect about 10% of pregnant women, most of these in the prenatal period. Those who have had UTIs previously are especially prone to recurrence during pregnancy. Cervicitis, vaginitis, obstruction of the flaccid ureters, vesicoureteral reflux, and the trauma of birth predispose the pregnant woman to UTI, generally from *Escherichia coli*. Women with chronic STDs, especially gonorrhea and chlamydia, also are at risk. Asymptomatic bacteriuria occurs in about 5% to 15% of all pregnant women. If untreated, pyelonephritis during gestation will develop in approximately 30% of these women. Premature labor and birth may be more common also.

Urine culture and sensitivity tests should be obtained early in pregnancy, preferably at the first visit, from a clean-catch urine specimen. If infection is diagnosed, treatment with an appropriate antibiotic drug for 2 to 3 weeks, together with increased fluids intake and urinary tract antispasmodic medication (e.g., belladonna derivatives), is recommended. Infections caused by the colon's aerogenic organisms generally respond well to sulfisoxazole (Gantrisin) or nitrofurantoin. Treatment should be continued for 2 to 3 weeks until two negative cultures are obtained, and the infant should be observed for hyperbilirubinemia. Retreatment of the mother may be necessary if there is a recurrence.

Postpartum Infections

Postpartum infection (puerperal sepsis, or childbed fever) is any clinical infection of the genital canal that occurs within 28 days after abortion or childbirth. Infections may result from bacteria commonly found within the vagina (endogenous) or from the introduction of pathogens from outside the vagina (exogenous). An episiotomy or lacerations of the vagina or cervix may open avenues for sepsis. Even more formidable, however, may be the large placental site. Here the denuded endometrium (decidua basalis) and residual blood after birth make the uterus an ideal site for a wound infection.

Puerperal sepsis occurs after about 6% of births in the United States and probably is the major cause of maternal morbidity and mortality throughout the world. The most common infecting organisms are the numerous streptococcal and anaerobic organisms. *Staphylococcus aureus,* gonococci, coliform bacteria, and clostridia are less common but serious pathogenic organisms that cause postpartum infection.

Commonly the infection is complicated by medical disorders such as anemia, malnutrition, and diabetes mellitus. Obstetric problems, including PROM, a long exhausting labor, instrument birth, hemorrhage, and retention of the products of conception, increase the likelihood and severity of puerperal sepsis.

Chorioamnionitis may be the cause of or the result of PROM. Chorioamnionitis may be followed by placentitis and fetal congenital pneumonia, omphalitis, or septicemia. Placentitis and chorioamnionitis may be followed by endometritis.

An *endometritis,* usually at the placental site, permits infection to begin. Localized infection may be followed by salpingitis, peritonitis, and pelvic abscess formation. Septicemia may develop. Secondary abscesses may arise in distant sites such as the lungs or liver. Pulmonary embolism or septic shock, often with DIC, from any serious genital infection may prove fatal. Postpartum femoral thrombophlebitis (milk leg) may result in a swollen, painful leg and, if untreated, may become septic thrombophlebitis (Fig. 21-19).

The symptoms of puerperal infection may be mild or severe. A temperature of 100.4° F (38° C) or more on 2 successive days, not counting the first 24 hours after birth, must be considered to have been caused by post-

during childbirth and the postpartum period is very important.

Infection control measures for cure and comfort are instituted. Fluid and electrolyte balance is vital. Broadspectrum antibiotics are administered intravenously until the infecting organism is identified. Then organismspecific antibiotic therapy is begun. Breastfeeding may continue, depending on the prescribed antibiotic regimen.

The virulence of the organisms, the resistance of the woman, and her response to treatment affect the prognosis. Prevention, supportive therapy, and prompt massive antibiotic administration have reduced the maternal mortality in the United States to less than 0.4%.

Bacteremic Shock

Critical infections, particularly those in which the causative bacteria release endotoxins, may precipitate **bacteremic (septic) shock.** Pregnant women, especially those with diabetes mellitus or women who are receiving immunosuppressive drugs, are at increased risk, as are those with endometritis during the postpartum period.

High, spiking fever and chills are pathophysiologic evidence of serious sepsis. An anxious mother may become apathetic. Body temperature often falls to slightly subnormal levels. The skin becomes cool and moist. Coloring becomes pale, and the pulse becomes rapid and thready. Marked hypotension and peripheral cyanosis develop. Oliguria occurs.

Laboratory findings reveal marked evidence of infection. Blood cultures show bacteremia, usually consisting of enteric gram-negative bacilli. Additional studies may reflect hemoconcentration, acidosis, and coagulopathy. An ECG may show changes indicative of myocardial insufficiency. Evidence of cardiac, pulmonary, renal, and neurologic hypoxia is notable.

Management focuses on antimicrobial therapy, as well as oxygen support to relieve tissue hypoxia and circulatory support to prevent vascular collapse. Heart function, respiratory effort, and kidney function are closely monitored. Prompt treatment of bacteremic shock has a good prognosis, and maternal morbidity and mortality are decreased by controlling respiratory distress, hypotension, and DIC.

Mastitis

Mastitis, or breast infection, affects about 1% of women soon after childbirth, most of whom are first-time mothers who are breastfeeding. Mastitis almost always is unilateral and develops well after the flow of milk has been established. The infecting organism generally is the hemolytic *S. aureus.* An infected nipple fissure usually is the initial lesion, followed by ductal system involvement. Inflammatory edema and engorgement of the breast soon obstruct the flow of milk in the lobes. Chills, fever, malaise, and local breast tenderness are noted. Without

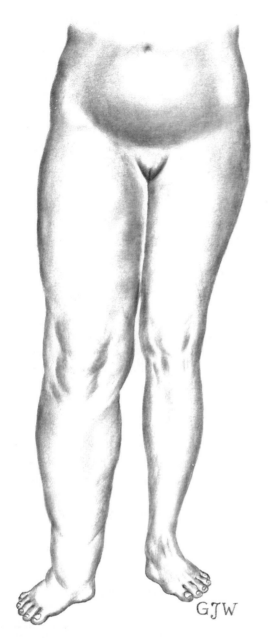

FIG. 21-19 Femoral thrombophlebitis (milk leg).

partum infection in the absence of convincing proof of another cause. The woman also may describe symptoms of fatigue and lethargy, lack of appetite, and chills. Perineal discomfort or lower abdominal distress, nausea, and vomiting may soon develop. Foul or profuse lochia is usually present. Intracervical or intrauterine bacterial cultures should reveal the offending pathogens within 36 to 48 hours.

The most effective and cheapest treatment of postpartum infection is prevention. Preventive measures include patient education regarding good prenatal nutrition to control anemia and intranatal hemorrhage. Also, good maternal perineal hygiene is emphasized. Strict adherence by all health care personnel to aseptic techniques

prompt treatment, a breast abscess will usually occur.

Interventions include intensive antibiotic therapy, support of breasts, local heat (or cold), and analgesics. Lactation is maintained (if desired) by emptying the breasts every 4 hours by manual expression or breast pump. Most women respond to treatment, and an abscess can be prevented.

Almost all instances of acute mastitis can be avoided by proper breastfeeding. Cleanliness practiced by all who have contact with the newborn and new mother also reduces the incidence of mastitis.

General Infections

Many infections place the woman at risk during the childbearing cycle. Following are some maternal infections the nurse may encounter.

Coxsackievirus B may cause mild illness in the mother. It is responsible for death, cardiovascular anomalies, myocarditis, and meningoencephalitis in the fetus.

Varicella (chickenpox) is highly contagious and is transmitted by direct contact with airborne virus. A maternal infection may appear as herpes zoster (shingles), especially in mothers with HIV. Severe, disseminated, epidemic type of varicella during pregnancy may be fatal for the mother (and fetus) because of necrotizing angitis (inflammation of blood and lymph vessels) and complications from varicella pneumonia. If maternal infection occurs within 20 days before birth, an infant should be considered possibly infectious and isolated from other infants (Fox, Strangarity, 1989).

Varicella-zoster immunoglobulin (VZIG) may be given prophylactically to exposed pregnant women. Severe varicella infections, especially if complicated by pneumonia, should be treated with intravenous acyclovir or vidarabine.

Influenza is caused by a virus. Maternal effects can be serious if complicated by pneumonia. Abortion and preterm labor may result.

Listeriosis is caused by the gram-positive bacterium, *Listeria monocytogenes*. This organism is harbored in the vagina or cervix by 4% of pregnant women. Listeriosis may exhibit influenza-like symptoms. It occurs most commonly in summer and fall. Other symptoms include vaginitis, UTI, and enteritis. This infection may result in abortion. Amnionitis or placentitis is evidenced by dirty brown amniotic fluid. Treatment with penicillin or erythromycin usually is successful. Unfortunately the diagnosis of listeriosis often is obscure or delayed; thus the prognosis for the fetus or newborn generally is poor.

Lyme disease is a tick-borne infection caused by the spirochete *Borrelia burgdorferi*. Infection is endemic in the Northeast, mid-Atlantic, parts of the Midwest, and West and peaks in the late spring and summer. Most infected persons develop a circular, expanding lesion (erythema chronicum migrans) at the site of the tick bite—usually groin, buttocks, axillae, trunk, upper part

of the arms, and legs. Viremic symptoms such as fatigue, headache, sore throat, fever, pain, and joint swelling also may develop; some persons remain free from symptoms.

The spirochete of Lyme disease, which closely resembles that of syphilis, crosses the placenta. Maternal effects include miscarriage, preterm birth, and stillbirth. Fetal and neonatal effects are not well documented because Lyme disease is still relatively new and frequently misdiagnosed. Birth defects are common, especially cardiac and neurologic defects. Treatment of choice for Lyme disease during pregnancy is amoxicillin or ceftriaxone.

Mumps (parotitis) occurs rarely in pregnant women. In the mother this virus may cause abortion or preterm labor. Fetal death may result. Congenital malformation such as endocardial fibroelastosis may be associated with this viral infection in survivors. Prophylaxis for epidemic parotitis is possible with administration of hyperimmune mumps gamma globulin.

Parvovirus B-19 is associated with a mild illness of childhood known as fifth disease or erythema infectiosum. Transmission occurs by droplets, and the primary symptoms are fever and a characteristic "slapped face" rash. Outbreaks usually occur in schools in the spring; adults who work with children are at increased risk. Maternal effects, in addition to fever and rash, include headache, malaise, and aching, swollen joints.

Rubeola, a viral infection also known as 2-week measles, is uncommon because most women have been immunized or have had the disease and are immune to it. Should the woman acquire rubeola during pregnancy, there are fetal and neonatal effects. Abortion or preterm labor may occur. The newborn may be born with a rash but generally survives, usually without developmental anomalies. Prophylactic gamma globulin may prevent the disease; measles vaccination of susceptible women before (not during) pregnancy is recommended.

Tuberculosis (TB) is caused by a gram-negative, acid-fast bacillus. Pulmonary TB does not jeopardize pregnancy, although urinary and CNS tuberculosis may. Pregnancy does not affect pulmonary tuberculosis adversely. Genital infection is rare. It may be sexually transmitted or result from primary lesions in the lungs. Spontaneous abortion occurs in 20% of infected women. Many pregnancies are ectopic, or the woman has impaired fertility with genital tuberculosis. Furthermore, TB is gaining increased attention as one of the opportunistic infections seen commonly in persons with AIDS.

Contraception is advocated for women with active TB; pregnancy is contraindicated until the woman has been free from the disease for 1½ to 2 years. All pregnant women should be evaluated for TB (tine test or PPD) early in pregnancy and again later if suspicion of the disease exists. If results of the tine test or PPD are positive, a chest film may be indicated to rule out active disease. Once born, the infant should have no intimate contact with the mother or others who may have the disease until contagion is no longer a problem. Therapeutic abortion rarely is indicated; cesarean birth is warranted only for obstetric indications.

Toxic shock syndrome (TSS) is a potentially life-threatening systemic disorder that has three principal clinical manifestations: fever of sudden onset, hypotension, and rash (Box 21-14). The erythematous macular desquamating rash is most prominent on palms and soles. The acute phase of TSS lasts about 4 to 5 days; the convalescent phase, about 1 to 2 weeks.

The CDC (1989) has established diagnostic criteria for TSS that include the aforementioned signs plus the following manifestations.

1. Involvement of three or more other organ systems:

System/Area	Manifestations
Gastrointestinal	Nausea, vomiting, diarrhea
Renal	Decreased urinary output; pyuria
Hepatic	Jaundice; abnormal values (increased transaminase)
CNS	Altered sensorium (decreased level of consciousness [LOC]); headache
Respiratory	Adult respiratory distress syndrome (ARDS)
Mucous membranes	Inflammation of vaginal, oropharyngeal, and conjunctival membranes
Muscular	Myalgia: weakness
Hematologic	Thrombocytopenia; DIC
Cardiac	Ischemic changes on ECG; decreased left ventricular contractility

2. Serologic laboratory test results for Rocky Mountain spotted fever, leptospirosis, and measles are negative. Cultures positive for *S. aureus* can be obtained from blood, urine, or stool. If primary site of infection is tampon related, positive cultures are obtained from the vagina and cervix.

A toxin (pyrogenic exotoxin C [PEC] or enterotoxin F) secreted by strains of *S. aureus* is the causative factor in TSS. About 9% of women harbor the organism normally in their vaginas; about 1% to 5% of sexually active males have urethral cultures that are positive for *S. aureus* without having the disease. Poor perineal hygiene and lack of hand washing before touching the perineal area may increase risk. Commonly associated conditions that may predispose the person to TSS by providing a

portal of entry into systemic circulation include the following:

1. Menstruation
2. Chronic vaginal infection (e.g., herpes)
3. Puerperal endometritis
4. Incisional or soft tissue abscess
5. Skin infection following a bee sting
6. IV injection of heroin
7. Use of high-absorbency tampons or barrier contraceptives (e.g., sponge, diaphragm) (Berkley et al, 1987; Wolf et al, 1987)
8. Neonatal infection concurrent with maternal infection.

The population at greatest risk is women between the ages of 15 and 24 who use tampons during menstruation. The three causes of mortality are (1) ARDS, (2) uncontrollable hypotension, and (3) DIC.

Most affected women have an uneventful recovery with no recurrence. Infection that recurs does so most often with the next menstrual cycle. Recurrence is most likely if the woman has not been treated with β-lactamase–resistant antibiotics.

Early identification of TSS is essential so that appropriate therapy can be initiated. Nursing care involves both prevention and treatment of TSS. Preventive care focuses on client education about the relationship of TSS to the use of tampons, diaphragms, cervical caps, and contraceptive vaginal sponges (see Teaching Approaches p. 607). Treatment in the acute care setting may include IV fluid replacement for dehydration related to vomiting or diarrhea, administration of antibiotics, administration of transfusions for low platelet counts, and medications to treat skin rashes and hypotension (Eschenbach, 1990).

CARE MANAGEMENT

✦ ASSESSMENT

Prevention, diagnosis, and treatment of maternal infections often create a complicated task. A comprehensive assessment focuses on some lifestyle issues that may be personal or sensitive. A nonjudgmental approach is essential for facilitating accurate data collection. Assessment includes the following key areas.

History

Factors that influence the development and management of STDs during pregnancy include a previous history of STD or PID, the number of current sexual partners, the frequency of intercourse per week, and anticipated sexual activity through the pregnancy. Lifestyle choices also may affect STD in the perinatal period. Mothers who are intravenous drug users or who have partners who use intravenous drugs are at risk. Other lifestyle factors that increase susceptibility to STD (through suppressive effects on the immune system) include smoking, alcohol use, in-

---

BOX 21-14

Warning Signs—Toxic Shock Syndrome (TSS)

1. Fever of sudden onset—over 102° F (38.9° C)
2. Hypotension—systolic pressure <90 mm Hg; orthostatic dizziness; disorientation
3. Rash—diffuse, macular erythrodema

adequate or poor nutrition, and high levels of fatigue or personal stress.

Preconception or antenatal factors that influence the development of vaginal or UTIs include a history of chronic UTIs or kidney infection and kidney stones; chronic conditions that impair kidney function (e.g., lupus, diabetes, sickle cell disease); chronic immunosuppressive states (e.g., steroid therapy, AIDS); poor fluid and nutritional status; failure to use condoms; and poor genital hygiene. Intrapartum events such as frequent catheterizations (especially with the use of epidural anesthesia); frequent vaginal examinations; prolonged second stage of labor; and birth trauma to the vagina, cervix, bladder, and urethra also may place the mother at greater risk for infection. Untreated or undertreated infections in the prenatal period may predispose mothers to postpartum infections. PROM and the length of time from rupture to birth also may be factors.

Physical Examination

Findings on examination vary. Some infections may be asymptomatic. Vaginal discharge may or may not be present, and vesicles or sores may be unnoticed. Fever or pain may be mild and therefore dismissed. A thorough symptom assessment, coupled with a complete history and physical examination is essential in identifying possible maternal infectious disease processes.

Laboratory Tests

Bacterial infections are easily determined from genital tract, urine, and blood studies. Viral agents also can be cultured but less successfully. An elevated white blood cell count may be of diagnostic help; other laboratory

TEACHING APPROACHES

PREVENTION OF TOXIC SHOCK SYNDROME

GENERAL INFORMATION

- Avoid the use of tampons, cervical caps, diaphragms, and contraceptive vaginal sponges during the postpartum period (6 weeks).
- Do not use any of the above if you have a history of TSS.
- Call your health care provider if you experience sudden onset of a high fever, vomiting, diarrhea, or skin rash.

TAMPON USE

- Insert only clean tampons with clean hands.
- Change tampons every 3 to 6 hours.
- Avoid use of superabsorbent tampons.
- Avoid overnight use of tampons by substituting other products such as sanitary napkins or minipads.

CONTRACEPTIVE VAGINAL SPONGE USE

- Insert only clean sponges with clean hands.
- Wet sponge with clean water only.
- Do not use the sponge during your menstrual period.

DIAPHRAGM OR CERVICAL CAP

- Insert clean diaphragm or cervical cap with clean hands.
- Do not use during your menstrual period.
- Remove within 6 hours after intercourse.

BOX 21-15

Assessment for the Woman at Risk for Sexually Transmitted Disease

HISTORY

Chief complaint

Description of the present illness, including symptoms, self-care treatment, use of prescribed or over-the-counter medications

Sexual history, including previous history of STD, number of current sexual partners, typical frequency of sexual activity

Lifestyle: use of intravenous drugs or partner who uses intravenous drugs; smoking, alcohol, poor nutrition, high level of stress

General health: date of last menstrual period, date of last Pap smear, history of contraception

PHYSICAL EXAMINATION

Inspection

Palpation

LABORATORY TESTS*

Saline wet preparation (*Trichomonas*)

Potassium hydroxide wet preparation (candidiasis, *Gardnerella*)

Urinalysis

Gonorrhea culture

Cervical culture

Herpes cervical culture

Pap smear

Complete blood cell count

VDRL test

Herpes simplex virus type 1 and 2 antibodies

Western blot—HIV

Chlamydia—culture or antigen detection test

Modified from Smith LS, Lauver D, Gray PA Jr: Sexually transmitted disease. In Fogel CI, Lauver D, editors: *Sexual health promotion*, Philadelphia, 1989, WB Saunders.
*Choice depends on specific STD.

tests are useful depending on what other infectious agents are suspected. Other laboratory data to assess include hematocrit, hemoglobin, proteinuria, and BUN. (Box 21-15 on p. 607 describes assessment for the woman suspected of having an STD.)

✤ NURSING DIAGNOSES

Nursing diagnoses are derived after carefully analyzing assessment findings and medical management directives. Nursing diagnoses for the patient at risk for infections include the following:

Pain/impaired tissue integrity related to
- Effects of infection process
- Scratching (excoriation) of pruritic areas
- Hygienic practices

Knowledge deficit related to
- Transmission/prevention of infection/reinfection
- Safer sex behaviors
- Management and course of infection

Anxiety/low self-esteem/body image disturbances related to
- Perceived effects on sexual relationships and family processes
- Possible effects on pregnancy/fetus
- Long-term sequelae to infection

High risk for altered parenting related to
- Fear of spread of infection to newborn

Altered patterns of urinary elimination related to
- Presence of edema and pain
- Impaired urinary function

Fear/anxiety related to
- Possible loss of pregnancy
- Preterm labor/birth

Altered family processes related to
- Unexpected complication to expected postpartum recovery
- Possible separation from newborn
- Interruption in process of realigning relationships after the addition of the new family member

✤ EXPECTED OUTCOMES

A plan of care is formulated that relates specifically to the physical and psychosocial needs of the woman. Goals are mutually determined with the woman. Expected outcomes include:

1. The women's infection will be cured.
2. She will experience absence or reduction of pain, her edema will be relieved, and excoriated areas will heal.
3. She will experience a return to her previous urinary function and pattern of elimination with no sequelae or recurrence of infection.

4. She will state that she is less anxious about losing the pregnancy or experiencing preterm labor/birth.
5. She will identify and be able to state the etiology, management, and expected course of the infection and its prevention.
6. The fetus will be born free from the infection and its sequelae, or will experience minimal sequelae.
7. She and her family verbalize acceptance of the unexpected events; they verbalize positive coping measures (e.g., arrangement for home health care).

✤ COLLABORATIVE CARE

Interventions include continuous assessment for signs and symptoms of infection, monitoring laboratory results, administering antimicrobial agents as ordered, and providing information to the mother and family as needed (Box 21-16). General care, such as adequate hydration, rest, and proper nutrition, also are implemented. Discussion of measures to avoid reinfection is essential. Topics of instruction should include proper medication administration; "safer" sex practices (see Box 21-12) and genital hygiene (see Box 21-13).

✤ EVALUATION

Evaluation of patient outcomes is a continuous process. To be effective, evaluation is based on patient-centered goals identified during the planning stage of nursing care. The nurse can be reasonably assured that care was effective to the extent that the expected outcomes have been met (see Plan of Care).

Infection Control

Infection control measures are essential to protect care providers and to prevent *nosocomial* infection of patients, regardless of the infectious agent. The risk of occupational transmission varies with the disease. Even if that

---

BOX 21-16

Prevention of Genital Tract Infections

Practice genital hygiene.
Choose underwear or hosiery with a cotton crotch.
Avoid tight-fitting clothing (especially tight jeans).
Select cloth car seat covers instead of vinyl.
Limit time spent in damp exercise clothes (especially swimsuits and leotards or tights).
Discontinue use of feminine hygiene deodorant sprays, if sensitive.
Use condoms.
Avoid douching.

PLAN OF CARE

Sexully Transmitted Disease

Case History

Elizabeth Cox, a 28-year-old married gravida 3, para 2-0-0-2, is at 25 weeks' gestation. She has been admitted to the antepartum unit with a primary diagnosis of pneumonia and a secondary diagnosis of chlamydial infection. Elizabeth's prenatal course is significant for a reactive HIV test at 22 weeks' gestation.

On physical assessment, the nurse observes that Elizabeth's skin is very warm and flushed but with normal skin turgor. Vital signs are temperature 101° F (39° C), pulse 110 beats/min (up from her normal rate of 80 beats/min), respirations 28/min (her usual rate is 22), and blood pressure 100/60 mm Hg (normal for her). Auscultation of Elizabeth's lungs reveals scattered basilar crackles (rales), and she reports a dry, persistent cough. Fetal heart tones are elevated to 170 beats/min.

Elizabeth is wearing a sanitary pad that shows purulent discharge containing small amounts of blood. Her labia are excoriated and tender to the touch. No uterine contractions are reported or palpated, and other physical findings are normal.

Laboratory results include a WBC of 9800/mm³ and urine and cervical cultures that are positive for chlamydia. Chest films show findings consistent with *Pneumocystis carinii* pneumonia. (*NOTE:* Patients with HIV and pneumonia frequently show a "normal" WBC. Because HIV infection represents an immunosuppressed state, the WBC may drop to 2500/mm³ in the presence of opportunistic infections.)

EXPECTED OUTCOMES	IMPLEMENTATION	RATIONALE	EVALUATION
Nursing Diagnosis: Altered respiratory function/ineffective breathing patterns related to infection*			
Elizabeth will reestablishe effective breathing patterns as evidenced by return of vital signs (including FHR) to WNL; improved/clear lung sounds; white blood cell count WNL.	Assess and document vital signs (including FHR). Monitor laboratory values, and report abnormalities. Assess and record presence and quality of cough or sputum; assess and record lung sounds. Administer IV therapy and antibiotics per care provider's order. Accurately record intake and output. Assess for adequate nutritional intake. Encourage fluid intake. Provide for sleep and rest as needed.	Ongoing assessment of vital signs, respiratory conditions, and laboratory values provides data used to plan and evaluate interventions.

Adequate fluid intake, a nutritious diet, and sleep/rest are important to support recovery. | Elizabeth reestablishes effective breathing; her work of breathing is decreased and she states that she is less fatigued. |
| **Nursing Diagnosis: Altered health maintenance related to lack of knowledge of prevention of STD** | | | |
| Elizabeth's restoration of health maintenance will be evident by her expressed understanding of STD transmission, causes, and symptoms and by her willingness to use practices to prevent STD transmission. | Assess Elizabeth's current knowledge of STD. Assess Elizabeth's readiness to learn. Provide factual information on STD transmission, causes, symptoms, and transmission. Discuss/display methods for protection during any sexual activity (see Box 21-12). | Assessment of Elizabeth's current knowledge provides an opportunity for the correction of misinformation and is the basis for the teaching plan. Factual, direct information, presented with consideration of education abilities, is necessary in the prevention and treatment of STDs. | Elizabeth's restoration of health maintenance is accomplished; Elizabeth verbalizes an understanding of STD transmission, causes, and symptoms; and states intent to prevent STD transmission. |

FHR, Fetal heart rate; *IV*, intravenous; *WNL*, within normal limits.
*Potential complications: pneumonia as collaborative diagnosis.

Continued.

PLAN OF CARE—cont'd

Sexully Transmitted Disease

EXPECTED OUTCOMES	IMPLEMENTATION	RATIONALE	EVALUATION
Nursing Diagnosis: Altered health maintenance related to lack of knowledge of prevention of STD—cont'd			
	Offer instruction in an open and nonjudgmental manner. Allow for Elizabeth's privacy. Discuss options for the notification of potentially infected sexual partners. Encourage Elizabeth to express her feelings and concerns; answer questions directly.	An open, nonjudgmental environment facilitates learning and promotes Elizabeth's self-esteem and self-worth. Sexuality and STDs are personal and sensitive topics.	
Nursing Diagnosis: Impaired tissue integrity related to irritation from vaginal discharge			
Elizabeth's tissue integrity will be restored as evidenced by replacement of damaged tissue with healthy tissue.	Assess, monitor, and record characteristics of the damaged area, including color, lesions, drainage, and edema. Instruct Elizabeth in genital hygiene practices (see Box 21-13).	Information on the characteristics of the affected area establishes the basis with which to plan and evaluate interventions. Meticulous genital hygiene prevents infection of damaged tissue from other organisms.	Elizabeth verbalizes understanding of hygiene and complies with prescribed treatment.
	Provide warm soaks or sitz baths. Instruct Elizabeth to dry the genital area with a blow dryer (with the temperature on a cool setting). Administer prescribed medications per care provider's order.	Comfort and healing are promoted.	Elizabeth's tissue integrity is restored.

risk is low, as it is with HIV, that any risk exists is significant to warrant reasonable precautions. Precautions against airborne disease transmission are available in all health care agencies. Universal precautions from the CDC are in Box 21-17.

Another consideration in the prevention of occupational disease transmission is that of cross-contamination. Health care providers may develop a false sense of security about the protection that gloves provide. For example, little is gained if gloves are worn to assess a newborn and those same gloved hands answer the telephone,

turn on a light, or document findings on the infant's chart.

Proper cleaning of contaminated surfaces is essential. The following guidelines are recommended: (1) cleanse washable surfaces with a solution of sodium hypochlorite (household bleach) and water (1 cup of household bleach to 9 cups of water); health care institutions often purchase commercial products to disinfect; (2) remove all blood or other fluids before disinfection to avoid neutralizing the bleach solution.

BOX 21-17

Universal Precautions

Medical history and examination cannot reliably identify all persons infected with HIV or other bloodborne pathogens. Thus blood and body fluid precautions should be used consistently for everyone. This approach should be used in the care of all persons, especially those in emergency care settings in which the risk of blood exposure is increased and the infection status of the person is usually unknown.

1. All health care workers should routinely use appropriate barrier precautions to prevent skin and mucous membrane exposure when contact with blood or other body fluids of any person is anticipated. *Latex gloves* should be worn for touching blood and body fluids, mucous membranes, or nonintact skin of all persons; for handling items or surfaces soiled with blood or body fluids; and for performing venipuncture and other vascular access procedures. Gloves should be changed after contact with each patient. *Masks and protective eyewear* or face shields should be worn during procedures that are likely to generate droplets of blood or other body fluids to prevent exposure of mucous membranes of the mouth, nose, and eyes. *Gowns or aprons* should be worn during procedures that are likely to generate splashes of blood or other body fluids.

2. Hands and other skin surfaces should be washed immediately and thoroughly if contaminated with blood or other body fluids. Hands should be washed immediately after gloves are removed.

3. All health care workers should take precautions to prevent injuries caused by needles, scalpels, and other sharp instruments or devices during procedures; when cleaning used instruments; during disposal of used needles; and when handling sharp instruments after procedures. *To prevent needlestick injuries,* needles should not be recapped, purposely bent or broken by hand, removed from disposable syringes, or otherwise manipulated by hand. After they are used, disposable syringes and needles, scalpel blades, and other sharp items should be placed immediately in puncture-resistant containers for disposal; the puncture-resistant containers should be located as close as practical to the use area.

4. Although saliva has not been implicated in HIV transmission, to minimize the need for emergency mouth-to-mouth resuscitation, mouthpieces, resuscitation bags, or other ventilation devices should be available for use in areas in which the need for resuscitation is predictable.

5. Health care workers who have exudative lesions or weeping dermatitis should refrain from all direct patient care and from handling patient care equipment until the condition resolves.

6. Pregnant health care workers are not known to be at greater risk of contracting HIV infection than health care workers who are not pregnant; however, if a health care worker develops HIV infection during pregnancy, the infant is at risk of infection resulting from perinatal transmission. Because of this risk, pregnant health care workers should be especially familiar with and strictly adhere to precautions to minimize the risk of HIV transmission.

PRECAUTIONS FOR INVASIVE PROCEDURES

An invasive procedure is defined as surgical entry into tissues, cavities, or organs or repair of major traumatic injuries (1) in an operating or birthing room, emergency department, or out-of-hospital setting, including both physicians' and dentists' offices and (2) a vaginal or cesarean birth or other invasive obstetric procedure during which bleeding may occur. The aforementioned universal blood and body fluid precautions, combined with the following precautions, should serve as minimum precautions for all such invasive procedures.

1. All health care workers who participate in invasive procedures must routinely use appropriate barrier precautions to prevent skin and mucous membrane contact with blood and other body fluids of all patients. Gloves and surgical masks must be worn for all invasive procedures. Protective eyewear or face shields should be worn for procedures that commonly result in the generation of droplets, splashing of blood or other body fluids, or the generation of bone chips. Gowns or aprons made of materials that provide an effective barrier should be worn during invasive procedures that are likely to result in the splashing of blood or other body fluids. All health care workers who perform or assist in vaginal or cesarean births should wear gloves and gowns when handling the placenta or the infant until blood and amniotic fluid have been removed from the infant's skin and should wear gloves during postnatal care of the umbilical cord.

2. If a glove is torn or a needlestick or other injury occurs, the glove should be removed and a new glove used as promptly as patient safety permits; the needle or instrument involved in the incident also should be removed from the sterile field.

KEY POINTS

- Hypertensive disorders during pregnancy are a leading cause of maternal and perinatal morbidity and mortality worldwide.
- The cause of preeclampsia is unknown, and there are no known reliable tests for predicting women at risk for developing preeclampsia-eclampsia.
- Preeclampsia-eclampsia is a multisystem disease, and the pathologic changes are present long before clinical manifestations, such as hypertension, are evident.
- Once preeclampsia becomes clinically evident, therapeutic interventions are palliative (e.g., bed rest, diet), which may slow the progression of the disease allowing the pregnancy to continue, but the underlying pathology continues.
- The HELLP syndrome, which may become apparent during the second trimester, is considered life threatening.
- Magnesium sulfate, the anticonvulsant of choice for preventing eclampsia, requires careful monitoring of reflexes, respirations, and renal function; its antidote, calcium gluconate, should be at the bedside.
- Intent of emergency interventions for eclampsia is to prevent self-injury, ensure adequate oxygenation, reduce aspiration risk, and establish control with magnesium sulfate.
- Blood loss during pregnancy should always be regarded as a warning sign until ruled out by the woman's health care provider.
- Ectopic pregnancy is a significant cause of maternal morbidity and mortality even in developed countries.
- Abruptio placentae and placenta previa are differentiated by type of bleeding, uterine tonicity, and presence or absence of pain.
- Clotting disorders are associated with many obstetric complications.

- Postpartum hemorrhage is the most common and most serious type of excessive obstetric blood loss.
- Hemorrhagic (hypovolemic) shock is an emergency situation in which the perfusion of body organs may become severely compromised and death may ensue.
- The physiologic adaptations of pregnancy mask warning signs and changes in vital signs during early shock states.
- The potential hazards of therapeutic interventions may further compromise the woman experiencing hemorrhagic disorders.
- Pregnancy confers no immunity against infection, and both mother and fetus must be considered when the pregnant woman contracts an infection.
- HIV is transmitted through blood, semen, and perinatal events.
- *C. trachomatis* is the most common sexually transmitted bacterial pathogen in the United States and is responsible for substantial morbidity, personal suffering, and heavy economic burden.
- STDs often occur in groups; what appear to be resistant infections actually may be multiple infections or reinfections.
- Abuse of alcohol and drugs compromises the body's immune system and increases the risk for AIDS and associated conditions.
- Because medical history and examination cannot reliably identify all persons with HIV or other blood-borne pathogens, blood and body fluid precautions should be consistently used for everyone.
- STDs and genital and perigenital infections are biologic events, for which all individuals have a right to expect objective, compassionate, and effective health care.

CRITICAL THINKING EXERCISES

1. Susan F. has been diagnosed with mild preeclampsia. She is resisting needed diet changes and bed rest. Role play a nurse attempting to provide teaching for the woman who resists dietary change and bed rest. Ask the group to suggest additional strategies.
2. Susan's condition has become worse, and she is hospitalized. She has been receiving magnesium sulfate IV for several hours for severe preeclampsia.
   a. Give rationale for the magnesium sulfate infusion.
   b. You assess her DTRs as 0 (no response). In order of priority, list four interventions, and specify rationale for each.
3. The charge nurse alerts you to the possibility that Susan could convulse anytime during labor or early postpartum.
   a. What assessment findings would indicate that a convulsion is imminent?
   b. In order of priority, list interventions during a convulsion, and specify rationale for each.
4. You are providing care for a 42-year-old nullipara admitted at 34 weeks' gestation with possible abruptio placentae. She has a history of cocaine use.
   a. What are the possible reactions of the woman to the situation?
   b. Examine your reactions to this assignment. What assumptions have you made? What do you need to verify?
   c. Analyze assessment findings to determine appropriate nursing diagnoses.
   d. Generate a plan of care for this woman.
   e. Evaluate the appropriateness of the proposed interventions for this woman.
5. You are assigned to a 22-year-old unmarried woman threatened with the loss of her first pregnancy at 14 weeks' gestation.
   a. What reactions might the woman have about her condition?
   b. What assumptions can you make about this patient situation?
   c. Identify ways to verify or negate your assumptions.
   d. How might these assumptions affect your plan of care?
6. Interview a woman who has experienced postpartum hemorrhage or other hemorrhagic disorder.
   a. Examine her reaction to the experience.
   b. Identify implications of her reactions on planning effective nursing care.
7. You are assigned to a single woman in labor who has a history of herpes simplex virus II (HSV II). Vaginal examination reveals an active lesion that appears to be a recurrence of HSV II on the cervix. The woman is told of the finding, and a cesarean birth is planned. You notice the father of the baby appears upset and angry. As you leave the room, you overhear him ask the woman why she did not tell him that she has herpes.
   a. What is your assessment of the situation? What further information do you need to verify your assumptions?
   b. What are some of the effects the situation may have on the relationship between the couple?
   c. Examine your personal reaction to working with this woman in light of this new information about the presence of an infection. How might these feelings affect your plan of care?
   d. Formulate a plan of care, and provide a rationale for your interventions.
8. You are assigned to a 19-year-old mother who has tested positive for HIV. She is being discharged home with her baby.
   a. Examine your personal reactions to this young mother and her baby.
   b. Generate possible reactions the young woman might have to her HIV status. Compare these reactions with your own.
   c. Analyze the significance of your reaction in terms of providing care to this young woman.
   d. Formulate a discharge teaching plan for the woman and her family that includes care and infection control.

REFERENCES

Hypertension

American College of Obstetricians and Gynecologists: Management of preeclampsia, *ACOG Tech Bull*, vol 91, 1986.

American College of Obstetricians and Gynecologists: Invasive hemodynamic monitoring in obstetrics and gynecology, *ACOG Tech Bull*, vol 175, 1992.

Brown M: Pregnancy-induced hypertension: pathogenesis and management, *Aust NZ J Med* 21:257, 1991.

Chesley LC: History and epidemiology of preeclampsia-eclampsia, *Clin Obstet Gynecol* 27:801, 1984.

Consensus Report of The National High Blood Pressure Education Program Working Group Report on High Blood Pressure in Pregnancy, 1990.

Cunningham FG, MacDonald PC, Gant NF: *Williams obstetrics*, ed 19, Norwalk, CT, 1993, Appleton & Lange.

Dildy N et al: Complications in pregnancy-induced hypertension. In Clark SL et al, editors: *Critical care obstetrics*, ed 2, Boston, 1991, Blackwell Scientific Publications.

Easterling TR, Benedetti TJ: Preeclampsia: a hyperdynamic disease model, *Am J Obstet Gynecol* 160:1447, 1989.

Egley CC, Gutliph J, Bowes WA: Severe hypoglycemia associated with HELLP syndrome, *Am J Obstet Gynecol* 152:576, 1985.

Fairlie FM, Sibai BM: Hypertensive diseases in pregnancy. In Reece EA et al, editors: *Medicine of the fetus and mother*, Philadelphia, 1993, JB Lippincott.

Fairlie FM: Doppler flow velocimetry in hypertension in pregnancy. *Clin Perinatol* 18:749, 1991.

Farmakides G et al, Coury A, Decavalas G: Pregnancy surveillance with Doppler velocimetry, *Female Patient* 15:49, 1990.

Farmakides G et al: Surveillance of the pregnant hypertensive patient with Doppler flow velocimetry, *Clin Obstet Gynecol* 35:387, 1992.

Gilbert ES, Harmon JS: *High-risk pregnancy and delivery: nursing perspectives*, St Louis, 1993, Mosby.

Guyton AC: *Human physiology and mechanisms of disease*, ed 5, Philadelphia, 1992, WB Saunders.

Harvey CJ, Burke ME: Hypertensive disorders in pregnancy. In Mandeville LK, Troiano NH, editors: *High-risk intrapartum nursing*, Philadelphia, 1992, JB Lippincott.

Iams JD, Zuspan FP, Quilligan EJ: *Zuspan and Quilligan's manual of obstetrics and gynecology*, ed 2, St Louis, 1990, Mosby.

Klonoff-Cohen HS et al: An epidemiologic study of contraception and preeclampsia, *JAMA* 262:3143, 1989.

Leduc L et al: Coagulation profile in severe preeclampsia, *Obstet Gynecol* 79:14, 1992.

Martin JN et al: Peripartal adult thrombotic thrombocytopenic purpura and hemolytic uremic syndrome. In Clark SL et al, editors: *Critical care obstetrics*, ed 2, Boston, 1991, Blackwell Scientific Publications.

Marx GF et al: Automated blood pressure measurements in laboring women: are they reliable? *Am J Obstet Gynecol* 168:796, 1993.

O'Brien WF: The prediction of preeclampsia, *Clin Obstet Gynecol* 35:351, 1992.

Perry KG, Martin JN: Abnormal hemostasis and coagulopathy in preeclampsia and eclampsia, *Clin Obstet Gynecol* 35:338, 1992.

Poole JH: Getting perspective on HELLP syndrome, *MCN* 13:432, 1988.

Poole JH: HELLP syndrome and coagulopathies of pregnancy, *Crit Care Nurs Clin North Am* 5:457, 1993.

Roberts JM et al: *New developments in preeclampsia* (NIH Grant HP 24180), San Francisco, 1990, University of California.

Saftlas AF et al: Epidemiology of preeclampsia and eclampsia in the United States, *Am J Obstet Gynecol* 163:460, 1990.

Schiff E et al: The use of aspirin to prevent pregnancy-induced hypertension and lower the ratio of thromboxane A_2 to prostacyclin in relatively high risk pregnancies, *N Engl J Med* 321:351, 1989.

Scott JR et al: *Danforth's obstetrics and gynecology*, ed 6, Philadelphia, 1990, JB Lippincott.

Sibai BM et al: Eclampsia III. Neonatal outcome, growth and development, *Am J Obstet Gynecol* 146:307, 1983.

Sibai BM et al: Maternal-perinatal outcome associated with the syndrome of hemolysis, elevated liver enzymes, and low platelets in severe preeclampsia-eclampsia, *Am J Obstet Gynecol* 155:501, 1986.

Sibai BM: Pitfalls in diagnosis and management of preeclampsia, *Am J Obstet Gynecol* 159:1, 1988.

Sibai BM: Eclampsia. IV. Maternal-perinatal outcome in 254 consecutive cases, *Am J Obstet Gynecol* 163:1049, 1990a.

Sibai BM: Magnesium sulfate is the ideal anticonvulsant in preeclampsia-eclampsia, *Am J Obstet Gynecol* 162:1141, 1990b.

Sibai BM: Preeclampsia-eclampsia: valid treatment approaches, *Contemp OB/GYN* 35:84, 1990c.

Sibai BM: The HELLP syndrome (hemolysis, elevated liver enzymes, and low platelets): much ado about nothing? *Am J Obstet Gynecol* 162:311, 1990d.

Sibai BM: Immunologic aspects of preeclampsia, *Clin Obstet Gynecol* 34:27, 1991a.

Sibai BM: Management of preeclampsia, *Clin Perinatol* 18:793, 1991b.

Sibai BM, Anderson GD: Hypertension. In Gabbe SG, Niebyl JR, Simpson JL, editors: *Obstetrics—normal and problem pregnancies*, ed 2, New York, 1991, Churchill Livingstone.

Sibai BM, Rodriguez JJ: Preeclampsia: diagnosis and management. In Reece EA et al, editors: *Medicine of the fetus and mother*, Philadelphia, 1992, JB Lippincott.

Smith CV et al: Reliability of compact electronic blood pressure monitors for hypertensive pregnant women, *J Reproduct Med* 35:399, 1990.

Villar MA, Sibai BM: Eclampsia. In Arias F, editor: High risk pregnancy, *Obstet Gynecol Cl Nor Am* 15(2):355 1988.

Walsh SW: Physiology of low-dose aspirin therapy for the prevention of preeclampsia, *Semin Perinatol* 14:152, 1990.

Weiner CP: Preeclampsia-eclampsia syndrome and coagulation, *Clin Perinatol* 18:713, 1991.

Willis DC, Blanco J: Preeclampsia-eclampsia. Benrubi GI, editor: *Contemporary issues in emergency medicine: obstetric emergencies*, New York, 1990, Churchill Livingstone.

Zuspan FP: New concepts in the understanding of hypertensive diseases during pregnancy: an overview, *Clin Perinatol* 18:653, 1991.

Hemorrhage

American College of Obstetrics and Gynecology: Management of gestational trophoblastic disease, ACOG Technical Bulletin #178, 1993.

Arias F: *Practical guide to high-risk pregnancy and delivery*, ed 2, St Louis, 1993, Mosby.

Baskett TF, Writer WDR: Postpartum hemorrhage. In Datta S, editors: *Anesthetic and obstetric management of high-risk pregnancy*, St Louis, 1991, Mosby.

Berman ML, DiSaia PJ: Pelvic malignancies, gestational trophoblastic neoplasia, and nonpelvic malignancies. In Creasy RK, Resnik R, editors: *Maternal-fetal medicine: principles and practice*, ed 2, Philadelphia, 1989, Saunders.

Carp H et al: Recurrent miscarriage: a review of current concepts, immune mechanisms, and results of treatment, *Obstet Gynecol Surv* 45:657, 1990.

Clark SL et al: Central hemodynamic assessment of normal term pregnancy, *Am J Obstet Gynecol* 161:1439, 1989.

Cunningham FG et al: *Williams obstetrics,* ed 19, Norwalk, CT, 1993, Appleton & Lange.

de Crespigny LC: The value of ultrasound in ectopic pregnancy, *Clin Obstet Gynecol* 30:136, 1987.

DePetrillo AD et al: Symposium: gestational trophoblastic disease: an update, *Contemp OB/GYN* 29(1):199, 1987.

Deutchman M: The problematic first-trimester pregnancy, *Am Fam Physician* 39(1):185, 1989.

Dorman KF: Hemorrhagic emergencies in obstetrics, *J Perinat Neonatal Nurs* 3(2):23, 1989.

Gilbert ES, Harmon JS: *High-risk pregnancy and delivery: nursing perspectives,* St Louis, 1993, Mosby.

Glass RH, Golbus MS: Habitual abortion. In Creasy RK, Resnik R, editors: *Maternal-fetal medicine: principles and practice,* ed 2, Philadelphia, 1989, WB Saunders.

Green JR: Placenta previa and abruptio placentae. In Creasy RK, Resnik R, editors: *Maternal-fetal medicine: principles and practice,* ed 2, Philadelphia, 1989, WB Saunders.

Iams JD, Zuspan FP, Quilligan EJ: *Zuspan and Quilligan's manual of obstetrics and gynecology,* ed 2, St Louis, 1990, Mosby.

Kulb NW: Abnormalities of the placenta and membranes. In Buckley K, Kulb NW, editors: *High risk maternity nursing manual,* Baltimore, 1990, Williams & Wilkins.

Lavery JP: Placenta previa, *Clin Obstet Gynecol* 33(3):414, 1990.

Lowe TW, Cunningham G: Placental abruption, *Clin Obstet Gynecol* 33(3):406, 1990.

McBride W: Spontaneous abortion, *Am Fam Physician* 43:175, 1991.

Mills JL et al: Incidence of spontaneous abortion among normal women and insulin-dependent diabetic women whose pregnancies were identified within 21 days of conception, *N Engl J Med* 319:1617, 1988.

Murahata SA: Third stage of labor and postpartum hemorrhage. In Frederickson HL, Wilkins-Haug L, editors: *OB/GYN Secrets,* St Louis, 1991, Mosby.

Nager CW, Murphy AA: Ectopic pregnancy, *Clin Obstet Gynecol* 33(3):403, 1991.

Robichaux AG, Stedman CM, Hammer C: Uterine activity in patients with cervical cerclage, *Obstet Gynecol* 76(7s):63, 1990.

Rosenak D et al: Cocaine: maternal use during pregnancy and its effect on the mother, the fetus, and the infant, *Obstet Gynecol Survey* 45(6):348, 1990.

Scott JR et al: *Danforth's obstetrics and gynecology,* ed 6, Philadelphia, 1990, JB Lippincott.

Simpson J: Genetic cause of spontaneous abortion, *Contemp OB/GYN* 35:25, 1990.

Stoval TG, Ling FW, Buster JE: Reproductive performance after methotrexate treatment of ectopic pregnancy, *Am J Obstet Gynecol* 162:1620, 1990.

Suresh MS, Kinch RA: Antepartum hemorrhage. In Datta S, editor: *Anesthetic and obstetric management of high-risk pregnancy,* St Louis, 1991, Mosby.

Zahn CM, Yeomans ER: Postpartum hemorrhage: placenta accreta, uterine inversion, and puerperal hematomas, *Clin Obstet Gynecol* 33(3):422, 1990.

Infections

American College of Obstetrics and Gynecology: Antimicrobial therapy for obstetric patients, *ACOG Tech Bull,* vol 117, 1988.

American College of Obstetrics and Gynecology: Human immunodeficiency virus infection, *ACOG Tech Bull,* vol 169, 1992a.

American College of Obstetrics and Gynecology: Group B streptococcal infections in pregnancy. *ACOG Tech Bull,* vol 170, 1992b.

American College of Obstetrics and Gynecology: Rubella and pregnancy, *ACOG Tech Bull,* vol 171, 1992c.

American College of Obstetrics and Gynecology: Hepatitis in pregnancy, *ACOG Tech Bull,* vol 174, 1992d.

American College of Obstetrics and Gynecology: Perinatal viral and parasitic infections, *ACOG Tech Bull,* vol 177, 1993.

Aral SO, Holmes KK: Epidemiology of sexual behavior and sexually transmitted diseases. In Holmes KK, editor: *Sexually transmitted diseases,* ed 2, New York, 1990, McGraw-Hill.

Bendell A, Efantis-Potter J: Acquired immune deficiency syndrome in pregnancy. In Mandeville LK, Troiano NH, editors: *High-risk intrapartum nursing,* Philadelphia, 1992, JB Lippincott.

Berkley SF et al: The relationship of tampon characteristics to menstrual toxic shock syndrome, *JAMA* 258:908, 1987.

Bourcier KM, Seidler AJ: Chlamydia and condylomata acuminata: an update for the nurse practitioner, *JOGNN* 16:17, 1987.

Boyer J et al: Factors predictive of maternal-fetal transmission of HIV-1, *JAMA* 271 (24): 1925, 1994.

Brown ZA, Baker DA: Genital herpes in pregnancy: risk factors associated with recurrences and asymptomatic viral shedding, *Am J Obstet Gynecol* 73:526, 1989.

Brunham RC, Holmes KK, Embree JE: Sexually transmitted diseases in pregnancy. In Holmes KK et al, editors: *Sexually transmitted diseases,* ed 2, New York, 1990, McGraw-Hill.

Center for Disease Control and Prevention: *1989 sexually transmitted disease treatment guidelines,* Atlanta, 1989, Public Health Services.

Center for Disease Control and Prevention: 1993 sexually transmitted disease treatment guidelines, *MMWR* 42 (RR-14): 1, 1993.

Corey L: Genital herpes. In Holmes KK et al, editors: *Sexually transmitted diseases,* ed 2, New York, 1990, McGraw-Hill.

Eschenbach DA: Pelvic infections and sexually transmitted diseases. In Scott JR et al, editors: *Danforth's obstetrics and gynecology,* ed 6, Philadelphia, 1990, JB Lippincott.

Ferenczy A: Treating genital condyloma during pregnancy with the carbon dioxide laser, *Am J Obstet Gynecol* 148:9, 1984.

Fox GN, Strangarity JW: Varicella-zoster virus infections in pregnancy, *Am Fam Physician* 39:89, 1989.

Francis DP, Chin J: The prevention of acquired immunodeficiency syndrome in the United States, *JAMA* 257:1357, 1987.

Friedland GH, Klein RS: Transmission of the human immunodeficiency virus, *N Engl J Med* 317:1125, 1987.

Hecht F: Counseling the HIV-positive woman regarding pregnancy, *JAMA* 257:3361, 1987.

Hill HR: Group B streptococcal infections. In Holmes KK et al, editors: *Sexually transmitted diseases,* ed 2, New York, 1990, McGraw-Hill.

Keeling RP: AIDS education: a mandate for schools of nursing, *Dean's Notes* 9:1, 1987.

Landesman S et al: Serosurvey of human immunodeficiency virus infection in parturients, *JAMA* 258:2701, 1987.

Marvin C, Slevin A: Chlamydia—cause, prevention, and cure, *MCN* 12:318, 1987.

McGregor JA: Chlamydial infection in women, *Obstet Gynecol Clin North Am* 16:565, 1989.

Minkoff HL et al: Pregnancies resulting in infants with acquired immunodeficiency syndrome: description of the antepartum, intrapartum, and postpartum course, *Obstet Gynecol* 69:285, 1987a.

Minkoff HL et al: Follow-up of mothers and children with AIDS, *Obstet Gynecol* 87:288, 1987b.

Oriel D: Genital human papillomavirus infection. In Holmes KK et al, editors: *Sexually transmitted diseases,* ed 2, New York, 1990, McGraw-Hill.

Rein MF, Müller M: *Trichomonas vaginalis* and trichomoniasis. In Holmes KK et al, editors: *Sexually transmitted diseases,* ed 2, New York, 1990, McGraw-Hill.

Schachter J: Why we need a program for the control of *Chlamydia trachomatis, N Engl J Med* 320:802, 1989.

Scott GB et al: Mothers of infants with the acquired immunodeficiency syndrome: evidence for both symptomatic and asymptomatic carriers, *JAMA* 253:363, 1985.

Shah KV: Biology of human genital tract papillomaviruses. In Holmes KK et al, editors: *Sexually transmitted diseases,* ed 2, New York, 1990, McGraw-Hill.

Spence MR: Epidemiology of sexually transmitted diseases, *Obstet Gynecol Clin North Am* 16:453, 1989.

Wolf PH et al: Toxic shock syndrome, *JAMA* 258:908, 1987.

BIBLIOGRAPHY

Acosta Y et al: HIV disease and pregnancy. Part 2. Antepartum and intrapartum care, *JOGNN* 21(2):97, 1992.

Bastian N et al: HIV disease and pregnancy. Part 3. Postpartum care of the HIV positive woman and her newborn, *JOGNN* 21(2):105, 1992.

Burke ME, Medford LK: Hypertension in pregnancy. In Harvey CJ, editor: *Critical care obstetrical nursing,* Gaithersburg, MD, 1992, Aspen.

Kelly K, Galbraith M, Vermund S: Genital human papillomavirus infection in women, *JOGNN* 21(6):503, 1992.

Knuppel R, Drukker J: *High risk pregnancy: a team approach,* ed 2, Philadelphia, 1993, WB Saunders.

Luegenbiehl D: Postpartum bleeding, NAACOG *Clin Issues Perinat Women Health Nurs* 2(3):402, 1991.

Martin JM, Troiano NH: Principles in hemodynamic monitoring, *NAACOG Clin Issues Perinat Women Health Nurs* 3(3):377, 1992.

Surratt N: Severe preeclampsia: implications for critical care obstetrics, *JOGNN* 22(6):500, 1993.

Tillman J: Syphilis: an old disease, a contemporary problem, *JOGNN* 21(3):209, 1992.

Tinkle M, Amaya M, Tamayo O: HIV disease and pregnancy. Part 1. Epidemiology, pathogenesis, and natural history, *JOGNN* 21(2):86, 1992.

Wheeler D: Intrapartum bleeding, *NAACOG Clin Issues Perinat Women Health Nurs* 2(3):381, 1991.

CHAPTER

22

Endocrine, Cardiovascular, and Medical-Surgical Problems during Pregnancy

KATHRYN RHODES ALDEN
CAROL FOWLER DURHAM

LEARNING OBJECTIVES

Define the key terms listed.

Differentiate the types of diabetes mellitus and their respective risk factors in pregnancy.

Summarize the effects of pregnancy on insulin requirements.

Discuss maternal and fetal risks and complications associated with diabetic pregnancy.

Discuss each step of the nursing process as it relates to diabetic pregnancy.

Explain the effects of hyperemesis gravidarum on pregnancy.

Describe the effects of thyroid disorders on pregnancy.

Review the management of pregnant women with cardiovascular disorders.

Discuss anemia during pregnancy.

Review the care of women whose pregnancies are complicated by autoimmune disorders.

Explain basic principles of care for a pregnant woman having abdominal surgery.

Identify priorities in assessment of the injured pregnant woman.

KEY TERMS

adult respiratory distress syndrome (ARDS)
autoimmune disease
cardiac decompensation
cholecystitis
cholelithiasis
gestational diabetes mellitus
glycosylated hemoglobin (Hgb A_{1c})
hydramnios
hyperemesis gravidarum
hyperglycemia
hyperthyroidism
hypertrophic cardiomyopathy (HCM)
hypoglycemia
hypothyroidism
idiopathic peripartum cardiomyopathy
infective endocarditis
ketoacidosis
macrosomia
mitral valve prolapse (MVP)
mitral valve stenosis
normoglycemia
peripartum heart failure
pregestational diabetes mellitus
rheumatic heart disease
sickle cell hemoglobinopathy
systemic lupus erythematosus (SLE)
thalassemia

RELATED TOPICS

Cesarean birth (Chap. 24) • Dystocia (Chap. 24) • Fetal assessment tests (Chap. 20) • Infants of diabetic mothers (Chap. 27) • Large for gestational age, small for gestational age infants (Chap. 27) • Maternal infections (Chap. 21) • Preeclampsia (Chap. 21) • Preterm birth (Chap. 24) • Spontaneous abortion (Chap. 21)

It is not uncommon for women with preexisting medical problems to become pregnant. Nor does pregnancy protect women from developing medical problems or sustaining injuries. The maternity nurse is challenged to provide sound, effective care that meets the unique maternal and fetal needs prompted by intervening medical conditions. The primary objective of nursing care must be to guide and support the woman and her family in achieving optimal pregnancy outcome for both the pregnant woman and the fetus. The nurse serves as teacher, counselor, and support person to assist the woman and her family in achieving the best possible outcome and to deal with the problems and disappointments that may arise.

This chapter focuses on endocrine disorders and cardiovascular disorders, with discussion of selected disorders of the respiratory, gastrointestinal, integumentary and central nervous systems. Some surgical procedures and injuries and the related nursing roles are also discussed.

Endocrine Disorders

DIABETES MELLITUS

Before the discovery of insulin in the early 1920s, diabetes and pregnancy were clearly incompatible. Many diabetic women of childbearing age were infertile or sterile, and the majority of those who became pregnant were unable to carry to term. Maternal and perinatal mortality was as high as 50%, with stillbirth the primary cause of perinatal death (Gabbe, 1992).

Over the last 70 years there have been remarkable improvements in the understanding and management of diabetic pregnancy. These advances in care have prompted substantial changes in maternal and perinatal outcomes. The current maternal mortality rate is approximately 0.5%; however, this rate is still five times that of nondiabetic pregnancies (Meyer, Palmer, 1990). The perinatal mortality rate has declined to less than 5%, compared with 1% to 2% in nondiabetic pregnancies (CDC, 1990). In well-managed cases the maternal and perinatal mortality rates are similar to those of the nondiabetic population.

Despite the advances in care, pregnancy complicated by diabetes is still considered high risk. It is most successfully managed with a multidisciplinary approach involving the obstetrician, endocrinologist, neonatologist, nurse, nutritionist, and social worker. Favorable outcome of diabetic pregnancy requires commitment and active participation by the woman. She must comply with a schedule of frequent prenatal visits, strict adherence to dietary regimen, regular self-monitoring of blood glucose level, frequent laboratory evaluation, intensive fetal surveillance, and possible hospitalization.

Care of the pregnant diabetic woman requires that the nurse fully understand the normal physiologic responses to pregnancy as well as the altered metabolism of diabetes. Furthermore, the nurse must understand the relationship between pregnancy and diabetes to accurately assess the woman, plan for her care, and intervene appropriately. An awareness of the psychosocial implications of diabetic pregnancy must guide the nurse in planning, implementing, and evaluating care of the woman and her family.

Pathogenesis

Diabetes mellitus is a systemic disorder of carbohydrate, protein, and fat metabolism. It is characterized by **hyperglycemia** (elevated blood glucose) resulting from inadequate production of insulin or ineffective use of insulin at the cellular level. Insulin, produced by the beta cells in the islets of Langerhans in the pancreas, is responsible for transporting glucose into the cell. When insulin is insufficient or ineffective, glucose accumulates in the bloodstream and hyperglycemia results. Hyperglycemia causes hyperosmolarity of the blood, which attracts intracellular fluid into the vascular system, resulting in cellular dehydration and expanded blood volume. Consequently, the kidneys excrete large volumes of urine *(polyuria)* in an attempt to regulate excess blood volume and to excrete the unusable glucose *(glycosuria)*. Cellular dehydration, in combination with polyuria, causes excessive thirst *(polydipsia)*.

The body compensates for its inability to convert carbohydrate (glucose) into energy by burning proteins (muscle) and fats. The end products of this metabolism are ketones and fatty acids, which in excess quantity produce **ketoacidosis.** Weight loss occurs due to the breakdown of fat and muscle tissue. This tissue breakdown causes a state of starvation that compels the individual to eat excessively *(polyphagia).*

Over time, diabetes causes significant vascular changes, primarily affecting the heart, eyes, and kidneys. Complications resulting from diabetes include premature atherosclerosis, retinopathy, and nephropathy.

Diabetes (types I and II) is typically regarded as a genetically determined syndrome. It is usually inherited as a recessive trait, but occurs as a dominant trait in some families. Inheritance of the genetic trait (genotype) for diabetes mellitus does not necessarily mean that the individual will demonstrate diabetic glucose intolerance (phenotype). Many people with the genotype do not show any evidence of diabetes until they experience one or more of a variety of stressors, or precipitating factors. Examples of such stressors are an increase in age, normal developmental periods of rapid hormonal change (menarche, pregnancy, menopause), obesity, infection, surgery, emotional crisis, and tumor or infection of the pancreas.

TABLE 22-1   National Institutes of Health Classification of Diabetes

CLASSIFICATION	PREVIOUS NAMES	DEFINITION
Type I: IDDM	Juvenile-onset diabetes Brittle diabetes	Insulin-dependent diabetes mellitus (IDDM); pancreatic beta cells in islets of Langerhans virtually do not produce insulin
Type II: NIDDM	Adult-onset diabetes	Non–insulin-dependent diabetes mellitus (NIDDM); pancreatic beta cells in islets of Langerhans are unable to meet increased demands for insulin over time or in times of stress
Type III: gestational diabetes	Gestational diabetes	Carbohydrate intolerance that develops during pregnancy, regardless of severity

TABLE 22-2   Classification of Diabetes during Pregnancy

CLASS	CHARACTERISTICS	IMPLICATIONS
Glucose intolerance of pregnancy	Abnormal glucose tolerance during pregnancy: postprandial hyperglycemia during pregnancy	Diagnosis before 30 weeks' gestation important to prevent macrosomia Treat with diet adequate in calories to prevent maternal weight loss Goal is postprandial blood glucose <130 mg/dl at 1 hour, or <105 mg/dl at 2 hours; if insulin is necessary, manage as in classes B, C, and D
A	Chemical diabetes diagnosed before pregnancy; managed by diet alone; any age at onset	Management as for glucose intolerance of pregnancy
B	Insulin treatment used before pregnancy; onset at age 20 or older; duration <10 years	Some endogenous insulin secretion may persist; fetal and neonatal risks same as in classes C and D, as is management
C	Onset at age 10 to 20, or duration 10 to 20 years	Insulin-deficient diabetes of juvenile onset
D	Onset before age 10, or duration >20 years, or chronic hypertension (not preeclampsia), or background retinopathy (tiny hemorrhages)	Fetal macrosomia or intrauterine growth retardation possible; retinal microaneurysms; dot hemorrhages, and exudates may progress during pregnancy, then regress after birth
F	Diabetic nephropathy with proteinuria	Anemia and hypertension common; proteinuria increases in third trimester, declines after giving birth. Fetal intrauterine growth retardation common; perinatal survival about 85% under optimum conditions; bed rest necessary
H	Coronary artery disease	Serious maternal risk
R	Proliferative retinopathy	Neovascularization, with risk of vitreous hemorrhage or retinal detachment; laser photocoagulation useful; abortion usually not necessary; with active process of neovascularization, prevent bearing-down efforts

From Benson RC, editor: *Current obstetric and gynecologic diagnosis and treatment,* ed 5, Los Altos, CA, 1984, Lange Medical Publications.

Classification

Diabetes has been classified into three major types by the National Institutes of Health (ADA, 1990) as shown in Table 22-1. Diabetes in pregnancy can be further categorized using White's classification system, based on age of onset of diabetes, its duration, and the severity of vascular changes that have occurred (White, 1978). This classification enables health care providers to identify those diabetic women who are at higher risk during pregnancy (Table 22-2).

Diabetes during pregnancy can also be classified according to whether the diabetes preceded the pregnancy or had its onset during gestation. **Pregestational diabetes** is the label given to type I or type II diabetes that existed prior to pregnancy, whereas **gestational diabetes** refers to glucose intolerance first recognized during the pregnancy.

Metabolic Changes during and after Pregnancy

Normal pregnancy has been labeled a diabetogenic state in which the need for glucose is increased. Maternal metabolism is altered to ensure a constant and adequate supply of glucose to the developing fetus. Maternal glucose is transported to the fetus by the process of facilitated diffusion. *Maternal insulin does not cross the placenta.* By the tenth week of gestation the fetus secretes his or her own insulin at levels adequate to use the glucose obtained from the mother.

During the first trimester of pregnancy, maternal glucose levels drop below nonpregnant values to between 55 and 65 mg/dl (Fig. 22-1, *A* and *B*). Due to the influence of estrogen and progesterone, the pancreas increases insulin production, which increases peripheral glucose utilization. At the same time, glucose utilization by the fetus is increasing, thus decreasing the maternal glucose levels. In addition, the first trimester is characterized by nausea, vomiting, and decreased food intake by the mother, further decreasing her glucose levels.

During the second and third trimesters, rising levels of human placental lactogen, estrogen, progesterone, cortisol, prolactin, and insulinase increase insulin resistance through their actions as insulin antagonists. Insulin resistance is a glucose-sparing mechanism that ensures an abundant supply of glucose for the fetus. The mother's need for insulin increases beginning in the second trimester. Insulin requirements may double or quadruple by term gestation (Fig. 22-1, *C* and *D*).

At birth, expulsion of the placenta prompts an abrupt drop in levels of circulating placental hormones, cortisol, and insulinase. Maternal tissues quickly regain their prepregnancy sensitivity to insulin. For the nonbreastfeeding mother, prepregnancy insulin-carbohydrate balance usually returns in about 7 to 10 days (Fig. 22-1, *E*). Lactation utilizes maternal glucose, so the breastfeeding mother's insulin requirements remain low for up to 9 months (Fig. 22-1, *F*). On completion of weaning, prepregnancy insulin requirement is reestablished (Fig. 22-1, *G*).

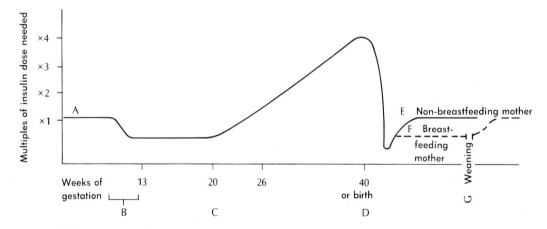

FIG. 22-1 **A,** Changing insulin needs during pregnancy caused by properties of placental hormones and enzyme (insulinase) and cortisol. **B,** Gestational period characterized by nausea, vomiting, and often decreased food intake by mother while glucose use of embryo-fetus increases. **C,** Increase in peripheral resistance to insulin (mother becomes less sensitive to insulin). **D,** Day of birth; maternal insulin requirements drop dramatically to about prepregnancy levels; she is now very sensitive to insulin. **E,** For nonbreastfeeding mother prepregnancy insulin-carbohydrate balance usually returns in about 7 to 10 days. **F,** For breastfeeding mother, her insulin requirements will remain low for 6 to 9 months. **G,** At weaning, woman's prepregnancy carbohydrate metabolism is reestablished.

Pregestational Diabetes

When a recognized diabetic woman becomes pregnant, she is known as a pregestational diabetic; that is, the diabetes existed before conception and will continue after the pregnancy. Pregestational diabetics may have either type I (insulin-dependent) or type II (non–insulin-dependent) diabetes, which may or may not be complicated by vascular disease, retinopathy, nephropathy, and other diabetic complications. Type II diabetics are considered insulin dependent during pregnancy because oral hypoglycemics must be discontinued due to potential effects on the fetus.

The reported incidence of insulin-dependent diabetes during pregnancy varies from 0.1% to 0.5% and accounts for approximately 10% of all diabetic pregnancies (CDC, 1990; Hagay, Reece, 1992).

The diabetogenic state of pregnancy imposed on the compromised metabolic system of the pregestational diabetic has significant implications. The normal hormonal adaptations of pregnancy affect glycemic control in the pregestational diabetic. Pregnancy may also accelerate the progress of vascular complications of diabetes.

During the first trimester, while maternal blood glucose levels are normally reduced and insulin response to glucose is enhanced, glycemic control is improved. Insulin dosage for the well-controlled diabetic may need to be adjusted to avoid **hypoglycemia** (low blood glucose). Hypoglycemic episodes are not uncommon in type I diabetics during early pregnancy (Meyer, Palmer, 1990).

As insulin requirements steadily increase after the first trimester, insulin dosage must be adjusted accordingly to prevent episodes of *hyperglycemia*. Insulin resistance begins as early as 14 to 16 weeks and continues to rise until leveling off during the last few weeks of pregnancy.

Whether pregnancy worsens diabetes-related vascular disease depends on the extent of this complication before pregnancy. The greater the degree of vascular involvement, the greater the likelihood of poor outcome for mother and infant. Women with atherosclerotic heart disease are at greatest risk. Pregnancy can contribute to worsening of retinal disease in women with a background of proliferative retinopathy, especially in the presence of hypertension (Jovanovic-Peterson, Peterson, 1991; Rosenn et al, 1992). In the majority of diabetic women, pregnancy is not associated with permanent deterioration in kidney functioning, provided that blood pressure and glucose levels are maintained within normal ranges (Jovanovic-Peterson, Peterson, 1992; Meyer, Palmer, 1990).

Preconceptional Counseling

Preconceptional counseling is recommended for all diabetic women of reproductive age and is associated with improved pregnancy outcome (Rosenn et al, 1991; Willhoite et al, 1993). Under ideal circumstances the prege-

stational diabetic woman is counseled before the time of conception in order to plan the optimal time for pregnancy, to establish glycemic control before conception, and to evaluate the woman for any evidence of vascular complications of diabetes. Diabetic women with preexisting vascular complications are informed that pregnancy may compound the problems of diabetic nephropathy, retinopathy, and other diabetic sequelae.

The diabetic woman and her partner should be included in the counseling process to assess their level of understanding related to the effects of pregnancy on the diabetic condition, and the potential complications of pregnancy due to diabetes. They should also be informed of the anticipated alterations in management of diabetes due to pregnancy.

Oral hypoglycemic agents may exert teratogenic effects on the fetus and should be discontinued in the preconceptional period in type II diabetic women who had previously used them for glucose control. These women are started on insulin injections before pregnancy when the pregnancy is planned and as soon as the pregnancy is diagnosed when it is unplanned.

Maternal Risks and Complications

The pregnant diabetic woman is at risk for the development of complications. The degree of risk is directly related to the woman's glucose control before conception and during pregnancy, and is influenced by the presence of preexisting diabetic complications. Maternal complications commonly occurring in association with diabetic pregnancy include the following:

Spontaneous abortion occurs more frequently among pregnant diabetic women and is related to poor glycemic control at the time of conception and in the early weeks of pregnancy (Combs, Kitzmiller, 1991; Rosenn et al, 1991).

Pregnancy-induced hypertension (PIH), or *preeclampsia,* occurs two times more frequently during diabetic pregnancy. The highest incidence occurs in women with preexisting vascular changes related to diabetes (Cunningham et al, 1993; Meyer, Palmer, 1990).

Hydramnios (polyhydramnios), amniotic fluid in excess of 2000 ml, occurs about 10 times more often in diabetic pregnancies than in nondiabetic pregnancies. Hydramnios, causing overdistention of the uterus, increases the risk of premature rupture of membranes, preterm labor, and postpartum hemorrhage.

Infections are much more common and serious in diabetic women who are pregnant. Vaginal infections, particularly monilial vaginitis, are more common. Urinary tract infections (UTIs), common during pregnancy, are more prevalent among pregnant diabetic women, possibly related to glycosuria. Infection in a diabetic woman is serious because it causes increased insulin resistance and may result in ketoacidosis. These infections can also precipitate preterm labor. The rate of postpartum infection among insulin-dependent diabetics has been reported five times greater than among nondiabetics (Stamler, 1990).

Ketoacidosis can be life threatening to the mother and to the fetus. It occurs most often during the second and third trimesters when the diabetogenic effect of pregnancy is the greatest as insulin resistance increases. Ketoacidosis, the consequence of untreated hyperglycemia, is commonly caused by maternal infection or illness, or inappropriate insulin doses. Hyperglycemia occurs when glucose cannot be transported into the cells due to a lack of insulin. Because the body cannot utilize glucose for energy, it begins to break down fat and muscle tissue.

As a result of fat metabolism, ketone bodies are produced by the liver, accumulate in the blood (ketosis), and are spilled over into the urine (ketonuria). As ketosis increases, metabolic acidosis develops from the pH-lowering effects of the ketones. Large amounts of fluid are lost due to osmotic diuresis resulting in dehydration and electrolyte imbalance. Prompt treatment is necessary to avoid maternal coma or death. Ketoacidosis occurring at any time during pregnancy can lead to intrauterine fetal death. Perinatal mortality may be as high as 50% to 80% with maternal ketoacidosis (Gabbe, 1990; Harvey, 1992) (Table 22-3).

Although strict glycemic control is the goal of management of diabetic pregnancy, the risk of *hypoglycemia* is increased (Langford, Bartholomew, 1992). Hypoglycemia is typically caused by overdose of insulin, late or skipped meals, or overzealous exercise. During the first trimester when blood glucose levels are characteristically

TABLE 22-3 Differentiation of Hypoglycemia (Insulin Shock) and Hyperglycemia (Diabetic Ketoacidosis)

	HYPOGLYCEMIA (INSULIN SHOCK)	HYPERGLYCEMIA (DIABETIC KETOACIDOSIS)
Causes	Excess insulin	Insufficient insulin
	Insufficient food (delayed or missed meals)	Excess or wrong kind of food
	Excessive exercise or work	Infection, injuries, illness
	Indigestion, diarrhea, vomiting	Emotional stress
Onset	Rapid (regular insulin)	Insufficient exercise
	Gradual (modified insulin or oral hypoglycemic agents)	Slow (hours to days)
Symptoms	Hunger	Thirst
	Sweating	Nausea or vomiting
	Nervousness	Abdominal pain
	Weakness	Constipation
	Fatigue	Drowsiness
	Blurred or double vision	Dim vision
	Dizziness	Increased urination
	Headache	Headache
	Pallor, clammy skin	Flushed, dry skin
	Shallow respirations	Rapid breathing
	Normal pulse	Weak, rapid pulse
	Laboratory values:	Acetone (fruity) breath odor
	Urine: negative for sugar and acetone	Laboratory values:
	Blood glucose: $\leq$ 60 mg/dl	Urine: positive for sugar and acetone
		Blood glucose: $\geq$ 250 mg/dl
Intervention	Notify primary health care provider	Notify primary health care provider
	Give low-fat milk	Administer insulin in accordance with blood glucose levels
	If orange juice is given for a fast supply of sugar, follow it later with milk	Give IV fluids such as normal saline or one-half normal saline; potassium when urinary output is adequate; bicarbonate for pH < 7.0
	If patient is unconscious, 50% dextrose IV push, 5% to 10% D/W IV drip, or glucagon	
	Obtain blood and urine specimens for laboratory testing	Monitor laboratory testing of blood and urine

D/W, Dextrose in water; *IV,* intravenous.

below normal, hypoglycemia frequently results. Later in pregnancy, as insulin doses are adjusted to maintain glycemic control, hypoglycemia may also occur. The effects of hypoglycemia on the fetus are usually minimal provided that the mother is treated appropriately. Severe maternal hypoglycemia during the first trimester may cause congenital defects in the fetus (Meyer, Palmer, 1990; Rotondo, 1990) (see Table 22-3).

Fetal/Neonatal Risks and Complications

From the moment of conception the infant of a diabetic mother faces increased risk of complications that may occur during the antenatal, intrapartal or neonatal periods. These complications may be mild and transient but are often life threatening and may result in death of the infant. Infant morbidity and mortality associated with diabetic pregnancy are significantly reduced with strict control of maternal glucose levels before and during pregnancy.

The incidence of *congenital anomalies* among infants of insulin-dependent diabetic women is two to eight times that of the general population. Up to 50% of all perinatal deaths among infants of diabetic mothers are the result of congenital malformations (Becerra et al, 1990; CDC, 1990). The risk of congenital anomalies is increased with poor glycemic control before conception and in the early weeks of pregnancy, during the period of organogenesis (Greene et al, 1989; Kitzmiller et al, 1991; Steele et al, 1990). Anomalies common to infants of diabetic mothers include neural tube defects, caudal regression syndrome, congenital cardiac and renal anomalies, and gastrointestinal malformations (Becerra et al, 1990; Cooper et al, 1992; Rizzo et al, 1991).

Macrosomia, infant weight greater than 4000 g, occurs in 25% to 42% of pregnancies complicated by diabetes as compared with 8% to 14% of nondiabetic pregnancies (Jovanovic-Peterson et al, 1991). The fetal pancreas begins to secrete insulin at 10 to 14 weeks' gestation. The fetus responds to maternal hyperglycemia by secreting large amounts of insulin (hyperinsulinism). Insulin acts as a growth hormone, causing the fetus to lay down excess stores of glycogen, protein, and adipose tissue, leading to increased fetal size, or macrosomia. These infants are considered *large for gestational age (LGA)*. Macrosomia is associated with dystocia, often resulting in operative vaginal birth (episiotomy and forceps), and is responsible for the increased rate of cesarean birth among diabetic mothers. The macrosomic infant may suffer from a fractured clavicle, liver or spleen laceration, brachial plexus injury, facial palsy, phrenic nerve injury, or subdural hemorrhage. Severe asphyxia may occur due to difficult, prolonged birth.

In the mother who has experienced vascular changes as a complication of diabetes, there may be compromised uteroplacental circulation. This decreases the amount of oxygen available to the fetus and may contribute to *intrauterine growth retardation (IUGR)*, resulting in a neonate who is *small for gestational age (SGA)*. Preterm birth, common to diabetic pregnancy, may also be related to fetal hypoxia (Matheson, Efantis, 1989).

Infants of diabetic mothers are at increased risk for respiratory distress syndrome (RDS) related to *hyaline membrane disease*. Hyperglycemia has been associated with delayed lung maturity due to interference with phosphatidylglycerol (PG) production (Piper, Langer, 1993). Also, in past years the incidence of hyaline membrane disease was greater as many infants were born before term in an attempt to prevent fetal demise. With advanced fetal surveillance techniques and improved maternal glycemic control, the incidence of preterm birth with resultant respiratory distress syndrome has declined.

For infants of diabetic pregnancy the transition to extrauterine life is often plagued with metabolic abnormalities. Within the first 30 to 60 minutes after birth neonatal hypoglycemia often occurs. The fetal pancreas has been programmed to produce large amounts of insulin in response to maternal hyperglycemia while in utero. With birth the glucose supply is abruptly interrupted, yet the neonatal pancreas continues to produce insulin at the previous rate. Glucose stores are quickly utilized, resulting in neonatal hypoglycemic episodes. *Hypocalcemia, hypomagnesemia, hyperbilirubinemia,* and *polycythemia* occur more frequently in infants of diabetic mothers and place the neonate at increased risk (Salveson, 1992; Samson, 1992).

Care Management—The Pregnant Diabetic Woman

✦ ASSESSMENT

History

Whenever a pregnant diabetic woman requests prenatal care, thorough evaluation of her health status is completed. In addition to routine prenatal assessment, the nurse obtains a detailed history regarding the onset and course of the diabetic condition, as well as the management of diabetes and the degree of glycemic control before pregnancy. Effective management of diabetic pregnancy depends on the woman's adherence to a plan of care. For the woman to care for her diabetes daily, she must have an adequate understanding of her condition and the prescribed regimen. Thus, with the initial prenatal visit, the nurse conducts a thorough assessment of the woman's knowledge regarding diabetes and pregnancy, potential maternal and fetal complications, and the plan of care. With subsequent visits, follow-up assessments are completed. Data from these assessments are used to identify the woman's specific learning needs.

The woman's emotional status is assessed to determine how she is coping with pregnancy superimposed on preexisting diabetes. Whereas normal pregnancy typically evokes some degree of stress and anxiety, pregnancy designated as high risk serves to compound anxiety and stress levels. Fear of maternal and fetal complications is a major concern. Strict adherence to the plan of care necessitates alterations in patterns of daily living and may be an additional source of stress.

The woman's support system is assessed to identify those persons significant to her and their role in her life. The support person's knowledge of diabetes is also assessed and teaching needs are identified. It is important to assess the family's/significant other's reaction to the pregnancy and the strict management plan, as well as their involvement in the treatment regimen. Research has shown that social support improves compliance. Socioeconomic factors are also reviewed. Any area of emotional stress is identified because such stress can precipitate complications (Leff et al, 1991; Ruggiero et al, 1993).

Physical Examination

At the initial visit a thorough physical examination is performed to assess the woman's health status. In addition to the routine prenatal examination, specific efforts are made to assess effects of diabetes on the pregnant woman. A baseline electrocardiogram (ECG) is done to assess cardiovascular status. Evaluation for retinopathy is done, with follow-up as needed by an ophthalmologist. Blood pressure is monitored carefully throughout pregnancy due to the increased risk for PIH. The woman's weight gain is also monitored at each visit. Fundal height is measured, noting any abnormal increase in size for dates, which may be indicative of hydramnios or fetal macrosomia. Leopold's maneuvers are also performed to check for fetal size and possible hydramnios.

Laboratory Tests

Routine prenatal laboratory examinations are performed. Baseline renal function is assessed with a 24-hour urine test for total protein excretion and creatinine clearance. Urine tests are performed at each prenatal visit to assess for urinary tract infection, glycosuria, ketonuria, and proteinuria. Thyroid function tests may also be done due to the risk of coexisting thyroid disease.

For the woman with pregestational diabetes, type I or II, laboratory tests are done to assess glycemic control. Glycemic control is evaluated based on **glycosylated hemoglobin (HbA$_{1c}$)** levels. This measurement is based on the fact that glucose attaches to hemoglobin A during its normal 120-day life span. In effect, glycosylated hemoglobin measures the level of hemoglobin A that has been "sugar coated." Therefore a test for glycosylated hemoglobin provides a measurement of glycemic control over the previous 4 to 6 weeks. Regular measurements

of glycosylated hemoglobin provide data for altering the treatment plan to promote glycemic control (Larsen et al, 1990). Values for the measurement of HbA$_{1c}$, the most commonly used index of glycosylated hemoglobin, are as follows (Pagano, Pagano, 1992):

Nondiabetic adult	2.2% to 4.8%
Good diabetic control	2.5% to 6%
Fair diabetic control	6.1% to 8%
Poor diabetic control	>8%

Fetal Surveillance

Diagnostic techniques for fetal surveillance are often performed during pregnancy complicated by diabetes to assess fetal growth and well-being. Efforts are made to determine the estimated date of birth (EDB). A baseline ultrasound is done to assess gestational age of the fetus. Follow-up ultrasound examinations are performed during the pregnancy, as often as every 4 to 6 weeks, to monitor fetal growth and development and to assess for congenital anomalies.

Because diabetic pregnancies are at greater risk for neural tube defects (e.g., spina bifida, anencephaly, microcephaly), measurement of maternal serum alpha-fetoprotein (AFP) is usually performed between 16 and 18 weeks' gestation. Amniocentesis may be done to diagnose congenital anomalies.

Fetal movement, or kick counts, is determined daily beginning around 24 weeks. Nonstress tests (NSTs) are often used weekly or more often during the third trimester to assess fetal well-being. Fetal biophysical profile monitoring may be used to evaluate both fetal well-being and uteroplacental adequacy. Fetal cardiac anomalies may be assessed by routine echocardiography (Jovanovic-Peterson, Peterson, 1992; Matheson, Efantis, 1989).

Determination of Birth Date

In the past, preterm birth was often elected to avoid the risk of intrauterine death. Today the majority of diabetic pregnancies are allowed to progress to term, provided the woman has maintained **normoglycemia** or good glycemic control. In women with vasculopathy or less than optimal glycemic control who have not adhered to the program of care or who have had a previous stillbirth, amniocentesis may be performed at 36 or 37 weeks to assess fetal lung maturity. For the fetus who has documented lung maturity and poor results of fetal surveillance testing, birth is accomplished immediately. Despite fetal lung immaturity, birth may be essential when testing suggests fetal compromise or if the pregnant woman develops PIH, rapidly worsening retinopathy, or renal failure (Jovanovic-Peterson, Peterson, 1992).

✦ NURSING DIAGNOSES

Each woman's experience of pregnancy that has been complicated by diabetes is unique to her and to her family. As a result of this, the nursing diagnoses must be carefully formulated so that they reflect the actual or potential altered health-related responses that could be influenced, improved, or alleviated by nursing intervention. The following section gives examples of possible nursing diagnoses for the patient who has pregestational diabetes during antepartum, intrapartum and postpartum.

Antepartum

Knowledge deficit related to
- Diabetic pregnancy, management, and potential effects on pregnant woman and fetus
- Insulin effects and its administration
- Hypoglycemia and hyperglycemia
- Diabetic diet

High risk for ineffective individual or family coping related to
- Woman's responsibility in managing her diabetes during pregnancy

Anxiety, fear, dysfunctional grieving, powerlessness, body image disturbance, situational low self-esteem, spiritual distress, altered role performance, and altered family processes related to
- Effects of diabetes and its potential sequelae on the pregnant woman and the fetus

High risk for injury to fetus related to
- Uteroplacental insufficiency

High risk for maternal injury related to
- Improper insulin administration
- Hypoglycemia and hyperglycemia

Altered nutrition: less or more than body requirements related to
- Diabetes and pregnancy

High risk for infection related to
- Hyperglycemia

High risk for noncompliance related to
- Lack of understanding about diabetes and pregnancy
- Lack of financial resources to purchase blood glucose or urine testing supplies

Intrapartum

High risk for maternal injury related to
- Hypoglycemia or hyperglycemia
- Preeclampsia

Altered cardiopulmonary tissue perfusion related to
- Supine hypotension

Postpartum

High risk for injury related to
- Fluctuating blood glucose levels after the infant's birth

High risk for injury related to
- Complications of involution (hemorrhage, infection)
- Postpartum appearance of preeclampsia

❖ EXPECTED OUTCOMES

Planning care for the diabetic pregnant woman and her family is given direction from identified nursing diagnoses and the plan for medical management of diabetic pregnancy. The plan is individualized, relating specifically to needs identified by the health care team and to those mutually identified by the woman, family, and the caregivers.

Expected outcomes for the pregnant diabetic include:
1. The woman and her family will demonstrate/verbalize understanding of diabetic pregnancy, plan of care, and importance of glycemic control.
2. The woman will comply with the plan of care.
3. The woman will achieve and maintain glycemic control.
4. The woman will demonstrate effective coping.
5. The woman will experience no complications; maternal morbidity/mortality will be prevented.
6. The infant will experience no complications; perinatal morbidity and mortality will be prevented.
7. The family will experience mutuality and support among its members.

❖ COLLABORATIVE CARE

As a vital member of the health care team ministering to the needs of the pregnant diabetic woman, the nurse assumes a variety of roles. Normal pregnancy is a maturational crisis for most women; those pregnancies complicated by diabetes may represent a situational crisis as well, due to the high risk nature of the condition. These women require individualized, in-depth nursing care throughout the pregnancy and in the postpartum period.

Assisting the woman with stress reduction is central to the care needed by women whose pregnancies are complicated by diabetes mellitus. Increased stress contributes to elevated blood glucose levels. Stress reduction and relaxation techniques are taught as needed. Space, privacy, and time are provided for the woman and her family to voice their feelings and questions, as well as to problem solve among themselves. The nurse acknowledges both positive and negative feelings about the pregnancy in seeking to improve the woman's motivation and understanding of diabetic management. Providing care that is sensitive to individual needs and based on a collaborative relationship with the woman and family fosters their physical and emotional well-being (Leff et al, 1991).

Fetal surveillance techniques may identify a congenital malformation incompatible with survival. Parents need supportive care as they consider the option of early pregnancy termination. The early detection of serious fetal malformations allows for exploration of various options in planning birth and immediate care of the newborn. The parents may also benefit from the time to prepare for the birth of a child with a congenital abnormality. Diagnostic tests for fetal malformations should be conducted under conditions that are both voluntary and informed. The risks, accuracy, and limitations of the tests should be discussed. The benefits of diagnosis and the options available when a positive diagnosis is obtained should be discussed in advance. In those instances when pregnancy loss occurs, the nurse is key in providing counseling for the woman and her family (Penha et al, 1993).

Engaging the woman as an active participant in the plan of care maintains or enhances her self-esteem and helps her to develop self-confidence that she will be able to care for herself and her baby. Open communication with members of the health care team is encouraged to facilitate her participation in self-care.

The nurse is most often the primary educator for the diabetic woman and her family. Through ongoing assessment, learning needs are identified. Teaching is instituted early in pregnancy and is continued throughout the period of gestation. Adequate understanding of diabetes and pregnancy, the treatment plan, and potential complications encourages patient compliance. It is only through compliance that strict glucose control can be maintained and maternal and fetal well-being are promoted.

Antepartum

Management of diabetic pregnancy is a complex process that requires the woman to be knowledgeable about the treatment regimen and astute to the changes that may occur so that she may respond appropriately. Even though the woman is likely to have some knowledge and experience with the various aspects of diabetic care—diet, insulin, exercise, blood glucose monitoring—she needs assistance from the nurse to understand the impact of pregnancy on diabetes to manage her care effectively.

Diet

The pregnant woman with pregestational diabetes has probably had nutritional counseling regarding management of the diabetes. Because pregnancy precipitates special nutritional concerns and needs, the woman must be educated and counseled to incorporate these changes into dietary planning. Nutritional counseling is usually provided by a registered dietitian. Pregnancy is an ideal time for the diabetic to fine-tune her self-management skills because self-motivation is typically high. It is essential that the woman understand the importance of maintaining normoglycemia during pregnancy.

Dietary management during diabetic pregnancy must be based on blood glucose (not urinary glucose) levels. The diet is individualized to allow for increased fetal and metabolic requirements, with consideration of such factors as prepregnancy weight and dietary habits, overall health, ethnic background and lifestyle, stage of pregnancy, knowledge of nutrition, and insulin therapy. The

dietary goal is to provide weight gain consistent with a normal pregnancy, to prevent ketoacidosis, and to minimize widely fluctuating blood glucose levels.

Energy needs are calculated on the basis of 30 to 40 calories per kilogram of ideal body weight, with the average diet including 2200 to 2400 calories. Total calories may be distributed among three meals and one evening snack, or more commonly three meals and at least two snacks. The woman may choose to divide the calorie intake among five to seven small meals per day. Meals should be eaten on time and never skipped. Snacks must be carefully planned in accordance with insulin therapy to avoid fluctuations in blood glucose levels. A large bedtime snack of at least 25 g of carbohydrate with some protein is recommended. To prevent blood glucose from dropping too low during the night, some women find that they need an additional snack of milk and crackers or fruit.

The ratio of carbohydrate, protein, and fat is important to meet metabolic needs of the woman and the fetus. Approximately 50% of the total calories should be carbohydrate, with a minimum of 250 g per day. Simple carbohydrates are avoided; complex carbohydrates that are high in fiber content are recommended because the starch and protein in such foods help to regulate the blood glucose level due to more sustained glucose release. Protein intake should constitute around 20% of the total calories, or about 100 to 200 g per day. Less than 30% of the daily caloric intake should come from fat, or no more than 80 g per day. Highly saturated fats are to be avoided. A registered dietitian determines the num-

HOME CARE

DIETARY MANAGEMENT OF DIABETIC PREGNANCY

- Follow the prescribed diet plan.
- Eat a well-balanced diet, including daily food requirements for a normal pregnancy.
- Divide daily food intake among three meals and two to four snacks, depending on individual needs.
- Eat a substantial bedtime snack to prevent a severe drop in blood glucose level during the night.
- Limit the intake of fats if weight gain occurs too rapidly.
- Take daily vitamins and iron as prescribed by the health care provider.
- Avoid foods high in refined sugar.
- Eat consistently each day; never skip meals or snacks.
- Reduce the intake of saturated fat and cholesterol.
- Eat foods high in dietary fiber.
- Avoid alcohol and caffeine.

ber of exchanges allowed for each meal and snack and helps the woman use the exchange list to plan daily intake.

In addition to sufficient calories, vitamins and minerals are necessary during pregnancy. These are usually provided as daily supplements to the diet (Worthington-Roberts, Williams, 1993) (see the Home Care box).

Monitoring Blood Glucose Levels

Blood glucose testing at home is the commonly accepted method for monitoring blood glucose levels. The preferred method of home glucose monitoring involves the use of a glucose reflectance meter (Fig. 22-2). Blood glucose levels are usually measured before meals and snacks, 2 hours after meals, and at bedtime, although more or

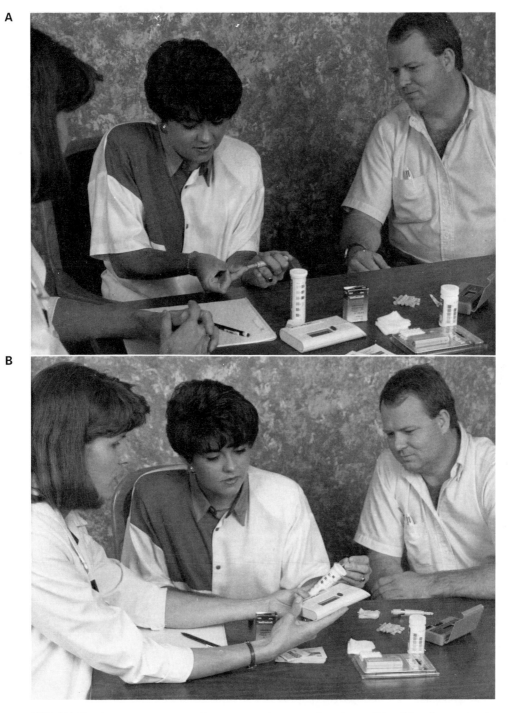

FIG. 22-2 **A,** Pregnant woman demonstrates how to collect drop of blood for glucose monitoring. **B,** Nurse assists woman and her husband in interpreting glucose values displayed by monitor. (Courtesy Jonas McKoy, University of North Carolina at Chapel Hill School of Nursing.)

less frequent testing may be done according to the woman's glycemic control. Women are encouraged to check glucose levels at any sign of hypoglycemia or hyperglycemia. Insulin dosage, diet, and other aspects of the daily management plan are adjusted in response to blood glucose levels, thus accuracy in testing and reporting is essential. Target ranges for blood glucose levels during pregnancy are as follows:

Target Ranges	Blood Glucose Levels (mg/dl)
Before breakfast	60 to 90
Before lunch, dinner, and bedtime	60 to 105
Two hours after meals	60 to 120

Urine Testing

Urine is tested for ketones upon awakening and whenever a meal or snack is delayed. When ketonuria occurs, carbohydrate intake should be cautiously increased, or another snack should be added to the daily meal plan (Jovanovic-Peterson, Peterson, 1992).

Insulin Therapy

Biosynthetic human insulin is recommended for pregnant women due to the unlikelihood of an allergic reaction as compared with the animal-base insulins. Rapid (regular) and intermediate-acting (NPH and lente) insulins are administered during pregnancy (Jovanovic-Peterson, Peterson, 1992).

The total daily dosage of insulin is determined based on the woman's gestational week and her body weight. This initial dosage calculation is then adjusted as needed according to blood glucose levels. Most insulin-dependent diabetic women require multiple daily injections during pregnancy. A combination of intermediate-acting and regular (short-acting) insulin before breakfast and at dinner time is a common regimen.

Although subcutaneous insulin injections are most commonly used, continuous insulin infusion systems may also be utilized during pregnancy (Fig. 22-3). The insulin pump infuses insulin at a set basal rate with a bolus dose to cover meals. The infusion tubing from this portable, battery-operated system can be left in place for several weeks without local complications. Insulin pumps are usually reserved for women whose diabetes cannot be controlled by multiple insulin injections and who are highly motivated because meticulous blood glucose monitoring is required (Tomky, 1989).

Exercise

Exercise during pregnancy complicated by diabetes is somewhat controversial, but it has been recognized that exercise enhances the utilization of glucose and decreases insulin need in type II and gestational diabetes (Artal, 1992; Winn, Reece, 1989). In type I diabetic women ex-

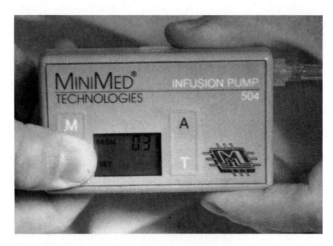

FIG. 22-3 Pregnant woman with diabetes sets basal rate on her insulin pump. (Courtesy Jonas McKoy, University of North Carolina at Chapel Hill School of Nursing.)

HOME CARE

EXERCISE FOR PREGNANT WOMEN WITH PREGESTATIONAL DIABETES

- Exercise plans are individualized and should be monitored by the health care provider.
- Select exercises that are enjoyable to foster regularity.
- Exercise does not have to be vigorous to be effective.
- Avoid exercising in a warm environment.
- The best time to exercise is after meals, when blood glucose is beginning to rise.
- Monitor blood glucose levels before, during, and after exercise to determine variations in glucose levels.
- Do not administer insulin into an extremity that is to be immediately involved in exercise.

---

ercise plans are prescribed judiciously and monitored closely by the health care providers. Particularly in those women with preexisting vascular changes, exercise may cause a redistribution of blood flow, which increases the potential for ischemic injury to already compromised organs and to the placenta (see the Home Care box above).

Supervision

Prenatal care for the pregnant diabetic woman typically assumes a more frequent schedule than that of the nondiabetic pregnant woman. It is essential that the woman understand the importance of early prenatal care and the need to keep all scheduled appointments. If there is any question about glycemic control, visits are scheduled a

ETHICAL CONSIDERATIONS

PREGNANT WOMEN WITH MEDICAL COMPLICATIONS

Ethical dilemmas can occur in patient care situations involving the risk/benefit ratio of care to the mother and fetus. One issue is forced maternal bed rest or hospitalization to treat an underlying medical problem such as diabetes or cardiac disease. Traditionally, care has been provided based on the one-patient model (maternal-fetal unit), but recently the two-patient model (pregnant woman and fetus) increasingly has been used to make treatment decisions. Maternal refusal or acceptance of treatment can be ethically analyzed using these models.

minimum of every 2 weeks for the first 32 weeks and then weekly until the birth.

Hospitalization

Despite advances in care, some women may require hospitalization for regulation of insulin dosage and stabilization of glucose levels. Hospitalization offers a controlled situation to regulate insulin therapy while providing opportunity for intensive education in self-administration of insulin and regulation of blood glucose (see Ethical Considerations box).

Complications

The woman is alerted to potential complications during pregnancy and is instructed about the need for prompt reporting of such problems as nausea, vomiting, and infections. It is essential that the woman and her family be knowledgeable about hypoglycemia and hyperglycemia, their causes, and symptoms as well as prevention and treatment measures (see Table 22-3).

To prevent complications, the woman should not engage in any long-term travel without first contacting the health care provider. Whenever she is away from home, she should carry along insulin, syringes, and fast-acting sugar. She should wear an identification bracelet at all times. It is also helpful to carry along an exchange list for dietary needs.

Intrapartum

During the intrapartum period the pregestational diabetic woman must be monitored closely to prevent complications related to dehydration, hypoglycemia, and hyperglycemia. Most women use large amounts of energy (calories) to accomplish the work and manage the stress of labor and birth; however, this calorie expenditure varies with the individual. Blood glucose levels and hydration must be carefully controlled during labor. To ac-

complish this, an IV line is inserted for infusion of a maintenance fluid, usually lactated Ringer's (LR) or 5% dextrose/lactated Ringer's (D5LR) solution. Insulin may be administered by continuous infusion or intermittent subcutaneous injection. Determinations of blood glucose are made every 1 to 2 hours while dextrose and insulin are titrated by calibrated pump to maintain blood glucose levels between 60 and 100 mg/dl. It is essential that these target glucose levels be maintained because hyperglycemia during labor can precipitate metabolic problems in the neonate, particularly hypoglycemia. Maternal hyperglycemia during labor can also lead to perinatal asphyxia (Matheson, Efantis, 1989; Palmer, Inturrisi, 1992).

Note: For the laboring diabetic woman a prescribed amount of insulin is usually mixed with 250 ml to 500 ml of normal saline or lactated Ringer's solution for IV administration. (Insulin, a protein, is attracted chemically to the plastic in the IV tubing. It leaves the solution and adheres to the lining of the tubing. Adherence to the tubing can be prevented by flushing the line first with 100 ml of normal saline and 10 units of insulin, which will completely coat the lining. Then the prescribed solution of insulin is begun and will remain stable. A protein [albumin] may be added to the solution instead; however, it is more expensive.)

During labor, continuous fetal heart monitoring is advised. The mother should assume an upright or a side-lying position during labor to prevent supine hypotension because of a large fetus or polyhydramnios. Labor is allowed to progress provided normal rates of cervical dilatation and fetal descent are maintained. Failure to progress may indicate a macrosomic infant and cephalopelvic disproportion (CPD), which necessitates cesarean birth. The woman is observed and treated during labor for diabetic complications such as hyperglycemia, ketosis, ketoacidosis, and glycosuria. A pediatrician may be present at birth to initiate neonatal assessment and care.

Postpartum

In the immediate postpartum period there is a substantial decrease in insulin requirements because the major source of insulin resistance, the placenta, has been removed. The type I diabetic woman may require only one half to two thirds of the prenatal insulin dose on the first postpartum day, provided she is eating a full diet. It takes several days after the birth to reestablish carbohydrate homeostasis (see Fig. 22-1). Blood glucose levels are monitored in the postpartum period and insulin dosage is adjusted accordingly. The insulin-dependent woman must realize the importance of eating on time even if the baby needs feeding or other pressing demands exist. Type II diabetic women often require no insulin in the postpartum period and are able to maintain normoglycemia through diet alone or with oral hypoglycemics.

Possible postpartum complications include preeclampsia-eclampsia, hemorrhage, and infection. The risk of preeclampsia-eclampsia is increased in the woman with preexisting vascular disease. Hemorrhage is a possibility if the mother's uterus was overdistended (hydramnios, macrosomic fetus), or overstimulated (oxytocin induction). Infections such as monilial vaginitis are more likely to occur in a postpartum woman with diabetes.

Diabetic mothers are encouraged to breastfeed. Besides the advantages of maternal satisfaction and pleasure, breastfeeding has an antidiabetogenic effect. Insulin requirements of the lactating diabetic mother are decreased due to the carbohydrate utilized in human milk production. Insulin dosage, which is decreased during lactation, must be recalculated at the time of weaning (Benz, 1992) (see Fig. 22-1, F to G).

The new mother needs information related to family planning and contraception. Whereas family planning is important for all women, it is essential for the diabetic woman to safeguard her own health and to promote optimal outcome in any future pregnancies. The woman and her partner should be informed that the risks associated with pregnancy increase with the duration and severity of the diabetic condition, and that pregnancy may contribute to vascular changes associated with diabetes. The risks and benefits of contraceptive methods are discussed. Use of oral contraceptives by diabetic women has been controversial, due to the risk of thromboembolic and vascular complications, and the effect on carbohydrate metabolism. Progestin-only pills and triphasic oral contraceptives are considered safer for diabetics than combined oral contraceptives.

Barrier methods such as the diaphragm or condom and spermicide pose the least risk to the diabetic woman. The problem with these methods, however, is the inconsistency of use which often leads to unplanned pregnancy. Intrauterine devices (IUDs) are associated with an increased risk of infection, especially during the first 4 months after insertion. In the presence of significant vasculopathy, surgical sterilization may be recommended (Jovanovic-Peterson, Peterson, 1992; Mestman, Schmidt-Sarosi, 1993).

✤ EVALUATION

Successful management of diabetic pregnancy involves a complex treatment plan and requires the participation and commitment of the pregnant woman as well as the direction and support of the health care team. Effectiveness of the plan of care is best measured in terms of pregnancy outcome for the mother and the neonate. Positive outcomes are closely associated with the degree of maternal metabolic control during pregnancy (see Plan of Care on p. 631).

Management of diabetic pregnancy has implications for future health of the pregestational diabetic woman.

During pregnancy, while motivation is high, the development and refinement of self-management skills are likely to occur. Ideally, the new skills and diabetic management techniques will continue to be utilized throughout the rest of her life, allowing the woman greater control over her diabetes with fewer long-term complications.

GESTATIONAL DIABETES MELLITUS (GDM)

Gestational diabetes mellitus (GDM) is defined as "carbohydrate intolerance of variable severity with onset or first recognition during the present pregnancy" (ADA, 1990). Although GDM generally disappears at the end of the pregnancy, there is a high probability that it will recur in subsequent pregnancies (Jovanovic-Peterson, Peterson, 1992; Philipson, Super, 1989). GDM occurs in approximately 2% to 6% of all pregnant women and accounts for 90% of cases of diabetes during pregnancy (Radak, 1991; Siddiq, 1989). Classic risk factors for gestational diabetes include obesity, family history of diabetes, family history of macrosomia, and previous poor obstetric history (Jovanovic-Peterson, Peterson, 1992). Estimates of ethnic prevalence are variable, although Asians, Hispanics, and African-Americans appear to be at increased risk (Berkowitz, 1992; Dooley et al, 1991; Hollingsworth, Vaucher, Yamamoto, 1991).

The diagnosis of GDM is usually made during the second half of pregnancy. As fetal nutrient demands rise during the late second and third trimester, maternal nutrient ingestion induces greater and more sustained levels of blood glucose. At the same time maternal insulin resistance is also increasing due to the insulin antagonistic effects of the placental hormones, cortisol, and insulinase. Consequently, maternal insulin demands rise as much as threefold. The majority of pregnant women are capable of increasing insulin production to compensate for the insulin resistance and maintain normoglycemia. When the pancreas is unable to produce sufficient insulin or if the insulin is not utilized effectively, GDM can result (Dickinson, Palmer, 1990).

Some women with GDM exhibit the classic symptoms of diabetes—excessive thirst, hunger, urination, and weakness. However, because approximately 70% of GDM occurs in an asymptomatic form, universal screening of all pregnant women is essential to diagnosis and treatment. The American Diabetes Association (ADA) recommends that all women who have not been identified as having impaired glucose tolerance before the twenty-fourth week be screened for GDM between the twenty-fourth and twenty-eighth weeks of pregnancy (ADA, 1990). This screening is accomplished by administering a 50-g oral glucose load, regardless of previous meal or time of day, followed by a plasma glucose deter-

PLAN OF CARE

Pregestational Diabetes

Case History

Linda James is a 27-year-old insulin-dependent diabetic at 4 weeks' gestation. This is her first prenatal visit.

Linda is in her second pregnancy. Her first pregnancy terminated in spontaneous abortion at 6 weeks. Because she is afraid this pregnancy will end in a miscarriage, she is anxious to begin prenatal care and expresses the desire to learn everything she can about diabetes and pregnancy so that she can take care of herself and the unborn baby.

Diagnosed with IDDM at age 17, Linda has been on a daily injection regimen of intermediate-acting insulin. Through the years she has maintained good glycemic control most of the time, but she reports that lately her blood glucose levels have bordered on hypoglycemia. Linda monitors her blood glucose levels with a reflectance meter and is able to demonstrate correct technique in doing so. Her dietary regimen before pregnancy was a 2000-calorie ADA diet. Because of nausea, she has found it difficult to maintain this intake since she became pregnant.

EXPECTED OUTCOMES	IMPLEMENTATION	RATIONALE	EVALUATION
Nursing Diagnosis: Knowledge deficit related to diabetes, its management, and potential effects on the pregnant woman and fetus			
Linda will verbalize understanding of diabetes, its management, and potential complications during pregnancy. Linda will comply with the plan of care. Linda and her fetus will not experience complications, or if complications occur, they will be minimized.	Assess Linda's knowledge of diabetic pregnancy and her understanding of the treatment plan. Review the pathophysiology of diabetes. Explain the effect of diabetes on pregnancy and the effect of pregnancy on the diabetes. Describe the potential sequelae of diabetes for mother and fetus. Discuss management of diabetic pregnancy. Stress the importance of strict adherence to the plan of care and the need for regular prenatal care. Encourage Linda to ask questions. Clarify misconceptions. Assist Linda in formulating questions for the primary health care provider. Ask Linda to repeat (paraphrase) information to validate her understanding.	Adequate understanding of diabetic pregnancy, its management, and potential sequelae will promote compliance with the plan of care. Understanding also helps to decrease fear and anxiety.	Linda verbalizes understanding of diabetic pregnancy, its management, and potential sequelae for herself and the fetus. Linda complies with the plan of care.

Continued.

EXPECTS OUTCOMES	IMPLEMETATION	RATIONALE	EVALUATION

Nursing Diagnosis: Fear/anxiety related to threat to maternal and fetal well-being

Linda will identify sources of fear and anxiety Linda will express concerns and feelings regarding diabetes and its potential sequelae for herself and the fetus. Linda will verbalize that she feels less fearful and anxious.	Promote an open, trusting relationship with Linda. Provide private area for conversation. Assess Linda's feelings regarding diabetic pregnancy. Convey acceptance of her fears and anxieties. Encourage Linda to differentiate between real and imagined threat to personal and fetal well-being. Review potential dangers to Linda and her fetus as a result of diabetes. Encourage Linda to share her concerns with the primary health care provider.	Verbalizing fears and concerns will help Linda to deal with them. It is important that fear and anxiety be reduced because they interfere with the woman's ability to cope and are a source of stress that can contribute to diabetic complications such as hyperglycemia.	Linda identifies that she is afraid this pregnancy will end in a miscarriage or that the baby may be malformed or mentally retarded. The nurse acknowledges her fears and provides her with factual information related to the chances of these problems actually occurring. Linda states she is less fearful after discussing these concerns with the nurse. Linda compiles a list of questions for the physician related to fetal risk.

Nursing Diagnosis: High risk for injury related to improper insulin dosage/administration

Linda will verbalize understanding of insulin needs and insulin therapy during pregnancy, including purpose, side effects, schedule for taking, and importance of taking as prescribed. Linda will demonstrate proper technique for withdrawal and mixing of insulin. Linda will describe proper method of insulin storage. Linda will demonstrate correct technique for administering insulin. Linda and the fetus will suffer no injury from improper insulin administration.	Assess Linda's understanding of insulin needs during pregnancy and insulin dosage/administration. Explain effect of insulin on the body and purpose of insulin therapy, as well as possible side effects. Describe changing insulin needs during pregnancy. Review peak action of insulin and signs of hypoglycemia. Stress importance of following prescribed regimen. Discuss importance of administration of correct dosage with appropriate syringe. Discuss storage of insulin. Explain technique for mixing insulin in the same syringe. Demonstrate correct withdrawal and administration of insulin. Discuss site rotation, and identify sites that can be used.	Adequate understanding of insulin, its purpose, and effects on the body are essential to proper management of diabetes. Administration of correct dosage of insulin by proper technique will minimize complications such as hypoglycemia.	Linda verbalizes a basic understanding of insulin therapy but is not familiar with changing insulin needs during pregnancy. Although she had administered insulin to herself since her diabetes was diagnosed, she is not experienced with mixing insulins in the same syringe. She uses proper technique for withdrawal and administration of insulin but admits that she is not consistent about site rotation. After teaching is completed, Linda verbalizes understanding of the information and states she feels comfortable with insulin therapy during pregnancy.

PLAN OF CARE—cont'd

Pregestational Diabetes

EXPECTED OUTCOMES	IMPLEMENTATION	RATIONALE	EVALUATION

Nursing Diagnosis: High risk for injury related to improper insulin dosage/administration—cont'd

| | Explain how to adjust insulin dosage based on self-monitoring of blood glucose.
Monitor Linda's self-administration of insulin until techniques are correctly demonstrated and understood. | | |

Nursing Diagnosis: High risk for injury related to hyperglycemia and hypoglycemia

| Linda will verbalize understanding of hyperglycemia and hypoglycemia, including causes, symptoms, treatment and prevention.
Linda will identify the potential consequences for herself and the fetus related to hyperglycemia and hypoglycemia.
Linda and her husband will promptly recognize signs and symptoms of hyperglycemia and hypoglycemia and will take appropriate measures.
Episodes of hyperglycemia and hypoglycemia will be prevented or minimized. | Assess Linda's knowledge of hyperglycemia and hypoglycemia.
Assess her husband's knowledge also, and include him in the teaching session.
Explain causes, symptoms, treatment, and prevention of hyperglycemia and hypoglycemia (Table 22-3).
Stress importance of calling the primary health care provider when signs and symptoms occur.
Stress importance of carrying insulin and syringes, as well as a fast-acting sugar, when away from home.
Give Medic-Alert information, and encourage Linda to wear bracelet or necklace.
Discuss relationship of exercise and diet and the effect of stress. | Hyperglycemia and hypoglycemia compromise maternal and fetal well-being and must be prevented. | Linda and her husband have a basic understanding of hyperglycemia and hypoglycemia, but request that the nurse review related information to ensure their understanding. At the conclusion of the teaching session, Linda and her husband state they understand the information.
Linda already carries insulin and candy with her when away from home.
She plans to obtain a Medic-Alert bracelet. |

mination 1 hour later. A glucose level of 140 mg/dl or greater is considered positive and should be followed by a 3-hour oral glucose tolerance test (GTT). The 3-hour GTT is administered after an overnight fast and at least 3 days of unrestricted diet (at least 150 g carbohydrate) and physical activity. A 100-g glucose load is given, followed by measurements of plasma glucose at 1, 2, and 3 hours. The test is deemed positive if two or more of the following values are met or exceeded (ADA, 1985; 1990):

Fasting	105 mg/dl
1 hour	190 mg/dl
2 hours	165 mg/dl
3 hours	145 mg/dl

If only one of the values is elevated, the 3-hour (100-g) GTT is repeated at 32 weeks. A repeat GTT is recommended at 32 to 34 weeks for those women who tested positive for the 50-g glucose test yet exhibited a normal GTT, if there are significant risk factors present (Howard, 1992).

As with pregestational diabetes, the key to positive pregnancy outcome for both mother and fetus is strict glycemic control instituted as early as possible during gestation. Women with gestational diabetes are at increased risk for preeclampsia and cesarean birth (Jacobson, Cousins, 1989). Perinatal morbidity and mortality are increased among gestational diabetic women with history of previous stillbirth, those who develop preeclampsia, and those who were diagnosed with GDM late in pregnancy. Infants of gestational diabetic women are at risk for fetal macrosomia, neonatal hypoglycemia, hypocalcemia, polycythemia, and hyperbilirubinemia (ADA, 1990).

Care Management—The Gestational Diabetic

In caring for the woman diagnosed as having GDM, the nursing role essentially mirrors that of pregestational diabetes. There is one distinct difference in that those nurses involved in prenatal care delivery in any setting can be instrumental in the identification of women at risk for the development of GDM.

✜ ASSESSMENT

In the early prenatal period a thorough history is necessary to identify any risk factors that may predispose the pregnant woman to GDM. A woman with any of the risk factors for GDM is alerted to the possibility of diabetes during pregnancy and is taught to report any symptoms that may represent onset of the condition (increased thirst, hunger, or urination; weakness). The women is instructed regarding screening measures for GDM.

With the initial prenatal interview and during subsequent visits, assessment of physical and/or emotional stress is important because stress is a factor known to precipitate diabetes in the individual prone to the disease. The diagnosis of GDM often represents a crisis to the pregnant woman and her family. Suddenly the pregnancy is labeled high risk, which evokes fear and anxiety related to the well-being of the mother and the fetus. Whereas the pregestational diabetic woman is usually familiar with necessary self-care skills, the gestational diabetic woman must learn about diabetic management and master the skills on short notice. Because the diagnosis of GDM is often crisis oriented, there may be barriers to learning and decision-making. The nurse is instrumental in assisting the pregnant woman and her family in overcoming these barriers through therapeutic communication and support, while providing the education necessary for diabetic control and self-care. Women with GDM who need insulin injections require additional support as they learn self-administration techniques (Keohane, Lacey, 1991).

Assessment of the woman's support system is an essential part of care planning. The family's reaction to the diagnosis and the necessary treatment regimen influences the woman's emotional response to the diagnosis and her compliance with the plan of care. Sources of physical and psychosocial stress are identified, with the recommendation that stress be avoided to prevent complications such as hyperglycemia (Ruggiero et al, 1990).

✜ NURSING DIAGNOSES

Based on assessment data and individual response to GDM, nursing diagnoses are identified. Those diagnoses

 CLINICAL APPLICATION OF RESEARCH

EFFECT OF FIBER-ENRICHED DIETS ON GLUCOSE LEVEL IN PREGNANCY

Diet therapy is standard treatment for patients with diabetes mellitus. Diabetic control has been improved in nonpregnant diabetic patients with fiber-enriched diets. Researchers have found that postprandial hyperglycemia decreases and insulin requirements are lower with increased fiber. In this study the researchers investigated whether high-fiber diets would lower blood glucose levels in women with GDM who do not require insulin. Fifty-one patients with GDM participated in the study. The fiber was given in divided amounts with half in fiber-containing foods and half as a high-fiber drink. Participants were in one of three groups depending on the amount of dietary fiber they consumed (group 1, 40 to 60 mg; group 2, 70-80 mg; group 3, 20 mg or less). Obstetric management and diabetes care were the same for all participants. The researchers found no differences in glucose control between the first two groups. At higher levels of fiber intake (over 80 mg), participants reported nausea, abdominal discomfort, dissatisfaction with taste, and poor compliance. Increased dietary fiber appears to reduce postprandial blood glucose levels in nonpregnant women but not in pregnant women with GDM. Dividing the dose of fiber makes it more tolerable. Until researchers find otherwise, the diabetic diet recommended by the American Diabetes Association is most appropriate for women with GDM. When an increase in fiber is recommended, dividing the dose makes it more acceptable.

Reference: Reece EA et al: Do fiber-enriched diabetic diets have glucose-lowering effects in pregnancy? *Am J Perinatol* 10:272, 1993.

appropriate for pregestational diabetic women generally apply to gestational diabetes as well (see p. 625).

✥ EXPECTED OUTCOMES

Expected outcomes are formulated based on identified nursing diagnoses and the medical plan of care. The pregnant woman and her support person(s) are involved with the nurse in the mutual establishment of goals.

In general, the expected outcomes of care for GDM are the same as for pregestational diabetes. The major difference is that the time frame for planning may be shortened with GDM because the diagnosis is usually made later in pregnancy. Planning and implementation of collaborative care must occur as soon as possible after diagnosis.

✥ COLLABORATIVE CARE

Antepartum

When the diagnosis of GDM is made, treatment begins immediately. This allows little or no time for the woman and her family to adjust to the diagnosis before they are expected to comply with the treatment plan. This is in contrast to the pregestational diabetic woman who may have had years to learn about the disease and adapt to dietary modifications, glucose self-monitoring, and insulin administration. With each step of the treatment plan it is important that the nurse and other health care providers educate the woman and her family, providing detailed and comprehensive explanations to ensure understanding, participation, and compliance with the necessary interventions. Potential complications resulting from noncompliance are discussed while reinforcing the need for maintenance of normoglycemia throughout the remainder of the pregnancy. It may be reassuring for the woman and her family to know that the diabetic condition typically disappears when the pregnancy is over.

Dietary modification is the mainstay of treatment for GDM. There are two main goals in diet therapy: maintenance of normal blood glucose levels (normoglycemia) and appropriate weight gain during the pregnancy. Nutritional counseling provided by a registered dietitian (RD) is instituted as soon as possible after the diagnosis is made. The dietary program is individualized according to the woman's needs and primary health care provider's orders. A typical GDM diet includes 2000 to 2200 calories per day consumed in three meals and three or four snacks, reduction of fat intake, exclusion of simple sugars, and increased intake of soluble dietary fiber and complex carbohydrates (see Clinical Application of Research box on p. 634). It is desired that the pregnant woman attain an ideal weight gain of 24 to 30 lb during pregnancy (average 0.9 lb per week the last two trimesters). For the obese woman caloric intake may be tailored to prevent excess weight gain

during pregnancy, while still meeting maternal and fetal requirements (Worthington-Roberts, Williams, 1993).

Daily *exercise* is an integral part of the treatment plan because it helps to lower blood glucose levels and may be instrumental in eliminating the need for insulin. Walking is often recommended and should be done at the same time each day. Exercise for the insulin-dependent GDM woman should be prescribed by the physician (Artal, 1992; Rosas, Constantino, 1992).

Approximately 10% to 15% of GDM women require *insulin* to maintain normoglycemia. Once the dietary regimen is implemented, weekly determinations of fasting and postprandial glucose levels are made. Indications for the initiation of insulin therapy include a fasting plasma or capillary glucose level in excess of 105 mg/dl or a postprandial plasma level greater than 120 mg/dl or a capillary level of 140 mg/dl 2 hours after a meal (ADA, 1985). A combination of regular and NPH insulin is administered in two or three injections per day, and dosage is adjusted based on self-determinations of blood glucose levels. Typically, two thirds of the total insulin dose is administered in the morning and the remaining one third is given in the evening (Chez et al, 1989; Landon, Gabbe, 1992).

The woman and her family are taught the necessary skills to manage insulin administration. In some instances hospitalization may be required to regulate blood glucose levels and to educate the pregnant woman about glycemic control with insulin, diet, and exercise.

Self-monitoring of blood glucose is a requirement for effective insulin therapy and is usually done four times daily—on rising and after meals. GDM women managed by dietary modification alone are also taught to measure blood glucose levels. Visually read reagent strips or a glucose reflectance meter may be used for self-monitoring of blood glucose. These women are also taught to measure urine ketone levels.

GDM women, particularly those on insulin therapy, are at risk for developing hypoglycemia and hyperglycemia. The woman and her family are taught signs and symptoms as well as causes, prevention, and treatment measures (see Table 22-3).

Women with GDM who maintain normoglycemia are allowed to progress to term birth, but should give birth by 42 weeks. If labor cannot be safely induced at 40 weeks, biophysical assessment or nonstress tests are done once or twice weekly. Fetal surveillance may begin at 30 weeks for those women with poor glycemic control, PIH, history of stillbirth, and those who required insulin in a prior gestation. The program of fetal surveillance is similar to that employed with pregestational diabetic women (Dickinson, Palmer, 1990).

Intrapartum

During the labor and birth process, blood glucose levels are monitored at least every 2 hours to maintain levels at 100 mg/dl or less. Glucose levels within this range decrease the severity of neonatal hypoglycemia. Intravenous fluids containing glucose are not given as a bolus to the GDM patient, although they may be necessary as maintenance fluids.

Postpartum

Approximately 98% of GDM patients revert to normoglycemia in the postpartum period. Six weeks after birth or when breastfeeding is stopped, a GTT is performed to ensure that the diabetes has disappeared. Those women with abnormal results are referred to a diabetologist for follow-up (Corcoy et al, 1992; Jovanovic-Peterson, Peterson, 1992).

In planning for future pregnancies it is important that the woman be aware that there is a 90% chance that GDM will recur. In addition, the woman who has experienced GDM is at risk for the development of overt diabetes in subsequent years. Obese women who remain overweight have a 60% chance of developing diabetes within 20 years. This risk can be reduced significantly if the obese woman reduces her weight and maintains it within a normal range. (Coustan et al, 1993; Damm et al, 1992).

HYPEREMESIS GRAVIDARUM

Hyperemesis gravidarum is defined as excessive or intractable vomiting during pregnancy, leading to dehydration, electrolyte disturbances, or nutritional deficiencies and weight loss. The incidence of this condition is approximately 3.5 per 1000 births. Although most cases are mild and resolve with time, one of every 1000 pregnant women will require hospitalization. Hyperemesis gravidarum is generally self-limiting, but recovery is slow and frequent relapses are common. It occurs most frequently among primigravidas and tends to recur in subsequent pregnancies. Other predisposing factors include maternal age less than 20, obesity, multifetal gestation, and trophoblastic disease (hydatidiform mole) (Feldman, 1989; Singer, Brandt, 1991).

The etiology of hyperemesis gravidarum remains obscure. Several theories have been proposed as to the cause, although none of them adequately explain the disorder (Abell, Riely, 1992). Possible causes of hyperemesis gravidarum include high levels of estrogen and hyperthyroidism, which may be caused by elevated levels of human chorionic gonadotropin (Chin et al, 1990; Goodwin Montero, Mostman, 1992). Psychologic factors may be instrumental in the development of hyperemesis gravidarum. Ambivalence toward the pregnancy and conflicting feelings regarding prospective motherhood, body changes, and lifestyle alterations may cause episodes of vomiting. Women whose normal reaction patterns to stress involve gastrointestinal disturbances are often affected. However, in some women psychologic causes cannot be identified.

In extreme cases of hyperemesis gravidarum persistent vomiting results in rapid weight loss and dehydration, which leads to fluid and electrolyte imbalances. Dehydration results in hypovolemia, which manifests as hypotension, tachycardia, increased hematocrit and BUN, and diminished urine output. Vomiting involves loss of gastric acid fluids as well as alkaline contents from deeper within the gastrointestinal tract. This leads to the development of metabolic acidosis. Extreme maternal nutritional deprivation, or starvation, causes hypoproteinemia and hypovitaminosis. Jaundice and hemorrhage secondary to vitamin C and B-complex deficiency and hypothrombinemia lead to bleeding from mucosal surfaces. In these extreme cases, the embryo or fetus may die, and the mother may die from irreversible metabolic alterations.

Conservative management of a woman experiencing hyperemesis gravidarum includes intravenous hydration, vitamin supplements, sedation, antiemetics, and in some cases psychotherapy. For more severe cases enteral or parenteral nutrition may be necessary to correct maternal nutritional deprivation (Charlin, 1993).

Care Management

Nursing care of the hyperemetic pregnant woman involves implementing the medical plan of care: initiating and monitoring intravenous therapy, administering pharmacologic agents and nutritional supplements, and monitoring the woman's response to interventions. The nurse observes the woman for any signs of complications, such as metabolic acidosis, jaundice, or hemorrhage and alerts the health care provider should these occur. Accurate intake and output, including the amount of emesis, is an important aspect of nursing care. Oral hygiene while the woman is on NPO status, and after episodes of vomiting, helps to allay associated discomforts. When the woman begins responding to therapy, limited amounts of oral fluids and bland foods such as crackers or toast are begun. The diet is progressed slowly as tolerated by the woman until she is able to consume a nutritionally sound diet. Promoting adequate rest is important for the woman with hyperemesis; the nurse can assist in coordinating treatment measures and periods of visitation to provide opportunity for rest periods. The nurse addresses the psychosocial status of the woman, recognizing that the condition is both physically and emotionally debilitating.

Usually hyperemesis gravidarum responds to therapy and the prognosis is good. The woman is discharged home when fluid and electrolyte balance is restored and weight gain begins (see Plan of Care on p. 637).

PLAN OF CARE

Hyperemesis Gravidarum

Case History

Carolyn Scott is a 20-year-old single, first-time mother at 6 weeks' gestation who has been admitted to the antepartum unit with a diagnosis of hyperemesis gravidarum.

The admission interview revealed that Carolyn has been vomiting for 2 days and has been unable to retain any food or fluids. She states that she feels miserable. Carolyn is very concerned about the well-being of her baby and keeps asking "Is my baby going to die?" During the physical examination of Carolyn, the nurse notes that her eyes appear sunken, her skin turgor is poor, and oral mucous membranes are dry. Carolyn has lost 5 pounds since her last prenatal visit 2 weeks ago. Assessment of vital signs reveals a pulse rate of 98 beats/min, up from her normal rate of 70 beats/min. Her blood pressure has dropped from her usual measurement of 118/70 to 100/60 mm Hg. A review of laboratory findings reveals elevated values for hematocrit, BUN, and urine specific gravity.

EXPECTED OUTCOMES	IMPLEMENTATION	RATIONALE	EVALUATION
Nursing Diagnosis: Fluid volume deficit related to abnormal fluid loss secondary to vomiting and inadequate fluid intake			
Carolyn's fluid and electrolyte balance will be restored as evidenced by normal skin turgor, moist mucous membranes, stable weight, vital signs WNL for her; serum electrolytes, hemoglobin, hematocrit, and urine specific gravity will be WNL. Carolyn will experience no further vomiting. Carolyn will resume adequate oral intake.	Assess and document skin turgor, condition of mucous membranes, vital signs, and urine specific gravity. Obtain weight daily. Monitor laboratory values and report abnormalities. Assess and record color, amount, and frequency of emesis. Maintain accurate intake and output record. Assist health care provider or initiate IV fluid therapy as ordered; monitor infusion carefully. Administer antiemetics as ordered. Maintain NPO status as ordered. When oral intake is allowed, offer Carolyn's preferred liquids. Encourage oral fluids, slowly increasing amount as tolerated.	Accurate assessment of fluid and electrolyte status provides basis for planning and evaluating interventions. Restoration of fluid and electrolyte balance requires parenteral therapy until Carolyn can tolerate oral intake. Fluid and electrolyte imbalance must be corrected to prevent severe complications such as metabolic acidosis and maternal or fetal death.	Carolyn received IV fluids for 3 days until all laboratory values had returned to normal. Her skin turgor, mucous membranes, and vital signs returned to previous levels. Carolyn lost 2 more pounds, but by discharge she had gained half a pound.

Continued.

PLAN OF CARE—cont'd

Hyperemesis Gravidarum

EXPECTED OUTCOMES	IMPLEMENTATION	RATIONALE	EVALUATION

Nursing Diagnosis: Altered nutrition: less than body requirements related to nausea and persistent vomiting

Carolyn will resume oral intake of nutritionally sound diet. Her nausea and vomiting will be alleviated. Carolyn will describe components of nutritionally sound diet and will verbalize willingness to follow that diet. Carolyn will tolerate prescribed diet. Carolyn will gain weight appropriately during pregnancy.	Begin oral intake as ordered by health care provider and tolerated by Carolyn. Provide small amounts of attractively served foods to fit her preferences. Increase amounts slowly as tolerated. Monitor and document oral intake. Have dietitian consult with Carolyn in developing a meal plan that meets nutritional requirements during pregnancy and that includes a schedule of meals, as well as Carolyn's food preferences and eating environment. Discuss with Carolyn the importance of adequate nutrition during pregnancy. Verify Carolyn's understanding of nutritional information. Assess her willingness to follow the prescribed diet plan, and encourage her compliance. Monitor Carolyn's weight gain.	Adequate maternal nutrition is necessary for the health of the mother and for growth and development of the fetus.	On the third day of hospitalization, Carolyn was tolerating oral fluids and slowly progressed to a regular diet by the day of discharge. She met with the dietitian on two occasions and stated she understood the dietary regimen as well as the importance of compliance. Carolyn had begun to gain weight before discharge.

THYROID DISORDERS
Hyperthyroidism

Hyperthyroidism affects approximately 1 or 2 of every 1000 pregnancies and is most often due to Graves' disease. Common symptoms of hyperthyroidism include nervousness, hyperactivity, weakness, fatigue, weight loss (or poor weight gain), diarrhea, tachycardia, shortness of breath, excessive perspiration, heat intolerance, and muscle tremors. Exophthalmos and enlargement of the thyroid gland (goiter) may also occur. Laboratory findings indicative of hyperthyroidism include an elevated free thyroxine (T_4) index and increased basal metabolic rate (Kaplan, 1992; Lazarus, 1993).

Hyperthyroidism in women may be responsible for anovulation and amenorrhea, but the disease is not a recognized cause of spontaneous abortion or fetal malformation. With inadequate control of hyperthyroidism during pregnancy, there is an increased risk of preterm birth and stillbirth. Infants of hyperthyroid mothers are often of low birth weight and may experience thyrotoxicosis in the neonatal period. While most cases of neonatal hyperthyroidism are transient, some may progress and ultimately impair central nervous system development (Davis et al, 1989).

The primary treatment of hyperthyroidism during pregnancy is drug therapy utilizing the thiouracils. The medication of choice is propylthiouracil (PTU) in the

PLAN OF CARE—cont'd

Hyperemesis Gravidarum

EXPECTED OUTCOMES	IMPLEMENTATION	RATIONALE	EVALUTION

Nursing Diagnosis: Fear related to effects of hyperemesis on fetal well-being

Carolyn will verbalize feelings and concerns about fetal well-being.	Convey acceptance of Carolyn's perception of fear. Encourage her to express feelings and concerns. Help Carolyn identify personal strengths and previous coping mechanisms. Provide Carolyn with information related to potential risks to fetus. Encourage Carolyn to discuss these concerns with the health care provider. Help her identify sources of support and mobilize support person/group of her choice. Arrange for psychology or social work consult as needed.	Acceptance of Carolyn's fears will encourage open communication regarding the source of fear. Knowledge of potential risks to fetus may help to allay her fear. Effective coping strategies are needed to enable Carolyn to deal with her illness and its effects.	Carolyn discussed her concerns with the nurse and stated that she felt relieved after discussion of the fetal risks related to hyperemesis gravidarum. Carolyn's mother was identified as her main source of support, and she was included in the discussion.

smallest effective dosage. Thiouracils readily cross the placenta and may induce fetal hypothyroidism, goiter, and subsequent mental and physical retardation. Radioactive iodine must not be used in diagnosis or treatment of hyperthyroidism because it may compromise the fetal thyroid (Cunningham et al, 1993; Hamburger, 1992).

In severe cases of hyperthyroidism subtotal thyroidectomy may be performed during the second or third trimester. Postoperative hypothyroidism is common, occurring in at least 20% of hyperthyroid women (Hamburger, 1992).

Hypothyroidism

Hypothyroidism during pregnancy is rare because women with this condition are often infertile. Hypothyroidism is usually due to Hashimoto's disease, thyroid gland ablation by radiation, previous surgery, or antithyroid medications. Reduced thyroid function due to hypothalamic or pituitary failure is rare, with only a few reported cases (Kaplan, 1992).

Characteristic symptoms of hypothyroidism include lethargy, weakness, anorexia, weight gain, cold intolerance, mental impairment, constipation, and headache. Dry skin, thin brittle nails, alopecia, poor skin turgor, and delayed deep tendon reflexes are also common. Laboratory findings of hypothyroidism include reduced triiodothyronine and thyroxine(T_3 and T_4 levels).

Pregnant women with hypothyroidism are at increased risk for spontaneous abortion in the first trimester. There is an increased incidence of preeclampsia and abruptio placentae among hypothyroid women, with a corresponding increase in low birth weight infants and stillbirth (Lazarus, 1993; Leung et al, 1993).

Thyroid hormone supplements are used to treat hypothyroidism. Levothyroxine (Synthroid) is most often prescribed during pregnancy. Serum thyroid-stimulating hormone (TSH) levels are monitored, and may take up to 2 months to reach normal levels. Thyroid supplements do not cross the placenta in any appreciable amount; thus treatment of the mother is considered safe for the fetus.

Cardiovascular Disorders

Every pregnancy taxes the cardiovascular system of the mother. The strain is present during pregnancy and continues for a few weeks after birth. The normal heart can compensate for the increased workload so that pregnancy and birth generally are well tolerated.

If the cardiovascular changes are not well tolerated, cardiac failure can develop during the last few weeks of pregnancy, during labor, or during the postnatal period (Cunningham et al, 1993). In addition, if myocardial disease develops, if valvular disease exists, or if a congenital heart defect is large, **cardiac decompensation** (inability of the heart to maintain a sufficient cardiac output) is anticipated.

Some degree of cardiac impairment affects 0.5% to 3% of pregnant women (McKeon, Perrin, 1989). Heart disease is the leading cause of nonobstetric maternal mortality. It ranks fourth overall as a cause of maternal death. A maternal mortality rate of 37% is expected in women who have myocardial infarctions during pregnancy (Clark, 1991; Graber, 1989). A perinatal mortality of up to 50% is anticipated with persistent cardiac decompensation.

The degree of dysfunction (disability) of the woman with cardiac disease often is more important in the treatment and prognosis of cardiac disease complicating pregnancy than is the diagnosis of the valvular lesion per se. The New York Heart Association's functional classification of organic heart disease, a widely accepted standard, is as follows:

Class I: asymptomatic at normal levels of activity
Class II: symptomatic with increased activity
Class III: symptomatic with ordinary activity
Class IV: symptomatic at rest

No classification of heart disease can be considered rigid or absolute, but this one offers a basic practical guide for treatment, assuming that frequent prenatal visits, patient compliance, and proper obstetric care occur. Medical therapy is conducted collaboratively with a cardiologist. The functional class of the disease is determined at 3 months and again at 7 or 8 months of gestation.

Spontaneous abortion is increased and preterm labor and birth are more prevalent in the pregnant woman with cardiac problems. In addition, *intrauterine fetal growth retardation (IUGR)* (impeded or delayed development of the fetus) is common, probably because of low oxygen pressure (Po_2) in the mother.

A cardiac diagnosis depends on the history, physical examination, x-ray findings, and, if indicated, ultrasonogram results. The differential diagnosis of heart disease also involves ruling out respiratory problems, as well as other potential causes of chest pain.

Care Management

✤ ASSESSMENT

The presence of cardiac disease makes the decision to become pregnant more difficult. Planned pregnancy requires that the woman understand the peripartum risks. In an unplanned pregnancy the nurse needs to explore the woman's desire to continue the pregnancy given all of the risks. The nurse should review with the woman any options for pregnancy termination if her cardiac status is tenuous.

The pregnant woman with cardiac disease requires detailed assessment to determine the potential for optimal maternal health and a viable fetus throughout the peri-

---

SIGNS OF POTENTIAL COMPLICATIONS

CARDIAC DECOMPENSATION

PREGNANT WOMAN: SUBJECTIVE SYMPTOMS

- Increasing fatigue or difficulty breathing, or both, with her usual activities
- Feeling of smothering
- Frequent cough
- Palpitations; feeling that her heart is racing
- Swelling of face, feet, legs, fingers (e.g., rings do not fit anymore)

NURSE: OBJECTIVE SIGNS

- Irregular weak, rapid pulse (≥ 100 beats/min)
- Progressive, generalized edema
- Crackles (rales) at base of lungs, after two inspirations and exhalations
- Orthopnea; increasing dyspnea
- Rapid respirations (≥25 breaths/min)
- Moist, frequent cough
- Increasing fatigue
- Cyanosis of lips and nail beds

---

partum period. If she chooses to continue the pregnancy, the woman's condition is assessed at weekly intervals.

The nurse assesses for factors that would increase stress on the heart, such as anemia, infection, or a home situation that includes responsibility for the house, other children, or extended family members. The woman is observed for signs of cardiac decompensation, that is, progressive generalized edema, crackles (rales) at the base of the lungs that persist after one or two deep inspirations, or pulse irregularity (see Signs of Potential Complications box above). Symptoms of cardiac decompensation may appear abruptly or gradually. Medical intervention must be instituted immediately to correct cardiac status. Unfortunately dyspnea, chest pain, palpitations, and syncope occur commonly in pregnant women and can mask the symptoms of a developing or worsening cardiovascular disorder.

The routine assessment continues for the antepartum period, including monitoring weight gain and pattern of weight gain, edema, vital signs, discomforts of pregnancy, urinalysis, and blood work. The nurse documents all medications taken by the woman—including supplemental iron—and is alert to their potential side effects and interactions.

During the *intrapartum period* assessment includes the routine assessments for all laboring women as well as assessments for cardiac decompensation (see Legal Tip on p. 641). The latter include measurements of the pulse and respiratory rate at least four times every hour during the first stage of labor and every 10 minutes during the second stage (Cunningham et al, 1993). *The health care provider is alerted if the pulse rate is 100 beats/min or greater or if respirations are 25 per minute or greater. Respiratory status* is checked constantly for developing dyspnea, coughing, or crackles (rales) at the base of the lungs. The color and temperature of the skin are noted. Pallor, cooling, and sweating may indicate cardiac shock. The laboring woman is carefully watched for symptoms of emotional stress.

The *immediate postpartum period* is hazardous for a woman with a compromised heart. Cardiac output remains elevated for at least 48 hours after giving birth. Venous return is increased as extravascular fluid is remobilized into the vascular compartment and pressure on the inferior vena cava is reduced. Stroke volume is increased and reflex bradycardia occurs. Some health care providers favor the application of the abdominal binder or alternating tourniquets on the extremities to minimize the effects of this rapid change in the early puerperium. By 2 to 3 weeks postpartum, these changes have returned to nonpregnant levels.

Cardiac monitoring for decompensation continues through the first weeks after birth because it has been known to occur as late as the sixth postpartum week. Routine assessment as for any postpartum woman is instituted; for example, vital signs, lochia, uterine contractility, urinary output, pain, rest, diet, and daily weight. Laboratory (e.g., hemoglobin, hematocrit, and urinalysis) results are noted and reported if indicated to the health care provider. It is important to assess the woman's support systems, since activity will be curtailed until the cardiac system is recovered. The family's response to the birth and infant needs to be observed because the mother may not be directly involved in the infant's care for a while (e.g., prematurity of infant, health of mother).

LEGAL TIP: **Cardiac and Metabolic Emergencies**

The management of emergencies such as maternal cardiopulmonary distress or arrest or maternal metabolic crisis should be documented in policies, procedures, and protocols in the health care setting providing maternity care. Any independent nursing actions appropriate to the emergency should be clearly identified.

Cardiopulmonary Resuscitation of the Pregnant Woman

Trauma, pulmonary embolism, anesthesia complications, drug overdose, hypovolemia, or septic shock may result in cardiopulmonary arrest. Preexisting disorders, such as heart or pulmonary disease, hypertension, or autoimmune collagen vascular disease, increase this risk (Troiano, 1989). Some modifications of the procedure for cardiopulmonary resuscitation (CPR) (see the Emergency box on p. 642) and the Heimlich maneuver are

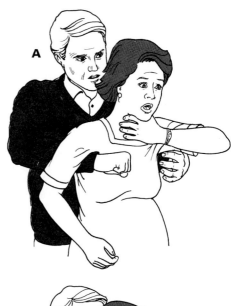

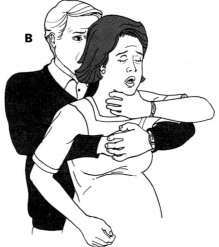

FIG. 22-4   Clearing airway obstruction on pregnant woman. **A,** Place top of clenched fist against middle of sternum; place other hand on top of clenched fist. Perform chest thrusts until obstruction is expelled or woman loses consciousness. **B,** If woman is unconscious, give chest compressions as for woman without pulse.

needed (Fig. 22-4). To prevent supine hypotension, the woman is positioned on a flat firm surface, with the uterus displaced laterally (manually or with a wedge or rolled towel under her right hip).

Complications may be associated with CPR of a pregnant woman. These complications include laceration of the liver, rupture of the uterus, hemothorax, and hemoperitoneum (Troiano, 1989). Fetal complications also may occur. These include cardiac arrhythmia or asystole related to maternal defibrillation and medications, central nervous system (CNS) depression related to antiarrhythmic drugs and inadequate uteroplacental perfusion, and onset of preterm labor.

After successful resuscitation, the woman and her fetus must receive careful monitoring for at least 24 hours. She remains at increased risk for recurrent pulmonary ar-

E M E R G E N C Y

CARDIOPULMONARY RESUSCITATION (CPR) FOR THE PREGNANT WOMAN

CPR

Airway

Determine unresponsiveness.

Activate emergency medical system.

Position woman on a flat firm surface with the uterus displaced laterally with a wedge (e.g., a rolled towel placed under her right hip) or manually.

Open airway with head tilt-chin lift maneuver.

Breathing

Determine breathlessness (look, listen, feel).

If the woman is not breathing, give two slow breaths.

Circulation

Determine pulselessness by feeling carotid pulse.

If there is no pulse, begin chest compressions at a rate of 80 to 100/minutes.

After four cycles of fifteen compressions and two breaths, check her pulse. If pulse is not present, then continue CPR.

HEIMLICH MANEUVER (FIG 22-4)

If the pregnant woman is unable to speak or cough, then perform chest thrusts. Stand behind the woman and place your arms under her armpits to encircle her chest. Press backwards with quick thrusts until the foreign body is expelled.

Reference: American Heart Association: *Basic life support, heart saver guide,* Dallas, 1993, AHA.

rest and arrhythmias (ventricular tachycardia, supraventricular tachycardia, bradycardia). Therefore her cardiovascular, pulmonary, and neurologic status should be assessed continuously. Uterine activity and resting tone must be monitored. Fetal status and gestational age should be determined. All assessment data influence both the medical and nursing plans of care.

✜ NURSING DIAGNOSES

Following are examples of nursing diagnoses that may be formulated. Individualization of diagnoses is vital.

Antepartum

Fear related to
- Increased peripartum risk

High risk for ineffective individual/family coping related to
- Woman's cardiac condition

High risk for altered tissue perfusion related to
- Hypotensive syndrome

High risk for activity intolerance related to
- Cardiac condition

Knowledge deficit related to
- Cardiac condition
- Requirements to alter self-care activities

High risk for self-care deficit related to
- Activity intolerance

Impaired home maintenance management related to
- Mother's confinement to bed and/or limited activity level

Intrapartum

Anxiety related to
- Fear for infant's safety

Fear of dying related to
- Perceived physiologic inability to cope with the stress of labor

High risk for impaired gas exchange related to
- Cardiac condition

High risk for fluid volume excess related to
- Extravascular fluid shifts

Postpartum

Self-care deficit related to
- Fatigue
- Need for bed rest

Situational low self-esteem related to
- Restriction placed on involvement in care of infant

Ineffective breastfeeding related to
- Fatigue from cardiac condition

High risk for altered parenting related to
- Inadequate bonding

✜ EXPECTED OUTCOMES

The mother with cardiovascular problems faces curtailment of her activities. The restrictions can have physical and emotional implications. The community health or home care nurse, social worker, and pediatrician are some of the resource people whose services may need to be incorporated into the plan of care. Expected outcomes such as the following might be appropriate.

1. Woman and family will verbalize knowledge of the disorder, management, and probable outcome.
2. Woman and family will describe their role in management, including when and how to take medication, adjust diet, and prepare for and participate in treatment.
3. Woman and family will cope with emotional reactions to pregnancy and infant at risk.
4. Woman will be able to withstand the physiologic stressors of pregnancy.
5. Woman will be able to carry pregnancy to term or the point of fetal viability.

✤ COLLABORATIVE CARE

Therapy is focused on minimizing stress on the heart. Factors that increase the risk of cardiac decompensation are treated and the woman is monitored closely for signs and symptoms of cardiac decompensation. The workload on the cardiovascular system is reduced by appropriate treatment of any coexisting emotional stress, hypertension, anemia, hyperthyroidism, or obesity.

Infections are treated promptly, since respiratory, urinary, and gastrointestinal tract infections can complicate the condition by accelerating heart rate and by direct spreading of organisms (e.g., *Streptococcus*) to the heart structure.

Sodium intake is restricted and accompanied by careful monitoring for hyponatremia. The woman's intake of potassium is monitored to prevent hypokalemia, which is associated with heart and other muscular weakness and dysfunction. Anticoagulant therapy, if used, is monitored. Tests for fetal maturity and well-being and placental sufficiency may be necessary. Other therapy, which follows, is directly related to the functional classification of heart disease.

Antepartum

The pregnant woman with class I heart disease should limit stress to protect against cardiac decompensation. Frequent evaluations and the early and effective treatment of respiratory and other infections should be stressed. Vaccines against pneumonococcal and influenza infections are recommended. Therapeutic abortion is never medically warranted.

A plan of care similar to that for class I should be followed for the pregnant woman with class II heart disease. However, the woman should be admitted to the hospital near term (if signs of cardiac overload or arrhythmia develop) for evaluation and treatment. Bed rest for much of each day is necessary for pregnant women with class III cardiac disease. About 30% of these women experience cardiac decompensation during pregnancy. With this possibility the woman may be hospitalized for the remainder of the pregnancy and the early puerperium. Early therapeutic abortion may be suggested, particularly if the woman experienced a previous episode of cardiac failure. A major initial effort must be made to improve the cardiac status of pregnant women with class IV cardiac disease because they can have decompensation even at rest. Early therapeutic abortion, although not without risk, may be feasible with regional anesthesia in some cases. Prophylactic antibiotic therapy may be ordered with the procedure.

Signs and symptoms of cardiac decompensation are reviewed with the pregnant woman and her family. The woman requires *adequate rest*. She should sleep 8 to 10 hours every day and 30 minutes after meals. Her activities are restricted; for example, if the woman is at home, she needs to limit housework, shopping, walking, and laundry to the amount allowed for her functional classification of heart disease. Nutrition counseling is necessary, optimally with the woman's family present. Adequate nutrition may be difficult to achieve, especially when someone else shops and cooks for her. The woman needs a diet high in iron and protein and adequate in calories to gain 10.8 kg (24 lb) during pregnancy. To prevent pyrosis (heartburn), the pregnant woman is advised to assume a semi-Fowler's or low Fowler's position after eating. Note that iron supplements tend to cause constipation. It is important for the pregnant cardiac woman to avoid straining during defecation. Straining or bearing down results in the *Valsalva maneuver* (forced expiration against a closed airway, which when released causes blood to rush to the heart and overload the cardiac system).

If anticoagulant therapy is required during pregnancy, heparin should be used because this large-molecule drug does not cross the placenta (Contemporary *OB/GYN*, 1990; Cunningham et al, 1993; Scott et al, 1990). The woman may need to learn to self-administer heparin. Even though heparin is the anticoagulant of choice during pregnancy, it is not without risk. Heparin use can result in maternal hemorrhage, preterm birth, and stillbirth. Oral anticoagulants, such as warfarin (Coumadin) compounds, cross to the fetus and may cause anomalies or hemorrhage in the infant (*Contemporary OB/GYN*, 1990). The pregnant woman is cautioned to avoid foods high in vitamin K, such as raw, deep green, leafy vegetables, which counteract the effects of the heparin. Therefore she will require a substitute source of folic acid in her diet.

Infection adds considerable stress to cardiac function. The pregnant woman should notify her health care provider at the first sign of infection or when she is exposed to infection. Hospitalization may be required until the infection is cured.

The nurse may need to reinforce the health care provider's explanation for the need for close medical supervision. Information about management of the woman's labor and her early postpartum period is reviewed. The woman and her family will need time to plan for the necessary extra care the mother will require.

Intrapartum

Nursing care during labor and birth focuses on the promotion of cardiac function. *Anxiety is alleviated* through maintaining a calm atmosphere and keeping the woman and her family informed. *Uterine perfusion* is facilitated by placing the woman in a side-lying position. *Cardiac function* is supported by keeping her head and shoulders elevated and body parts resting on pillows. Bearing down (Valsalva maneuver) must be avoided, since this reduces diastolic ventricular filling and obstructs left ventricular outflow (Scott et al, 1990). Since pain can contribute to cardiovascular stress, discomfort is relieved with medication and supportive care. For birth the nurse assists in the administration of pharmacologic relief of discomfort. Epidural regional anesthesia provides better pain relief than narcotics and fewer alterations in hemodynamics (Cunningham et al, 1993; Gilbert, Harmon, 1993). *Hypotension must be avoided.*

For the woman with cardiac disease, vaginal birth is recommended, if there are no obstetric problems. This is accomplished using epidural or pudendal block anesthesia with forceps for shortening the second stage of labor. Penicillin prophylaxis of nonsensitized pregnant women against bacterial endocarditis in labor and during early puerperium may be ordered. Mask oxygen and pudendal block anesthesia are important. Ergot products should not be used because they tend to increase blood pressure. Dilute intravenous oxytocin immediately after birth may be employed to prevent hemorrhage.

Vaginal birth is accomplished with the woman in a side-lying position, or if placed in the supine position, a pad is positioned under the hip to minimize the danger of supine hypotension. The knees are flexed, and the feet are flat on the bed. Stirrups are not used to prevent compression of popliteal veins and an increase in blood volume in the chest and trunk as a result of the effects of gravity. An episiotomy and the use of outlet forceps also decrease the work of the heart.

Beta-adrenergic agents (e.g., ritodrine and terbutaline) should not be used for tocolysis. These agents are associated with myocardial ischemia. *Syntocinon*, a synthetic oxytocin, can be used for induction of labor. This drug does not appear to cause significant coronary artery constriction in dosage prescribed for labor induction or control of postpartum uterine atony.

Postpartum

Care in the postpartum period is tailored to the woman's functional capacity. The woman must be *protected from infection.* A private room is one method to restrict traffic into her room. Positioning in bed is the same as that for the labor; that is, the head of the bed is elevated and the woman is encouraged to lie on her side. Bed rest may be ordered with or without bathroom privileges. The nurse may need to help the woman meet her grooming and hygiene needs and even help her with turning in bed, eating, and other activities. Boredom and respiratory and circulatory sequelae to immobility must be addressed. Progressive ambulation may be permitted as tolerated. The nurse assesses the woman's pulse, skin, and affect before and after walking.

Bowel and bladder elimination require special attention. Bowel movements without stress or strain are promoted with stool softeners, diet, and fluids, plus mild analgesia and local anesthetic spray. Overdistention of the bladder is prevented, because a distended bladder can result in an atonic uterus. Hemorrhage can occur, resulting in anemia, adding stress to cardiac function. Rapid

emptying of the bladder is avoided, however, since rapid decompression of the bladder results in a precipitous drop in intraabdominal pressure, leading to *splanchnic engorgement* and generalized hypotension.

Although breastfeeding is often not advised for class III and class IV mothers, it is not contraindicated (Lawrence, 1994). The woman can conserve her energy by breastfeeding in a resting position and by having others bring the baby to her for feedings.

Mother-child interactions receive special planning. The interactions should not stress the mother. The mother may direct care of the infant by a designated family member. The baby can be brought regularly to the mother, held at her eye level and by her lips, and brought to her fingers so that she can establish an emotional bond with her baby with a low expenditure of her energy. At the same time, involving the mother passively in her infant's care helps the mother feel important—as she is—to the infant's well-being (e.g., "You can do something no one else can: provide your baby with your sounds, touch, and rhythms that are so comforting"). Perhaps the mother can be encouraged to make a tape recording of her talking, singing, or whispering, to be played for the baby in the nursery, to help the infant feel her presence and be in contact with her voice.

Before discharge the nurse assesses the home support for the woman and infant. Preparation for discharge is carefully planned with the woman and family. Provision of help in the home for the mother by relatives, friends, and others must be addressed. If necessary, the nurse refers the family to community resources (e.g., for homemaking services). Rest and sleep periods, activity, and diet must be planned. The couple will want information about reestablishing sexual relations and contraception (possibly sterilization of the man or the woman).

Potential hazards of a subsequent pregnancy need to be examined by the woman and her partner. If sterilization is selected as a method of contraception, the risks of surgery, especially for the class III or IV woman need to be explained. Oral contraceptives are often contraindicated because of the risk of thromboembolism (Gilbert, Harmon, 1993). Both the woman and her partner need to be involved in the decision-making process.

✣ EVALUATION

The nurse uses the following criteria as *overall indications* for the success of therapy.

- The woman adapts to the physiologic stressors of pregnancy; for example, she does not develop cardiac decompensation during the postpartum period.
- The home situation is controlled, with assistance provided as necessary.
- The mother and family accept the limitations imposed on the woman by the presence of heart disease.

PLAN OF CARE

Pregnant Woman with Heart Disease

Case History

Sarah Hargrove is a 24-year-old married woman in her first pregnancy. She has a history of rheumatic heart disease. Sarah works full time and also cares for her elderly mother-in-law who lives with Sarah and her husband. Sarah comes to the clinic for her regular prenatal visit at 28 weeks of gestation.

Sarah complains of shortness of breath during her regular activities and of increased fatigue. She says she has trouble keeping up with her work and with household demands. Physical assessment reveals that Sarah's pulse rate is 100 beats/min, respirations are 26/min, rales are present in the base of her lungs, and there is edema of the lower extremities. A review of laboratory results reveals that hematocrit and white blood cell levels are within normal limits; urine specific gravity is increased.

EXPECTED OUTCOMES	IMPLEMENTATION	RATIONALE	EVALUATION
Nursing Diagnosis: Activity intolerance related to the effects of pregnancy in the presence of cardiac condition			
Sarah will monitor activity tolerance/intolerance and will take appropriate actions to avoid further development of cardiac decompensation. Sarah will reduce physical activities, sleep at least 8 hours a night, and take rest periods during the day; she will experience less shortness of breath and fatigue by the next clinic visit.	Assist Sarah to restructure her daily activities to include adequate rest/sleep periods. Teach Sarah to assess for signs of worsening cardiac condition.	Activity is limited to the extent of the cardiac disease. Adequate rest and sleep minimize cardiac stress and conserve energy. Development of signs indicate a worsening of the woman's condition.	Sarah reported that she got 8 hours of sleep at night and rested after meals. Sarah reduced her work hours and did only essential housework. At her next clinic visit, Sarah reported less fatigue and shortness of breath. Sarah will continue to need close assessment for respiratory and/or circulatory impairment for the remainder of her pregnancy.
Nursing Diagnosis: Ineffective individual coping related to inability to meet role expectations secondary to pregnancy and its effects on her cardiac condition			
Sarah and her family will verbalize understanding of Sarah's physical limitations and identify effective coping techniques.	Encourage Sarah's husband to accompany her to clinic. Provide information about effects of pregnancy on women with cardiac disease and the need to limit activities. Encourage verbalization of feelings. Offer information about community resources.	Including family in clinic visits promotes their understanding of the woman's disease and impresses on them the necessity of limiting physical activities. Information can help families determine if and how needs can be met by resources outside the family.	Sarah's husband accompanies her to clinic. He verbalizes understanding of the need for Sarah to cut back on her work hours and to have help at home. A home health aide is employed to assist Sarah's mother-in-law three times a week. Sarah states she feels supported and better able to cope with her limitations.

Continued.

PLAN OF CARE—cont'd

Pregnant Woman with Heart Disease

EXPECTED OUTCOMES   IMPLEMENATION   RATIONALE   EVALUATION

Nursing Diagnosis: High risk for alteration in tissue perfusion related to cardiac condition secondary to increased circulatory needs during pregnancy

Sarah's BP, pulse, ABG and WBC values will be WNL. The fetus will be reactive with FHR WNL.	Monitor BP, pulse. Assess for signs of decompensation and hypoxia. Review signs of cardiac failure with Sarah. Monitor laboratory values, especially WBC, Hb/HCT, ABG. Assess FHR, perform NST as indicated.	Tachycardia and increased BP may indicate early heart failure/hypoxia. These are late signs of hypoxia and may indicate severe cardiac compromise. Uteroplacental insufficiency causes hypoxia, resulting in decreased fetal activity. Normal ABG values reflect adequate ventilation and oxygenation; anemia can reduce oxygen-carrying power of the blood; infections can increase the metabolic rate and oxygen needs.	Sarah's condition does not worsen. Her BP and pulse remain WNL as do her laboratory values. Sarah reports her fetus is active, and NST results are reactive. Sarah will continue weekly clinic visits for close supervision of her cardiac status and fetal status until the birth.
	Provide information on using a modified upright position for sleeping.	Eases respiratory rate by decreasing pressure of uterus on diaphragm and increases lung expansion.	

Nursing Diagnosis: High risk for alteration (decompensation) in cardiac output related to increased circulatory volume secondary to pregnancy

Sarah will maintain adequate perfusion and will not experience fluid overload as exhibited by stable BP, clear lung fields, and regular pulse rate between 60 and 100 beats/min. Sarah will exhibit no edema and will have adequate urine output. The fetus will be reactive, and FHR will be in normal range.	Provide information about adequate rest, especially in the left lateral position. Assess for edema; teach Sarah to elevate her legs when sitting. Assess intake and output. Administer medications if ordered. Evaluate fetal status (FHR, daily fetal movement counts, NST results).	Tachycardia and increased BP may be related to early cardiac decompensation. Rest minimizes cardiac stress; lateral position increases uterine blood flow and also prevents supine hypotension. Elevating the legs promotes venous return. Cardiac disease may cause kidney problems (anuria, oliguria); intake and output should be about the same. Fetal hypoxia can occur, causing bradycardia or tachycardia and decreased fetal activity.	Sarah does not develop cardiac decompensation. Her BP and pulse remain WNL; her intake and output are about the same, and no oliguria is present. Sarah states that "the baby moves a lot!" and nursing assessments of FHR range from 140-150 beats/min. Sarah gets 8 hours of sleep at night and rests after meals with her feet elevated. Sarah's condition will need continued assessment for the duration of pregnancy.

ABG, Arterial blood gases; *BP,* blood pressure, *FHR,* fetal heart rate; *Hb,* hemoglobin; *HCT,* hematocrit; *NST,* nonstress test; *WBC,* white blood cell count, *WNL,* within normal limits.

- The parent-child relationship is fostered by the family.
- The woman and family verbalize understanding of the disorder, management, and probable outcome.
- The woman and family describe their role in management, including when and how to take medication, adjust diet, and prepare for treatment.
- The woman and family participate in treatment.
- The woman and family cope with emotional reactions to pregnancy and an infant at risk.
- The woman is able to carry pregnancy to term or the point of viability of the fetus.

See the Plan of Care for a pregnant woman with heart disease.

SPECIFIC CARDIOVASCULAR CONDITIONS

Care of the woman with cardiovascular disorders combines routine peripartum care with care specific for the cardiac diagnosis. Cardiac conditions vary in their impact on pregnancy because of acuteness or chronicity. The following discussion focuses on peripartum heart failure, rheumatic heart disease, infective endocarditis, mitral valve prolapse, Marfan's syndrome, and cerebrovascular accidents.

Peripartum Heart Failure

Peripartum heart failure (failure of the heart to maintain an adequate circulation of blood) can result from an underlying chronic hypertension, previously unrecognized mitral valve stenosis, obesity, viral myocarditis, or idiopathic peripartum cardiomyopathy (Cunningham et al, 1993). In addition, anemia and infection can predispose the pregnant woman to congestive heart failure.

Peripartum heart failure from an explainable cause such as an underlying heart disease usually responds well to therapy. The typical response is rapid reversal of heart failure with furosemide (Lasix), diuresis, and correction of associated obstetric complications (Cunningham et al, 1993). Within days the heart size of these women returns to normal; their long-term prognosis depends on the underlying heart disease (e.g., hypertrophic cardiomyopathy).

Hypertrophic cardiomyopathy (HCM) is a primary disease, classified on the basis of its structural abnormality and function. In this disorder the muscle tissue of the heart walls and the septum are hypertrophied, leaving relatively small chambers. HCM usually is asymptomatic until late adolescence or early adulthood or more rarely, in middle age. Symptoms include angina, exertional dyspnea, dizziness, syncope, ventricular arrhythmias, S_3 gallop, and mild cardiomegaly. Propranolol (Inderal), a beta-blocker, is given if symptoms develop (Cunningham

et al, 1993). HCM is associated with sudden death, unrelated to functional status. HCM may be precipitated by physical or emotional stress, and the myocardial ischemia resulting from stress may promote ventricular fibrillation.

Idiopathic peripartum cardiomyopathy comprises a syndrome of heart failure (1) occurring during the peripartum period, (2) with no previous history of heart disease, and (3) with no specific etiologic factors. Autoimmune factors may be implicated (Lee, Cotton, 1989).

The incidence of peripartum cardiomyopathies has been reported as 1 in 4000 to 15,000 pregnancies (Lang and Borow, 1991). It occurs more often in multiparous women. Maternal mortality has been estimated in the range of 30% to 60%, whereas infant mortality is approximately 10%. Clinical findings are those of congestive heart failure (left ventricular failure). Signs include breathlessness, tachyarrhythmias, and edema with radiologic findings of cardiomegaly (Fig. 22-5). The prognosis is good if cardiomegaly does not persist after 6 months. The prognosis for women whose hearts remain enlarged after 6 months of bed rest is not as favorable. Future pregnancies usually result in some cardiac failure (50% to 88%). In subsequent pregnancy, mortality has been estimated as high as 60%. Sterilization should be considered. Oral contraceptives are contraindicated because of the risk of thromboembolism.

During pregnancy, bed rest is prescribed from the onset of the disease until 3 months after the heart returns to normal size. The rationale for instituting bed rest is to decrease the heart rate, stroke volume, and arterial pressure—the overall work of the heart. Prevention and treatment of arrhythmias are major goals. Antiarrhythmic drugs or beta-adrenergic or calcium channel blockers are used. Digitalis and nitrates are contraindicated in the obstructive form of HCM.

Low sodium intake (1.5 to 2 g per day) is ordered for pregnant women with severe congestive heart failure. During labor the avoidance of intravenous fluid overload is important. Because all women experience some rise in blood pressure at the onset of lactation, suppression of lactation may be recommended to minimize stress.

The nursing care of pregnant women with peripartum cardiomyopathies is essentially the same as for those with other types of cardiac problems. The necessity for prolonged bed rest can pose social and economic hardships for the family; therefore referral to community resources for assistance may be necessary. Because sudden death is a possibility with this condition, the family needs to be trained in CPR.

Rheumatic Heart Disease

Rheumatic fever usually develops suddenly, several symptom-free weeks after an inadequately treated group A beta-hemolytic streptococcal infection. Episodes of

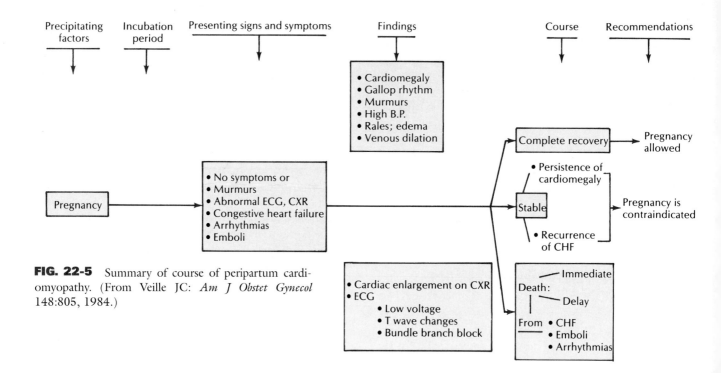

FIG. 22-5 Summary of course of peripartum cardiomyopathy. (From Veille JC: *Am J Obstet Gynecol* 148:805, 1984.)

rheumatic fever create an autoimmune reaction in the heart tissue, leading to permanent damage of heart valves (usually the mitral valve) and the chorda tendineae cordis. This damage is referred to as **rheumatic heart disease.** Rheumatic heart disease may be evident during acute rheumatic fever or discovered years later. Heart murmurs, resulting from stenosis, valvular insufficiency, or thickening of the walls of the heart, characterize rheumatic heart disease. Abnormal pulse rate and rhythm, as well as congestive heart failure, are common.

Mitral valve stenosis (narrowing of the opening of the mitral valve due to stiffening of valve leaflets, obstructing flow of blood from atrium to ventricles) accounts for 90% of rheumatic heart disease seen in pregnancy (Scott et al, 1990) and is the most important lesion hemodynamically (Brady, Duff, 1989). A tight stenosis, plus the increase in blood volume and cardiac output of normal pregnancy (see Chapter 5), may cause ventricular failure and pulmonary edema; hemoptysis may occur. Atrial fibrillation is common because of the enlarged left atrium. Cardiac failure occurs for the first time during pregnancy in 25% of women with mitral valve stenosis. Digoxin prophylaxis may be warranted. Atrial fibrillation also predisposes the woman to thromboembolism, especially in cerebral vessels (Brady, Duff, 1989), necessitating the use of heparin therapy. The care of the pregnant woman with mitral stenosis typically is managed by reducing her activity and increasing bed rest. Prophylaxis for intrapartum endocarditis and pulmonary infections usually is provided. Epidural anesthesia for labor and avoidance of intravenous fluid overload are appropriate (Cunningham et al, 1993). Mitral valvotomy

during pregnancy often brings dramatic relief of congestive heart failure that has been unresponsive to medical treatment.

Infective Endocarditis

Infective endocarditis (inflammation of the lining of the heart due to invasion of microorganism) is an uncommon condition during pregnancy (Cox, Leveno, 1989). It is seen commonly in women taking illicit drugs intravenously. Bacterial endocarditis, leading to incompetence of heart valves and cerebral emboli, can result in death. Treatment is the same as for the nonpregnant woman.

Mitral Valve Prolapse

Mitral valve prolapse (MVP) is a common, usually benign, condition occurring in nearly 10% of women of reproductive age (Cunningham et al, 1993). The mitral valve leaflets prolapse into the left atrium during ventricular systole, allowing some backflow of blood. Midsystolic click and late systolic murmur are hallmarks of this syndrome. Most cases are asymptomatic. A few women have atypical chest pain (sharp and located in the left side of the chest) that occurs at rest, unrelated to exercise, and does not respond to nitrates. Pregnancy usually is well tolerated unless bacterial endocarditis occurs.

Marfan's Syndrome

Marfan's syndrome is an autosomal dominant disorder characterized by general weakness of connective tissue. About 90% of individuals with this symptom have mitral valve prolapse, and 25% have aortic insufficiency. There is an increased risk of *aortic dissection* and rupture during pregnancy, and maternal mortality is reported at 25% to 50% (Scott et al, 1990). Management during pregnancy is by restricted activity and propranolol therapy.

Cerebrovascular Accidents

Ischemia of the brain tissues, or *cerebrovascular accidents* (CVAs), occurs from occlusion of blood vessels that normally perfuse the area. It results from a cerebral hemorrhage or an embolus. Uncontrolled hypertension during pregnancy can cause cerebral hemorrhages (Cunningham et al, 1993). CVAs have been reported to occur in 1 in 6000 pregnancies (Simolke et al, 1991). The extent of damage depends on the location and the extent of ischemia.

Medical Disorders during Pregnancy

Medical conditions may complicate pregnancy. The most common of these is anemia, especially anemia caused by iron or folic acid deficiency, sickle cell trait or disease, and thalassemia. Pulmonary, gastrointestinal, integumentary, neurologic, and autoimmune disorders also may be encountered. Pregnancy-related aspects of these conditions are addressed in the following sections.

ANEMIA

Anemia, the most common medical disorder of pregnancy, affects at least 20% of pregnant women. These women have a higher incidence of puerperal complications, such as *infection,* than do pregnant women with normal hematologic values.

Anemia results in reduction of the oxygen-carrying capacity of the blood; the heart tries to compensate by increasing the cardiac output. This effort increases the workload of the heart and stresses ventricular function. Therefore anemia that occurs with any other complication (e.g., preeclampsia) may result in congestive heart failure.

An indirect index of the oxygen-carrying capacity is the packed red blood cell volume, or hematocrit level. The normal hematocrit range in nonpregnant women is 37% to 47%. However, normal values for pregnant women with adequate iron stores may be as low as 33%. This has been explained by hydremia (dilution of blood), or the physiologic anemia of pregnancy.

At or near sea level, during the first trimester, the pregnant woman is anemic when her hemoglobin level is less than 11 g/dl or her hematocrit level falls below 37%. She is anemic in the second trimester when the hemoglobin level is less than 10.5 g/dl or the hematocrit level falls below 35%; and she is anemic in the third trimester when the hemoglobin level is less than 10 g/dl

or the hematocrit level is less than 33%. In areas of high altitude, much higher values indicate anemia, for example, at 1500 m (5000 ft) above sea level, a hemoglobin level less than 14 g/dl indicates anemia.

When a woman has anemia during pregnancy, the loss of blood at birth, even if minimal, is not well tolerated. She is at an increased risk for requiring blood transfusions. About 80% of cases of anemia in pregnancy are of the iron deficiency type (Arias, 1993). The remaining 20% of cases embrace a considerable variety of acquired and hereditary anemias, including folic acid deficiency, sickle cell anemia, and thalassemia.

Nursing care of the anemic pregnant woman requires that the nurse be able to distinguish between the normal physiologic anemia of pregnancy and the disease states. (See section on physiologic anemia of pregnancy, p. 100 and 178.) During the prenatal visits the nurse should take a diet history and provide dietary teaching as appropriate. The effects of pregnancy for a woman with anemia may cause increased fatigue, stress, and financial difficulties as she copes with her activities of daily living. The nurse should assess the pregnant woman's needs and provide her with appropriate resources.

Iron Deficiency Anemia

Without iron therapy even pregnant women who enjoy excellent nutrition will conclude pregnancy with an iron deficit. Diet alone cannot replace gestational iron losses. Inadequate nutrition without therapy will certainly mean iron deficiency anemia during late pregnancy and the puerperium.

Successful iron therapy during pregnancy can be carried out in most cases with oral iron supplements (e.g., ferrous sulfate, 0.3 g, three times a day). It is important to teach the pregnant woman the significance of iron therapy (see Chapter 8). In addition, it is necessary to instruct the woman in dietary ways to decrease the gastrointestinal side effects of iron. Some pregnant women cannot tolerate the prescribed oral iron. In such cases the woman should receive parenteral iron such as an iron-dextran complex (Imferon).

Folic Acid Deficiency Anemia

Folic acid deficiency anemia occurs in at least 2% of pregnant women in North America, an incidence much higher than that suspected even 5 years ago. Anemia compromises the women's defenses, and it makes her more vulnerable to urinary tract infections and hemorrhage.

Poor diet, cooking with large volumes of water, or home canning of food (especially vegetables) may lead to folate deficiency. Also, malabsorption may play a part in the development of anemia caused by a lack of folic acid.

During pregnancy the recommended daily intake of folate is 0.4 mg folic acid. In folate deficiency a dosage of about 5 mg per day orally for several weeks should ensure a remission. A generous maintenance dose each day should prevent a relapse. Because iron deficiency anemia may also accompany folate deficiency, augmented iron intake should be provided.

Sickle Cell Hemoglobinopathy

Sickle cell hemoglobinopathy is a disease caused by the presence of abnormal hemoglobin in the blood. *Sickle cell trait* (SA hemoglobin pattern) is sickling of the red blood cells (RBCs) but with a normal RBC life span and usually causes only mild clinical symptoms. *Sickle cell anemia* (sickle cell disease) is a recessive, hereditary, familial hemolytic anemia that affects those of African-American or Mediterranean ancestry. These individuals usually have abnormal hemoglobin types (SS or SC). Persons with sickle cell anemia have recurrent attacks (crises) of fever and pain in the abdomen or extremities beginning in childhood. These attacks are attributed to vascular occlusion (from abnormal cells), tissue hypoxia, edema, and RBC destruction. Crises are associated with normochromic anemia, jaundice, reticulocytosis, positive sickle cell test, and the demonstration of abnormal hemoglobin (usually SS or SC).

Almost 10% of African-Americans in North America have the sickle cell trait, but less than 1% have sickle cell anemia. The anemia often is complicated by iron and folic acid deficiency.

Pregnancy usually results in a worsening of most aspects of the disease (Scott et al, 1990). The anemia that occurs in normal pregnancies may aggravate sickle cell anemia and bring on more crises. Pregnant women with sickle cell anemia are prone to pyelonephritis, leg ulcers, bone infarction, cardiopathy, congestive heart failure, and preeclampsia. Urinary tract infection (UTI) and hematuria are common. An aplastic crisis may follow serious infection. Medical therapy, including transfusions to maintain the hematocrit level at least at 30%, is essential. Cesarean birth is warranted only for obstetric indications. Oral contraceptives are contraindicated.

Table 22-4 identifies some potential problems faced by the woman with sickle cell disease and some preventive and maintenance interventions.

Thalassemia

Thalassemia (Mediterranean or Cooley's anemia) is a relatively common anemia in which an insufficient amount of globin is produced to fill the red blood cells. Thalassemia is a hereditary disorder that involves the abnormal synthesis of the alpha- or beta-chains of globin. Beta thalassemia is the more common variety in the United States and is often diagnosed in individuals of Italian, Greek, or southern Chinese descent. The unbalanced synthesis of globin leads to premature red blood cell death resulting in severe anemia. Thalassemia major is the homozygous form of the disorder; thalassemia minor is the heterozygous form.

Thalassemia major may complicate pregnancy. Preeclampsia is more common in women with thalassemia major. Thalassemia major may be associated with low-birthweight infants and increased fetal wastage. Placental weight often is increased, perhaps as a result of maternal anemia. The frequency of fetal distress from hypoxia is greater than in normal pregnant women. Therefore pregnant women with thalassemia major should be monitored more closely than normal pregnant women.

Regular transfusion may be necessary. Folic acid should be given to avoid folate deficiency. Partial exchange transfusion may be warranted in severe thalassemia. Splenectomy may be necessary if enlargement and pain occur. Women with thalassemia major may die of chronic infection or progressive hepatic or cardiac failure, the result of excessive iron deposition.

Persons with *thalassemia minor* have a mild persistent anemia, but the RBC may be normal or even elevated. However, no systemic problems are caused by the anemia that is a part of the minor form of the disease. Thalassemia minor must be distinguished principally from iron deficiency anemia.

Pregnancy will neither worsen thalassemia minor nor will it be compromised by the disease. The anemia will not respond to iron therapy. Prolonged parenteral iron can lead to harmful, excessive iron storage. Infants born to parents with thalassemia will inherit the disorder. Persons with thalassemia minor should have a normal life span despite a moderately reduced hemoglobin level.

PULMONARY DISORDERS

As pregnancy advances and the uterus moves upward in the abdominal cavity and displaces the diaphragm in the thoracic cavity, any pregnant woman may experience increased respiratory difficulty. This difficulty will be compounded by pulmonary disease.

A pregnant woman with a pulmonary disorder requires assessment, planning, and interventions specific to the disease process, in addition to the routine peripartum care. The nurse also must be alert to pulmonary complications precipitated by the pregnancy.

Bronchial Asthma

Bronchial asthma is an acute respiratory illness caused by allergens, marked change in ambient temperature, or emotional tension. In many cases the actual cause may be unknown. A family history of allergy is likely in about 50% of all persons with asthma. In response to stimuli, there is widespread but reversible narrowing of the hyperreactive airways, making it difficult to breathe. The clinical manifestations are expiratory wheezing, productive cough, thick sputum, and dyspnea.

The effect of pregnancy on asthma is unpredictable. Physiologic alterations induced by pregnancy do not make the pregnant women more prone to asthmatic at-

TABLE 22-4 Sickle Cell Anemia: Potential Problems, Prevention, and Maintenance

POTENTIAL PROBLEM	PREVENTION AND MAINTENANCE
1. Inadequate oxygen to meet needs of labor and prevent sickling	1. a. Monitor Hb level and HCT to maintain Hb at ≥ 7 g and HCT at $\geq 20\%$ b. Have typed and crossmatched blood available c. Assist with transfusions d. Administer oxygen continuously during labor e. Coach for relaxation and to lessen anxiety
2. Infection resulting from anemia: urinary tract infection, pyelonephritis, pneumonia	2. a. Continue actions as under no. 1 b. Maintain adequate hydration c. Administer antibiotics, as ordered d. Maintain strict asepsis e. Encourage frequent voiding to keep bladder empty
3. Sequestration crisis caused by need for and destruction of RBCs	3. Administer folic acid supplement (15-30 mg) to decrease erythropoietic demands and reduce probability of capillary stasis
4. Crisis caused by hypoxia, hypotension, acidosis, dehydration, exertion, sudden cooling, low-grade fever	4. a. Continue actions as under no. 1 b. Avoid supine hypotension c. Maintain adequate hydration d. Maintain comfortable room temperature: use warm blankets or cool cloths as needed e. Assist with analgesia and anesthesia
5. Pseudotoxemia (hypertension, and proteinuria; *no* large weight gain); often accompanies bone pain crisis	5. a. If true PIH occurs, care is the same as for PIH b. Monitor blood pressure and urine c. Administer heparin, as ordered
6. Thromboembolism (from increased blood viscosity)	6. a. Monitor for positive Homans' sign b. Initiate bed rest if Homans' sign is positive or if reddened, warm areas, or a lump is found c. Maintain adequate hydration d. Administer heparin, as ordered e. Apply warm compresses f. Apply antiembolism stockings
7. Congestive heart failure	7. a. Assess pulse, respiratory rate every 15 min b. Auscultate for crackles (rales) frequently c. Place in semirecumbent position d. Administer oxygen and medications (e.g., digitalis, antibiotics, diuretics, analgesics) e. Prevent bearing down: reassure woman about low forceps birth under anesthesia (local or regional)
8. Pulmonary infarction (hemoptysis, cough, temperature to 102° F [38.9° C], friction rub)	8. Assess for this possible complication to facilitate early diagnosis
9. Postpartum hemorrhage (resulting from heparin therapy)	9. Administer ordered oxytocic medication

Hb, Hemoglobin; *HCT,* hematocrit; *PIH,* pregnancy-induced hypertension; *RBCs,* red blood cells.

tacks. Asthma increases the incidence of abortion and preterm labor, but the fetus per se is unaffected. In severe cases asthma may be life threatening for the pregnant women. The prognosis for both mother and fetus is good in most cases.

Therapy for bronchial asthma has two objectives: (1) relief of the acute attack and (2) prevention or limitation of later attacks. In all persons with asthma, known allergens should be eliminated and a comfortable home temperature maintained. Respiratory infections should be treated and mist or steam inhalation employed to aid expectoration of mucus. Bronchial asthma therapy is initiated. Acute episodes may require steroids, aminophylline, oxygen, and correction of fluid-electrolyte imbalance. Precautions specific for obstetrics include the following:

- Do not use morphine in labor because it may cause bronchospasm: meperidine (Demerol) usually will relieve bronchospasm.
- Avoid or limit the use of ephedrine and corticotropin (pressor drugs) in preeclampsia and eclampsia.
- Choose vaginal birth with use of local or regional anesthesia, whenever possible.

Adult Respiratory Distress Syndrome

Adult respiratory distress syndrome (ARDS), or shock lung, occurs when the lungs are unable to maintain levels of oxygen and carbon dioxide within normal limits. Marked tachycardia, dyspnea, and cyanosis that do not respond to nasal oxygen or intermittent positive pressure breathing are the most noted signs. ARDS is not a condition specific to pregnancy; it also can result from chest trauma, drug ingestion, or pneumonia. When ARDS is associated with pregnancy, pulmonary or amniotic fluid embolism, disseminated intravascular coagulation (DIC), and aspiration pneumonia are the precipitators.

The postpartum incidence of ARDS is not affected by the means of birth but by the amount of trauma experienced during pregnancy and birth that leads to sepsis. It also may occur after spontaneous or medically induced abortion.

Laboratory reports are important in identifying the origin of acute pulmonary problems. The important observations for the nurse to note are vital signs, signs of thromboembolism, and hemorrhage. During the postpartum period, apprehension, distended neck veins, cyanosis, diaphoresis, and pallor provide clues. Mental confusion or disorientation also may be noted.

Temperature elevation may indicate the development of thrombophlebitis. The pulse rate increases to compensate for respiratory insufficiency of any origin. The severity of the pulmonary problem increases as the pulse rate rises. An initial rise in blood pressure occurs as cardiac output increases in an attempt to supply the tissue with oxygen. When lung damage is severe, the blood pressure drops.

Respiratory changes are the most important indicators of ARDS. The rate, depth, respiratory pattern, symmetry of chest movement, and use of accessory muscle should be noted; therefore observation of respiratory characteristics after activity is important. If there is any indication of abnormality, respirations are counted for a full minute; an error of plus or minus 4 may be highly significant. On auscultation, crackles (rales), rhonchi, wheezes, or a pleural friction rub should be reported, especially when they have occurred since an earlier normal assessment. The pregnant woman should be positioned for breathing comfort. Oxygen and emergency equipment should be available. The woman should be reassured and coached in relaxation techniques so that her anxiety is lessened.

The lower extremities need to be checked for swelling, pain, inflammation, venous distention, and Homans' sign. If thrombophlebitis is suspected, the woman should be maintained on bed rest. Sudden movement or straining can dislodge a clot and lead to pulmonary embolism.

Alterations in vein distensibility have been noted, possibly because of softening of collagen induced by hormonal influences. The combination of vein distensibility and obstruction of venous blood return from the lower extremities (caused by fetal pressure on veins, especially in the last trimester) predisposes a woman to pooling of blood. In addition, hypercoagulation and pooling may lead to thrombophlebitis. Thrombophlebitis can result in ARDS (emboli from thromboembolism cause obstruction in the pulmonary circulation).

It has been noted that during pregnancy there is an increase in some of the coagulation factors. This increase in coagulation results in shortening of the partial thromboplastin time (PTT). This state predisposes the woman to an increase in rapidity of blood clotting and an increased tendency to form blood clots (hypercoagulability). Petechiae, ecchymosis, hematuria, and epistaxis are important indications of DIC. Replacement of clotting factors and heparin therapy may be required for DIC. Sources of trauma should be identified and eliminated so that outside causes of hemorrhage are avoided.

Aspiration pneumonia can be caused by changes in the gastrointestinal system during pregnancy. Progesterone has been known to relax smooth muscles. When the resting tone is lowered, the cardiac sphincter becomes weak and reflux of the stomach contents can easily occur. Increased intraabdominal pressure (because of fetal growth) further predisposes the mother to gastric reflux.

Food eaten as long as 24 to 48 hours before labor can be vomited and then aspirated. Aspiration of solid foods and liquids may cause bronchial obstruction leading to bronchoconstriction, which in turn can result in ARDS. Large particles can be removed by coughing, suctioning, or bronchoscopy, but liquids are harder to remove. The hydrochloric acid in the aspirated stomach contents may cause an asthmalike syndrome with necrotizing bronchitis. For this reason an antacid is given before cesarean birth as a prophylactic measure.

ARDS carries a high rate of mortality (50% to 70%) (Dorman, 1991). The prognosis is good if the woman is otherwise healthy and if ventilatory support can be maintained until the underlying disease can be treated (Cunningham et al, 1993).

Cystic Fibrosis

Improvements in diagnosis and treatment of cystic fibrosis have allowed an increasing number of females to survive to adulthood. Most women diagnosed with cystic fibrosis are infertile; however, pregnancy is not uncommon. The pregnancy is often complicated by chronic hypoxia and frequent pulmonary infections. Women with cystic fibrosis show a decrease in their residual volume during pregnancy, as do normal pregnant women. However, persons with cystic fibrosis are unable to maintain vital capacity. Presumably, the pulmonary vasculature cannot accommodate the increased cardiac output of pregnancy. The results are decreased oxygen to the myocardium, decreasing cardiac output, and an increase in hypoxemia. Increased maternal and perinatal mortality is related to severe pulmonary infection.

During labor, monitoring for fluid and electrolyte balance is required. The amount of sodium lost through sweat can be significant, and hypovolemia can occur. Conversely, if the woman has any degree of cor pulmonale, she must be guarded against fluid overload. Oxygen is freely given during labor. Epidural or local anesthesia is the method of choice for birth.

The woman should know that her child will be heterozygous for cystic fibrosis, even if it is not homozygous. This in turn is likely to increase the genetic pool in the community (Creasy, Resnick, 1989).

The baby of a woman with cystic fibrosis should be breastfed only after the sodium content of her milk has been estimated. If normal levels of sodium are present, breastfeeding is considered safe (Creasy, Resnik, 1989; Lawrence, 1994).

GASTROINTESTINAL DISORDERS

Compromise of gastrointestinal function during pregnancy is apparent to all concerned. Obvious physiologic alterations, such as the greatly enlarged uterus, and less apparent changes, such as hormonal differences and hypochlorhydria (deficiency of hydrochloric acid in the stomach's gastric juice), require understanding for proper diagnosis and treatment. Gallbladder disease and inflammatory bowel disease are two gastrointestinal disorders that may occur during pregnancy.

Cholelithiasis and Cholecystitis

Women are four times more likely to have **cholelithiasis** (presence of gallstones in the gallbladder) than are men (Creasy, Resnik, 1989). Maternal adaptation significantly alters gallbladder function (Scott et al, 1990). Pregnancy seems to make the woman more vulnerable to gallstone formation. Decreased muscle tone allows gallbladder distention, thickening of the bile, and prolonged emptying time. Increased progesterone levels result in a slight hypercholesterolemia. However, **cholecystitis** (inflammation of the gallbladder) does not commonly occur during pregnancy.

Inflammatory Bowel Disease

Inflammatory bowel disease can be acute or chronic. Chronic inflammatory bowel disease can be classified as *regional enteritis* (Crohn's disease) or *ulcerative colitis*.

Chronic inflammatory bowel diseases are prone to periods of exacerbation and remission. The cause is unknown. The clinical manifestations for this chronic disorder are liquid diarrhea, urgency of defecation, and crampy lower abdominal pain. Blood, mucus, and pus may be seen in the stool.

Treatment and therapy are the same for the pregnant woman as for the nonpregnant woman. Medications include sulfasalazine and prednisone. Folic acid and vitamin supplementation is especially important because of the problems with malabsorption and malnutrition associated with chronic inflammatory bowel disease.

The effect of inflammatory bowel disease on pregnancy is minimal unless there is marked debilitation, whereupon spontaneous abortion, fetal death, or preterm birth may occur. In general, when pregnancy coincides with active ulcerative colitis, most women will experience a severe exacerbation of the disease. When pregnancy occurs during a period of inactivity of the disorder, a flareup is unlikely.

INTEGUMENTARY DISORDERS

Dermatologic disorders induced by pregnancy include melasma (chloasma), herpes gestationis, noninflammatory pruritus of pregnancy, vascular spiders, palmar erythema, and pregnancy granuloma (including epulides). Skin problems generally aggravated by pregnancy are acne vulgaris (acne) (in the first trimester), erythema multiforme, herpetiform dermatitis (fever blisters and genital herpes), granuloma inguinale (Donovan bodies), condylomata acuminata (genital warts), neurofibromatosis (von Recklinghausen's disease), and pemphigus. Dermatologic disorders usually improved by pregnancy include acne vulgaris (in the third trimester), seborrhea dermatitis (dandruff), and psoriasis. An unpredictable course during pregnancy may be expected in atopic dermatitis, lupus erythematosus, and herpes simplex.

Elective abortion or early birth may be justified for some dermatologic conditions. These conditions include disseminated lupus erythematosus, neurofibromatosis, and herpes gestationis. Herpes gestationis (not a viral induced disorder) is a rare blistering skin disease of pregnancy. Prednisone usually brings prompt relief and inhibits development of new lesions. The process may recur in subsequent pregnancies (Cunningham et al, 1993).

Isotretinoin (Accutane), commonly prescribed for cystic acne, is highly teratogenic. There is a risk for craniofacial, cardiac, and CNS malformations in exposed fetuses.

Explanation, reassurance, and common sense measures should suffice for normal skin changes. In contrast, disease processes during and soon after pregnancy may be extremely difficult to diagnose and treat.

NEUROLOGIC DISORDERS

The pregnant woman with a neurologic disorder needs to deal with potential teratogenic effects of prescribed medications, changes of mobility during pregnancy, and ability to care for the baby. The nurse should be aware of all drugs the pregnant woman is taking and the associated potential for producing congenital anomalies. As the pregnancy progresses, the woman's center of gravity shifts and causes balance and gait changes. The nurse needs to advise the woman of these expected changes and to suggest safety measures as appropriate. Familial and community resources should be assessed to provide child care for the neurologically impaired woman.

Epilepsy

Epilepsy may result from developmental abnormalities or injury. Epilepsy seriously complicates about 1 in 1000 gestations. Convulsive seizures may be more frequent or severe during complications of pregnancy, such as edema, alkylosis, fluid-electrolyte imbalance, cerebral hypoxia, hypoglycemia, and hypocalcemia. On the other hand, the effects of pregnancy on epilepsy are unpredictable. Seizure frequency remains the same in about 50% of the women, with 25% experiencing a decrease and 25% experiencing an increase in seizure activity (Krumholz, 1992).

The differential diagnosis of epilepsy vs. eclampsia may pose a problem. Epilepsy and eclampsia can coexist. However, a history of seizures and a normal plasma uric acid level, as well as the absence of hypertension, or proteinuria, point to epilepsy. Electroencephalography rarely is diagnostic.

Pregnancy usually alters pharmacokinetics. In addition, nausea and vomiting may interfere with ingestion and absorption of medication. Diazepam (Valium) crosses the placenta and accumulates in fetal circulation. Cleft lip or cleft palate or other malformations may be associated with its use (Mattison et al, 1989). Although diazepam and chlordiazepoxide (Librium) are safe analeptic drugs, they may cause respiratory depression in the newborn. Phenytoin (Dilantin) and its analogues may be fetotoxic.

Grand mal seizures can be controlled by intravenous sodium amobarbital or magnesium sulfate. Epilepsy is not an indication for therapeutic abortion or cesarean birth.

Multiple Sclerosis

Multiple sclerosis (MS), a patchy demyelinization of the spinal cord and CNS, may be a viral disorder. Women are affected twice as often as men, with the most common onset occurring between the ages of 20 and 35. It is common to have an interaction between MS and pregnancy. MS may occasionally complicate pregnancy, but exacerbations and remissions are unrelated to the pregnant state. For this reason medically indicated therapeutic abortion is illogical. The burden of pregnancy and subsequent child care may warrant early interruption of pregnancy and sterilization in extreme cases. Nursing care of the pregnant woman with MS is similar to the care of the normal pregnant woman. The incidence of MS in the offspring is about 3% to 5% (Rudick, Birk, 1992). During the first 3 months after birth 20% to 40% of MS patients experience a clinical relapse or worsening of the disease (Rudick, Birk, 1992).

Bell's Palsy

An association between idiopathic facial paralysis and pregnancy was first cited by Bell in 1830. Bell's palsy occurs in about 1 in 2000 pregnancies. Incidence peaks during the third trimester and the puerperium (Cherry, Merkatz, 1991). A causative relationship does not seem to exist between the appearance of Bell's palsy and any of the complications of pregnancy.

No effects of maternal Bell's palsy have been observed in infants. Maternal outcome is generally good. In most affected women, 90% or more of facial function can be expected to return (Cunningham et al, 1993; Scott et al, 1990). Supportive care includes prevention of injury to the exposed cornea, facial muscle massage, careful chewing and manual removal of food from inside the affected cheek, and reassurance that return of total neurologic function is likely.

AUTOIMMUNE DISORDERS

Autoimmune disorders comprise a large group of diseases that disrupt the function of the immune system of the body. In these types of disorders the body develops antibodies that attack its normally present antigens. Autoimmune disorders have a predilection for women in their reproductive years; therefore associations with pregnancy are not uncommon (Scott et al, 1990). Pregnancy may affect the disease process. Some disorders adversely affect the course of pregnancy or are detrimental to the fetus. Autoimmune disorders include rheumatoid arthritis, systemic lupus erythematosus, myasthenia gravis, and immunologic thrombocytopenic purpura. Autoantibodies from rheumatoid arthritis do not cross the placenta; those of the other disorders do. The woman with immunologic thrombocytopenic purpura may give birth to a child who demonstrates thrombocytopenia. Petechiae and bleeding into the gastrointestinal and genitourinary tracts and into the brain may be evident. If the mother has myasthenia gravis, the newborn may exhibit a weak cry, sucking mechanism, and facial muscles and may have respiratory problems.

Rheumatoid Arthritis

Most women with rheumatoid arthritis (RA) find that the severity of symptoms decreases during pregnancy (Buchanan, Needs, Brooks, 1992). For this reason many affected women attempt to become pregnant as often as possible; however, many are subfertile because of the RA. During pregnancy, women with RA experience an increase in alpha$_2$-glycoprotein. In addition, total plasma and free cortisol (especially estrogens and progesterone) show an increase. This combination apparently leads to depressed cellular immunity (Buchanan, Needs, Brooks, 1992). Women in whom the rheumatoid factor (autoantibodies found in the synovial fluid) decreases during pregnancy report improvement in their symptoms. Researchers are now investigating the possibility of a positive effect on RA associated with the use of oral contraceptives.

The woman with RA needs to be informed of the positive and negative aspects that accompany pregnancy. She must be cautioned that, although symptoms may subside during pregnancy, she should anticipate a return of her symptoms after giving birth. Exacerbations often recur about a month after birth (Buchanan, Needs, Brooks, 1992).

Management of RA during pregnancy includes an appropriate balance of rest and exercise, heat and physical therapy, and salicylates. Aspirin probably remains the safest and most useful antiinflammatory drug for these women. Mild hemostatic changes in the newborn, an increase in the average length of gestation, and possibly premature closure of the ductus arteriosus are attributed to maternal ingestion of large doses of aspirin (Cunningham et al, 1993).

Systemic Lupus Erythematosus

One of the most common serious disorders of childbearing age, **systemic lupus erythematosus (SLE)** is a chronic multisystem inflammatory disease. The condition is not rare; more than 250,000 persons are known to have SLE, with an estimated 50,000 new cases per year. Although the antibody may be formed in response to a virus, a familial tendency seems to be involved.

The vague early symptoms, such as fatigue, may be overlooked. Eventually all organs become involved. The condition is characterized by a series of exacerbations and remissions.

If the diagnosis has been established and the woman desires a child, she is advised to wait for 2 years. At that time, if the disease has been controlled well on low doses of corticosteroids, pregnancy may be reasonably considered (Blackburn, Loper, 1992; Scott et al, 1990). Postpartum exacerbation may represent a rebound phenomenon as suppression of cell-mediated activity, normal during pregnancy, is terminated. Oral contraceptives are contraindicated; diaphragms and condoms are the preferred methods of fertility management if pregnancy is desired in the future. Sterilization is suggested if no more children are wanted. The outlook for persons with SLE has improved markedly in the past few years. Persons diagnosed with SLE have a 5-year survival rate of more than 90%, and more than 80% survive for 10 years or more.

The effect of pregnancy on SLE seems inconsistent. The rate of spontaneous abortion is high. Maternal complications correlate with the degree of cardiac or renal involvement (Blackburn, Loper, 1992; Scott et al, 1990). Renal failure, hypertension, and death are associated with diffuse proliferative lupus glomerulonephritis. When the kidneys are involved, women are subject to superimposed preeclampsia, stillbirths, preterm birth, and small-for-gestational age infants. However, if the disease is stable during pregnancy, the risk that the disease will worsen with gestation is only slight.

The relationship of immunosuppressive drugs (such as corticosteroids) and infection must be acknowledged. Infection is now a leading cause of death among persons with SLE.

Although the antibodies cross the placenta, the amount varies so that the effect on the fetus also varies. The most severely affected newborns suffer from discoid lupus, anemia, neutropenia, thrombocytopenia, and congenital complete heart block.

Myasthenia Gravis

Myasthenia gravis, an autoimmune motor (muscle) end plate disorder that involves acetylcholine use, affects the motor function at the myoneural junction. Muscle weakness, particularly of the eyes, face, tongue, neck, limbs, and respiratory muscles, results. The peak prevalence of myasthenia gravis is about 25 years of age. Pregnancy may complicate the disorder, although some women experience a remission during gestation. Pregnancies in women with this disease can be carried to safe birth if certain precautions are taken (Cartlidge, 1991). Therefore the disorder is not an indication for elective abortion.

The health care providers should be alert to symptoms, which include easy fatigue, intermittent double vision, upper eyelid drooping, and facial muscle weakness. In more serious cases upper arm weakness and breathing difficulty are seen. Infections may precipitate the onset or relapse and must be treated aggressively during pregnancy.

Women with myasthenia gravis usually tolerate labor well because they already have some degree of muscle relaxation. During the second stage, some women may show impairment of voluntary expulsive efforts. Meperidine is the obstetric analgesic of choice. Local anesthesia is preferred. Oxytocin may be given, but scopolamine and muscle relaxants (e.g., magnesium sulfate) are contraindicated. After birth, women must be carefully supervised, because relapses often occur during the puerperium.

All infants of myasthenia gravis mothers should be closely monitored for muscle weakness (e.g., weak cry, respiratory distress, poor Moro reflex, difficulty in feeding). In 12% of the babies born to myasthenic mothers, transient muscle weakness occurs within the first few days after birth. Symptoms may persist from 1 to 2 months. Of the infants that show myasthenic signs, three fourths require anticholinesterase medications. The response of the infant to the medications is usually good (Cartlidge, 1991).

ABDOMINAL SURGERY DURING PREGNANCY

The need for immediate abdominal surgery occurs as frequently among pregnant women as among nonpregnant women of comparable age. However, diagnosis is more difficult in the pregnant woman. An enlarged uterus and displaced internal organs may prevent adequate palpation and may alter the position of the surgical procedure (Sibai, 1992). The health care provider is confronted with both a surgical and an obstetric problem.

Laparotomy or laparoscopy may be required. Hazards of these procedures include abortion and preterm labor. However, surgical or anesthetic intervention does not affect the incidence of congenital malformations.

Appendicitis

Acute suppurative appendicitis complicates about 1 in 1000 pregnancies. This disorder poses the following special problems during gestation.

1. Appendicitis is more difficult to diagnose during pregnancy. The appendix is carried high and to the right, away from McBurney's point, by the enlarged uterus (Fig. 22-6).
2. Appendiceal rupture and peritonitis occur two to three times more often in pregnant women than in nonpregnant women.

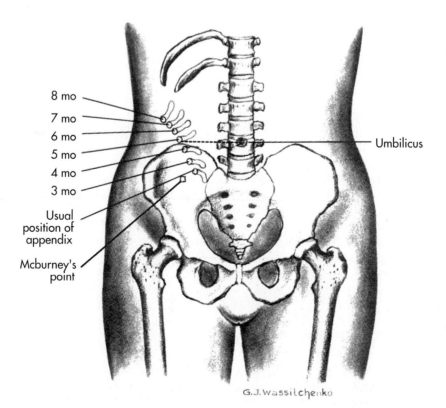

G.J. Wassilchenko

FIG. 22-6 Change in position of appendix during pregnancy.

3. Maternal and perinatal morbidity and mortality are greatly increased when appendicitis occurs during pregnancy.

Most cases of acute appendicitis occur during the first 6 months of gestation, with decreasing frequency through the third trimester, labor, and puerperium. The differential diagnosis of appendicitis during pregnancy is complicated by gastrointestinal or genitourinary problems that may be confused with appendicitis. A high level of suspicion is important in the diagnosis of appendicitis.

Gynecologic Problems

Ovarian cysts and twisting of ovarian cysts or adnexal tissues may occur. Pregnancy predisposes a woman to ovarian problems, especially during the first trimester. Conditions include retained or enlarged cystic corpus luteum of pregnancy, ovarian cyst, and bacterial invasion of reproductive or other intraperitoneal organs.

Laparotomy or laparoscopy may be required to discriminate between ovarian problems and early ectopic pregnancy, appendicitis, and other infectious processes.

Care Management

Fetal vital signs and activity and uterine contractility (labor may have begun) are monitored, and constant vigilance for symptoms of impending obstetric complications is maintained. The woman and her family may have heightened concerns regarding effects of the procedure and medication on fetal well-being and the course of pregnancy. The extent of preoperative assessment is determined by the immediacy of surgical intervention and the specific condition that requires surgery (Phipps, Long, 1993).

Preoperative care for a pregnant woman differs from that of a nonpregnant woman in one significant aspect: the presence of at least one other person—the fetus. Food by mouth is restricted for several hours before a scheduled procedure or surgery. Even if she has had nothing by mouth and especially if the surgery is unexpected the woman is in danger of vomiting and aspirating, thus special precautions are taken before anesthesia is administered (p. 653). Note that maternal ketosis and hypoglycemia rapidly occur in both the woman and fetus (Shaver, 1992). If the woman experiences a prolonged NPO status, IV fluids with dextrose should be given.

General preoperative and postoperative observations and ongoing care are the same as for any surgery. Examples of these are monitoring vital signs and fluid and electrolyte balance, providing for safety, comfort, and rest, as well as monitoring for complications. Because of the decreased respiratory excursion associated with the enlarged uterus, the pregnant woman is at greater risk of postoperative atelectasis and pulmonary complications

(Shaver, 1992). The important addition to the postoperative care of the pregnant patient is that of fetal surveillance. If intrauterine pregnancy continues, monitoring of fetal heart rate and activity, as well as uterine activity, is continued.

Discharge Planning

Planning for discharge begins when the pregnant woman first enters the health care system. The extent to which the preoperative expected outcomes of care can be met are reviewed, and adjustments are made accordingly. For example, if the surgery was an emergency, such as for appendicitis, there is little time for preoperative preparation. After the woman has recovered from the effects of surgery, the nurse needs to take time to encourage her to voice her fears, concerns, and questions. She may have questions regarding the effect of the surgery and anesthesia on the fetus. If she is unable to express these concerns to the surgeon, the nurse acts as patient advocate and informs the health care provider.

The participation of the woman and her family in discharge planning is necessary to individualize the care to fit with the available family support systems, the home situation, and the facilities. The woman may demonstrate symptoms of grief and loss, and her participation in discharge planning may be minimal. She may need assistance coping with these feelings.

The woman may need referral service to various community agencies for evaluation of the home situation, child care, home health care, and financial or other assistance. All arrangements for her return home and for convalescent care should be completed as early as possible before her expected date of discharge (Box 22-1).

BOX 22-1

Discharge Teaching for Home Care

- Care of incision site
- Diet and elimination related to gastrointestinal function
- Signs and symptoms of developing complications: wound infection, thrombophlebitis, pneumonia
- Equipment needed and technique for assessing temperature
- Recommended schedule for resumption of activities of daily living
- Treatments and medications ordered
- List of resource persons and their telephone numbers
- Schedule of follow-up visits

If birth has not occurred:
- Assessment of fetal activity (kick counts)
- Signs of preterm labor

TRAUMA DURING PREGNANCY

Minor injury during pregnancy is common; most trauma (more than 50%) occurs during the third trimester. A change in the woman's center of gravity as well as other changes in pregnancy are responsible for syncope, loss of balance, and general clumsiness. Discomfort such as a contracting uterus or vigorous fetal movement may be distracting while the woman is driving or working. It is interesting, that the leading cause of death in women of reproductive age is trauma and not neoplasms or obstetric complications (Daddario, 1989; Troiano, 1991).

Care Management

The woman's condition is the initial concern. The injury sustained determines the type and extent of assessment conducted. Attention is focused first on the basic ABCs: airway, breathing, and circulation. The woman's abdomen is assessed for ruptured uterus and for uterine activity. The fetus is then assessed for heart rate and activity. An individualized health assessment is performed and the woman's prenatal record is reviewed when available.

Findings from the injury must not be confused with the normal physiologic changes during pregnancy. The

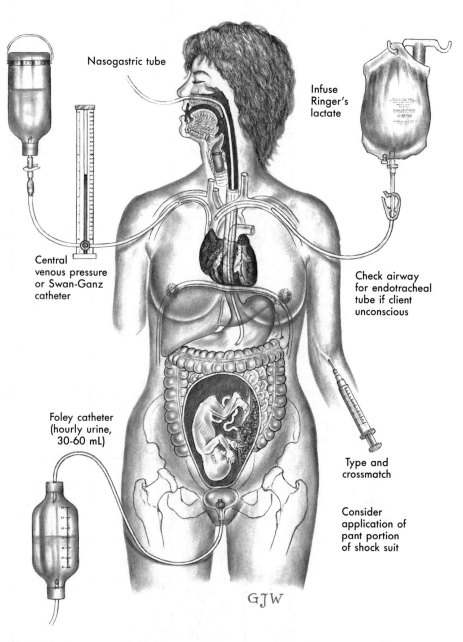

Nasogastric tube

Infuse Ringer's lactate

Central venous pressure or Swan-Ganz catheter

Check airway for endotracheal tube if client unconscious

Foley catheter (hourly urine, 30-60 mL)

Type and crossmatch

Consider application of pant portion of shock suit

GJW

FIG. 22-7 Summary of technique used for resuscitation. Trauma care should begin in field where injury occurred, always with attention to basic ABCs: airway, breathing, and circulation.

usual signs of organ rupture—for example, guarding, rebound tenderness, and rigidity—may be only responses to stretching of the abdominal wall. An examination of the woman in a supine position results in hypotension and a systolic value as low as 80 mm Hg; changing her to a lateral position or simply moving the fetus raises the systolic value to more than 100 mm Hg. A silent abdomen, a sign of bowel trauma, may be a normal finding because of the decreased motility that occurs during pregnancy. Delayed emptying time of the stomach during pregnancy poses a threat of vomiting and possible aspiration if the woman has eaten within the last several hours.

During pregnancy the woman may sustain a significant blood loss (approximately a 30% reduction of circulating blood volume) without the usual signs and symptoms of hypovolemia. Pelvic blood vessels (retroperitoneal and parametrial arteries) enlarge greatly during pregnancy; thus they are more easily damaged and potentially ruptured. The large uterus can compartmentalize and hide hemorrhage originating in the liver and spleen. A rapid pulse may reflect only the usual increase of 10 to 15 beats/min, or it may be a sign of hypovolemia.

Laboratory and diagnostic tests are determined by the type of injury. Appropriate blood studies include tests for serum amylase and blood gases; baseline bleeding profile; and complete blood cell count, typing, and crossmatching. In normal pregnancies a WBC of 18,000/mm^3 in the last trimester and 25,000/mm^3 during labor is usual; however, these same values also indicate intraabdominal hemorrhage. DIC can complicate severe trauma, placental abruption, and sepsis.

An indwelling urinary bladder catheter for drainage facilitates management of fluid therapy and aids diagnosis (Fig. 22-7). For example, difficulty in passing the catheter suggests urethral disruption, and hematuria suggests a ruptured bladder. The catheter also provides access for retrograde cystogram x-ray examination.

Intraperitoneal hemorrhage must be detected. Radiology, real-time ultrasound, and computed tomography scan are useful diagnostic modalities. The physician places a peritoneal lavage catheter for detecting intraperitoneal hemorrhage. The procedure is performed through a small incision into the peritoneum, with the woman under local anesthesia. The test result is positive for bleeding if the aspirate exceeds 10 ml nonclotting blood or if, after instillation of 1 L lactated Ringer's solution, bloody fluid is recovered. Radiographic studies may be necessary to guide management.

Intervention begins with prevention. The pregnant woman is counseled to discontinue activities requiring balance and coordination, to use car seat restraints appropriately, to recognize early adverse symptoms, and to seek therapy immediately. If the woman is hospitalized only for observation, she is involved in assessment for signs and symptoms of complications.

In case of minor trauma the woman is hospitalized and evaluated for the following: vaginal bleeding, uterine irritability, abdominal tenderness, abdominal pain or cramps, evidence of hypovolemia, a change in or absence of fetal heart rate, fetal activity, leakage of amniotic fluid, and the presence of fetal cells in maternal circulation.

Immediate trauma care consists of attention to the ABCs. While hypoxia and hypovolemia are being corrected, the woman should be transferred to a trauma center with obstetric and neonatal back-up, if possible. During transfer, attendants must remember the aortocaval (supine hypotension) syndrome. The woman should be positioned on her side, or the uterus should be displaced laterally by a uterine displacer or by a pillow placed under the woman's right hip. Hypotension must be avoided to prevent compromise of cardiac output followed by decrease of blood flow to the uterus.

A nasogastric tube is inserted, if indicated, because delayed gastric emptying time and increased intestinal transit time increase the risk of vomiting and aspiration. Mouth care and reassurance are used to counter any irritation caused by the tube. Fluid and electrolyte replacement is instituted and monitored. Oxygen needs are met.

Penetrating abdominal wounds, internal hemorrhage, and ruptured uterus are all indications for immediate surgical intervention. Wounds high in the abdomen have most likely penetrated a vital structure because organs such as the bowel, liver, and spleen have been displaced upward by the enlarging uterus (see Fig. 22-7).

Posttraumatic Uterine and Fetal Surveillance

When the mother's condition has been stabilized, attention is turned toward monitoring the fetus and monitoring for preterm labor and placental abruption. Usually, if these complications occur, they happen within 24 to 48 hours after the accident (Smith, Phelan, 1991). Uterine rupture can occur at the site of a previous scar or over the site of implantation, which is weakened by increased vascularity at the site. Expulsion of the uterine contents into the abdominal cavity may occur and usually is followed by massive hemorrhage.

KEY POINTS

- Lack of maternal glycemic control before conception and in the first trimester of pregnancy may be responsible for fetal congenital malformations.
- Maternal insulin does not cross the placenta; the fetus begins to secrete its own insulin by the tenth week of gestation.
- After the tenth week of gestation, fetal hyperinsulinism results from maternal hyperglycemia.
- Maternal insulin requirements increase as the pregnancy progresses and may quadruple by term as a result of insulin resistance created by placental hormones, insulinase, and cortisol.
- Poor glycemic control before and during pregnancy is responsible for maternal complications such as spontaneous abortion, infection, pregnancy-induced hypertension, and dystocia (difficult labor) caused by hydramnios and macrosomia.
- Home monitoring of blood glucose levels, multiple doses or constant infusion of insulin, and dietary counseling are being used to create a normal intrauterine environment for fetal growth and development in the pregnancy complicated by diabetes mellitus.
- In most cases, GDM is asymptomatic, thus reinforcing the need for routine screening of all pregnant women.
- The woman with hyperemesis gravidarum is discharged home when fluid and electrolyte balance is restored and weight gain begins.

- Thyroid dysfunction during pregnancy requires close monitoring of thyroid hormone levels to regulate therapy and prevent fetal insult.
- The stress of the normal maternal adaptations to pregnancy on a heart whose functions are already taxed may cause cardiac decompensation.
- Anemia, the most common medical disorder of pregnancy, affects at least 20% of women.
- The chance of developing adult respiratory distress syndrome increases with the amount of trauma experienced during pregnancy or birth.
- Autoimmune disorders (e.g., systemic lupus erythematosus, myasthenia gravis) show a predilection for women in their reproductive years; therefore associations with pregnancy are not uncommon.
- Trauma during pregnancy has the potential to affect both the mother and the fetus; assessment after trauma is more difficult because of the normal physiologic changes of pregnancy.
- In the pregnant woman an enlarged uterus, displaced internal organs, and altered laboratory values may confound differential diagnosis when the need for immediate abdominal surgery occurs.
- Preoperative care for a pregnant woman differs from that for a nonpregnant woman in one significant aspect: the presence of at least one other person—the fetus.

CRITICAL THINKING EXERCISES

1. Interview several diabetic mothers in the clinic and postpartum period. Determine their feelings about the number and inconvenience of prenatal visits, home care or hospitalizations before birth, tests undergone, and medication costs. In group discussion, present this information and discuss and compare the mothers' perceptions of their experiences.
   a. How did this exercise affect your perception of their experiences?
   b. Identify at least three interventions (e.g., physical care, teaching) that you would modify in a nursing plan of care because of your new perceptions. Justify your decisions and actions.

2. You are assigned to a woman who has a history of class III cardiovascular disorder (New York Heart Association classification). She has come to the clinic, where she is diagnosed to be at 8 weeks' gestation. She has a 2-year-old at home and her husband, who is not present today, thinks she is healthy and does not need any help with household or child care activities during pregnancy.

   a. Examine the options for this woman given this situation. What are the pros and cons of each?
   b. Select one option. Justify your choice; identify nursing diagnoses; formulate a plan of care.

3. Mrs. S. was admitted to the ICU after sustaining multiple injuries in an automobile accident. She is at 30 weeks' gestation and is being maintained on life support measures to keep the fetus alive until it can be born as close to term as possible. Mr. S. has been at his wife's side since she was admitted.
   a. What are the critical issues to be addressed by the nursing staff in this situation?
   b. How can the wishes of the husband/family be incorporated into the care of Mrs. S.?
   c. What are the pros and cons of maintaining Mrs. S. on life support for the sake of the fetus?
   d. Examine what your reactions would be if you were asked to care for Mrs. S.

References

Abell TL, Riely CA: Hyperemesis gravidarum, *Gastroenterol Clin North Am* 21(4):835, 1992.

American Diabetes Association: Position statement: office guide to diagnosis and classification of diabetes mellitus and other categories of glucose intolerance, *Diabetes Care* 13(suppl 1):3, 1990.

American Diabetes Association: Summary and recommendations of the second international workshop-conference on gestational diabetes mellitus, *Diabetes* 34(suppl 2):123, 1985.

Anticoagulants: how safe are they during pregnancy? *Contemp OB/GYN* 35(1):182, 1990.

Arias F: *Practical guide to high-risk pregnancy and delivery*, St Louis, 1993, Mosby.

Artal R: Exercise and pregnancy, *Clin Sports Med* 11(2):363, 1992.

Becerra JE et al: Diabetes mellitus during pregnancy and the risks for specific birth defects: a population-based case-control study, *Pediatrics* 65(1):1, 1990.

Benz J: Antidiabetic agents and lactation, *J Hum Lact* 8(1):27, 1992.

Berkowitz GS et al: Race/ethnicity and other risk factors for gestational diabetes, *Am J Epidemiol* 135(9):965, 1992.

Blackburn ST, Loper DL: *Maternal, fetal and neonatal physiology: a clinical perspective*, Philadelphia, 1992, WB Saunders.

Brady K, Duff P: Rheumatic heart disease in pregnancy, *Clin Obstet Gynecol* 31(1):21, 1989.

Buchanan WW, Needs CJ, Brooks PM: Rheumatic diseases: the arthropathies. In Gleicher N et al, editors: *Principles and practice of medical therapy in pregnancy*, Norwalk, CT, 1992, Appleton & Lange.

Cartlidge NEF: Neurologic disorders. In Barron WM, Lindheimer MD, editors: *Medical disorders during pregnancy*, St Louis, 1991, Mosby.

Centers for Disease Control: Perinatal mortality and congenital malformations in infants born to women with insulin dependent diabetes mellitus—U.S., Canada, and Europe, 1940-1988, *JAMA* 264(4):437, 1990.

Charlin V et al: Parenteral nutrition in hyperemesis gravidarum, *Nutrition* 9(1):29, 1993.

Cherry SH, Merkatz IR: *Complications of pregnancy: medical, surgical, gynecologic, psychosocial, and perinatal*, ed 4, Baltimore, 1991, Williams & Wilkins.

Chez RA et al: Meeting the challenge of gestational diabetes, *Contemp OB/GYN* 34(3):120, 1989.

Chin RK et al: A longitudinal study of changes in erythrocyte concentration in hyperemesis gravidarum, *Gynecol Obstet Invest* 29(1):22, 1990.

Clark SL: Cardiac disease in pregnancy, *Obstet Gynecol Clin North Am* 18(2):237, 1991.

Combs S, Kitzmiller J: Spontaneous abortion and congenital malformations in diabetes, *Baillieres Clin Obstet Gynecol* 5(2):315, 1991.

Cooper MJ et al: Asymmetric septal hypertrophy in infants of diabetic mothers, *Am J Dis Child* 146(2):226, 1992.

Corcoy R et al: Gestational diabetes: what are the implications, *Postgrad Med* 91(5):393, 1992.

Coustan DR et al: Gestational diabetes: predictors of subsequent disordered glucose metabolism, *Am J Obstet Gynecol* 168(4):139, 1993.

Cox SM, Leveno KJ: Pregnancy complicated by bacterial endocarditis, *Clin Obstet Gynecol* 31(1):48, 1989.

Creasy RK, Resnik R: *Maternal-fetal medicine: principles and practice,* ed 2, Philadelphia, 1989, WB Saunders.

Cunningham FG et al: *Williams obstetrics,* ed 19, Norwalk, CT, 1993, Appleton & Lange.

Daddario JB: Trauma in pregnancy, *J Perinat Neonat Nurs* 3(2):14, 1989.

Damm P et al: Prediction factors for the development of diabetes in women with previous gestational diabetes mellitus, *Am J Obstet Gynecol* 167(2):607, 1992.

Davis LE et al: Thyrotoxicosis complicating pregnancy, *Am J Obstet Gynecol* 160:63, 1989.

Dickinson JD, Palmer SM: Gestational diabetes: pathophysiology and diagnosis, *Semin Perinatol* 14(1):2, 1990.

Dooley SL et al: The influence of demographic and phenotypic heterogeneity on the prevalence of gestational diabetes mellitus, *Int J Gynaecol Obstet* 35(1):13, 1991.

Dorman K: Acute pulmonary insults during pregnancy. In Harvey CJ, editor: *Critical care obstetrical nursing,* Gaithersburg, MD, 1991, Aspen.

Feldman M: Nausea and vomiting. In Sleisenger MH, Fordtran JS, editors: *Gastrointestinal disease,* ed 4, Philadelphia, 1989, WB Saunders.

Gabbe SG: A story of two miracles: the impact of the discovery of insulin on pregnancy in women with diabetes mellitus, *Obstet Gynecol* 79(2):295, 1992.

Gilbert E, Harmon J: *Manual of high risk pregnancy and delivery,* St Louis, 1993, Mosby.

Goodwin TM, Montero M, Mostman JH: Transient hyperthyroidism and hyperemesis gravidarum: clinical aspects, *Am J Obstet Gynecol* 167(3):148, 1992.

Graber EA: When an OB patient has coronary disease, *Contemp OB/GYN* 33:56, 1989.

Greene MF et al: First trimester hemoglobin A1 and risk for major malformations and spontaneous abortion in diabetic pregnancy, *Teratology* 39:225, 1989.

Hagay Z, Reece EA: Diabetes mellitus in pregnancy and periconceptual genetic counseling, *Am J Perinatol* 9(2):87, 1992.

Hamburger JI: Diagnosis and treatment of Grave's disease in pregnancy, *Thyroid* 2(3):219, 1992.

Harvey MG: Diabetic ketoacidosis during pregnancy, *J Perinat Neonat Nurs* 6(1):1, 1992.

Hollingsworth DR, Vaucher Y, Yamamoto TP: Diabetes in pregnancy in Mexican-Americans, *Diabetes Care* 14(7):695, 1991.

Howard ED: Gestational diabetes mellitus screening tests: a review of current recommendations, *J Perinat Neonat Nurs* 6(1):37, 1992.

Jacobson JD, Cousins L: A population-based study of maternal and perinatal outcomes in patients with gestational diabetes, *Am J Obstet Gynecol* 161(4):981, 1989.

Jovanovic-Peterson L et al: Maternal postprandial glucose levels and infant birth weight: the diabetes in early pregnancy study, The National Institute of Child Health and Human Development, *Am J Obstet Gynecol* 64:103, 1991.

Jovanoic-Peterson L, Peterson C: Diabetic retinopathy, *Clin Obstet Gynecol* 34(3):516, 1991.

Jovanovic-Peterson L, Peterson C: Pregnancy in the diabetic woman, *Endocrinol Metab Clin North Am* 21(2):433, 1992.

Kaplan M: Assessment of thyroid function during pregnancy, *Thyroid* 2(1):57, 1992.

Keohane NS, Lacey LA: Preparing the woman with gestational diabetes for self-care: use of a structured teaching plan by nursing staff, *JOGNN* 20(3):189, 1991.

Kitzmiller JL et al: Preconception care of diabetes: glycemic control prevents congenital anomalies, *JAMA* 265(6):731, 1991.

Krumholz A: Epilepsy in pregnancy. In Goldstein PJ, Stern BJ, editors: *Neurological disorders of pregnancy,* Mount Kisco, NY, 1992, Futura Publishing.

Landon MB, Gabbe SG: Diabetes mellitus and pregnancy, *Obstet Gynecol Clin North Am* 19(4):633, 1992.

Lang RM, Borow KM: Heart disease. In Barron WM, Lindheimer MD, editors: *Medical disorders during pregnancy,* St Louis, 1991, Mosby.

Langford H, Bartholomew S: Severe hypoglycemia in diabetic pregnancy, *VA Med Q* 119(3):172, 1992.

Larsen ML, Horder M, Mogensen EF: Effect of long-term monitoring of glycosylated hemoglobin levels in insulin-dependent diabetes mellitus, *N Engl J Med* 323(15):1021, 1990.

Lawrence R: *Breastfeeding: a guide for the medical profession,* ed 4, St Louis, 1994, Mosby.

Lazarus JH: Treatment of hyper- and hypothyroidism in pregnancy, *J Endocrinol Invest* 16(5):391, 1993.

Lee W, Cotton DB: Peripartum cardiomyopathy: current concepts and clinical management, *Clin Obstet Gynecol* 31:54, 1989.

Leff EW, Gagne MP, Jeffries SC: Type I diabetes and pregnancy . . . are we hearing women's concerns, *MCN* 16(2):83, 1991.

Leung AS et al: Perinatal outcome in hypothyroid pregnancies, *Obstet Gynecol* 81(3):349, 1993.

Matheson D, Efantis J: Diabetes and pregnancy: need and use of intensive therapy, *Diabetes Educ* 15(3):242, 1989.

Mattison D et al: Pharmacology: effects of drugs and chemicals on the fetus, *Contemp OB/GYN* 33:97, 1989.

McKeon VA, Perrin KO: The pregnant woman with myocardial infarction: nursing diagnosis, *Dimens Crit Care Nurs* 8(2):92, 1989.

Mestman JH, Schmidt-Sarosi C: Diabetes mellitus and fertility control: contraception management issues, *Am J Obstet Gynecol* 168(6 Pt 2):2012, 1993.

Meyer BA, Palmer SM: Pregestational diabetes, *Semin Perinatol* 14(1):12, 1990.

Pagano K, Pagano T: *Mosby's diagnostic and laboratory test reference,* St Louis, 1992, Mosby.

Palmer DG, Inturrisi M: Insulin infusion therapy in the intrapartum period, *J Perinat Neonat Nurs* 6(1):25, 1992.

Penha ML et al: Diabetic mothers and pregnancy loss: implications for diabetes educators, *Diab Educ* 19(1):35, 1993.

Philipson EH, Super DM: Gestational diabetes mellitus: does it recur in subsequent pregnancy? *Am J Obstet Gynecol* 100(6):1324, 1989.

Phipps WJ, Long BC, Woods NF: *Medical-surgical nursing: concepts and clinical practice,* ed 5, St Louis, 1993, Mosby.

Piper JM, Langer O: Does maternal diabetes delay fetal pulmonary maturity? *Am J Obstet Gynecol* 168(3 Pt 1):783, 1993.

Radak JT: Why worry about gestational diabetes, *Diabetes Forecast* 44(4):27, 1991.

Rizzo G, Arduini D, Romanini C: Cardiac function in fetuses of type I diabetic mothers, *Am J Obstet Gynecol* 164(3):837, 1991.

Rosas T, Constantino N: Exercise as a treatment modality to maintain normoglycemia in gestational diabetes, *J Perinat Neonat Nurs* 6(1):14, 1992.

Rosenn B et al: Preconception management of insulin-dependent diabetes: improvement of pregnancy outcome, *Obstet Gynecol* 77(6):847, 1991.

Rosenn B et al: Progression of diabetic retinopathy in pregnancy: association with hypertension in pregnancy, *Am J Obstet Gynecol* 166(4):1214, 1992.

Rotondo LM: Diabetes mellitus: impact on pregnancy, *NAACOG's Clin Issu Perinat Womens Health Nurs* 1(2):133, 1990.

Rudick RA, Birk KA: Multiple sclerosis and pregnancy. In Goldstein PJ, Stern BJ, editors: *Neurological disorders of pregnancy,* Mount Kisco, NY, 1992, Futura Publishing.

Ruggiero L et al: Impact of social support and stress on compliance in women with gestational diabetes, *Diabetes Care* 13:441, 1990.

Ruggiero L et al: Self-reported compliance with diabetes self-management during pregnancy, *Int J Psychiatry Med* 23(2): 195, 1993.

Salveson DR, Brudenell MJ, Nicolaides KH: Fetal polycythemia and thrombocytopenia in pregnancies complicated by maternal diabetes mellitus, *Am J Obstet Gynecol* 166(4): 1287, 1992.

Samson LF: Infants of diabetic mothers: current perspectives, *J Perinat Neonat Nurs* 6(1):61, 1992.

Scott JR et al: *Danforth's obstetrics and gynecology,* ed 6, Philadelphia, 1990, JB Lippincott.

Shaver DC: Complications of operative obstetrics. In Gleicher N et al, editors: *Principles and practice of medical therapy in pregnancy,* Norwalk, CT, 1992, Appleton & Lange.

Sibai BM: Surgery during pregnancy. In Gleicher N et al, editors: *Principles and practice of medical therapy in pregnancy,* Norwalk, CT, 1992, Appleton & Lange.

Siddiq YK: Management of diabetes during pregnancy, *J Med Assoc Ga* 78(11):745, 1989.

Simolke GA, Cox SM, Cunningham FG: Cerebrovascular accidents complicating pregnancy and the puerperium, *Obstet Gynecol* 78:37, 1991.

Singer AJ, Brandt LJ: Pathophysiology of the GI tract during pregnancy, *Am J Gastroenterol* 86(12):1695, 1991.

Smith CV, Phelan JP: Trauma in pregnancy. In Clark SL, editor: *Critical care obstetrics,* Boston, 1991, Blackwell Scientific Publications.

Stamler EF et al: High infectious morbidity in pregnant women with insulin dependent diabetes: an understated complication, *Am J Obstet Gynecol* 163(4 Pt 1):1217, 1990.

Steele JM et al: Can pre-pregnancy care of diabetic women reduce the risk of abnormal babies, *Br Med J* 301:1070, 1990.

Tomky D: Tapping the full power of insulin pumps, *RN* 52(6):46, 1989.

Troiano NH: Cardiopulmonary resuscitation of the pregnant woman, *J Perinat Neonat Nurs* 3(2):1, 1989.

Troiano NH: Trauma during pregnancy. In Harvey CJ, editor: *Critical care obstetrical nursing,* Gaithersburg, MD, 1991, Aspen.

White P: Classification of obstetrics diabetes, *Am J Obstet Gynecol* 130:228, 1978.

Willhoite MB et al: The impact of preconception counseling on pregnancy outcomes, the experience of the Maine Diabetes in Pregnancy Program, *Diabetes Care* 16(2):450, 1993.

Winn HN, Reece EA: Integrating management of diabetic pregnancies, *Contemp OB/GYN* 33(1):91, 1989.

Worthington-Roberts B, Williams SR: *Nutrition in pregnancy and lactation,* ed 5, St Louis, 1993, Mosby.

Bibliography

Austin D, Davis P: Valvular disease in pregnancy, *J Perinatol Neonat Nurs* 5(2):13, 1991.

Birk K et al: The clinical course of multiple sclerosis during pregnancy and the puerperium, *Arch Neurol* 47:738, 1990.

Bourgeois FJ, Duffer J: Outpatient management of women with type I diabetes, *Am J Obstet Gynecol* 163(3):1065, 1990.

Capeless EL, Clapp JF: When do cardiovascular parameters return to their preconception values? *Am J Obstet Gynecol* 165(4 Pt 1):883, 1991.

Donaldson JO: The pregnant epileptic: fetal risks from anticonvulsant therapy, *JAMA* 264:1044, 1990.

Dunn PA et al: Assessing a pregnant woman after trauma, *Nursing90* 20:53, 1990.

Harvey M, Troiano N: Trauma during pregnancy, *NAACOG's Clin Issu Perinat Womens Health Nurs* 3(3):521, 1992.

Kjaer K et al: Infertility and pregnancy outcome in an unselected group of women with insulin dependent diabetes mellitus, *Am J Obstet Gynecol* 166(5):1412, 1992.

Lavery JP: Treating asthma in pregnancy, *Contemp OB/GYN* 36:121, 1991.

Mandeville L: Diabetic ketoacidosis, *NAACOG's Clin Issu Perinat Womens Health Nurs* 3(3):514, 1992.

Mitchell PJ, Bebbington M: Myasthenia gravis in pregnancy, *Obstet Gynecol* 80(2):178, 1992.

Montoro MN et al: Outcome of pregnancy in diabetic ketoacidosis, *Am J Perinatol* 10(1):17, 1993.

Newman V, Fullerton J, Anderson P: Clinical advances in the management of severe nausea and vomiting during pregnancy, *JOGNN* 22(6):483, 1993.

Reece EA, Homko CJ: Diabetes-related complications of pregnancy, *J Natl Med Assoc* 85(7):537, 1993.

Resnik R: Managing SLE during pregnancy, *Contemp OB/GYN* 35:67, 1990.

Roth CK, Riley B, Cohen SM: Intrapartum care of a woman with aortic aneurysms, *JOGNN* 21(4):310, 1992.

Simpson K, Moore K, LaMartina M: Acute fatty liver of pregnancy, *JOGNN* 22(3):213, 1993.

Sipes SL, Malee MP: Endocrine disorders in pregnancy, *Obstet Clin North Am* 19(4):655, 1992.

Smith JE: Pregnancy complicated by thyroid disease, *J Nurse Midwife* 35(3):143, 1990.

Tarkington MA, Gilbert RN, Bresette JF: Reducing iatrogenic ureteral injury, *Contemp OB/GYN* 37:93, 1992.

Troiano N, Harvey C, editors: Critical care obstetrics, *NAACOG's Clin Issu Perinat Womens Health Nurs* 3(3): 1992.

CHAPTER

23

Psychosocial Problems

BARBARA J. LIMANDRI

LEARNING OBJECTIVES

Define the key terms listed.

Review the care of women experiencing emotional complications during the childbearing cycle.

Discuss the care of pregnant women who use, abuse, or are dependent on drugs such as alcohol, opioids, and cocaine.

Discuss violence against women as it occurs during pregnancy.

Assess the effects of poverty on the childbearing cycle.

KEY TERMS

attachment (bonding) behaviors
depressive reactions
drug dependence (addiction)
family violence
intimate partner abuse
intoxication
invisible poverty
manic reactions
mood disorders
postpartum blues
postpartum depression
postpartum psychosis
psychoactive substances
schizophrenia
toxicology screen
visible poverty
withdrawal (drug)

RELATED TOPICS

Abruptio placentae *(Chap. 21)* • Teratogens *(Chap. 4)* • Maternal-infant attachment *(Chap. 17)* • Preterm labor *(Chap. 24)* • Infants of substance abusing mothers *(Chap. 27)*

Psychosocial conditions have implications for the health of the mother and newborn. These conditions can interfere with family integration and restrict attachment to the newborn. Some may threaten the safety and well-being of the mother and newborn. This chapter explores emotional disorders, psychoactive substance use (drug dependency), and poverty. The nursing process with affected women and their families is emphasized.

EMOTIONAL COMPLICATIONS

Mental health problems can complicate pregnancy, childbirth, and the postpartum period. Developmental and personality disorders generally begin in childhood or adolescence. They usually persist into adulthood (Stuart,

Sundeen, 1991). Mental retardation, autism, and disruptive behavior disorders are examples. Mental health disorders generally predate pregnancy. Sleep and arousal disorders, schizophrenic disorders, delusional (paranoid) disorders, and anxiety disorders are a few behavioral categories.

Pregnancy per se is not a cause of psychiatric illness. The psychologic and physical stresses relating to pregnancy or to the new obligations of motherhood may, however, bring on an emotional crisis (Affonso, 1984). The principal emotional disturbances complicating gestation are mood (affective) disorders and schizophrenia. Organic mental syndromes and disorders (non–substance-induced) also may be seen. The mood disturbances include depression or depression with manic episodes (bipolar disorders). Paranoia or other disorganizational problems may characterize schizophrenic disorders. Toxic delirium associated with substance abuse, excessive analgesia, or serious metabolic disorders is not common. Psychoactive substance-induced organic mental disorders are seen more often today. They are discussed later in this chapter.

No one single factor has been isolated as responsible for precipitating postpartum mental illness. Emotional illnesses arising during the puerperium are diagnosed by their initial features: affective, schizophrenic, or organic. Those illnesses that do not meet the criteria for any of these disorders are designated "postpartum psychoses" (American Psychiatric Association, 1994).

Mood Disorders

Although the cause of **mood disorders** is not fully understood, the family history may reveal that one or more adults have had this problem. Moreover, women who have psychiatric complications during the course of pregnancy often have had preexisting psychiatric illness (Marks et al, 1992a). More than 50% of pregnancy-related mental illnesses are affective reactions. Of these, about 10% are prenatal manic or depressive states; the remainder occur in the postnatal period. Younger women seem more prone to manic reactions, but depression is the more common problem for most women.

Difficulty bonding between the mother and infant is a prominent feature of mood disorders. Sometimes the mother may be obsessed by the notion that the offspring may take her place in her partner's affections. In other instances, guilt regarding aversion to pregnancy, attempted abortion, or other personal conflicts may be the basic problem.

Manic reactions often occur during the first or second week of the puerperium, perhaps after a brief depression (Marks et al, 1992a). Agitation, excitement, and volubility (ready and continuous flow of words; talkativeness), often with rhyming or punning, develop. The woman becomes disinterested in personal care and food. Because dehydration or exhaustion may occur, prompt and effective supportive treatment is essential.

Psychiatric therapy may include a tranquilizer with a significant sedative effect, for example, promethazine (Phenergan). Lithium may be given later for more prolonged control. Psychotherapy is essential. The usual duration of the manic state is 1 to 3 weeks. The prognosis for mother and infant is good after initial separation and gradual reunion.

Depressive reactions are far more common than manic reactions. The stress of pregnancy is both biologic and psychologic. During the postpartum period, women often experience many emotional reactions (Laizner, Jeans, 1990). Four aspects after birth demand significant coping abilities: physical adjustment, initial insecurities, support systems, and loss of previous identity. Some mothers are unable to adjust and become depressed or experience other emotional upheaval (Nicolson, 1990).

The emotional disorders of the postpartum period can be grouped into three categories: postpartum blues, nonpsychotic postpartum depression, and postpartum psychosis.

Postpartum Blues

Postpartum blues are usually transient and may affect 75% to 80% of women giving birth (Hansen, 1990; Jones 1990). The significance of such transition-related depression has prompted the addition of a specific diagnosis in the upcoming edition of the *Diagnostic and Statistical Manual of Mental Disorders,* called postpartum onset (of depression and mania) (American Psychiatric Association, 1994). The blues may elicit crying spells, feelings of loneliness or rejection, anxiety, confusion, restlessness, exhaustion, forgetfulness, and inability to sleep (Hansen, 1990; Jones, 1990). These reactions may occur any time after birth but often appear on the third or fourth day and peak between the fifth and fourteenth postpartum days. Diagnosing and categorizing the blues have been difficult because of the lack of standard assessment instruments. However, Kennerley and Gath (1989a) describe a reliable and valid instrument that measures the seven symptoms of postpartum blues: mood swings, feeling "low," anxiety, feeling overemotional, tearfulness, fatigue, and confused or muddled thinking.

Predisposing factors of postpartum blues may include biologic changes, stress, normal responses, or social or environmental causes. Biologic theorists have studied the hormonal fluctuations and attribute some affective reactions to changes in progesterone, estradiol, cortisol, and prolactin levels (Ehlert et al, 1990; Harris et al, 1989; Majewski, Ford-Rice, Falkey, 1989). Stress theory supporters propose that any stressful event (e.g., surgery) can trigger reactions such as the blues (Iles, Gath, Kennerley, 1989). Others view the blues as a normal physiologically based response that increases mothering instincts and protectiveness toward the infant (Majewski, Ford-Rice, Falkey, 1989). Social and environmental issues such as strained marital and family relations, a history of premenstrual syndrome (PMS), anxiety, fear of labor and depression during the pregnancy, and poor social adjustment may be predisposing factors (Kennerley, Gath, 1989b).

Postpartum Depression

The frequency of **postpartum depression** varies from 5% to more than 25% of women giving birth (Daw, 1988; Steiner, 1990). The criteria for classifying postpartum depression vary but often are limited to affective syndromes that occur within 6 months of childbirth. The depressive episode may be minor or major without psychotic features (Jones, 1990; Troutman, Cutrona, 1990). Loss of sexual interest and fatigue occur commonly in all postpartum women. However, those experiencing depression also demonstrate poor concentration, feelings of guilt, loss of energy, and lack of interest in usual activities (Hopkins, Campbell, Marcus, 1989). The symptoms of postpartum depression last longer than the blues. In addition, the woman may experience weight changes (loss or gain), social withdrawal, inability to cope, and concern about mothering skills to care for the infant. If major depression continues, hospitalization may be required. Support from groups may be needed, as well as individual therapy and administration of antidepressants such as fluoxetine (Prozac), sertraline (Zoloft), and bupropion (Wellbutrin) (Busch, Perrin, 1989; Harding, 1989; Martell, 1990; Taylor, 1989). Such drugs, however, are not recommended for breast-feeding women.

Predisposing factors may be hormone-related, stress-related, or infant-related. As with postpartum blues, some researchers have identified a link between hormonal levels and postpartum depression (Harris et al, 1989; Smith et al, 1990). Prolactin and progesterone levels are found to be significantly related to depression. Environmental and family stress issues may be linked to postpartum depression. Women who experience depression often have fewer support systems, more stressful life events, and poor personal resources with which to combat these events. Predictive factors for postpartum depression that may assist the nurse in assessing potential problems include low income, absence of a confidant for support, meager or absent social support, and stressful life events (e.g., single parenthood, divorce, or recent death of a parent or child) (Auerbach, Jacobi, 1990; Stein et al, 1989). There may be a correlation between the infant's behavior and the mother's depression. Maternal depression is associated with a range of adverse outcomes for the newborn, such as newborn irritability (Zuckerman et al, 1990) and low birth weight (McAnarney, Stevens-Simon, 1990). Infants who had a difficult temperament and were unpredictable and less adaptable often had mothers who were depressed. However, the mothers rarely attributed their depression to the infant, rather they blamed themselves for their lack of skill in providing for the baby (Whiffen, Gotlib, 1989).

Postpartum Psychosis

The most severe psychiatric crisis is that of **postpartum psychosis.** Symptoms often begin as postpartum blues or postpartum depression. Delusions, hallucinations, confusion, delirium, and panic may occur (Metz, Sichel, Goff, 1988). The woman may manifest symptoms resembling schizophrenia or schizoaffective disorder (Marks et al, 1992a; Steiner, 1990). Hospitalization for several months usually is required. Suicide or danger to the infant, or both, are the greatest hazards of postpartum psychosis (Goldstein, 1989; Hamilton, 1989).

Schizophrenia

Schizophrenia, or schizophrenic reactions, may be a disorder of cerebral metabolism and/or structural changes.

Schizophrenia affects adolescents and younger adults more often than older people. Abnormal thought processing features such as concrete thinking, marked distractibility, and intense suspiciousness are common (American Psychiatric Association, 1994). Antipsychotic medications like trifluoperazine (Stelazine) and haloperidol (Haldol) are useful. Transfer of the woman to an in-hospital setting usually is necessary. A good prognosis is likely with the first psychotic episode, especially if it occurs unexpectedly during the puerperium. (Miller et al, 1990).

Care Management

✦ ASSESSMENT

Recognition of the symptoms of mood disorders is essential for the perinatal nurse. The nursing plan of care must reflect the expected behavioral responses of the particular disorder. The individualized plan is based on the woman's characteristics and her specific circumstances. The woman's partner, the father of the baby, or another family member also may experience emotional upheaval as a result of the woman's behavior.

✦ NURSING DIAGNOSES

Nursing diagnoses relevant to any emotional illness that complicates pregnancy may include the following:

High risk for injury to the fetus related to
- Psychotropic medication
- Maternal suicide

High risk for injury to the newborn related to
- Unmet needs (e.g., hygiene, nutrition) and safety precautions
- The mother's poor impulse control

Ineffective family coping related to
- Increased care needs of the mother-fetus/newborn

Impaired home maintenance management related to
- Increased care needs of the mother-fetus/newborn

High risk for altered parenting related to
- Lack of opportunities for attachment to the infant

High risk for altered growth and development of the infant related to
- Lack of intellectual stimulation
- Unmet needs (hygiene, nutrition) and safety precautions

✦ EXPECTED OUTCOMES

Planning focuses on the mother's dependency needs, attachment to the infant, family integration, parenting skills and care of the infant, and home maintenance management. Supervision of the mother and family in the home is a prime concern (Martell, 1990). Patient-centered expected outcomes include the following:

- The mother's and infant's physical well-being will be maintained.
- The mother and family will cope effectively.
- Each family member will continue healthy growth and development.

✤ COLLABORATIVE CARE

Community resources such as the community health nurse, homemaker service, or foster care are utilized as necessary. Discharge planning, carefully developed with the family in collaboration with a hospital-community health care team, is vital.

Antepartum Hospitalization

In-hospital psychiatric treatment often is required to treat psychotic pregnant women. Maternal physiologic adaptations and fetal movement often result in intensification of delusional ideas in the schizophrenic woman. Women with bipolar mood disorders may respond well during pregnancy and childbirth. After the birth, however, these women are prone to worsening of psychotic symptoms and depression (Marks et al, 1992b; Spielvogel, Wile, 1986). Hospitalized women present treatment challenges in three areas: psychotropic medication, legal sanctions, and management in an acute hospital setting. A brief overview of these difficulties is given here. Psychiatric textbooks must be consulted for specific details.

Psychotropic Medications

All psychotropic medications pass through the placenta to the fetus and through breast milk to the infant. The risks of medication are weighed against the risks of maternal agitation and potentially self-destructive behavior. Infants exposed to psychotropics between 8 and 10 weeks' gestation show a higher rate of congenital anomalies (5.4%) than does the population with no such exposure (3.2%) (Edlund, Craig, 1984). A higher perinatal death rate and an increased incidence of an extrapyramidal syndrome consisting of "tremors, hypertonia, weakness, and poor sucking and other reflexes" complicate the neonatal period (Hauser, 1985). Medication dosage is balanced between the mother's needs and fetal response determined by nonstress tests (NSTs). Some medications may be behavioral teratogens with short-term and long-term effects (Cook et al, 1990).

Bipolar disorders often are treated with *lithium*. A high incidence of fetal cardiovascular abnormalities is linked to lithium taken during the first trimester. Maternal shifts in fluid balance may require doubling the lithium dose to achieve a therapeutic level (Spielvogel, Wile, 1986). Fetal lithium toxicity may cause polyhydramnios. Fetal toxicity can result if the lithium dose is not decreased by at least 50% 1 week before birth, that is if the date can be correctly anticipated. Regardless of dose and the mother's plasma level, the neonate may show signs of toxicity: cyanosis, lethargy, low Apgar

scores, and absent Moro's reflex (Krause, Ebbesen, Lange, 1990).

Legal Sanctions

Women with mental health problems who can provide self-care may be unable to care for themselves *and* the fetus. Hospital care may be mandated during pregnancy. Delusions about the pregnancy and its medical monitoring may necessitate legal intervention. Other legal issues arise closer to the birth. These issues surround the care of the mother and her infant and fertility management (Spielvogel, Wile, 1986).

In-Hospital Management

Pregnant women with schizophrenia often experience an intensification of their disorder. These women usually remain ambivalent toward the fetus and resist examination and procedures. Because they seem unaware of signs of labor, staff members must be keenly alert to behavioral and physical indicators of labor. Even though disorganization often diminishes, specific delusions may persist. The new mother may not be able to be close to her baby or to recognize or meet the baby's needs. A more positive outcome and recovery is expected when partners and family members remain supportive and noncritical throughout the pregnancy (Marks et al, 1992b).

Pregnant women with bipolar disorders usually respond well to pregnancy, the fetus, and the birth. The new mother's responses may not be consistent or appropriate to the baby, however. After the birth psychotic symptoms or depression worsens. Mothers need to be supervised carefully when visiting with their babies in order to ensure their babies' safety.

Postpartum Mental Illness

In caring for a woman experiencing postpartum depression, the nurse must be aware of the effect on the family. If the mother is feeling inadequate, is unable to cope with herself or the infant, is withdrawn, or is severely fatigued, then the family is affected. Stressors are magnified, which can result in isolation of the mother and family, a change in relationship with the partner, or a negative impact on parenting. The nurse must be alert for these signs of dysfunction and be prepared to help promote attachment between mother and baby, referral of the mother and family for support services and counseling, and assisting the family in prioritizing and performing necessary family functions (Martell, 1990).

Most treatment programs for postpartum depression tend to be reactive rather than predictive. Nicolson (1990) reports that a more effective approach would be to assess postnatal depression not as an individual illness or vulnerability rather as a normal grief reaction and part of every postnatal profile. Interpretation by the mother regarding her experience may be the key to more appropriate treatment. Nurses could help mothers recognize that the experience is not always happy, positive, and a gain. Many mothers grieve over the loss of their former selves (figures, lifestyles, sexual attractiveness) and experience upheaval and extreme stress. The nurse can help the mother acknowledge her new self and new role, as well as accept the knowledge that depression and a grief reaction may be normal and not permanent.

The nurse's role varies with the type of postpartum depression. With the baby blues or mild depression, the nurse can refer the woman to peer support groups or workshops that may help her with specific problems, such as assertiveness. In more severe depression a nurse-practitioner or psychiatric specialist could provide specialized counseling, or a referral for psychiatric counseling may be needed. In the most extreme cases, in-hospital management may be required.

The onset of postpartum psychosis usually is abrupt and occurs within days of childbirth. The symptoms center around the mother's relationship with the baby. The mother's response may be of an overprotective or of a rejecting nature (Hurt, Ray, 1985). The mother may be convinced that someone is trying to take her baby from her, so she clutches her baby protectively. Or she may believe that the baby is dead or defective or that God is caring for it, so the baby does not need care.

The presenting symptoms form the basis for management. A major depressive condition is one that continues for more than 2 weeks and includes at least four of the following symptoms: change in appetite, change in sleep, psychomotor agitation, loss of interest in usual activities, decrease in sexual drive, increased fatigue, feelings of guilt or worthlessness, slowed thinking or impaired concentration, and possible suicidal ideation (American Psychiatric Association, 1994). Schizophrenia-like symptoms are treated with psychotropic medications. Lithium may be prescribed with or without psychotropic medications for bipolar affective disorders. A phenothiazine type of tranquilizer, for example, chlorpromazine (Thorazine), will be useful. Depression may be treated with psychotherapy and electroconvulsive therapy if suicidal or infanticidal thoughts are identified. Women may need assistance for alterations in patterns of sleep-rest, self-care (basic hygiene), nutrition and fluid balance, elimination, self-esteem, and family coping processes. Discharge planning focuses on preparation for meeting the demands of an infant while the mother is still integrating her experience with psychosis, supporting the partner, and exploring the effects of the illness on their family (Hurt, Ray, 1985).

The mother's depression or psychosis prevents her from engaging in the mutual interaction with the baby that is needed for acquaintance and subsequent attachment (bonding). If the mother wants to breastfeed, nurses can assist with the same techniques used for any new mother. It is important to maintain and support the maternal role (Auerbach, Jacobi, 1990). Within the hospital setting the reintroduction of the mother and baby

can occur at the mother's own pace. During these interactions the mother's readiness to care for the baby after discharge is evaluated. The interactions are carefully supervised and guided. A schedule is set for increasing hours over 3 to 4 days, culminating in the infant's admission to the unit for an overnight stay. The overnight stay allows the mother to experience the infant's being there and giving up sleep for the baby, a situation difficult for new mothers under ideal conditions. During this time the nurses observe the woman for **attachment,** or **bonding behaviors.** Attachment behaviors are defined as eye-to-eye contact (*en face* position), physical contact of holding, touching, cuddling, talking to the baby and calling the baby by name, as well as initiating care for the baby when appropriate. A staff member is assigned to keep the baby within sight at all times. Indirect teaching, praise, and encouragement are designed to bolster the mother's self-esteem and self-confidence. Staff work with the father is provided concurrently. Administrative and clinical support in the psychiatric unit has facilitated comprehensive care to women who develop a psychosis in the puerperium and to their families.

A good prognosis is likely with the first psychotic episode, especially if it occurs unexpectedly during the puerperium. The child probably will never suffer from schizophrenia, despite speculation regarding hereditary tendencies.

❖ EVALUATION

Evaluation is based on the patient's progress toward meeting the expected outcomes established (p. 666). The nurse can be assured that care has been effective if the physical well-being of the mother and infant is maintained, the mother and family are able to cope effectively, and each family member continues in a healthy growth and development pattern.

PSYCHOACTIVE SUBSTANCE USE

The use of **psychoactive** (mind-altering) **substances** is pandemic in the United States and other industrialized countries. In this discussion, substance abuse is defined as the use of any mind-altering agent to such an extent that it interferes with the individual's biologic, psychologic, or sociocultural integrity (Stuart, Sundeen, 1991). Interference with biologic integrity might be exemplified during pregnancy in poor nutrition leading to poor weight gain, anemia, and a predisposition to infection and pregnancy-induced hypertension. Poor hygiene and multidrug use may compound and confuse the signs and symptoms (Little et al, 1990; Lynch, McKeon, 1990). Some drugs (morphine, heroin, diazepam, and others) induce platelet disorders that predispose the woman to hemorrhage (Scott et al, 1990). Psychologic consequences may include acute psychosis in a pregnant teenager who has been taking phencyclidine (PCP) or the inability of a new mother to attach to her infant (see previous discussion of emotional disturbances).

Expectant and new mothers using psychoactive substances receive negative feedback from society, as well as from health care providers who condemn them for endangering the unborn and newborn infant and who may withhold support. **Drug dependence (addiction)** is the physical or psychologic dependence, or both, on a substance. Pregnant women who are drug dependent often do not seek prenatal care until labor begins (Burkett, Yosin, Palow, 1990; Cordero, Custard, 1990). Pregnant women often have little understanding of the effects of these substances on themselves, their pregnancies, or their babies. They may take the drug just before seeking admission; therefore withdrawal symptoms can be delayed for 6 to 12 hours. **Withdrawal** refers to the psychologic and physical symptoms that occur after removal of the substance in the substance-dependent person.

Substance abuse during pregnancy imposes severe risks to both the mother and infant. Complications for the infant include prematurity, abruptio placentae, growth retardation, intrauterine fetal death, and neonatal drug withdrawal (Keith et al, 1989). To the mother, substance abuse during pregnancy is often accompanied by domestic violence, suicidal tendencies, and depression (Amaro et al, 1990; Berenson et al, 1991).

The care of the substance-dependent, pregnant woman is based on historic data, symptoms, physical findings, and laboratory results. Because the woman may be defensive and deny her substance abuse, history taking has to be done in a sensitive and competent manner.

The woman dependent on a drug tends to exhibit a passive response to life and its responsibilities. She may show a high degree of depression. Substance use has meant a way for her to relieve psychologic distress, to encourage social interaction, and to blunt the feelings of loneliness and emptiness that are part of depression. Pregnancy usually is not planned. It occurs as an "accidental" phenomenon. In contrast, pregnancy may serve as a positive event, confirming her worth as a woman.

After birth, however, the woman is faced with the parental tasks of caring for and nurturing a completely dependent infant and of forming a warm, close, intimate relationship with the child. Care of the woman addicted to a drug offers a tremendous nursing challenge. The difficulty of this challenge soon becomes apparent. The demands of motherhood are being made of a person who is herself dependent and focused on taking and receiving rather than giving. Most substance-dependent people have difficulty establishing positive, intimate relationships and lack a meaningful support system.

With the advent of very early discharge, often within 24 hours after birth, assessment becomes extremely difficult and an increasing challenge to health care professionals. The mother's ability to care for her infant after discharge from the hospital should be assessed by frequent observations, including some observations made in the home setting. The woman should be referred to a chemical dependency treatment center before discharge.

Although many substances are abused, this discussion focuses on the use and abuse of alcohol, heroin, cocaine, and methamphetamine. The amount of care needed by these individuals varies with the particular circumstances and the substance being abused; however, the nursing process is similar for all patients.

Alcohol

Identification of the woman with an alcohol problem may be difficult. Denial of the problem or its consequences is almost universal and a key element of the disease. Underreporting of alcohol use in pregnancy is a major concern of health care workers. A concerned, nonjudgmental, matter-of-fact approach is used to encourage the woman to disclose her alcohol problem, if it exists. Inability to form positive relationships often results from manipulative behavior. A low tolerance for frustration or anxiety and expressions of guilt related to alcoholic behavior patterns may be evident. Physical signs and symptoms also may be present (Table 23-1). During withdrawal, central nervous system (CNS) agitation is expressed as fatigue, insomnia, agitation, restlessness, and belligerence. Bruises, rashes, and other injuries may be observed. Poor physical hygiene and malnutrition are potential problems, especially in the chronic alcohol abuser. Assessment for maternal and fetal well-being follows the protocols discussed for other patients. Women who smoke, are unmarried, less educated, and younger (i.e., younger than 25 years of age) are at the highest risk for alcohol abuse in pregnancy and should be the prime targets of educational efforts of health workers.

Cocaine

The cocaine abuser often has a constellation of cocaine-related problems: family problems, employment difficulties, various health issues, psychologic stress, guilt, and anger (Landry, Smith, 1987). Coexisting psychiatric disorders cloud differential diagnosis. Cocaine raises *norepinephrine* and *serotonin* levels rapidly and then depletes them abruptly. Drug use may mimic serious mental illnesses. The biochemical systems of norepinephrine, serotonin, and dopamine play a vital role in mood regulation and mental health; all three systems are affected by cocaine. Those with schizophrenia, for example, display excessive dopamine levels in some areas of the brain. Decreased amounts of norepinephrine and serotonin have been implicated in people with biologically based depression. Dysfunction of serotonin metabolism is seen in manifestations of violence, rage, and maladaptive behavior.

TABLE 23-1 Psychoactive Substance Effects

DRUG	PSYCHOLOGIC SIGNS	PHYSIOLOGIC SIGNS
ALCOHOL		
Intoxication*	Mood lability or change	Slurred speech
	Impaired attention or memory	Flushed face
	Irritability	Incoordination, unsteady gait
	Talkativeness	Nystagmus
Withdrawal	Anxiety	Nausea and vomiting
	Depressed mood or irritability	Malaise or weakness
	Maladaptive behavior	Hyperactivity
		Coarse tremor of hands, tongue, eyelids
		Orthostatic hypotension
COCAINE ("CRACK")		
Intoxication*	Psychomotor agitation	Tachycardia
	Elation	Pupillary dilation
	Grandiosity; talkativeness	Hypertension
	Hypervigilance	Perspiration; chills
	Maladaptive behaviors	Nausea; vomiting
Withdrawal	Depressed mood	Fatigue
	Disturbed sleep	Headache
	Increased dreaming	Convulsions (seizure)
HEROIN		
Intoxication*	Euphoria, dysphoria	Pupillary constriction
	Psychomotor retardation	Drowsiness
	Apathy	Slurred speech
	Maladaptive behavior	
	Impaired attention or memory	
Withdrawal	Insomnia	Lacrimation, rhinorrhea
		Pupillary dilation
		Sweating
		Diarrhea
		Yawning
		Mild hypertension
		Tachycardia
		Fever
METHAMPHETAMINE ("ICE")		
Intoxication*	Hyperactivity	Tachycardia, palpitations
	Insomnia	Tachypnea
	Restlessness	Nausea, vomiting
	Irritability	Constipation
	Aggressiveness	Impotence
Withdrawal	Depression	Headache
	Increased sleeping	Nausea, vomiting
	Lethargy	Muscle pain
		Weakness
PHENCYCLIDINE (PCP)	Euphoria	Vertical or horizontal nystagmus
	Psychomotor agitation	Hypertension
	Increased anxiety	Increased heart rate
	Emotional lability	Numbness
	Grandiosity	Decreased response to pain
	Sensation of slowed time	Ataxia; dysarthria
	Synesthesias	
	Maladaptive behaviors	

*State of inebriation due to excessive consumption of alcohol, drugs, or other toxic substances.

The effects of cocaine are similar to those of amphetamines (p. 672), with short-term CNS stimulation. There is a blockage of re-uptake of catecholamines, resulting in high levels of norepinephrine, serotonin, and dopamine. This leads to the hyperaroused state found in cocaine abusers (Janke, 1990).

The increase in the use of cocaine and the even more addictive "crack" among childbearing women has been phenomenal in the past few years (Tracy, 1988). Crack is cocaine mixed with baking soda and heated until it reaches its purest form. It is sold in the form of "rocks," which are smoked in pipes. Whereas its use may cross all cultural groups, its inexpensiveness and availability are making it the drug of choice among poorer populations (Lynch, McKeon, 1990). Because crack is highly addictive, it poses new problems to health care providers who may first see the pregnant addict in the labor and birthing area.

Diagnostic protocol to distinguish between drug use and drug addiction requires considerable knowledge and is beyond the scope of this text. An appropriate plan of care is designed depending on the diagnosis (i.e., substance use problems or addiction disease). The focus of this section is the identification of the pregnant cocaine user and the effects of cocaine on the pregnancy.

The nurse or health care provider takes a history of the drug abuse (95% also are addicted to heroin or methadone), type of drug and mode of administration, and participation (if any) in drug programs; assesses the woman's feelings and plans for this pregnancy (infant); and determines the expected date of birth. The social worker or psychiatric social worker is brought in to evaluate the woman's social, economic, home, and ethnic problems; welfare requirements; and educational or vocational status and needs.

Medical Complications

Pregnancy is compromised by cocaine-related medical complications that are encountered by the infrequent, as well as frequent, high-dose user. A variety of less serious medical problems is seen, including lack of energy, insomnia, nasal sinus problems, nose bleeds, sore throat, and decreased libido. More serious problems develop as general health deteriorates. The nasal septum perforates. Cardiovascular stress increases and tachycardia, systemic hypertension, ventricular arrhythmias, sudden coronary artery spasm, and myocardial infarction develop. Cocaine-associated complications also include liver damage, intestinal ischemia, seizures, hemorrhagic bronchitis, headaches, and death. Needle-borne diseases such as hepatitis B and acquired immunodeficiency syndrome (AIDS) are common. "Tracks," septic phlebitis, cellulitis, and superficial abscesses are seen in intravenous drug users. Many users are poorly nourished and commonly have sexually transmitted diseases (STDs). Pulmonary disease with acute pulmonary edema is a commonly encountered complication. A **toxicology** (urine) **screen** (for the presence of abused substances) or other laboratory tests for liver damage and anemia may be ordered when drug use is suspected (see Legal Tip).

LEGAL TIP: **Urine Drug Testing**

In some of the states in the United States a woman who has a positive urine drug test at the time of labor and birth can be referred to the child welfare agency. If the mother is not in a drug treatment program or is assessed to be unable to provide adequate care for the newborn, the infant may be placed in foster care. However, no state requires a caregiver to test either the mother or newborn for the presence of drugs.

An assessment of the woman's support system adds valuable data for developing a plan of care. The presence of any of the medical complications, results of laboratory tests, or signs and symptoms of intoxication or withdrawal (Table 23-1) assist in the identification of substance use problems and addictive disease.

Ingestion of crack cocaine during pregnancy has detrimental effects on both the mother and the developing fetus. A significant number of crack cocaine babies are born prematurely or are small for gestational age (Burkett, Yasin, Palow, 1990). There is also a higher percentage of placental abruption, spontaneous abortion, and fetal death (Gilbert, Harmon, 1993). These infants are very irritable with neurologic problems and congenital abnormalities (Burkett, Yasin, Palow, 1990).

Cocaine users typically mediate the side effects of cocaine by a CNS depressant such as alcohol (Landry, Smith, 1987; Matera et al, 1990). Thus the woman and her fetus are exposed to the risks of cocaine and alcohol. In some areas of the United States it is estimated that 10% of pregnant women use cocaine (Lynch, McKeon, 1990).

Cocaine produces tachycardia and a rise in blood pressure by increasing the levels of catecholamines (Woods, Plessinger, Clark, 1987). During pregnancy, uterine blood vessels are maximally dilated, but they vasoconstrict readily in the presence of catecholamines. Separation of the placenta (abruption) or acute onset of preterm labor, with long, hard contractions and precipitous birth after intravenous cocaine administration, probably is secondary to acute spasm of uterine blood vessels (Adams, Eyler, Behnke, 1990; Chisum, 1990; Janke, 1990; Woods, Plessinger, Clark, 1987). Use of the drug during pregnancy can lead to small-for-gestational-age newborns and fetal death (Chasnoff, 1989). Newborn addiction is discussed in Chapter 27.

Heroin

Assessment of heroin use is similar to that for alcohol and cocaine use. Interview and open discussion may disclose the problem and its extent (e.g., length of addiction, amount needed in cost per day). Physical examination reveals intravenous tracks, cellulitis, and surface abscesses at the administration sites. Further assessment of the peripheral vascular system may reveal burning paresthesia or decreased or absent peripheral pulses (or both) in the extremity used for self-injection. Signs of STDs and urinary tract infections often are present.

Laboratory tests are ordered for toxicology, STDs, hepatitis B, and antibodies to human immunodeficiency virus (HIV). Determinations of blood urea nitrogen, serum creatinine, total protein levels, albumin-to-globulin ratio, total iron-binding capacity, hemoglobin, and hematocrit values are obtained. Chest x-ray study may be ordered for pulmonary disease. Hilar lymphadenopathy in 95% of addicted persons, pulmonary edema, bacterial pneumonia, and foreign body emboli (from the substances used to "cut" street drugs) may be revealed.

Initial and serial ultrasound studies are used to determine gestational age because amenorrhea, common among drug users, precludes dating by history of last menstrual period. However, nonstress and stress testing are not significantly helpful in assessing fetal well-being. The addicted fetus is nonreactive. The heroin-addicted woman is more likely to experience premature rupture of membranes and preterm labor (Ney et al, 1990).

Methamphetamine

The active metabolite of methamphetamine is *amphetamine*, a CNS stimulant. Powdered methamphetamine is known as "speed" and "meth". Methamphetamine-exposed pregnant women have higher rates of preterm births and neonates with intrauterine growth retardation and smaller head circumferences than those of a drug-free comparison group (Oro, Dixon, 1987). Neonatal behavioral patterns are altered. They are characterized by abnormal sleep patterns, poor feeding, tremors, and hypertonia. These behaviors are seen if the fetus was exposed to cocaine, methamphetamine, or their combination (Cook et al, 1990; Oro, Dixon, 1987). The addition of cocaine significantly increases the rate of placental hemorrhage and stillbirth. Other neonatal behaviors include state disorganization and decreased sleep. Feeding may be prolonged and accompanied by disorganized rooting and sucking. Tube feeding may be required. Withdrawal symptoms may be treated with phenobarbital or opium tincture (Paregoric).

Ice

The crystalline form of methamphetamine is known as "ice." This smokable form is odorless. It gives users a very long steady high, is more addictive that heroin, and

is more potent than crack cocaine (*San Francisco Chronicle*, 1989a). Ice enables a person to go without rest or food for 24 hours, only to "crash" for the next 24 hours. Common signs include tachycardia, tachypnea, paranoid delusions, and violent behavior. Symptoms of amphetamine abuse appear after 2 years of use: paranoia and delusional, irrational, and illogical behavior. Convulsions, coma, and death follow overdose (*San Francisco Chronicle*, 1989b).

The drug is very popular with young women who want to lose weight rapidly and also with teenagers who want to stay up all night. Drug dependency has serious consequences for the pregnant woman. The drug causes convulsions in the mother and the newborn. Other effects on the fetus/newborn are thought to be similar to those experienced by the fetus/newborn exposed to powdered methamphetamine.

Marijuana

Marijuana may be the most common illicit drug used in pregnancy (Feng, 1993). Marijuana can be smoked in cigarettes, pipes, water pipes, or mixed into food and eaten. It provides an intoxicating and sensory-distorting "high." Marijuana smoke has the characteristics of tobacco smoke and has similar dangers (Cook et al, 1990). Marijuana readily crosses the placenta. Both cigarettes and marijuana increase carbon monoxide levels in the mother's blood, which can reduce oxygen in fetal blood. Research findings regarding marijuana effects on pregnancy are inconsistent. That is, maternal use did not consistently increase the incidence of spontaneous abortion or stillbirths. Neonatal effects also vary and may include altered sleep and arousal patterns and tremulousness. Reasons for the inconsistent results may reflect variations in composition of the drug, other maternal factors (e.g., lifestyle, health), problems of unreporting of marijuana use, or methodologic issues (Cook et al, 1990). Women who abuse marijuana are more likely to bear children with features compatible with fetal alcohol syndrome. This finding supports the possibility that marijuana may have a synergistic effect on alcohol and other substances (Cook et al, 1990). Marijuana rapidly passes into breast milk. Because the effects on the newborn of marijuana-contaminated breast milk are unknown, breastfeeding by these mothers is not recommended. Postnatal effects of prenatal exposure to marijuana have not as yet been identified.

Phencyclidine (PCP)

PCP is a synthetic drug known by various names (peace pill, angel dust, hog). Its effects are unpredictable and include hostility, aggressiveness, and other bizarre behavior (Cook et al, 1990). Because some effects mimic schizophrenia, a user may be admitted to a psychiatric unit. After use, PCP persists in the brain and body fat for an extended period. It crosses the placenta and tends to be found in higher concentration in fetal tissue than in maternal tissue. Inasmuch as PCP tends to be used in various combinations of alcohol, cocaine, and marijuana, specific effects on pregnancy, the fetus, and the neonate have not been identified (Cook et al, 1990).

Smoking

Women who smoke tobacco cigarettes place themselves and their fetuses at risk for various problems during pregnancy. They place themselves at risk for ectopic pregnancy and spontaneous abortion in early pregnancy. In late pregnancy they are at risk for abruptio placentae, placenta previa, premature rupture of membranes, and intrauterine growth retardation. Nicotine and carbon monoxide are thought to be the main ingredients of cigarette smoke that cause these adverse effects. Nicotine causes vasoconstriction of the placental vessels and carbon monoxide inactivates the maternal and fetal hemoglobin essential to the transport of oxygen to the fetus.

The fetus is at risk for being small for gestational age, with a birth weight of up to 200 g less than that of infants of nonsmokers (American College of Obstetrics and Gynecologists, 1993). The fetus is also at risk for being born preterm, especially if the woman smokes more than one pack per day (American College of Obstetrics and Gynecologists, 1993). Sudden infant death syndrome (SIDS) in white infants has also been linked to maternal smoking during pregnancy (Li, Daling, 1991).

Care Management

✤ ASSESSMENT

Each patient is assessed for signs and symptoms of psychoactive substance use through interview, physical examination, and laboratory tests (see discussions of substances and Table 23-1). Psychologic and physiologic symptoms are described and reported. Nurses may use the CAGE questionnaire (Box 23-1) as a simple set of interview questions that they can remember to provide a basic, quick assessment for alcohol abuse. The Drug Assessment Screening Test (Box 23-2) is a longer and easily scored questionnaire that can be included in a complete health history.

✤ NURSING DIAGNOSES

The following are examples of nursing diagnoses formulated from the assessment data:

High risk for fluid volume deficit and altered nutrition, less than body requirements related to
- Effects of excessive use of psychoactive drugs
High risk for injury to self, fetus, or newborn related to
- Sensory effects of drug

High risk for infection related to
- Lifestyle
- Dehydration and malnutrition
- Method of administration of drug or effects of drug
Self-care deficit, bathing/hygiene related to
- Effects of substance
Denial, related to
- Lack of understanding of disease process
- Effects of psychoactive drug on developing fetus and pregnancy
Ineffective individual coping related to
- Lack of support system
- Low self-esteem
- Lack of healthy mechanisms for recognition and release of anger
High risk for violence related to
- Maintenance of drug habit
- Effects of substance used

✤ EXPECTED OUTCOMES

Planning for care must be accomplished with recognition of the woman's lifestyle and habits. The ideal long-term expected outcome would be total abstinence. However, the woman may be unable to face that level of commitment at this time. The thought of giving up the substance forever is anxiety provoking. It is rare for a substance-dependent person to stop use of that substance suddenly. Short-term expected outcomes are necessary. The woman must participate in the decision-making process in formulating the expected outcomes.

BOX 23-1

The CAGE Questionnaire

1. Have you ever felt you ought to **C**ut down on your drinking?
2. Have people **A**nnoyed you by criticizing your drinking?
3. Have you ever felt bad or **G**uilty about your drinking?
4. Have you ever had a drink first thing in the morning, to steady your nerves or get rid of a hangover? i.e. **E**ye-opener

APPLICATION:

First ask if the client uses alcohol and if affirmative ask the CAGE questions. If negative ask if ever and when the client stopped. A single positive response warrants investigation, 2 out of 4 suggests alcohol dependence and 4 out of 4 is positive for alcoholism.

From Ewing J: Detecting alcoholism: the CAGE questionnaire, *JAMA* 252(14):1905, 1984.

BOX 23-2

The Drug Abuse Screening Test (DAST)

(*Items 4, 5, and 7 are scored in the "no" or false direction.)

1. Have you used drugs other than those required for medical reasons?
2. Have you abused prescription drugs?
3. Do you abuse more than one drug at a time?
4. Can you get through the week without using drugs (other than those required for medical reasons)?*
5. Are you always able to stop using drugs when you want to?*
6. Do you abuse drugs on a continuous basis?
7. Do you try to limit your drug use to certain situations?*
8. Have you had "blackouts" or "flashbacks" as a result of drug use?
9. Do you ever feel bad about your drug abuse?
10. Does your spouse (or parents) ever complain about your involvement with drugs?
11. Do your friends or relatives know or suspect you abuse drugs?
12. Has drug abuse ever created problems between you and your spouse?
13. Has any family member ever sought help for problems related to your drug use?
14. Have you ever lost friends because of your use of drugs?
15. Have you ever neglected your family or missed work because of your use of drugs?
16. Have you ever been in trouble at work because of drug abuse?
17. Have you ever lost a job because of drug abuse?
18. Have you gotten into fights when under the influence of drugs?
19. Have you ever been arrested because of unusual behavior while under the influence of drugs?
20. Have you ever been arrested for driving while under the influence of drugs?
21. Have you engaged in illegal activities to obtain drugs?
22. Have you ever been arrested for possession of illegal drugs?
23. Have you ever experienced withdrawal symptoms as a result of heavy drug intake?
24. Have you had medical problems as a result of your drug use (e.g., memory loss, hepatitis, convulsions, or bleeding)?
25. Have you ever gone to anyone for help for a drug problem?
26. Have you ever been in the hospital for medical problems related to your drug use?
27. Have you ever been involved in a treatment program specifically related to drug use?
28. Have you been treated as an outpatient for problems related to drug abuse?

Scoring: A score of greater than five requires further evaluation for substance abuse problems.

From Skinner HA: The drug abuse screening test, *Addict Behav* 7(4):363, 1982.

It is particularly important that the expected outcomes be phrased so that it is clear that the woman has responsibility for her behavior. The expected outcomes may be written into a contract signed by the woman and the nurse (or health care provider). One copy is kept by the woman.

Short-term expected outcomes include the following:
- The woman's physiologic status will be stabilized.
- The woman will keep appointments for prenatal and postpartum care for herself and her infant.
- Fetal effects will be minimized; the baby will remain safe and receive care.

Long-term expected outcomes include the following:
- The woman will voluntarily become involved in long-term medical, social (e.g., Alcoholics Anonymous, withdrawal [methadone] program), psychiatric, and vocational rehabilitation.

✤ COLLABORATIVE CARE

A multidisciplinary approach is needed to plan for the care of the expectant mother. In increasing numbers, pregnant psychoactive drug users are seen on maternity units. Hospitals are reporting an increase of three to four times as many drug-related births since 1985 (Janke, 1990). The needs of these mothers present special challenges to nurses. A standardized nursing care plan of care may be best developed by the total team of nurses on the maternity unit. A starting point in the development of a care plan may need to be a values clarification experience. It is not uncommon for nurses to harbor negative feelings about the behavior of psychoactive drug users. Collaboration with psychiatric nurses may be necessary to strengthen the maternity nurse's therapeutic potential with these patients. Comprehensive care involves many organizations, child protective services, human resource agencies, and the community health department (Mondanaro, 1987).

The need for *biologic support* may be related to overdose, withdrawal, allergy, or toxicity. Physical deterioration results from the harmful effects of drugs, including conditions such as malnutrition, dehydration, and various infections. The acute physical condition takes priority over the woman's other health needs.

ETHICAL CONSIDERATIONS

DRUG SCREENING

Nurses face an ethical dilemma in situations where fetal injury can occur because of the mother's drug use. Although no specific law against drug use in pregnancy exists, it has been suggested that all pregnant women be screened routinely for illegal drug use. It has been further suggested that those women who test positive be reported to state child protective agencies, placed in jail, or placed in an inpatient psychiatric setting to protect the fetus. Fear of prosecution can prevent women from getting prenatal care and can increase the risk to the fetus.

Interactive interventions are initiated as soon as appropriate. The intervention is directed toward reducing the stressors that apply to each individual and is identified in the nursing diagnoses. Examples of interactive interventions include group support, patient education, or individual counseling. Psychiatric nurses are skilled in intervening in denial, dependency, manipulation, and anger. Other required skills include establishing behavioral contracts and increasing self-esteem. The primary focus of care is the woman. Usually she is already acutely aware of the dangers to the fetus resulting from her behavior. Emphasis on the fetus's well-being instead of on her own may add to her guilt, frustration, and low self-esteem.

Social support systems are mobilized. Family counseling, self-help groups, transitional living programs, and community treatment programs are involved. Some social service agencies remove the child from the home. Others focus on assisting troubled parents in learning to solve their problems with the child in the home. Employee assistance programs are now available in many industries, including hospitals.

Labor nurses need to work out a standardized plan for care. Typically the woman displays poor control over her behavior and a low threshold for pain, which is especially noticeable when she is in labor. Increased dependency needs are apparent. **Intoxication** (state of inebriation due to excessive consumption of alcohol) or withdrawal signs and symptoms of the mother and fetus (Table 23-1) may challenge staff members. Staffing should be sufficient to ensure strict surveillance of visitors to prevent unsupervised drug administration.

Advice regarding breastfeeding is individualized. All abused substances appear in breast milk, some in greater amounts than others. Some substances (e.g., methadone) may cause newborn depression and failure to thrive (Lawrence, 1994). The baby's eating and safety needs must of course be considered. Breastfeeding necessitates a closeness between the mother and child, and the baby may be more irritable and difficult to console. These women, who are already in a fragile state with depleted energy reserves and coping capability, commonly experience severe emotional decompensation. This can be aggravated by breastfeeding and care of the infant, which are exhausting even under ideal circumstances. For some women the need to breastfeed and care for the infant provides the impetus to break the drug dependency habit. Community health agencies may be mobilized for home supervision or guidance in antepartum care and infant care or for putting the infant up for adoption. Day/night-center care programs or halfway houses may be indicated.

The substitution of methadone for heroin is still a controversial issue. If women withdraw from heroin during pregnancy, blood flow to the placenta is impaired. To prevent this, methadone is used to assist in withdrawal from heroin. Some experts advocate complete withdrawal without methadone use, despite the risk of interrupted blood flow to the placenta. Others contend that use of methadone to withdraw from heroin is good for the mother; however, methadone withdrawal for the infant may be worse after birth (Edeline et al, 1988).

Unfortunately less than one fourth of the women who smoke will give it up during pregnancy. Successful interventions for pregnant women should focus on programs to help the woman stop smoking rather than only focusing on antismoking advice. The expected outcomes are to help women stop or cut down on their smoking during pregnancy and to avoid relapse after giving birth. The use of nicotine patches and gum is contraindicated in pregnancy. Benowitz (1991) suggests nicotine replacement therapy may benefit women who smoke more than 20 cigarettes a day and proposes clinical research in this area.

Discharge planning begins with the first contact with the woman. When the woman and newborn are ready for discharge, several nursing actions may be employed. The patient is involved in decision making whenever possible. The mother is involved with the care of her infant when she is willing. Mother-child attachment is promoted. Angry, argumentative encounters between the mother and nurse are avoided; the nurse needs to respond with patience, sympathy, consistency, and at times, with firmness. The mother's positive maternal responses and feelings are supported even if she is relinquishing her infant for adoption.

✦ EVALUATION

Evaluation is difficult because the long-range effects cannot be projected. Short-term positive achievements are indicators of success (e.g., if the mother keeps her appointments or improves her nutrition and personal hygiene or learns to diaper the baby). It is not reasonable to expect to see evidence of significant strides, such as complete abstinence from drugs and assumption of mature adult behaviors within a short period (see Plan of Care).

Case History

Joy Taylor is a 19-year-old, single, primigravida who is at 32 weeks of gestation. She is admitted to the perinatal unit in preterm labor (PTL) and admits to "occasional" snorting of cocaine.

Admitting history included the following data: Joy has tried to stop use of cocaine during her pregnancy but still "binges" at least every weekend and sometimes during the week. Joy states, "I know I shouldn't use it, but everyone was, and I was so upset that Joe was gone!" The baby's father has just left her without providing any emotional or financial support. She will soon have to quit her job as a receptionist and rely on welfare and food stamps. Her vital signs are all elevated above her normal baseline: pulse 108 beats/min, respirations 20/min, temperature 99.3° F (37.4° C), blood pressure 140/98 mm Hg. She has gained only 15 lb during her pregnancy. Her pupils are dilated, and she seems agitated. The monitor displays a fetal heart rate (FHR) of 158 beats/min, and the fetus is active. Joy is experiencing mild contractions every 5 to 6 minutes. Her blood and urine test results are negative for infection and preeclampsia.

EXPECTED OUTCOMES	IMPLEMENTATION	RATIONALE	EVALUATION
Nursing Diagnosis: High risk for injury to fetus related to preterm labor (PTL)			
Joy's preterm labor will be suppressed.	Monitor IV tocolytic therapy. Monitor maternal and fetal status for response to therapy.	Close monitoring is essential to determine effectiveness and to identify early signs of toxicity.	Joy's PTL is suppressed without occurrence of toxicity.
	Encourage decision making about bed rest, diversion, hygiene.	Shows respect for Joy's ability to make decisions so that she will feel less powerless.	Joy is able to comply with bed rest.
	Prepare Joy for discharge: provide education in oral administration and in recognition of recurrence of PTL; what and how to report; resource persons to call as needed.	Knowledge provides a basis for decision making; process assists in developing new coping skills; nurse's trust helps Joy develop self-esteem that may carry over into other facets of her life.	Joy takes oral medication as instructed; PTL does not recur.
Nursing Diagnosis: Ineffective individual coping related to lack of support system			
Joy will express positive attitude toward self.	Encourage recognition of personal strengths.	Decreases reliance on inappropriate peer dominance.	Joy is able to use positive "I" statements.
Joy will carry pregnancy to term without use of cocaine.	Help develop problem-solving strategies.	Encourages involvement in planning care and activities.	Joy helps develop appropriate plan of care for full-term birth.
	Explore resources for decreasing use of substances.	Joy will need help and support to "kick the habit" and remain drug free for rest of pregnancy and as new mother.	Joy attends rehabilitation program; discusses problem issues with clinic nurse and/or community health nurse, and remains drug free for remainder of pregnancy.
Nursing Diagnosis: Nutrition, less than body requirements related to drug use/lack of knowledge			
Mother (and fetus) will maintain adequate nutritional status.	Counsel Joy on nutrition for pregnant woman and fetus. Mutually develop meal plan to include schedule, environment, likes/dislikes.	Joy has poor understanding of nutritional requirements for pregnancy. Substance abusers often forget to eat or acknowledge personal preferences.	Joy's nutritional status and intake are appropriate for third trimester. Joy follows meal plan and includes personal preferences in meal selection.

VIOLENCE AGAINST WOMEN

The frequency with which women are battered and abused, and its consequent serious repercussions for women, their families, and society combine to make this one of the leading health care problems in the United States. The following is offered as a foundation for caring for the pregnant woman who may be in an abusive relationship. One in three women is physically abused (McFarlane, 1989) with 4% to 8% of pregnant women experiencing battering (Campbell et al, 1992). Statistics, however, depend on reporting by the victim or by observers. Without direct and routine assessment for interpersonal violence, women do not easily disclose the violence they are experiencing. Abuse is seen as a personal stigma that must be kept concealed so that others will not think that the woman is contributing to her abuse.

The concept of domestic violence has remained confusing both because of the taboo about discussing interpersonal violence and because of the imprecise language used to identify the phenomenon. **Family violence** is a general term to refer to all varieties of interpersonal violence including child, elder, sibling, and spouse abuse. Domestic violence has referred specifically to violence between intimate adults and is sometimes erroneously called wife abuse. To more adequately identify the parties involved in the abuse, a better term might be **intimate partner abuse.** This term focuses on the specific relationship, permits the wide variety of relationship configurations (e.g., heterosexual and homosexual partners, married or unmarried couples), and avoids the gender stereotyping of women as victims and men as perpetrators.

Abuse comes in many forms. Since physical assault is the easiest to measure, it is the type of abuse most discussed. Additionally, emotional or psychologic abuse, characterized by intimidation and assaults on self-esteem, has immense concealed harmful effects. Although sexual abuse is receiving more attention, many women still do not identify their forced sexual compliance within their marriage as rape. Social abuse occurs when a person controls and interferes with the partner's social network and contact with family or attempts to isolate the partner in other ways.

Dynamics of Abuse

Although the vehicles for imposing abuse may be physical and verbal intimidation, the underlying motive is to have power over another. Often times such power is evident in physical size and strength. When a woman becomes pregnant, her partner may perceive a loss of personal power in the relationship and resort to abuse as a way to restore that power. Pregnancy presents a time of transition in many ways. These changes may feel threatening and imposing. Therefore it is not surprising to find that the chance of abuse increases by 60% when a woman becomes pregnant (see Clinical Application of Research). Usually the abuse occurs in the first trimester with the incidence decreasing with each succeeding trimester (Amaro et al, 1990; Helton, McFarlane, Anderson,

---

 CLINICAL APPLICATION OF RESEARCH

PHYSICAL AND EMOTIONAL ABUSE IN PREGNANCY

Significant numbers of women experience violence, including physical and mental abuse. Abuse appears to escalate during pregnancy. Teenagers in intimate relationships also experience violence. This study compared adult and teenage pregnant women on the amount of physical and mental abuse that they experienced. The sample consisted of 691 pregnant women, of whom 214 (31%) were teenagers. The sample included 27% white, 34% Hispanic, and 38% African-American women. The majority of participants (95%) lived below the poverty level. Data were collected using the Abuse Assessment Screen, the Index of Spouse Abuse, and the Conflicts Tactics Scale. The Danger Assessment Screen was given to women who reported abuse. All new prenatal patients were assessed in English or Spanish, as preferred by the women. If the woman reported abuse, she received information, counseling, and referral to services for abused women. Researchers found that the time of the first prenatal visit was similar for both teenaged and adult women, but that abused women sought prenatal care later in pregnancy.

At their first visit 181 women (26%) reported abuse within the last year. More teenagers (31.6%) than adults (23.6%) reported abuse. During interviews later in their pregnancy, 29% of nonabused women reported abuse since their first visit. Abuse during pregnancy was calculated to be 15.9% for adult women and 21.7% for teenagers. Adults reported more mental abuse than teenagers. Nurses who provide care for women must use opportunities during prenatal and other visits to assess for abuse. A cue to screen carefully for abuse is when a woman initiates prenatal care late in her pregnancy. Nurses need to be knowledgeable about screening for abuse and assessing for danger once abuse has been detected. They must know of referral resources so that the woman's safety is ensured. Concerted efforts must be directed toward intervention with teenagers to break the cycle of violence.

Reference: Parker B et al: Physical and emotional abuse in pregnancy: a comparison of adult and teenage women, *Nurs Res* 42:173, 1993.

BOX 23-3

ABUSE ASSESSMENT

These questions may help you when assessing female patients for abuse. For some women, answering "sometimes" to abuse questions is easier than *yes* or *no*.

1. Do you know where you could go or who could help you if you were abused or worried about abuse?
   Yes _____ No_____
   If yes, where _____

2. Are you in a relationship with a man who physically hurts you?
   Yes _____ No_____ Sometimes_____

3. Does he threaten you with abuse?
   Yes _____ No _____ Sometimes_____

4. Has the man you are with hit, slapped, kicked or otherwise physically hurt you?
   Yes _____ No _____ Sometimes_____

For Pregnant Patients ⟨

5. If yes, has he hit you since you've been pregnant?
   Yes _____ No _____ Not Applicable_____

6. If yes, did the abuse increase since you've been pregnant?
   Yes_____ No _____ Not Applicable_____

7. Have you ever received medical treatment for any abuse injuries?
   Yes _____ No_____ Not Applicable_____

8. If you've been abused, remembering the last time he hurt you, mark the places on the body map where he hit you.

9. Were you pregnant at the time?
   Yes _____ No_____ Not Applicable_____

When assessing for abuse, some women may be uncomfortable with the topic and may exhibit some of the behaviors below. For some women these behaviors may be suggestive of abuse and disclosure of battering may follow at a later date.

Actions Suggestive of Abuse

1. Laughing/"tittering" ....yes   no
2. No eye contact (not applicable in some cultures) ....yes   no
3. Crying ....yes   no
4. Sighing ....yes   no
5. Minimizing statements ....yes   no
6. Searching/engaging eye contact (fear) ....yes   no
7. Anxious body language ....yes   no
   (standing to leave, dropped shoulders, depressed)
8. Anger, defensiveness ....yes   no
9. Comments about emotional abuse ....yes   no
10. Comments about a "friend" who is abused ....yes   no

EVALUACION DE ABUSO

1. ¿Conoce Ud. adonde y con quién una mujer maltratada o preocupada con la posibilidad de ser maltratada podria recurrir?
   si_____ no_____
   Si s dónde y con quién?_____

2. ¿Tene Ud. una relación con un compañero o esposo que la maltrata fisicamente?
   si _____ no_____ a veces_____

3. ¿Su esposo o companñero la ha amenazado? (Ha dicho que le va a pegar o maltratar?)
   si_____ no _____ a veces_____

4. ¿Ud. ha sido golpeada, bofeteada o le ha dado palmazos en la cara su esposo o compañero?
   si_____ no _____ a veces_____

Para Pacientes ⟨ Embarazadas

5. ¿Él la ha golpeado o maltratado desde su embarazo?
   si_____ no_____ no aplica_____

6. Se ha incrementado el maltrato desde que se embarazó?
   si_____ no_____ no aplica_____

7. Alguna vez, ¿Ud. ha recibido tratamiento médico (cuarto de emergencia, hospital o doctor) por injurias causados por el maltrato?
   si_____ no_____ no aplica_____

8. Si la ha maltratado, por favor, marque en esta hoja los lugares donde fue golpeada la última vez.

9. Durante esa última vez, ¿estaba Ud. embarazada?
   si_____ no_____ No aplica_____

1987). The decrease, however, may be due to the abused partner leaving the relationship. Studies indicate that health care providers rarely assess for family violence, and it is rarer still that health care providers give women appropriate referrals if abuse is identified (McFarlane, 1989; Tilden, Shepherd, 1987). Fear and shame tend to restrain women who have been abused from seeking help or from acknowledging the abuse to a helper (Limandri, 1989).

NURSING CONSIDERATIONS

The most significant intervention for intimate partner abuse is the assessment. Just being asked about being hurt or frightened by her partner permits the woman to disclose her experience. In a research study women said that they had frequently gone to their health care provider with bruises and injuries that seemed obvious. These women had waited for someone to ask about the bruises and injuries because they were too ashamed to volunteer the information. Their greatest disappointment was that no one asked (Limandri, 1987).

A simple abuse assessment and body map (see Box 23-3 and Fig. 23-1) can help the nurse gather sufficient information in a nonthreatening and nonjudgmental way. It is important to provide privacy for this assessment and to be sure that her partner is not present, in order to permit her to be honest without fearing reprisal later. If the woman has not experienced violence in her relationship, she will at the least be surprised by the question and at the most be educated that abuse is important enough to inquire about routinely.

To the nurse who is inexperienced in dealing with family violence, it can be disconcerting or uncomfortable to have the patient acknowledge abuse. It is important to have a list of community resources available for abused women including shelters, safe homes, crisis lines, and counselors. Many communities have this information available on small business cards that are easy to slip into a pocket. To find information about intimate partner abuse, the nurse may call the local battered women's organization in the closest community and ask for assistance from their staff. The nurse can respond to the woman's disclosure by acknowledging that it must be difficult for her to talk about her experiences, and that she does not deserve to be treated like that. Women most fear that disclosure will result in being told that she must leave her abuser in order to receive further help. Such advice only alienates the woman who is socially and economically trapped in the relationship. It is least likely that she can leave the relationship while she is pregnant or has a newborn. Instead the nurse may offer resources for the woman's safety, places to call for emotional support, and counseling to help her clarify what she wants and needs (Limandri, 1987). The nurse does not have to res-

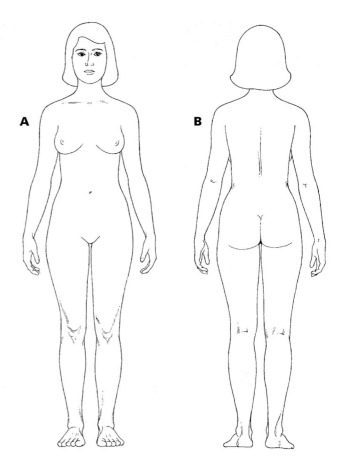

FIG. 23-1   Body maps for abuse assessment.

cue the abused woman. What the abused woman most often wants is sensitivity, acceptance, and guidance regarding where she can seek additional help when she is ready (see Plan of Care on p. 680).

POVERTY

The very poor—the social class of people who consistently live at or below the poverty level—are in a perpetual state of despair. Their limited skills give them no bargaining power in the job market. Education needed to improve their status is beyond them. The poor desire a better life for their children but are trapped in a circular pattern that perpetuates their condition. Their powerlessness to control their fate or condition is a source of fatalism and resignation that is characteristic of the group in general. This fatalistic attitude is a significant impediment to occupational and educational aspirations and to seeking health care. A newer phenomenon in today's economic situation is that of the "new" poor who are educated but have lost their jobs as a result of economic and social conditions. These persons comprise an entirely different group of patients with whom the nurse may work.

PLAN OF CARE

The Pregnant Battered Woman

Case History

Susan, a 22-year-old woman, brought her 2-year-old and 3-year-old to her prenatal visit. Her partner, David, reads a magazine as she watches the children. When the nurse approaches them, David steps forward and says he wants to come with Susan. In the interview David corrects Susan frequently, and she looks to him before she answers questions. The nurse asked Susan to accompany her to the bathroom for a urine sample and while en route gives Susan an abuse questionnaire to complete and leave in the bathroom with her specimen. Susan's responses to the questionnaire indicate that she was hit and slapped by David throughout her previous pregnancies and recently in this pregnancy. She does not want David to know that she told this and says she is afraid of David but loves him and needs his support for the children. On subsequent visits the nurse has private time with Susan during which she assessed that Susan is quite depressed. She used alcohol in the past to deal with the depression but will not during her pregnancy. Because David controls her friendships and contact with family members, Susan feels isolated and believes she deserves what she gets from David because he also cares for her.

EXPECTED OUTCOME	IMPLEMENTATION	RATIONALE	EVALUATION
Nursing Diagnosis: High risk for violence by other (partner) related to domestic violence			
Susan will develop a safety plan and use as needed.	Provide materials about abuse and discuss them with Susan.	Knowledge of available resources can assist in problem-solving, provide some relief of her tension, and provide her with concrete ways to avoid the next abusive episode.	Susan identifies the risk of violence in her situation.
	Encourage Susan to develop and plan to get herself and her children out of the situation as she perceives danger or abuse occurring.		Susan describes her safety plan and how and when she would implement it.
	Provide a telephone number of an abused women's hotline and services.		Susan memorizes the phone number for the women's crisis services.
	Discuss and role play ways to handle escalating tension leading to violence.		

The term *poverty* implies both visible and invisible impoverishment. **Visible poverty** refers to lack of money or material resources, which includes insufficient clothing, poor sanitation, and deteriorating housing. **Invisible poverty** refers to social and cultural deprivation such as limited employment opportunities, inferior educational opportunities, lack of (or inferior) medical services and health care facilities, and an absence of public services (Spector, 1979).

Factors Related to Poverty

One factor that notably affects women is *employment and wage discrimination*. Poverty and undue stress are responses to the discrimination and exploitation that women experience in the workplace. Most seriously af-

fected are the growing numbers of single-parent families headed by women (Griffith-Kenney, 1986).

Throughout the United States are geographically segregated groups of people, who constitute what is known as "pockets of poverty." They are seen in the dense urban areas, such as the ghettos, and many rural areas, especially those that are geographically isolated from needed facilities and services. The nonurbanized regions identified as poverty areas in the United States are Appalachia, the deep South, the lower Southwest, and northern New England (Spector, 1979).

Certain *ethnic or racial groups* are overrepresented in the impoverished population. The most obvious of these are African-Americans, Mexican-Americans, Mexican immigrants, and Native Americans.

PLAN OF CARE—cont'd

The Pregnant Battered Woman

EXPECTED OUTCOME	IMPLEMENTATION	RATIONALE	EVALUATION
Nursing Diagnosis: Chronic low self-esteem with respect to persistent partner abuse			
Susan will more realistically value self.	Provide realistic positive feedback. Refer her to an abused women's support group. Teach Susan ways to self-nurture. Refer her to counseling if necessary.	A supportive environment can assist one to promote positive self-esteem.	Susan identifies that self-esteem is unrealistic. Susan joins a support group. Susan becomes more self-assured.
Nursing Diagnosis: Risk for injury with respect to alcohol abuse			
Susan will refrain from drinking alcohol during her pregnancy.	Reinforce Susan's understanding about effects of alcohol on fetal development. Discuss the use of alcohol as a medication for her anxiety and mood. Discuss an alternative way to deal with her emotions. Teach stress management skills and have her return the demonstration of skills.	A supportive environment and taking positive action (e.g., developing a safety plan) may assist her to manage stress without using alcohol during pregnancy.	Susan avoids using alcohol or other nonprescribed drugs during her pregnancy. Susan uses other means of reducing stress and elevating her mood.

Migrant Families

Migrant farm workers and their families are among the most disadvantaged groups. The low position of these families on the economic scale and their rootless, mobile existence subject them to inadequate sanitation, substandard housing, social isolation, and lack of educational opportunities and medical services. This is especially harmful to the mothers and children. Health care generally is inadequate. Families are apt to live in a number of localities in the course of a year, without continuity of whatever health care is available. Pesticides and herbicides have been identified as mutagenic and teratogenic. Because both parents work in the fields, both are exposed to potential mutagens; the women may be exposed to teratogens during pregnancy. Accident rates are high, and meals may be erratic.

Some migrants have a home base to which they return at the end of a growing season; others travel continuously, migrating north in summer and south in winter. With most there is little if any integration into the dominant culture; therefore migrant groups suffer social isolation. Groups who travel together, especially those with the same ethnic background, develop a cohesiveness and form their own set of values and customs. Sometimes a migrant family will leave the migration stream and become a part of a permanent community. However, this involves adaptation to a new environment and lifestyle that can be stress provoking to these families.

Preventive Health Care

The vulnerability of economically and socially deprived people in our society to health problems is apparent across the spectrum of health care from prevention to rehabilitation. Preventative health care is more than the prevention of disease states. It involves those factors in a person's life that protect the individual and allow for growth and development of potential. Adequate clothing and shelter, proper nutrition, education, a safe environment—all taken for granted by the economically advantaged—are noticeably lacking in the health experience of many low-income groups.

The concept of preventive health often is missing. The development of a concept of preventive health begins in childhood as the child is directed and encouraged to "eat your dinner and grow up to be a strong boy," "brush your teeth," "go to the doctor for a checkup," and "get enough sleep." These repeated admonitions eventually result in a concept of health care that includes prevention as well as cure. For women who have experienced this introduction, acceptance of the necessity for prenatal care comes more readily. For those women who have gone to a health care provider only when they were very ill, the relative health of the pregnant state precludes full use of care available. For some low-income women a choice between prenatal care (preparation for birth) and providing their families with necessities results in their foregoing prenatal care.

In some communities, clinics have been established specifically for high-risk mothers and their infants. Adolescent mothers and preterm infants make up a large part of the patient population at these clinics. Although prevention of the problem is probably the best approach, follow-up care is of great importance. Helping mothers develop parenting skills will do much to promote the optimum growth and development of these disadvantaged children.

In England, Olds and Kitzman (1990) demonstrated a marked improvement in health-related behaviors during pregnancy with home visitation programs and education. Nursing and nurse-researchers, are in the forefront of efforts to provide care for childbearing families. The Children's Defense Fund reported that the increasing maternal and infant mortality rates can be blamed in part on poor health care related to poverty and lack of medical insurance and publicly financed health services (*San Francisco Chronicle*, 1990).

The national concern over infant mortality and access to health care has led to an increase in some areas of medicaid assistance for prenatal care. However, increased medicaid coverage alone cannot increase use of early prenatal care or improve birth outcomes. Reasons include the difficulties in enrolling in the medicaid program, lack of additional social support, and reluctance of many health care providers to accept medicaid patients. A newly restructured system may be necessary to address the multiple issues involved rather than only an increase in financial aid (Guyer, 1990; Piper, Ray, Griffin, 1990).

The following reasons provide additional explanations for delayed care: (1) lack of acceptance of pregnancy (denial of or unwanted pregnancy, psychologic problems of depression, or anxiety); (2) fear of hospitals or health care workers, problems with making and keeping appointments, and feeling that there is no need for prenatal care; (3) financial issues such as lack of knowledge of availability of care; and (4) family responsibilities, including conflict with the father, baby-sitting problems, other family crises, or geographic moves (Young et al, 1989). Parity, availability of clinics, and public transportation may be of more importance than are financial barriers (St. Clair et al, 1990).

Reproductive Experience

Low-income women tend to begin reproducing at an earlier age and to stop reproducing at a later age than do other women. In addition, they have many pregnancies, and these are adversely affected by the close spacing of the gestations. In 1970 Birch and Gussons described this phenomenon as "too young, too old, and too often." This has not changed in recent years. Maternal age and parity are implicated in perinatal mortality. There is increased risk to the fetus, infant, and mother when the mother is at either extreme of age or parity. The quality of prenatal care has a significant impact on birth weight and optimal birth outcomes (Poland et al, 1990). Preterm birth, low birth weight, and their complications remain the chief causes of perinatal mortality. Low-income mothers are more likely to give birth to preterm infants than are mothers in the population at large. Social support, often unavailable to the poor, is essential to enable people to cope with life's stresses. There is a correlation between life stresses during pregnancy and the outcome of that pregnancy (Norbeck, Anderson, 1989).

Pregnancy Outcomes

The differences in pregnancy outcomes related to socioeconomic class have been well documented for more than half a century. Studies have consistently demonstrated a relationship between economic class and maternal and infant morbidity and mortality. These discrepancies have been of major concern to nursing groups as they have attempted to improve the health and well-being of all individuals in society.

Complications

Low-income mothers are more predisposed to illness and obstetric complications during pregnancy. Obstetric complications such as placenta previa, abruptio placentae, and placental insufficiency often result in preterm births, intrauterine growth retardation, and low-birth-weight or small-for-gestational-age newborns and subsequent infant difficulties (Wen et al, 1990). Many obstetric complications have life-threatening consequences for both the mother and the infant. Examples of complications include hemorrhage, cardiac disease, or uncontrolled infection.

The problems faced by low-income mothers have direct implication for nursing service. Much of our current knowledge could be used to minimize or prevent the occurrence of the problems. One of the prerequisites to providing assistance to the low-income mother is to find better and more effective ways to deliver safe and meaningful care to her.

Infants born to homeless women are at very high risk as a result of poor prenatal care and nutritional status of the mother, low-birth-weight, inadequate infant nutrition, and respiratory and ear infections (Damrosch et al, 1988). Nurses must realize that they cannot provide all the solutions needed for the problems of homelessness and poverty. However, a connection exists between health and other conditions that affect those involved. Nurses can assist families by helping them to improve their self-esteem and develop and use skills that will help them to move out of the poverty cycle. Peer and professional support can be great assets for these families, as can information on stress management. Nurses can help most by using their influence to develop and shape political policies that deal with the issues of the poor and homeless (Berne et al, 1990). Primary, secondary, and

tertiary measures must be included in the care of these patients. Involvement of the family, interdisciplinary team support, and community resources are all required to provide long-term care for both the mother and newborn.

KEY POINTS

- Psychosocial problems that may complicate childbearing can interfere with family integration and restrict bonding with the infant.
- Involvement of the family, an interdisciplinary team approach, and community resources are required to provide long-term care for both the mother and the newborn.
- Values clarification for the health care workers may be necessary to assist them in providing nonjudgmental care for substance abusers.

- Perpetuation of violence against women is influenced by the historical and societal norm of valuing women.
- Nurses must explore their values and beliefs concerning violence against women in order to identify and intervene effectively.
- Low-income mothers are more predisposed to intercurrent illness and obstetric complications during the childbearing cycle.
- The nurse must be aware of community health resources for low-income patients.

CRITICAL THINKING EXERCISES

1. Visit a high-risk, part-pay, or county-supported clinic. Assess the risk factors for the patients.
   a. What is the reproductive history for the low-income patient?
   b. What nursing actions may alleviate potential complications for the low-income patient? Justify your answers.
   c. What criteria must the patient meet to be eligible for service?

2. Through research of charts from medical records and interviews, determine what percentage of the women giving birth at your hospital have had no prenatal care.
   a. Compare risk factors identified in these women to those found in women who sought care early in the prenatal period and had excellent prenatal supervision.
   b. Make and check inferences based on data.

References

Adams C, Eyler FD, Behnke M: Nursing interventions with mothers who are substance abusers, *J Perinat Neonat Nurs* 3:43, April 1990.

Affonso D: Postpartum depression. In Fields P, editor: *Recent advances in perinatal nursing,* New York, 1984, Churchill Livingstone, Inc.

Amaro H et al: Violence during pregnancy and substance use, *Am J of Public Health* 80(5):575, 1990.

American College of Obstetricians and Gynecologists: Smoking and reproductive health, *Int J Gynaecol Obstet* 43:75, 1993.

American Psychiatric Association: *Diagnostic and statistical manual of mental disorders,* ed 4, Washington DC, 1994, The Association.

Auerbach KG, Jacobi AM: Postpartum depression in the breastfeeding mother, *NAACOG's Clin Issu Perinat Womens Health Nurs* 1(3):375, 1990.

Benowitz NL: Nicotine replacement therapy during pregnancy, *JAMA* 266(22):3174, 1991.

Berenson AB et al: Drug abuse and other risk factors for physical abuse in pregnancy among white non-hispanic, black, and hispanic women, *Am J Obstet Gynecol* 164(6 Part 1):1491, 1991.

Berne AS et al: A nursing model for addressing the health needs of homeless families, *Image J Nurs Sch* 22:8, Jan 1990.

Birch HG, Gussons JD: *Disadvantaged children: health, nutrition, and future,* New York, 1970, Harcourt Brace & World.

Burkett G, Yasin S, Palow D: Perinatal implication of cocaine exposure, *J Reprod Med* 35(1):35, Jan 1990.

Busch P, Perrin K: Postpartum depression: assessing risk, restoring balance, *RN* 52:46, 1989.

Campbell JC et al: Correlates of battering during pregnancy, *Res Nurs Health* 15(3):219, 1992.

Chasnoff LJ: Cocaine, pregnancy, and the neonate, *Women Health* 15(3):23, March 1989.

Chisum GM: Nursing interventions with the antepartum substance abuser, *J Perinat Neonat Nurs* 3:26, April 1990.

Cook PS et al: *Alcohol, tobacco, and other drugs may harm the unborn,* Rockville, MD, 1990, US Public Health Service.

Cordero L, Custard M: Effects of maternal cocaine abuse on perinatal and infant outcome, *Ohio Med* 86:410, 1990.

Damrosch SP et al: On behalf of homeless families, *MCN* 13:259, July/Aug 1988.

Daw JL: Postpartum depression, *South Med J* 81:207, 1988.

Edeline KC et al: Methadone maintenance in pregnancy: consequences to care and outcome, *Obstet Gynecol* 71:399, 1988.

Edlund MJ, Craig TJ: Antipsychotic drug use and birth defects, an epidemiologic reassessment, *Compr Psychiatry* 25:32, 1984.

Ehlert U et al: Postpartum blues: salivary cortisol and psychological factors, *J Psychosom Res* 34:319, 1990.

Feng T: Substance abuse in pregnancy, *Curr Opin Obstet Gynecol* 5:16, 1993.

Gilbert E, Harmon J: *Manual of high risk pregnancy and delivery*, St Louis, 1993, Mosby.

Goldstein RL: The psychiatrist's guide to right and wrong, III, postpartum depression and the "appreciation" of wrongfulness, *Bull Am Acad Psychiatry Law* 17:121, 1989.

Griffith-Kenney J: *Contemporary women's health: a nursing advocacy approach*, Menlo Park, CA, 1986, Addison-Wesley.

Guyer B: Medicaid and prenatal care: necessary but not sufficient, *JAMA* 264:2264, 1990.

Hamilton JA: Postpartum psychiatric syndromes, *Psychiatr Clin North Am* 12:89, 1989.

Hansen C: Baby blues: identification and intervention, *NAACOG's Clin Issu Perinat Womens Health Nurs* 1(3): 369, 1990.

Harding JJ: Postpartum psychiatric disorders: a review, *Compr Psychiatry* 30:109, 1989.

Harris B et al: The normal environment of postnatal depression, *Br J Psychiatry* 154:660, 1989.

Hauser LA: Pregnancy and psychiatric drugs, *Hosp Community Psychiatry* 36:817, 1985.

Helton AS, McFarlane J, Anderson ET: Battered and pregnant: a prevalance study, *Am J Public Health* 77:1337, 1987.

Hopkins J, Campbell S, Marcus M: Postpartum depression and postpartum adaptation: overlapping constructs? *J Affect Discord* 17:251, 1989.

Hurt LD, Ray CP: Postpartum disorders: mother-infant bonding on a psychiatric unit, *J Psychosoc Nurs Ment Health Serv* 23(2):15, 1985.

"Ice" drug now used at work, officials say, *San Francisco Chronicle*, Oct 25, 1989a.

Iles S, Gath D, Kennerley H: Maternity blues: a comparison between post-operative women and post-natal women, *Br J Psychiatry* 155:363, 1989.

Janke JR: Prenatal cocaine use: effects on perinatal outcome, *J Nurse Midwifery* 35:74, March/April 1990.

Jones LC: Postpartum emotional disorders, *ICEA Rev* 14(4):21, Nov 1990.

Keith LG et al: Substance abuse in pregnant women: recent experience at the Perinatal Center for Chemical Dependence of Northwestern Memorial Hospital, *Obstet Gynecol*, 73 (Pt 1):715, 1989.

Kennerley H, Gath D: Detection and measurement by questionnaire, *Br J Psychiatry* 155:356, 1989a.

Kennerley H, Gath D: Maternity blues: association with obstetric psychological and psychiatric factors, *Br J Psychiatry* 155:367, 1989b.

Krause S, Ebbesen F, Lange AP: Polyhydramnios with maternal lithium treatment, *Obstet Gynecol* 75(3):504, 1990.

Laizner AM, Jeans ME: Identification of predictor variables of postpartum emotional reactions, *Health Care Women Int* 11:191, 1990.

Landry M, Smith DE: Crack: anatomy of an addiction, II, *Calif Nurs Rev* 9(3):28, 1987.

Li DK, Daling JR: Maternal smoking, low birth weight, and ethnicity in relation to sudden infant death syndrome, *Am J Epidemiol* 134:958, 1991.

Limandri BJ: Disclosure of stigmatizing conditions: the discloser's perspective, *Arch Psychiatr Nurs* 3(2):69, 1989.

Limandri BJ: The therapeutic relationship with abused women, *J Psychosoc Nurs Ment Health Serv*, 25(2):9, 1987.

Little BB et al: Patterns of multiple substance abuse during pregnancy: implications for mother and fetus, *South Med J* 83:507, 1990

Lynch M, McKeon VA: Cocaine use during pregnancy: research findings and clinical implications, *JOGNN* 19:283, 1990.

Majewski MD, Ford-Rice F, Falkey G: Pregnancy-induced alterations of GABAA receptor sensitivity in maternal brain: an antecedent of postpartum blues, *Brain Res* 482:397, 1989.

Marks MN et al: Contribution of psychological and social factors to psychotic and non-psychotic relapse after childbirth in women with previous histories of affective disorder, *J Affect Disord* 24(4):253, 1992a.

Marks MN et al: Women whose mental illnesses recur after childbirth and partners' levels of expressed emotion during late pregnancy, *Br J Psychiatry* 161:211, 1992b.

Martell LK: Postpartum depression as a family problem, *MCN* 15:90, March/April 1990.

Matera C et al: Prevalence of use of cocaine and other substances in an obstetric population, *Am J Obstet Gynecol* 163:797, 1990.

McAnarney ER, Stevens-Simon C: Maternal psychological stress, depression and low birth weight. Is there a relationship? *Am J Dis Child* 144(7):789, 1990.

McFarlane J: Battering during pregnancy: tip of an iceberg revealed, *Women Health* 15(3):69, 1989.

Metz S, Sichel F, Goff C: Postpartum panic disorder, *J Clin Psychiatry* 49:278, 1988.

Miller WH et al: The pregnant psychiatric inpatient: a missed opportunity, *General Hospital Psychiatry*, 12(6):373, 1990.

Mondanaro J: Strategies for AIDS prevention: motivating health behavior in drug dependent women, *J Psychoactive Drugs* 19(2):113, 1987.

New drug "ice" called worse peril than crack, *San Francisco Chronicle*, Aug 31, 1989b.

Ney JA et al: The prevalence of substance abuse in patients with suspected preterm labor, *Am J Obstet Gynecol* 162:1362, 1990.

Nicolson P: Understanding postnatal depression: a mother-centered approach, *J Adv Nurs* 15(6):689, 1990.

Norbeck JS, Anderson NJ: Psychosocial predictors of pregnancy outcomes in low-income black, Hispanic and white women, *Nurs Res* 38:204, July/Aug 1989.

Olds D, Kitzman H: Can home visitation improve the health of women and children at environmental risk? *Pediatrics* 86:108, 1990.

Oro AS, Dixon SD: Perinatal cocaine and methamphetamine exposure: maternal and neonatal correlates, *J Pediatr* 111:571, 1987.

Piper JM, Ray WA, Griffin MR: Effects of Medicaid eligibility expansion on prenatal care and pregnancy in Tennessee, *JAMA* 264:2219, 1990.

Poland ML et al: Quality of prenatal care: selected social, behavioral, and biomedical factors, and birth weight, *Obstet Gynecol* 75:607, 1990.

Scott JR et al: *Obstetrics and gynecology*, ed 6, Philadelphia, 1990, JB Lippincott Co.

Smith R et al: Mood changes, obstetric experiences, and alterations in plasma cortisol beta-endorphin and corticotrophin-releasing hormone during pregnancy and the puerperium, *J Psychosom Res* 34:53, 1990.

Spector RE: *Cultural diversity in health and illness*, New York, 1979, Appleton-Century-Crofts.

Spielvogel A, Wile J: Treatment of the psychotic pregnant patient, *Psychosomatics* 27(7):487, 1986.

St. Clair PA et al: Situational and financial barriers to prenatal care in a sample of low-income, inner-city women, *Public Health Res* 105:264, 1990.

Stein A et al: Social adversity and perinatal complications: their relation to postnatal depression, *Br Med J* 2928:1073, 1989.

Steiner M: Postpartum psychiatric disorders, *Can J Psychiatry* 35:89, 1990.

Stuart GW, Sundeen SJ: *Principles & practice of psychiatric nursing,* ed 5, St Louis, 1995, Mosby.

Taylor E: Postnatal depression: what can a health visitor do? *J Adv Nurs* 14:877, 1989.

Tilden VP, Shepherd P: Battered women: the shadow side of families, *Holistic Nursing Practice,* 1(2):25, 1987.

Tracy CE: Women suffer most from drugs, *The Philadelphia Inquirer,* p 7E, Nov 27, 1988.

Troutman B, Cutrona C: Nonpsychotic postpartum depression among adolescent mothers, *J Abnorm Psychol* 99:69, 1990.

Wen SW et al: Intrauterine growth retardation and preterm delivery: prenatal risk factors in an indigent population, *Am J Obstet Gynecol* 162:213, 1990.

Whiffen V, Gotlib I: Infants of postpartum depressed mothers: temperamental and cognitive status, *J Abnorm Psychol* 98:274, 1989.

Woods JR, Plessinger MA, Clark KE: Effect of cocaine on uterine blood flow and fetal oxygenation, *JAMA* 257:957, 1987.

Young C et al: Maternal reasons for delayed prenatal care, *Nurs Res* 38:242, July/Aug 1989.

Zuckerman B et al: Maternal depressive symptoms during pregnancy and newborn irritability, *J Dev Behav Pediatr* 11(4):190, April 1990.

Bibliography

American College of Obstetricians and Gynecologists: Cocaine in pregnancy, *Cocaine Opinion: Committee on Obstetrics: Maternal and Fetal Medicine* 114, Washington DC, 1993, ACOG.

Affonso D et al: Pregnancy and postpartum depressive symptoms, *J of Women's Health,* 2(2):157, 1993.

Barbour BC: Alcohol and pregnancy, *J Nurse Midwifery* 35:78, March/April 1990.

Beck CT: The lived experience of postpartum depression: a phenomenological study, *Nurs Res* 41(3), May/June 1992.

Berchtold N, Burrough M: Reaching out: depression after delivery support group network, *NAACOG's Clin Issu Perinat Womens Health Nurs* 1:385, 1990.

Boyer DB: Prediction of postpartum depression, *NAACOG's Clin Issu Perinat Womens Health Nurs* 1:395, 1990.

Casiano ME: Outpatient medical management of postpartum psychiatric disorders, *NAACOG's Clin Issu Perinat Womens Health Nurs* 1:395, 1990.

Duncan GJ, Hoffman SF: Teenage welfare receipt and subsequent dependence among black adolescent mothers, *Fam Plann Perspect* 22:16, Jan 1990.

Fried P: Marijuana use during pregnancy: consequences for the offspring, *Semin Perinatol* 15:280, 1991.

Gotlib IH et al: Prospective investigation of postpartum depression: factors involved in onset and recovery, *J Abnorm Psychol* 100:122, 1991.

Ginzberg E: Access to health care for Hispanics, *JAMA* 265:238, 1991.

Grossman LK, Harter C, Kay A: The effect of postpartum lactation counseling on the duration of breast-feeding in low-income women, *Am J Dis Child* 144:471, 1990.

Hansen CH: Baby blues: identification and intervention, *NAACOG's Clin Issu Perinat Womens Health Nurs* 1:369, 1990.

Kumar R: An overview of postpartum psychiatric disorders, *NAACOG's Clin Issu Perinat Womens Health Nurs* 1:351, 1990.

Levy M, Koren G: Obstetric and neonatal effects of drugs of abuse, *Emerg Med Clin North Am* 8:633, 1990.

Lia-Hongberg B et al: Barriers and motivators to prenatal care among low-income women, *Soc Sci Med* 30:487, 1990.

Mastrogiannis DS: Perinatal outcome after recent cocaine usage, *Obstet Gynecol* 76:8, 1990.

Matti L, Caspersen V: Prevalence of drug use among pregnant women in a rural area, *JOGNN* 22(6):510, 1993.

Mullen P, Carbonari J, Glenday M: Identifying pregnant women who drink alcoholic beverages, *Am J Obstet Gynecol* 165:1429, 1991.

Noel N, Yam M: Domestic violence: the pregnant woman, *Nurs Clin North Am* 27(4):871, 1992.

Schneck ME et al: Low-income pregnant adolescents and their infants: dietary findings and health outcomes, *J Am Diet Assoc* 90:555, 1990.

Starn J et al: Can we encourage pregnant substance abusers to seek prenatal care? *MCN* 18(3):148, 1993.

Suitor CW, Gardner JD, Feldstein ML: Characteristics of diet among a culturally diverse group of low-income pregnant women, *J Am Diet Assoc* 90:543, 1990.

Sullivan J, Bondreaux M, Keller P: Can we help the substance abusing mother and infant? *MCN* 18(3):153, 1993.

Wasserman GA et al: Psychosocial attributes and life experiences of disadvantaged minority mothers: age and ethnic variations, *Child Dev* 61:566, 1990.

24 Labor and Birth at Risk

DEITRA LEONARD LOWDERMILK

Define key terms listed.

Identify assessments for women experiencing different types of dystocia.

Formulate nursing diagnoses based on assessment of dystocia.

Describe interventions for different types of abnormal labor and birth problems related to dystocia: trial of labor, induction of labor, forceps-assisted birth, vacuum extraction, cesarean birth, and vaginal birth after cesarean.

Discuss criteria for evaluating nursing care of women experiencing dystocia.

Compare nursing assessment and care management of women with preterm labor at home and in the hospital setting.

Describe assessment and care management of women experiencing postterm pregnancy.

amniotomy (artificial rupture of membranes [AROM])
augmentation of labor
Bishop score
cephalopelvic disproportion (CPD)
cesarean birth
dysfunctional labor
dystocia
external cephalic version (ECV)
forceps-assisted birth
hypertonic uterine dysfunction
hypotonic uterine dysfunction
induction of labor
multifetal pregnancy
oxytocin
postterm birth
precipitous labor
preterm birth
prostaglandins
therapeutic rest
tocolytic agents
trial of labor (TOL)
vacuum extraction
vaginal birth after cesarean (VBAC)

Amniocentesis *(Chap. 20)* • Epidural anesthetic *(Chap. 10)* • Biophysical profile *(Chap. 20)* • Care of preterm infants *(Chap. 27)* • Essential factors of labor *(Chap. 9)* • Fetal monitoring *(Chap. 11)* • Loss and grief *(Chap. 28)* • Magnesium sulfate *(Chap. 21)* • Multifetal pregnancy *(Chap. 4)* • Normal labor and birth *(Chap. 12)* • Placenta previa *(Chap. 21)* • Preterm labor recognition *(Chap. 7)* • Prostaglandins *(Chap. 3)* • Respiratory distress syndrome *(Chap. 27)* • Risk scoring system for preterm labor *(Chap. 7)*

When complications arise during labor and birth, perinatal morbidity and mortality increase. Some complications are anticipated, especially if the mother is identified at high risk during the antepartum period; others are unexpected or unforeseen. The woman, her family, and the labor nurse can feel devastated when things go wrong. These feelings must be recognized if nurses are to provide effective support. It is crucial for nurses to understand the normal birth process to prevent and detect deviations from normal labor and birth and to implement nursing measures when complications arise. Optimum care of the laboring woman, fetus, and family experiencing complications is possible only when the nurse and other members of the obstetric team use their knowledge and skills in a concerted effort for the provision of care.

DYSTOCIA

Dystocia is defined as long, difficult, or abnormal labor and is caused by various conditions associated with the five essential factors of labor. Any of the following can cause dystocia:

1. *Dysfunctional labor* resulting in ineffective uterine contractions or maternal bearing-down efforts (the powers)
2. *Alterations in the pelvic structure* (the passage)
3. *Fetal causes* including abnormalities of presentation or position, anomalies, excessive size, and number of fetuses (the passengers)
4. *Maternal position* during labor and birth
5. *Psychologic responses* of the mother to labor related to past experiences, preparation, culture and heritage, and support system

These five factors are interdependent. In assessing the woman for an abnormal labor pattern the nurse considers the interactions of these factors and how they influence the labor process. Dystocia is suspected when there is a lack of progress in the rate of cervical dilatation, a lack of progress in fetal descent and expulsion, or an alteration in the characteristics of uterine contractions.

Dysfunctional Labor

Dysfunctional labor is described as abnormal uterine contractions that prevent normal progress of cervical dilatation, effacement (primary powers), and/or descent (secondary powers).

Dysfunction of uterine contractions can be further described as being primary or secondary. The woman who experiences *primary dysfunctional labor,* or **hypertonic uterine dysfunction,** often is an anxious first-time mother who is having painful contractions. These contractions are out of proportion to their intensity and do not cause cervical dilatation or effacement. They usually occur in the latent stage (cervical dilatation <4 cm) and are usually uncoordinated and frequent (Fig. 24-1).

Women experiencing hypertonic uterine dysfunction may be exhausted and express concern about loss of control because of the intense pain and lack of progress. Management of primary uterine dysfunction is by **therapeutic rest,** which is achieved through the administration of effective analgesics such as morphine or meperidine to reduce the pain and encourage sleep. Often these women will awaken with normal uterine activity.

The second and more common type of uterine dys-

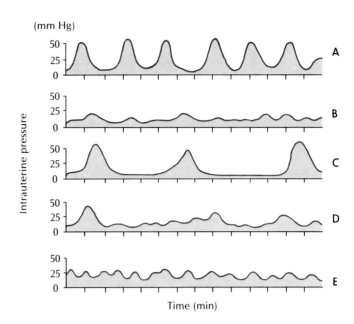

FIG. 24-1   Uterine contractility patterns in labor. **A,** Typical normal labor. **B,** Subnormal intensity, with frequency greater than needed for optimum performance. **C,** Normal contractions, but too infrequent for efficient labor. **D,** Incoordinate activity. **E,** Hypercontractility.

function is *secondary uterine inertia,* or **hypotonic uterine dysfunction.** The woman, who may be either in her first or a subsequent pregnancy, initially makes normal progress into the active stage of labor; then the contractions become weak and inefficient or stop altogether (Fig. 24-1). The uterus is easily indentable even at the peak of contractions. Cephalopelvic disproportion and malpositions are common causes.

Women experiencing hypotonic uterine dysfunction may become exhausted and are at risk for infection. Medical management usually includes ruling out cephalopelvic disproportion by ultrasound or x-ray examination followed by augmentation of dysfunctional labor with oxytocin (see p. 699; Bowes, 1989). *Secondary powers* or bearing-down efforts can be compromised by large amounts of analgesic, administration of anesthetic, maternal exhaustion, inadequate hydration, and maternal position. Table 24-1 summarizes dysfunctional labor.

Alterations in Pelvic Structure
Pelvic Dystocia

Pelvic dystocia can occur with contractures of the pelvic diameters that reduce the capacity of the bony pelvis, including the inlet, mid pelvis, outlet, or any combination of these planes. Pelvic contractures may be caused by congenital abnormalities, maternal malnutrition, neoplasms, and lower spinal disorders. Immature pelvic size predisposes some adolescent mothers to pelvic dystocia. Pelvic deformities may be the result of automobile or other accidents.

Inlet contracture occurs in 1% to 2% of term births and is diagnosed when the diagonal conjugate is less than 11.5 cm. The incidence of face and shoulder presentation continues to increase. These presentations prevent engagement and fetal descent, thereby increasing the risk of prolapse of the umbilical cord. Inlet contracture is associated with maternal rickets and a flat pelvis. Weak uterine contractions may be noted during the first stage of labor.

Midplane contracture, the most common cause of pelvic dystocia, is diagnosed when the sum of the interischial spinous and posterior sagittal diameters of the midpelvis is 13.5 cm or less. Fetal descent is arrested (transverse arrest of the fetal head) because the head cannot rotate internally. Cesarean birth is the usual management, but vacuum extraction has been used safely if the cervix is fully dilated. Midforceps-assisted birth usually is avoided because of increased perinatal morbidity associated with this intervention.

Outlet contracture exists when the interischial diameter is 8 cm or less. It rarely occurs without midplane contracture. Outlet contracture is associated with a long, narrow pubic arch and an android pelvis. Fetal descent is arrested. Maternal complications include extensive perineal lacerations during vaginal birth because the fetal head is pushed posteriorly.

Soft Tissue Dystocia

Soft tissue dystocia results from obstruction of the birth passage by an anatomic abnormality other than that of

TABLE 24-1 Dysfunctional Labor: Primary and Secondary Powers

HYPERTONIC UTERINE DYSFUNCTION	HYPOTONIC UTERINE DYSFUNCTION	INADEQUATE VOLUNTARY EXPULSIVE FORCES
DESCRIPTION		
Usually occurs before 4 cm dilation; cause not yet known, may be related to fear and tension (primary powers) (Fig. 24-1)	Cause may be contracture and fetal malposition, overdistention of uterus (twins), or unknown (primary powers) (Fig. 24-1)	Involves abdominal and levator ani muscles Occurs in second stage of labor; cause may be related to conduction anesthetic, heavy analgesic, exhaustion
CHANGE IN PATTERN OF PROGRESS		
Pain out of proportion to intensity of contraction Pain out of proportion to effectiveness of contraction in effacing and dilating the cervix Contractions increase in frequency Contractions uncoordinated Uterus is contracted between contractions, cannot be indented	Contractions decrease in frequency and intensity Uterus easily indentable even at peak of contraction Uterus relaxed between contractions (normal)	No voluntary urge to push or bear down or else inadequate/ineffective pushing
POTENTIAL MATERNAL EFFECTS		
Loss of control related to intensity of pain and lack of progress Exhaustion	Infection Exhaustion Psychologic trauma	Spontaneous vaginal birth prevented
POTENTIAL FETAL EFFECTS		
Fetal asphyxia with meconium aspiration	Fetal infection Fetal and neonatal death	Fetal asphyxia
MEDICAL MANAGEMENT		
Rule out cephalopelvic disproportion Oxytocic stimulation of labor (p. 698)	Analgesic (e.g., morphine, meperidine) if membranes not ruptured or cephalopelvic disproportion not present Relief of pain permits mother to rest; when she awakens, normal uterine activity may begin	Coach mother in bearing down with contractions Position mother in favorable position for pushing Low forceps or vacuum extraction if assistance for vaginal birth is needed Cesarean birth only if nonreassuring fetal status occurs

the bony pelvis. The obstruction may result from placenta previa (low-lying placenta) that partially or completely obstructs the internal os of the cervix. Other causes, such as leiomyomas (uterine fibroids) in the lower uterine segment, ovarian tumors, and a full bladder or rectum, may prevent the fetus from entering the pelvis. Occasionally, *cervical edema* occurs in labor when the cervix is caught between the presenting part and the symphysis, preventing complete dilatation.

Bandl's ring, a pathologic retraction ring (see Fig. 9-10), is associated with prolonged rupture of membranes and protracted labor (Cunningham et al, 1993).

Fetal Causes

Dystocia of fetal origin may be caused by anomalies, excessive size and malpresentation, malposition, or multifetal pregnancy. Complications associated with dystocia of fetal origin include neonatal asphyxia, fetal injuries or fractures, and maternal vaginal lacerations. Although spontaneous vaginal birth is possible, fetal dystocia often leads to low forceps, vacuum extraction, or cesarean births.

Anomalies

Gross ascites, abnormal tumors, myelomeningocele, and hydrocephalus are fetal anomalies that can cause dystocia. These anomalies can affect the relationship of fetal anatomy to the maternal pelvic capacity, resulting in failure of the fetus to descend through the birth canal.

Cephalopelvic Disproportion

Cephalopelvic disproportion (CPD), or *fetopelvic disproportion (FPD)* related to excessive fetal size (4000 g [8 lb 13½ oz] or more) occurs in about 5% of term births. Excessive fetal size, or macrosomia, is associated with maternal diabetes mellitus, obesity, multiparity, or the large size of one or both parents. Shoulder dystocia, a condition in which the head is born but the anterior shoulder cannot pass under the pubic arch, can occur with macrosomia. When this occurs in a vaginal birth, the mother must be placed in a position to free the shoulders. The McRoberts maneuver, a maneuver in which the mother's legs are flexed with her knees on her abdomen, may be implemented (O'Leary, 1992). This maneuver causes the sacrum to straighten, and the symphysis pubic rotates toward the mother's head; the angle of pelvic inclination is decreased, freeing the shoulder (Fig. 24-2).

Malposition

The most common fetal malposition is persistent occipitoposterior position [right occipitoposterior (ROP) or left occipitoposterior (LOP); see Fig. 9-2], occurring in about 25% of all labors. Labor is prolonged, especially the second stage; the mother complains of severe back pain from the pressure of the fetal head against her sacrum. Counterpressure to the sacral area and frequent position changes may decrease the pain. The hands and knees or lateral position has been used to facilitate rotation of the fetus from a posterior to an anterior position (Biancuzzo, 1991; Fenwick, Simkin, 1987).

Fetal Malpresentation

Breech presentation is the most common example of malpresentation, occurring in 3% to 4% of all births and in up to 25% of preterm births. Four main types of breech presentation exist: frank breech (thighs flexed, knees extended); complete breech (thighs and knees flexed); incomplete breech, in which the foot extends below buttocks; and incomplete breech, in which the knee extends below buttocks (Fig. 24-3). Breech presentations are associated with multifetal gestation, preterm birth, fetal and maternal anomalies, hydramnios, and oligohydramnios. Diagnosis is made by abdominal palpation and vaginal examination and is usually confirmed by ultrasound scan.

During labor, fetal descent may be slow because the breech is not as good a dilating wedge as the fetal head, but labor usually is not prolonged. There is a risk of prolapsed cord if membranes rupture in early labor. Presence of meconium in amniotic fluid is not necessarily a sign of fetal distress because it results from pressure on the fetal abdominal wall as the fetus traverses the birth canal. Fetal heart tones are best heard at or above the umbilicus. Vaginal birth is accomplished by mechanisms related to emergence of the buttocks and lower extremities (Fig. 24-4). Piper forceps are sometimes used to deliver the head (see Fig. 24-8).

Breech presentation births are associated with birth trauma, asphyxiation, preterm birth, and congenital anomalies, which result in higher neonatal and perinatal morbity and mortality rates, as well as neurologic abnormalities later in life than occur in vertex presentation births (Englinton, 1988). Alternatives to vaginal birth of the fetus in breech presentation are *external cephalic version* (ECV), in which the fetus is turned to a vertex presentation by exerting pressure on the fetus externally through the maternal abdomen, and *cesarean birth,* in which the fetus is born through an abdominal incision.

Although options vary, cesarean birth (p. 702) is commonly performed for women with fetuses estimated to be larger than 3800 g (8 lb 6 oz) or smaller than 2000 g (4 lb 4 oz), or if labor is ineffective or complications occur (Bowes, 1989). Although cesarean birth reduces the risks to the fetus, maternal risks increase. External cephalic version (p. 696) also poses risks and is not always successful. Women with a breech presentation late in pregnancy need to be informed about their birth options, as well as the risks associated with each.

Face and brow presentations (Fig. 24-5) are uncommon and are associated with fetal anomalies, pelvic contractures, and fetopelvic disproportion. Vaginal birth is

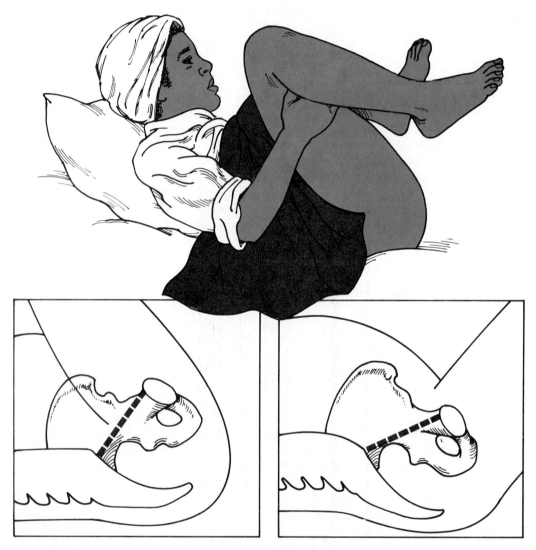

FIG. 24-2 McRoberts maneuver. (Modified from Gabbe S, Niebyl J, Simpson J: *Obstetrics, normal and problem pregnancies,* New York, 1986, Churchill-Livingstone).

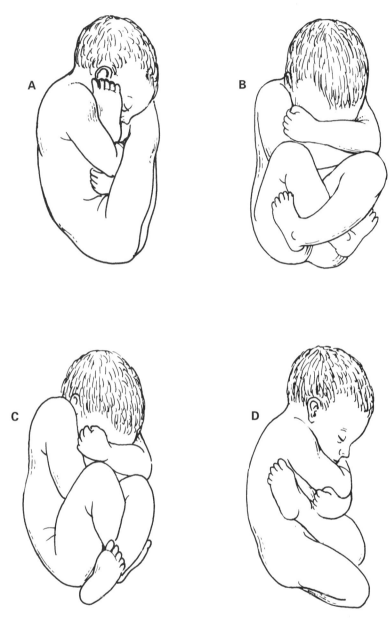

FIG. 24-3 Types of breech presentation. **A,** Frank breech: thighs are flexed on hips; knees are extended. **B,** Complete breech: thighs and knees are flexed. **C,** Incomplete breech: foot extends below buttocks. **D,** Incomplete breech: knee extends below buttocks.

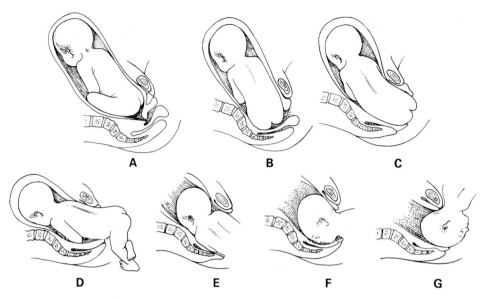

FIG. 24-4 Birth of infant in breech position. **A,** Breech before onset of labor. **B,** Engagement and internal rotation. **C,** Lateral flexion. **D,** External rotation or restitution. **E,** Internal rotation of shoulders and head. **F,** Face rotates to sacrum when occiput is anterior. **G,** Head is born by gradual flexion during elevation of fetal body.

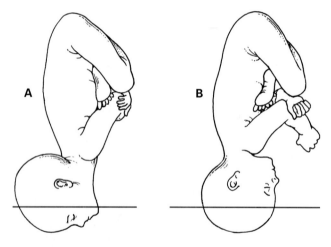

FIG. 24-5 Extension of normally flexed head. **A,** Face presentation. **B,** Brow presentation.

possible if the fetus flexes to a vertex presentation, although forceps often are used. Cesarean birth is indicated when the presentation persists, if there is fetal distress, or if labor progress stops.

Shoulder presentations, in which the fetus is in a transverse lie, usually require cesarean birth, although external cephalic version may be attempted after 38 weeks' gestation (Cunningham et al, 1993) (see Clinical Application of Research; see Fig. 9-3).

Multifetal Pregnancy

Multifetal pregnancy is the gestation of twins, triplets, quadruplets, or more infants. Infants of multifetal preg-

nancies account for 2% to 3% of all viable births and are associated with more complications, including dysfunctional labor, than are single births. The high incidence of complications and risk of perinatal mortality are primarily related to low-birth-weight (LBW) infants resulting from preterm birth and intrauterine growth retardation. In addition, fetal complications such as congenital anomalies and abnormal presentations can cause dystocia and increased incidence of cesarean birth. For example, only half of all twin pregnancies will have both fetuses presenting in the vertex position, the most favorable for vaginal birth; one third may present as one twin in vertex and one in breech. to accomplish a vaginal birth of both twins, an intrapartum external version may be attempted for the twin in a nonvertex position when the presenting twin's position is vertex. If the presenting twin is not in a vertex position, a cesarean birth is usually performed (Acker, Sachs, 1989; Adams, Chervenak, 1990).

Position of the Mother

The functional relationships between the uterine contractions, the fetus, and the mother's pelvis are altered by maternal positioning. In addition, positioning can provide either a mechanical advantage or disadvantage to the mechanisms of labor by altering the effects of gravity and the relationships among body parts that are significant to labor progress (Gilbert, Harmon, 1993). Discouraging maternal movement or restricting labor to the recumbent or lithotomy position may compromise labor. The incidence of dystocia increases, resulting in an increased need for augmentation of labor, use of forceps,

CLINICAL APPLICATION OF RESEARCH

ACCURACY OF LEOPOLD'S MANEUVERS IN SCREENING FOR MALPRESENTATION

Leopold's maneuvers, the systematic palpations of the abdomen, are used to determine the presentation of the fetus (i.e., cephalic, breech, or shoulder presentation) in the uterus. Knowledge of fetal presentation can provide the caregiver the opportunity to try to turn the fetus to a more favorable presentation or to prepare for a complicated birth. It is important that such a screening test be sensitive so that problems are identified and specific, and so that misdiagnosis is minimized. Ultrasound is an accurate, but expensive and not universally available diagnostic alternative. Concerns have been expressed about the safety of ultrasound.

The purpose of this study was to assess the accuracy of Leopold's maneuvers in screening for malpresentation. For the study, four nurse-midwives, who averaged 14 years of experience, performed Leopold's maneuvers on 150 women before giving the women ultrasound examinations. They found that 26 of the 150 women had fetal malpresentation. The nurse-midwives had identified 23 of the 26 malpresentations (88%) by using Leopold's maneuvers. In 116 of 124 cases (94%) the fetal presentation was correctly observed to be in the cephalic presentation. These results indicate that Leopold's maneuvers effectively test for fetal malpresentation. Nurses with less experience may not obtain similar results. Nurses who work with pregnant women need to practice Leopold's maneuvers until they become proficient. Leopold's maneuvers can be used as a low-cost, noninvasive, safe method of diagnosing fetal malpresentation.

Reference: Lydon-Rochelle M et al: Accuracy of Leopold maneuvers in screening for malpresentation: a prospective study, *Birth* 20(3):132, 1993.

vacuum extraction, and cesarean birth (Andrews, Chrzanowski, 1990).

Psychologic Response

Hormones released in response to stress can cause dystocia. Sources of stress vary for each individual, but pain and the absence of a support person are two accepted factors. Confinement to bed and restriction of maternal movement add a potential psychologic stress to compound the physiologic stress of immobility in the unmedicated laboring woman. When anxiety is excessive, it can inhibit normal cervical dilatation, resulting in *prolonged labor* and increased pain perception. Anxiety also causes increased levels of stress-related hormones (β-endorphin, adrenocorticotropic hormone [ACTH], cortisol, and epinephrine). The labor-inhibiting effects of excessive levels of these hormones are well documented (Simkin, 1986) and may be associated with dystotic labor patterns (Liu, 1989).

Abnormal Labor Patterns

Abnormal labor patterns occur in 8% of pregnancies, with the highest incidence among nulliparous women (Friedman, 1989). These patterns may result from the various causes previously described (ineffective uterine contractions, pelvic contractures, cephalopelvic disproportion, abnormal fetal presentations or position, early use of analgesics, conduction anesthesia, and anxiety and stress. Progress in either the first or second stage of labor can be protracted (delayed) or arrested. Abnormal progress can be recognized when cervical dilatation is plotted on a labor graph and compared with a normal labor curve. Fig. 24-6, *A* is a graphic representation of normal labor progress of a first-time mother.

The *latent phase* includes that portion of the first stage between the onset of labor contractions and the acceleration in rate of cervical dilatation. The upswing in the curve denotes the onset of the *active phase* of the first stage of labor, which is divided into an acceleration phase, a phase of maximum slope, and a deceleration phase. Compare these normal phases with Fig. 24-6, *B*, which shows major types of deviation from normal progress of labor. These can be detected by noting the dilatation of the cervix at various intervals after labor begins. If a woman exhibits an abnormal labor pattern as depicted by the broken lines, then the primary health care provider is notified.

Six abnormal labor patterns have been identified and classified by Friedman (1989) according to cervical dilatation and fetal descent. A prolonged latent phase is one that exceeds 20 hours or longer in nulliparous women and 14 hours or longer in the multiparous woman. The active phase of labor can also be complicated. In a protracted active phase, the cervix dilates less than 1.2 cm/hr in the nulliparous woman and less than 1.5 cm/hr in the multiparous woman. Arrest of the active phase is determined when neither the nulliparous nor multiparous woman demonstrates progress for more than 2 hours.

Descent of the presenting part also can be protracted or arrested in the active phase of labor. Active descent generally begins when cervical dilatation reaches the slope of maximum phase, with the rate of descent reaching its maximum at the beginning of the deceleration phase (about 9 cm). A protracted descent pattern is one in which the rate of descent is less than 1 cm/hr in the nulliparous woman and less than 2 cm/hr in the multiparous woman. Arrest of descent is the lack of progress

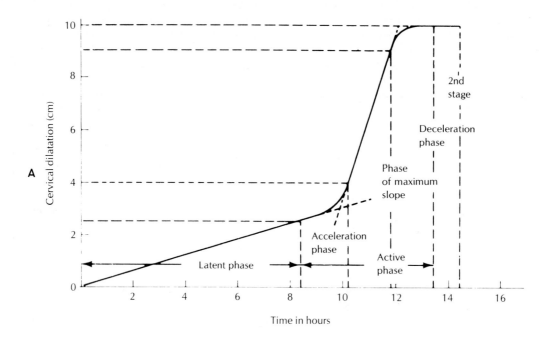

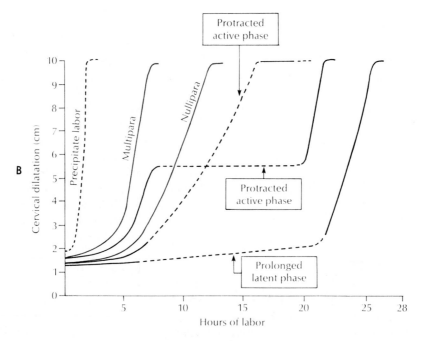

FIG. 24-6 **A,** Partogram of a normal labor. **B,** Major types of deviation from normal progress of labor may be detected by noting dilatation of cervix at various intervals after labor begins. If a woman exhibits an abnormal labor pattern as depicted by broken lines, then the health care provider should be notified immediately.

for more than 1 hour in both nulliparous and multiparous women. Failure of descent is a lack of descent of the presenting part during the deceleration phase and the second stage.

Fetal mortality increases sharply after 15 hours of the active first stage of labor. Maternal morbidity and mortality may occur as a result of uterine rupture, infection, serious dehydration, and postpartum hemorrhage. A long difficult labor also can have an adverse psychologic effect on the mother, father, and family. Management of prolonged labor depends on the cause and can include therapeutic rest, augmentation with oxytocin, forceps birth, vacuum extraction, and cesarean birth (Bowes, 1989).

Precipitous labor is defined as labor that lasts less than 3 hours from onset of contractions. Hypertonic uterine contractions may result in precipitous labor, characterized by tetanic-like contractions. Because labor is rapid, maternal and fetal complications can occur. Maternal complications include uterine rupture, lacerations of the birth canal, amniotic fluid embolism, and postpartum hemorrhage. Fetal complications include hypoxia caused by decreased periods of uterine relaxation between contractions and intracranial hemorrhage related to rapid birth (Cunningham et al, 1993). A summary of normal and abnormal labor patterns is given in Table 24-2.

TABLE 24-2 Labor Patterns in Normal and Abnormal Labor

NORMAL LABOR

1. Dilatation: continues
   a. Latent phase: <4 cm and low slope
   b. Active phase: >5 cm or high slope
   c. Deceleration phase: ≥9 cm
2. Descent: active at ≥9 cm dilatation

ABNORMAL LABOR

PATTERN	NULLIPARAS	MULTIPARAS
Prolonged latent phase	>20 hr	>14 hr
Protracted active phase dilatation	<1.2 cm/hr	<1.5 cm/hr
Secondary arrest: no change	≥2 hr	≥2 hr
Protracted descent	<1 cm/hr	<2 cm/hr
Arrest of descent	≥1 hr	≥½ hr
Failure of descent	no change during deceleration phase and second stage	
Precipitous labor	>5 cm/hr	>10 cm/hr

Care Management

✦ ASSESSMENT

Risk assessment is a continuous process. Review of the initial *interview* conducted at the woman's admission to the labor unit and ongoing observations of her psychologic response to labor reveal factors that can cause dysfunctional labor, for example, anxiety or fear, presence of a complication of pregnancy, or previous labor complications. The initial *physical assessment* data and ongoing assessments provide information about the frequency, duration, and intensity of uterine contractions, cervical status, fetal heart rate (FHR), presentation and station of the fetus, and status of membranes. *Laboratory data* such as scalp pH can identify fetal distress; ultrasound findings can identify potential dysfunctional labor problems related to the fetus or maternal pelvis. All these assessments contribute to accurate identification of potential and actual nursing diagnoses related to dystocia and maternal-fetal compromise.

✦ NURSING DIAGNOSES

Nursing diagnoses vary with the type of dystocia, as well as with the individual needs of the woman and her family. Potential or actual nursing diagnoses that might be identified for women experiencing dystocia include the following:

Anxiety related to
  ▪ Slowed labor progress
Pain related to
  ▪ Dystocia
  ▪ Obstetric procedures
High risk for fetal injury related to
  ▪ Fetal compromise
High risk for maternal injury related to
  ▪ Interventions implemented for dystocia
Powerlessness related to
  ▪ Loss of control
High risk for infection related to
  ▪ Rupture of membranes, operative procedures
Fatigue related to
  ▪ Prolonged labor
Fear related to
  ▪ Real or potential threat to self or fetus
Impaired tissue integrity related to
  ▪ Operative procedures
High risk for altered parenting related to
  ▪ Unplanned cesarean birth
Altered sensory perception overload related to
  ▪ Numerous interventions for dystocia
Ineffective individual coping related to
  ▪ Disappointment
  ▪ Pain
  ▪ Fear

- Exhaustion
- Lack of support system

Knowledge deficit related to
- Procedures, positioning, relaxation techniques, etc.

Situational low self-esteem related to
- Inability to labor and give birth as expected

Fluid volume excess related to
- Intravenous infusion with oxytocin

Fluid volume deficit related to
- NPO status

❖ EXPECTED OUTCOMES

Nursing diagnoses provide direction for care. During this important step, expected outcomes are set in patient-centered terms and then prioritized. Nursing actions are selected with the patient, as appropriate, to meet the expected outcomes.

Expected outcomes for the woman who experiences dystocia include the following:

- She will understand the causes and treatment of dysfunctional labor.
- She will utilize positive patterns of coping to maintain a positive self-concept.
- She will demonstrate diminished or minimal anxiety.
- She will express relief of pain.
- She will experience labor and birth with minimal or no complications such as infection, injury, or hemorrhage.
- She will give birth to a healthy infant who has not experienced fetal distress.

❖ COLLABORATIVE CARE

Nurses assume many caregiving roles when labor is complicated. Knowledge of medical management for each condition is essential to implementing the nursing process. This knowledge enables the nurse to work collaboratively with other health care providers and to meet the woman's knowledge and emotional needs. Interventions include external cephalic version, trial of labor, induction/augmentation with oxytocin, amniotomy, and operative procedures such as forceps-assisted birth, vacuum extraction, and cesarean birth.

External Cephalic Version

External cephalic version (ECV) is the attempt to turn the fetus from a breech or shoulder presentation to a vertex presentation for birth. ECV may be attempted in a labor and birth setting after 37 weeks' gestation. Before attempting ECV, ultrasound scanning is used to determine the fetal position in order to rule out placenta previa, and assess the amount of amniotic fluid, the fetal age, and the presence of any anomalies. A non-stress test is performed to ensure fetal well-being.

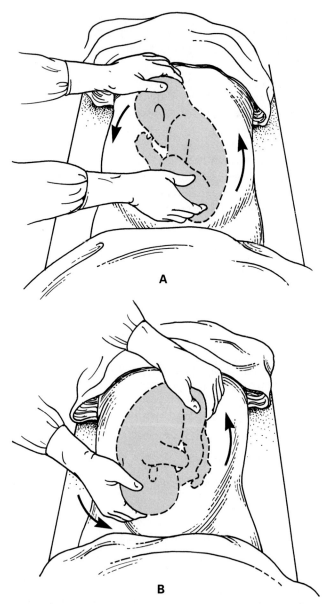

FIG. 24-7 External version of fetus from breech to vertex presentation. This must be achieved without force. **A,** Breech is pushed up out of pelvic inlet while head is pulled toward inlet. **B,** Head is pushed toward inlet while breech is pulled upward.

Informed consent is obtained. The ECV is accomplished by gentle, constant pressure accompanied by continuous fetal heart surveillance (Fig. 24-7). A tocolytic agent, such as ritodrine or terbutaline (p. 715), may be given intravenously to relax the uterus and facilitate the maneuver. Ultrasound may be used to identify potential problems such as cord entanglement and placental separation (Englinton, 1988).

During an attempted ECV, the nurse continuously monitors the FHR, especially for bradycardia, checks maternal vital signs frequently, and assesses the woman's level of comfort because the procedure may cause discomfort. After the procedure is completed, the nurse continues to monitor maternal vital signs, uterine activity, and FHR. The nurse also assesses for vaginal bleeding until the woman's condition stabilizes.

Trial of Labor

A **trial of labor (TOL)** is a reasonable period (4 to 6 hours) of active labor. It allows assessment of the possibility for a safe vaginal birth for both the mother and the infant. TOL may be initiated when the mother's pelvis is of questionable size or shape, when she wishes to have a vaginal birth after a previous cesarean birth, and when the fetus shows an abnormal presentation. Fetal sonography and/or maternal pelvimetry is used before a TOL to rule out fetopelvic disproportion. The cervix must be soft and dilatable. During TOL, the woman is evaluated for active labor, including adequate contractions, engagement and descent of the presenting part, and effacement and dilatation of the cervix. Induction of labor is seldom implemented.

LEGAL TIP: **Standard of Care-Labor and Birth at Risk**

Document all assessments, interventions, and patient responses on patient record and monitor strips.

Assess whether the woman is fully informed about the procedures for which she is consenting.

Maintain safety in correctly administering medications and treatments.

Get verbal orders signed as soon as possible.

Provide care at the acceptable standard (e.g., according to hospital protocols).

If short staffing occurs in the unit and the nurse continues the present assignment, then the nurse should document that rejecting the assignment would have placed the patient in danger as a result of abandonment.

Maternal and fetal monitoring continues until birth even when a decision for cesarean birth is made.

The nurse assesses uterine activity, cervical changes, maternal vital signs, and fetal status during this TOL. If maternal or fetal complications are identified, the nurse is responsible for initiating appropriate actions, including notifying the health care provider and evaluating and documenting the maternal or fetal response to the interventions.

Induction of Labor

Induction of labor is the initiation of uterine contractions before their spontaneous onset for the purpose of bringing about the birth. Induction may be indicated for a variety of medical and obstetric reasons, including

TABLE 24-3   Bishop Score

	SCORE			
	0	1	2	3
Dilatation (cm)	0	1 to 2	3 to 4	5 to 6
Efface-ment (%)	0 to 30	40 to 50	60 to 70	80
Station (cm)	−3	−2	−1	−1
Cervical consis-tency	Firm	Medium	Soft	
Cervix posi-tion	Posterior	Midline	Anterior	

pregnancy-induced hypertension, diabetes mellitus and other maternal medical problems, postterm gestation, suspected fetal jeopardy (e.g., intrauterine growth retardation), logistic factors (e.g., rate of rapid birth, distance from the hospital, and fetal death). Under such conditions childbirth is less of a risk for the newborn or fetus than is the continuation of pregnancy (Dunn, 1990).

Both chemical and mechanical methods are used to induce labor. Intravenous oxytocin and amniotomy are the most common methods used in the United States. Less commonly used methods of induction include nipple stimulation, ingestion of castor oil, soapsuds enema, stripping of membranes, and acupuncture (Tal et al, 1988; ACOG, 1991).

Success rates for induction of labor are higher when the cervix is favorable or inducible. A rating system such as the **Bishop score** (Table 24-3) can be used to evaluate inducibility. For example, a score of nine or more on this 13-point scale indicates that the cervix is soft, anterior, 50% effaced, and dilated 2 cm or more; the presenting part is engaged. Induction of labor is more likely to be successful if the score is five or more for multiparas and nine or more for nulliparas.

Cervical Ripening Methods

Different **prostaglandins** (hormones) have been applied to the cervix before induction to induce or "ripen" (soften and thin) the cervix. PGE_2 gel was approved in 1993 by the FDA as a cervical ripening agent in the United States. The gel may be administered through a catheter into the cervical canal or applied to a diaphragm that is placed next to the cervix. Additional doses may be reapplied every 4 to 6 hours. Two to three doses are usually sufficient. Oxytocin induction usually is not started until 4 to 6 hours later to avoid hyperstimulation (ACOG, 1993). Side effects of PGE_2, which include vomiting, fever, diarrhea, and hyperstimulation of the uterus, are uncommon with gel applications (Husslein, 1991; Sokol, Brindley, 1990).

Nursing assessments after the gel has been administered are similar to those performed for women whose labor is induced with oxytocin.

Laminaria tents (natural cervical dilators made from seaweed) and synthetic dilators are also effective in ripening the cervix. The dilators are inserted into the cervix. As the dilators absorb cervical fluids, they expand and cause cervical dilatation (Blumenthal, Ramanauskas, 1990).

Amniotomy

Amniotomy (artificial rupture of membranes [AROM]) can be used to stimulate labor when the condition of the cervix is favorable. Labor usually begins within 12 hours of the rupture; however, if amniotomy does not stimulate labor, prolonged rupture may lead to infection. For this reason, amniotomy is often used in combination with oxytocin induction. Before the procedure, the nurse gives the woman an explanation of what to expect and assures her that the procedure is painless for her and her fetus. The membranes are ruptured with an amnihook or other sharp instrument; amniotic fluid is allowed to drain slowly. The fluid is assessed for color, odor, and consistency (i.e., absence of meconium or blood). The time of rupture is recorded. The fetal heart rate (FHR) is assessed before and after the procedure to detect changes that may indicate presence of cord compression or prolapse. The patient's temperature should be checked at least every 2 to 4 hours to rule out possible infection. The primary care provider is notified if the temperature is greater than 100.4° F (38° C). Comfort measures, such as changing the patient's underpads frequently, should be implemented, since the amniotic fluid will continue to leak from the vagina after rupture of the membranes.

Oxytocin

Oxytocin, a hormone normally produced by the posterior pituitary gland, stimulates uterine contractions. Oxytocin may be used either to induce the labor process or to augment a labor that is progressing slowly because of inadequate uterine contractions.

The *indications* for oxytocin induction of labor may include, but are not limited to, the following:
- Suspected fetal jeopardy
- Need to stimulate the uterus
- Premature rupture of membranes (PROM)
- Postterm pregnancy (42 to 43 weeks)
- Maternal medical problems (e.g., diabetic mother or mother with severe Rh isoimmunization)
- Pregnancy-associated hypertensive diseases
- Multiparous women with a history of precipitous labor who live far away from the hospital

The management of stimulation of labor is the same

regardless of indication. Because of the potential dangers associated with the use of injectable oxytocin in the prenatal and intranatal periods, the FDA has placed restrictions on its use.

Contraindications to oxytocic stimulation of labor include, but are not limited to, the following:
- Cephalopelvic disproportion (CPD)
- Nonreassuring FHR
- Placenta previa
- Prior classic uterine incision or uterine surgery
- Active genital herpes infection

Oxytocin can present hazards to both mother and fetus. Maternal hazards include tumultuous labor and tetanic contractions, which may cause premature separation of the placenta, rupture of the uterus, laceration of the cervix, or postbirth hemorrhage. These complications can cause infection, disseminated intravascular coagulation, and amniotic fluid pulmonary embolism. Women also may become anxious or fearful if the induction is not successful because of concerns they may have about the method of birth.

Fetal hazards include fetal asphyxia and neonatal hypoxia from too frequent and prolonged uterine contractions, physical injury, and prematurity, if the estimated date of birth is inaccurate.

Initiation of induction or augmentation of labor with oxytocin is the responsibility of the primary health care provider, although the medication often is administered by a nurse. A written protocol for the preparation and administration of oxytocin should be established by the obstetric department in each institution. Until recently,

E M E R G E N C Y

UTERINE HYPERSTIMULATION WITH OXYTOCIN

SIGNS

Uterine contractions >90 seconds, occurring in intervals every 2 minutes
Uterine resting tone >20 mm Hg
Nonreassuring FHR
—Abnormal baseline rate
—Absent variability
—Repeated late decelerations or prolonged decelerations

INTERVENTIONS

Maintain woman in side-lying position
Turn off oxytocin; keep maintenance IV line open; increase rate
Start oxygen via face mask
Notify primary health care provider
Continue monitoring of FHR and uterine activity
Document responses to actions

the aim of induction with oxytocin was to achieve a contraction pattern that simulated the active phase of labor as quickly as possible. Recent research on uterine tolerance to oxytocin has shown that lower doses given at longer intervals are as effective as previous protocols and are less likely to cause uterine hyperstimulation and dysfunctional labor (Brodsky, Pelzar, 1991; Mercer, Pilgrim, Sibai, 1991).

Another method under study that uses less oxytocin without loss of effectivenss is pulsatile oxytocin administration. Oxytocin is given in 10-second pulses every 8 minutes. The initial dose is 1 mU/pulse, and is doubled every 24 minutes until reaching a maximum dose of 32 mU/pulse (Cummiskey, Dawood, 1990).

After the woman has been evaluated for induction, the following recommended procedures are performed in a labor and birth setting (ACOG, 1991; Association of Women's Health, Obstetric and Neonatal Nurses, 1993; Davis, 1992):

- A primary intravenous infusion of a physiologic electrolytic fluid is started. Intravenous medications other than oxytocin can be administered through this line. The nurse explains the procedure, the rationale, and what to expect (uterine contractions will become stronger and will occur more often and more regularly).
- A secondary intravenous infusion containing dilute oxytocin (usually 10 U/1000 ml) is added to the main line. This line should be connected close to the primary venipuncture site. No medication except oxytocin should be given through this line. Oxytocin should be administered through a pump delivery system to ensure accurate dose and safe administration.
- Oxytocin is administered according to prescribed orders or protocol. Initial dosages of 0.5 to 3 mU/min, with increases of 1 to 2 mU/min, may be administered at 15-minute to 60-minute intervals until the desired contraction pattern is achieved. That is, contractions are of 40 to 90 seconds' duration and 2 to 3 minutes apart; intensity is 40 to 90 mm Hg if intrauterine pressure is being monitored internally.
- Once the cervix is dilated 5 to 6 cm and labor is established, the oxytocin dose can be reduced by similar decrements.
- Usually no more than 20 mU oxytocin per minute are needed to achieve progressive cervical dilatation. In many cases, less than 4 mU/min are needed (Sokol, Brindley, 1990).
- The FHR; uterine resting tone; and frequency, duration, and intensity of contractions are monitored continuously (electronic fetal-maternal monitoring is suggested), intrauterine monitoring is often instituted using an intrauterine pressure catheter); and maternal blood pressure and pulse are monitored at 30-minute to 60-minute intervals and/or when doses are changed.
- The nurse assesses intake and output to prevent water intoxication. The intravenous intake usually is limited to 1000 ml in 8 hours (125 ml/hr); urine output should be 120 ml or more in 4 hours.
- The nurse also assesses for side effects of nausea, vomiting, headache, or hypotension.
- *Oxytocin is discontinued immediately and the primary health care provider notified of uterine hyperstimulation or nonreassuring FHR.* With the latter, other nursing interventions, such as administration of oxygen by face mask and positioning the woman on her side, are implemented immediately (see Emergency box).
- Documentation of maternal and fetal assessments is necessary in the medical record and on the fetal monitor tracing. In addition, the woman and her support persons are kept informed of her progress.

Augmentation

Augmentation of labor is the stimulation of uterine contractions after labor has started spontaneously, yet progress is unsatisfactory. Augmentation usually is implemented for hypotonic dysfunctional labor. The procedures and nursing assessments used are the same as those used for oxytocin induction of labor.

Some health care providers advocate active management of labor, that is, intervention with augmentation of labor as soon as labor is not progressing at least 1 cm/hr. Advocates of active management indicate that intervening early with aggressive use of oxytocin (increases of 6 mU/min) shortens labor (usually 12 hours or less) and reduces the incidence of cesarean birth (Akoury et al, 1988; Akoury et al, 1991; Turner, Brassil, Gordon, 1988). These practices are currently under study in the United States to determine the effectiveness and impact on perinatal morbidity and mortality.

The Protocol box found on p. 700 summarizes the nursing responsibilities for induction of labor by oxytocin administration.

Forceps-Assisted Birth

In **forceps-assisted birth,** two instruments with curved blades are used to assist in the birth of the fetal head. The cephalic-like curve of the commonly used forceps is similar to the shape of the fetal head. A pelvic curve of the blades conforms to the pelvic axis. The blades are joined by a pin, screw, or groove arrangement. These locks prevent the forceps from compressing the fetal skull. Maternal indications for forceps-assisted birth include the need to shorten the second stage in dystocia (difficult labor) or to correct the mother's deficient expulsive efforts (e.g., she is tired or has been given spinal or epidural anesthesia), as well as to reverse a dangerous condition (e.g., cardiac decompensation).

Fetal indications include birth of a fetus in distress, in certain abnormal presentations, or in arrest of rotation, as well as to birth an aftercoming head in a breech presentation (Dennan, 1989).

Certain conditions are required for a successful forceps-assisted birth. The woman's cervix must be fully dilated to avoid lacerations and hemorrhage. The presenting part must be engaged, and a vertex presentation is desired. Membranes should be ruptured so that the position of the fetal head can be determined and so that a firm grasp of the forceps on the head during birth can be ensured. Cephalopelvic disproportion (CPD) should not be present. To avoid lacerations and injury, the woman's bladder should not be distended, and an episiotomy may be performed to facilitate placement of the forceps (Sokol, Brindley, 1990).

There are different definitions of forceps applications. According to ACOG (1988), *outlet* forceps are appropriate when the fetal scalp is visible on the perineum without manually separating the labia. Outlet forceps are used to shorten the second stage of labor. *Low* forceps is the term used when forceps are applied to the fetal head that is at least at +2 station. *Midforceps* are defined as forceps applied when the fetal head is engaged (no higher than station 0) but above a +2. There are no circumstances when forceps should be applied to an unengaged presenting part.

Nursing Considerations

The nurse obtains forceps designated by the physician (Fig. 24-8). The FHR is checked, reported, and recorded *before* forceps are *applied*. The mother is informed that

PROTOCOL
Induction of Labor with Oxytocin

OXYTOCIN ADMINISTRATION

Patient/Family Teaching:

Explain technique, rationale, and reactions to expect:
- Route and rate
  What "piggyback" is for
- Reasons for use:
    Induce labor
    Improve labor
- Reactions to expect concerning the nature of contractions. The intensity of contraction increases more rapidly, holds the peak longer, and ends more quickly. The contractions will begin to come regularly and more often.
- Monitoring to anticipate:
    Maternal: blood pressure, pulse, uterine contractions, uterine tone
    Fetal: heart rate, activity
- Success to expect: a favorable outcome will depend on inducibility of the cervix (Bishop score of nine or more for nullipara; five or more for multipara)

Administration:

Position woman in side-lying position.
Prepare solutions and administer according to prescribed orders with pump delivery system:
- Infusion pump and solution is set up
- Piggyback solution is connected to IV line
  Solution with oxytocin is flagged with a medication label
  Begin induction at 0.5 to 1.0 mU/min
  Increase dose 1 to 2 mU/min at intervals of 30 to 60 minutes for up to 20 mU/min or 300 montevideo units are reached

Maintain dose when:
- Intensity of contractions results in intrauterine pressures of 40 to 90 mm Hg (by internal monitor)
- Duration of contraction is 40 to 90 sec
- Frequency of contractions is 2 to 3 min intervals

Maternal/Fetal Assessments:
- Monitor blood pressure and pulse every 30 to 60 minutes
- Monitor contraction pattern every 15 minutes
- Assess intake and output; limit IV intake to 1000 ml/8 hr; output should be 120 ml or more every 4 hours.
- Monitor for nausea, vomiting, headache, hypotension.
- Assess fetal status according to hospital protocol; electronic fetal monitoring is recommended

Reportable Conditions:
- Uterine hyperstimulation
- Nonreassuring FHR/pattern
- Suspected uterine rupture

Emergency Measures:

Discontinue use of oxytocin per hospital protocol:
- Turn woman on her side
- Increase primary IV rate up to 200 ml/hr unless patient has water intoxication; in presense of water intoxication, rate will be decreased to a rate that keeps the vein open
- Give woman oxygen by face mask at 8 to 10 L/min

Documentation:
- Medication: kind, amount, time of beginning, increasing dose, maintaining dose, and discontinuing medication in patient record and on monitoring strip
- Reactions of mother and fetus:
    Pattern of labor
    Progress of labor
    FHR
    Maternal vital signs
    Nursing interventions and woman's response
- Notification of primary health care provider

the forceps blades fit like two tablespoons around an egg. The blades come over the baby's ears. The FHR is rechecked, reported, and recorded *before traction* is applied after application of forceps. Compression of the cord between the fetal head and the forceps would cause a drop in FHR. The physician would then remove and reapply the forceps.

After birth, the mother is assessed for vaginal and cervical lacerations (bleeding occurs even with a contracted uterus) and urine retention, which may result from bladder injuries. The infant should be assessed for bruising or abrasions at the site of the blade applications, facial palsy resulting from pressure of the blades on the facial (Cranial VII) nerve, and subdural hematoma. Newborn and postpartum caregivers should be informed that a forceps-assisted birth was performed.

Vacuum Extraction

Vacuum extraction is a birth method involving the attachment of a vacuum cup to the fetal head, using negative pressure. It is a popular alternative to forceps birth in Europe and is gaining popularity in the United States. Indications for the use of vacuum extraction are similar to those for outlet forceps, but it is especially appropriate in cases of failure to rotate and arrest of the second stage of labor (Galvan, Broekhuizen, 1987). Prerequisites for use include a vertex presentation, ruptured membranes, and absence of fetopelvic disproportion.

The woman is prepared for a vaginal birth in the lithotomy position to allow for sufficient traction. The cup is applied to the fetal head, and a caput develops inside the cup as the pressure is initiated (Fig. 24-9). Traction is then applied to facilitate descent of the fetal head. As the head crowns, an *episiotomy* is performed if necessary and the vacuum cup is released and removed after birth of the head. If vacuum extraction is unsuccessful, a forceps-assisted or cesarean birth should be performed.

Risks to the newborn include cephalhematoma, scalp lacerations, and subdural hematoma. Maternal complications are uncommon but can include perineal, vaginal and cervical lacerations.

Nursing Considerations

The nurse's role for the woman who has given birth by use of vacuum extraction is one of support person and educator. The nurse can prepare the woman for birth and encourage her to remain active in the birth process by

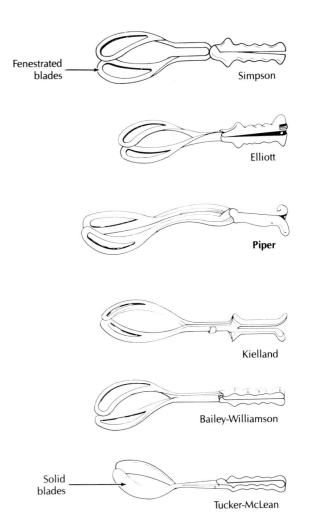

FIG. 24-8 Types of forceps. Piper forceps are used to assist birth of the aftercoming head in breech birth.

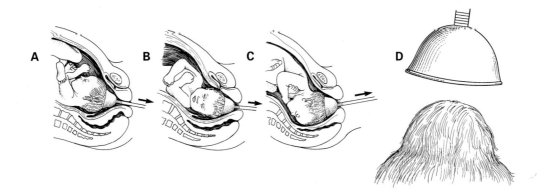

FIG. 24-9 Use of vacuum extraction to rotate fetal head and assist with descent.

pushing during contractions. Also, the FHR should be assessed frequently during the procedure. After birth, the newborn should be observed for signs of infection at the application site and cerebral irritation (e.g., poor sucking, listlessness). The parents may need to be reassured that the caput succedaneum will begin to disappear in a few hours. Neonatal caregivers should be alerted that the birth was by vacuum extraction.

Cesarean Birth

Cesarean birth is the birth of a fetus through a transabdominal incision of the uterus. Although the myth persists that Julius Caesar was born in this manner, the derivation of the term is more likely from the Latin word *caedo* meaning "to cut." Whether cesarean birth is planned (scheduled) or unplanned (emergency), the woman's loss of the experience of giving birth to a child in the traditional manner may have a negative effect on her self-concept. An effort is made to maintain the focus on the *birth* of a child rather than on the operative prodcedure. The mother experiences abdominal rather than vaginal birth.

The basic purpose or use of cesarean birth is to perserve the life or health of the mother and her fetus. The use of cesarean birth is based on evidence of maternal or fetal stress. Maternal and fetal morbidity and mortality have decreased since the advent of modern surgical methods and care. However, cesarean birth still poses threats to the health of both mother and infant (see Ethical Considerations). The technique of cesarean surgery has changed. Today incisions into the lower uterine segment rather than into the muscular body of the uterus permit a more effective healing.

The incidence of cesarean births has increased dramatically in the last 25 years. From the mid-1960s to the late 1980s, the cesarean birth rate in the United States increased from less than 5% to almost 24% (Taffel, Placek, Kosary, 1992). Reasons cited for this increase include increased use of electronic fetal monitoring, an increase in the number of first-time pregnancies, as well as pregnancy at an older age, and the high incidence of repeat cesarean births (Dunn, 1990; Martel et al, 1987; Silver, Wolfe, 1989). In 1992 this rate dropped slightly to 22.6% (Public Citizen, 1994). This decline may be attributed, in part, to more attempts at having a vaginal birth after giving birth by cesarean.

Indications

There are few absolute indications for cesarean birth. Today most cesarean births are performed for the benefit of the fetus. Four diagnostic categories are responsible for 75% to 90% of cesarean births: dystocia, repeat cesarean, breech presentation, and fetal distress (Marieskind, 1989). Other indications for the procedure include active herpes viral infection, prolapsed umbilical cord, medical complications such as pregnancy-induced hypertension, placental abnormalities such as placenta previa and premature separation (abruption), malpresentations such as shoulder presentation, and fetal anomalies such as hydrocephaly.

Surgical Techniques

The two main types of cesarean operation are *classic* and *lower segment* cesarean births. Classic cesarean birth is rarely performed today; however, it may be used when rapid birth is necessary and in some cases of shoulder presentation and placenta previa. The incision is vertical into the upper body of the uterus (Fig. 24-10, *A*). This procedure is associated with a higher incidence of blood loss, infection, and uterine rupture in subsequent pregnancies than is lower segment cesarean birth.

Lower segment cesarean birth can be performed through a vertical (Sellheim) or transverse (Kerr) incision (Fig. 24-10, *B* and *C*). The transverse incision is more popular because it is easier to perform, is associated with less blood loss and fewer postoperative infections, and is less likely to rupture in subsequent pregnancies (Cunningham et al, 1993; Dunn, 1990). Vaginal birth after cesarean is contraindicated with classic incisions.

Complications/Risks

Cesarean births are not without complications for both the mother and the fetus. Maternal complications occur in 25% to 50% of births and include aspiration, pulmonary embolism, wound infection, wound dehiscence, thrombophlebitis, hemorrhage, urinary tract infection, injuries to bladder or bowel, and complications related to anesthesia. There are also risks that the fetus will be born prematurely if gestational age is not accurately assessed and that fetal injuries can occur during surgery (Dunn, 1990). In addition, the woman is at economic

ETHICAL CONSIDERATIONS

FORCED CESAREAN BIRTH

Refusal of a cesarean birth for fetal reasons by a woman is often described as a maternal-fetal conflict. Health care providers are ethically obliged to protect the well-being of both the mother and the fetus; it is difficult to make a decision for one without affecting the other. If a woman refuses a cesarean that is needed, health care providers need to make every effort to find out why she is refusing and provide information to persuade her to change her mind. If the woman continues to refuse surgery, then health care providers must decide if it is ethically right to force her to make the decision and to try and get a court order for the surgery. Every effort should be made to avoid this legal step.

risk because the cost of a cesarean birth is higher than that of vaginal birth, and a longer recovery period may require additional expenditures.

Many women who experience cesarean birth speak of feelings that interfere with their maintenance of an adequate self-concept. These feelings include fear, disappointment, frustration at losing control, anger (the "why me" syndrome), and loss of self-esteem related to a change in body image. Success in mothering activities and in the recovery process can do much to restore these women's self-esteems. Some women see the scar as mutilating, and worries concerning sexual attractiveness may surface. Some men are nervous about resuming intercourse because of the fear of hurting their mates. Parents will wonder if a cesarean birth was absolutely necessary. Such feelings may surface even years later.

Anesthesia

Spinal, epidural, and general anesthetics are used for cesarean births. Since the 1970s, epidural blocks have increased in popularity because women have wanted to be awake for and aware of the birth experience. However, the choice of anesthetic depends on several factors. The

mother's medical history or present condition, such as a spinal injury or hemorrhage, may contraindicate the use of regional anesthesia. Time is another factor, especially if an emergency arises and the life of the mother or infant is at stake. Then general anesthetic will most likely be used. The woman herself is a factor. She may not know all the options, or she may have fears about "a needle in her back" or about being awake and feeling pain. The woman needs to be fully informed about the risks and benefits of the different types of anesthesia so that she can participate in the decision whenever there is a choice.

Scheduled Cesarean Birth

Women face scheduled or planned cesarean birth when labor is contraindicated (e.g., placenta previa), when birth is necessary but labor is not inducible (e.g., hypertensive states that cause a poor intrauterine environment that threatens the fetus), or when a decision is made between the health care provider and the woman (e.g., a repeat cesarean birth). These women usually have time for psychologic preparation, although they may have concerns about surgery, as well as being able to cope with infant care in addition to recovering from surgery.

Emergency Cesarean Birth

Women having emergency or unplanned cesarean births share with their families abrupt changes in their expectations for birth, postbirth care, and the care of the new baby at home. This may be an extremely traumatic experience. The woman usually approaches surgery tired and discouraged after a fruitless labor. She is worried about her own and her infant's condition. She may be dehydrated and have low glycogen reserves. All preoperative procedures must be done quickly and competently. The time for explanation of procedures and of the operation is short. Because maternal and family anxiety levels are high, much of what is said is forgotten or misconstrued. After surgery, time must be spent reviewing the events preceding the operation and the operation itself to ensure that the woman understands what has happened. Fatigue is often noticeable in these women. They need much supportive care.

Prenatal Preparation

Concerned professional and lay groups in the community have established councils for cesarean birth to meet the needs of these women and their families. Such groups advocate the inclusion of preparation for cesarean birth in all parenthood preparation classes. No woman can be guaranteed a vaginal birth, even if she is in good health and there is no indication of danger to the fetus before the onset of labor. Every woman needs to be aware of and prepared for this possibility. The unknown and unexpected are ego weakening.

Childbirth educators stress the importance of empha-

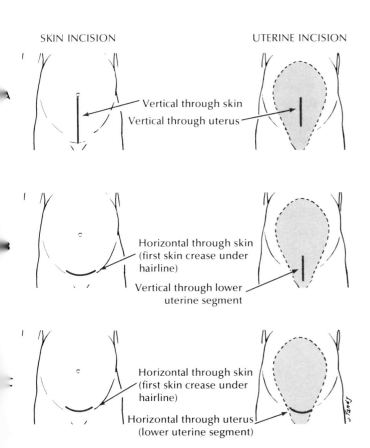

SKIN INCISION   UTERINE INCISION

Vertical through skin
Vertical through uterus

Horizontal through skin
(first skin crease under hairline)
Vertical through lower uterine segment

Horizontal through skin
(first skin crease under hairline)
Horizontal through uterus
(lower uterine segment)

FIG. 24-10   Cesarean birth: skin and uterine incisions. **A,** Classic: vertical incisions of skin and uterus. **B,** Low cervical: horizontal incision of skin; vertical incision of uterus. **C,** Low cervical: horizontal incisions of skin and uterus.

sizing both the similarities and differences between cesarean and vaginal birth. Also, in support of the philosophy of family-centered birth, many hospitals have policies that permit fathers to share in these births as they have in vaginal ones. Women undergoing cesarean birth agree that the continued presence and support of their partners have helped them respond positively to the entire experience (Fawcett, Henklein, 1987).

Care during Cesarean Birth

The goal for the woman and her family is family-centered care for a cesarean birth. The *preparation* of the woman for cesarean birth is the same for either elective or emergency surgery. The obstetrician discusses the need for the cesarean birth and the prognosis for mother and infant with the woman and her family. The anesthesiologist assesses the woman's cardiopulmonary system and presents the options for types of anesthesia. Informed consent is obtained for the procedure.

Maternal vital signs and blood pressure and FHR continue to be assessed per hospital routine until the operation begins. Physical preoperative preparation usually includes an abdominal-mons shave or clipping of pubic hair (Gallup, 1988), inserting a retention catheter to keep the bladder empty, and administration of prescribed preoperative medications. An antacid is often prescribed to prevent aspiration of acidic gastric secretions into the patient's lungs. Intravenous fluids are started to maintain hydration and to provide an open line for administration of blood or medications if needed. Blood and urine samples are collected and sent to the laboratory for analysis. Laboratory tests, usually ordered to establish baseline data, include a complete blood cell count and chemistry, type and cross-matching, and urinalysis.

Dentures and nail polish are removed, but removal of jewelry may be optional depending on hospital policies. If the patient wears glasses and is going to be awake, the nurse should make sure her glasses accompany her to the operating room so she can see her infant. If the patient wears contact lenses, the nurse can find out whether they can be worn for the birth.

During preoperative preparation the support person is encouraged to remain with the woman as much as possible to provide continuing emotional support (Shearer Shiono, Rhoads, 1988). During the preoperative preparation the nurse provides essential information about the procedures. Although the nursing actions may be carried out quickly when the cesarean birth is unplanned, verbal communication, particularly explanations, is important. Silence can be frightening to the woman and her support person. The nurse's use of touch can communicate feelings of care and concern for the patient.

The nurse should assess the woman's and her partner's perceptions about the cesarean birth. As the woman expresses her feelings, the nurse may identify potential for disturbance in self-concept during the postpartum period. For example, the woman may feel that she is a failure because she did not have a vaginal birth, and that this was her fault.

If there is time before the birth, the nurse can teach the woman about postoperative expectations, pain relief, turning, coughing, and deep breathing.

Once the woman has been taken to surgery, her care becomes the responsibility of the obstetric team, surgeon, anesthesiologist, pediatrician, and surgical nursing staff (Fig. 24-11). If possible, the father, gowned appropriately, accompanies the mother to the surgical unit and remains close to her so that he can continue to provide support and comfort.

The nurse, who is circulating, may assist with positioning the woman on the birth (surgical) table. It is important to position her so that the uterus is displaced laterally to avoid compressing the inferior vena cava, which causes decreased placental perfusion (Bowes, 1989).

If the father is not allowed or chooses not to be present during the cesarean birth, the nurse can stay in communication with him and give progress reports when possible. If the mother is awake during the birth, the nurse can tell her what is happening and provide support. The mother may be anxious about the sensations she is experiencing, such as cold solutions used to prepare the abdomen and pressure or pulling during the actual birth of the infant. She also may be apprehensive because of the bright lights, unfamiliar equipment present, and masked and gowned personnel in the room (see Clinical Application of Research).

Care of the infant is delegated to a pediatrician and a nurse who is skilled in neonatal resuscitation because these infants are considered to be at risk until there is evidence of physiologic stability after the birth.

A crib with resuscitative equipment is readied before surgery. Those responsible for care are expert in resuscitative techniques, as well as in observational skills for detecting normal infant responses. After birth, if the infant's condition permits, the baby can be given to the father to hold. If the mother is awake, she can see and touch the baby (Fig. 24-12, *A*). The infant whose condition is compromised is transported immediately to the nursery for observation and appropriate interventions. In some hospitals the father may accompany the infant; if not, personnel keep the family informed of the infant's progress, and parent-infant contacts are initiated as soon as possible.

If the family-oriented approach is not feasible, then the family is directed to the surgical waiting room. The health care provider reviews with the family members the condition of the mother and infant after the birth is completed. Family members may accompany the infant to the nursery. This gives the family an opportunity to see and admire the new baby.

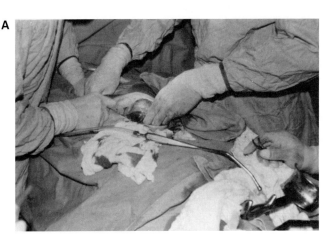

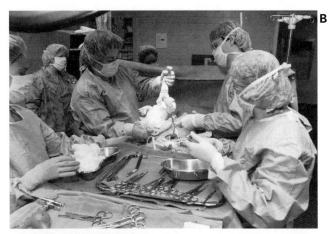

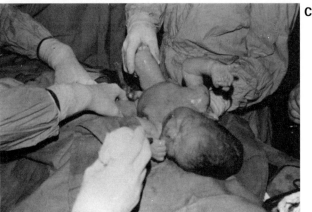

FIG. 24-11 Cesarean birth. **A,** "Bikini" incision has been made, the muscle layer is separated, the abdomen entered, the uterus has been exposed and incised; suctioning of amniotic fluid continues as head is brought up through the incision. Note small amount of bleeding. **B,** The neonate's birth through the uterine incision is complete. **C,** A quick assessment while neonate's mouth and nares are suctioned with bulb syringe; note extreme molding of head resulting from cephalopelvic disproportion. (**A** and **C** courtesy Majorie Pyle, RNC, *Lifecircle,* Costa Mesa, CA; **B** courtesy St. John's Mercy Medical Center, St Louis, MO.)

 CLINICAL APPLICATION OF RESEARCH

CESAREAN BIRTH RATE AND NURSES' CARE DURING LABOR

The cesarean birth rate in the United States was 23.5% in 1990, a rate higher than most other countries. Nursing care has been shown to influence use of analgesic, length of labor, and psychologic outcomes. There have been no studies of the influence of nurses' care on the cesarean birth rate.

This study examined the influence of individual nurses on the rate of abdominal birth. Nurses working in labor and birth units were grouped according to cesarean birth rates. The study compared nurses who gave care to the greatest number of patients, whose pregnancies resulted in cesarean births, to those who gave care to patients with the fewest cesarean births. Data were collected from birth logs and medical records. Radin et al performed five analyses to determine whether differences could be attributed to factors other than the nursing care; however, the large differences between the groups, could

only be explained by the nursing care experiences. In addition, they found that nurses in the low cesarean rate group used more psychosocial data in their care and their patients had fewer forceps or vacuum-assisted births.

Nurses working with women in labor *can* influence the outcome of the birth. They should examine their own philosophies and practices including supportive care provided to laboring women and their families. They can examine the rate of cesarean birth and other events surrounding childbirth over which they may have influence. It is imperative that nurses implement appropriate changes in their practice and keep up-to-date through continuing education or other activities, such as review of the literature.

Reference: Radin TG, Harmon JS, Hanson DA: Nurses' care during labor: its effect on the cesarean birth rate of healthy, nulliparous women, *Birth* 20(1):14, 1993.

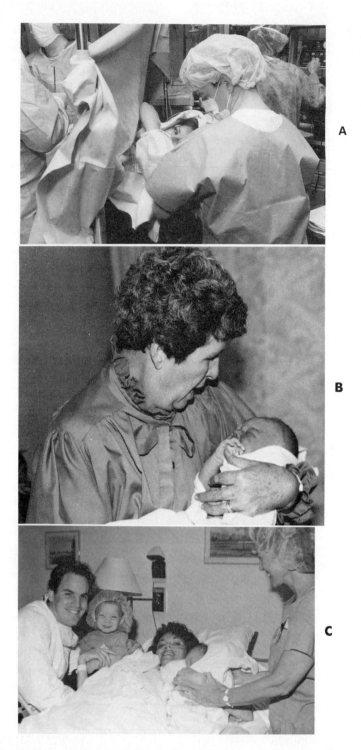

FIG. 24-12 **A,** Parents and their newborn. The health care provider manually removes the placenta, suctions the remaining amniotic fluid and blood from the uterine cavity, and closes the uterine incision, peritoneum, muscle layer, fatty tissue, and finally the skin, while the new family shares some private time. **B,** The grandmother begins bonding and attachment as the mother's postsurgery recovery begins. **C,** Older siblings are reassured by a visit with their mother after surgery; this provides the older siblings an introduction to the newest member of the family while being held in the security of the father's arms. **A** courtesy St. John's Mercy Medical Center, St Louis, MO. **B** courtesy Barbara Kalmen, Edwards Air Force Base, CA, **C** courtesy Marjorie Pyle, RNC, *Lifecircle,* Costa Mesa, CA.)

Postpartum Care

The care of the woman after cesarean birth combines surgical and maternity nursing. Once surgery is completed, the mother is transferred to a recovery area. Nursing assessments in this immediate postbirth period include degree of recovery from anesthetic effects, postoperative and postbirth status, and degree of pain. A patent airway is maintained, and the woman is positioned to prevent possible aspiration. Vital signs are taken every 15 minutes for 1 to 2 hours, or until the woman is stable. The condition of the incisional dressing, the fundus, and the amount of lochia are assessed, as well as intake and output. The nurse helps the woman turn and do deep breathing and leg exercises. Medications for pain may be administered.

If the baby is present, the mother and father are given some time alone to facilitate bonding and attachment with the infant. Breastfeeding can be initiated if the mother feels like trying. The woman usually is transferred to the postpartum unit after 1 to 2 hours, or when her condition is stable (see Care Path for cesarean birth).

The attitude of the nurse and other health team members can influence the woman's perception of herself after a cesarean birth. The caregivers should stress that the woman is a new mother first and a surgical patient second. This attitude will help the woman perceive herself as having the same problems and needs as other new mothers.

Physiologic concerns the first few days may be dominated by pain at the incision site and from intestinal gas and the need for pain relief. Pain medications usually are ordered every 3 to 4 hours, but patient-controlled analgesia (PCA) or epidural narcotics may be ordered instead. Other comfort measures such as position changes, splinting the incision with pillows, heat to the abdomen, and relaxation techniques may also be implemented. Ambulation and avoiding gas-forming foods and carbonated beverages may relieve gas pains (see Teaching Approaches above at right).

Daily care includes perineal care, breast care, and routine hygienic care, including showering after the dressing has been removed (if showering is within the woman's cultural prescription). During each shift the nurse assesses vital signs, the incision, fundus, and lochia. Breath sounds, bowel sounds, Homans' sign, and urinary and bowel elimination also are assessed.

During the postpartum period the nurse can provide care that meets psychologic and teaching needs of mothers who have had cesarean births. The nurse can explain postpartum procedures to help the woman cooperate in her recovery from surgery. The nurse can also help the woman plan care and visits from family and friends that will provide her with adequate rest periods. Information and assistance with infant care can facilitate the adjustment to the mothering role. The woman's partner can be included in infant teaching sessions and explanations

TEACHING APPROACHES

POSTPARTUM PAIN RELIEF AFTER CESAREAN BIRTH

INCISIONAL

Splint incision with a pillow when moving or coughing.

Use relaxation techniques such as music, breathing, and dim lights.

Apply a heating pad to the abdomen.

GAS

Walk as often as possible.

Do not eat or drink gas-forming foods, carbonated beverages, or whole milk.

Do not use straws for drinking fluids.

Lie on the left side to expel gas.

Use rocking chair.

about her recovery. The couple should be encouraged to express their feelings about the birth experience. Some parents are angry, frustrated, or disappointed about not having had a vaginal birth. Some women express feelings of low self-esteem or negative self-image. It may be helpful to have the nurse, who was present during the birth, visit and help fill in "gaps" about the experience.

Discharge teaching includes information about diet, exercise and activity restrictions, breast care, sexual activity and contraception, medications, signs of complications (see Teaching Approaches below), and infant care. The nurse assesses the need for continued support or counseling to facilitate the mother's emotional recovery from the birth. Referral to support groups or to community agencies may be indicated.

Vaginal Birth after Cesarean

The incidence of primary cesarean birth is 17.4% (National Center for Health Statistics, 1989). Indications for

TEACHING APPROACHES

SIGNS OF POSTOPERATIVE COMPLICATIONS AFTER DISCHARGE

REPORT THE FOLLOWING SIGNS TO THE HEALTH CARE PROVIDER:

Fever greater than 100.4° F (38° C)

Painful urination

Lochia heavier than a normal menstrual period

Wound separation

Redness or oozing at the incision site

Severe abdominal pain

CARE PATH

Mother-Baby Cesarean Birth without Complications Expected Length of Stay—4 Days

	Immediate Post-Op Cesarean	By 4th Hour after Admission to PP Unit	1st Day with Baby	1st PP Day
ABDOMINAL INCISION	Dressing dry and intact	Dressing dry and intact		Dressing dry and intact
ACTIVITY	Bedrest	Bedrest	Assisted to comfortable position for holding and feeding the baby	OOB X3 with help ADLs assisted
PULMONARY CARE	Patent airway; 0² d/c'd	TCDB every 2 hours with splinting; incentive spirometry every 1 hour if ordered; lungs clear		TCDB every 2 hours while awake; lungs clear
MEDICATIONS	Oxytocin added to IV; pain control: analgesics, IV or epidural narcotic	Oxytocin continued; pain control: analgesics—PCA, IM, PO		Oxytocin discontinued; pain control: IM, PO analgesics; PCA d/c'd
TEACHING/DISCHARGE PLAN	Breastfeeding; positioning; leg exercises	Verbalize understanding of unit routines, how to achieve rest, TCDB, involution, and pain control	Handwashing, infant, safety, positioning for feeding and burping; if breastfeeding, then positioning baby, latching-on, timing, removing from breast	Comfort measures and care; reinforce TCDB and positioning; introduce teaching videos, lactation suppression or promotion
ASSESSMENTS:	Recovery room/PACU admission assessment completed	PP admission assessment and care plan completed		
Vital signs	every 15 min times 1 hour; every 30 min times 4; WNL	Every hour times 3; WNL		Every 8 hours; WNL
Postpartum assessment	Every 15 min times 1 hour; WNL	Every 1 hour times 3; WNL		Every 8 hours; WNL
Genitourinary	Retention catheter output ≥ 30 ml/hour	Retention catheter output >30 ml/hour		Catheter d/c'd output >100 cc/void
Gastrointestinal		BS-absent or hypoactive		Hypoactive to active BS
Muscoskeletal	Alert or easily aroused; can move legs	Alert and oriented; moving all extremities		Ambulating with help

PP, postpartum; *d/c'd*, discontinued; *TCDB*, turn, cough, deep breathe; *CBC*, complete blood count; *Post-op*, post-operative; *IV*, intravenous solution; *WNL*, within normal limits; *IM*, intramuscular; *PO*, oral; + *flatus*, passing flatus; + *BM*, passed bowel movement; *OOB*, out of blood; *PCA*, patient controlled analegesia; *ADLs*, activities of daily living; *ad lib*, as desired; *BS*, bowel sounds; *PP Hct*, postpartum hematocrit; *BM*, bowel movement; *PNV*, prenatal vitamin.

CARE PATH—cont'd

Mother-Baby Cesarean Birth Without Complications Expected Length of Stay—4 Days

2nd Day with Baby	2nd PP Day	3rd Day with Baby	3rd PP Day	Discharge Day
	Dressing off or changed; incision intact		Incision intact; assessment WNL	Staples out; steri-strips in place; incision WNL
Holds baby comfortably	Ambulates without assistance, ADLs unassisted		Activity ad lib	
	Lungs clear			
	Stool softener PNV PO Analgesics			Prescriptions filled or given to take home
Bonding; parent concerns; feeding	Diet; activity/rest; bowel/bladder function	Infant bath; cord care; need for car seat; newborn characteristics; circumcision care, if needed; answer questions; return demonstration for diaper change and feeding	Home care—signs of complications (infection, bleeding), normal psychologic adjustments, resumption of normal activities of daily living, resumption of sexual activities, contraception; identification of support system at home; self concept issues related to cesarean birth	Return demonstration infant care; reinforce use of booklets for infant and self care; inform whom to call if problems; review need for follow-up appointment; provide information about community resources; discuss immunization needs; provide a copy of home care instructions.
	Every 8 hours; WNL		Every 8 hours; WNL	
	Every 8 hours; WNL		Every 8 hours; WNL	
	Urine output > 240 ml/8 hours			
	Active BS; + flatus		Active BS; + flatus; + BM	
	Ambulating unassisted		Ambulating ad lib	

Continued.

CARE PATH—cont'd

Mother-Baby Cesarean Birth without Complications Expected Length of Stay—4 Days

	Immediate Post-Op Cesarean	By 4th Hour after Admission to PP Unit	1st Day with Baby	1st PP Day
Bonding	Evidence of parent/infant bonding; first breastfeeding, if desired		Parent/infant bonding continues	
Laboratory tests		Intrapartal CBC results on chart/computer; determine Rh status and need for anti-Rh globulin; check for rubella immunity		PP HCT WNL; all lab results on chart
INTERVENTIONS:				
IV	IV continues	IV continues		May be discontinued
diet	NPO	Ice chips Sips of clear liquids		Clear liquids
perineal		Perineal care by nurse		Self perineal care
referral/consult				

primary cesarean birth, such as dystocia, breech presentation, or fetal distress, are often nonrecurring. Therefore a woman who has had a cesarean birth may subsequently become pregnant and not have any contraindications to labor and vaginal birth.

The continued practice of "once a cesarean, always a cesarean" is no longer recommended by most obstetricians. A trial of labor and **vaginal birth after cesarean (VBAC)** are now recommended as routine procedures by ACOG (1988) for women who have had one previous cesarean birth by low transverse incision. In 1992, 25.4% of women who had a previous cesarean birth, had a vaginal birth with their second pregnancy (Public Citizen, 1994). Studies have shown that vaginal birth is relatively safe with only a 0.5% risk of uterine rupture through a lower uterine segment scar (Knuppel, Drukker, 1993). Labor and vaginal birth are not recommended if contraindications such as a previous fundal classic cesarean scar or evidence of cephalopelvic disproportion are present.

According to Scott et al (1990), 60% to 75% of women can give birth vaginally after a trial of labor (p. 697). A trial of labor is recommended for women who meet the requirements for VBAC. During the antepartal period, the woman should be given information about VBAC and be encouraged to choose VBAC as an alternative to repeat cesarean if no contraindications occur. VBAC support groups and prenatal classes can help prepare the pregnant woman psychologically for labor and vaginal birth.

This labor should occur in a hospital facility that has the equipment and personnel available within 30 minutes from the time a decision is made for cesarean birth to the beginning of the procedure. Ideally, the woman is admitted to the labor and birth unit at the onset of spontaneous labor. In the latent phase of labor, the nurse encourages normal activities such as ambulation. In the active phase of labor, FHR and uterine activity usually are monitored electronically, and intravenous access, such as a heparin lock, may be established. Collaboration among the woman in labor, the nurse, and other health care providers often results in a successful VBAC.

There is no evidence that administering oxytocin to induce or augment labor or the use of an epidural anesthetic is contraindicated, although some health care providers may not elect these procedures (Flamm et al, 1987; 1988).

Attention should be given to the woman's psychologic, as well as physical, needs during the trial of labor. Anxiety can inhibit release of oxytocin, delaying the labor progress and leading to failure and repeat cesarean birth. The nurse can encourage the woman to use breathing and relaxation techniques and to change position to promote labor progress. The husband or support person can be encouraged to provide comfort measures and emotional support (Fawcett, Tulman, Spedden, 1994). If a trial of labor does not result in progression, the woman will need support, as well as encouragement to express her feelings about once again not achieving her desired outcome.

CARE PATH—cont'd

Mother-Baby Cesarean Birth Without Complications Expected Length of Stay—4 Days

2nd Day with Baby	2nd PP Day	3rd Day with Baby	3rd PP Day	Discharge Day
Parent/infant bonding progressing				
	Give anti-Rh globulin if indicated		PP Hct WNL	Give Rubella vaccine if indicated
	Regular diet			
	Sitz bath, if ordered			
	Assess need for referral/consults (e.g., social work, lactation consultant)		Referral as needed before discharge	Refer to community agency as needed

❖ EVALUATION

To evaluate the effectiveness of nursing care for a woman experiencing dystocia, the nurse reviews the goals and expected outcomes that were met and assesses the woman's and her family's level of satisfaction with the care they received. Expected outcomes include the following:

- The woman demonstrates an understanding of the causes and treatment of dysfunctional labor.
- She expresses decreased anxiety and fear about her condition and the status of the fetus.
- She does not exhibit signs of complications such as infection, hemorrhage, and fetal distress.
- She verbalizes decreased pain.
- She states satisfaction with her participation in decision making about her care options.
- She verbalizes positive feelings about herself.
- She gives birth to a healthy infant.

See the Plan of Care for an example of a situation in which the woman experiences dystocia.

PRETERM LABOR AND BIRTH

Preterm birth occurs after 20 weeks' gestation but before the beginning of week 37. The overall incidence of preterm birth in the United States ranges from 250,000 to 400,000 per year, or approximately 9% of births (Creasy, Merkatz, 1990). Preterm birth accounts for almost two thirds of infant deaths; one half of these deaths are associated with infants weighing 1500 g or less.

Etiologic Factors

In approximately 50% of preterm births the cause can not be identified. However, one third of preterm labors occur after premature rupture of membranes (PROM). Other complications of pregnancy associated with preterm labor include multifetal gestation, hydramnios, incompetent cervix, premature separation of the placenta, and certain infections (e.g., polynephritis and chorioamnionitis (Andersen, Merkatz, 1990).

Risk factors for preterm labor and birth have been identified, and certain categories of these risk factors are generally agreed upon by health care professionals. These categories include demographic risks, medical risks, current pregnancy risks, and behavioral and environmental risks (Institute of Medicine, 1985; Knuppel, Drukker, 1993; Neal, Bockman, 1992) (see Box 24-1).

Uterine irritability and events that trigger uterine contractions such as sexual activity, progesterone deficiency, inadequate plasma volume, and certain infections such as *Chlamydia* may be involved in the onset of preterm labor. The impact of these factors is not clearly understood (Bennett, Botti, 1989; Brustman et al, 1989; Main, 1988).

PLAN OF CARE

Patient with Dysfunctional Labor

Case History

Maggie Vadis is a married, 21-year-old nullipara at 38 weeks' gestation who has been admitted to the labor unit in active labor. She is accompanied by her husband, Tom. Maggie's physical examination reveals that her cervix is dilated 5 cm, 90% effaced; the fetus is at station 0; mild uterine contractions are occurring every 4 to 6 minutes and lasting 40 seconds; FHR is 148 beats/min, with good beat-to-beat variability and accelerations with fetal movements.

After 3 hours, assessment of Maggie reveals no change in labor pattern or in cervical dilatation. Maggie is showing signs of fatigue. Augmentation of labor with intravenous oxytocin was prescribed and implemented. After 2 hours of augmentation, Maggie is crying and asking for something for the pain and is no longer using her breathing and relaxation techniques.

EXPECTED OUTCOMES	IMPLEMENTATION	RATIONALE	EVALUATION
Nursing Diagnosis: High risk of maternal injury related to dysfunctional labor			
Labor pattern will be sufficient to produce dilatation, and birth will be accomplished without maternal complications.	Assess frequency of uterine contractions. Encourage ambulation or position changes. Encourage Maggie to void every 1 to 2 hours. Monitor for progressive cervical dilatation and effacement. Administer oxytocin as ordered (see Protocol, p. 700). Monitor intake and output. Assess for dehydration.	Early recognition of dysfunctional labor pattern may prevent complications; actions may stimulate uterine activity and normal labor pattern.	Maggie's vital signs remain within normal limits; signs of infection do not develop. Maggie's labor does not progress satisfactorily; her labor is augmented with oxytocin. Although maternal complications do not develop, Maggie gives birth by cesarean because of fetal distress.
Nursing Diagnosis: Ineffective coping related to prolonged labor, pain, and fatigue			
Effective coping techniques will be identified and used by Maggie.	Encourage relaxation and position changes. Give factual information about what is happening. Offer comfort measures such as massage and warm blankets. Acknowledge reality of pain.	Relaxation and decreased level of anxiety facilitate positive coping with the situation. Providing information and support may enhance coping.	Maggie again tries to use relaxation techniques and states that back massage is somewhat helpful. She continues to complain of pain. Other interventions are needed.
Nursing Diagnosis: Anxiety related to lack of progress, feelings of failure, and the need for induced labor			
Anxiety will be diminished or managed. Maggie will verbalize feelings of vulnerability and participate in the decision-making progress.	Give encouragement; keep informed of progress. Provide information about procedures. Encourage verbalization of feelings. Present options in care when possible. Listen to Maggie's comments that may indicate loss of self-esteem.	Reassurance and information can decrease anxiety and enhance understanding; this may increase Maggie's feelings of being in control of the situation.	Maggie states that she understands the reason for labor augmentation and feels less anxious.

PLAN OF CARE—cont'd

Patient with Dysfunctional Labor

EXPECTED OUTCOMES	IMPLEMENTATION	RATIONALE	EVALUATION

Nursing Diagnosis: Pain related to intensity of uterine contractions

Maggie's pain will be managed or relieved effectively.	Encourage use of relaxation techniques. Review breathing techniques. Encourage position changes. Provide comfort measures. Provide quiet environment. Administer pain medications as ordered.	Breathing and relaxation techniques, comfort measures, quiet environment, and pain medications may decrease pain or enhance Maggie's coping response to pain.	Maggie states pain is decreased after implementation of comfort measures and epidural analgesic.

Nursing Diagnosis: High risk for fetal injury related to hypoxia

Nonreassuring fetal status will not occur or will be managed and the infant will be born safely.	Assess reaction of FHR to contractions, noting decelerations or bradycardia. If nonreassuring fetal status occurs, position Maggie on her side, turn off oxytocin, increase maintenance IV, start oxygen, and notify the primary health care provider.	Assessment will determine fetal well-being; hypoxia is prevented or managed.	Nonreassuring fetal status does occur; male infant is born by cesarean birth in satisfactory condition; resuscitation is not needed. Tom and Maggie hold their infant in the recovery unit.

BOX 24-1

Risk Factors for Preterm Labor

DEMOGRAPHIC RISKS
Race (African-American)
Age (<17, >40 years old)
Low socioeconomic status
Unmarried
Low education level

MEDICAL RISKS
Previous preterm labor or birth
Second-trimester abortion (more than two spontaneous or elective)
Uterine anomalies
Medical diseases (e.g., diabetes, hypertension)
Current pregnancy risks
  Multifetal pregnancy
  Hydramnios
  Poor weight gain
  Placental problems (e.g., placenta previa, abruptio placentae)
  Abdominal surgery
  Infections (e.g., pyelonephritis, recurrent UTIs*)
  Incompetent cervix
  Spontaneous premature rupture of membranes
  Fetal anomalies

BEHAVIORAL AND ENVIRONMENTAL RISKS
Poor nutrition
Smoking (more than 10 cigarettes a day)
Alcohol and other substance abuse (e.g., cocaine)
DES† exposure and other toxic exposures
Little or no prenatal care

POTENTIAL RISK FACTORS
Stress
Uterine irritability
Events triggering uterine contractions
Cervical changes before onset of labor
Inadequate plasma volume expansion
Progesterone deficiency
Infections (e.g., mycoplasma, *Chlamydia trachomatis*)

---

*UTIs, urinary tract infections.
†DES, Diethylstilbestrol.

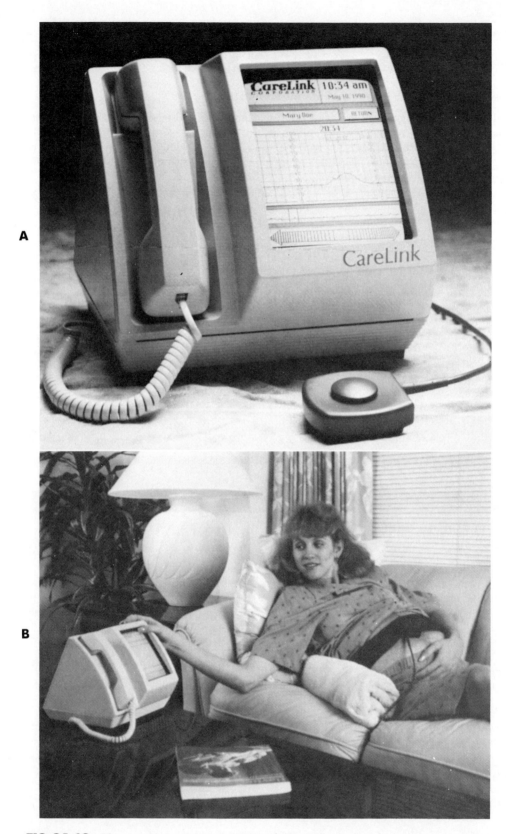

FIG. 24-13 Home uterine activity monitoring. **A,** Recording unit and transmitter. **B,** Toko-dynamometer in place at center of the abdomen below the umbilicus. (Courtesy Carelink Home Perinatal Services.)

Care Management

✤ ASSESSMENT

Management of preterm birth involves early detection of preterm labor, suppressing uterine activity, and improving intrapartum care of the fetus destined to be born early.

All pregnant women are screened according to risk factors associated with preterm labor at their initial prenatal visit. Many risk-scoring systems have been developed to assist in identifying women who might be at high risk for preterm labor. Women need to be reassessed each subsequent visit. Those who are considered at high risk are followed-up more closely, for example, on a weekly basis. They receive education in the symptoms of preterm labor (see guidelines in Chapter 7), as well as instruction in palpation, timing, and reporting of uterine contractions.

Home uterine monitoring with an ambulatory tokodynamometer device (Fig. 24-13) may be implemented to detect excessive uterine contractions before contractions can be perceived by the woman herself. The woman records uterine activity twice a day; the data are transmitted by telephone to the hospital or to a monitoring service for analysis. Appropriate therapy is instituted if labor is suspected (Hill et al, 1990). Although some studies show that the use of home uterine activity monitoring is associated with lower incidence of preterm birth, others speculate that the decrease is related to more frequent contact with health care providers (Creasy, Merkatz, 1990; Dyson et al, 1991; Hill et al, 1990). Continued study is needed.

✤ NURSING DIAGNOSES

The common nursing diagnoses for the woman with preterm labor include the following:

Knowledge deficit related to
- Recognition of preterm labor and/or management of preterm labor

High risk for maternal or fetal injury related to
- Preterm labor and birth

Anxiety related to
- Possible preterm birth

Impaired physical mobility related to
- Prescribed bed rest

Anticipatory grieving related to
- Potential loss of fetus

Situational low self-esteem related to
- Inability to carry pregnancy to term

✤ EXPECTED OUTCOMES

The nurse develops a plan of care based on whether the woman's care is managed at home or in the hospital. Common *expected outcomes* include the following:

- The woman will demonstrate compliance with prescribed activity limitations, medication schedules, or both.
- She will not experience complications from prescribed drug management.
- She will carry her pregnancy to term or near term.
- She will give birth to a healthy, mature infant.

✤ COLLABORATIVE CARE

Pregnant women should be told to notify the health care provider if they have symptoms of preterm labor, particularly uterine contractions occurring more frequently than every 10 minutes. If the woman is active, it may be helpful if she lies on her side and drinks fluids to increase blood flow to the uterus, in order to correct myometrial hypoxia and to decrease uterine activity. If the woman continues to have uterine contractions after 1 hour of implementing these interventions, she is usually instructed to come to the health care provider's office or to the hospital for further evaluation. The woman lies on her side, and an external fetal and uterine monitor is applied to assess uterine activity and FHR. An intravenous fluid may be started to provide additional hydration. A sterile speculum examination is usually performed to obtain cervical and/or vaginal cultures to detect the presence of an infection such as β-streptococcus. A clean-catch or catheterized urine specimen is obtained and examined for the presence of a urinary tract infection. A cervical examination is performed to assess for dilatation and/or effacement.

The diagnosis of preterm labor includes both uterine and cervical changes in effacement and dilatation (Andersen, Merkatz, 1990). If uterine activity subsides and dilatation and effacement do not change from the initial examination, then the woman may be discharged to return home. She may be given instructions regarding limitations of activities (see Home Care) and medications for the prevention of preterm labor. If labor continues, care will continue in the hospital setting until the woman's condition stabilizes. Then she can go home with limitations placed on her activity and/or with medications, in order to prevent recurrence of preterm labor or until the infant is born.

Suppression of Uterine Activity

If uterine contractions persist, or if cervical changes occur, tocolytic treatment may be used to stop labor. **Tocolytic agents** are drugs that inhibit uterine contractions. The agents used include β-adrenergic drugs such as ritodrine or terbutaline, and magnesium sulfate (Andersen, Merkatz, 1990).

Ritodrine

Ritodrine (Yutopar) was the first, and remains the only β-sympathomimetic drug approved by the FDA for use in the United States to inhibit preterm labor (Cunningham et al, 1993). Ritodrine acts on type II β-adrenergic receptors, which cause uterine muscle relaxation, vasodilation, bronchodilation, and muscle glycogenolysis. Decrease in serum potassium levels may cause arrhythmias. The initial dose is usually given intravenously. After the woman's condition stabilizes, intramuscular therapy and/or oral therapy follows. The dose is determined by the health care provider and the woman's response to the medication.

Contraindications for use include maternal diseases such as cardiovascular disease, severe preeclampsia, severe antepartum hemorrhage, chorioamnionitis, and hyperthyroidism. Fetal death and gestational age of fewer than 20 weeks, which has been confirmed by an ultrasound scan, are two fetal-related contraindications.

Cardiopulmonary complications are possible, therefore, careful assessment and monitoring are essential. Because of the possible cardiopulmonary effects, an electrocardiogram may be ordered before treatment. A cardiac monitor for the mother may be used to maintain continuous assessment for *tachycardia* and *arrhythmia* (see Emergency box).

Terbutaline

Terbutaline (Brethine) is another β-adrenergic agent often used for preterm labor. The administration and contraindications of terbutaline are similar to those described for ritodrine; however, terbutaline is more frequently given either subcutaneously or orally.

Prolonged and continuous high-dose treatment with ritodrine or terbutaline causes desensitization of β-adrenergic receptors. Preterm labor usually recurs as a result of tocolytic breakthrough. The use of subcutaneous terbutaline by pump infusion for long-term tocolysis has been effective in preventing this recurrence (Iams et al, 1988). The pump therapy decreases desensitization by delivering a continuous low-dose infusion, with intermittent bolus doses at times when uterine activity is known to occur in the individual patient. The average daily dose by pump is 3 to 4 mg terbutaline administered subcutaneously; a daily oral dose is 30 to 60 mg (Gill, Smith, McGregor, 1989; Sala, Moise, 1990.)

Women who use the terbutaline pump (Fig. 24-14) require instruction in the operation of the pump and self-injection techniques. In addition, they need to know the signs of preterm labor, how to palpate uterine contractions, recognize warning signs and symptoms of terbutaline toxicity (see Signs of Potential Complications), and follow activity precautions. Nursing assessments for women who are at home or in the hospital may include determinations of vital signs; weight gain; breath sounds; FHR and fetal movement; fundal height; urine checks for glucose, protein, and ketones; cervical examination to detect changes; uterine activity monitoring; gastrointestinal function; deep tendon reflexes and edema; and psychosocial adaption (Eganhouse, Burnside, 1992; Gill, Smith, McGregor, 1989).

Nursing Considerations. Nursing interventions for women receiving ritodrine or terbutaline depend on whether the drug is administered intravenously, subcutaneously, or orally. Before intravenous therapy, the woman may receive hydration with 500 ml isotonic crystalloid within 30 minutes. The drug is then administered via pump infusion. The dose is increased in increments as ordered, using the minimum amount of the drug that will stop the uterine contractions. After 12 to 24 hours of successful therapy, oral therapy is usually instituted (ACOG, 1989).

During intravenous therapy the nurse monitors uterine activity and FHR continuously. FHR should not exceed 180 beats/min. Maternal vital signs, including

---

HOME CARE

HOME MANAGEMENT OF PRETERM LABOR

Remain on bed rest in a side-lying position as instructed.
Assess for fetal activity daily.
Monitor for uterine contraction activity daily.
Practice relaxation techniques.
Eat well-balanced meals.
Drink 8 to 10 (8 oz) cups of fluids a day.
Report rupture of membranes, vaginal bleeding, signs of labor (menstrual-like cramps, pelvic pressure, low backache, uterine contractions) to your health care provider.
Avoid or limit activities that could stimulate labor as instructed (e.g., sexual intercourse, breast stimulation).
Take medications as prescribed. Report side effects to your health care provider.
Keep appointments with your health care provider.

E M E R G E N C Y

PULMONARY EDEMA CAUSED BY RITODRINE THERAPY

SIGNS
Dyspnea
Crackles (rales)

INTERVENTIONS
Discontinue drug immediately.
Start oxygen.
Give diuretics as ordered.
Restrict fluids.

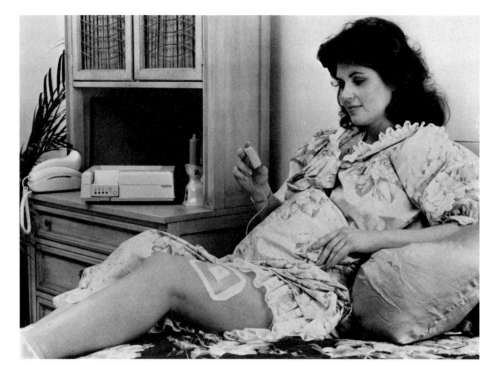

FIG. 24-14 Subcutaneous terbutaline pump attached to woman. (Courtesy Healthdyne Perinatal Services, Marietta, GA.)

blood pressure, are assessed per protocol. The woman's pulse should not exceed 140 beats/min. Breath sounds are assessed and lungs auscultated every 8 to 12 hours. The nurse assesses the woman for other signs of drug side effects such as fluid overload, pulmonary edema, and cardiac arrhythmias. If any side effects are noted, the medication is stopped and the health care provider is notified. An *antidote,* a β-blocking agent such as *propranolol* (Inderal), may be prescribed. The maximum intravenous fluid rate is 100 ml/hr. Blood samples may be drawn for laboratory analysis of glucose and potassium levels to detect hypokalemia or hyperglycemia. The woman is maintained on bed rest in a side-lying position to optimize placental perfusion and to decrease pressure on the cervix. Intake and output, as well as daily weights are monitored to detect overhydration. The woman should be told about the potential side effects in order to prevent undue stress if they should occur (Caritis et al, 1988).

If the woman is on an oral or a subcutaneous therapy regimen, maternal vital signs, FHR, fetal activity, and uterine activity are assessed per hospital routine or as ordered. Medications need to be given on time every 4 to 6 hours in order to prevent recurrence of uterine activity.

Magnesium Sulfate

Magnesium sulfate decreases uterine activity. It is being used as a tocolytic agent because it is safer for the woman than ritodrine. It is usually given intravenously, but intramuscular and oral routes may be used (Anderson,

SIGNS OF POTENTIAL COMPLICATIONS

SIDE EFFECTS OF TERBUTALINE

MATERNAL

Central Nervous System
Severe dizziness, drowsiness, headache, nervousness, restlessness

Blood Pressure
Slight hypertension or increase in systolic with decrease in diastolic pressure

Heart Rate
Continuous palpitations, chest pain, tachycardia ≥140 beats/min

Musculoskeletal
Severe muscle cramps and weakness

Gastrointestinal
Continuous nausea and vomiting

Respiratory
Shortness of breath, coughing, respirations, > 24/min, pulmonary edema (life-threatening)

Metabolic
Hyperglycemia, hypokalemia

FETAL
Tachycardia >180 beats/min

Merkatz, 1990). However, if administered orally, magnesium oxide or gluconate is used . Diarrhea is the primary side effect (Caritis et al, 1988; Creasy, 1989).

For intravenous therapy, magnesium sulfate is mixed with normal saline, and a 4 g dose is infused over a 20-minute period. The drug is then infused via a pump at 1 to 2 g/hr and increased per protocol (usually 0.5 g/hr every 15 to 30 minutes) until contractions stop. After 12 hours of successful therapy, oral tocolytic therapy may be started.

Nursing Considerations. Nursing assessments during intravenous administration of magnesium sulfate therapy include monitoring blood pressure, pulse, and respiratory rates; checking deep tendon reflexes; measuring intake and output; assessing level of consciousness; and checking laboratory results for therapeutic levels of magnesium (4 to 8 g/dl) and calcium levels for hypocalcemia. Calcium gluconate should be available to reverse serious side effects. Uterine activity and FHR also are monitored.

Other Drugs

Other drugs being investigated for treatment of preterm labor include prostaglandin antagonists, indomethacin, nonsteroidal inflammatory agents (naproxen and salicylates), and calcium channel blockers (nifedipine). Although these drugs are effective in relaxing the uterus, concern about potential effects on the fetus and bleeding have limited their use (Brown, 1989; Creasy, 1989).

Promotion of Fetal Lung Maturity

Respiratory distress syndrome (RDS) is common in small preterm infants who have fetal lung immaturity. The incidence and severity of RDS has been found to be reduced if glucocorticoids (e.g., betamethasone) are administered to the mother at least 24 to 48 hours before the birth. The fetus must be at less than 34 weeks of gestation. The administration must be made at least 24 hours before birth and no longer than 7 days before birth. Neither the use of tocolytics nor steroidal therapy is universally recommended for preterm labor after premature rupture of membranes (Anderson, Merkatz, 1990).*

Care during Preterm Labor and Birth

If labor cannot be stopped, the health care provider makes every attempt to help the mother give birth to the preterm infant safely and without trauma. If time permits, usually the woman will be transferred to a center

with facilities to care for her preterm infant. During labor, drugs such as narcotics or barbiturates that can depress the fetus are avoided. An epidural analgesic is commonly used during labor, but pudendal block or local anesthetic may be administered for the birth instead. An episiotomy is often performed to shorten the second stage of labor and to reduce excessive pressure on the fragile fetal head. The route of birth is controversial, but cesarean birth may be performed for malpresentation and maternal or fetal distress (Anderson, Merkatz, 1990).

Parental concern for the well-being of the infant is apparent during labor. Parents need to be aware of the interest and support of staff members. However, false assurance of fetal health must be avoided. Some parents do not appreciate the reality of the situation until they see their newborn in the intensive care unit. For others who experience fetal or newborn death, the loss intensifies once the stress of labor and childbirth is over.

During the postpartum period physical care of the mother is similar to that required after any vaginal birth; however, the family will be anxious concerning the health and prognosis of their infant. Nursing care of the preterm infant involves not only medical and nursing personnel but also the parents' participation. The nurse must be aware of the impact that preterm birth may have on family dynamics (Richardson, 1987). Parents must accept that their infant has special needs, and that they must learn to meet these needs before discharge so that they will have more realistic expectations when they are at home (Weingarten et al, 1990).

❖ EVALUATION

Evaluation of the effectiveness of nursing care for women with preterm labor is based on the expected outcomes. These may include that the woman verbalizes an understanding of her treatment, complies with her prescribed treatment, develops no complications related to drug therapy, and gives birth at or near term to a healthy, mature infant.

POSTTERM LABOR AND BIRTH

Postterm birth is the birth of an infant beyond the end of week 42 of gestation, or 294 days from the first day of the last menstrual period. The incidence of postterm gestation is estimated to be between 3.5% and 15%; only about 4% of pregnancies terminate after 42 weeks (Resnik, 1989; Spellacy, 1990).

Maternal risks are related to the birth of an excessively large infant. The woman is at increased risk for dysfunctional labor, induction of labor, forceps-assisted birth, lacerations related to vaginal birth, and cesarean birth (Boyd et al, 1988; Spellacy, 1990).

Fetal risks appear to be twofold. The first relates to

---

*ALERT: The woman who has received tocolytics, as well as glucocorticoids to stimulate fetal lung maturity is at risk for cardiac decompensation. Therefore the nurse must be vigilant in monitoring the woman for signs of cardiac decompensation (see Signs of Potential Complications, p. 640).

the possibility of birth trauma and asphyxia through fetopelvic disproportion. The second risk results from the compromising effects on the fetus of an "aging" placenta. Spellacy (1990) notes that placental function decreases after 40 weeks of gestation and amniotic fluid volume declines to approximately 250 to 300 ml. Oligohydramnios is associated with fetal distress related to cord compression. If placental insufficiency is present, then there is a high incidence of fetal distress during labor. Neonatal problems may include asphyxia, meconium aspiration syndrome, and respiratory distress. Postterm babies also have increased mortality, increased feeding and sleeping problems, more illness, and low developmental and mental scores (Asher et al, 1988; Beckmann, 1990; Spellacy, 1990).

The management of postterm pregnancy is still controversial. Induction of labor at 42 weeks is suggested by some authorities. Others allow pregnancy to proceed to 43 weeks as long as tests of fetal well-being are performed and results are normal. Antepartum assessments for postterm pregnancy may include daily fetal movement counts (at least 10 in a 12-hour period) and abdominal girth measurements (to detect oligohydramnios). Nonstress test should be performed at least weekly. The biophysical profile may be the best indication of fetal well-being because it combines nonstress testing with real-time ultrasound scanning to assess fetal movements, fetal breathing movements, and amniotic fluid volume (AFV). Determining the amount of AFV is critical because decreased AFV has been associated with nonreassuring fetal status in postterm pregnancies (Spellacy, 1990).

Cervical checks are performed weekly after 40 weeks' gestation to assess if the condition of the cervix is favorable for induction (Table 24-3). Amniocentesis or amnioscopy may be performed to detect meconium in the amniotic fluid (Resnik, 1989; Spellacy, 1990).

HOME CARE

POSTTERM GESTATION

Perform daily fetal movement counts.
Assess for signs of labor.
Call your health care provider if your membranes rupture.
Keep appointments for fetal assessment tests or cervical checks.
Come to the hospital soon after labor begins.

Nursing Considerations

During the postterm period the woman is encouraged to assess fetal activity daily, assess for signs of labor, and keep appointments with her health care provider (see Home Care). The woman should be instructed to go to the hospital soon after labor begins.

Labor of a woman with a postterm fetus should be monitored for signs of nonreassuring fetal status. The woman is encouraged to come to the hospital in early labor so the fetus can be monitored electronically for more accurate assessment of the FHR pattern. Nurses may need to assist with fetal scalp pH sampling or send a cord blood sample for determining pH levels after birth. If variable decelerations occur or thick meconium is present after rupture of the membranes, a saline amnioinfusion may also be initiated (Gilbert, Harmon, 1993). Accurate assessment of the woman's labor pattern also is important because dysfunctional labor is common in this complication (Spellacy, 1990).

Emotional support is essential for the postterm woman and her family. A vaginal birth is anticipated, but the couple should be prepared for a forceps-assisted birth (or vacuum extraction) or for cesarean birth if complications arise.

KEY POINTS

- Dystocia results from differences in the normal relationships among any of the five essential factors of labor.
- The differences between dystocia and normal labor relate to changes in the pattern of progress in labor.
- The functional relationships between the uterine contractions, the fetus, and the mother's pelvis are altered by maternal positioning.
- Uterine contractility is increased by oxytocin and prostaglandin and is decreased by tocolytic agents.
- All expectant parents benefit from learning about operative obstetrics (e.g., use of forceps and cesarean birth) and preterm labor during the prenatal period.

- The basic purpose of cesarean birth is to preserve the life or health of the mother and her fetus.
- Unless contraindicated, vaginal birth is possible after previous cesarean birth.
- The pregnant woman and her family can be taught to treat preterm labor at home with bed rest, tocolytics, and avoidance of activities that stimulate the uterus.
- In-hospital treatment for preterm labor involves the use of tocolytics and pharmacologic stimulation of fetal lung maturity.
- Postterm birth poses a risk to both the mother and the fetus.

CRITICAL THINKING EXERCISES

1. You are assigned to a woman experiencing preterm labor at 32 weeks' gestation. Her previous labor was also preterm and the infant died at 3 days of age. This is the woman's third admission for preterm labor this pregnancy.
   a. What impact might her history have on the nursing care she receives this time?
   b. What approach to this woman will best meet her needs for this admission?
   c. Discuss pros and cons of home management for prevention of preterm birth for this woman.
   d. Develop a plan of care for prevention of preterm birth based on the above discussion.

2. You are preparing a woman for an unplanned cesarean birth for failure to progress.
   a. Examine possible reactions of the woman to this situation. How would these affect the effectiveness of nursing care?
   b. Examine your feelings as you think about how to prepare the woman for surgery. How would these feelings affect your care?
   c. How would your preparation differ from preparing a woman for a planned cesarean? Explain differences in postpartum needs between the woman who had a planned cesarean and the woman who experienced an unplanned one.

References

Acker DB, Sachs BP: Twin gestation in labor. In Cohen WR et al, editors: *Management of labor,* ed 2, Rockville, MD, 1989, Aspen.

Adams DM, Chervenak FA: Intrapartum management of twin gestation, *Clin Obstet Gynecol* 33:42, 1990.

Akoury HA et al: Active management of labor and operative delivery in nulliparous women, *Am J Obstet Gynecol* 158:255, 1988.

Akoury HA et al: Oxytocin augmentation of labor and perinatal outcome in nulliparas, *Obstet Gynecol* 78:227, 1991.

American College of Obstetricians and Gynecologists: (ACOG committee opinion No 64) *Guidelines for vaginal delivery after a previous cesarean birth,* Washington, DC, October 1988, ACOG.

American College of Obstetricians and Gynecologists: Technical bulletin No. 133: *Preterm labor,* Washington, DC, 1989, ACOG.

American College of Obstetricians and Gynecologists: Technical bulletin No. 157: *Induction and augmentation of labor,* Washington, DC, 1991, ACOG.

American College of Obstetricians and Gynecologists: *Prostaglandin E2 gel for cervical ripening* (ACOG committee opinion No. 123). Washington, DC, 1993, ACOG.

Andersen HF, Merkatz IR: Preterm labor. In Scott JR et al: *Danforth's obstetrics and gynecology,* ed 6, Philadelphia, 1990, JB Lippincott.

Andrews CM, Chrzanowski: Maternal position, labor, and comfort, *Appl Nurs Res* 3:7, Feb 1990.

Asher RH et al: Assessment of fetal risk in postdate pregnancies, *Am J Obstet Gynecol* 158:259, 1988.

Association of Women's Health, Obstetric and Neonatal Nurses: *Cervical ripening and induction and augmentation of labor: practice resource,* Washington, DC, 1993, AWHONN.

Beckmann CA: Postterm pregnancy: effects on temperature and glucose regulation, *Nurs Res* 39:21, Jan/Feb 1990.

Bennett NL, Botti JJ: New strategies for preterm labor, *Nurs Pract* 14(4):27, April 1989.

Biancuzzo M: The patient observer: does the hands and knees position during labor help to rotate the occiput posterior fetus? *Birth* 18(1):40, 1991.

Blumenthal P, Ramanauskas R: Randomized trial of dilapan and laminaria as cervical ripening agents before induction of labor, *Obstet Gynecol* 75:365, 1990.

Bowes WA: Clinical aspects of normal and abnormal labor. In Cohen WR et al, editors: *Management of labor,* ed 2, Rockville, MD, 1989, Aspen.

Boyd ME et al: Obstetric consequences of postmaturity, *Am J Obstet Gynecol* 158:334, 1988.

Brodsky P, Pellzar E: Rationale for the revision of oxytocin administration protocols, *JOGNN* 20(6):440, 1991.

Brown JJ: Calcium: channel blockers for tocolysis. In Parer JJ, editor: *Antepartum and intrapartum management.* Philadelphia, 1989, Lea & Febiger.

Brustman LE et al: Changes in the pattern of uterine contractility in relationship to coitus during pregnancies at low and high risk for preterm labor, *Obstet Gynecol* 73:166, 1989.

Caritis SN et al: Pharmacologic treatment for preterm labor, *Clin Obstet Gynecol* 31:635, 1988.

Creasy RK: Preterm labor and delivery. In Creasy RK, Resnik R: *Maternal-fetal medicine: principles and practice,* ed 2, Philadelphia, 1989, WB Saunders.

Creasy RK, Merkatz IR: Prevention of preterm birth: clinical opinion, *Obstet Gynecol* 76(suppl 1):25, 1990.

Cummiskey K, Dawood M: Induction of labor with pulsatile oxytocin, *Am J Obstet Gynecol* 163:1868, 1990.

Cunningham FG et al: *Williams obstetrics,* ed 19, Norwalk, CT, 1993, Appleton & Lange.

Davis LK: Protocol for the nursing management of the patient requiring oxytocin for induction and augmentation of labor. In Mandeville L, Troiano N: *High-risk intrapartum nursing,* Philadelphia, 1992, JB Lippincott.

Dennan PC: *Dennan's forceps deliveries,* ed 3, Philadelphia, 1989, Davis.

Dunn LJ: Cesarean section and other obstetric operations. In Scott JR et al: editors: *Danforth's Obstetrics and Gynecology,* ed 6, Philadelphia, 1990, JB Lippincott.

Dyson DC et al: Prevention of preterm birth in high risk patients: the role of education and provider contact versus home monitoring, *Am J Obstet Gynecol* 164:756, 1991.

Eganhouse DJ, Burnside SM: Nursing assessment and responsibilities in monitoring the preterm pregnancy, *JOGNN* 21(5):355, 1992.

Englinton CS: External version in modern obstetrics. In Phelan JP, Clark SL, editors: *Cesarean delivery,* New York, 1988, Elsevier.

Fawcett J, Henklein J: Antenatal education for cesarean birth: extending a field test, *JOGNN* 16:61, Jan-Feb 1987.

Fawcett J, Tulman L, Spencer J: Responses to vaginal birth after cesarean section, *JOGNN* 23(3):253, 1994.

Fenwick L, Simkin P: Maternal positioning to prevent or alleviate dystocia in labor, *Clin Obstet Gynecol* 30:83, Jan 1987.

Flamm BL et al: Oxytocin during labor after previous cesarean section: results of a multicenter study, *Obstet Gynecol* 70:709, 1987.

Flamm BL et al: Vaginal birth after cesarean section: results of a multidimensional study, *Am J Obstet Gynecol* 158:1079, 1988.

Friedman EA: Normal and dysfunctional labor. In Cohen WR et al, editors: *Management of Labor,* ed 2, Rockville, MD, 1989, Aspen.

Gallup DG: Opening and closing the abdomen. In Phelan JP, Clark SL, editors: *Cesarean delivery,* New York, 1988, Elsevier.

Galvan BJ, Broekhuizen FF: Obstetric vacuum extraction, *JOGNN* 16:242, July/Aug 1987.

Gilbert ES, Harmon JS: *Manual of high risk pregnancy & delivery,* St Louis, 1993, Mosby.

Gill P, Smith M, McGregor C: Terbutaline by pump to prevent recurrent preterm labor, *MCN* 14:163, May/June 1989.

Hill WC et al: Home uterine activity monitoring is associated with a reduction in preterm birth, *Obstet Gynecol* 76(suppl1):13s, 1990.

Husslein P: Use of prostaglandins for induction of labor, *Semin Perinat* 15(2):173, 1991.

Iams JD, Johnson FF, Creasy RK: Prevention of preterm birth, *Clin Obstet Gynecol* 31:599, 1988.

Institute of Medicine (Committee to Study the Prevention of Low Birthweight): *Preventing low birthweight,* Washington, DC, 1985, National Academy Press.

Knuppel RA, Drukker JE: *High-risk pregnancy: a team approach,* ed 2, Philadelphia, 1993, WB Saunders.

Liu YC: The effects of the upright position during childbirth, *Image: J Nurs Scholar* 21(1):14, Jan 1989.

Main DM: Epidemiology for preterm birth, *Clin Obstet Gynecol* 31:521, 1988.

Marieskind H: Cesarean section in the United States: has it changed since 1979? *Birth* 16:196, 1989.

Martel M et al: Maternal age and primary cesarean rates: a multivariate analysis, *Am J Obstet Gynecol* 156:305, 1987.

Mercer B, Pilgrim P, Sibai B: Labor induction with continuous low-dose oxytocin infusion: a randomized trial, *Obstet Gynecol* 77:659, 1991.

National Center for Health Statistics: *Vital and health statistics: detailed diagnosis and procedures, National hospital discharge survey, 1987 (Series 13 No. 100),* Washington, DC,

March 1989, U.S. Department of Health and Human Services.

Neal A, Bockman V: Preterm labor and preterm premature rupture of membranes. In Mandeville L, Troiano N, editors: *High-risk intrapartum nursing,* Philadelphia, 1992, JB Lippincott.

O'Leary JA: *Shoulder dystocia and birth injury: prevention and treatment,* New York, 1992, McGraw Hill.

Public Citizen Health Research Group: Fewer c-sections, *USA Today,* May 19, 1994.

Resnik R: Postterm pregnancy. In Creasy RK, Resnik R, editors: *Maternal-fetal medicine: principles and practice,* ed 2, Philadelphia, 1989, WB Saunders.

Richardson P: Women's important relationships during pregnancy and the preterm labor event, *West J Nurs Res* 9:203, 1987.

Sala DJ, Moise KJ: The treatment of preterm labor using a portable subcutaneous terbutaline pump, *JOGNN* 19:108, March/April 1990.

Scott JR et al: *Danforth's obstetrics and gynecology,* ed 6, Philadelphia, 1990, JB Lippincott.

Shearer E, Shiono P, Rhoads G: Recent trends in family centered maternity care for cesarean birth families, *Birth* 15:3, Jan 1988.

Silver L, Wolfe SM: *Unnecessary cesarean section: how to cure a national epidemic,* Washington, DC, 1989, Public Citizens Health Research Group.

Simkin P: Stress, pain and catecholamines in labor. I. A review, *Birth* 13(8):234, 1986.

Sokol RI, Brindley BA: Practical diagnosis and management of abnormal labor. In Scott JR et al, editors: *Danforth's obstetrics and gynecology,* ed 6, Philadelphia, 1990, JB Lippincott.

Spellacy WN: Postdate pregnancy. In Scott JR et al, editors: *Danforth's obstetrics and gynecology,* ed 6, Philadelphia, 1990, JB Lippincott.

Taffel S, Placek P, Kosary C: U.S. cesarean section rates 1990: an update, *Birth* 19(1):21, 1992.

Tal Z et al: Breast electrostimulation for the induction of labor, *Obstet Gynecol* 72:671, 1988.

Turner MJ, Brassil M, Gordon H: Active management of labor associated with a decrease in the cesarean rate of nulliparas, *Obstet Gynecol* 71:150, 1988.

Weingarten CT et al: Married mothers perceptions of their premature or term infants and the quality of their relationships with their husbands, *JOGNN* 19(1):64, 1990.

Bibliography

Clark S et al: *Critical care obstetrics,* ed 2, Boston, 1991, Blackwell Scientific Publications.

Day M, Snell B: Use of prostaglandins for induction of labor, *J Nurse Midwifery* 38(2 Suppl):425, 1993.

Fawcett J, Pollio N, Tully A: Women's perceptions of cesarean and vaginal delivery: another look, *Research in Nursing & Health* 15:436, 1992.

Johnson S: Ethical dilemma: a patient refuses a life-saving cesarean, *MCN* 17(3):121, 1992.

Lake M: Prolonged pregnancy. In Mandeville L, Troiano N, editors: *High-risk intrapartum nursing,* Philadelphia, 1992, JB Lippincott.

Lyman L, Miller M: Mothers and nurses' perceptions of the needs of women experiencing preterm labor, *JOGNN* 21(2):126, 1992.

May K: Impact of maternal activity restriction for preterm labor on the expectant father, *JOGNN* 23(3):246, 1994.

Penney D, Perlis D: Shoulder dystocia: when to use suprapubic or fundal pressure, *MCN* 17(1):34, 1992.

Poziac S: Induction and augmentation of labor. In Mandeville L, Troiano N, editors: *High-risk intrapartum nursing,* Philadelphia, 1992, JB Lippincott.

Tauer C: When pregnant patients refuse interventions, *AWHONN's Clin Issu in Perinat and Womens Health Nursing* 4(4):596, 1993.

Thomas L et al: The effects of rocking, diet modifications, and antiflatulent medication on postcesarean section gas pain, *J Perinat Neonat Nurs* 4(3):12, 1990.

CHAPTER

25 Adolescent Sexuality, Pregnancy, and Parenthood

PHYLLIS A. JOHNSON

LEARNING OBJECTIVES

Define the key terms listed.
Discuss the dynamics of adolescent sexual development.
Examine the incidence and cost of adolescent pregnancy and parenthood.
Discuss societal and cultural factors related to adolescent sexual activity.
Compare the developmental tasks of adolescence, pregnancy, and parenthood.
Identify teaching strategies for discussing sexuality and contraception.
Compare the nutritional needs of the nonpregnant, pregnant, and lactating adolescent.
Discuss the similarities and differences in planning care for the adolescent who decides to terminate her pregnancy and the one who chooses to carry her pregnancy to term.
Describe the application of the nursing process in planning care for the adolescent father.
Discuss the application of the nursing process in planning care for the grandparents-to-be.

KEY TERMS

adolescence
developmental tasks of adolescence
developmental tasks of parenthood
developmental tasks of pregnancy
psychologic sexual self-concept and identity
risk taking
sexual decision making
sex education
sexual history
sexuality

RELATED TOPICS

Maternal and fetal nutrition *(Chap. 8)* • Contraception *(Chap. 18)* • Substance abuse *(Chap. 23)* • Family dynamics *(Chap. 6 and 17)* • Violence *(Chap. 23)* • Loss and grief *(Chap. 28)* • Abortion *(Chap. 30)*

ADOLESCENT DEVELOPMENT, SEXUALITY, AND PREGNANCY

The term *adolescent* comes from the Latin *ad alescere*, which means "to grow up." Throughout this developmental phase, a number of physical, social, and psychologic issues combine to create unique characteristics, behaviors, and needs.

Health strategies planned and implemented on the basis of an understanding of adolescent development are more successful than those that are not. Health professionals working with adolescents need to understand the cognitive-developmental levels, cultural environment, value systems, and biologic functioning of adolescents in order to successfully plan and implement health care strategies.

The growing number of adolescent pregnancies means that most perinatal nurses will care for pregnant adolescents or their infants at some time. This chapter provides some of the information necessary to improve the health of pregnant adolescents.

Adolescence and Development

Adolescence is the period of time during which an individual transforms from a child to an adult. During this time the individual asks and answers the question "who am I?"

Developmental Tasks of Adolescence

Children must accomplish **developmental tasks of adolesence** before becoming mature adults. These tasks vary from culture to culture and with individual adolescents and their goals. These general tasks include: (1) acceptance of body image, (2) acceptance of sexual identity, (3) development of a personal value system, (4) preparation for making a living, (5) independence from parents, (6) development of decision-making skills, (7) development of an adult identity. Adolescence is characterized by the onset of the physical changes of puberty and by the psychosocial development of the ego, which helps the individual achieve a sense of self.

Certain physical developments, behaviors, and concerns are commonly noted at different ages during adolescence. However, each adolescent is different and develops at his or her own rate. In addition to biologic changes, each adolescent's development is influenced by the family, society, peer group, religion, and socioeconomic condition.

The period of adolescence may be divided into three stages: early, middle, and late (see Box 25-1). The higher the developmental level, the greater the readiness to accept responsibility for self and others. Early adolescents (ages 10 to 14) have only a vague sense of self. They are unable to relate their own behavior with the consequences of that behavior. Middle adolescents (ages 15 to 16) struggle with feelings of dependence vs. independence as peers replace parents; they are more likely to demonstrate wide variations in their emotions. Early and middle adolescents learn and retain information but are incapable of applying this information to their own lives. They frequently operate by trial and error without considering the consequences. Late adolescents (ages 17 to 21) have a firmer sense of self and can clearly relate abstract information to their own lives. Effective interaction with adolescents requires an understanding of the level of psychosocial development and the tasks of this age group. One important task for adolescents is to develop decision-making abilities. Decisions about sexual activity, pregnancy, and parenthood also face adolescents (Fig. 25-1).

Another task of adolescence is to establish an adult identity. The combination of dramatic bodily changes, sexual maturation, movement from concrete to abstract thought, emancipation from parents, and growing in-

---

BOX 25-1

Adolescent Development

EARLY ADOLESCENCE (AGES 10 TO 14)

1. Thinking is concrete.
2. Major interests are in same sex peers, but interest in the opposite sex is beginning.
3. There are conflicts with parents.
4. The adolescent behaves as a child one minute and as an adult the next.

MIDDLE ADOLESCENCE (AGES 15 TO 16)

1. Peer group acceptance is the major issue and often determines self-esteem.
2. The adolescent engages in daydreams, fantasies, and magical thinking.
3. The adolescent struggles for independence from parents.
4. The adolescent exhibits idealistic and narcissistic behaviors.
5. The adolescent exhibits emotional lability, frequent outbursts, and mood swings.
6. Heterosexual relationships are important.

LATE ADOLESCENCE (AGES 17 TO 21)

1. The adolescent begins to go steady with the opposite sex.
2. The adolescent develops abstract thinking.
3. The adolescent begins to develop plans for the future.
4. The adolescent seeks emotional and financial independence from parents.
5. Love is part of intimate, heterosexual relationships.
6. Decision-making ability has developed.
7. A firm sense of self as an adult is developed.

---

volvement with peers can all create a sense of confusion about who they are. The peer group functions as the mechanism by which adolescents can alleviate their anxieties about separating themselves from their parents and becoming adults. Identity formation gives the ego strength and helps adolescents recognize their sex roles. By identifying their sex roles, adolescents are able to engage in sexual intimacy with another individual without losing their own identity (Erikson, 1968).

One challenge of adolescence is the establishment of sexual identity. Sexual identity refers to an individual's inner sense and self-perception of femaleness or maleness, which have developed over time. The onset of puberty produces drastic changes in the adolescent's physical growth, normal functioning, and sexual tension. Sexual tension subsides with behavior such as masturbation, sexual intercourse, or the unconscious equivalent (e.g., nocturnal emission). These experiences are new to the young adolescent. Group pressure from peers may

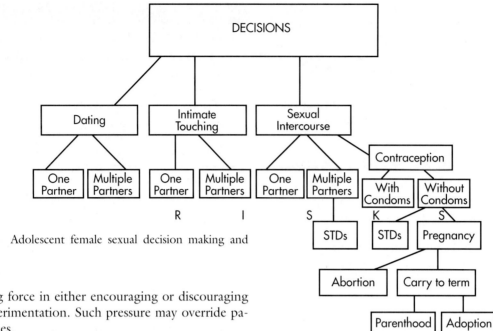

FIG. 25-1 Adolescent female sexual decision making and risks.

be a strong force in either encouraging or discouraging sexual experimentation. Such pressure may override parental wishes.

Sexual decision making for the adolescent includes choosing whether or not to be sexually active with one or more partners, whether or not to use some form of contraception to prevent pregnancy, and whether or not to use condoms to decrease the risk of sexually transmitted diseases (STDs). If pregnancy should occur, decisions must be made about abortion or carrying the pregnancy to term. If pregnancy is chosen, the adolescent must decide whether to keep the infant or place the baby for adoption (Fig. 25-1). The adolescent's level of cognitive development, value system, perception of external controls, and self-identity all influence sexual decision making. The nurse who recognizes these influences must understand these processes in order to help the adolescent develop more effective reasoning about sexuality.

Cognitive and Moral Development

Cognitively the pregnant early adolescent is a concrete thinker with limited or nonexistent reasoning capabilities. She is unable to conceptualize what could "possibly" happen. She fails to relate how the sex act tonight can result in a child's birth in 9 months. Only through abstract thinking (formal operations) is she able to solve problems by evaluating "if-then" alternatives. The development of morality depends on this cognitive development. Most middle adolescents follow rules for the purpose of gaining approval from others (conventional level of morality). As late adolescents mature cognitively and gain life experiences with right and wrong, they develop their own moral code (postconventional morality) (Kohlberg, 1980).

Physiologic Development

The neuroendocrine interaction of hormones stimulates the onset of puberty. As the brain matures, stimulation of the hypothalamus leads to the secretion of gonadotropin-releasing hormones. These hormones induce the anterior pituitary to release gonadotropins (follicle-stimulating hormone and luteinizing hormone), which stimulate the gonads to mature and release ova in the female or to produce and release sperm in the male. These changes prepare the adolescent for reproduction.

The release of growth hormone from the hypothalamus triggers the onset of rapid physical growth (Greydanus, Shearin, 1990). This accelerated growth continues over a 3-year period and occurs approximately two years earlier in females than in males. Physical size of adolescents should not be used as the only basis for planning care.

As children move through adolescence to become adults, they must complete the necessary processes of biologic, cognitive, and psychosocial development (see Box 25-1). *Each adolescent must be assessed individually* to ascertain her or his maturational status, since each person matures at a different rate.

Adolescence is a developmental process that must be completed. Life events may force a young person into adult roles before completing this adolescent period, but an adolescent cannot change the prescribed order and "grow up" because he or she will soon be a parent.

ADOLESCENT SEXUALITY

Effective approaches to solving the problem of adolescent pregnancy begin with a definition of that problem. Redefining adolescent pregnancy as a social problem "of" society rather than "in" society may lead to more comprehensive solutions. There is a pervasive moralism in American society that views adolescent sexual activity as unacceptable. Sex outside of marriage, regardless of age, is unacceptable to many individuals. In the United States opinions differ as to whether the primary issue in adolescent pregnancy is a lack of access to contraception or one of inappropriate premarital sexual activity. Some people are concerned that providing sex education and contraceptives gives permission for or encourages sexual activity.

Sexuality is an integral component of personal identity that evolves and matures throughout a person's life. Sexuality is not synonymous with sex, rather it is the interaction of biology, personal psychology, and environmental factors. Biologic functioning refers to the individual's ability to give and receive pleasure and to reproduce. **Psychologic sexual self-concept and identity** refer to the individual's internal meaning of sexuality such as body image, identification with being either male or female, and learning masculine or feminine roles. Sociocultural values or rules help shape how individuals relate to the world, and how they choose relationships of shared sexuality with other people.

Sexual Behavior

Many adolescents in the United States are sexually active and at risk for pregnancy. Each year more than one million American teenagers become pregnant. The United States has higher adolescent pregnancy, birth, and abortion rates than most other developed countries. The National Centers for Health Statistics (1993) reported that 86% of adolescent males and 75% of adolescent females had become sexually active before the age of 19. The greatest increase in live births per 1,000 women is found in early adolescents. Almost half of today's 14-year-olds will become pregnant before reaching the age of 20. Most young girls have their first sexual encounter in their home. The most frequent season for the initiation of sexual intercourse is during the summer months. In addition, 22% of high school students in the United States reported that they had had at least four sex partners (Centers for Disease Control and Prevention, 1991). Sexually experienced adolescents are unlikely to abstain from continued sexual activity. About 63% of all cases of STDs occur among people younger than 24 years of age (Tyre, Rothbart, Anderson, 1990). A review of records of adolescents 15 years of age or younger, who have attended a family planning clinic, revealed that 41% had had their first sexual experience (i.e., intercourse) between 12 and 13 years of age, 18% between the ages of 14 and 15, and remainder before the age of 12. Although more than 7% of these teenagers reported having been sexually abused or raped, an additional 19% described situations in the home or exhibited symptoms associated with a history of sexual abuse, 11% had had a history of

two or three different STDs, and 26% had contracted three or more STDs (Swenson, 1992).

Behaviors associated with the major causes of adolescent morbidity and mortality share a common theme—risk taking. **Risk taking** is defined as intentional behaviors with uncertain outcomes (Irwin, 1989). Teenagers say that they take risks because risks are enjoyable, the consequences do not seem that great, and everybody else is taking chances. Risk-taking behaviors are associated with adolescent pregnancy. Although many healthy, happy adolescents enjoy an active sex life, are responsible, and are aware of the implications of their sexual expression, *the United States has one of the highest rates of adolescent pregnancy and childbearing in the industrialized world.*

The media (television, music, movies, radio, videos, and print) influence adolescents' ideas about sexuality. Sexual themes and activities have increased 103% in soap operas since 1980 (Fine, Mortimer, Roberts, 1990). The conflicting messages given by the media place pressure on adolescents who do not wish to be sexually active. Two reasons young adolescents choose to become sexually active are because of increased sexual desires and the earlier onset of menarche, which now occurs between the ages of 10 and 12. Sexual abuse or incest must be suspected in early adolescents who become sexually active. A study of 14-year-old, African-American, pregnant girls revealed that sexual decision making was related to four key factors: attempts to establish a relationship based on trust, their it-can't-happen-to-me attitude toward becoming pregnant, their family structure, and their beliefs about the alternatives available if pregnancy occurs (Pete, Desantis, 1990).

Adolescent boys express their sexuality in a number of ways. The average male has intercourse for the first time when he is 15.7 years of age. Male adolescents often brag about their sexual conquests. An adolescent boy may not want to carry the stigma of being the only virgin in his group. As a result, when sexually inexperienced adolescents listen to these tales of sexual adventures, they have no way of knowing that many of these stories were invented to impress the listeners. Many adolescent boys become sexually active, not from sexual desire, rather from the need to belong to the group (Adler et al, 1990).

Contraception

Adolescents who are sexually active often do not use contraceptives consistently and correctly. Recent data suggest an encouraging increase in the use of condoms among adolescents. However, more than half of sexually active female adolescents do not use condoms during their first intercourse (Forest, Singh, 1990). On the average, adolescents become sexually active 15 months before initiating regular contraceptive use. According to White and Kellinger (1989), most adolescents discontinue contraceptive use within the first year after its initiation. Girls "forget" to take their birth control pills or hide them; they do not want pills to "pollute" their bodies. Adolescent boys often carry condoms in their wallets merely as a symbol. Adolescents say that they do not use contraceptives because they do not think that they will become pregnant, or they do not anticipate having intercourse. Many girls are afraid they will be considered "bad girls" if they use contraceptives, because having contraceptives means that they have planned for sexual intercourse.

Since adolescent males are unable to think abstractly or see situations from another person's perspective, they may have difficulty understanding the importance of contraceptive use. Adolescent females frequently romanticize their boyfriends' decisions not to use contraceptives by perceiving unprotected intercourse as an affirmation of love or commitment.

When advising teenagers about contraception, the nurse should consider the adolescent's maturity level, motivation to avoid pregnancy, moral and religious beliefs, frequency of intercourse, regularity of menses, and risk of contracting STDs.

More adolescents use oral contraceptives than condoms, which are the second most popular method. Young teenagers and women in their early 20s have the lowest risk of severe complications from oral contraceptive use. There is no evidence that 13- or 14-year-old girls have special problems with oral contraceptives. Earlier concerns that oral contraceptives would cause premature epiphyseal closure have been disproved. Nevertheless, it is preferable for the young adolescent to have had up to 12 months of regular menstrual cycles before initiating oral contraceptive use.

Adolescents should be educated about all contraceptive methods, including abstinence. The method chosen should reflect the teenager's lifestyle. Adolescents should also know that the simultaneous use of oral contraceptives and condoms will help to protect them from STDs.

Abortion

Approximately 39% of all adolescent pregnancies are terminated by induced abortion; approximately one third of all abortions in the United States are performed on adolescents (McAnarney, Hendee, 1989a). The educational level of the adolescent's parent is a factor concerning whether she will have an abortion. This is true for African-Americans, whites, and Hispanics. The higher the parent's level of education, the less likely the pregnancy will be carried to term (Cooksey, 1990). In a national study conducted in states without parental involvement laws in effect, 61% of adolescents who had an abortion said that one or both of their parents (usually their mother) knew about the abortion (Henshaw, Kost, 1992). The most common reasons adolescents gave for not telling their parents were wanting to preserve their

relationships with their parents and wanting to protect their parents from stress and conflict. Approximately one third of teenagers who did not tell their parents had experienced or feared family violence. Teenagers who have more than one abortion during adolescence may have needs that require referral for psychologic counseling. Because of their developmental status, teenagers usually need more intensive counseling than adult women when coping with an abortion. If the issue is inadequately resolved, adolescents may have problems with sexuality and parenting issues later in life. The physical and psychologic consequences of abortion among adolescents are unclear because of a lack of scientific studies and follow-up investigations.

Sex Education

Past **sex education** strategies focused on reproductive anatomy and physiology and on teaching behaviors typical of middle-class American family life. More recently, sex education began addressing problems of human sexuality faced by teenagers. For example, programs now focus on helping teens "say no." Opponents of school-based sex education programs believe that explicit discussions about sexuality increase teenagers' sexual activity and undermine the role of the parents. Proponents cite the absence of such discussions by parents and their failure to provide their children with needed information have actually served as barriers to the prevention of adolescent pregnancy. The roles of the family, church, and school are complex and controversial with respect to sex education.

Parents may not involve themselves in the sex education of their children for several reasons, such as the following: (1) parents may not have adequate information, (2) parents may be uncomfortable with the topic of sex, and (3) adolescents may be uncomfortable when parents discuss sex. Some parents find it difficult to acknowledge that their "child" is a sexual person with sexual feelings and behaviors. Parental refusal to discuss sexual behavior with their adolescent daughter may cause her to keep her sexual activity a secret and may interfere with efforts to seek help.

National surveys of parents reveal greater support for the inclusion of comprehensive sex education in school curricula and also for beginning sex education at an earlier age (Centers for Disease Control and Prevention, 1991; Donovan, 1989; Rosoff, 1989). Sex education programs should begin before puberty, and some people suggest that it begin as early as kindergarten. These programs should provide adolescents with experience in personal decision making and practice in applying this information to their lives. Programs should address how to handle peer pressure, focus on both females and males, and involve parents in order to enhance parent-adolescent communication and to strengthen family ties. Community institutions (e.g., churches, local lay groups, and professional groups) should also become involved and lend support to these sex education programs. Such support may be in the form of financial help or volunteers. These programs must be based on a clearly communicated set of values (Lockhart, Wodarski, 1990). For example, abstinence-*based* vs. abstinence-*only* curricula may be more acceptable to more individuals and groups. As yet, systematic research regarding the effects of sex education remain inconclusive.

Sexually Transmitted Diseases and Human Immunodeficiency Virus

The incidence of STDs has risen more rapidly among teenagers than in the general population (Brown, 1989). Young adolescents are at the lowest risk for sexual exposure to the human immunodeficiency virus (HIV) unless they are sexually abused by an adult who is HIV positive. Teenaged prostitutes are at greater risk. Teenagers who may have acquired HIV through transfusion for the treatment of hemophilia or other blood-related conditions, through intravenous drug use or through sexual activity should be counseled about the potential for infecting a sexual partner. The highest incidences of gonorrhea and syphilis have occurred in the 15- to 19-year-old age group. For children younger than 15 years of age who are HIV positive, death from HIV infection and its complications is greater than 70%. Researchers predict that HIV will increasingly be found in the adolescent population. Therefore sex education programs must make the link between the prevention of AIDS and the prevention of other STDs.

ADOLESCENT PREGNANCY

Pregnancy in adolescence interrupts work on identity formation and developmental tasks. Trying to simultaneously accomplish the developmental tasks of both pregnancy and normal adolescence may be overwhelming. The psychologic burden may lead to depression and to postponement in attaining an adult identity.

Primary, secondary, and tertiary prevention are needed to prevent adolescent pregnancy. Primary intervention includes, but is not limited to, teaching young children about sexuality. In addition, society must address inequities in opportunities that place females and ethnic minorities at higher risk for becoming victims of social problems such as adolescent pregnancy. Comprehensive health care services for adolescents must be available. Secondary prevention must include accessible contraceptive services for sexually active teenagers. Finally, tertiary prevention must include easily accessible prenatal care, family planning, and follow-up care for infants and children of adolescents (McAnarney, Hendee, 1989b).

Many risk factors are associated with teenage pregnancy, including low socioeconomic status, ethnic minority status, growing up in a single-parent household, low educational achievement, low occupational aspirations, and growing up in a neighborhood characterized by a high incidence of all these factors. Adolescents who become pregnant before graduating from high school are on average two years behind their grade level at the time of pregnancy. Adolescents younger than 16 years of age are at greatest risk for pregnancy (McAnarney, Hendee, 1989b). Pregnant adolescents may not be as socially competent or as proficient in their problem-solving skills as their nonpregnant peers (Passino et al, 1993).

Pregnant teenagers often prolong the period of time between suspecting and confirming their pregnancy, usually because they are in denial. Since teenagers may not volunteer that they suspect pregnancy, health care providers should directly ask adolescents about their sexual activity and discuss the importance of early testing if pregnancy is suspected (Bluestein, Rutledge, 1992).

Developmental Tasks of Pregnancy

When an adolescent becomes pregnant, she faces certain **developmental tasks of pregnancy.** These tasks include the following:

1. *Accepting the biologic reality of pregnancy* — Most adolescents do not expect to become pregnant. They may deny it until the signs are so obvious that they can no longer be ignored by their family members. It is common for teenagers to diet and wear constricting clothes in an attempt to hide their pregnancy. Some girls succeed in hiding their pregnancy until it is quite advanced, sometimes until the birth. The level of denial in some teenagers and their families can be quite high.

    In their study Young et al (1989) found that concealment of the pregnancy was the primary reason younger adolescents failed to seek prenatal care before the third trimester. In contrast, poor motivation was frequently the reason given by older adolescents.

2. *Accepting the reality of the unborn child* —The adolescent may accept only the fantasy of having a cute, happy, healthy baby whom she can dress up and play with like a doll. She does not accept the reality that the infant will grow and develop into an older child.

3. *Accepting the reality of parenthood* —Being a parent implies being loving, concerned, and capable of providing the nurturing care that an infant needs. Although they usually *desire* to be good parents, adolescent mothers and fathers have limited life experiences. They neglected their own needs to grow, and, therefore, developed little ability to

cope with abstractions and solve problems.

The amount and type of support available to adolescent parents can significantly influence the accomplishment of these tasks.

Cultural Influences

The pregnancy rate for low-income, ethnic minority adolescents is high. Poverty and societal racism have a harmful effect on family and community life. Minority adolescents tend to become sexually active at an earlier age and to have less access to birth control information than do white adolescents. A lack of social and family support, nurturance, and supervision coupled with fewer opportunities to accomplish social and educational goals, place these teenagers at greater risk for adolescent pregnancy. Cultural differences exist with respect to knowledge and beliefs about sexuality, pregnancy, and prevention. For example, many Native Americans believe that intrauterine devices (IUDs) might mark the baby if pregnancy occurs. African-American teenagers consider birth control pills and IUDs unacceptable. The beliefs and preferences of white teenager tend to vary along religious lines. Mexican-American and Central/South American girls are more likely to use effective birth control than are Puerto Rican, Cuban, or other Hispanic girls (Durant et al, 1990).

Nurses must be aware of differences in cultural beliefs in order for open communication to occur. By assessing and incorporating these beliefs into a plan of care, nurses can provide more appropriate care, and more effective programs for pregnancy prevention may result.

Family Reactions to Adolescent Pregnancy

One of the most difficult tasks facing the pregnant adolescent is telling her parents. She may not talk about her pregnancy until it becomes obvious. Her mother usually finds out first and may attempt to protect the adolescent's father from discovering their daughter's pregnancy.

Initial reactions of grandparents-to-be are usually shock, anger, shame, guilt, and sorrow. The nurse must assess any disharmony within the family. The nurse should also assist as family members adapt to their decision regarding pregnancy, adoption, or abortion. The stereotype of the low-income family accepting the pregnant daughter and her newborn unequivocally is not verified. Mothers of low-income African-American, pregnant adolescents often become angry and disappointed, because they wanted their daughters to have a better chance in life than they themselves had.

Adolescent Fathers

Teenage fathers are more likely to be children of teenage parents than their peers who are not fathers. Conse-

quently, they may not see pregnancy as a disruption to their young lives. In some low-income communities an adolescent's ability to impregnate is viewed with a sense of pride and as a sign of manhood (Marsiglio, 1993).

Adolescent fathers are more likely to be poorer and less educated than boys who do not become fathers at an early age. Contrary to popular belief, pregnant adolescent couples do not have transient relationships, rather many of these relationships tend to be ongoing. According to Elsters, Lamb, and Kimmerly (1989) fewer than 9% of pregnant adolescents knew their partners fewer than 6 months before conception and more than 50% knew their partners for 2 years or longer. Most adolescent fathers try to provide some support for their partners such as money, gifts, and transportation (Sander, Rosen, 1989). They also want to be involved in the decision-making process concerning options regarding the pregnancy. However, families of the adolescent couple frequently exclude the adolescent father from this decision-making process because of anger about the pregnancy, or because they believe he is incapable of making such a decision. Frequently adolescent fathers think that their partners do not really need them for support; as a result, some adolescent fathers do not believe they are neglecting their partners.

If the adolescent couple does not marry, contact diminishes significantly over time; if they marry, marital satisfaction tends to be low. The nurse should assess the adolescent couple's relationship when planning care for the pregnant adolescent and her partner. The nurse must be familiar with state and federal law to ensure that the patient's rights are protected with respect to legal issues associated with pregnant adolescents (see Legal Tip).

LEGAL TIP: **Care of Adolescents**

Legal Issues Related to Pregnant Adolescents

Emancipated minors. Minors who are married, who are in the military service, or who are living away from home and are self-supporting may give their own medical consent. Parents have no legal responsibility for the medical bill.

Confidentiality. The Constitution protects an adolescent's right to privacy. Parents who give consent for and pay for a minor's health care are entitled to information about his or her care and may request and receive the adolescent's medical records.

Contraception and abortion. In most states it is legal to provide contraceptive services to minors. A minor's consent to abortion varies across states. Some state statutes may require parental consent; others require parental notification before an unemancipated minor may obtain an abortion. Sterilization law also varies from state to state. Some states prohibit the elective sterilization of anyone younger than 18 years of age.

Retaining child custody. The birth mother can authorize or refuse medical treatment for her infant regardless of whether she is married or unmarried to the child's father.

Adoption. State law determines the procedures for adoption. Options available to the mother vary by type of agency (i.e., public vs. private) and by type of arrangements (i.e., no sharing of any identifying information between parties vs. open adoption in which the birth mother may visit her child regularly).

ADOLESCENT PARENTHOOD

The transition to parenthood may be difficult for adolescent parents. Coping with the developmental tasks of parenthood is often complicated by the unmet developmental needs and tasks of adolescence. They may experience difficulty accepting a changing self-image and adjusting to new roles related to the responsibilities of infant care. They may feel "different" from their peers, excluded from "fun" activities, and prematurely forced to enter an adult social role. The conflict between their own desires and the infant's demands, in addition to the low tolerance for frustration that is typical of adolescence further contribute to the normal psychosocial stress of childbirth.

Some differences between adolescent and adult mothers have been observed. For example, adolescent mothers provide warm and attentive physical care; however, they use less verbal interaction than do older parents, and adolescents tend to be less responsive to their infants than older mothers. Although some observations suggest that some adolescents may use more aggressive behaviors, a higher incidence of child abuse has not been documented. In comparison to adult mothers, teenage mothers have a limited knowledge of child development. They tend to expect too much of their children too soon and often characterize their infants as being fussy. This limited knowledge may cause teenagers to respond to their infants inappropriately.

Developmental Tasks of Parenthood

The **developmental tasks of parenthood** include the following: (1) reconciling the imagined child with the actual child, (2) becoming adept in caregiving activities, (3) being aware of the infant's needs, (4) and incorporating the infant into the family. Although it is biologically pos-

sible for an adolescent girl to become a parent, her egocentrism and concrete thinking interfere with her ability to parent effectively. The early adolescent is inexperienced and not prepared to recognize early signs of illness, potential danger, or household hazards. Infants may inadvertently be neglected. Infants of adolescents are nine times more likely to die from accidents and violence than infants who have older mothers (McAnarney, Greydanus, 1989). These higher infant mortality rates are attributed to the inexperience, lack of knowledge, and immaturity of the adolescent mother, which results in her inability to recognize a problem and obtain the necessary resources. Nevertheless, in most instances, with adequate support and developmentally appropriate teaching, adolescents can learn effective parenting skills.

Maintaining a relationship with the baby's father is beneficial for both the mother and the child. The father's involvement directly corresponds with appropriate maternal behaviors (Ruff, 1990), the mother's increased sense of confidence and security, and the child's healthy sense of trust, self-esteem, and social skills (Sander, Rosen, 1989).

The Extended Family

Childbearing in low-income families often occurs without the supporting presence of the newborn's father. For early adolescents another member of the family may assume a significant role in the infant's care. Frequently the baby's grandmother supports, coaches, or supervises the adolescent mother as she learns her maternal role. Often times the grandmother assumes the primary caregiver's role if she thinks that her daughter is too immature or lacks the necessary judgment for the caregiver's role.

RISKS AND CONSEQUENCES OF PREGNANCY

The effects of young maternal age on obstetric and neonatal outcome are often difficult to separate from the influences of low socioeconomic status, ethnic background, educational disadvantage, substance abuse, overcrowded living conditions, STDs, marital status, and lack of social support. The young adolescent is at greater risk for being affected by one or more of these influences. These influences, not the adolescent's age, may increase her risk during pregnancy. Nevertheless, because young maternal age is associated with a higher risk for adverse maternal and neonatal outcomes, the relationship between age and pregnancy outcomes is addressed.

Physiologic Maternal Risk

In the past people believed that adolescents were more likely than adults to experience pregnancy-induced hypertension and cephalopelvic disproportion (CPD). Although a higher incidence of abruptio placentae for early adolescents has also been reported, adolescents who receive early and adequate prenatal care should have no greater risk of experiencing an adverse obstetric outcome than adult women of a similar sociodemographic background. Pregnancy-induced hypertension is believed to be related to the fact that mothers younger than 16 years of age are more likely to be African-American and first-time mothers. More recent studies have not confirmed the findings of earlier reports that note an increased risk of CPD among pregnant adolescents in comparison to adults (McAnarney, Hendee, 1989a). In fact, assisted operative births are more often related to low-birth-weight (LBW) infants than to CPD.

Iron deficiency anemia is a potential problem in all pregnant women. The adolescent who is already anemic when she begins her pregnancy is at greater risk and must be followed-up closely and carefully counseled regarding nutrition during pregnancy.

Other problems found in adolescents are cigarette smoking and substance abuse. Fetal damage from maternal smoking or drug use may already have occurred by the time pregnancy is confirmed.

Physiologic Neonatal Risk

As maternal age increases, the risk of having an LBW infant decreases. Multiparous adolescents and early adolescents are more likely to bear LBW infants. Their infants are also at greater risk of dying within the first 28 days of life. This higher mortality rate is primarily due to the higher incidence of LBW infants born to these teenagers. Prenatal care appears to reduce this morbidity and mortality. Early adolescent parents experience higher postneonatal mortality rates, higher rates of sudden infant death syndrome (SIDS), and a greater number of childhood illnesses and injuries.

Socioeconomic Risks

Teenage pregnancy remains the number one cause for adolescent girls to terminate their education prematurely. Leaving school early is associated with unemployment and poverty. As a result, adolescent parents often fail to complete their basic education, have fewer opportunities for employment and career advancement, and have limited earning potential. More young mothers than older mothers live in families with annual incomes near the poverty level. Payments from Aid to Dependent Children (ADC) rarely provide adequate support for the optimal development of young children. Adolescent mothers tend to have more children than they desire, and their children tend to be closely spaced. All these factors result in limited resources that can impair optimal parenting.

Abandonment, child abuse, separation, and divorce occur two-to-four times more often among women who married as teenagers than among those who married in their 20s. In addition to the stress of the transition to marriage, family instability is also related to a low level of education, low level of employment, and lack of support systems.

The Pregnant Early Adolescent

Early adolescents are at greatest risk for problems in pregnancy and childbirth. The incidence of LBW infants, infant mortality, and abortion is two to three times greater in this age group than for women older than 25 years of age (National Center for Health Statistics, 1993).

Since early adolescents tend to begin prenatal care later than older adolescents and women, they are especially at high risk. Entering prenatal care later may result in inadequate time before the birth to attend to correctable problems. These adolescents are also at higher risk for conditions associated with first pregnancy (e.g., pregnancy-induced hypertension). When prenatal care is early and consistent, and high-risk factors (e.g., socioeconomic factors) are accounted for, the risks for both mother and infant are equal to those of older pregnant women. To reduce risks and consequences of adolescent pregnancy, nurses need to encourage early and continued prenatal care and, if necessary, to refer the adolescent to appropriate social support services that can help correct a negative socioeconomic environment.

Care Management—Sexually Active Adolescents

When adolescents choose to engage in sexual activity, they become at risk for a number of health problems. The nurse can work effectively with sexually active adolescents to achieve optimal health outcomes.

❖ ASSESSMENT

The nurse should conduct a thorough health history interview (including menstrual, sexual, and dietary factors), with a review of body systems, a complete physical examination (including a breast and pelvic examination), and laboratory tests. In addition, assessment of the psychosocial (e.g., sexual identity, body image, self-concept), cognitive-developmental stage, and support systems are also essential. Careful assessment is needed to identify the adolescent's learning and care needs. When conducting the health history interview, the nurse should use a quiet, private room and the adolescent should be fully clothed. An unhurried, nonjudgmental attitude encourages patient relaxation. Interviews should begin with nonthreatening questions followed by more sensitive questions in order to establish a rapport with the adolescent. During the interview, the nurse needs to be aware of culturally unacceptable verbal and nonverbal responses, as well as use direct language such as "sexual intercourse" instead of "making love." Docu-

---

BOX 25-2

Elements Essential to a Sexual History

LIFESTYLE FACTORS

History of chronic illnesses (e.g., diabetes)
Past or current STDs or chronic vaginitis
Regularity of menses
Drug or alcohol use
Type and frequency of contraceptive use (e.g., with or without condoms)
Previous abortions
Types of sexual activities
Number and gender of sexual partners
Past or current physical or sexual abuse, rape, or incest

KNOWLEDGE

Knowledge of safer sex practices and STDs
Sources of sex education

ATTITUDE

Sexual self-concept, body image, and gender identity
Satisfaction with sex and sexual partner(s)
Attitude toward current intimate relationship

---

mentation of the adolescent's **sexual history** is essential. Box 25-2 lists the essential elements of a **sexual history.**

In addition to the interview, a thorough physical examination is also necessary. The nurse should be alert for possibilities of sexual abuse in young adolescents. This is because they have little experience with what normal body functions are, so STDs may go unnoticed and unreported to health care providers for treatment. In the presence of severe pleuritic pain with right-upper-quadrant tenderness under the rib cage, the sexually active adolescent should be assessed for Fitz-Hugh and Curtis syndrome. Fitz-Hugh and Curtis syndrome is a localized peritonitis involving the anterior surface of the liver and the adjacent peritoneum of the anterior abdominal wall. This syndrome accompanies perihepatitis that is secondary to gonococcal or nongonococcal pelvic inflammatory disease (PID). Pelvic ultrasound may help to distinguish the masses of pelvic infection from those of other conditions such as ectopic pregnancy (Tierney et al, 1993). Heavy menstrual bleeding or other abnormal bleeding in adolescents may be related to abortion, trauma, endocrinologic diseases, infection, oral contraceptives, as well as other causes (Hilliard, Rebar, 1990).

A pelvic examination is essential for any teenager who sexually active and for those considering oral contraceptives. During puberty the vaginal epithelium is thin, which makes it more vulnerable to irritation and infection. Contact vaginitis can result from the use of per-

fumed soap, powders, sprays, and wearing tight jeans or other garments. Adolescent girls are modest and usually tense during the pelvic examination, which they find distasteful and anxiety provoking. If sexual abuse has occurred, the examination is even more threatening. An appropriate expected outcome should be to help the adolescent feel in control and not embarrassed. The adolescent should be asked to decide whether her mother may remain in the room during the examination. Before a first pelvic examination, instruction in relaxation techniques is helpful. Lidocaine ointment may be used as a lubricant. The anxious adolescent may feel more comfortable using a mirror so that she can participate in the examination. If she finds the examination too painful and is unable to cooperate, then the examination may either be performed under anesthesia (Hilliard, Rebar, 1990) or deferred.

Although breast disease is uncommon in adolescent girls, anxiety about symptoms, such as swelling, is common. Breast findings in teenagers are frequently hormone-related and commonly occur during the surge of puberty. Swelling of the breasts may also occur during pregnancy and with substance abuse. The teenager should be reassured that breast swelling will decrease spontaneously when the hormone surge regresses (Beach, 1990).

Laboratory studies may include a complete blood count, rubella antibody test, HIV antibody test, urinalysis, urine culture and sensitivity, Papanicolaou's (Pap) test, wet smear, cervical culture, hemoglobin and hematocrit levels, blood typing, gonorrhea and *Chlamydia* cultures, and serologic test for syphilis (STS).

❖ NURSING DIAGNOSES

The nurse formulates appropriate nursing diagnoses after reviewing the assessment findings from the interview, physical examination, and laboratory/diagnostic tests. Nursing diagnoses may include the following:

Body image disturbance related to
  ▪ Lack of knowledge regarding puberty changes
Knowledge deficit related to
  ▪ STDs
  ▪ Fertility and contraception
High risk for pregnancy complications related to
  ▪ Unsafe sexual practices
  ▪ Noncompliance

❖ EXPECTED OUTCOMES

The nurse bases the plan of care on the adolescent's health care needs. The *expected outcomes* for care, mutually determined by the adolescent and the nurse, are stated in patient-centered terms. Examples of expected outcomes include the following:

- The adolescent will experience a therapeutic relationship with her health care providers.
- The adolescent will be able to relax or experience no trauma during the pelvic examination.
- The adolescent will describe the biologic events occurring throughout the menstrual cycle.
- The adolescent will dispel myths and misunderstandings about contraception and sexual behaviors.
- The adolescent will identify safer sex behaviors.

✤ COLLABORATIVE CARE

Health education must be conducted at the primary, secondary, and tertiary levels of prevention. At the primary prevention level, health education provides information about good hygiene, the menstrual cycle, and STDs. Secondary prevention includes education about appropriate protective barriers during sex. Tertiary prevention includes proper treatment of current STDs, as well as prevention of sequelae and further exposure. Health education strategies need to be creative and developmentally, culturally, educationally, and linguistically appropriate. Education should be appropriate for low-risk groups, high-risk groups, and parents or partners of adolescents.

Adolescents, because of their risk-taking behavior, are expected to be the next group that becomes hardest hit by the HIV epidemic. Treatment for AIDS or HIV infection will be difficult for adolescents with no usual source of health care (e.g., uninsured, homeless, or runaway adolescents). On the basis of the nursing diagnoses, the nurse may need to refer the adolescent to a nurse practitioner, physician, nurse-midwife, counselor, social worker, or legal service organization.

Oral contraceptives do not reduce the risk of contracting STDs. However, oral contraceptives can reduce the adolescent's risk by 50% that certain STDs, such as gonorrhea and chlamydial infection, will escalate into pelvic inflammatory disease (PID).

The condom, when used with a spermicide, is the next-best contraceptive choice for teenagers. In addition to preventing pregnancy, the latex condom and spermicide help protect against STDs.

Adolescents frequently misuse and misunderstand the "rhythm" method ("fertility-awareness" method), thus making this method ineffective for this age group. They often are unaware that ovulation occurs approximately 14 days *before* the first day of the next menstrual period. In order to effectively use this method, the adolescent needs to be taught the complex process of determining her individual fertility status so that she abstains from sexual intercourse for the entire time that sexual intercourse is considered to be "unsafe." This method is even less effective for adolescents who have irregular menstrual cycles (Tyre, Rothbart, Anderson, 1990).

✤ EVALUATION

The nurse can be reasonably assured that care has been effective if the expected outcomes of care have been achieved; that is, if the adolescent experiences a therapeutic relationship with health care providers. Outcome criteria may include the following: the adolescent is able to relax during pelvic examinations; understands the menstrual cycle; dispels myths and misunderstandings regarding contraception and sexual behaviors; identifies safer sex behaviors, and avoids pregnancy and STDs.

Care Management— during Pregnancy

Many interacting biologic and social factors affect the quality of human reproduction. These, in turn, are influenced by the preconceptional, maternal, and neonatal care made available. The adolescent and her offspring are particularly vulnerable to the risks inherent in pregnancy and parenthood because of circumstances characteristic of her age group. These circumstances include the adolescent's cognitive-developmental level, psychologic immaturity, economic dependency, and delayed health care. The multifaceted and complex needs of adolescents are most effectively addressed by a multidisciplinary team of nurses, health care providers, registered dietitians, and social workers.

✤ ASSESSMENT

Interview

Before becoming pregnant the early adolescent usually received her medical care from a pediatric health care provider. With her pregnancy, the emphasis of care shifts to a far more intimate and sexual nature. The nurse needs to obtain the adolescent's thorough health history with a review of systems in addition to her sexual history (p 842). The nurse also needs to know the health status of the father-to-be (American Academy of Pediatrics, 1989). If possible, it should be determined if the pregnant adolescent is the victim of sexual abuse or incest, which are the most common causes of pregnancy in early adolescents.

During this examination nurses should conduct vision and dental screenings, as well as assess the adolescent's immunization status. Immunizations such as those against diphtheria, tetanus (every 10 years), polio, measles, mumps, and rubella may need to be renewed. The nurse should also screen for tuberculosis, since the poor economic conditions that increase crowding and homelessness are making tuberculosis more common in low-income populations.

In early pregnancy, vaginal bleeding may be mistaken for menstrual bleeding and delay the diagnosis of pregnancy. As a result, if the date of the last menstrual period (vaginal bleeding) is the only factor used to date the pregnancy, then this date may be inaccurate and result in a delay of prenatal care.

Nutrition Assessment

Prepregnancy weight-for-height is used to determine gestational weight gain. Usually maternal characteristics that increase the risk of low gestational weight gain (e.g., <7 kg, or 16 lb) and preterm births occur in combination. These characteristics include low family income, African-American race, young age, unmarried status, and low educational level (Institute of Medicine, 1990).

Diet evaluation using 24-hour recall can be easily performed anywhere, and it provides a base for assessing the nutrients consumed. Nurses should ask adolescents about athletic participation, dance classes, and other vigorous activities that could alter calorie requirements. The high fat content of food served in school cafeterias and the accepted practice of eating a lot of fast foods place adolescents at greater nutritional risk. Beverage intake should also be assessed. Adolescents may inadvertently consume excessive amounts of caffeine in soft drinks and other beverages. In addition, lifestyle behaviors such as frequent dieting, eating disorders, alcohol abuse, smoking, and substance abuse affect nutritional status and should be assessed.

Current studies show significant substance abuse among pregnant adolescents, and indicate that adolescents underestimate their own abuse (Kokotailo, Adger, 1991). Pregnant adolescents with a history of combined physical and sexual assault tend to abuse substances more often than adolescents without a history of assault (Berenson, San-Miguel, Wilkinson, 1992). The fact that the use of substances during pregnancy drops significantly has implications for intervention programs and prevention. Nurses should also determine the adolescent's pattern of abuse. Young adolescents are most likely to drink on weekends with the intent of "getting drunk." Weekend binge drinking patterns may cause fetal alcohol syndrome.

Early adolescents have more nutritional needs than women whose growth is complete. Although the Recommended Dietary Allowance (RDA) is based on chronologic age, it provides the best available figures to use for pregnant adolescents who are still growing. Adolescents tend to have inadequate diets that are especially deficient in iron and folic acid (Jackson, Mathur, 1991). Many pregnant teenagers, particularly low-income teenagers (Schneck et al, 1990), are nutritionally at risk. These adolescents require nutrition intervention early and throughout their pregnancies. Hematocrit values of adolescents show them to be at risk for nutritional anemia.

Health care providers should measure the adolescent's weight and height. These measurements should then be compared with accepted normal parameters, such as standard weight-for-height, to establish weight gain goals and to monitor weight gain over the course of pregnancy (Institute of Medicine, 1990).

Psychosocial Status

Psychosocial screening includes assessment for the adolescent's response to pregnancy, depression, or suicide. In addition, the nurse assesses the adolescent's cognitive-developmental level, literacy, problem-solving ability, time orientation, body image, dependency, and peer and partner relationships.

Knowledge Base and Perceived Needs

The adolescent is assessed for her knowledge of reproduction, sexual functioning, and her own sexuality. A basic knowledge of these factors helps the pregnant adolescent more readily understand the additional changes occurring during her pregnancy. The assessment of these perceived learning needs elicits valuable information that may be used as the basis for planning and intervention (see Clinical Application of Research).

Support Systems

Emotional support, particularly from the adolescent's family, and financial support are extremely important to the pregnant adolescent. People within her support system (especially her parents, boyfriend, or husband) can significantly influence pregnancy outcome. The nurse assesses the level of support received by the adolescent, as well as how the pregnant adolescent perceives her own role and the roles of others in her support system.

Many pregnant teenagers come from socially and economically deprived families. Appropriate use of health care resources and compliance with preventive health care measures may not be a part of their health value system. The nurse can help these at-risk adolescents change their own behavior so that the health care delivery system and its resources can enhance their health and well-being. A support plan that effectively combines informal and societal supports offers the best probability for successful pregnancy outcome.

Physical Examination and Laboratory Tests

Physical assessment for the pregnant adolescent is the same as that for the sexually active adolescent (see p. 730). Careful determination of baseline blood pressure is necessary since teenagers have lower systolic and diastolic pressures than older women. A pregnant teenager could be in serious jeopardy for eclampsia with a blood pressure reading of 140/90 mm Hg. Screenings such as the laboratory tests listed in Box 25-3 are also necessary.

CLINICAL APPLICATION OF RESEARCH

SELF-DESCRIBED LEARNING NEEDS OF PREGNANT TEENS

The increasing number of adolescent pregnancies is creating a strain on the health care services available to teenagers. With shortened hospital stays, the maternity staff has fewer opportunities to provide health education to this high-risk population.

This descriptive study investigated the learning needs and preferred teaching methods of a group of adolescents, who were either pregnant or new parents, who attended a school program for pregnant girls. This weekly, 2-hour health education class was taught by registered nurses, who were students in a baccalureate nursing program. The *Learning Needs Assessment* was completed by 121 participants and the *Evaluation of Health Class* was filled-out by 83 participants. Both tools were developed by the researcher. The researcher found that the adolescent's greatest learning needs concerned complications during pregnancy, labor, and birth. Other learn-

ing needs included adoption, abortion, and newborn care. Of the least interest were topics related to drugs and alcohol, breastfeeding, and AIDS. A field trip to the hospital was the preferred teaching method; the least liked teaching method was lecture. Audiovisual materials were well received. By using appropriate teaching methods for teenagers and by including content that teenagers find important and interesting, the needs of this high-risk population can effectively be met. Also, linking nursing education with community needs benefits both the nursing students and the community. Such cooperation may help bring needed education and services to communities in spite of reductions in federal, state, or local education funding.

Reference: Bachman JA: Self-described learning needs of pregnant teen participants in an innovative university/community partnership, *Matern Child Nurs J* 21(2):65, 1993.

BOX 25-3

Initial Laboratory Tests for Pregnant Adolescents

Hemoglobin and hematocrit levels
White blood cell count and differential
Blood types, Rh factor
Antibody rubella titer
VDRL and fluorescent treponemal antibody absorption test (FTA-ABS)
Urinalysis, urine culture, and renal function tests: blood urea nitrogen, creatinine, electrolytes, creatinine clearance, and total protein excretion
PAP test, vaginal, or rectal smear for *Neisseria gonorrhea,* beta-streptococcal, and *Chlamydia* infections
Tuberculin skin testing
In some settings cardiac evaluation may be conducted to include: ECG, chest x-ray film, and echocardiogram
Adolescent pregnancies should be dated by both ultrasound scanning and Dubowitz assessment of the newborn

Reference: Stevens-Simon, Roghman, McAnarney, 1991.

✤ NURSING DIAGNOSES

The nurse analyzes information gathered during the assessment and the laboratory data. This information provides the basis for formulating nursing diagnoses. Nursing diagnoses relevant to the pregnant adolescent may include the following:

High risk for fetal injury related to
- Inadequate placental perfusion secondary to preeclampsia

Knowledge deficit related to
- Nutritional needs of the mother and fetus during pregnancy
- Infant growth and development

Altered health maintenance related to
- Socioeconomic deficits

Altered nutrition (e.g., less than body requirements) related to
- High fat, inadequate protein, vitamin and mineral intake

✤ EXPECTED OUTCOMES

The plan of care reflects the pregnant adolescent's need for increased observation, compliance with health care measures, and feelings of personal and social integrity. The care begins as early as possible in the prenatal period and extends through the formative period of the new family.

Whenever possible expected outcomes for care are mutually determined. These expected outcomes may include the following:

- The adolescent will actively participate in her own prenatal care.
- She will return for regular prenatal visits as scheduled.
- She will utilize medical, psychosocial, parenting, and social services to maximize the potential for optimal pregnancy outcome.

- She will experience a physically safe and emotionally satisfying pregnancy, as well as promote optimum health for her child.
- She will acquire knowledge and skills that enhance her decision-making abilities.
- She will show effective use of support systems.

If appropriate, the grandparents-to-be and the father of the adolescent's baby should help set the expected outcomes.

✜ COLLABORATIVE CARE

Health care professionals who work with pregnant adolescents must come to terms with their own sexuality in order to be able to maintain a nonjudgmental approach. They should be enthusiastic, warm, caring individuals who are genuinely interested in the adolescent and able to view her with respect and dignity.

When working with an adolescent, the nurse must be able to listen and to respond with honest answers. If possible, the nurse should be available to the adolescent by telephone. An environment of trust will enable the adolescent to discuss her true feelings, and help the health care professional determine the adolescent's real problems and set realistic goals. With knowledge of adolescent development, the nurse can accept normal adolescent behavior, rather than see it as "acting out."

Nurses need to be adept in using various teaching strategies. Group discussions meet the adolescent's strong need for peer contact and acceptance; however, the nurse may need to act as the group leader because of the participants' immaturity. Anonymous questions and quizzes can be used to identify knowledge deficits or myths. Demonstrations by the nurse with return demonstrations by the teenagers facilitate the assessment of each teenager's abilities. It is important to use simple, concrete, direct language rather than subtlety. Teenage slang should be used by the nurse only if these words are part of the nurse's usual vocabulary. By using correct terminology for body parts and giving direct answers to questions, the nurse communicates respect. Because early adolescents have short attention spans, stimulation of more than one of the senses through the use of multimethod approaches and active participation by the adolescents are helpful. For example, the use of visual models, films, charts, and role playing helps to reinforce learning and fits the concrete way in which early adolescents think (Fig. 25-2). Written instructional materials, such as brochures and visual teaching aids, should be attractive, brightly colored, and use more pictures than words. The comic book format may appeal to the early adolescent. Adolescents are more likely to read materials that resemble regular school assignments.

Because the young adolescent tends to be narcissistic, focusing on the needs of her fetus tends to be less suc-

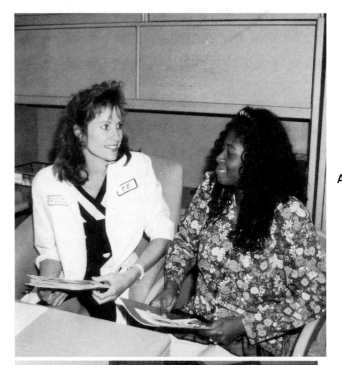

A

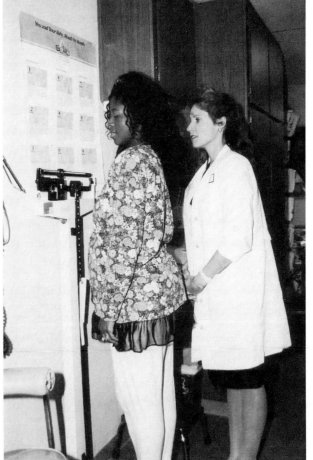

B

FIG. 25-2   Teenage expectant mothers learn about maternal adaptations to pregnancy. **A,** Expectant mother and nurse discuss prenatal care concerns. **B,** Weighing-in during a clinic visit. (Courtesy Marjorie Pyle, RNC, *Lifecircle,* Costa Mesa, CA.)

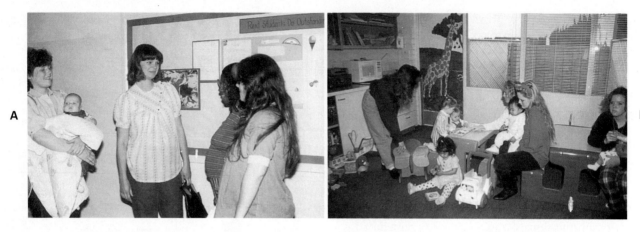

FIG. 25-3   A support and information group meeting for pregnant and parenting adolescents. **A,** Sharing experiences in prenatal clinic may help anxiety for teenage mothers. **B,** Teenage mothers learn child care in a day-care facility. (Courtesy Marjorie Pyle, RNC, *Lifecircle,* Costa Mesa, CA.)

cessful than focusing on her own needs. Nurses need to help the adolescent improve her decision-making ability, explore the risks and consequences of her actions, and assume responsibility for her behavior. Some of the techniques used to encourage growth in these areas include having the adolescent select a menu for her infant, choose appropriate types of clothing for her infant for a certain temperature, and discuss solutions to real problems. The nurse can also help the adolescent separate herself from her baby so that she can see the child's unique needs. Information relative to child development and to infant caregiving is basic to attaining this expected outcome.

Antepartum Care

The adolescent is considered to be at risk during her pregnancy, and an increased number of prenatal visits are scheduled. Prompt clinic attendance is encouraged; missed appointments should be followed up by telephone calls or personal contacts. Adolescents are likely to obtain better care if the prenatal site provides comprehensive services (Stevens-Simon, Fullar, McAnarney, 1992), if the site is attractive and inviting, and if special efforts are made to register and retain them in care. (Cartoof, Klerman, Zazueta, 1991).

When choosing the content of prenatal classes, the nurse should keep the adolescent's needs and developmental level in mind. The nurse needs to use concrete examples of "what to do" and "what not to do" when discussing maternal adaptation during pregnancy. Prenatal education requires creativity, flexibility, humor, and a strong ego. The nurse should avoid treating the adolescent like a child. Nevertheless, typical content and methods of presentation for adult women may be ineffective for adolescents. For example, if the teenager does not

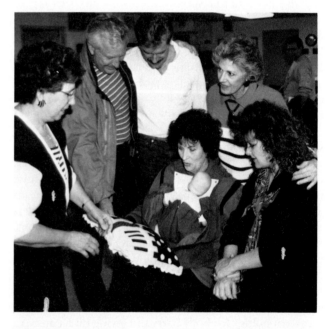

FIG. 25-4   Grandparent classes help grandparents-to-be update their knowledge and skills, such as teaching about infant stimulation (pillow is designed for infant stimulation). Grandparents discuss how best to help their adolescents with the developmental tasks of adolescence, pregnancy, and parenthood. (Courtesy Marjorie Pyle, RNC, *Lifecircle,* Costa Mesa, CA.)

have a partner, she may be "turned off" by films depicting a loving couple.

Support and Information Groups

Most of the prenatal care services discussed earlier in the chapter are offered in clinics or hospitals. In addition to these services, a variety of self-help groups are available for pregnant teenagers and their families. These pro-

TABLE 25-1   Sample Menus for Pregnant Adolescents

	DAY 1	DAY 2
BREAKFAST	1 cup unsweetened, ready-to-eat cereal with 1 cup 2% milk ¾ cup orange juice	2 pancakes, 1 medium waffle, or 1 slice French toast 2 Tbsp syrup 1 cup 2% milk
SNACK	1 blueberry muffin 1 cup 2% milk	2 graham crackers 1 6-oz can apple juice
LUNCH	1 cheeseburger (fast food) 1 banana Carrot sticks 1 cup 2% milk	3 slices pizza 1 apple Small salad 1 Tbsp dressing 1 cup 2% milk
SNACK	1 apple 3 Tbsp peanut butter Caffeine-free soda*	½ cup cottage cheese dip Raw vegetables Caffeine-free soda*
DINNER	1 cup spaghetti with meat sauce Salad 2 Tbsp dressing 1 roll ½ cup chocolate pudding 1 glass water†	3 oz baked chicken 1 cup rice 1 cup green beans 1 roll 1 ice cream sandwich 1 glass water†
SNACK	1 slice angel-food cake ½ cup fresh or frozen fruit, no sugar added Calories = 2525‡	3 cups popcorn 1 glass ginger ale Calories = 2568‡

*Sample diets should include foods that patients normally eat and, therefore, provide teaching opportunities about better choices (example: cola vs. caffeine-free drink).
†Encourage adequate water consumption daily—6 to 8 glasses.
‡Calorie calculations are based on the maximum allowance for growth; however, the best indication that a pregnant adolescent is eating sufficient Calories is to monitor weight gain throughout pregnancy. If inadequate or excess weight gain occurs, consultation with a registered dietitian is recommended.

grams vary in structure and content depending on the organization or agency sponsoring the program. Some of these groups focus on the pregnant adolescent and her self-care, on teenage parenting (whereby teens and their infants may attend together [Fig. 25-3], and on support for parents of the pregnant teen). In a special support group, parents of pregnant teenagers learn how to cope and adapt to the experience better (Fig. 25-4). Generally, group meetings are held weekly or monthly. Such programs have proven highly effective in helping pregnant teenagers and their families cope with the experiences associated with pregnancy and parenting (see Appendix H).

Nutrition Counseling

Nutrition counseling helps adolescents learn about nutrients, as well as plan, select, and prepare optimally nutritious foods for herself and her family. The nutritional needs of teenagers can best be met by eating foods with a high concentration and balance of nutrients (Table 25-

1). The nutritional needs of the older pregnant adolescent approach the nutritional needs required by pregnant adults. Additional amounts of vitamins, minerals, and calories are needed to meet the growth needs of pregnant adolescents and their infants, as well as to correct deficiencies resulting from inadequate intake of nutrients before, during, and after pregnancy. Iron supplements are needed to provide for the growing muscle mass and blood volume increase in pregnant teenagers (Story, 1990). Most adolescent females consume between one and seven snacks daily. Snacks often contribute more than "empty calories." Many snacks eaten by adolescent females contribute approximately half the RDA of the riboflavin, vitamin C, and thiamin that they need.

As an integral part of a health care program for a pregnant teenager, the nutrition consultant must be able to establish a rapport and develop a relationship within which to counsel her in the nutritional aspects of reproduction. Counseling includes working with the pregnant adolescent to set a weight gain goal preferably at the initial prenatal examination, and to explain the importance of weight gain. Additional strategies include building on cultural practices; for example, categorizing nutrition practices as beneficial, neutral, or harmful, and reinforcing positive eating practices while encouraging change in harmful eating practices. In order to have a significant and lasting effect on the future of both the parents and the child, counseling should continue into the postpartum period.

Because energy expenditure for pregnant adolescents varies, the best assurance of adequate intake is a satisfactory weight gain. The recommended range for an adolescent's total weight gain and pattern of gain should be based on her prepregnancy weight-for-height. For women with a normal prepregnancy body mass index, a recommended gain of approximately 0.4 kg (<1 lb) per week during the second and third trimesters of pregnancy is advised (Gutierrez, King, 1993). Young adolescents and African-American women are encouraged to target their weight gain for the higher end of the appropriate range. Weight gain recommendations begin at 40 lb for an underweight adolescent, 35 lb for an adolescent of normal weight, and 25 lb for an overweight adolescent. All pregnant women should have 30 mg of ferrous iron daily. If the adolescent has an inadequate diet, she may need multivitamins and folate. If she consumes less than 600 mg of calcium daily (two cups of milk contain 698 mg), then calcium supplements would be necessary (Institute of Medicine, 1990).

Adolescents frequently begin their pregnancy with depleted body reserves, or else they are still growing. Additional energy intake is probably unnecessary during the first trimester; however, young adolescents may require higher energy intakes later in their pregnancy. In general, pregnant adolescents should consume at least 2000 calories per day; in many cases, higher calorie intakes are needed. Table 25-2 includes the recommended caloric intakes for pregnant and lactating adolescents.

By improving her own diet and that of her family the young mother helps to build the foundation for a healthier beginning for generations to follow. Referral to the Women, Infants, and Children program (WIC), or other food supplementation programs, can ensure that nutritious food is available in the home during pregnancy and throughout the infant's first year.

Newborn Feeding

Many adolescents initially respond negatively to the idea of breastfeeding. They may fear a permanent alteration of the breasts, may think that breastfeeding is "dirty," may lack breastfeeding role models, or may receive negative reactions from peers. These misconceptions, situations, and responses contribute to the low number of adolescents who choose to breastfeed. Thus bottle-feeding is often the feeding method chosen among teenage mothers (see Fig. 25-5). The nurse may help the ado-

TABLE 25-2 Recommended Daily Dietary Allowance in Calories (Kilocalories)* for Females

AGE (YR)	WEIGHT		HEIGHT		CALORIES PER KG	CALORIES PER DAY
	KG	LB	CM	IN		
11 to 14	46	101	157	62	47	2200
15 to 18	55	120	163	64	40	2200
19 to 24	58	128	164	65	38	2200
25 to 50	63	138	163	64	36	2200
51+	65	143	160	63	30	1900
Pregnant						
First trimester						+0†
Second trimester						+300‡
Third trimester						+300‡
Lactating						
First 6 mo						+500§
Second 6 mo						+500§

From Subcommittee on the Tenth Edition of the RDAs, Food and Nutrition Board, Commission on Life Sciences, National Research Council—10th rev ed: *Recommended dietary allowances,* Washington, DC, 1989, National Academy Press.
*Based on light to moderate activity.
†If weight is at or above standard for height and age.
‡Based on pregnancy gain of 12.5 kg and infant birth weight of 3.3 kg.
§Plus 650 calories if weight is below standard for age and height.

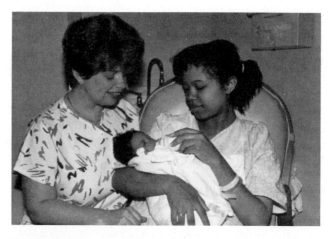

FIG. 25-5 Young mother bottle-feeding her newborn. (Courtesy Caroline E. Brown, Hershey, PA.)

lescent weigh the realities of breastfeeding, such as its being a 24-hour commitment, with the realities of continuing her education. For successful breastfeeding the adolescent's family and school must work together. When counseling needs are beyond the nurse's scope, the adolescent should be referred to a counselor who works well with teenagers.

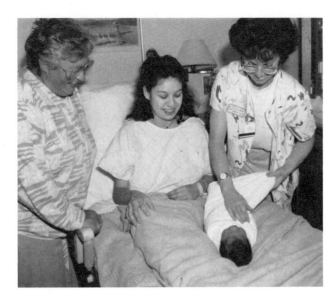

FIG. 25-6   Role modeling by the nurse and grandparent supports the adolescent's transition into parenthood. (Courtesy Marjorie Pyle, RNC, *Lifecircle,* Costa Mesa, CA.)

Labor and Birth

The early adolescent may be frightened by needles, pelvic examinations, noises from other women in labor, medical equipment, and birthing rooms. Single, private rooms should be provided whenever possible. The adolescent in labor should have the support of a knowledgeable coach, whether the coach is her husband, friend, parent, or nurse.

Many teenagers come to labor unprepared. Often they are fearful and alone. If the adolescent is admitted early in the first stage of labor, then the nurse has time to teach her how to relax with contractions, as well as teach her the benefits of ambulation, side-lying positions, and comfort measures. The adolescent is more concerned with how the baby will get out than with fetal well-being.

Even though she may show an intense response to the contractions, the adolescent is trusting and will follow suggestions. Labor often progresses quickly. Anticipatory guidance and explanation of all procedures before they are administered should always be a part of the nurse's care.

Many adolescents keep their infants and are responsive to the staff members' sharing in their delight about the infant. For these young parents, efforts to promote parent-child attachment are particularly important.

Postpartum Care

Physically, the adolescent mother requires the same care as an adult who has given birth. Explicit directions for self-care and infant care are required. Most adolescents view the infant's care as their primary concern. The need for continued assessment of the new mother's parenting abilities during this postbirth period is essential. In ad-

dition, continued support should be provided by involving the grandparents (Fig. 25-6) and other family members, as well as through home visits and group sessions for discussion of infant care and parenting problems. Outreach programs concerned with self-care, parent-child interactions, child injuries, and failure to thrive, in addition to programs that provide prompt and effective community intervention, prevent more serious problems from occurring.

Postpartum contraception is a priority for early adolescents. The risk of repeat pregnancy in adolescence is high, and the accompanying risks of adolescent pregnancy increase with each subsequent pregnancy. Almost universally, postpartum adolescents say they will never have sex again and, therefore, "need no birth control." Nevertheless, adolescents need to leave the hospital with a knowledge of contraception methods and how and when to use their chosen method. Early adolescents may be too shy or embarrassed about touching their genitals to use the barrier method; in addition, they are unlikely to anticipate intercourse. For these reasons some adolescents choose oral contraceptives or injectible or subdermal hormone implants. The decision must be based on the individual and her life situation. Adolescent partners need to be considered and included in any interventions in sexual education, family planning, and parent education when possible.

The adolescent needs support if she is considering adoption for her child. It is important to protect the patient who has not made a decision about adoption yet. Avoid using phrases that give negative connotations to the adoption process. Phrases such as "put up for adoption" or "give up for adoption" implies a callous, uncaring, insensitive biologic parent. The terms "real" or "natural parents" should not be used exclusively for the genetic parents. The adoptive parents are the "real parents," because they care for the child. Neutral language, such as "arranging for an adoption," "biologic parent," "birth mother," and "adoptive parent" are preferable. The mother is given the option to either remain on the postpartum floor or be transferred to another unit. She should be assured that she will have as much access to the baby as she desires.

Grief results from a change or from an actual or perceived loss. The adolescent may experience grief brought on by the contemplation of adoption, by the birth of a preterm infant who may be in the intensive care unit, or by the infant's death. The nurse may help the birth mother move through this grieving process. The adolescent who gives birth to a preterm infant or an infant who is small for gestational age may find it difficult to reconcile this tiny, scrawny infant with her fantasized "Gerber" baby. She may experience fear at the thought of caring for her infant in the intensive care unit. The confidence and trust in her abilities that were built up so trustingly in the prenatal period may be replaced by feelings of being overwhelmed and incompetent. The consequent alienation of the mother from her infant may never be overcome. Intensive teaching and continuous support programs are essential if the young mother and her vulnerable infant are not to become estranged.

Many young mothers pattern their maternal role on what they themselves experienced. Therefore it is vital to determine the kind of support that people close to the young mother are able and prepared to give, as well as the kinds of community aid available to supplement this support. As the adolescent performs her mothering role within the framework of her family, she may need to address dependency vs. independency issues. The adolescent's family members may also need help adapting to their new roles.

The Adolescent Father

Nursing care includes the father of the child. As with the mother, the nurse must be aware of the male adolescent's cognitive-developmental levels, values, and culture. More successful outreach programs address cultural diversity in teenage fathers.

The adolescent father and mother face immediate developmental crises, which include: completing the developmental tasks of adolescence, making a transition to parenthood, and sometimes adapting to marriage. These transitions can be stressful. The nurse may initiate interaction with the adolescent father by asking his pregnant partner to bring him to the clinic with her so that he may participate in the birth. With the pregnant adolescent's agreement, the father may be contacted directly. The decision to include the young father in all aspects of the care is based on assessment in the following four areas: (1) the couple's relationship, (2) levels of stress, concern, and coping, (3) educational and vocational goals, and (4) the level of health education knowledge. Adolescent fathers, as do all fathers, need support to discuss their emotional responses to the pregnancy. The nurse's nonjudgmental attitude is essential for open communication. The father's feelings of guilt, powerlessness, or bravado should be recognized because of their negative consequences for both the parents and the child. Counseling needs to be reality oriented. Topics such as finances, child care, parenting skills, and the father's role in the birth experience need to be discussed. Teenage fathers also need to know about reproductive physiology and birth control options.

The adolescent mother's partner and her family affect how she will deal with her pregnancy, labor, birth, and subsequent parenthood. The adolescent partner may continue to be involved in an ongoing relationship with the young mother. In many instances he plays an important role in the decisions she faces during her pregnancy. He may influence her decision to continue the pregnancy, have an abortion, keep the child, or arrange for the child's adoption.

The nurse supports the young father by helping him develop realistic perceptions of his role as "father to a child." The nurse encourages him to use coping mechanisms that are not detrimental to his own, his partner's, and his child's well-being. The nurse enlists support systems, parents, and professional agencies on his behalf. The father is encouraged to be involved in decisions regarding future contraception and safer sex practices.

✤ EVALUATION

Perinatal nurses need to evaluate the care they provide to adolescent patients, in order to determine the effectiveness of their nursing actions. Nurses can be reasonably assured that care was effective to the extent that the expected outcomes of care have been met:

- The adolescent received early and continued prenatal care.
- She received comprehensive medical, psychosocial, parenting, and social services.
- She received creative, developmentally appropriate health care.
- She experienced a physically safe and emotionally satisfying pregnancy and promoted optimal child health.
- She acquired knowledge and skills that enhanced her decision-making abilities.
- She exhibited an increased awareness and made effective use of her support systems (e.g., baby's grandparents, baby's father, her friends).

Care Management— for Parenthood

An adolescent may choose to carry her pregnancy to term and keep the baby. As with all parents, the adolescent's parenting ability is based on her sensitivity to her infant's needs. Many factors can affect sensitivity, including stress, level of cognitive development, knowledge, infant responses, and support systems. The age and educational level of the adolescent mother influence her behavior toward her infant. Even though many books have been written and much advice has been given about parenting, no household perfectly models this parenting advice, nor are the suggestions and recommendations given always appropriate. Parenting is a complex process that depends on the decision-making of the adolescent parent within her unique situation.

✤ ASSESSMENT

In assessing the adolescent's parenting abilities, the nurse must evaluate the following: the adolescent's ability to empathize with her child, her self-concept, her definition of and identification with the maternal role, her ability to solve problems and consider the child within the context of the future, and the adolescent's support system. In addition, the nurse should assess the adolescent's ability to perform caregiving tasks such as feeding, stimulating, diapering, and nurturing her infant. This should be done regardless of whether the infant is in good health or is sick.

The amount of stress experienced by the adolescent directly affects her ability to function in a mothering role. Adolescents are exposed to many stresses as they undertake the tasks and responsibilities of parenthood. Because stress can make the adolescent insensitive to another person's needs, the nurse must assess the type of stressors, the adolescent's reactions to the actual or perceived stress, her problem-solving ability, and her support system.

✤ NURSING DIAGNOSES

Many nursing diagnoses may evolve from the assessment data, including the following:

Anxiety or ineffective individual coping related to
- Inadequate knowledge of the labor and birth process
- Lack of support from significant others/family

Situational low self-esteem related to
- Perception of behavior or performance during labor and birth
- Judgmental attitude of those who surround the adolescent during labor and birth

Pain related to
- Inadequate knowledge of self-care techniques

Impaired communication related to
- Age difference between her and her health care providers

Family coping and potential for growth related to
- Individualized nursing plan of care
- Involvement of grandparents and significant others

✤ EXPECTED OUTCOMES

Mutual expected outcomes should be developed on the basis of the adolescent's health care needs. Expected outcomes are stated in patient-centered terms and may include the following:
- The adolescent mother will respond appropriately to her newborn's cues.
- The adolescent mother will state that she is satisfied with her family's support.
- The adolescent mother will make positive statements about her infant and herself as a mother.
- The adolescent mother will demonstrate appropriate infant-care and self-care techniques.

✤ COLLABORATIVE CARE

Since most adolescents may resent the attention paid to their new babies, the nurse needs to show the adolescent mother that she is still important. This will help establish the necessary trust and cooperation for future interaction and teaching.

Before discussing infant care topics, the nurse should ask the adolescent about herself, her friends, her school, and her social life. The nurse should encourage the adolescent to discuss her feelings and responses to the labor and birth process, too.

The nurse can serve as a positive role model for adolescent parents with respect to caring for themselves and their infants. Healthy lifestyles, cleanliness, and good eating habits are especially important to model and emphasize to the adolescent mother. Physical assessment skills can be taught to the adolescent so that she becomes more knowledgeable about her child's needs. An early adolescent usually lacks the knowledge and maturity to provide continuous care to her child. A high-risk, LBW, or preterm infant requires even more care from his/her mother than a normal infant.

The adolescent's egocentricity makes it difficult for her to separate her own thoughts, feelings, and needs from those of her baby. She may attribute sophisticated thought processes to her infant. It is not uncommon for the adolescent to make statements such as, "he doesn't like breast milk," "he is just crying to get attention," or "she is just doing that to make me stay home." The nurse should demonstrate the limited capacity of the infant to engage in sophisticated thought. The adolescent may try to feed her infant foods that she herself likes to eat (e.g., pizza, soda, or potato chips) thereby placing her child in danger of choking. A list of foods that should and should not be fed to the infant is helpful.

Adolescent mothers tend to be less sensitive and less communicative with their infants than adult mothers. As a result, interventions that emphasize verbal and nonverbal communication skills between mother and child are important. Such intervention strategies must be concrete and specific because of the cognitive level of adolescents. The neonatal behavior assessment scale developed by Brazelton (1973) helps parents become aware of the way their infants communicate need and satisfaction and to see their newborn as an interactive partner. Physical self-care and infant care are essential topics that must be covered in direct language. For example, some adolescents need to learn a lot about good hygiene. In addition to addressing specific topics, demonstrations of baby care techniques with return demonstrations are also essential.

Family members may share or take on the role of the infant's primary caregiver either with or without the adolescent mother's permission. It is important to assess the adolescent's feelings about this situation and to facilitate family discussions about such arrangements in order to encourage open communication and a positive experi-

CLINICAL APPLICATION OF RESEARCH

GRANDMOTHER SOCIAL SUPPORT, ADOLESCENT MOTHERING, AND INFANT ATTACHMENT

The number of adolescent mothers is growing. These mothers face the tasks of adolescence in addition to the challenges of parenthood. Adolescents are at high-risk for parenting problems. Social support may facilitate successful parenting and promote infant attachment.

Researchers observed 197 adolescent mothers with their 1-year-old children. Of these participants, 68 lived with the infants' grandmothers, 64 lived with their partners, and 65 either lived alone or with someone other than the grandmother or partner. The participants were observed both in the laboratory playroom and in their homes during an interview. Researchers gathered data by using the *Strange Situation* to assess infant attachment, the *Quick Test* to measure the adolescent's intellectual ability, the *Arizona Social Support and Interview Schedule* to measure social support, the *Demographics and Living Arrangements Interview,* the *Home Observation for Measurement of the Environment* to evaluate the home environment, and the *Nursing Child Assessment Teaching Scale* to measure mother-child interaction.

The researchers found that the more secure infants lived with their mothers and a partner and had supportive grandmothers. The environment was better when the adolescent lived with either her partner or the infant's grandmother. Having a second caregiver in the home appeared to be beneficial for the infant's development. When the adolescent lived with the infant's grandmother, she was more likely to remain in school, but she did not develop parenting skills as quickly as adolescent mothers who had other living arrangements. Nurses working with adolescents can discuss optimal living arrangements with the young mothers, their partners, and the infants' grandmothers. Nurses can also provide counseling in child-care skills to enhance the infants' development.

Reference: Spieker SJ, Bensley L: Roles of living arrangements and grandmother social support in adolescent mothering and infant attachment, *Dev Psychol* 30(1):102, 1994.

PLAN OF CARE

Teenage Pregnancy

Case History

Jane Brady is a 16-year-old, single primigravida who is 28 weeks' pregnant. Despite encouragement to bring a support person with her to the clinic, she always comes alone. Jane's parents are divorced, and she lives with her mother and older sister.

The admission interview shows that Jane has missed several prenatal care appointments at the clinic. She says that she does not have transportation to the clinic because her mother and sister both work full-time. Her mother and sister have expressed an interest in assisting with child-care but Jane says, "sometimes I want to keep the baby and sometimes I don't." During the assessment interview the nurse discovers that Jane has several close friends but feels embarrassed and "different" around her peers at school because of her "big belly." During Jane's physical examination the nurse notes that her blood pressure has remained within her usual range of 100/70 to 106/72. Her pulse rate is 76, and her laboratory tests are within normal limits.

EXPECTED OUTCOMES	IMPLEMENTATION	RATIONALE	EVALUATION
Nursing Diagnosis: High risk for injury (maternal and fetal) related to several missed prenatal appointments			
Jane will attend all scheduled prenatal care appointments and will have a safe and healthy pregnancy and birth.	Identify transportation problems to the clinic and suggest solutions. Schedule appointments around school activities. Examine Jane's feelings or concerns about the prenatal visits. Create a safe, stable environment. Provide a consistent caregiver. Explain the need to closely monitor the pregnancy.	Accurate identification and elimination of barriers to prenatal care increase the probability of optimal pregnancy outcome.	Jane attends her scheduled prenatal visits. Jane identifies her feelings. Jane verbalizes her understanding of the need for prenatal care.

PLAN OF CARE—cont'd

Teenage Pregnancy

EXPECTED OUTCOMES	IMPLEMENTATION	RATIONALE	EVALUATION

Nursing Diagnosis: Situational low self-esteem related to altered body image and altered role performance because of pregnancy and middle-stage adolescence

EXPECTED OUTCOMES	IMPLEMENTATION	RATIONALE	EVALUATION
Jane will discuss her feelings and concerns and will actively participate in school activities with peers and with the nursing plan of care.	Take unhurried time to discuss Jane's concerns and feelings. Encourage Jane to discuss her thoughts with her close friends. Identify Jane's expected outcomes in life and suggest ways to meet those expected outcomes (e.g., Who am I?). Encourage participation in known problem solving. Compliment Jane on her general appearance, verbalization of fears, and participation in care. Help Jane identify her support system, including outside resources (AFDC, WIC, home health care, child care, psychologists, guidance counselors, and tutors). Refer Jane to her guidance counselor if she needs tutoring to achieve her educational needs. Encourage Jane to choose one person who will attend prenatal care, assist in childbirth, and participate in child care activities with her.	Jane's developmental need for a sense of identity is enhanced by the nurse's caring attitude and the involvement of Jane's support system.	Jane discusses her concerns and feelings. Jane participates in problem-solving. Jane continues her education during pregnancy. Jane brings a support person to prenatal visits. Jane appears clean and well-groomed. Jane utilizes community resources as needed.

AFDC, Aid to families with dependent children; *WIC,* Women, infants, and children.

Continued.

PLAN OF CARE—cont'd

Teenage Pregnancy

EXPECTED OUTCOMES	IMPLEMENTATION	RATIONALE	EVALUATION

Nursing Diagnosis: High risk for ineffective individual coping related to knowledge deficit for making a decision regarding parenthood and adoption issues

EXPECTED OUTCOMES	IMPLEMENTATION	RATIONALE	EVALUATION
Jane will make an informed decision. Jane will increase her problem-solving skills as evidenced by her identifying several options for action and choosing from among them.	Evaluate Jane's feelings regarding parenthood and adoption and avoid sending verbal or nonverbal messages that could influence her. Discuss the pros and cons of parenthood and adoption with Jane. Encourage questions and answer these questions honestly. Clarify misconceptions. Suggest solutions to problems, such as financial support or educational needs, that may be of concern to Jane in evaluating parenthood. Refer Jane to a licensed adoption agency for specific questions regarding the adoption process. Encourage Jane to discuss her decision with her family, but stress that she alone can make the decision. Evaluate Jane's feelings regarding seeing her child after birth or knowing its sex if adoption is chosen. Until adoption papers are signed, Jane should know that she can change her mind about her decision.	Exploring feelings and providing accurate, honest information will enhance Jane's ability for optimal decision-making.	Jane makes an informed decision regarding parenthood or adoption. Jane's problem-solving skills improve.

ence for everyone involved (see Clinical Application of Research).

✛ EVALUATION

Nurses can be reasonably assured that care has been effective to the extent that the expected outcomes of care have been achieved:

- The adolescent mother responds appropriately to her newborn's cues.
- She states that she is satisfied with her family's support.
- She makes positive statements about herself as a mother and about her infant.
- She exhibits appropriate infant-care and self-care techniques (see Plan of Care)

KEY POINTS

- Adolescents see their world in far different terms than do adults; their major tasks are the development of cognitive ability and identity formation.
- Cognitive development influences sexual decision making.
- Poverty, lifestyle, and risk-taking behaviors are implicated in adolescent morbidity, resulting in sequelae of pregnancy and other major health problems.
- The physiologic consequences and the personal and public costs of adolescent pregnancy and parenthood are staggering.
- The developmental tasks of adolescents are interrupted by pregnancy.

- Poor nutrition and poverty have been implicated in physiologic consequences to the adolescent mother, her fetus, and her newborn.
- Adolescents' reactions to perceived stress depend on the quality of their support systems, their self-esteem, and their problem-identification and problem-solving skills.
- Adolescents usually have a limited knowledge of child development.
- Standard approaches to prenatal and postpartum teaching are inappropriate or unappealing to most adolescents.

CRITICAL THINKING EXERCISES

You are assigned to care for Lisa, a 14-year-old girl who is pregnant and attending the prenatal clinic for the first time.

1. Identify your feelings about adolescent pregnancy. What assumptions did you make about Lisa? How can you verify or negate these assumptions?
2. Examine pregnancy from Lisa's viewpoint by using the theories found in this chapter. Where do your perceptions differ?

3. Design a teaching plan to meet Lisa's cognitive level and her learning needs with respect to prenatal care.
4. Observe the attitudes of the prenatal clinic's staff toward Lisa. Analyze the impact of these attitudes on the service she receives.

References

Adler N, et al: Adolescent contraceptive behavior: an assessment of decision processes, *J Pediatr* 116(3):463, 1990.

American Academy of Pediatrics: Committee on adolescence: care of adolescent parents and their children, *Pediatrics* 83:138, 1989.

Beach R: Breast exam: protect, reassure, educate, *Contemp OB/GYN*, 35(2):41, 1990.

Berenson A, San-Miguel VV, Wilkinson GS: Violence and its relationship to substance use in adolescent pregnancy, *J Adolesc Health* 13(6):470, Sept 1992.

Bluestein D, Rutledge CM: Determinants of delayed pregnancy testing among adolescents, *J Fam Pract* 35(4):406, Oct 1992.

Brazelton TB: *Neonatal behavioral assessment scale,* London, 1973, Spastics International Medical Publication.

Brown H: Recognizing common STDs in adolescents, *Contemp OB/GYN* 33(3):47, 1989.

Cartoof V, Klerman L, Zazueta V: The effect of source of prenatal care on care-seeking behavior and pregnancy outcomes among adolescents, *J Adolesc Health Care* 12(2):124, 1991.

Centers for Disease Control and Prevention (CDC): *Survey: teen health and sex habits,* Atlanta, September 1991, Centers for Disease Control and Prevention.

Cooksey E: Factors in the resolution of adolescent premarital pregnancies, *Demography* 27(2):207, Feb 1990.

Donovan P: *Risk and responsibility: teaching sex education in America's schools today,* New York, 1989, Alan Guttmacher Institute.

Durant R, et al: Contraceptive behavior among sexually active Hispanic adolescents, *J Adolesc Health Care* 11(6):490, 1990.

Elsters A, Lamb M, Kimmerly N: Perceptions of parenthood among adolescent fathers, *Pediatrics* 83(5):758, 1989.

Erikson E: *Identity, youth, and crisis,* New York, 1968, WW Norton.

Fine G, Mortimer J, Roberts D: Leisure, work and the mass media. In Feldman S, Elliott G, editors: *At the threshold: the developing adolescent,* Cambridge, MA, 1990, Harvard University Press.

Forest JD, Singh S: The sexual and reproductive behavior of American women, 1982-1988, *Fam Plan Perspect* 22:206, 1990.

Greydanus D, Shearin R: *Adolescent sexuality and gynecology,* Philadelphia, 1990, Lea & Febiger.

Gutierrez Y, King JC: Nutrition during teenage pregnancy, *Pediat Ann,* 22(2):99, Feb 1993.

Henshaw S, Kost K: Parental involvement in minors' abortion decisions, *Fam Plann Perspect* 24(5):196, Sept-Oct 1992.

Hilliard P, Rebar R: Abnormal uterine bleeding needs a special approach, *Contemp OB/GYN* 35(5):51, 1990.

Institute of Medicine: *Nutrition During Pregnancy. Part I: Weight Gain. Part II: Nutrient Supplements,* Washington, DC, 1990, National Academy Press.

Irwin C: Risk-taking behaviors during the second decade of life, *Proceedings from the 1989 Adolescent Health Coordinators*

Conference, Washington, DC, 1989, National Center for Education in Maternal and Child Health.

Jackson E, Mathur K: Adolescent pregnancy: effects of nutrients on hematocrit and birth weight, *J S C Med Assoc* 87(1): 8, Jan 1991.

Kohlberg L: Stage and sequence: the cognitive developmental approach to socialization. In Nadien MB, editor: *The child's psychosocial development: from birth to adolescence,* Wayne, NJ, 1980, Avery Publishing Group Inc.

Kokotailo P, Adger J: Substance use by pregnant adolescents, *Clin Perinatol* 18(1):125, 1991.

Lockhart L, Wodarski J: Teenage pregnancy: implications for social work practice, *Family Therapy* 17(1):29, 1990.

Marsiglio W: Adolescent males' orientation toward paternity and contraception, *Fam Plann Perspect* 25(1):22, Jan-Feb 1993.

McAnarney E, Greydanus D: Adolescent pregnancy and abortion. In Hofman A, Greydanus D, editors: *Adolescent Medicine,* Norwalk, CT, 1989, Appleton & Lange.

McAnarney E, Hendee W: Adolescent pregnancy and its consequences, *JAMA* 262:74, 1989a.

McAnarney E, Hendee W: The prevention of adolescent pregnancy, *JAMA* 262:78, 1989b.

National Center for Health Statistics: *Advance Report of the Monthly Vital Statistics. United States Department of Health and Human Services,* 1990, 41(9) supplement, Hyattesville, MD, 1993, US Department of Health and Human Services.

Passino AW, et al: Personal adjustment during pregnancy and adolescent parenting, *Adolescence* 28(109):97, Spring 1993.

Pete J, Desantis L: Sexual decision making in young black adolescent females, *Adolescence* 25(97):145, Spring 1990.

Rosoff J: Sex education in the schools: policies and practice, *Fam Plan Perspect,* 21(2):52, March/April 1989.

Ruff C: Adolescent mothering: assessing their parenting capa-

bilities and their health education needs, *J Natl Black Nurses Assoc* 4(1):55, Jan 1990.

Sander J, Rosen J: Teenage fathers: working the neglected partner in adolescent childbearing, *Fam Plann Perspect* 21:6, Jan/Feb 1989.

Schneck M et al: Low-income pregnant adolescents and their infants: dietary findings and health outcomes, *J Am Diet Assoc* 90(4):555, 1990.

Stevens-Simon C, Roghman K, McAnarney E: Early vaginal bleeding, late prenatal care, and misdating in adolescent pregnancies, *Pediatrics* 87:838, 1991.

Stevens-Simon C, Fullar S, McAnarney E: Tangible differences between adolescent-oriented and adult-oriented prenatal care, *J Adolesc Health Care* 13(4):298, Jun 1992.

Story M, editor: *Nutrition management of the pregnant adolescent—a practical reference guide* (March of Dimes), Washington, DC, 1990, US Department of Health and Human Services, US Department of Agriculture.

Swenson IE: A profile of young adolescents attending a teen family planning clinic, *Adolescence* 27(107):647, Fall 1992.

Tierney L et al, editors: *Current Medical Diagnoses and Treatment,* Norwalk, CT, 1993, Appleton & Lange.

Tyre L, Rothbart B, Anderson K: Helping adolescents make the right contraceptive choice, *Contemp OB/GYN* 35(3):37, March 1990.

White J, Kellinger K: Teenagers' perceptions of unplanned adolescent pregnancies and oral contraceptive use, *J Am Acad Nurse Pract* 1(2):55, Feb 1989.

Young C et al: Adolescent third-trimester enrollment in prenatal care, *J Adolesc Health Care* 10(5):393, 1989.

Bibliography

ACOG: Cocaine in pregnancy, *Committee Opinion: Committee on Obstetrics: Maternal and Fetal Medicine* 114, 1993, ACOG.

Christmon K: Parental responsibility of African-American unwed adolescent fathers, *Adolescence* 25(49):645, Fall 1990.

Church C: Neonatal implications of adolescent pregnancy, *NAACOG's: Clin Issu Perinat Womens Health Nurs* 2(2): 245, 1991.

Fleming BW et al: Assessing and promoting positive parenting in adolescent mothers, *MCN* 18(1):32, Jan/Feb 1993.

Foodym D: *Contraception for special populations: teenagers and women over thirty-five*, Palo Alto, CA, 1992, Syntex Labs.

Podgurski M: School-based adolescent pregnancy classes, *AWHONN's Clinical Issu in Perinat and Womens Health* 4(1):80, 1993.

Reedy N: The very young pregnant adolescent, *NAACOG's: Clin Issu Perinat Womens Health Nurs* 2(2):209, 1991.

Seven

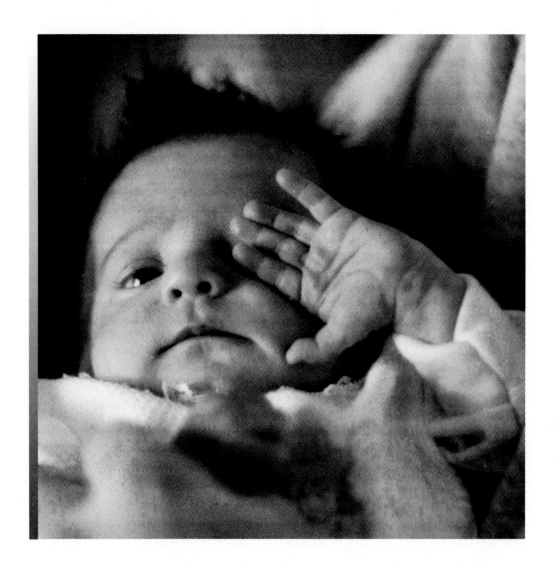

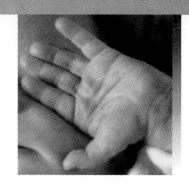

Complications of the Newborn

26 The Newborn at Risk

27 Specific Problems of the Newborn at Risk

28 Loss and Grief

26 The Newborn at Risk

LILA PARAM

LEARNING OBJECTIVES

Define the key terms listed.
Describe a "Quick Check" assessment of a compromised newborn.
Outline a head-to-toe assessment of a newborn in distress.
Explain the importance of thermoregulation in the newborn.
Describe stabilization of the compromised newborn.
Explore the emotional aspects of care for the compromised newborn.

KEY TERMS

asphyxia
acrocyanosis
plethora
grunting (expiratory)
flaring (of nares)
retraction of chest wall
neutral thermal environment (NTE)
pulse oximetry

RELATED TOPICS

Apgar scoring *(Chap. 14)* · Caput succedaneum *(Chap. 13)* · Cephalhematoma *(Chap. 13)* · Dysmature infant *(Chap. 27)* · Fetal circulation *(Chap. 4)* · Meconium aspiration syndrome *(Chap. 27)* · Normal variations of the newborn *(Chap. 13)* · Persistent pulmonary hypertension *(Chap. 27)* · Postterm infant *(Chap. 27)* · Thermoregulation *(Chap. 14)* · Loss and grief *(Chap. 28)*

One of the most difficult components of the maternity/well-baby nurse's role is caring for the unexpected high-risk newborn. An environment geared to the healthy, uncomplicated birth experience may leave the health care provider unprepared for the "crash and burn" situations these infants present. Acute assessment skills, knowledge, and appropriate, functioning equipment are the maternity/well-baby nurse's most important tools under these circumstances. This chapter provides a basic understanding of the most common problems that nurses encounter when caring for newborns.

The optimum site for the care of compromised newborns is in a newborn intensive care unit, where specialized personnel and equipment are available. Hospitals unequipped to care for the high-risk mother and her fetus or newborn must arrange for their immediate transfer to a specialized perinatal or regional tertiary care center. Community hospital nurses have the responsibility

of caring for the compromised fetus or newborn until the transfer can be arranged. These nurses must have the necessary skills, medical back-up, and equipment for emergency interventions to stabilize the infant's physical condition until the transport can occur.

It is crucial that a relationship exist between the community hospital and the regional center before a crisis occurs. Health care providers at a community hospital need to know whom to call at the regional center when questions arise in the stabilization process. The regional center has a responsibility to its community to provide consultation under these circumstances. Most regional centers have an outreach department that acts as a liaison to facilitate communication between the community and the regional center. If community hospital based nurses are unsure of whom to call, then they should call the nearest regional center and ask for the intensive care nursery. The key is to *know what resources are available*.

All health care providers involved in the birth of newborns should be familiar with the transport system within their own community. In addition, they should be able to answer the following questions:

- Who should make the initial call and to whom?
- Will the regional center come for the infant or will the community hospital have to manage the transport?
- If the community hospital is responsible for the transport, who will go with the infant, and how is the appropriate transportation mobilized?

The time involved in finding the answers to these questions may affect the outcome of the infant.

When possible, maternal transports (i.e., transports of pregnant women) are preferable to neonatal transports (i.e., transports of newborns). Transfer of the mother before birth has two distinct advantages: (1) neonatal morbidity and mortality decrease, and (2) the mother and infant will not be separated at birth. With maternal transport, the infant does not experience the stresses of transport, rather, the infant is born at a regional center that is staffed and equipped to address the special needs of the compromised newborn.

TRANSITION TO EXTRAUTERINE LIFE

Normal Transition

Historically, labor and birth have been seen from the mother's perspective—her discomfort, her joy, her experience. Only recently has the father's experience been explored. What has not been as well documented is the birth experience from the perspective of the fetus/newborn.

In utero the fetus is contained in a small, dark, warm, fluid, gravity-free environment with muffled sounds and no pain. After birth this environment changes dramatically to that of a bright, cold, gravity-filled, loud, perhaps painful, open space. With the possible exceptions of dying or giving birth, being born is arguably the moment of greatest physiologic change a human ever experiences. A documented pattern of normal transition exists within the body of knowledge of the cardiovascular-pulmonary and bio-chemical changes essential for survival at birth. Any deviation from this pattern alerts the nurse to potential problems.

Dysfunctional Transition

The first few moments in an infant's life are critical. At this time the infant abruptly moves from the mother's uterus to the extrauterine environment.

Asphyxia most often occurs during the immediate period after birth and creates a need for resuscitation. **Asphyxia** is the interruption of either placental or pulmonary gas exchange, which results in hypercarbia, hypox-

TABLE 26-1 Neonatal Resuscitation Supplies and Equipment

SUCTION EQUIPMENT

Bulb syringe
Mechanical suction
Suction catheters 5 (or 6), 8, 10 French
8 French feeding tube and 20 ml syringe
Meconium aspirator

BAG-AND-MASK EQUIPMENT

Infant resuscitation bag with a pressure-release valve or pressure gauge; the bag must be capable of delivering 90% to 100% oxygen
Face masks—newborn and premature sizes (cushioned-rim masks preferred)
Oral airways—newborn and premature sizes
Oxygen source with intact flowmeter and tubing

INTUBATION EQUIPMENT

Laryngoscope with straight blades—No. 0 (premature) and No. 1 (term newborn)
Extra bulbs and batteries for laryngoscope
Endotracheal tubes—sizes 2.5 mm, 3.0 mm, 3.5 mm, and 4.0 mm
Stylet
Scissors
Gloves

MEDICATIONS

Epinephrine 1:10,000, 3 ml or 10 ml ampules
Naloxone hydrochloride 0.4 mg/ml in 1-ml ampules or 1.0 mg/ml in 2-ml ampules
Volume expander—one or more
  Whole blood
  Fresh frozen plasma
  Albumin (5%)/saline solution
Sodium bicarbonate 4.2% (5 mEq/10 ml) in 10 ml ampules
Dextrose 10%-250 ml
Sterile water-30 ml
Normal saline-30 ml

OTHER EQUIPMENT AND SUPPLIES

Radiant warmer
Stethoscope
Blood pressure monitor with transducer (desirable)
Adhesive tape—½-inch or ¾ -inch width
Syringes—1 ml, 3 ml, 5 ml, 10 ml, 20 ml, and 50 ml
Needles—25-gauge, 21-gauge, and 18-gauge
Alcohol sponges
Umbilical artery catheterization tray
Umbilical tape
Umbilical catheters—3½, 5 French
3-way stopcocks
5 French feeding tube
Cardiotachometer with ECG oscilloscope (desirable)
Pressure transducer and monitor (desirable)

Modified from American Heart Association/American Academy of Pediatrics: *Textbook of neonatal resuscitation*, Dallas, 1991, American Heart Association.

emia, and acidosis. In turn, these cause profound changes in the distribution of the blood flow so that blood is diverted to the head, heart, and adrenals and away from the systemic circulation and lungs. If blood is diverted from the lungs, it can not become oxygenated. The infant will die without appropriate and timely resuscitation. Therefore the management of an asphyxiated infant during the first minutes of life can affect the quality of that infant's life and can have consequences lasting a lifetime (American Heart Association/American Academy of Pediatrics, 1991).

Successful transition to extrauterine life requires the following sequence of cardiovascular and pulmonary events:

1. The lungs expand with air down to the terminal airways (alveoli).
2. The alveoli become oxygenated.
3. The pulmonary vasculature dilates in response to lung expansion and alveolar oxygenation.
4. In response to pulmonary vasodilation, cardiac output to the lungs changes from about 7% in the fetus to approximately 100% in the newborn.
5. The onset of continuous breathing begins.

When this sequence of events is disrupted or does not occur, the infant becomes asphyxiated.

Health care providers must be skilled in the resuscitation of newborns. In addition, the resuscitation of newborns requires teamwork and the availability of the proper equipment in the birthing room. Table 26-1 includes a list of neonatal resuscitation supplies and equipment.

LEGAL TIP: Negligence during Neonatal
Emergencies—Use of Malfunctioning
Equipment

Missing, malfunctioning, or broken equipment in an emergency situation may result in a charge of nursing negligence.

At birth the newborn is placed under a heat source, dried off, positioned on the back or side, suctioned through the mouth and the nose, and given gentle stimulation. Then the infant is assessed for respiratory effort. Figure 26-1 shows the decision tree used in this assessment and in further resuscitation efforts. The American Heart Association/American Academy of Pediatrics *Textbook of Neonatal Resuscitation* provides in-depth information regarding neonatal resuscitation.

The health care provider assigns the infant's Apgar score at 1 and 5 minutes. If the infant had low scores at these times, then an Apgar score is also assigned at 10 minutes. Zero is assigned only to stillborn infants. Resuscitation efforts must not be delayed until this score is obtained at 1 minute. This delay could have a negative affect on the outcome of the compromised infant.

Care Management

✦ ASSESSMENT DURING THE TRANSITIONAL PERIOD

Accurate assessment of the newborn in the first 12 to 24 hours of life is based on the knowledge of "normal" transitional patterns. Heart rate and sound, respiration, and motor activity all follow distinct patterns that may be abnormal at other age periods but are normal during specific time intervals in the transitional period. Fig 26-2 shows a schematic of these normal variations. Any aberration in these values or observations is cause for further assessment and close attention to the infant's physiologic support.

Quick Check

When caring for a newborn in distress, the nurse needs to make a quick assessment. The "Quick Check," found in Box 26-1, provides adequate information to begin immediate planning and interventions. In this instance CPR stands for color, perfusion, and respiratory effort. These assessments take 5 seconds or less.

Color. Color is a good indication of the infant's cardiac output and respiratory status. Cyanosis is an indicator of impaired oxygenation. Cyanosis occurs only when there are 3 to 5 mg/dl of unsaturated hemoglobin, regardless of the total hemoglobin concentration. Therefore a polycythemic infant with a high hemoglobin concentration will exhibit cyanosis at higher oxygen tensions in the arterial system (PaO_2), whereas the anemic infant will not appear cyanotic until the actual oxygen content of arterial blood becomes quite low. Compounding this effect, fetal hemoglobin (Hgb F), which comprises 70% to 90% of the newborn's red blood cell (RBC) mass, has a greater affinity for oxygen than adult hemoglobin and does not release oxygen into the tissues as readily as adult hemoglobin. This accounts for the left shift on the oxyhemoglobin disassociation curve (Fig. 26-3).

It is important to distinguish between central cyanosis and acrocyanosis or peripheral cyanosis. **Acrocyanosis** or *peripheral cyanosis* is cyanosis of the extremities and can be either pathologic or physiologic. Hypothermia can cause peripheral cyanosis. During transition the vasomotor instability of the normal newborn can appear as peripheral cyanosis; however, the underlying cause may be sepsis, shock, and other pathologic processes. Warming of one extremity will clear physiologic peripheral cyanosis but have no effect on pathologic peripheral cyanosis.

Central cyanosis is usually pathologic. The best indicator of central cyanosis is cyanosis of the tongue and mucous membranes. Central cyanosis is commonly due to respiratory or cardiac disease. Infants with central cyanosis require immediate medical attention.

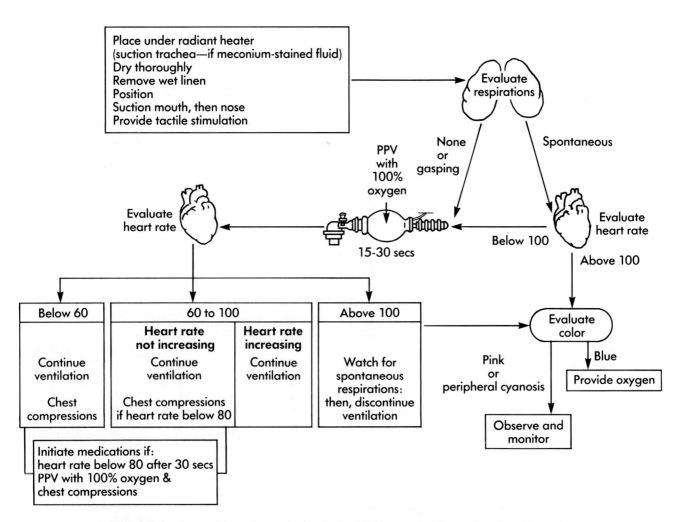

FIG. 26-1 An overview of resuscitation in the birthing room. (From American Heart Association/American Academy of Pediatrics: *Textbook of neonatal resuscitation,* Dallas, 1991, American Heart Association).

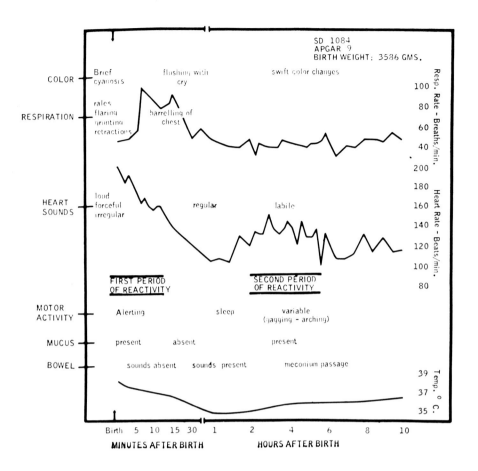

FIG. 26-2 The normal transition period. (From Desmond M, Rudolph A, Phitakspharai-
wan P: *Pediatr Clin North Am* 13:651, 1966.)

BOX 26-1

Quick Check = CPR

C = COLOR

Pass = pink, may have acrocyanosis during transition, but assess for possible pathology
Fail = cyanosis, pallor, mottling, plethoric at any
  time, or jaundice in the first 24 hours of life

P = PERFUSION

Pass = capillary fill time (CFT) of 2 to 3 seconds
  centrally (may have delayed transit time peripherally during transition)
Fail = delayed CFT (> 3 seconds centrally)

R = RESPIRATORY EFFORT

Pass = no grunting, flaring, or retracting; has symmetrical chest wall movement
Fail = any grunting, flaring, or retracting; asym-
  metrical chest wall movement

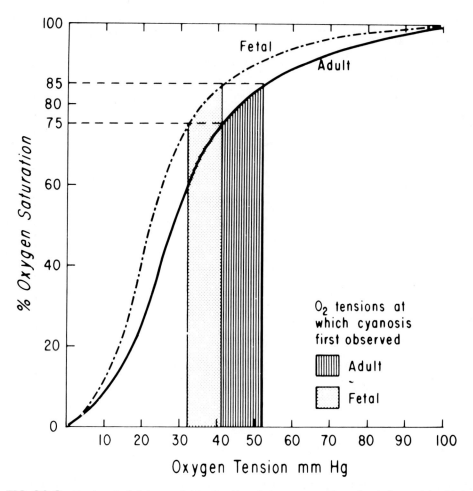

FIG. 26-3 Fetal and adult hemoglobin-O_2 dissociation curves. Note that infants with a high proportion of fetal hemoglobin will have a very low PaO_2 (33 to 42 mm Hg) before cyanosis is observed.

Pallor may be due to loss of RBC mass, hemolysis, or underproduction of RBC mass. *Mottling* indicates vasoconstriction and is seen in hypothermia, shock, and sepsis. The *plethoric* newborn is ruddy in color, especially when crying. This color can indicate polycythemia, or an RBC mass that is too high. This may precipitate hyperviscosity of the circulating blood volume and require partial exchange transfusion to correct. *Jaundice* may be physiologic in the first week of life, however, jaundice in the first 24 hours of life is considered a pathologic hemolytic process requiring immediate attention.

Perfusion. Capillary fill time is the easiest assessment of perfusion to the tissues. To assess capillary fill time, press the infant's skin on the sternum gently until it blanches, then count the seconds it takes for the skin to regain its color. Normal capillary fill time is 2 to 3 seconds centrally. More than 3 seconds indicates a delayed capillary fill time and a decreased perfusion at the tissue level (Rudolph, 1991).

Respiratory Effort. Newborn respiratory effort should be unlabored at a rate of 30 to 60 breaths per minute. In the "Quick Check," the nurse only assesses respiratory effort. Any unusual effort required to maintain respiration is cause for further assessment. Grunting, flaring, and retracting are all signs that the newborn is resorting to compensatory mechanisms in order to maintain normal ventilation.

A **grunting** sound is made as the infant breathes out against a partially closed glottis and vocal cords. This creates continuous positive airway pressure and is an attempt to hold alveoli open at the end of expiration. If the alveoli collapse during the expiratory phase of respiration, then the pressure required to open the alveoli up during the next inspiration increases.

The widening of the nares with inspiration is called **flaring.** This effectively decreases airway resistance. With flaring of the nostrils, the infant is able to take deeper breaths, thereby increasing oxygenation and decreasing the work of breathing.

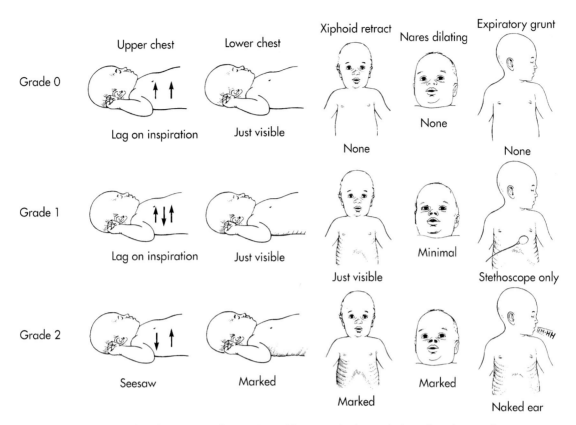

Upper chest   Lower chest   Xiphoid retract   Nares dilating   Expiratory grunt

Grade 0

Lag on inspiration   Just visible   None   None   None

Grade 1

Lag on inspiration   Just visible   Just visible   Minimal   Stethoscope only

Grade 2

Seesaw   Marked   Marked   Marked   Naked ear

FIG. 26-4 The observation of retractions. Silverman-Anderson index of respiratory distress is determined by grading each of five arbitrary criteria: *grade 0* indicates no difficulty; *grade 1* indicates moderate difficulty; and *grade 2* indicates maximum respiratory difficulty. The retraction score is the sum of these values. A total score of 0 indicates no dyspnea, whereas a total score of 10 denotes maximum respiratory distress. (Modified from Silverman W, Anderson D: *Pediatrics* 17:1, 1956.)

Retraction of the chest wall indicates the increased work of breathing. The negative intrapleural pressures necessary to inflate the lungs is determined by a combination of the diaphragm's force, the lung's mechanical properties, and the chest wall's stability. The neonatal chest wall is extremely pliant. The retraction of the chest wall occurs when higher negative intrapleural pressures are needed to open the lung during inspiration (Fanaroff, Martin, 1992). Figure 26-4 shows a grading scale of this phenomenon.

In summary, the "Quick Check" provides the nurse with immediate information to identify nursing diagnoses and develop expected outcomes for the compromised newborn. Following this abbreviated assessment the nurse must proceed to stabilization and further assess the compromised newborn by systems.

Assessment of the Compromised Newborn by Systems

This assessment provides a point-in-time evaluation of the infant's condition, as well as a baseline for evalua-

BOX 26-2
Skin
normal = warm, dry, pink, no anomalies or lesions, good tissue turgor

tion of any change in the infant's condition. The equipment necessary for this assessment includes a stethoscope, tape measure, thermometer, blood pressure device, and *warm, clean hands.* Gloves should be worn if the infant has not had an initial bath. The assessment should be performed in a warm, safe, and comfortable environment.

The following assessment presents the normal assessment followed by questions the nurse must ask in order to identify potential or actual nursing problems. Chapter 27 discusses specific problems and diseases that are common to the compromised newborn.

Integumentary System

Questions Nurses Should Ask Themselves

1. *Is the baby cyanotic or dusky?* (See previous discussion of cyanosis p. 753).

2. *Is the baby plethoric or jaundiced?* **Plethora** refers to the ruddy color exhibited by polycythemic infants, especially when they cry. An assessment of the hematocrit is necessary to diagnose polycythemia. Definitions of polycythemia vary from institution to institution, but generally fall in the 65% to 67% range for central venous hematocrit. Polycythemia results in the hyperviscosity of the blood. This thick, sludgy blood is unable to flow normally through the capillary bed and adequately oxygenate the tissues. Treatment consists of a partial exchange transfusion to dilute the blood without depleting the total blood volume. This procedure involves the removal of the infant's blood in small amounts with simultaneous equal infusion of 5% salt poor albumin, plasma protein fraction USP (Plasmanate), or fresh frozen plasma.

3. *Is the baby mottled?* Mottling is the bluish lacy pattern seen in the vasoconstricted infant. Possible causes of mottling include, but are not limited to, hypothermia, sepsis, or decreased perfusion from shock.

4. *Is the baby pale?* Pallor may be because of blood loss related to:
   - Hemorrhage prior to birth (e.g., twin to twin transfusion)
   - Complications during birth (e.g., abruptio placentae, placenta previa)
   - Internal hemorrhage (e.g., intracranial hemorrhage, giant cephalhematoma)
   - Excessive blood sampling
   or because of hemolysis related to:
   - Isoimmunization (e.g., Rh disease or ABO incompatibility)
   - Congenital defects of the RBC (e.g., G6PD deficiency)
   - Acquired defects of the RBC (e.g., infections, drugs)
   or because of under production of RBCs related to anemia of prematurity.

5. *Are there any lesions, bruises, birth marks, rashes, incisions?* Refer to Chapter 13 for a discussion of normal variations in newborn skin. Any unusual lesions or rashes call for further assessment. Incisions must be assessed for any sign of impaired healing.

6. *Is the skin macerated or meconium-stained?* If the skin is meconium-stained, it has been exposed to meconium in utero for an extended period of time. These infants are at risk for meconium aspiration syndrome and persistent pulmonary hypertension of the newborn. For a discussion of postterm, dysmature infants, see Chapter 27.

7. *Is there edema (i.e., fluid overload) or tenting (i.e., dehydration)?* Assessment of tissue turgor gives an indication of hydration. The nurse tests the skin's elasticity by *gently* pinching a fold of skin between the thumb and forefinger. When released, the skin should spring back to its original shape. When the skin remains in the same position after release, it is called "tenting" (i.e., remaining in the shape of a tent). Edema in newborns is usually generalized and not pitting.

8. If a peripheral intravenous (PIV) access device is used, then the nurse should ask:
   - Is the site soft and easy to flush?
   - Is the PIV patent?
   - Is the site puffy, red, and infiltrated?

Infants are particularly at risk for localized necrosis of tissue from intravenous extravasation. Recently the use of hyaluronidase has been shown to decrease this necrosis and the resulting need for skin grafts. Hyaluronidase is an enzyme that breaks down the connective tissue. This allows the extravasated solution to disperse over a larger area and effectively dilute it, thereby diminishing its effect on local tissue (Fig. 26-5).

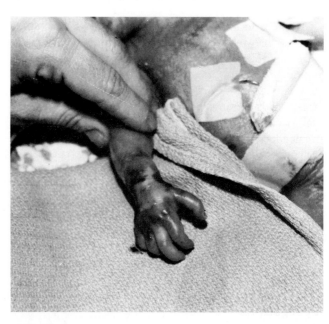

FIG. 26-5 Intravenous infiltration in small infants can cause severe ischemia. (Courtesy Mount Zion Hospital and Medical Center, San Francisco, CA.)

BOX 26-3

Nervous System

normal = the anterior fontanel is soft and flat; reflexes are intact; the baby has a vigorous cry, is active, has good muscle tone, and can move all extremities

Nervous System

Questions Nurses Should Ask Themselves

1. *Is the anterior fontanel depressed? dehydrated? firm, even bulging?* This may indicate increased intracranial pressure.

2. *Are the cranial sutures overlapping, approximated, or separated?* Normal newborns have approximated or transiently overlapping cranial sutures. Separated cranial sutures may indicate increased intracranial pressure.

3. *Are there any bumps on the scalp? caput succedaneum or cephalhematoma?*

4. *Is there limited range of motion?* A limited range of motion may be caused by birth trauma, which could cause nerve damage or palsy. Birth defects may be present that affect the infant's limbs. The infant's arm may be restrained on an arm board.

5. *Is the cry weak, high-pitched, or difficult to elicit?* This may occur if the mother used drugs, or it may indicate a problem with the newborn's central nervous system (CNS).

6. *Is the baby lethargic?* Nurses must act quickly if the baby is lethargic. Lethargy is one of the first subtle signs of many problems such as sepsis or necrotizing enterocolitis (NEC). It should *always* alert the nurse to the need for further assessment.

7. *Is the infant's body flaccid, or does the newborn have poor muscle tone?* This may be the result of CNS depression or the infant may be sedated and/or paralyzed with Pavulon.

8. *Is the baby making any rhythmic movements suggestive of seizures?* Seizures usually signal a life-threatening, underlying disease or disorder that can produce irreversible brain damage. (Fanaroff, Martin, 1992). Infants usually do not exhibit the organized pattern of seizure activity seen in older children or adults. Abnormal movements or alterations of tone in the body and extremities (e.g., bicycling movements of the legs, extension of the extremities), facial or oral movements (e.g., sucking, grimacing, or lip smacking), ocular movements (e.g., staring or tonic, horizontal eye deviations), and autonomic manifestations (e.g., apnea, changes in the heart rate, blood pressure, and pupillary size) can all be signs of seizures in the newborn.

9. *How does the infant respond to stimulation or handling?* The term, healthy newborn maintains all body subsystems with handling. The stressed and/or preterm infant may decompensate with handling, as evidenced by apnea, color change, and decreased heart rate (see Clinical Application of Research).

CLINICAL APPLICATION OF RESEARCH

PAIN ASSESSMENT IN PREMATURE INFANTS

Premature infants, who are cared for in neonatal intensive care units, experience many painful diagnostic procedures and interventions. The most premature and sickest infants experience the most painful procedures. Although researchers have studied term infants' responses to pain, little is known about premature infants' physiologic and behavioral responses to pain.

The purposes of this study were to describe the physiologic and behavioral responses of premature infants to a painful stimulus and to determine whether the responses were affected by the infant's state and severity of illness. The sample included 40 premature infants between 32 and 34 weeks' gestational age who were less than 5 days postbirth. Data were collected for each infant before, during, and after a routine heelstick. Physiologic data (i.e., oxygen saturation, heart rate, and intracranial pressure) were sampled on a second-to-second basis and fed into a computer. Behavioral data (i.e., facial expressions and crying) were obtained by videotape and audiotape.

Researchers found that the heart rate and intracranial pressure increased, and that the oxygen saturation decreased during the stick and squeeze phases of the heelstick. The facial actions common to full-term infants in pain were most prevalent in the stick and squeeze phases. Crying occurred more often in the stick phase than in the squeeze phase. An infant's state affected behavioral responses but not physiologic responses; infants who were active and awake showed more facial action. The infants' cries were affected by the severity of their illnesses, but not their physiologic responses or facial expressions.

The researchers concluded that the responses of premature infants to a painful stimulus are similar to those of full-term infants. Nurses providing care for premature infants often inflict pain during procedures. Nurses must learn to recognize the behavioral and physiologic responses of infants to pain; with this information, nurses can better assess and manage the pain.

Reference: Stevens BJ, Johnston CC, Horton L: Multidimensional pain assessment in premature neonates: a pilot study, *JOGNN* 22:531, 1993.

Respiratory System
Questions Nurses Should Ask Themselves

1. *Is there unequal chest wall movement?* It may be difficult to ascertain unequal chest wall movement while looking down at the infant's chest. Instead, with the infant at eye level, look across the chest from side to side and from head to toe. Unequal chest wall movement may indicate pneumothorax, congenital diaphragmatic hernia, or another pathologic process that impedes lung expansion on one side.
2. *Are there unequal breath sounds? Are these sounds diminished in any lobe?* Unequal breath sounds are produced by any process that impedes lung expansion unilaterally or in a particular lobe.
3. *Are rales, rhonchi, or wheezing sounds audible?* These sounds may indicate that any number of problems may be occurring, such as respiratory distress syndrome (RDS), pneumonia, meconium aspiration, congestive heart failure (CHF), pulmonary edema, or that the airway needs suctioning.
4. *Any grunting, flaring, or retracting* (see the discussion grunting, flaring, and retracting)?
5. *Is the respiratory rate outside normal parameters (30 to 60 breaths/min)?*
   - Tachypnea (i.e., respiratory rate >60 breaths/min)—Tachypnea may indicate hyperthermia, transient tachypnea of the newborn (TTNB), respiratory distress syndrome (RDS), pneumonia, and/or that the $PaCo_2$ is too high.
   - Respiratory rate <30 breaths/min—may indicate that breathing was not counted for a full minute during periodic breathing, or the $PaCo_2$ is too low.
   - Apnea (Cessation of breathing for more than 15 to 20 seconds)—Apnea results from multiple reasons such as stress, sepsis, airway obstruction, or apnea of prematurity.
6. *Does the infant require assisted ventilation?* If so, the nurse and respiratory therapist share the responsibility for regularly noting the following:
   - FiO_2—the fraction of inspired oxygen, or the amount of oxygen being given to the infant.

- PIP—PIP is the positive inspiratory pressure or the volume of air being delivered with each mechanical breath on inspiration.
- PEEP (or CPAP)—positive end expiratory pressure or continuous positive airway pressure is the pressure used to keep the lungs open at the end of expiration.
- IT—IT refers to inspiratory time or the amount of time air is pushed into the lungs on each mechanical inspiration.
- I:E Ratio—the ratio of inspiratory time to expiratory time is called the I:E Ratio. Expiratory time should be longer then inspiratory time in order to avoid "stacking" breaths.
- Flow—this refers to the flow of air in liters that is given to the infant; the higher the flow, the more barotrauma to the airway.
- MAP—this refers to the mean airway pressure; the higher the mean airway pressure, the greater barotrauma to the airway.
- Temperature of air—all air given to the infant should be warmed and humidified to prevent excessive cooling and drying of the mucous membranes.
- Arterial or capillary blood gases—capillary blood gases are obtained by heel stick and provide accurate measurement of Co_2, pH and bicarbonate levels within the tissues, but are not accurate in measuring oxygenation (see the discussion on p. 763 regarding arterial blood gases).
- Oxygen saturation (see the discussion on p. 765).
- Transcutaneous Co_2 monitor—Co_2 tension is measured by using an electrode placed on the skin that heats the area under the probe and causes certain physiologic changes. The Co_2 is diffused through the heated skin and is measured by the electrode with the value digitally displayed on the monitor. These monitors require frequent calibrations. The site of the electrode should be changed every 2 to 4 hours, depending on the fragility of the infant's skin. It is important that the infant does not lie on the electrode, because this increases the pressure on the underlying capillaries and results in a falsely low reading. Discomfort and skin breakdown can develop from the excessive pressure of the electrode against the infant's skin.

BOX 26-4

Respiratory System

normal = equal chest wall movement; clear and equal breath sounds that are audible in all lobes; no grunting, flaring, or retracting (GFR); breathing without assistance with a respiratory rate of 30 to 60 breaths/min; and maintaining arterial blood gases within normal limits

---

Cardiovascular System
Questions Nurses Should Ask Themselves

1. *Is there an abnormal rate or rhythm?* Benign and pathologic arrhythmias exist in the newborn (Table 26-2).
2. *Is there an active precordium?* An active precordium means that the nurse can see the heart beat-

ing through the chest wall. This indicates that the heart is working too hard. It is a sign of patent ductus arteriosus (PDA), which often occurs in preterm infants in the middle of their first week of life.

3. *Are peripheral pulses unequal, weak, or bounding?* Assess the radial, brachial, femoral, and posttibial pulses. If both the upper and the lower pulses are unequal, obtain 4-limb blood pressures. If the systolic blood pressure in the upper extremities is greater than that found in the lower extremities (by >15 mm Hg), then the nurse should suspect coarctation of the aorta (Merenstein, Gardner, 1993). If pulses are weak, the nurse should be concerned about cardiac output or shock. If the pulses are too full or bounding, the nurse should worry about pulmonary artery (PA) run off, as in a PDA.

4. *Is the capillary fill time more than 3 seconds centrally?* (See the previous discussion of CFT).

5. *Is the mean blood pressure outside the normal parameters for the infant's weight?*

6. *Is the hematocrit too high or too low?* If the hematocrit is too high, then polycythemia is indicated and the nurse should refer to skin assessment. If the hematocrit is too low, then anemia is indicated and the nurse should also refer to skin assessment.

Gastrointestinal/Renal Systems
Questions Nurses Should Ask Themselves

1. *Is the abdomen distended?* Infants normally have a soft, rounded abdomen. Distention has a fuller, tenser appearance and may indicate delayed peristalsis or a pathologic process of abnormal gas formation. The only way to know that the abdomen is getting larger is to measure it regularly over the same area before feeding. Any distention must be reported to the primary health care provider in order to determine if feeding should proceed. Measure the abdominal girth either above or below the umbilicus, and chart where the abdomen was measured for later reference.

Other worrisome abdominal signs include visible loops of bowel and a bluish tinge demarcated at the rib cage and groin. These signs are ominous, may indicate necrotizing enterocolitis (NEC), and require immediate attention.

2. *Is the umbilicus inflamed or draining?* Omphalitis is potentially lethal, but easily prevented with thorough hand washing and proper caregiver techniques.

3. *Are bowel sounds hypoactive, hyperactive, or absent?* Abnormal bowel sounds require further assessment.

4. *Are stools heme positive or Clinitest positive?* Heme or occult positive stools may be normal if the stool is meconium. It could indicate a simple anal fissure, or it could be an ominous sign of NEC. Clinitest positive stools indicate the presence of carbohydrate in the stool, as well as possible abnormal absorption in the intestines.

5. *Is there any emesis, especially bilious emesis?* Bilious emesis may indicate bowel obstruction or NEC.

6. *Are there excessive residuals (half or more of previous feedings) and what do these residuals look like?* Small amounts of partially digested formula or breast milk are normal; large amounts or discoloration indicate that *something is wrong.*

7. *Are chemstrips too high or too low?* (See the dis-

TABLE 26-2 Common Arrhythmias in Newborns

BENIGN ARRHYTHMIAS	PATHOLOGIC ARRHYTHMIAS
sinus bradycardia	supraventricular tachycardia (SVT)
sinus tachycardia	atrial flutter and fibrillation
sinus arrhythmias	Wolff-Parkinson-White syndrome, ventricular tachycardia, and atrioventricular blocks

Modified from Fanaroff, Martin: *Neonatal-perinatal medicine: diseases of the fetus and infant,* ed 5, St Louis, 1992, Mosby.

BOX 26-5
Cardiovascular System

normal = normal sinus rhythm; a rate of 120 to 160 beats/min; no murmur (although an intermittent murmur *may* be normal during transition); peripheral pulses are 2+, strong, and equal bilaterally in both the upper and the lower extremities; capillary fill time (CFT) is 2 to 3 seconds centrally and peripherally; and mean arterial or blood pressure is appropriate for the infant's weight

BOX 26-6
Gastrointestinal/Renal Systems

normal = soft round abdomen, stable girth, no visible loops of bowel, healing umbilicus, active bowel sounds, tolerating feedings, stable chemstrips (glucose 80 to 120 mg/dl), appropriate stools, urinary output is ≥2 ml/kg/hr, intake is appropriate ml/kg/day and cal/kg/day

cussion of hypoglycemia in the stabilization section).

8. *Is the urinary output <2 ml/kg/hr?* This may indicate renal failure. To calculate the urinary output/kg/hr, divide the total output by the infant's weight, then divide this by the number of hours the output is counted. For example, an infant's urinary output since midnight is 52 ml. It is now 7 a.m., and the infant weighs 3500 g (3.5 kg).

$$52 \text{ (ml urine output)} \div 7 \text{ (hr)} \div 3.5 \text{ (kg)} = 2.1 \text{ ml/kg/hr}$$
urine output since midnight

9. *Is the urine specific gravity too low (<1.005) or too high (>1.015)?* Preterm infants have a decreased ability to concentrate urine and are at risk for abnormal fluid losses.

10. *Is fluid intake too high or too low for an infant on a given day, when considering its gestational and corrected age, weight, and overall physiologic condition?**

✤ NURSING DIAGNOSES

Analyses of the significance of findings collected during a "Quick Check" or systemic assessment leads to the establishment of nursing diagnoses. Possible nursing diagnoses for the compromised newborn include the following:

High risk for ineffective airway clearance related to
- Secretions
- Newborn anatomy
- Immaturity or congenital disorder

Ineffective breathing pattern related to
- Immaturity
- Cold stress

Ineffective thermoregulation related to
- Physiologic immaturity
- Large surface area to body mass ratio
- Congenital disorder

Altered nutrition, less than body requirements related to
- Immaturity
- Respiratory disorder
- Congenital disorder

High risk for altered parenting related to
- Infant's physical condition at birth
- Separation from infant

✤ EXPECTED OUTCOMES

During this important step, expected outcomes are identified to meet the unique needs of the compromised newborn during transition. These expected outcomes should be patient-centered and involve the parents as much as the infant's condition and parental readiness allow. These expected outcomes include the following:
- The newborn's airway will remain will be patent.
- The newborn's respirations will be maintained.
- The newborn will maintain an axillary temperature between 97.8° and 98.6° F (36.6° and 37° C).
- The newborn's respiratory needs of all tissues will be met (e.g., blood gases and acid-base balance will be maintained within their normal limits).
- The newborn's metabolic needs will be met by adequate nutritional intake.
- The parent-newborn relationship will develop.

✤ COLLABORATIVE CARE

Stabilization

Stabilization is necessary to maintain the infant within normal physiologic parameters. Table 26-3 lists six areas of concern when stabilizing a newborn.

Hypothermia

When faced with the compromised newborn, the nurse must take extraordinary measures to maintain the neu-

TABLE 26-3 Six Areas of Concern when Stabilizing a Newborn	
FIVE "Hs" & AN "A" OF STABILIZATION	**THE STABILIZED INFANT HAS**
Hypothermia	Axillary temperature of 97.8° and 98.6° F (36.6° to 37° C).
Hypoxemia-the definitions of hypoxemia are controversial and may differ among medical texts, health care providers, and medical institutions.	PaO_2 of 50 to 70 mm Hg if birth weight < 1000 g and FiO_2 > 0.21% PaO_2 of 50 to 80 mm Hg if birth weight > 1000 g and FiO_2 > 0.21% *Please note that an appropriate PaO_2 for a term infant will depend on the infant's underlying condition.*
Hypercarbia	$PaCo_2$ of 35 to 45 mm Hg
Hypoglycemia	Blood glucose *above 40 mg/dl*
Hypotension	Mean arterial pressure or blood pressure is appropriate for the infant's weight (1 kg = about 30 mm Hg).
Acidosis	Blood pH 7.35 to 7.45

*FiO_2, fraction of inspired oxygen; PaO_2, partial pressure of oxygen in arterial blood; $PaCO_2$, partial pressure of carbon dioxide with arterial blood.
Modified from Roberts D: Neonatal resuscitation, a practical guide, New York, 1981, Academic Press.*

*For more information about the intricacies of fluid and electrolyte balances in the newborn, see Chapter 22 of Fanaroff, Martin: *Neonatal-perinatal medicine: diseases of the fetus and infant,* ed 5, 1992, Mosby.)

tral thermal environment (NTE) for that infant. The NTE is that environmental temperature at which a particular infant will maintain a normal core temperature without expending excessive energy to do so. Hypothermic infants increase their metabolic rate to raise their temperatures to within normal range. Increasing the metabolic rate requires the use of additional oxygen and glucose. If not corrected, this may lead to hypoglycemia and hypoxemia. Hypothermia can exacerbate respiratory distress or other pathologic conditions since the infant "wastes" energy just to stay warm. The consequences of hypothermia can be severe, resulting in significant morbidity or even death.

Measures used to maintain the ideal NTE include radiant warmers or double-walled isolettes that are set at the appropriate temperature. Several NTE charts are available and one should be posted in every nursery. Table 26-4 shows an example of an NTE chart.

Wool or double-thickness cotton or acrylic hats are another thermoregulatory measure that should be used for infants since their head comprises about one fourth of their body weight and surface areas. Swaddling the infant with warm blankets is not always possible if continuous assessment of the infant's respiratory status is required, or if various lines and monitors are in use. Booties can be used unless an umbilical arterial catheter (UAC) is in low placement. UAC internal placement is either above the diaphragm (high placement) at T8 or between L3 (third lumbar spine) and L4 (fourth lumbar spine) on an x-ray examination. When the UAC is in low placement, the catheter may cause vasospasm of one femoral artery and decrease perfusion of that extremity. Blanching of the affected leg's toes or foot is the first sign of complication. Booties covering the foot delay assessment and treatment and can lead to necrosis of the distal extremity.

"Warm" water gloves have been used to increase the cold infant's environmental temperature. These *warm* gloves are often *hot* water gloves and can cause severe burns, even though the infant is wrapped in blankets or diapers. Alternative methods include using plastic, sterile irrigation bottles, commonly used in surgery. These bottles are kept in a warmer that is set at 102.2° to 104° F (39° to 40° C). The nurse wraps these bottles with a diaper or blanket and places them close to, but not touching, the infant. Disposable chemical mattresses are now available. These mattresses warm up to 104° F (40° C) and last between 4 and 6 hours. They are invaluable in the stabilization of the hypothermic newborn.

LEGAL TIP: **Negligence during Neonatal Emergencies—Use of Warming Equipment**
Any adverse sequelae, especially burns, resulting from the inappropriate use of warming equipment, may lead to a charge of nursing negligence.

Other warming measures include, but are not limited to, the following:
1. Heat shields that decrease the environment's size thereby decreasing radiant heat loss
2. Keeping the infant away from drafts and high-traffic areas
3. Plastic wrap blankets for intubated infants (Since these blankets are placed over the entire infant, suffocation can occur unless the infant's air supply comes from an external source).
4. Heated water mattress, K-pads, and other devices set at 100.4° F (38° C) or warmer, as ordered by the primary health care provider (To protect the infant from possible burns, a blanket or diaper must completely cover the surface of the warming devices that touch the infant. Nurses must frequently monitor the temperature of these devices.)

Thermoregulation of the infant is limited only by the resources available and the creativity of the nurse caring for the hypothermic newborn.

Hypoxemia

In utero the normal fetus is exposed to lower oxygen levels than at any other period of life. The fetus thrives with a PaO_2 (oxygen tension in the arterial system) of 20 mm Hg to low 30 mm Hg (Fanaroff, Martin, 1992). At birth the exposure of the newborn to room air, which has an FiO_2 of about 21%, increases the infant's arterial oxygen levels to between 80 and 100%. Administering oxygen to the newborn can increase these levels to well above 100%. The term newborn appears to tolerate these higher levels for limited periods without residual detrimental effects. In contrast, premature infants who have not vascularized their retina are at risk for retinopathy of prematurity (ROP) when exposed to high oxygen tensions within their arterial systems. The appropriate level of PaO_2 in premature infants is controversial.

To maintain the appropriate oxygen tensions in the blood stream, oxygen administration may be required. This can be achieved with "blow by" oxygen, a temporary means of administering oxygen by a mask or a tube that is held close to the infant's mouth and nose. If the nurse uses a tube with flow from a 100% oxygen source, then the concentration of oxygen delivered will depend on the distance that the tube is held from the infant's mouth and nose. If the tube is held 2 inches away, the amount of oxygen delivered will equal room air (21%). Oxygen can also be delivered by a hood. With this method, the infant's head is covered by a clear plastic device and oxygen is directed into the hood. Oxygen may also be delivered with positive pressure ventilation, either with hand ventilation or on a ventilator. Whenever oxygen is delivered to an infant, the oxygen must be heated, humidified, and *continuously* monitored.

Arterial blood gases (ABGs) are excellent tools for assessing the arterial levels of PaO_2, $PaCO_2$, pH, and bicarbonate. However, these tools are invasive, require

TABLE 26-4 Neutral Thermal Environmental Temperatures

AGE AND WEIGHT	STARTING TEMPERATURE (°C)	RANGE OF TEMPERATURE (°C)	AGE AND WEIGHT	STARTING TEMPERATURE (°C)	RANGE OF TEMPERATURE (°C)
0-6 HOURS			**72-96 HOURS**		
Under 1200 gm	35.0	34.0-35.4	Under 1200 gm	34.0	34.0-35.0
1200-1500 gm	34.1	33.9-34.4	1200-1500 gm	33.5	33.0-34.0
1501-2500 gm	33.4	32.8-33.8	1501-2500 gm	32.2	31.1-33.2
Over 2500 (and >36 weeks)	32.9	32.0-33.8	Over 2500 (and >36 weeks)	31.3	29.8-32.8
6-12 HOURS			**4-12 DAYS**		
Under 1200 gm	35.0	34.0-35.4	Under 1500 gm	33.5	33.0-34.0
1200-1500 gm	34.0	33.5-34.4	1501-2500 gm	32.1	31.0-33.2
1501-2500 gm	33.1	32.2-33.8	Over 2500 (and >36 weeks)	31.0	29.5-32.6
Over 2500 (and >36 weeks)	32.8	31.4-33.8	4-5 days		
			5-6 days	30.9	29.4-32.3
			6-8 days	30.6	29.0-32.2
12-24 HOURS			8-10 days	30.3	29.0-31.8
Under 1200 gm	34.0	34.0-35.4	10-12 days	30.1	29.0-31.4
1200-1500 gm	33.8	33.3-34.3			
1501-2500 gm	32.8	31.8-33.8	**12-14 DAYS**		
Over 2500 (and >36 weeks)	32.4	31.0-33.7	Under 1500 gm	33.5	32.6-34.0
			1501-2500 gm	32.1	31.0-33.2
			Over 2500 (and >36 weeks)	30.1	29.0-31.4
24-36 HOURS					
Under 1200 gm	34.0	34.0-35.0	**2-3 WEEKS**		
1200-1500 gm	33.6	33.1-34.2	Under 1500 gm	33.1	32.2-34.0
1501-2500 gm	32.6	31.6-33.6	1501-2500 gm	31.7	30.5-33.0
Over 2500 (and >36 weeks)	32.1	30.7-33.5			
			3-4 WEEKS		
36-48 HOURS			Under 1500 gm	32.6	31.6-33.6
Under 1200 gm	34.0	34.0-35.0	1501-2500 gm	31.4	30.0-32.7
1200-1500 gm	33.5	33.0-34.1			
1501-2500 gm	32.5	31.4-33.5	**4-5 WEEKS**		
Over 2500 (and <36 weeks)	31.9	30.5-33.3	Under 1500 gm	32.0	31.2-33.0
			1501-2500 gm	30.9	29.5-32.2
48-72 HOURS					
Under 1200 gm	34.0	34.0-35.0	**5-6 WEEKS**		
1200-1500 gm	33.5	33.0-34.0	Under 1500 gm	31.4	30.6-32.3
1501-2500 gm	32.3	31.2-33.4	1501-2500 gm	30.4	29.0-31.8
Over 2500 (and >36 weeks)	31.7	30.1-33.2			

Modified from Fanaroff AA, Martin RJ, editors: *Neonatal-perinatal medicine: diseases to the fetus and infant,* ed 5, St Louis, 1992, Mosby.
Data from Scopes JW, Ahmed I: Minimal rates of oxygen consumption in sick and premature infants, *Arch Dis Child* 41:407, 1966; Scopes JW, Ahmed I: Range of critical temperatures in sick and premature newborn babies, *Arch Dis Child* 41:407, 1966. For his table, Scopes had the walls of the incubator 1° to 2° warmer than the ambient air temperatures.
Generally speaking, the smaller infants in each weight group require a temperature in the higher portion of the temperature range. Within each time range, the younger the infant, the higher the temperature required.

blood removal, and are painful when obtained by arterial puncture. Nurses need to remember that these are point-in-time measurements, reflecting only on what is happening while the ABG is being drawn. Trends of oxygen saturation and transcutaneous CO_2 may be as, if not more, useful in the management of the compromised newborn.

Oxygen saturation monitors, also called **pulse oximetry,** continuously monitor oxygen levels by detecting the amount of light absorbed by the oxygen-carrying hemoglobin. This method has the distinct advantage of being noninvasive and does not require the use of heat. A small sensor placed on the finger, hand, foot, or toe accomplishes the task. One side of the sensor is a light source: the other side is a photoreceiver. The sensor must be placed so that the light source and the photoreceiver are either aligned or directly opposite each other in order to detect the pulse and the amount of light absorbed by the hemoglobin as it passes through a vascular bed (Merenstein, Gardner, 1993).

Hypercarbia

The stabilized infant has an arterial or capillary heel stick blood gas value of 35 to 45 torr of CO_2. High CO_2 levels indicate hypoventilation. Hand ventilation, with a bag and mask, or intubation and mechanical ventilation may be required to correct hypercarbia.

Hypoglycemia

The definition of hypoglycemia, like that of hypoxemia, remains controversial. For the purpose of this discussion serum blood glucose values of less than 40 mg/dl define hypoglycemia (Fanaroff, Martin, 1992). Clinical signs of hypoglycemia are subtle and nonspecific. Jitteriness is the classic sign nurses use to identify hypoglycemic infants; however, hypocalcemia and drug exposure/withdrawal may also produce jitteriness. Table 26-5 lists other clinical signs associated with hypoglycemia.

TABLE 26-5 Clinical Signs Often Associated with Neonatal Hypoglycemia*

Apneic spells
Cardiac arrest
Cardiac failure
Cyanotic spells
High-pitched or weak cry
Hypothermia
Irritability
Lethargy or stupor
Limpness
Refusal to feed
Seizures
Tremors or jitteriness

From Fanaroff AA, Martin RJ, editors: *Neonatal-perinatal medicine: diseases of the fetus and infant,* ed 5, St Louis, 1992, Mosby.
*The clinical sign should be alleviated with concomitant correction of the glucose level.

Hypotension

Blood pressure is the one vital sign parameter that nurses frequently overlook in the newborn. The golden standard of blood pressure measurement is obtained by transducing the arterial system, such as with an umbilical arterial catheter. Blood pressure measurement can also be obtained by electronic devices such as for indirect noninvasive automatic mean arterial pressure (DINAMAP). These machines are commonly found on adult units and can easily be adapted for use in the newborn by changing the cable and using an appropriately sized cuff. Too wide a cuff gives a falsely low reading; too narrow a cuff gives a falsely high reading. Nurses should base a newborn's normal blood pressure on the infant's weight, not on the gestational age.

Nursing Care of the Family

With the birth of a compromised newborn, parents must readjust their expectations. They need to grieve for the loss of the "perfect" baby they had anticipated, and they may have difficulty becoming attached to their infant. Misinterpretation of their emotional cues by the health care professional can further damage this process.

Socioeconomic and cultural differences can influence parental behavior and needs. In some cultures the husband must make all decisions and attempts to include the mother can undermine the integrity of the family. Other cultures do not name their infant until 31 days after birth, which could be misinterpreted as a lack of attachment. Non-English-speaking parents often encounter the additional difficulty of a language barrier with the health care providers.

Parents need to see and touch their compromised baby as soon as possible. They also need consistent information regarding their infant's condition. All members of the health care team must coordinate communication so that the parents hear the same message from several sources. Other interventions to assist the parents depend, in part, on the infant's condition. Parents of preterm infants can quite possibly look forward to a "normal" child whereas parents of infants with significant birth defects probably cannot. Normalizing the parents' interactions with their sick infant helps them accomplish the difficult task of parental attachment in the face of overwhelming grief.

✤ EVALUATION

The newborn's successful transition to extrauterine life, as defined by the chart in Fig. 26-2 on p. 755, and the development of a parent-newborn relationship assures the nurse that the expected outcomes have been achieved.

KEY POINTS

- The aim of transporting high-risk infants to regional centers is to provide access to the required level of care.
- Newborns are at more risk for asphyxia then any other age group.
- Normal transition to extrauterine life follows a defined pattern.
- The nurses' primary contribution to the welfare of the newborn begins with early observation, in addition to the accurate recording of and prompt reporting of signs that indicate deviations from normal.
- High-risk infants have special problems caused by immaturity, as well as alterations in the functioning of their systems and metabolic balances.
- A neutral thermal environment is essential for metabolic homeostasis.
- Parents need assistance with real or anticipated loss and grief.

CRITICAL THINKING EXERCISES

1. "Buddy up" with an ICN/NICU nurse for 1 clinical day. The clinical observation day should follow an orientation to the unit so that the student can focus on the experience to be described.
   a. Why is this suggestion made?
   b. What implications underlying this suggestion can you apply to parents viewing their infant in the ICN for the first time?
2. Choose any of the following:
   a. Observe a complete physical assessment. Compare with the routine physical assessments in the well-baby nursery.
   b. Describe the infant's willingness to interact with caregivers and to engage in eye-to-eye contact. Note your reactions to the neonate. Discuss implications for nursing care of the neonate and family, based on your findings.
   c. Calculate the percentage of weight gain and loss for three high-risk neonates. Identify probable causes and describe nursing actions.
   d. Observe nursing care related to maintenance of respirations, temperature, and nutrition and elimination. Compare with the care given in the well-baby nursery.

References

American Heart Association/American Academy of Pediatrics: *Textbook of neonatal resuscitation*, Dallas, 1991, American Heart Association.

Fanaroff AA, Martin RJ, editors: *Neonatal-perinatal medicine: diseases of the fetus and infant*, ed 5, St Louis, 1992, Mosby.

Merenstein GB, Gardner SL: *Handbook of neonatal intensive care*, ed 3, St Louis, 1993, Mosby.

Rudolph AM: *Pediatrics*, ed 19, Norwalk, CT, 1991, Appleton & Lange.

Bibliography

Crane LD et al: Effects of transcutaneous carbon dioxide tension in neonates with respiratory distress, *J Perinatal* 10:35, 1990.

Kenner C, Brueggemeyer A, Genderson LP: *Comprehensive neonatal nursing*, Philadelphia, 1993, WB Saunders.

Monett ZJ, Monihan PJ: Cardiovascular assessment of the neonatal heart, *J Perinat Neonat Nurs* 5(2):50, 1991.

Pettit J, Hughes K: Intravenous extravasation: mechanisms, management, and prevention, *J Perinat Neonat Nurs* 6(3): 69, 1993.

Polin RA, Fox WW: *Fetal and neonatal physiology*, Philadelphia, 1992, WB Saunders.

Sonesso G: Are you ready to use pulse oximetry? *Nursing 91* 21(8):60, 1991.

Tappero EP, Honeyfield ME: *Physical assessment of the newborn: a comprehensive approach to the art of physical examination*, Petaluma, CA, 1993, NICU Ink Book Publishers.

Thomas K: Thermoregulation in neonates, *Neonatal Network* 13(2):15, 1994.

Whitney JD: The measurement of oxygen tension in tissue, *Nurs Res* 39:203, 1990.

CHAPTER

27

Specific Problems of the Newborn at Risk

LILA PARAM

LEARNING OBJECTIVES

Define key terms listed.

Discuss nursing care of newborns who vary in gestational age.

Identify the clinical characteristics of transient tachypnea of the newborn.

Develop a nursing care plan for an infant with fetal alcohol syndrome.

Describe the pathophysiology of respiratory distress syndrome and current treatments for it.

Describe the assessment of the newborn for infection.

Review prenatal diagnosis of neonatal disorders.

Describe the pathophysiology of persistent pulmonary hypertension and the current treatments for it.

Describe the assessment of an intrauterine growth retarded infant.

Discuss discharge planning and teaching for compromised newborns and their families.

KEY TERMS

ABO incompatibility
appropriate for gestational age (AGA)
bronchopulmonary dysplasia (BPD)
fetal alcohol syndrome (FAS)
hydramnios
hydrocephalus
inborn errors of metabolism
infants of diabetic mothers (IDMs)
intrauterine growth retardation (IUGR)
kernicterus
large for gestational age (LGA)
low birth weight (LBW)
macrosomia
meconium aspiration syndrome (MAS)
necrotizing enterocolitis (NEC)
postmature
postterm (postdate)
premature
preterm
respiratory distress syndrome (RDS)
retinopathy of prematurity (ROP)
sepsis neonatorum
small for gestational age (SGA)
spina bifida
term
TORCH
very low birth weight (VLBW)

RELATED TOPICS

Alpha-fetoprotein *(Chap. 20)* • Asphyxia *(Chap. 26)* • Fetal circulation *(Chap. 13)* • Gestational age assessment *(Chap. 14)* • Infant CPR *(Chap. 14)* • Loss and grief *(Chap. 28)* • Phototherapy *(Chap. 14)* • Sensory behaviors *(Chap. 13)* • Thermoregulation *(Chap. 26)* • Universal precautions *(Chap. 21)* • Maternal substance abuse *(Chap. 23)*

Nurses must always be prepared to provide immediate and emergency care to newborns who are born with or develop problems during the newborn period. Nurses assist in the stabilization of the infant before transporting the infant to a regional intensive care nursery. They deal with parents who are trying to cope with the birth of a baby who does not meet their expected ideal. In this chapter some of the problems encountered during the newborn period are discussed, and nursing care of compromised infants is described.

TRANSIENT TACHYPNEA OF THE NEWBORN

Transient tachypnea of the newborn (TTNB) is common in the term and near-term infant and is thought to be a result of delayed absorption of fetal lung fluid. It is seen more commonly after cesarean birth, apparently because the thorax of the fetus was not exposed to the vaginal squeeze during the birth process. This vaginal squeeze appears to expel a significant amount of fetal lung fluid during the transition through the vagina. Milner's studies of gas volume measurements in the newborn showed the mean thoracic gas volume after vaginal birth to be 32.7 ml/kg; after cesarean birth it was only 19.7 ml/kg even though chest circumferences were the same in both groups (Fanaroff, Martin, 1992). It is thought that infants who have not been exposed to vaginal compression have excessively high volumes of interstitial and alveolar fluid during the first few hours of life so that thoracic gas volume is reduced, but overall thoracic volume remains the same.

TTNB shares many clinical features with other respiratory problems caused by surfactant deficiency. This syndrome typically presents as respiratory distress in non-asphyxiated term or near-term infants. Signs include grunting, flaring, retracting, tachypnea and varying degrees of hypoxemia in the first hours of life. Chest roentgenogram is necessary to differentiate TTNB from other forms of respiratory disease in the newborn. The characteristic finding is prominent perihilar streaking and fluid in the interlobar fissures.

TTNB may last anywhere from 12 to 24 hours in the milder forms to in excess of 72 hours in severe cases. Transient tachypnea of the newborn is self-limiting with no risk of recurrence or residual pulmonary dysfunction; however, transient tachypnea must be distinguished from other causes of neonatal respiratory distress. For example, it may be difficult to distinguish this disorder from respiratory distress syndrome (RDS) or group B streptococcal pneumonia, both of which can cause significant morbidity or mortality. Evaluation, monitoring, and basic supportive care must cover all these contingencies.

SEPSIS NEONATORUM

Sepsis neonatorum, or neonatal septicemia, is defined as bacterial infections of the bloodstream in infants during the first 4 weeks of life. Incidence of sepsis varies from nursery to nursery and ranges from 1 in 500 to 1 in 600 live births. The incidence for the very low–birth-weight premature infant (<1500 g) increases to 1 in 250. Sepsis is associated with fatality rates of 13% to 50% and possible substantial morbidity for survivors (Fanaroff, Martin, 1992).

Factors affecting sepsis in the newborn can be divided into three categories: maternal factors, environment factors, and host factors. Maternal factors include prolonged rupture of membranes, preterm labor, clinical amnionitis, maternal fever, excessive manipulation during labor, and prolonged labor. Environmental influences that can predispose the newborn to sepsis include, but are not limited to, poor hand washing and caregiver techniques, arterial and venous umbilical catheters, peripheral IVs, hyperalimentation, central lines, indwelling catheters of any kind, endotracheal tubes, any invasive technology, and formula feeding. Host factors include male sex, premature infant, low birth weight, and impaired host defense mechanisms.

The pathophysiologic process in sepsis begins with bacterial invasion and systemic contamination. Bacterial release of endotoxin causes alteration in myocardial function, alteration in oxygen uptake and utilization, inhibition of mitochondrial function, and progressive metabolic derangements. In fulminant (sudden, severe) sepsis activation of the complement cascade accounts for much of the cell death and damage seen. The outcome of fulminant, overwhelming sepsis is decreased tissue perfusion, metabolic acidosis, and shock leading to disseminated intravascular coagulation (DIC) and death.

Clinical manifestations of sepsis begin with subtle, "soft" signs. *The key to diagnosis is noting a change in the condition of the infant.* Lethargy, irritability, and poor feeding may be the first signs. Temperature instability (usually hypothermia), mottling of the skin, delayed capillary fill time, and changes in the heart rate and respiratory status become evident as the disease progresses. One of the most reliable indicators of sepsis in the newborn is that the nurse or the mother says the infant is not doing as well as before. This is not because nurses or mothers have any unusual intuition in these circumstances, but because the nurse or mother has been constantly observing the infant and is able to notice subtle changes that may not be apparent to the health care provider, who sees the infant sporadically.

Other manifestations of sepsis in the newborn include unstable chem-strips, (especially hypoglycemia), hypocalcemia, thrombocytopenia, and neutropenia. The diagnosis is confirmed by positive blood cultures. Since these cultures take 48 hours to complete and the course of sepsis can result in mortality in a few hours, it is important to start antibiotic therapy as soon as possible. Antibiotics can be discontinued if the cultures prove negative and the infant no longer exhibits clinical signs of sepsis.

Treatment of sepsis in the nursery includes acute observation of the infant, early identification, the septic workup (Box 27-1), treatment with antibiotics, close monitoring of all systems, and support of the 5 *H*s and *A* of Stabilization (see Table 26-2).

OTHER INFECTIONS IN THE NEWBORN POPULATION
TORCH Infections

The occurrence of certain maternal infections during early pregnancy is well known to be associated with vari-

ous congenital malformations and disorders. The most common and best understood infections are represented by the acronym **TORCH,** for *t*oxoplasmosis, *o*ther, *ru*bella virus, *c*ytomegalovirus, and *h*erpes simplex (Box 27-2). Herpes simplex may result in a severe, often fatal, systemic illness in newborns. Survivors of herpetic infection may have residual neurologic defects and chorioretinitis. The other congenital infections also may result in an encephalopathy with various anomalies, including microcephaly, chorioretinitis, intracranial calcifications, microphthalmos, and cataracts. To a certain extent the varied clinical manifestations of these infections overlap, but a specific diagnosis can be made by the constellation of clinical findings, as well as specific antibody studies (Fanaroff, Martin, 1992).

Toxoplasmosis

Toxoplasmosis is a multisystem disease caused by the protozoan *Toxoplasma gondii.* Cats who hunt infected birds and mice harbor the parasite and excrete the infective oocysts in their feces. Human infection follows hand-to-mouth contact, such as after disposal of cat litter or after handling or ingesting raw meat from cattle or sheep that grazed in contaminated fields.

About 30% of women who contract toxoplasmosis during gestation transmit the disease to their offspring. The mother often has no symptoms. The diagnosis of toxoplasmosis in the newborn is supported by elevated levels of cord blood serum IgM.

More than 70% of affected newborns are free of symptoms. The clinical features of toxoplasmosis resemble cytomegalic inclusion disease in mother and infant. Both diseases are responsible for serious perinatal mortality and morbidity: 10% to 15% die; 85% have severe psychomotor problems or mental retardation by 2 to 4 years; and 50% have visual problems by 1 year.

Severe toxoplasmosis is associated with preterm birth, growth retardation, microcephaly or hydrocephaly, microphthalmos, chorioretinitis, CNS calcification, thrombocytopenia, jaundice, and fever. Some clinical manifestations do not develop until later in life.

BOX 27-1

The Septic Workup

COMPLETE BLOOD COUNT (CBC) WITH DIFFERENTIAL

The most important value in the CBC is the white blood cell (WBC) count. Septic infants usually show a decreased WBC count of <5000 mm³. The differential will show the amount of immature WBCs in the bloodstream. A large number of immature WBCs in relation to the total WBC count is an indication that the infant has had to mount a significant immune response.

PLATELETS

Normally 150,000 to 300,000 mm³. In sepsis the platelet count drops.

STAT GRAM STAIN AND BLOOD CULTURE/ SENSITIVITY

Results of the stat gram stain should be available within a few hours and will tell the number and kind of bacteria present (e.g., gram-positive or gram-negative rods). The blood culture/sensitivity takes 24 to 48 hours to develop and identify invading pathogens and their susceptibility to antibiotic therapy.

LUMBAR PUNCTURE FOR CULTURE AND SENSITIVITY OF CEREBRAL SPINAL FLUID

See blood cultures.

URINE CULTURE

Urine for latex agglutination and cultures may also be included.

SURFACE CULTURE

Surface cultures fell out of favor as they identify only colonization and not bacterial invasion.

BOX 27-2

TORCH Infections Affecting Newborns

T   Toxoplasmosis
O   Other: syphilis, varicella, group B beta-hemolytic streptococcus, chlamydial infections, hepatitis B, HIV
R   Rubella
C   CMV infections or cytomegalic inclusion disease (CMID)
H   Herpes simplex

Treatment of toxoplasmosis during pregnancy is problematic. Pyrimethamine is the first-choice drug against *T. gondii*. However, it may be teratogenic, especially during the first trimester (Fanaroff, Martin, 1992). Sulfonamide therapy is effective, but the drug must be discontinued before birth and exchange transfusion of the newborn may be necessary to avoid kernicterus. This may occur because sulfa drugs have a greater albumin-binding affinity than does bilirubin, which may rise after birth to critical levels. The newborn may be treated with pyrimethamine, as well as oral sulfadiazine, but folinic acid supplement will be required to prevent anemia. Encysted (intramuscular) forms of *T. gondii* cannot be eradicated by any therapy and they may cause recurrence of the disease.

Hepatitis B Virus Infection

Hepatitis B virus (HBV), the most common etiologic agent of viral hepatitis, is implicated in 24% to 40% of cases. HBV infection during pregnancy is *not* associated with an increase in malformations, stillbirths, or IUGR; however, there is about a 32% increase in risk for preterm birth (Fanaroff, Martin, 1992). The transmission rate of HBV to the newborn is as high as 90% (Hodson, Truog, 1989). Transmission occurs transplacentally, serum to serum, and by contact with contaminated urine, feces, saliva, semen, or vaginal secretions during birth. Infants are most commonly infected during birth or in the first few days of life. The rate of transmission is highest when the mother contracts the virus immediately before birth. Transmission may possibly occur through breast milk, but antigens also develop in formula-fed infants at the same or higher rate. Diagnosis is made by viral culture of amniotic fluid, as well as the presence of hepatitis B surface antigen and IgM in the cord or baby's serum.

Neonatal and fetal effects are serious. Infants may be symptom free at birth or show evidence of acute hepatitis with changes in liver function. Infants are at high risk for chronic hepatitis, cirrhosis of the liver, or liver cancer even years later (Fanaroff, Martin, 1992).

Infants whose mothers have antibodies for hepatitis B surface antigen (HBsAg) or who have developed hepatitis during pregnancy or the postpartum period should be treated with hepatitis B immune globulin (HBIG), 0.5 ml intramuscularly, as soon as possible after birth—within the first 12 hours of life. Concurrently, but at a different site, the vaccine also should be given (Fanaroff, Martin, 1992). The second dose of vaccine is given at 1 month, and the third dose is given at 6 months. The vaccine should protect the child for up to 9 years. After the newborn has been cleansed thoroughly and has received the vaccine, breastfeeding may be allowed.

The Public Health Service defines women at high risk for hepatitis B as those who are Indochinese refugees, of Asian descent, or born in Haiti or South Africa; women with a history of liver disease; women who have occupational exposure to the HBV, such as laboratory technologists, nurses, and physicians; and women who work with mentally retarded individuals. Intravenous drug abusers, prostitutes, and household contacts of hepatitis B carriers also are at high risk (Merenstein, Gardner, 1993).

In 1988 the Centers for Disease Control (CDC) recommended that all pregnant women be screened for HBsAg at an early prenatal visit (Fanaroff, Martin, 1992).

Syphilis

Congenital and neonatal syphilis has reemerged in recent years as a significant health problem.

Fetal infestation with the spirochete *Treponema pallidum* is blocked by Langhans' layer in the chorion until this layer begins to atrophy between 16 and 18 weeks' gestation. If spirochetemia is untreated, it will result in fetal death by midtrimester abortion or stillbirth in one of four cases. All newborns in whom the infection occurs before 7 months' gestation are affected. Only 60% are affected if the infection occurs late in pregnancy. If maternal infection is treated adequately before the eighteenth week, newborns seldom demonstrate signs of the disease. Although treatment after the eighteenth week may cure fetal spirochetemia, pathologic changes may not be prevented completely.

Because the fetus becomes infected after the period of organogenesis (first trimester), maldevelopment of organs does not result. Congenital syphilis may stimulate preterm labor, but there is no evidence that it causes IUGR. Stigmas of congenital syphilis (Fig. 27-1) may include inflammatory and destructive changes in the placenta, in organs such as the liver, spleen, kidneys, adrenal glands, and in bone covering and marrow. Disorders of the CNS, teeth, and corneas may not become evident until several months after birth.

The most severely affected newborns may be *hydropic* (edematous) and *anemic,* with enlarged liver and spleen. Later in the newborn period, early signs, such as poor feeding, slight hyperthermia, and snuffles, may be nonspecific. *Snuffles* refers to the copious clear scrosanguineous mucous discharge from the obstructed nose. Laboratory tests may show a pleocytosis (usually lymphocytosis) and elevated cerebrospinal fluid (CSF) protein levels.

By the end of the first week of life in untreated cases a copper-colored maculopapular *dermal rash* appears. The rash is characteristically first noticeable on the palms of the hands, soles of the feet, the diaper area, and around the mouth and anus. The maculopapular lesions may become vesicular and confluent and extend over the trunk and extremities. *Condylomas* (elevated wartlike lesions) may be seen around the anus. Rough, cracked mucocutaneous lesions of the lips heal to form circumoral radiating scars known as *rhagades.*

If the mother was adequately treated before giving

birth and serologic testing of the newborn does not show syphilis, generally the newborn is not treated with antibiotics. In this case the newborn is checked for antibody titer (received from the mother via the placenta) every 2 weeks for 3 months, at which time the test result should be negative. Some health care providers recommend antibiotic therapy for asymptomatic or inconclusive cases.

Rubella Infection

Congenital rubella infection is a major concern. Since vaccination was begun in 1969, congenital rubella cases have been reduced drastically. Rubella immunity should be confirmed in all women before pregnancy. Confirmation is determined either by verification of rubella immunization or by serologic determination of rubella-specific IgM in cord or neonatal serum because history of rubella infection is unreliable. Diagnosis is possible with viral cultures of amniotic fluid, placenta or neonatal throat, urine, or spinal fluid.

More than two thirds of infected infants show no apparent involvement at birth, but consequences develop years later. Central and peripheral hearing defects, the most common result, appear to be progressive after birth. The major teratogenic effects of rubella involve the cardiovascular system (pulmonary artery hypoplasia, patent ductus arteriosus, and coarctation of the aortic isthmus), and cataract formation. Multiple other abnormalities commonly occur (Fig. 27-2). Anomalies are most severe if the mother contracts the virus during the first trimester. Severe infections may result in fetal death.

The rubella virus has been cultured in babies for up

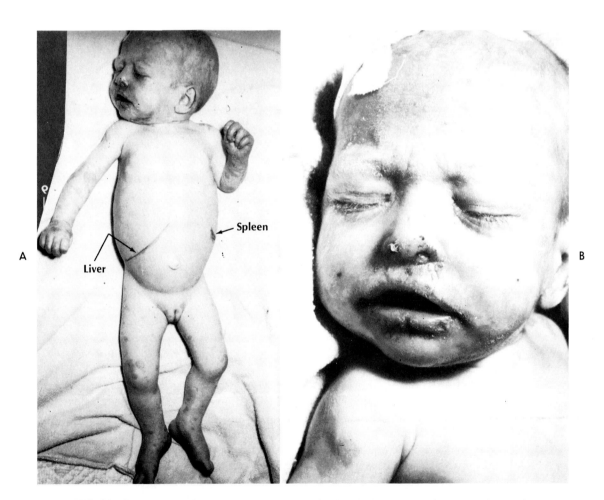

FIG. 27-1 Early congenital syphilis apparent at birth, which corresponds to secondary syphilis in the adult. (Late congenital syphilis, corresponding to tertiary syphilis, becomes apparent after 2 years of age.) **A,** Cutaneous lesions of congenital syphilis. Lines drawn on body indicate hepatosplenomegaly. No destruction of bridge of nose (common finding in congenital syphilis) is noted on this infant. **B,** Rhinitis (snuffles) resulting in rhagades and excoriation of upper lip. Red rash is around mouth and on chin. (From Shirkey HC, editor: *Pediatric therapy,* ed 6, St Louis, 1980, Mosby.)

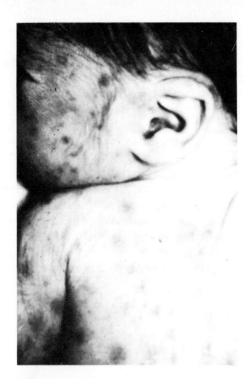

FIG. 27-2 Newborn with congenital rubella syndrome, showing multiple purpuric lesions over face, trunk, and upper arm. (From Fanaroff AA, Martin RJ, editors: *Neonatal-perinatal medicine: diseases of the fetus and infant,* ed 5, St Louis, 1992, Mosby.)

to 18 months after their birth. Extended pediatric isolation is mandatory until the noncontagious stage of rubella has been reached (the newborn should be isolated until pharyngeal mucus and urine are free from virus).

Cytomegalovirus Infection

Cytomegalic inclusion disease (CMID) is a disorder caused by one or more of at least six strains of cytomegalovirus (CMV). CMV is a deoxyribonucleic acid (DNA) virus of the herpes family. Maternal viremia during pregnancy may result in abortion, stillbirth, or congenital or neonatal CMID in a live-born infant. It is the most common cause of congenital viral infections in humans, occurring in 1% of all newborns (Fanaroff, Martin, 1992). It is always a severely crippling disease of the infant.

Maternal infection with CMV may begin as a mononucleosis-like syndrome. Respiratory transmission is the major vector, but the virus has been recovered from semen, vaginal secretions, urine, and feces, as well as from bank blood. Many women have antibody evidence of CMID. Women at risk for CMV infection include those who work in, or have children in, day-care centers, institutions for the mentally retarded, and certain health fields (nursery, dialysis, laboratories, oncology).

The newborn with classic, full-blown CMID displays IUGR and has microcephaly. The neonate also has a petechial rash, jaundice, and hepatosplenomegaly. Anemia, thrombocytopenia, and hyperbilirubinemia are to be expected. Intracranial, periventricular calcification often is noted on x-ray films. Inclusion bodies (owl's eye figures) in cells sedimented from freshly voided urine or in liver biopsy specimens are typical. Elevated levels of cord blood IgM are suggestive of disease. The virus may be isolated from urine or saliva of the newborn.

Despite the extensive, endemic nature of the disease in women and men and its potential for havoc in perinatal life, critically affected newborns are only occasionally born. Milder forms of the disease often may result when the fetus is affected late in pregnancy. CMV can be transmitted through breast milk while the mother is experiencing acute CMV syndrome. Severe mental and physical handicaps mark virtually all infants who survive CMID. Infants without symptoms at birth are at risk for late sequelae.

No reasonable prevention or specific therapy exists for mother or infant (Fanaroff, Martin, 1992). Repeated pregnancies may be complicated by CMV infection. Pregnant health care personnel who have contact with infants suspected of having CMV must be sure to maintain strict universal precautions.

Herpes Simplex Virus Infection

Herpes simplex virus (HSV) infections among newborns are being diagnosed more frequently (Fig. 27-3). HSV infection is estimated to occur in as many as 1 in 2000 to 1 in 5000 births (Fanaroff, Martin, 1992).

The herpes viruses belong to a group of DNA viruses that cause latent infection, last for the lifetime of the individual, and result in periodic recurrences. Pregnancy increases both the frequency of infection and the persistence of the virus. The newborn may acquire the virus by any of four *modes of transmission:*

- Transplacental infection
- Ascending infection by way of the birth canal
- Direct contamination during passage through an infected birth canal
- Direct transmission from infected personnel or family

Transplacental transmission of HSV infection to the newborn may occur during maternal viremia. An ascending transcervical infection first involves the intact fetal membranes, causing chorioamnionitis. Ascending transcervical infection of intact membranes may account for the high rate of spontaneous abortions in the first 20 weeks of gestation associated with genital HSV infections, the development of neonatal infections despite cesarean birth with intact membranes, and the high rate of preterm birth (Brown et al, 1987). Fetal monitoring electrodes break the fetal skin barrier and increase the risk of infection.

Congenital infection is rare and is marked by in utero destruction of normally formed organs. Most infants are

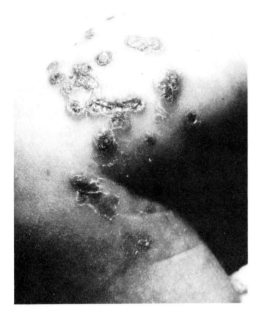

FIG. 27-3   Neonatal herpesvirus infection. (From Fanaroff AA, Martin RJ, editors: *Neonatal-perinatal medicine: diseases of the fetus and infant,* ed 5, St Louis, 1992, Mosby.)

infected directly during passage through the birth canal. The risk of infection during vaginal birth in the presence of genital herpes has not been clearly delineated. It may be as high as 40% to 60%, with active infection at term. Primary maternal infections after 32 weeks' gestation carry a higher risk for the fetus and newborn than do recurrent infections (Fanaroff, Martin, 1992). The transmission rate of chronic vaginal herpes from the pregnant woman to her newborn is low, 8% or less (Bennett, 1987; Prober, 1987). If the mother is symptom free at birth, detectable infection may not be found in the infant.

Postnatal acquisition of the virus and spread within a nursery have been documented by DNA analysis. Both the mother and father, as well as maternal breast lesions, have been implicated in neonatal infections. There also is concern regarding symptomatic and asymptomatic shedding among hospital personnel. Nursery personnel with cold sores should practice strict hand washing and wear a mask, but there is no evidence to require their actual removal from the nursery unless they have a herpetic whitlow (primary herpes simplex infection of the terminal segment of a finger) (Fanaroff, Martin, 1992; Frigoletto, Little, 1988).

Care of all newborn infants begins with parental prevention of genital infections. Spermicidal foams kill the virus, and condoms offer some protection against direct contact with lesions in the sexual partner. Although maternal ingestion of oral or intravenous acyclovir shortens the viral shedding time, its effect on fetal safety is unknown. Therefore this agent is not recommended during pregnancy (Fanaroff, Martin, 1992).

The best time and route of birth are still controver-

sial factors. There is consensus that infants should be born by cesarean surgery when an active herpes infection is present at the onset of labor and the amniotic membranes have been ruptured less than 4 hours, regardless of whether the infection is primary or recurrent. Because of the possibility of transplacental and ascending transcervical infection, the mother must be informed that even cesarean birth gives no guarantee that the baby will be free from infection (Fanaroff, Martin, 1992). Fetal scalp electrode monitoring is avoided.

During the postpartum period the nurse teaches the mother about the disease—recognition of lesions and prevention of its transmission during care of the infant. People should wear gloves when in contact with infants.

The newborn's eyes, oral cavity, and skin are inspected carefully for the presence of any lesions. Culture specimens are obtained from the mouth, the eyes, and any possible lesions. Circumcision, if performed, is delayed until the infant is ready to be discharged. The infant may be discharged with the mother if the infant's cultures are negative for the virus. As long as there are no suspicious lesions on the mother's breasts, breastfeeding is allowed. For the infant at risk, prophylactic topical eye ointment (vidarabine) administered for 5 days for prevention of keratoconjunctivitis. If herpetic lesions first occur after 6 weeks of life, the risk of dissemination and severe illness is very low (Fanaroff, Martin, 1992).

Therapy includes general supportive measures, as well as treatment with vidarabine or acyclovir. The earliest possible institution of therapy is recommended. Continuing therapy may be required in case of recurrence. Ophthalmic ointment should be administered simultaneously (Fanaroff, Martin, 1992).

Acyclovir has now become the most commonly used drug for neonatal infections. It is considered to be a safe drug because only viral replication is inhibited, although long-term sequelae are not yet known. Acyclovir is easier to administer and has been demonstrated to be more effective than vidarabine for herpes encephalitis. Clinical trials indicate no significant differences in outcome between the two drugs. The current recommended dosage of acyclovir is 10 mg/kg/day intravenously every 8 hours for at least 14 days (Fanaroff, Martin, 1992).

Chlamydia Infection

Chlamydia trachomatis is an intracellular bacterium that causes neonatal conjunctivitis and pneumonia. The conjunctivitis (congestion and edema), with minimal discharge, develops 5 days to 2 weeks after birth. If chlamydial disease is not treated, chronic follicular conjunctivitis, with conjunctival scarring and corneal neovascularization, may result. Newborns with pneumonia exhibit prolonged staccato cough, tachypnea, mild hypoxemia, and eosinophilia (Merenstein, Gardner, 1993).

If prenatal screening reveals infection with *C. trachomatis,* antepartum treatment of the mother with erythromycin or sulfisoxazole appears to improve pregnancy outcome. The newborn also is treated with oral erythromycin for 2 to 3 weeks, along with irrigation of the eye with saline or buffered ophthalmic solution daily. A topical antibiotic is not necessary. Silver nitrate is not effective against *C. trachomatis,* but erythromycin or tetracycline ointment may prevent ophthalmic infection (Fanaroff, Martin, 1992).

Human Immunodeficiency Virus—Acquired Immunodeficiency Syndrome

Transmission of HIV from the mother to the infant occurs transplacentally at various gestational ages, perinatally via maternal blood and secretions, and postnatally through breast milk (Fanaroff, Martin, 1992; Pyun et al, 1987). Although the transmission rate of HIV infections has been reported by some authors to be as high as 50% to 60% in infants born to mothers infected with HIV, most researchers cite a transmission rate between 20% and 35% (Cherry, Merkatz, 1991; Merenstein, Gardner, 1993). Pediatric acquired immunodeficiency syndrome (AIDS) accounts for 2% of reported AIDS cases in the United States, and 80% of these children acquired infection in the perinatal period. The incidence is likely to increase. The blood supply in the United States is now screened for HIV, thus decreasing the chance of transmission by this route. However, the number of women of childbearing age infected with HIV is increasing.

Diagnosis of HIV infection in the newborn is the subject of intense research. Pyun et al (1987) studied specific antibody responses by the neonate. Pregnant women infected with HIV produce IgG antibodies. The IgG crosses the placenta to the fetus. Therefore cord blood is positive for antibody when tested by enzyme-linked immunosorbent assay (ELISA) or Western blot techniques. Because of their physiologically depressed immune response, newborns generally produce a less vigorous and more limited antibody response to HIV infection.

Every baby born to a mother who is seropositive for HIV will have HIV antibody at birth. Uninfected infants lose this maternal antibody during the first 8 to 15 months of life. Most infected infants begin to develop their own antibodies and remain seropositive (Cherry, Merkatz, 1991; Fanaroff, Martin, 1992; Harnish et al, 1987; Johnson, Nair, Alexander, 1987).

The occurrence of an opportunistic infection in the newborn may alert the caregiver to the presence of HIV infection or assist in the confirmation of the diagnosis of HIV infection. In pediatrics the presence of lymphoid interstitial pneumonitis is now considered a criterion for diagnosis (Fanaroff, Martin, 1992). The presence of oral candidiasis (thrush) that is refractory to treatment with topical antifungal agents carries a high index of suspicion for HIV infection (Prenatal care and HIV screening, 1987).

Infants who exhibit signs of HIV infection at birth tend to die within a month. The disease progression has been slower and the mortality lower in infants with a later onset.

Management begins by implementing universal precautions and precautions for invasive procedures to prevent further transmission of HIV (Fanaroff, Martin, 1992). Circumcision in males is avoided. Umbilical cord stumps are cleaned meticulously every day until healing is complete. Therapy includes prophylactic gamma globulin, antimicrobial medications specific for the infections encountered, and corticosteroids in the presence of lymphoid interstitial pneumonitis. Zidovudine (AZT) and ribavirin cross the brain barrier and may result in increase in weight and in the number of helper T-lymphocytes. For general care of the compromised newborn, see Chapter 26.

Some parents are opting to place the infected infants in foster homes despite the low risk for transmission among members of the same household. Social services are required in these cases. If the parent chooses to keep the infant, home health care is arranged. For more information and updated information, parents are offered the following resource: the National AIDS Hotline, 1-800-342-AIDS.

The family must be counseled about vaccinations. Children with symptomatic or asymptomatic HIV infection should receive all routine vaccines except oral polio virus vaccine. The family should be advised that household contacts should not receive oral polio vaccine because the virus can be transmitted to the immunocompromised child. Inactivated poliomyelitis vaccine can be given (Whaley, Wong, 1995).

Candidiasis

Candida infections, also known as moniliasis, are not uncommon in the newborn. *Candida albicans,* the organism usually responsible, may cause disease in any organ system. It is a yeastlike fungus (producing yeast cells and spores) that can be acquired from a maternal vaginal infection during birth, by person-to-person transmission, or from contaminated hands, bottles, nipples, or other articles. It usually is a benign disorder in the neonate, often confined to the oral and diaper regions (Whaley, Wong, 1995).

Oral candidiasis (*thrush,* or mycotic stomatitis) is characterized by the appearance of white plaques on the oral mucosa, gums, and tongue. The white patches are easily differentiated from milk curds; the patches cannot be removed and tend to bleed when touched. In most cases the infant does not seem to be discomforted by the infection. A few newborns seem to have some difficulty swallowing.

Infants who are sick, debilitated, or receiving antibiotic therapy are more susceptible. Those with conditions such as cleft lip or palate, neoplasms, and hyperparathyroidism seem to be more vulnerable to mycotic infection.

Candidal diaper dermatitis appears on the perianal area, inguinal folds, and lower portion of the abdomen. The affected area is intensely erythematous, with a sharply demarcated, scalloped edge, frequently with numerous satellite lesions that extend beyond the larger lesion. The source of the infection is through the gastrointestinal tract. Treatment consists of applications of an anticandidal ointment, such as nystatin (Mycostatin), with each diaper change. The infant also may be given an oral antifungal preparation to eliminate any gastrointestinal source of infection (Whaley, Wong, 1995).

The objectives of management are to eradicate the causative organism, to control exposure to *C. albicans,* and to improve the infant's resistance. Interventions include maintenance of scrupulous cleanliness to prevent reinfection (nursery personnel, parents, others.) Good hand-washing technique is always essential. Clean surfaces should be provided for newborns (the newborn is never placed directly on sheets on which the mother has been sitting). If the infant is breastfeeding, the mother also is treated with topical nystatin.

Medications are administered as ordered. Aqueous solution of gentian violet (1% to 2%) is applied with a swab to oral mucosa, gums, and tongue (guard against permanent stain on skin, clothes, equipment. Warn parents about purple staining of baby's mouth).

Nystatin is instilled into the newborn's mouth with a medicine dropper after the infant is given sterile water to wash out any residual milk. Nystatin also may be swabbed over mucosa, gums, or tongue.

Gonorrhea

The incidence of gonococcal infection in pregnant women has ranged from 2.5% to 7.3% in recent studies (Fanaroff, Martin, 1992). With this high incidence, it is not surprising that neonatal infection with *Neisseria gonorrhoeae* occurs frequently. After rupture of membranes, ascending infection can result in orogastric contamination of the fetus. The organism also may invade mucosal surfaces such as the conjunctiva (ophthalmia neonatorum), rectal mucosa, and pharynx. Contamination may occur as the infant passes through the birth canal, or it may occur postnatally from an infected adult. Neonatal gonococcal arthritis, septicemia, meningitis, vaginitis, and scalp abscesses also can develop.

Endocervical cultures for *N. gonorrhoeae* should be obtained routinely during pregnancy and appropriate treatment instituted when necessary to prevent fetal-neonatal infection. The newborn with a mild infection often recovers completely with appropriate treatment. Occasionally infants die of overwhelming infection in the early neonatal period. Erythromycin (0.5%) ophthalmic ointment is effective against gonococcal ophthalmia neonatorum. For newborns with extraocular site infection or suspected septicemia, ceftriaxone is recommended for treatment.

GESTATIONAL AGE AND BIRTHWEIGHT

Modern technology and good nursing care have contributed significantly to improved health and overall survival of infants at risk because of gestational age or birth weight. However, the survival of infants born significantly before term has resulted in the development of conditions that may negatively affect the quality of their lives. These conditions include necrotizing enterocolitis, bronchopulmonary dysplasia, and retinopathy of prematurity. Classification of newborns according to *gestational age* is as follows:

Preterm or **premature.** Born before completion of 37 weeks' gestation, regardless of birth weight

Term. Born between the beginning of week 38 and the end of week 42 of gestation

Postterm (postdate). Born after completion of week 42 of gestation

Postmature. Born after completion of week 42 of gestation, having undergone the effects of progressive placental insufficiency

The cause of preterm and postterm birth is largely unknown; however, the incidence of preterm birth is highest among low socioeconomic groups. This is likely a result of the lack of comprehensive prenatal health care. Other factors found to be associated with preterm birth include preeclampsia, multifetal pregnancy, and placental accidents.

The birth weight of the newborn has a normal range for each gestational week (Fig. 27-4). Classification of newborns by weight is as follows:

Large for gestational age (LGA). Weight is above the 90th percentile (or two or more standard deviations above the norm) at any week.

Appropriate for gestational age (AGA). Weight falls between the 10th and 90th percentile for infant's age.

Small for gestational age (SGA). Weight is below the 10th percentile (or two or more standard deviations below the norm).

Low birth weight (LBW). Weight of 2500 g or less at birth. These newborns are considered to have had either less than the expected rate of intrauterine growth or a shortened gestation period. Preterm birth and LBW commonly occur together (e.g., <32 weeks and <1200 g birth weight). **Intrauterine growth retardation (IUGR)** is the term used to describe the fetus whose rate of growth does not meet expected norms.

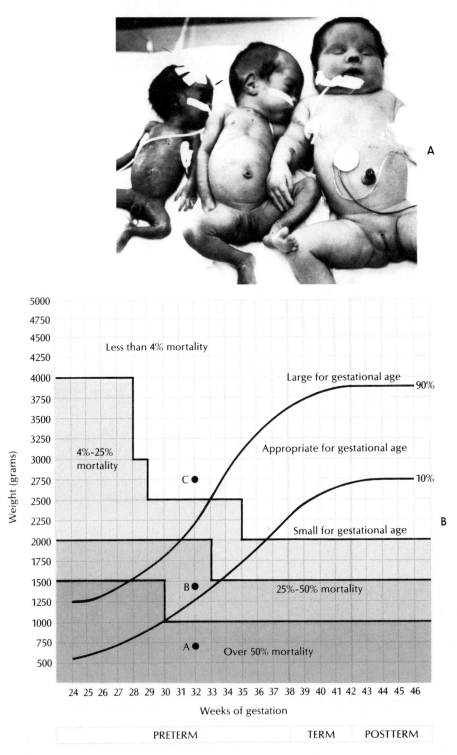

FIG. 27-4 Three babies of same gestational age, with weights of 600, 1400, and 2750 g, respectively, from left to right. (From Korones SB: *High-risk newborn infants: the basis for intensive nursing care,* ed 4, St Louis, 1986, Mosby.)

Very low birth weight (VLBW). Weight of 1500 g or less at birth

Common causes of LGA newborns include glucose intolerance of pregnancy, true maternal diabetes mellitus, maternal overnutrition, and heredity. SGA newborns may be affected by maternal smoking, hypertensive states, undernutrition, anemia, or nephritis. In addition, the birth of an SGA newborn may be associated with multifetal gestation, a discordant twin pregnancy, or congenital anomalies. High altitude, rubella, or intrauterine infection may predispose a woman to the birth of an SGA newborn. Fetal malnutrition, IUGR, and chronic fetal distress are other processes that may result in the birth of SGA infants.

Infant Mortality and Morbidity

Preterm birth is responsible for almost two thirds of infant deaths. The infant born before term does not possess the growth and development necessary for uncomplicated adjustment to extrauterine life, and prospects for survival or good health may be severely compromised. Infants weighing more than 2500 g (5½ lb) and born after 37 weeks of pregnancy have the best prospects of survival. There is a dramatic reduction in mortality in infants, regardless of weight, who are born after week 36 of gestation. The prognosis for LBW infants weighing more than 1800 g (4 lb) is more favorable than for those weighing 1500 to 1800 g (3 to 4 lb). The mortality is less than 5% if the pregnancy has progressed to 35 weeks and the fetus weighs more than 2000 g (4½ lb).

Children and adults who were LBW infants are more likely to have major problems such as cerebral palsy, mental retardation, sensory and cognitive disabilities, and a diminished ability to successfully adapt socially, psychologically, and physically to an increasingly complex envi-

ronment (Fanaroff, Martin, 1992). In addition to the human tragedy, the fiscal impact of this problem on our society is estimated to be in the billions of dollars each year (see the Ethical Considerations box).

The Premature or Preterm Infant

The preterm infant is at risk because of immaturity of organ systems and lack of reserves. The morbidity and mortality rate for preterm infants is higher by three to four times than that of older infants of comparable weight. The potential problems and care needs of the preterm infant of 2000 g differ from those of the term, postterm, or postmature infant of equal weight (Philip, 1987).

Preterm infants are at a distinct disadvantage when they face the transition from intrauterine to extrauterine life. The degree of disadvantage depends primarily on their level of maturity (Box 27-3). Physiologic disorders

---

BOX 27-3

Differences in Borderline, Moderately, and Extremely Premature Infants

BORDERLINE PREMATURE INFANT
37 weeks' gestation
2500 to 3250 g
16% of all live births
Usually normal
Problems
    Temperature instability
    Feeding difficulties
    Jaundice
    Respiratory distress syndrome
     (RDS) possible
Appearance
    Fewer creases on feet
    Smaller breasts
    Fuzzy hair
    Lanugo
    Less developed genitalia

MODERATELY PREMATURE INFANT
31 to 36 weeks' gestation
1500 to 2500 g
6% to 7% of all live births
Problems
    Temperature instability
    Glucose regulation
    Fluid balance
    RDS
    Jaundice
    Anemia
    Infections
    Feeding difficulties
Appearance
    As for borderline premies, but exaggerated
    Skin is thinner, more vascular

Continued.

 ETHICAL CONSIDERATIONS

RESUSCITATION OF EXTREMELY PREMATURE INFANTS

There are many different opinions about resuscitation of extremely preterm infants weighing between 500 and 750 g. Ethical issues that nurses are confronted with about this issue include:
    Whether or not to resuscitate?
    Who should decide?
    Is the cost of resuscitation justified?
    Do the benefits of technology outweigh the burdens in relation to the quality of life?
All individuals involved (health care providers and parents) should be involved in discussions that lead to resolution of these controversial issues.

BOX 27-3

Differences in Borderline, Moderately, and Extremely Premature Infants—cont'd

EXTREMELY PREMATURE INFANTS

24 to 30 weeks' gestation
500 to 1400 g
0.8% of all live births, but almost all neonatal deaths and neurologic deficits not attributable to birth defects or birth trauma
Problems
    Everything
Appearance
    Tiny, no fat, extremely thin skin
    Eyes may be fused

and anomalous malformations affect their response to treatment as well. In general, the closer they are to the normal term infant in gestational age and birth weight, the easier will be their adjustment to the external environment.

Care Management

✢ ASSESSMENT

Potential Problems of Preterm Newborn

In assessing the preterm infant, the health care provider follows a systematic approach. The response of the preterm infant to extrauterine life is different from that of the term infant. Knowing the physiologic basis of these differences helps the nurse assess these infants, understand the response of the preterm infant, and determine which potential problems are most likely to occur.

Respiratory Function

Just as with the term infant, initial assessment begins with respiratory function, observing the infant's ability to make the pulmonary transition from intrauterine to extrauterine life. The preterm infant is likely to have difficulty making this transition because of numerous deficits in the respiratory system:

- Decreased number of functional alveoli
- Deficient surfactant levels
- Smaller lumen in the respiratory system
- Greater collapsibility or obstruction of respiratory passages
- Insufficient calcification of the bony thorax
- Weak or absent gag reflex
- Immature and friable capillaries in the lungs

In combination, these deficits severely hinder the infant's respiratory efforts and result in respiratory distress or ap-

nea. The health care provider needs to be prepared to provide oxygen and ventilation, as necessary (Merenstein, Gardner, 1993).

Cardiovascular Function

After respiratory assessment the health care provider assesses the cardiovascular system and its ability to provide perfusion to essential tissues and organs. The health care provider must be prepared to intervene if symptoms of hypovolemia or shock, or both, are present. These symptoms include decreased blood pressure, slow capillary refill, and continued respiratory distress despite provision of oxygen and ventilation.

Maintaining Body Temperature

As a result of numerous factors, the preterm infant is susceptible to temperature instability. *Heat loss is great because of the large surface area in relation to body weight.* Other factors include the following:

- Minimal insulating subcutaneous fat
- Limited stores of *brown fat* (an internal source for generation of heat present in normal term infants)
- Decreased or absent reflex control of skin capillaries (shiver response)
- Inadequate muscle mass activity (therefore the preterm infant will be unable to produce his or her own heat)
- Friable (easily damaged) capillaries
- Immature temperature regulation center in the brain

To contend with the preterm infant's temperature instability, the health care provider performs ongoing assessment of temperature and provides a regulated, external source of heat.

Central Nervous System Function

The preterm infant's central nervous system (CNS) is susceptible to injury from various sources:

- Birth trauma with damage to immature structures
- Bleeding from fragile capillaries
- Impaired coagulation process, including prolonged prothrombin time
- Recurrent anoxic episodes
- Predisposition to hypoglycemia

The nurse assesses CNS function by checking the infant's ability to coordinate suck and swallow and by monitoring for impairment in the CNS control of respiratory and cardiovascular systems (apnea and bradycardia) (Merenstein, Gardner, 1993).

Maintaining Adequate Nutrition

Maintenance of adequate nutrition in the preterm infant is complicated by problems of intake and of metabolism. With regard to intake, the preterm infant has the following disadvantages: weak or absent suck, swallow, and gag reflexes, a small stomach capacity, and weak abdominal muscles. The preterm infant's metabolic functions are weakened by a limited store of nutrients, a decreased ability to digest proteins or absorb nutrients, and immature enzyme systems.

The nurse provides ongoing assessment of the infant's ability to take in and digest nutrients. The health care provider needs to be prepared to provide nourishment to the preterm infant by means other than the oral route (e.g., gavage or intravenous).

Maintaining Renal Function

The preterm infant's immature renal system is unable (1) to adequately excrete metabolites and drugs, (2) to concentrate the urine, and (3) to maintain balances in acid-base, fluids, or electrolytes. The nurse assesses intake and output, as well as specific gravity; monitors laboratory values for acid-base and electrolyte balance; and observes for symptoms of drug toxicity.

Maintaining Hematologic Status

Compared with the term infant, the preterm infant is predisposed to hematologic problems as a result of the following factors:

- Increased capillary friability
- Increased tendency to bleed (low plasma prothrombin levels)
- Slowed development of red blood cells
- Increased hemolysis
- Loss of blood from frequent laboratory tests

The nurse assesses for any evidence of bleeding, observing for symptoms of disseminated intravascular coagulation (DIC) (bleeding from puncture sites, gastrointestinal tract, CNS, or skin) (Merenstein, Gardner, 1993).

Resisting Infection

The preterm infant is at increased risk for infection because of a shortage of stored maternal immunoglobulins, an impaired ability to make antibodies, and a compromised integumentary system (thin skin and fragile capillaries).

Growth and Development Potential

Although it is impossible to predict with complete accuracy the growth and development potential of each preterm newborn, some findings support an anticipated favorable outcome. The growth and development landmarks are corrected for gestational age.

The age of a preterm newborn is corrected by adding the gestational age and the postnatal age. For example, if an infant was born at 32 weeks' gestation 4 weeks ago, the infant would be considered 36 weeks of age. The child's corrected age 6 months after the birth date is 4 months. Responses are evaluated against the norm expected for a 4-month-old infant.

Favorable findings that support the prediction of a growth and development pattern within the norm include certain measurable factors. At discharge from the hospital, which usually occurs between 37 and 40 weeks after the woman's last menstrual period (LMP), the infant exhibits the following characteristics. (1) The baby is able to raise the head when prone and is able to hold the head parallel with the body when tested for head lag response. (When the infant is pulled up by the hands, the infant's head lags, but then the head and chest will be in line as the upright position is reached. This alignment will be held momentarily before the head falls forward [pull-to-sit or traction reflex]). In addition, the infant (2) cries with vigor when hungry, (3) shows appropriate weight gain and pattern of weight gain according to growth grid, and (4) has neurologic responses appropriate for corrected age. Also, the retinas appear normal.

At *39 to 40 weeks* the infant is able to focus on the examiner's or parent's face and is able to follow with her or his eyes.

At the *corrected ages of 6 and 12 months* the infant is assessed again for age-appropriate responses. The infant who displays any of the following behaviors may have problems: was and continues to be a poor eater; is irritable; displays sensory, perceptual, intellectual, or motor deviations in development; or displays or develops hypertonia or hypotonia.

These behaviors must be interpreted with caution, and the infant requires reevaluation by an interdisciplinary team at frequent intervals. Parents will need continued support and attention should these signs appear. Minor behavioral deviations also are diagnosed so that the parents can be assisted in their understanding and acceptance of the child. Deviations such as clumsiness, varying degrees of incoordination, slowness in reading and writing, and similar problems may be distressing to the child, parents, and other family members.

Parental Adaptation to Preterm Infant

Parents who experience the preterm birth of their infant have a different experience from parents giving birth to a full-term infant (Sammons, Lewis, 1985). Because of this difference, parental attachment and adaptation to the parental role also are different.

Parental Tasks

Parents face a number of psychologic tasks before effective relationships and parenting patterns can evolve. These tasks include the following:

- *Anticipatory grief over the potential loss of an infant.* The parent grieves in preparation for the infant's possible death, although the parent clings to the hope that the child will survive. This begins during labor and lasts until the infant dies or shows evidence of surviving.
- *Acceptance by the mother of her failure to give birth to a healthy, full-term infant.* Grief and depression typify

this phase, which persists until the infant is out of danger and is expected to survive.

- *Resumption of the process of relating to the infant.* As the baby begins to improve—gains weight, feeds by nipple, and is weaned from the incubator—the parent can begin the process of developing attachment to the infant that was interrupted by the infant's precarious condition at birth (Als, Brazelton, 1981).
- *Learning how this baby differs in special needs and growth patterns.* Another parental task is to learn, understand, and accept this infant's caregiving needs and growth and development expectations (Sammons, Lewis, 1985).
- *Adjusting the home environment to the needs of the new infant.* Grandparents and siblings also react to the birth of the preterm infant. Parents must reconcile the grief of grandparents and the bewilderment and anger of brothers and sisters at the disproportionate amount of parental time absorbed by the newborn.

Parental Responses

Two different approaches noted by Newman (1980) are *coping through commitment* and *coping through distance*. With the first approach parents take each day as it comes, recognizing and accepting the lessened responses of their infant and noting the gradual progress in their child's condition. With the second approach the parents pull away from emotional attachment to the infant; they postpone becoming attached until the infant is in better health.

Parents have been observed to progress through stages as they spend more time with their infants. In the first stage they maintain an *en face* position, stroking and touching their infant (Fig. 27-5). In the second stage they assume some child care activities—feeding, bathing, changing the infant. In the third stage the infant becomes a person and is seen as a whole child (Schraeder, 1980). Sosa and Grua (1982) reported a personal communication with Brazelton in which he correlated parental behaviors with the previously noted three stages. In the first stage parents ask about *chemical data*, such as "What is his bilirubin today?" In the second stage they note their baby yawning, sneezing, hiccoughing, *reflexes* that mark their infant as human. At this time the infant is still not "claimed." In later stages they note their infant's *responses* to them and begin to feel that "this child is mine" and part of their family. Parents take on the role of advocate for their child.

Infant Responsiveness

The preterm infant's states of consciousness are more labile than the term infant's. The quiet alert state is less evident and unpredictable. Field (1979) noted that if a mother concentrated her interactions on imitation of the infant's behavior, the infant was increasingly attentive and interested. Too-active an involvement in child care tended to result in the infant's becoming disinterested and glancing away (gaze aversion).

❖ NURSING DIAGNOSES

To formulate nursing diagnoses, the nurse must analyze data obtained from continuous monitoring of the infant and from observation of and discussions with the parents. The diagnoses may be physical, cognitive, or psychologic, for example:

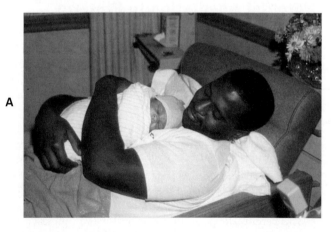

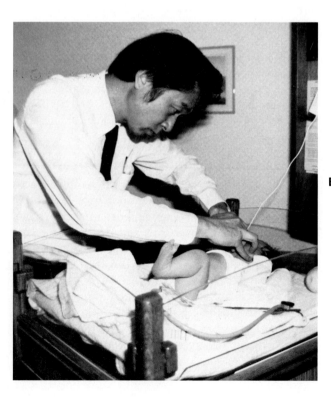

FIG. 27-5 Fathers interact with their newborns. **A,** Father spending the night with his newborn in the LDRP. **B,** Engrossment. Father looking at and touching his newborn. (Courtesy Marjorie Pyle, RNC, *Lifecircle,* Costa Mesa, CA.)

Ineffective breathing pattern related to
- Inadequate chest expansion, secondary to infant's position

Parental anxiety related to
- Knowledge deficit regarding infant's cues
- Knowledge deficit regarding feeding the infant

Situational low self-esteem related to
- Parent's feelings of inadequacy in caring for the infant

✤ EXPECTED OUTCOMES

The nursing plan of care for the preterm infant is dictated by the physiologic needs of immature systems, often involving emergency treatments and procedures. During this time, nursing care is a critical element in the infant's chances for survival. In addition to meeting the infant's physical needs, nursing care is planned in conjunction with parents to promote parent-infant attachment and interaction. Expected outcomes are presented in patient-centered terms.

The infant will achieve the following:
1. Maintain physiologic functioning
2. Maintain adequate nutrition
3. Experience no or minimal hematologic problems
4. Not develop infection
5. Not develop retinal problems
6. Not suffer trauma to immature musculoskeletal system
7. Experience parent-infant attachment

The parents will achieve the following:
1. Perceive the child as potentially normal (if this is medically substantiated)
2. Provide care comfortably
3. Experience pride and satisfaction in the care of the infant
4. Organize their time and energies to meet the love, attention, and care needs of the other members of the family as well as their own

✤ COLLABORATIVE CARE

The best environment for fetal growth and development is in the uterus of a healthy, well-nourished woman for 38 to 42 weeks. The extrauterine environment of the preterm newborn must approximate a healthy intrauterine environment for the normal sequence of growth and development to continue. The provision of such an environment is the basis for care of the preterm infant. Medical and nursing personnel and respiratory therapists work as a team to provide the intensive care needed. The nurse acts as a constant presence in the infant's support system.

Nursing actions are based on knowledge of the *physiologic problems* imposed on the preterm infant and on the infant's need to conserve energy for repair, maintenance,

and growth. Nursing care is conscientiously centered on the continuous assessment and analysis of physiologic status. Nurses fulfill many roles in providing the intensive and extended care that these infants require. Nurses continuously gather data regarding the infant's physiologic status. They make decisions and initiate therapies based on their interpretation of these data. In addition, nurses are the support persons and teachers during the first phase of the parents' adjustment to the birth of the preterm infant.

The nurse uses many technologic support systems to monitor body responses and maintain body function in the infant. Gentle touch, concern for the traumatic effects of harsh lighting, and control of machinery noise are interwoven with the technical skill of the nurse in the intensive care nursery.

Complications Common to Preterm Infants

Respiratory Distress Syndrome

Respiratory distress syndrome (RDS) (also known as idiopathic respiratory distress syndrome) is a collection of clinical, radiologic, and histologic findings that result primarily from immature lungs with small respiratory units that inflate with difficulty and do not remain gas filled between respiratory efforts. The term *hyaline membrane disease (HMD)* often is used interchangeably with RDS but actually refers to the specific lung injury involved—formation of hyaline membranes that are plasma clots containing fibrin, other plasma constituents, and cellular debris.

In addition to the anatomic structures, biochemical substances are also imperative to the survival of the infant at birth. The most important one for the fetal lung is *surfactant*. This is a surface-active lipoprotein mixture that coats the alveoli and prevents their collapse at the end of expiration. The alveoli can be thought of as spheres that tend to collapse in on themselves. If the alveoli collapse on expiration, they will require much higher pressures to open up on inspiration. Surfactant acts to reduce the surface tension of the alveoli, thereby reducing the pressure required to hold them open during expiration.

At approximately 16 to 20 weeks' gestation some of the epithelial cells lining the airway begin to differentiate into type II cells. These cells are responsible for production and synthesis of surfactant. Although they begin producing surfactant this early in gestation, they do not appear to release it into the alveolar lining until about 10 weeks later. Thus the healthy, nonasphyxiated infant born at about 30 weeks' gestation has a lower chance of acquiring lung disease then do infants born at an earlier gestation. Fig. 27-6 describes the pathophysiology of RDS.

Clinically the infant with RDS presents with tach-

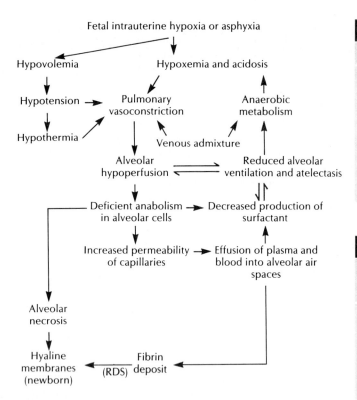

FIG. 27-6 Development of respiratory distress syndrome. (Courtesy A. Hacket, Stanford University Medical Center, Stanford, CA.)

ypnea, nasal flaring, subcostal and intercostal retractions, and an expiratory grunt in the first few hours of life. These are also signs of other clinical problems such as hypothermia, hypoglycemia, and polycythemia. Additionally, these conditions can be superimposed on RDS, complicating the picture further. Other signs of RDS include hypoxemia, hypercarbia, and respiratory or mixed acidosis. Clinical signs of RDS are listed in Box 27-4.

The typical, uncomplicated course of RDS is characterized by a "honeymoon" period in the first hours of life, followed by progressive worsening of signs for the next 2 or 3 days, then onset of recovery at about 72 hours of life. The progressive worsening of the disease coincides with fluid shifting within the extracellular compartments. As fluid shifts from the interstitial space to the vascular space and the kidneys begin to eliminate this extra fluid, it becomes easier to ventilate the lungs.

Vigilant attention to stabilization parameters is central to the care of the infant with RDS. Close attention to thermoregulation, glucose management, blood pressure maintenance, and normalization of blood gas values are necessary to support the infant in this delayed transition to extrauterine life.

In 1989 the Federal Drug Administration approved the use of exogenous surfactant in the treatment of RDS in infants. In the first year this treatment modality was approved, the infant mortality rate attributable to RDS was significantly decreased. Exogenous surfactant is administered through an endotracheal tube. Careful attention to the ventilation requirements is imperative as the surfactant may increase compliance of the lung rapidly. Delay in decreasing ventilation (particularly the pressures) can lead to pulmonary air leaks. Since oxygen therapy is likely to be used in the treatment of RDS, it is crucial that the nurse monitors the F_{IO_2} as well as oxygen saturation values. Optimal O_2 saturation values are shown in Box 27-5.

Positioning the infant on the abdomen with legs tucked up and arms flexed will help achieve better ventilation. Building a nest of blanket rolls or diapers around the infant decreases heat loss (there will be less surface area to lose heat from), lowers oxygen and glucose consumption (a quiet, warm infant has a lower metabolic rate), and presumably promotes comfort (the boundaries replicate the contained space of the intrauterine environment).

The infant needs periods of rest to recover from the stresses of RDS, but this condition necessitates repeated noxious interventions. Multiple examinations, obtaining blood for blood gases and other laboratory values, suctioning the endotracheal tube, administration of medications and perhaps blood products all interfere with this rest. *Care clustering* is used to provide uninterrupted periods of rest. This term describes the organization of nursing and medical care to allow the infant periods of uninterrupted rest.

CLINICAL APPLICATION OF RESEARCH

NIPPLE-FEEDING FOR PRETERM INFANTS WITH BRONCHOPULMONARY DYSPLASIA

Infants in the chronic stage of bronchopulmonary dysplasia (BPD) require good nutrition for tissue repair and growth of organs. When infants start to become physiologically stable, oral feedings are started. Nipple-fed infants may or may not meet recommended levels of caloric intake. The purpose of this study was to explore the effects of the physical condition of preterm infants with BPD on nipple-feeding practices and to examine the relationship of the age of the infant when feeding completely by nipple to caloric intake and growth outcomes. Participants were 55 infants who were 32 weeks' or less gestation at birth, appropriate for gestational age, and who had BPD and required supplemental oxygen more than 3 weeks. Infants were cared for in one of two level III nurseries. Data were collected by a retrospective review of medical records of infants who were hospitalized over a 6-year period. After determining that there were no significant differences in variables among the 6 years of the study or between the two nurseries, data were combined for subsequent analyses. The researchers found that infant weight was the best predictor of when

nipple-feeding was introduced, although gestational age, days of mechanical ventilation, and receiving supplemental oxygen or continuous positive airway pressure also contributed to the prediction. Neither feeding practices nor physical condition of the infants affected caloric intake. Infants who were older when completely fed by nipple and who received supplemental oxygen longer had less weight gain between the time they were completely fed by nipple and hospital discharge. Nurses need to assess behavioral cues related to hunger and readiness to feed as well as weight gain in determining when preterm infants are ready for nipple-feeding. Skill in caring for difficult-to-feed infants must be acquired by nurses so that adequate intake is ensured. Continuity and consistency of caregivers for these infants may ensure that cues of readiness to feed are recognized. Nurses must strive to standardize decision-making criteria in relation to initiation of nipple-feeding for preterm infants.

Reference: Pridham KF et al: Nipple feeding for preterm infants with bronchopulmonary dysplasia, *JOGNN* 22:147, 1993.

Oxygen-Associated Complications

Bronchopulmonary dysplasia (BPD) and retinopathy of prematurity (ROP) are diseases of preterm birth secondary to oxygen therapy (Bancalari, Gerhardt, 1986). Both conditions are relatively new disorders, recognized since the advent of methods of administering high concentrations of oxygen beginning in the 1940s. Although oxygen therapy may be lifesaving and occasionally must be given in high concentrations for extended periods, it also is potentially hazardous and must be administered cautiously. In addition to BPD and ROP, other conditions have become apparent. The mechanical creation of positive pressure in the lungs has increased the incidence of air leaks. Use of an oxygen apparatus also has resulted in nasal, tracheal, and pharyngeal perforation and inflammation (Whaley, Wong, 1995).

Bronchopulmonary Dysplasia. Bronchopulmonary dysplasia (BPD) is a common concomitant of lung disorders in infants, primarily preterm infants, in which focal areas of emphysema develop in the lungs. The cause is unknown, but the condition may develop as a sequela to alveolar damage caused by lung disease, use of high oxygen concentrations, and the prolonged use of continuous positive airway pressure (CPAP) or positive endexpiratory pressure (PEEP) (Bancalari, Gerhardt, 1986).

Symptoms of respiratory distress, tachypnea, and increased effort appear. It is difficult to wean the infant from the positive pressure ventilator. This finding may

be the first indication of the disease process.

The first sign that the infant is recovering from BPD is a decreasing dependence on oxygen therapy. Recovery may take several months (see the Clinical Application of Research box above). The mortality rate is between 30% and 50%; death may occur after the infant has been discharged from the hospital.

Retinopathy of Prematurity. The retinal changes in **retinopathy of prematurity (ROP)** were first described in 1942. Originally ROP was considered a disorder caused by prolonged exposure to high levels of oxygen. ROP is now thought to be a complex, multicausal disease of preterm birth (Whaley and Wong, 1995). Judicious use of oxygen therapy and monitoring of arterial oxygen pressure (Pao_2) levels have reduced the incidence of ROP, but the disease has not been eliminated.

Prevention of ROP is a fundamental concept for the nursing care of infants receiving oxygen. Close monitoring of oxygen regulation and infant status will facilitate therapeutic and safe oxygen administration. The most crucial period for toxic levels to occur is during the recovery phase from RDS and other respiratory distress. The exact level at which Pao_2 becomes toxic and causes ROP is unknown.

Oxygen tensions that are too high for the level of retinal maturity initially result in vasoconstriction. After oxygen therapy is discontinued, neovascularization occurs in the retina and vitreous, with capillary hemorrhages, fibrotic resolution, and possible retinal detachment. Cicatricial (scar) tissue formation and consequent visual impairment may be mild or severe. The entire disease process in severe cases may take as long as 5 months to evolve. Examination by an ophthalmologist before discharge and a schedule for repeat examinations thereafter are recommended for the parents' guidance.

Patent Ductus Arteriosus

Patent ductus arteriosus (PDA) is a common complication of prematurity. The ductus is a fetal shunt necessary for routing the majority (about 90%) of the cardiac output from the right side of the heart away from the developing lungs. It connects the main pulmonary artery with the aorta. During normal transition to extrauterine life this shunt (along with the foramen ovale) should close, routing all the output from the right side of the heart to the now functional lungs. The ductus arteriosus should functionally close by 12 to 24 hours of life in response to higher aortic oxygen levels and metabolism of circulating prostaglandins. A delay in the closure decreases oxygenation to the systemic circulation and predisposes the infant to disorders related to decreased oxygenation.

Fluid overload during the first few days of life is associated with increased incidence of symptomatic PDA. Fluid overload inhibits the natural shifting of fluids from the interstitial spaces into the vascular system and interferes with the necessary diuresis of this excess fluid.

Treatment for PDA can be medical or surgical. Intravenous indomethacin is the current drug of choice to medically close a patent ductus arteriosus. The efficacy of this treatment is well documented; however, its use poses the potential complications of decreased renal and mesenteric artery perfusion. Surgical ligation of the ductus poses the threats inherent to any surgical procedure.

Necrotizing Enterocolitis

Necrotizing enterocolitis (NEC) is a multifactorial disorder involving ischemic necrosis of the alimentary tract in the absence of predisposing anatomic or functional abnormalities. It is probably one of a limited number of potential final responses that the immature gastrointestinal (GI) tract may express after one or more stresses. The most common site for NEC is the terminal ileum and proximal colon. The overall incidence of NEC is between 1% and 5% of all neonatal intensive care unit admissions. It affects predominantly premature infants, although approximately 10% of those affected are term neonates. Incidence is increased at lower gestational age (Fanaroff, Martin, 1992).

The exact pathogenesis of NEC is unknown, but several factors seem to play a role in its development. GI immaturity in the face of mucosal injury from hypoxic, ischemic events seems to predispose the infant to this catastrophic event. These and other risk factors are listed in Box 27-6.

BOX 27-6

Proposed Risk Factors for NEC

Asphyxia
Respiratory distress syndrome
Umbilical artery catheter
Exchange transfusion
Early enteral feedings
Patent ductus arteriosus
Congenital heart disease
Polycythemia
Anemia
Shock

The signs and symptoms of NEC are quite variable, ranging from feeding intolerance to evidence of fulminant intraabdominal catastrophe with sepsis, shock, peritonitis, and death. The usual presentation includes abdominal distention, gastric aspirates, bilious vomiting, and bloody stools. Lethargy, apnea, and hypoperfusion also may be prominent features. Physical findings noted on serial examination include progressive abdominal tenderness, muscular guarding, and abdominal wall erythema.

Treatment for NEC includes discontinuing enteral feedings, resting the gut, antibiotic therapy, and acute attention to stabilization parameters. Frequent abdominal assessment (especially careful attention to increasing abdominal girths) and serial x-rays of the gut to identify any perforation are the additional cornerstones of managing NEC. Perforation is a surgical emergency. Outcome depends on how much of the gut can be saved in surgery.

Developmental Considerations in the Care of the Preterm Infant

These fragile infants are ill equipped to deal with normal transition to extrauterine life, much less the stresses they must endure in the environment of the neonatal intensive care unit. The nursing care of the premature infant must take into account the maintenance and support of normal growth and development. The groundbreaking work of Brazelton, Als, and Lawhon in the 1980s provides a basis for assessing and understanding the behavior of the premature infant. The *synactive theory of infant development* provides the framework for this understanding. In this theory the infant's behavior is viewed as subsystems of functioning. Each subsystem can be described independently yet functions in relation to the other subsystems. This process of subsystem interaction or synaction is combined with the infant's continuous interaction with the environment to formulate the synactive theory of infant development.

The identified subsystems are autonomic, motor, attentional, and self-regulatory. Any immaturity or disorganization of one subsystem causes an imbalance or dis-

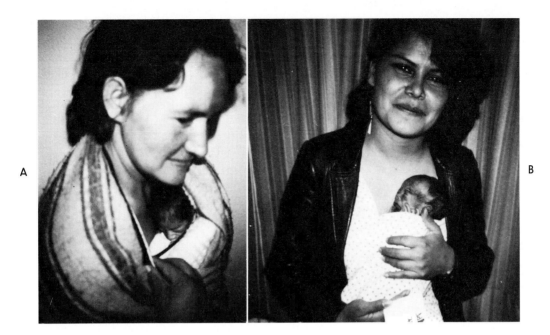

FIG. 27-7 Kangaroo method. **A,** Infant snuggled inside wrap. **B,** Infant inside mother's blouse in skin-to-skin contact (originally used in Bogota, Colombia. (Courtesy Vivian Wahlberg, Gothenberg, Stockholm.)

organization of the others. This theory provides for individualization of care for each infant, based on the infant's responses (Angelini et al, 1986).

Kangaroo care, or skin-to-skin contact, describes the practice of holding the preterm infant dressed only in a diaper on the mother's (or father's) bare chest (Fig. 27-7). Pioneered in Bogota, Colombia, as a replacement for incubators and radiant warmers, this intervention has recently gained acceptance in developed countries as an adjunctive therapy (Anderson, 1991).

✢ EVALUATION

Multidimensional evaluation of the care given to preterm infants and their families is required. In some families the infant dies despite all medical and nursing knowledge and skill. In other families the sequelae of preterm birth result in infants who will face disability throughout their lives. For these families, evaluation criteria concern loss, grief, and self-concept (see Chapter 28). For many other infants and their families the immediate threat to their well-being is overcome by intensive neonatal care.

The nurse can be reasonably assured that care was effective if the following *expected outcomes* regarding the *physical aspects of care are achieved:*

- Respirations are initiated and maintained.
- Body temperature is maintained.
- The infant is adequately nourished.
- CNS trauma is prevented or minimized.
- Infection is prevented.

POSTTERM AND POSTMATURE INFANTS

Postterm, or *postdate,* infants are those whose gestation is prolonged beyond 42 weeks, regardless of birth weight. These infants may be LGA or SGA, but most often their weight is AGA. Commonly these infants have little vernix caseosa other than in the skin creases, and that may be stained yellow or green. The cause of prolonged pregnancy is unknown. Certain groups are more likely to have gestations longer than 42 weeks, including first-time mothers, multiparous women (four or more children), and women with a history of a postdate pregnancy.

Postmaturity implies progressive placental insufficiency, resulting in a dysmature newborn. It is important to note that *not all postterm infants are postmature.*

In the SGA postterm infant, fetal malnutrition and hypoxia occur as a result of deteriorating metabolic exchange in the aging placenta. The depletion of subcutaneous fat produces the wasted appearance of the dysmature infant.

Perinatal mortality is significantly higher in the postterm fetus and neonate. During labor and birth, increased oxygen demands of the postmature fetus cannot be met. Insufficient gas exchange by the postmature placenta causes an increased incidence of intrauterine hypoxia and subsequent meconium aspiration. Of all the deaths of postterm newborns, one half occur during labor and birth, about one third occur before the onset of labor, and one sixth occur during the puerperium.

❖ ASSESSMENT

Most postterm and postmature infants are oversized but otherwise normal, with advanced development and bone age.

A postmature infant will have some but not necessarily all of the following physical characteristics:

- Generally has normal skull, but reduced dimensions of rest of body make skull look inordinately large
- Dry, cracked skin (desquamation), parchmentlike at birth
- Nails of hard consistency extending beyond fingertips
- Profuse scalp hair
- Subcutaneous fat layers depleted, leaving skin loose and giving an "old person" appearance
- Long and thin body contour
- Absent vernix
- Often meconium staining (golden yellow to green) of skin, nails, and cord
- May have an alert, wide-eyed appearance symptomatic of chronic intrauterine hypoxia

Persistent Pulmonary Hypertension of the Newborn (PPHN)

This term is applied to the combination of pulmonary hypertension, right-to-left shunting, and a structurally normal heart. PPHN may present either as a single entity or as the main component of meconium aspiration syndrome, congenital diaphragmatic hernia, RDS, hyperviscosity syndrome, or neonatal pneumonia or sepsis. PPHN is also called *persistent fetal circulation (PFC)* because the syndrome includes reversion to fetal pathways for blood flow.

A brief review of fetal blood flow can help visualize the problems with PPHN (Fig. 13-1 illustrates fetal circulation). In utero, oxygen-rich blood leaves the placenta via the umbilical vein, goes through the ductus venosus, and enters the inferior vena cava. From here it empties into the right atrium and is mostly shunted across the foramen ovale to the left atrium, effectively bypassing the lungs. This blood enters the left ventricle, leaves via the aorta, and preferentially perfuses the carotid and coronary arteries. Thus the heart and brain receive the most oxygenated blood. Blood drains from the brain into the superior vena cava, reenters the right atrium, proceeds to the right ventricle, and exits via the main pulmonary artery. The lungs are a high-pressure circuit, needing only enough perfusion for growth and nutrition. The ductus arteriosus (connecting the main pulmonary artery and the aorta) is the path of least resistance for the blood leaving the right side of the fetal heart, shunting most of the cardiac output away from the lungs and toward the systemic system. This *right-to-left shunting* is the key to fetal circulation.

After birth both the foramen ovale and ductus arteriosus close in response to various biochemical processes, pressure changes within the heart, and dilatation of the pulmonary vessels. This dilatation allows virtually all of the cardiac output to enter the lungs, become oxygenated, and provide oxygen-rich blood to the tissues for normal metabolism. Any process that interferes with this transition from fetal to neonatal circulation may precipitate PPHN. PPHN characteristically proceeds into a downward spiral of exacerbating hypoxia and pulmonary vasoconstriction. Prompt recognition and aggressive intervention are required to reverse this process.

The infant with PPHN is typically born at term or postterm and presents with tachycardia and cyanosis. Management depends on the underlying etiology of the persistent pulmonary hypertension. The recent development of extracorporeal membrane oxygenation (ECMO) has improved the survival of these infants. This process is similar to the heart-lung bypass used in intracardiac surgery. Large catheters are placed in the carotid artery and jugular vein, blood is siphoned off, oxygenated, then returned to the body. This process rests the lungs, allowing time for healing and vasodilatation. This treatment is a maximum intervention, used after conventional treatments have failed. Salvaging the carotid artery is possible with vascular microsurgery after decannulation.

Another mode of treatment for PPHN and other respiratory disorders of the newborn is high-frequency ventilation, a group of assisted ventilation methods that deliver small volumes of gas at high frequencies and limit the development of high airway pressure, thus reducing barotrauma (Fanaroff, Martin, 1992).

Meconium Aspiration Syndrome

Meconium staining of the amniotic fluid can be indicative of fetal distress. It appears in about 8% to 20% of all births. Many infants with meconium staining exhibit no signs of depression at birth; however, the presence of meconium in the amniotic fluid necessitates careful supervision of labor and close monitoring of fetal well-being. The presence of a team skilled at neonatal resuscitation is required at the birth of any infant with meconium stained amniotic fluid. The mouth and nares of the infant should be suctioned on the perineum before the infant's first breath. With thick or particulate meconium the standard of care is to intubate the infant at birth and suction any meconium visualized below the vocal cords. Appropriate management of the airway at birth can largely prevent **meconium aspiration syndrome (MAS).**

If meconium is not removed from the airway at birth, it can migrate down to the terminal airways, causing mechanical obstruction. It is also possible that the fetus aspirated meconium in utero. Meconium aspiration can cause a chemical pneumonitis. These infants may develop PPHN, further complicating their management.

LEGAL TIP: Standard of Care—Meconium Aspiration

When there are particles of meconium in the amniotic fluid, the standard of care is that the infant should be suctioned below the vocal cords immediately after birth. The nurse's responsibility is to notify the appropriate personnel to be at the birth and have suctioning equipment available.

SMALL-FOR-GESTATIONAL-AGE, INTRAUTERINE GROWTH RETARDED, AND DYSMATURE INFANTS

Infants whose birth weight falls below the 10th percentile expected at term, for reasons other than heredity, are considered at high risk (mortality greater than 10%) (Korones, 1986).

Various conditions can affect and impede growth in the developing fetus. The cause, severity, and the gestational age at which the insult occurs determine how fetal growth is affected and what problems will be present in the newborn. Conditions occurring in the first trimester, which affects all aspects of fetal growth (infections, teratogens, and chromosomal abnormalities), result in *symmetric* IUGR. Conditions causing symmetric growth retardation result in a short, SGA infant, usually with a smaller head circumference and reduced brain capacity.

Growth retardation in later stages of pregnancy, as a result of maternal or placental factors, results in *asymmetric* growth retardation (with respect to gestational age, weight will be ≤10th percentile whereas length and head circumference will be ≥10th percentile). Asymmetric growth retardation occurs as a result of the fetus receiving inadequate supplies of oxygen and nutrients (placental insufficiency). Conditions that cause placental insufficiency include maternal hypertension (preeclampsia and essential hypertension), smoking, malnutrition (undernutrition) and varied forms of maternal vascular and renal diseases (Creasy, Resnik, 1989). Infants with asymmetric IUGR have the potential for normal growth and development. Abnormal fetal size may indicate an adaptive response, with diminished fetal weight-sparing brain growth (Creasy, Resnik, 1989).

✣ ASSESSMENT

Several physical findings are characteristic of the *growth-retarded neonate:*

- Generally has normal skull, but reduced dimensions of rest of body make skull look inordinately large
- Reduced subcutaneous fat

- Loose and dry skin
- Diminished muscle mass, especially over buttocks and cheeks
- Sunken abdomen (scaphoid) as opposed to being normally well rounded
- Thin, yellowish, dry, and dull umbilical cord (normal cord is gray, glistening, round, and moist)
- Sparse scalp hair
- Wide skull sutures (inadequate bone growth)

SGA infants are likely to experience perinatal asphyxia, meconium aspiration syndrome, hypoglycemia, and heat loss.

Common Problems
Perinatal Asphyxia

Commonly, SGA infants have been exposed to chronic hypoxia for varying periods before labor and birth. Labor is a stressor to the normal fetus; it is an even greater stressor for the growth-retarded fetus. The chronically hypoxic infant is severely compromised by even a normal labor and has difficulty compensating after birth. The alert, wide-eyed appearance of the newborn is attributed to prolonged prenatal hypoxia. Appropriate management and resuscitation are essential for the depressed infant.

The birth of SGA babies with perinatal asphyxia may be associated with a maternal history of heavy cigarette smoking, preeclampsia, low socioeconomic status, multifetal gestation, gestational infections such as rubella, cytomegalovirus, and toxoplasmosis, advanced diabetes mellitus, and cardiac problems. When a woman with this background arrives in labor, the nursing staff must be alert to and prepared for possible perinatal asphyxia. Sequelae to perinatal asphyxia include meconium aspiration syndrome and hypoglycemia.

Meconium Aspiration Syndrome

See the section on postmaturity in this chapter.

Hypoglycemia

Stressed infants are at risk for the development of hypoglycemia (Merenstein, Gardner, 1993). Stress may include perinatal asphyxia and IUGR. Symptoms of hypoglycemia include cyanosis, apnea, tachypnea, and irregular respirations and diaphoresis. CNS symptoms can include jitteriness, weak cry, lethargy, floppy posture, convulsions, and coma. Diagnosis is confirmed by blood glucose determinations (<40 mg/dl) by laboratory or by on-unit visual methods with reagent strips such as Chemstrip-BG or Dextrostix.

Heat Loss

As a result of a number of factors, SGA infants require particular attention to maintain thermoneutrality. These infants have less muscle mass, less brown fat (an internal fuel source for generation of heat found in large amounts in normal term infants), less heat-preserving subcutaneous fat, and little ability to control skin capillaries. Nursing considerations focus on maintenance of thermoneutrality to support recovery from perinatal asphyxia; cold stress jeopardizes recovery from asphyxia.

INFANTS OF DIABETIC MOTHERS

No single physiologic or biochemical event can explain the diverse clinical manifestations seen in the **infants of diabetic mothers (IDMs)** or *infants of gestational diabetic mothers (IGDMs)*. A better understanding of maternal and fetal metabolism, resulting in stricter control of maternal diabetes and improved obstetric and neonatal intensive care, has led to a decrease in perinatal mortality in diabetic pregnancy from over 10% to under 4% in the last 25 years. Congenital anomalies are observed in IDMs two to six times more often than in the general population (Cherry, Merkatz, 1991; Creasy, Resnik, 1989). The mechanism of the process that leads to problems from conception through birth is as follows.

In early pregnancy, fluctuations in blood glucose levels and episodes of ketoacidosis are believed to cause congenital anomalies. Later in pregnancy, when the mother's pancreas cannot release sufficient insulin to meet increased demands, maternal hyperglycemia results. The high levels of glucose cross the placenta and stimulate the fetal pancreas to release insulin. The combination of the increased supply of maternal glucose and other nutrients and increased fetal insulin results in excessive fetal growth called *macrosomia*. Fetal hyperinsulinemia accounts for most of the problems seen. In addition, poor diabetic control, maternal vascular involvement, or superimposed maternal infection adversely affects the fetus. *Normally, maternal blood has a more alkaline pH than does fetal blood* (with its excess of carbon dioxide). This phenomenon encourages exchange of oxygen and carbon dioxide across the placental membrane. When the maternal blood is more acidotic than the fetal blood, no carbon dioxide or oxygen exchange occurs at the level of the placenta. The mortality for the unborn baby resulting from an episode of maternal ketoacidosis may be as high as 50% or more (Fanaroff, Martin, 1992). There is some indication that some neonatal conditions—macrosomia, hypoglycemia, hypocalcemia, hyperbilirubinemia, and perhaps fetal lung immaturity—may be eliminated or the incidence decreased by maintaining control over maternal glucose levels within narrow limits (Creasy, Resnik, 1989).

Care Management

Perinatal management focuses on maternal hydration-calorie-insulin balance, adequate fetal perfusion and oxy-

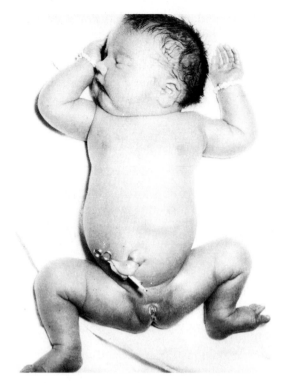

FIG. 27-8 "During their first 24 or more extrauterine hours they lie on their backs, bloated and flushed, their legs flexed and abducted, their tightly closed hands on each side of their head, the abdomen prominent and their respiration sighing. They convey a distinct impression of having had so much food and fluid pressed upon them by an insistent hostess that they desire only peace so that they may recover from their excesses." (From Shirkey HC, editor: *Pediatric therapy*, ed 6, St Louis, 1980, Mosby. Quotation in Whaley LF, Wong DF: *Essentials of Pediatric Nursing*, ed 3, St Louis, 1989, Mosby.)

genation, and prevention of maternal stress. Fetal hypoxia and acidosis can initiate or aggravate RDS. Careful assessment of labor identifies a dystotic labor early so that appropriate interventions may be implemented for a safe vaginal or abdominal birth. Infusions given to the mother that contain dextrose require insulin to minimize the risk of fetal postnatal hypoglycemia and hyperbilirubinemia (Polin, Fox, 1992).

Once the infant is born, the same management principles apply for the conditions already described and those that follow, whether they occur in the IDM or any other newborn. These conditions include macrosomia and birth trauma, congenital anomalies, hypoglycemia, hypocalcemia, lung immaturity, hyperbilirubinemia, hyperviscosity of blood, and cardiomyopathy.

✦ ASSESSMENT

Observation and physical examination of the newborn reveal the conditions associated with pregnancies complicated by diabetes mellitus. Appropriate laboratory tests are performed.

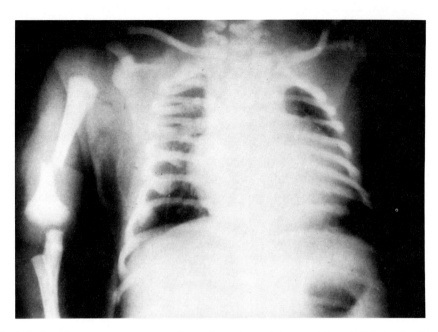

FIG. 27-9   Chest roentgenogram of a vaginally born full-term infant (4.7 kg) of a diabetic mother. The infant had cardiomegaly, hepatomegaly, congested lung fields, and fractures of the right humerus and left clavicle. (From Fanaroff AA, Martin RJ, editors: *Neonatal-perinatal medicine: diseases of the fetus and infant,* ed 5, St Louis, 1992, Mosby.)

Macrosomia

At birth the typical LGA infant has a round, cherubic ("tomato" or cushingoid) face, chubby body, and plethoric, or flushed, complexion (Fig. 27-8). These are the characteristics of **macrosomia.** The infant has enlarged viscera (hepatosplenomegaly, splanchnomegaly, cardiomegaly) and increased body fat (Fig. 27-9). The placenta and umbilical cord are larger than average. The brain is the only organ that is not enlarged. IDMs may be LGA but physiologically immature.

Insulin has been implicated as the primary growth hormone for intrauterine development. Maternal diabetes results in elevated maternal levels of amino acids and free fatty acids along with hyperglycemia. As the nutrients cross the placenta, the fetal pancreas responds by producing insulin to match the fuel supply. The resulting accelerated protein synthesis, together with a deposition of excessive glycogen and fat stores, is responsible for the typical macrosomic infant. This is the infant most at risk for the neonatal complications of hypoglycemia, hypocalcemia, hyperviscosity, and hyperbilirubinemia. The excessive amounts of metabolic fuels presented to the fetus from the mother and the consequent fetal hyperinsulinism are now understood to represent the basic pathologic mechanism in the diabetic pregnancy (Fanaroff, Martin, 1992).

Macrosomia (LGA infants) is particularly common in class A, B, and C diabetic pregnancies. Clinical efforts can focus only on the control of maternal plasma glucose concentrations. With good prenatal care and control of diabetes mellitus, the incidence of macrosomia can be decreased. The excessive size of these infants can and often does lead to dystocia because of fetopelvic disproportion. These infants, who may be born vaginally or by cesarean birth after a trial of labor, may incur birth trauma.

Birth Trauma and Perinatal Asphyxia

Birth injury (resulting from macrosomia or method of birth) and perinatal asphyxia occur in 20% of IGDMs and 35% of IDMs. Examples of birth trauma include cephalhematoma, paralysis of the facial nerve (seventh cranial nerve), fracture of the clavicle or humerus, brachial plexus paralysis, usually Erb-Duchenne (upper right arm) paralysis, and phrenic nerve paralysis, invariably associated with diaphragmatic paralysis.

Congenital Anomalies

Congenital anomalies occur in about 7% to 10% of IDMs. Their incidence is two to four times that for normal infants. The incidence is greatest among the SGA newborns. IUGR leading to SGA infants is seen in IDMs with severe vascular disease. The most commonly occurring anomalies involve the CNS (anencephaly, encephalocele, meningomyelocele, hydrocephalus) and caudal regression syndrome (sacral agenesis, with weakness or deformities of the lower extremities, malformation and fixation of the hip joints, and shortening or deformity of the femurs) (Fig. 27-10); tracheoesophageal fistula; and congenital heart malformations or cardiomyopathy. Hypertrichosis on the pinnae (excessive hair grown on the external ear) has been added to the list of characteristic clinical features (Fanaroff, Martin, 1992).

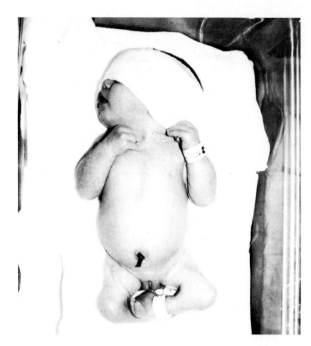

FIG. 27-10 Infant of diabetic mother with caudal regression syndrome (sacral agenesis). (From Fanaroff AA, Martin RJ, editors: *Neonatal-perinatal medicine: diseases of the fetus and infant,* ed 5, St Louis, 1992, Mosby.)

Cardiomyopathy

The incidence of congenital heart lesions in these infants is five times higher than in the general population. Other lesions include transposition of the aorta and pulmonary artery, ventricular septal defects, and coarctation of the aorta. Maternal diabetic control is correlated with the incidence of lesions. Poor control is defined as maternal blood glucose greater than 300 mg/dl, with glycosuria, ketonuria, or occasional ketoacidosis. Good control is defined as the maintenance of maternal blood glucose between 100 and 120 mg/dl. Careful diabetic management, especially in the second and third trimesters, decreases the severity of these lesions.

All IDMs need careful observation for cardiomyopathy; 30% to 50% of IDMs have cardiomegaly or congestive heart failure within 7 days of birth. Two types of cardiomyopathy can occur. Thus clinicians must be alert to identify correctly the type of lesion so that appropriate therapy is instituted. Both types are associated with respiratory symptoms and congestive heart failure.

Hypoglycemia and Hypocalcemia

In hypoglycemia and hypocalcemia, separation of the placenta suddenly interrupts the constant infusion of glucose. The high level of circulating glucose at the time the umbilical cord is severed falls rapidly in the presence of fetal hyperinsulinism. Asymptomatic or symptomatic hypoglycemia occurs within the first 1 to 3 hours after birth. Hypocalcemia occurs in 30% of IDMs. In addition, hypocalcemia is associated with preterm birth, birth trauma, and perinatal asphyxia. Symptoms of hypocalcemia, a prevalent finding in IDMs and IGDMs, are similar to those of hypoglycemia, but they occur between 24 and 36 hours of age. However, hypocalcemia must be considered if therapy for hypoglycemia is ineffective.

Respiratory Difficulty

IDMs and IGDMs manifest a greater incidence of RDS than is found in normal infants of comparable gestational age. Synthesis of surfactant may be delayed because of the high fetal serum level of insulin (Philip, 1987). Fetal lung maturity, as evidenced by a lecithin/sphingomyelin (L/S) ratio of 2 to 1, is not reassuring if the mother has diabetes mellitus or gestation-induced diabetes mellitus. For the infants of such mothers an L/S ratio of 3:1 or more, or the presence of phosphatidylglycerol in the amniotic fluid, is more indicative of adequate lung maturity.

Respiratory distress without RDS also occurs. Transient tachypnea, or wet lung syndrome, is a cause of respiratory distress (Fanaroff, Martin, 1992).

Hyperbilirubinemia

Hyperbilirubinemia develops in 50% of newborns of 32 to 34 weeks' gestation, and 15% of infants born at 37 weeks' gestation manifest this condition. Many newborns are plethoric because of polycythemia. *Polycythemia* increases blood viscosity, thereby impairing circulation. In addition, this increased number of red blood cells to be hemolyzed increases the potential bilirubin load that the newborn must clear. The excessive red blood cells are produced in extramedullary foci (liver and spleen) in addition to the usual sites in bone marrow. Therefore both liver function and bilirubin clearance may be adversely affected.

✤ NURSING DIAGNOSES

Following are examples of relevant nursing diagnoses.

Newborn

High risk for injury related to
- Metabolic effects of maternal condition
- Hypoglycemia, hypocalcemia, hyperbilirubinemia, hyperviscosity of blood
- Birth trauma

High risk for ineffective gas exchange related to
- Lung immaturity
- Cardiomyopathy

Ineffective thermoregulation related to
- Physiologic immaturity

PLAN OF CARE

Infant of a Gestational Diabetic Mother

Case History

Jason, born at 38 weeks' gestation by elective cesarean, is the first child for Judy Miller. Jason weighed 8 lb 10 oz (4763 g) at his birth 30 minutes ago. Judy's gestational diabetes mellitus was only moderately well controlled.

Initial physical examination revealed the following: Apgar scores of 8 at 1 minute and 9 at 5 minutes of age; LGA; no apparent congenital anomalies or birth trauma; and no meconium aspiration; amniotic fluid clear; skin, nails, and cord clear. Currently, Jason is under a radiant warmer with a thermistor probe attached. Judy has many questions about the possible effects of her condition on Jason.

EXPECTED OUTCOMES	IMPLEMENTATION	RATIONALE	EVALUATION
Nursing Diagnosis: Altered breathing pattern related to secretions in airway after cesarean birth			
Jason will maintain open airway and show no signs of respiratory distress.	Monitor closely for signs of respiratory distress, per hospital protocol.	Early identification is necessary for timely intervention.	Jason maintains an open airway and respiratory distress does not occur.
	Maintain body temperature; prevent cold stress.	Cold stress can result in respiratory distress.	
	Position Jason on side, with head slightly lower and neck slightly extended.	Facilitates mucus drainage and prevents aspiration of mucus from nasopharynx.	
	Suction mouth and nose as needed.		
	Ensure availability of resuscitation and oxygen equipment.	Saves time in event of respiratory distress.	
	Regard infant as preterm regardless of birth weight/size until gestational age and respiratory maturity are established.	Lung maturity is delayed when pregnancy is complicated by diabetes.	
Nursing Diagnosis: High risk for injury related to hypoglycemia/hypocalcemia secondary to maternal gestational diabetes			
Jason will maintain acceptable blood glucose levels and remain free from signs of hypoglycemia/hypocalcemia.	Assess for blood glucose levels per hospital protocol; for a term infant, levels of 40 mg/dl are within normal limits for first 3 days.	Jason's hyperinsulinism can lead rapidly to hypoglycemia after birth when maternal supply through the placenta stops.	Jason's blood glucose remained well above 40 mg/dl at each testing.
	Observe for and report signs of hypoglycemia.	Hypoglycemia can result in brain damage.	Jason did not show any signs of hypoglycemia.
	If suck/swallow reflexes are intact, feed per hospital protocol.	Maintains blood glucose within normal limits; prevents aspiration.	
	Assess for hypocalcemia if therapy for hypoglycemia is ineffective.	Hypocalcemia jeopardizes neonatal well-being, e.g., edema, apnea, intermittent cyanosis, abdominal distention and tetany can occur.	Jason had no episodes of hypocalcemia.

Continued.

PLAN OF CARE—cont'd

Infant of a Gestational Diabetic Mother

EXPECTED OUTCOMES	IMPLEMENTATION	RATIONALE	EVALUATION

Nursing Diagnosis: Anxiety (grieving, powerlessness, situational low self-esteem, spiritual distress, ineffective individual or family coping, altered family processes) related to having a newborn with a disorder or a potential disorder

Parents will verbalize understanding of effects of maternal diabetes on their child's well-being. Parents will verbalize feelings and concerns regarding their infant.	Explain effects of maternal diabetic condition on newborn. Explain all procedures to parents. Answer questions and correct misconceptions. Encourage open communication. Demonstrate child care activities. Observe parent-infant interactions. Schedule appointments for laboratory studies and follow-up physical examination. Refer to outside resources (child care, homemaker, clergy, home health).	Knowledge relieves fear of the unknown and supports coping and self-esteem. Encouraging and answering questions demonstrate respect and understanding for parents. Fosters parent-infant bonding/attachment.	Parents verbalize understanding of instructions.. Parents learn how to care for their child. Parents express feelings and concerns about their infant Parents express love for infant, call him by name, and participate in his care.

Parents/Family

Anxiety, fear, or powerlessness related to
- Uncertainty regarding neonate's prognosis

Self-esteem disturbance related to
- Experience of an abnormal pregnancy and compromised neonate

Anxiety related to knowledge deficit related to
- Neonate's condition, management, and prognosis

✤ EXPECTED OUTCOMES

Ideally, planning for the IDM begins during the antenatal period. Pediatric staff members are present at the birth. For each child an individualized plan of care is developed.

Expected outcomes for the infant include:
1. The infant will not develop respiratory distress.
2. The infant will maintain blood glucose levels within normal limits.
3. The infant will maintain temperature stability.

Expected outcomes for the family may include:
1. The family will understand effects of diabetes mellitus or the birth injury.
2. The family will willingly comply with management.

3. If the newborn exhibits a disorder or dies, the family will exhibit appropriate grief reactions

✤ COLLABORATIVE CARE

Implementation of care depends on the neonate's particular problems. General care of the compromised newborn is addressed in Chapter 26. If the maternal blood glucose level was well controlled throughout the pregnancy, the infant may require only monitoring. Because euglycemia is not always possible, the nurse must promptly recognize and treat any consequences of maternal diabetes that arise.

✤ EVALUATION

The nurse can be assured that care has been effective if the expected outcomes are achieved. That is, the newborn has a birth without trauma or injury and a neonatal period without sequelae of trauma or pregnancy complicated by maternal diabetes; the family has an understanding of diabetes or any birth injury and they willingly comply with management; and if the newborn exhibits a disorder or dies, the family initiates the grieving process (see Plan of Care on p. 791).

HYPERBILIRUBINEMIA

The yellow discoloration of the skin and other organs caused by accumulation of bilirubin is termed *jaundice* or *icterus.* Jaundice in the newborn, a common sign of potential trouble, is caused primarily by unconjugated bilirubin, a breakdown product of hemoglobin (Hb), after its release from hemolyzed red blood cells (RBCs). The challenge of neonatal jaundice is to distinguish physiologic jaundice from a serious clinical pathologic condition.

A variety of etiologic factors cause hyperbilirubinemia. The main focus of this section is isoimmune hemolytic disease of the newborn secondary to Rh or ABO incompatibility.

Rh Incompatibility

Soon after the Rh factor was reported, it was found that erythroblastosis fetalis, hydrops fetalis, and icterus gravis—variations of hemolytic disease of the newborn—are the results of the hemolysis of fetal Rh-positive RBCs by specific antibodies from an Rh-negative mother. Between 10% and 15% of white couples and about 5% of African-American couples have Rh incompatibility. It is rare that an Asian couple will be similarly affected. Not all Rh-positive men are homozygous for the Rh factor, nor will all children of Rh-positive men with Rh-negative partners be Rh positive. About 50% of the children of Rh-positive men who are heterozygous will be Rh positive; the remainder will be Rh negative. Rh-negative offspring are in no danger because their blood types are compatible with that of their mothers.

During first pregnancies with an Rh-positive fetus there usually is no effect on the fetus as a result of isoimmunization. Placental separation allows the transfer of fetal blood to maternal circulation, which stimulates maternal antibody production. Effects of sensitization are seen in subsequent pregnancies with an Rh-positive fetus when the maternal antibodies to Rh-positive RBCs enter the fetal circulation.

Severe Rh incompatibility results in marked fetal hemolytic anemia. The placenta clears the released blood pigments fairly well, however, so that only in extreme cases (such as icterus gravis) is the fetus icteric (yellow, or jaundiced). The marked anemia leads to cardiac decompensation, cardiomegaly, hepatomegaly, and splenomegaly. Edema, ascites, and hydrothorax develop. Severe anemia may lead to hypoxia. Intrauterine or early neonatal death may occur.

Once birth has occurred, the erythroblastotic newborn becomes icteric (in severe cases, this occurs within 30 minutes after birth) because the newborn cannot excrete the considerable residue of RBC hemolysis. Yellowish pigmentation of cerebrobasal nuclei, hippocampal cortex, and subthalamic nuclei often develop (kernicterus).

ABO Incompatibility

ABO incompatibility is more common than Rh incompatibility, but the effects generally are less severe in the affected infant. ABO incompatibility occurs when the fetal blood type is A, B, or AB and the maternal type is O. Naturally occurring anti-A and anti-B antibodies are transferred across the placenta to the fetus. First-born infants may be affected. The newborn may show a weakly positive direct *Coombs' test* result. Cord bilirubin usually is less than 4 mg/dl, and any resulting hyperbilirubinemia usually can be treated with phototherapy. Exchange transfusions are required only in occasional cases. Ongoing hemolysis may cause anemia, jaundice, and kernicterus and justifies serial hematocrit studies until the infant is stable.

Kernicterus

Kernicterus refers to bilirubin encephalopathy that results from the deposit of bilirubin, especially within the brainstem and cerebrobasal nuclei. The yellow staining (jaundice of the brain tissue) and necrosis of neurons result from toxic levels of unconjugated bilirubin. If not bound to proteins, unconjugated bilirubin is readily capable of crossing the blood-brain barrier because of its high lipid solubility. Kernicterus may occur in certain newborns with no apparent clinical jaundice but is generally directly related to the total serum bilirubin level. In a full-term infant, a serum bilirubin level of 20 mg/dl is considered the upper limit before brain damage begins.

Only one sequela in those infants who survive is specific: choreoathetoid cerebral palsy. Other sequelae, such as mental retardation and serious sensory disabilities, may reflect hypoxic, vascular, or infectious injury that often is associated with kernicterus. About 70% of newborns who develop kernicterus die during the neonatal period.

The perinatal events that reinforce the development of hyperbilirubinemia also increase the likelihood that kernicterus will develop, even in the presence of mild to moderate unconjugated hyperbilirubinemia. These perinatal events include hypoxia, asphyxia, acidosis, hypothermia, hypoglycemia, bacterial infection, certain maternal medications, and hypoalbuminemia. These conditions interfere with conjugation or compete for albumin-binding sites.

CONGENITAL ANOMALIES

The desired and expected outcome of every wanted pregnancy is a normal, functioning infant with good intellectual potential. Fulfillment of this hope depends on numerous factors, both hereditary and environmental. Probably all human characteristics have a genetic component, including those that produce undesirable symptoms or unwelcome physical abnormalities that impair the fitness of the individual. Some diseases occur through the action of a single gene or the combined action of many genes inherited from the parents; others are the result of the action of the environment on the genetic composition of the individual. A disease or disorder that can be transmitted from generation to generation is termed *genetic* or *hereditary*. A ***congenital disorder*** is one that is present at birth and can be caused by genetic or environmental factors, or both.

Each year 250,000 infants are born with significant structural and functional disorders. Major congenital defects are now the leading cause of death in infants younger than 1 year of age in the United States. With the fall in other causes of neonatal mortality, these defects now account for about 20% of those deaths.

The seriousness of this community health problem is reflected in the more than 6 million hospital days and $200 billion a year allocated to the care and treatment of these neonates. Prevention and detection procedures are being improved continuously. Methods of promoting the availability of these services to populations at risk challenge the community health care systems. An interdisciplinary team approach is vital in providing holistic care: surgery, rehabilitation, and education of the child and social, as well as psychologic and financial, assistance to the parents. Parental disappointment and disillusion, societal stigmatization of, or any negative feelings the nurse may have toward the infant's disorder add to the complexity of nursing care.

Prenatal Diagnosis

Refined testing procedures have become available to monitor the development of the fetus. Prenatal diagnostic techniques such as amniocentesis, ultrasound, alpha-fetoprotein measurements, chorionic villus sampling, percutaneous umbilical cord blood sampling, and gene probes contribute to the data base. Although they comprise a valuable adjunct to prenatal care, these tests do not achieve 100% accuracy in detecting congenital defects (Brambati et al, 1991; Greene, Benacerraf, 1991; Lemna et al, 1990; Wenstrom et al, 1991; Wolfe et al, 1990; Zacharias, 1990).

Despite the status and availability of current technology, not all congenital disorders are or can be anticipated. The historic and medical information in the prenatal record is reviewed for factors that are associated with congenital disorders. These factors include various medical and surgical conditions and their treatments (see Chapter 22), maternal infection (see Chapter 21), maternal endocrine and metabolic disorders (see Chapter 22), and infection and drug dependence in the newborn.

Perinatal Diagnosis

Many congenital anomalies require intervention soon after birth. Careful observations in the birth room or nursery will identify most of these conditions.

Volume of Amniotic Fluid

An excessive amount of amniotic fluid, **hydramnios,** is commonly associated with congenital anomalies in the newborn. The infant should be examined closely at the earliest possible time. In the presence of hydramnios, any of the following may be suspected:

1. Cephalocaudal malformations, such as hydrocephaly, microcephaly, anencephaly, and spina bifida
2. Orogastrointestinal malformations, such as cleft palate, esophageal atresia with or without a tracheal fistula, pyloric stenosis, volvulus, and imperforate anus
3. Miscellaneous conditions, such as Down syndrome, congenital heart disease, deformed extremities, and infants of diabetic or prediabetic mothers
4. Preterm birth

Oligohydramnios (an insufficient amount of amniotic fluid) is associated primarily with those anomalies of the urinary tract that prevent normal micturition in utero. As a rule, renal agenesis or renal dysplasia is involved.

1. Urethral stenosis has been reported to be associated with oligohydramnios.
2. Anomalies of the earlobes, rather than agenesis of the ear, sometimes are associated with renal abnormalities and are not direct results of oligohydramnios.
3. Potter's syndrome (renal agenesis) is the classic example of an association between oligohydramnios and renal anomalies. It includes atypical facies that involve abnormal earlobes.

Postnatal Diagnosis

An Apgar score and minimal assessment are completed for all neonates after birth. Any deviations from normal are reported to the primary health care provider immediately.

Respiratory System

Screening for congenital anomalies of the respiratory tract is necessary even for the infant who is apparently normal at birth. Respiratory distress at birth or shortly thereafter may be the result of lung immaturity or anomalous development. Congenital laryngeal web and bilateral choanal atresia (Fig. 27-11) are readily apparent at birth. Both require emergency surgery. Respiratory distress caused by diaphragmatic hernia and tracheoesophageal fistula appear immediately or may be delayed, depending on the severity of the defect.

Neurologic System

Neurologic signs may reflect hidden congenital anomalies, as well as numerous other conditions. Many neonatal responses are nonspecific. Each sign, such as high-pitched cry, hypotonia, jitteriness, low-set ears, and microcephaly or hydrocephaly, must be evaluated carefully before appropriate therapy can be instituted.

Some neural tube defects are obvious at first glance. The three main defects are anencephaly, spina bifida (which includes occult and visible meningocele and mye-lomeningocele), and encephalocele. These are defects in midline closures. If a neural tube defect is identified, the infant may have one or more of the other malformations in this group: cleft lip and palate, tracheoesophageal fistula, and diaphragmatic hernia.

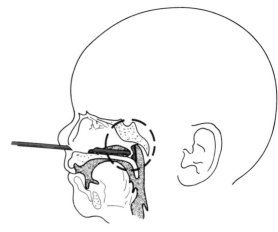

FIG. 27-11 Choanal atresia. Posterior nares are obstructed by membrane or bone either bilaterally or unilaterally. Infant becomes cyanotic at rest. With crying, newborn's color improves. Nasal discharge is present. Snorting respirations often are observed with increased respiratory effort. Newborn may be unable to breathe and eat at same time. Diagnosis is made by noting inability to pass small feeding tube through one or both nares. (Courtesy Ross Laboratories, Columbus, OH.)

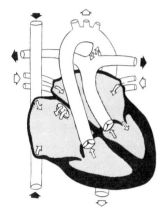

Complete transposition
of great vessels

The anomaly is an embryologic defect caused by a straight division of the bulbar trunk without normal spiraling. As a result, the aorta originates from the right ventricle, and the pulmonary artery from the left ventricle. An abnormal communication between the two circulations must be present to sustain life.

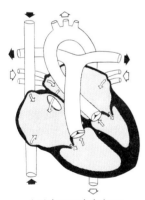

Atrial septal defects

An atrial septal defect is an abnormal opening between the right and left atria. Basically, three types of abnormalities result from incorrect development of the atrial septum. An incompetent foramen ovale is the most common defect. The high ostium secundum defect results from abnormal development of the septum secundum. Improper development of the septum primum produces a basal opening known as an ostium primum defect, frequently involving the atrioventricular valves. In general, left to right shunting of blood occurs in all atrial septal defects.

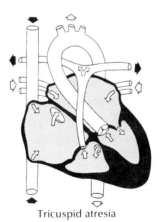

Tricuspid atresia

Tricuspid valvular atresia is characterized by a small right ventricle, large left ventricle, and usually a diminished pulmonary circulation. Blood from the right atrium passes through an atrial septal defect into the left atrium, mixes with oxygenated blood returning from the lungs, flows into the left ventricle, and is propelled into the systemic circulation. The lungs may receive blood through one of three routes: (1) a small ventricular septal defect, (2) patent ductus arteriosus, (3) bronchial vessels.

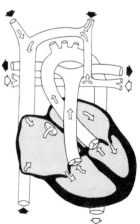

Anomalous venous return

Oxygenated blood returning from the lungs is carried abnormally to the right heart by one or more pulmonary veins emptying directly, or indirectly, through venous channels into the right atrium. Partial anomalous return of the pulmonary veins to the right atrium functions the same as an atrial septal defect. In complete anomalous return of the pulmonary veins, an interatrial communication is necessary for survival.

FIG. 27-12 Congenital heart abnormalities. (Courtesy Ross Laboratories, Columbus, OH.)

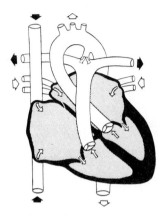

Patent ductus arteriosus

The patent ductus arteriosus is a vascular connection that, during fetal life, short circuits the pulmonary vascular bed and directs blood from the pulmonary artery to the aorta. Functional closure of the ductus normally occurs soon after birth. If the ductus remains patent after birth, the direction of blood flow in the ductus is reversed by the higher pressure in the aorta.

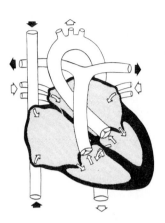

Ventricular septal defects

A ventricular septal defect is an abnormal opening between the right and left ventricle. Ventricular septal defects vary in size and may occur in either the membranous or muscular portion of the ventricular septum. Due to higher pressure in the left ventricle, a shunting of blood from the left to right ventricle occurs during systole. If pulmonary vascular resistance produces pulmonary hypertension, the shunt of blood is then reversed from the right to the left ventricle, with cyanosis resulting.

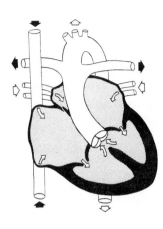

Truncus arteriosus

Truncus arteriosus is a retention of the embryologic bulbar trunk. It results from the failure of normal septation and division of this trunk into an aorta and pulmonary artery. This single arterial trunk overrides the ventricles and receives blood from them through a ventricular septal defect. The entire pulmonary and systemic circulation is supplied from this common arterial trunk.

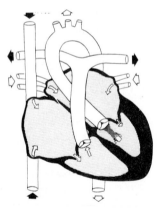

Subaortic stenosis

In many instances, the stenosis is valvular with thickening and fusion of the cusps. Subaortic stenosis is caused by a fibrous ring below the aortic valve in the outflow tract of the left ventricle. At times, both valvular and subaortic stenosis exist in combination. The obstruction presents an increased work load for the normal output of the left ventricular blood and results in left ventricular enlargement.

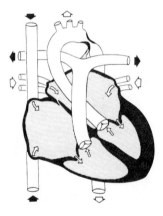

Coarctation of the aorta

Coarctation of the aorta is characterized by a narrowed aortic lumen. It exists as a preductal or postductal obstruction, depending on the position of the obstruction in relation to the ductus arteriosus. Coarctations exist with great variation in anatomic features. The lesion produces an obstruction to the flow of blood through the aorta causing an increased left ventricular pressure and work load.

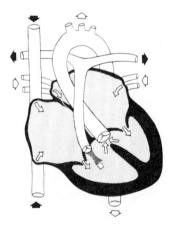

Tetralogy of Fallot

Tetralogy of Fallot is characterized by the combination of four defects: (1) pulmonary stenosis, (2) ventricular septal defect, (3) overriding aorta, (4) hypertrophy of right ventricle. It is the most common defect causing cyanosis in patients surviving beyond two years of age. The severity of symptoms depends on the degree of pulmonary stenosis, the size of the ventricular septal defect, and the degree to which the aorta overrides the septal defect.

FIG. 27-12, cont'd   For legend see p. 795.

Cardiovascular System

Congenital cardiovascular disorders are divided into two major types: cyanotic and noncyanotic. Severe congenital cardiovascular disorders often are evident immediately after birth, for example, severe cyanotic heart disease (Fig. 27-12). These infants usually are transferred directly to special nurseries or pediatric units. Some problems, such as a small patent ductus arteriosus or a minimal coarctation of the descending aorta, become apparent only as the infant is exposed to stresses such as growth demands of later infancy and early childhood or to infection. In about 75% of cases, cardiovascular anomalies are unexpected.

Cardiovascular defects occur in 4 to 10 in 1000 births (Hoffman, 1990). Congenital heart disease is implicated in approximately 50% of deaths from malformations during the first year of life. The etiologic factors are still unclear, although a familial tendency is evident in many cases. Coexisting congenital defects are common in newborns with cardiovascular anomalies. Maternal diseases such as rubella, alcoholism, and insulin-dependent diabetes during pregnancy, as well as maternal age over 40 years, have been implicated. Symptoms characteristically are first evident after the umbilical cord is severed. The infant's *cry* is weak and muffled or loud and breathless. The newborn may be *cyanotic*. Cyanosis usually is generalized, increases in the supine position, and often is unrelieved by oxygen. It usually deepens with crying. The gray dusky color may be mild, moderate, or severe. Other infants may be *acyanotic* and pale, with or without mottling on exertion (such as crying).

The newborn's *activity level* varies from restless to lethargic. The infant may be unresponsive except to pain. The arms may be flaccid while the infant is being fed. *Posturing* is significant. Hypotonia and flaccidity may be evident, even during sleep. There may be hyperextension of the neck or opisthotonos. The newborn may be dyspneic when supine. Persistent *bradycardia* (below 120 beats/min or less than 30 beats/min from the normal baseline for 10 minutes or more) or persistent tachycardia (160 beats/min or more) may be noted. The cardiac rhythm may be abnormal, and cardiac murmurs are heard in some infants. Signs of congestive heart failure, diminished cardiac output, and decreased tissue perfusion may be evident.

Respirations are counted when the newborn is asleep. Findings may include tachypnea (60 respirations per minute or more), retractions with nasal flaring or tachypnea, and dyspnea with diaphoresis or grunting. Diaphoresis is an uncommon response in the normal newborn. Respirations may be gasping, followed in 2 or 3 minutes by respiratory arrest without prompt treatment. Grunting may occur with or without exertion.

These findings must be reported immediately. Newborns showing these types of signs require prompt definite diagnosis and immediate appropriate therapy in a tertiary care neonatal intensive care unit or pediatric unit.

Gastrointestinal System

Screening for gastrointestinal tract malformations is performed on a routine basis for all infants. Abdominal wall defects are apparent at birth (omphalocele is discussed on p. 800). Intestinal obstruction, which occurs in about 1 in 3000 newborns, may occur in the presence of diaphragmatic hernia. A scaphoid (sunken) abdomen usually indicates a diaphragmatic hernia. A distended abdomen is particularly noteworthy in H-type tracheoesophageal fistula. These conditions require immediate surgery and are discussed later in this chapter.

Urogenital System

Careful notation of perinatal events and observations such as oligohydramnios and absence of voiding aid in the identification and confirmation of existing congenital anomalies. In cases of ambiguous genitals identification of the infant's sex must be established as quickly as possible to facilitate initiation of a positive parent-child relationship. Assessment to determine a gender assignment consists of several studies (Whaley, Wong, 1995), history (e.g., ingestion of steroids, relatives with ambiguous genitalia), physical examination, chromosomal analysis (results available in 2 to 3 days), endoscopy, ultrasonography, and radiographic contrast studies, biochemical tests (e.g., 17-ketosteroids), and laparotomy or gonad biopsy.

Exstrophy of the bladder or the cloaca is rare (p. 804).

Some infants have multiple congenital anomalies. A syndrome refers to a recognized pattern of malformations. The most familiar is Down syndrome (Fig. 27-13). Diagnosis is confirmed early in the neonatal period.

Genetic Diagnosis

Most diagnostic procedures for detection of genetic disorders are implemented after birth at any time from the postnatal period through adulthood. The number and variety of these tests are extensive. The most commonly employed are biochemical tests, cytologic studies, and dermatoglyphics.

Biochemical Tests

The most widespread use of postbirth testing for genetic disease is the routine screening of newborns for inborn errors of metabolism such as phenylketonuria (PKU), which is mandatory in most states. **Inborn errors of metabolism** is a term applied to a large group of disorders caused by a metabolic defect that results from the absence of or change in a protein, usually an enzyme, because of gene action. These defects can involve any substrate produced from protein, carbohydrate, or fat metabolism. Inborn errors of metabolism are recessive disorders and, as such, require that the individual receive a defective gene from each parent. The parents usually are unaffected because their normal, dominant gene directs the synthesis of sufficient protein to meet their metabolic

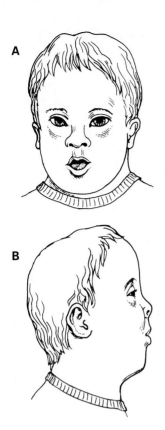

FIG. 27-13   Clinical features of Down syndrome.

needs under normal circumstances. With new biochemical techniques it is now possible to detect the presence of the abnormal gene in an increasing number of these disorders.

PKU results from a deficiency of the enzyme phenylalanine dehydrogenase. The test for PKU is not valid until the newborn has ingested an ample amount of the amino acid phenylalanine, a constituent of both human and cow milk. A diet low in phenylalanine is ordered to prevent the severe mental retardation and bizarre behavior seen in untreated cases.

Galactosemia, caused by a deficiency of the enzyme galactose-1-phosphate uridyltransferase, results in the inability to convert galactose to glucose. Galactosemia can be detected by measuring blood levels of galactose in the urine of affected newborns who have ingested milk containing galactose. Failure to thrive, mental retardation, cataracts, jaundice, hepatomegaly, and cirrhosis of the liver are manifestations in untreated cases. Therapy consists of the elimination of galactose from the diet.

In recent years many states in the United States have required routine screening for *hypothyroidism.* Thyroxine (T_4) is measured from a drop of blood obtained from a heel stick at 2 to 5 days of age. At this time the normally expected increase in T_4 is lacking in newborns with hypothyroidism. Cretinism develops in untreated affected individuals. The same blood sample can be used to test for all three of these metabolic disorders—PKU, galactosemia, and hypothyroidism (see Appendix F).

Cytologic Studies

In most instances disorders resulting from chromosomal abnormalities can be diagnosed by clinical manifestations alone. Occasionally an infant is born whose clinical appearance is only suggestive of a problem. In these cases cytologic studies may be carried out to confirm or to rule out a tentative diagnosis. Sometimes all that is required are sex chromatin or fluorescent staining techniques. These stains can be prepared from any cells in the body. The most easily obtained and therefore the most commonly used are mucosal cells scraped from the inside of the cheek, which are placed on a glass slide, prepared, and stained (buccal smear).

Preparation of a karyotype requires cells in the process of cell division. The most commonly used cells are those obtained from bone marrow, skin, or peripheral blood. The cells are grown in culture media. Division is arrested at the stage when cells are best visualized, then stained, photographed, and arranged in a karyotype for assessment. A karyotype also is requested in cases in which the sex of the infant is in doubt because the assignment of a gender constitutes a social emergency.

Two examples of chromosome abnormalities are Turner's and Klinefelter's syndromes. The child with *Turner's syndrome* is a female with the genetic designation of 45 X. She has short stature, webbed neck, low posterior hairline, shield-shaped chest with widely spaced nipples, lymphedema of hands and feet, and is sterile. The child with *Klinefelter's syndrome* is a male whose genetic designation may be 47 XXY or 48 XXYY. This boy is tall with long legs, has hypogenitalism, and is sterile. He may have deficient male secondary sexual characteristics and may demonstrate aberrant behavior.

Dermatoglyphics

The pattern formed by dermal ridges early in development is largely genetically determined by many genes on many chromosomes. Therefore addition or deletion of genetic material will produce alterations in the loops, swirls, and arches of the finger and toe prints, in the palm lines, and in the flexion creases on palms of the hands and soles of the feet. Characteristic dermatoglyphic patterns have been noted in almost all the chromosomal abnormalities such as Down syndrome. Certain fingerprint patterns may be found in persons who have cardiac valvular problems later in life.

Many other diagnostic studies may be performed in the neonatal period to detect or rule out genetic defects, for example, x-ray studies for a variety of structural defects of bone and for gastrointestinal, renal, and neurologic disorders. Meconium ileus in the newborn often is the first manifestation of cystic fibrosis.

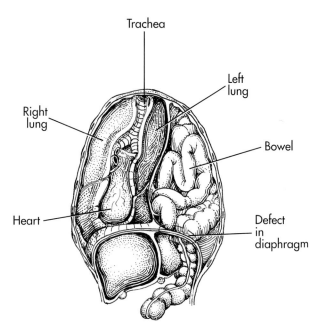

FIG. 27-14   Diaphragmatic hernia. (Courtesy Ross Laboratories, Columbus, OH.)

Common Surgical Emergencies

The following five congenital anomalies account for more than 90% of surgical emergencies of the newborn: diaphragmatic hernia, tracheoesophageal anomalies, omphalocele, intestinal obstruction, and imperforate anus.

Diaphragmatic Hernia

Diaphragmatic hernia is the most urgent of the neonatal emergencies. Incomplete embryonic development of the diaphragm allows herniation of abdominal viscera into the thoracic cavity (Fig. 27-14). The defect and herniation may be minimal and easily repairable, or the defect may be so extensive that the viscera present in the thoracic cavity during embryonic life prevented the normal development of pulmonary tissue. Most cases involve a posterolateral defect, usually on the left. The extent of the defect and the severity and timing of the symptoms determine the seriousness of the problem.

Signs that might indicate extensive diaphragmatic herniation can be assessed by the nurse. They include constant respiratory distress from birth that becomes increasingly severe as intestines fill with air, heart sounds heard in right side of the chest, large or asymmetric chest contour, dullness to percussion on the affected side, scaphoid abdomen, bowel sounds heard in the thoracic cavity, and diminished breath sounds.

Preoperative care focuses on decompression of the intestines to prevent further pressure on the heart and lungs. Positioning of the head and chest higher than the abdomen and with the affected side down and placement of a nasogastric or orogastric tube open to air or on intermittent low suction will accomplish this. These infants should not be mask ventilated because this will push air into the intestines. If they require assisted ventilation, endotracheal intubation is preferred.

Prompt surgical repair is imperative. The prognosis depends largely on the degree of pulmonary development and the success of diaphragmatic closure. Prognosis in severe cases is guarded. Extracorporeal membrane oxygenation (ECMO) may be indicated after surgery in infants who do not respond to conventional medical therapy for circulatory and respiratory complications (Polin, Fox, 1992).

Tracheoesophageal Anomalies

Esophageal atresia is an urgent congenital anomaly. Various types are recognized, depending on the presence or absence of an associated *tracheoesophageal fistula,* the site of the fistula, and the point and degree of esophageal obstruction (Fig. 27-15). Moderate hydramnios is common with esophageal atresia and tracheoesophageal fistula. About half of these newborns have associated anomalies, including congenital heart defects and genitourinary and gastrointestinal malformations.

The following signs suggest atresia, with or without tracheoesophageal fistula: excessive oral secretions with drooling, progressive respiratory distress as unswallowed secretions spill over into trachea, and feeding intolerance. In feeding intolerance, choking, coughing, and cyanosis follow even a small amount of fluid taken by mouth. Soon after the first feeding is initiated, there is regurgi-

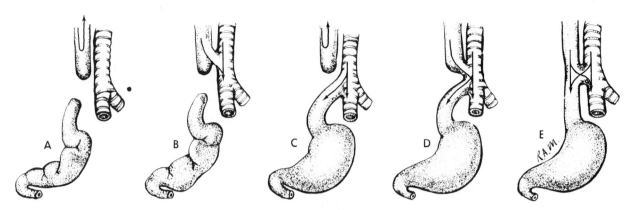

FIG. 27-15 Congenital atresia of esophagus and tracheoesophageal fistula. **A,** About 8%. Upper and lower segments of esophagus end in blind sac. **B,** Less than 1%. Upper segment of esophagus ends in atresia and connects to trachea by fistulous tract. Infant may drown with first feeding. **C,** About 87%. Upper segment of esophagus ends in blind pouch; lower segment connects with trachea by small fistulous tract. **D,** Less than 1%. Both segments of esophagus connect by fistulous tracts to trachea. Infant may drown with first feeding. **E,** About 4%. Esophagus is continuous but connects by fistulous tract to trachea; known as *H*-type. (From Whaley LF, Wong DL: *Nursing care of infants and children,* ed 4, St Louis, 1991, Mosby.)

tation of unaltered formula or colostrum (unmixed with stomach secretions or bile).

Nursing actions are supportive. In the presence of excessive oral secretions and respiratory distress, *the infant should not be fed orally* before the primary health care provider is consulted. In the presence of abdominal distention, the newborn is placed in semi-Fowler's position, and the head is raised 30 degrees or more (infant seat may be used). This position facilitates respiratory efforts and discourages reflux (spillage) of stomach secretions into the respiratory tree, with resultant chemical bronchitis and pneumonitis. On physician's order or per standing orders, a suction tube is inserted into the blind pouch, and the tube is connected to low, intermittent suction.

Surgical correction of the anomaly is mandatory. After the surgery, oropharyngeal suctioning is permitted only to a length of 8 cm or to the length of the endotracheal tube if one is present. This prevents damage to the anastomosis from the catheter. The prognosis depends on the degree of maturity of the newborn and the presence of a fistula or pneumonia.

Omphalocele

Omphalocele is a herniation noted at birth in which part of the intestine protrudes through a defect in the abdominal wall at the umbilicus (Fig. 27-16). Failure of migration of the midgut in embryonic development probably is responsible for omphalocele. The protruding bowel is covered only by a thin, transparent membrane composed of amnion.

Prompt closure of defects of less than 5 cm in diameter usually is successful. Larger defects may require clo-

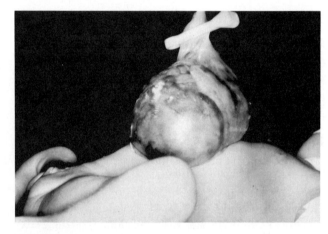

FIG. 27-16 Omphalocele containing liver. (Courtesy John R Campbell, MD, University of Oregon Health Sciences Center, Portland.)

sure in stages. The general prognosis is related to associated anomalies.

There usually is only a short time span between the infant's birth and surgical intervention. Planning support for the parents is an essential aspect of nursing care. In addition to the usual preoperative orders, preparation of the infant for surgery includes insertion of an orogastric tube, aspiration of stomach contents, insertion of an intravenous line in an upper extremity, immediate administration of antibiotics, and protection of the defect from infection, rupture, and drying.

The infant is placed in a sterile plastic bag with a drawstring. These bags can usually be found in surgery, where they are used for sterile specimens. The bag completely covers the omphalocele with the drawstring pulled

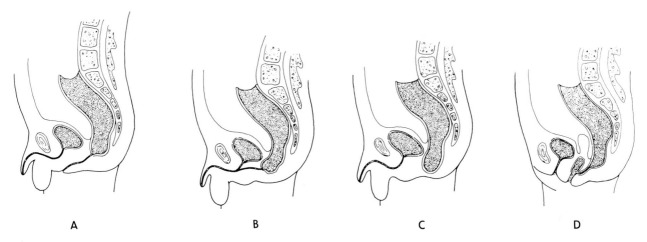

FIG. 27-17   Types of imperforate anus. Anal sphincter muscle may be present and intact. **A,** High lesion opening onto perineum through narrow fistulous tract. **B,** High lesion ending in fistulous tract to urinary tract. **C,** Low lesion in bowel passes through puborectal muscle. **D,** High lesion ending in fistulous tract to vagina.

snugly above the site and is left in place until surgery. Although the infant will void and possibly pass meconium into the bag, it is not changed because urine and meconium are assumed to be sterile and surgery should occur within 24 hours. Another method to protect the omphalocele until surgery involves sterile warm saline soaks, which are enclosed in plastic wrap to prevent heat and moisture loss.

Intestinal Obstruction

Congenital jejunal or ileal obstruction is suspected when distention and bile-stained or fecal vomiting occur in a newborn in the first 24 to 48 hours of life. Normal meconium stool is not passed. Although this condition is uncommon, preterm infants and those with other anomalies may be affected.

Nursing care is supportive.
- Stop oral feedings and monitor intravenous therapy and electrolyte replacement.
- Prevent aspiration, and suction gastric contents on physician's order (indwelling catheter to low, intermittent suction may be ordered).
- Place infant in semi-Fowler's position to facilitate respiration.

Prompt surgery usually provides good results.

Imperforate Anus

Imperforate anus is a term used to describe a wide variety of congenital disorders that are more common in male than in female infants (Fig. 27-17). About 85% of affected girls will have developed a small fistula, but this is rare in boys. The obstruction may be of the low type (anal membrane) or the high type (anal or rectal atresia).

Because lifetime continence may depend on coexisting sacral anomalies and proper corrective surgery, a pe-

diatric surgeon is consulted at once. Surgery may be as simple as an incision of an anal membrane. With anorectal agenesis, a prompt colostomy is necessary.

Common Malformations
Meningomyelocele

Meningomyelocele, a neural tube defect, is a herniation of part of the meninges (containing cerebrospinal fluid [CSF] and CNS tissue) through a defect in the vertebral column or skull. The defect often occurs in the lower portion of the back (Fig. 27-18). In the accompanying spinal malformation, **spina bifida,** the meningomyelocele extrudes through the opening of the spinal column. The opening is the result of a congenital absence of one or more vertebral arches. Occasionally a familial history (5% recurrence rate) of this anomaly is identified. Most cases are of unknown (infectious?) origin. A *meningocele* is also a herniation of the meninges. A meningocele contains CSF but does not contain CNS tissue (cord or nerve roots). Prenatal diagnosis of neural tube defects (meningomyelocele, meningocele, anencephaly) is now possible using analysis of alpha-fetoprotein (AFP) levels in the amniotic fluid and fetal ultrasound.

If the neonate is born with a large defect, the nurse aids in preventing the rupture and infection of any meningomyelocele sac before surgery. Protection of the defect includes the following actions:
1. Position infant with care.
   a. Position infant prone or side-lying with rolled towels to prevent pressure or injury to defect, thereby preventing portal of entry for infectious agents.
   b. Change position every hour to prevent pressure areas.
   c. If infant can be held, exercise caution to avoid injury to defect.

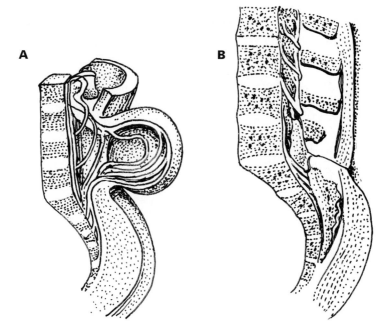

FIG. 27-18 **A,** Myelomeningocele. Note absence of vertebral arches. **B,** Dermal sinus tract with dermoid cyst, often associated with spina bifida occulta. Note also tuft of hair.

2. Provide skin care: skin around defect is cleansed and dried carefully to prevent breakdown, which would establish a portal of entry for infectious agents. Apply ordered dressings, ointments, and so on.

The nurse assists in the diagnosis of hidden defects (e.g., *spina bifida occulta*) (Fig. 27-18, *B*). The nurse assesses neurologic function and notes the following: paralysis of lower extremities, flaccidity and spasticity of muscles below defect, and sphincter control (character and number of voidings and stools; leakage of urine and stool).

Surgical repair often can be performed in the neonatal period. If other anomalies, such as hydrocephalus, are present, delayed correction may be elected. Permanent impairment of neuromuscular function below the level of the defect depends on the amount of CNS tissue involved. In severe cases, voluntary and involuntary functions are absent. The prognosis is guarded. Only about 60% of cases are operable. Many of these children die or achieve only partial function. Hydrocephalus ultimately develops in virtually all of these infants.

The parents will need considerable support and instruction regarding the infant's care. In some instances parents may require assistance in placing the child in a special care facility.

Congenital Hydrocephalus

Congenital **hydrocephalus** is macrocephaly caused by abnormal enlargement of the cerebral ventricles and skull. This disorder has many causes. Head enlargement is the result of increased intraventricular CSF pressure.

This condition is accompanied by enlargement of the head, prominence of the forehead, setting sun sign of the eyes, atrophy of the brain, weakness, and convulsions as the condition worsens. Congenital hydrocephalus is encountered in approximately 1 in 2000 fetuses (about 12% of all malformations). Several types are known. Spina bifida occurs in approximately one third of infants born with hydrocephalus.

Surgery may be performed in utero but usually is performed soon after birth. If surgical shunting is not accomplished, increasing intracranial pressure—evidenced by palpably widening fontanel and sutures, lethargy, irritability, vomiting, or high-pitched shrill cry—results in irreversible neurologic damage.

Nursing actions appropriate to the needs of a newborn with hydrocephalus include careful documentation of ongoing observations. Meticulous skin care is necessary to prevent pressure areas and infection of the skin of the head. Lamb's wool, sheepskin, or a flotation mattress is used under the infant. Frequent position changing and keeping the newborn clean and dry help maintain skin integrity and health.

The newborn's heavy head is supported carefully when being held or turned. The method, amount, and frequency of feeding are chosen to accommodate the infant's tolerance and energy level. Care is taken to prevent vomiting and subsequent aspiration. Nonnutritive sucking, touching, and cuddling needs are met.

Damaged or destroyed brain tissue cannot be restored. Spontaneous arrest of hydrocephalus may occur, but often surgical shunting may be required to eliminate

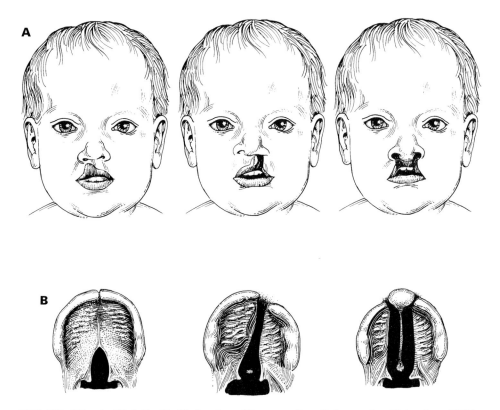

FIG. 27-19 **A,** Cleft lip. **B,** Cleft palate. (Courtesy Ross Laboratories, Columbus, OH.)

excess CSF. Despite arrest of the process, serious mental retardation and neurologic sequelae are common.

Anencephaly and Microcephaly

Anencephaly and microcephaly are congenital fetal deformities in which the head is considerably smaller than normal. In anencephaly there is complete or partial absence of the brain and of the overlying skull. Because the pituitary gland is absent or vestigial, the adrenal cortex is diminutive (for lack of adrenocorticotropic hormone [ACTH] stimulation). About 70% of anencephalic infants are girls. This condition commonly is accompanied by hydramnios. The cause of anencephaly is unknown, but multiple environmental factors have been postulated. A 3% recurrence rate has been noted in familial histories. Anencephaly is incompatible with life; warmth and fluids are provided until the neonate's death, which usually occurs before the end of the first 24 hours after birth.

In microcephaly the head generally is well formed but small. X-ray exposure of the woman may result in fetal microcephaly. Rubella, CMV, and perhaps other infectious processes are the causes in some cases. Microcephalic infants require specific nursing care and medical observation to appraise the extent of psychomotor retardation that almost always accompanies this abnormality. The nurse's supportive role with parents is considerable.

Cleft Lip or Palate

Cleft lip or palate is a common congenital midline fissure, or opening, in the lip or palate; one or both deformities may occur (Fig. 27-19). The incidence is approximately 1 in 700 white newborns and 1 in 2000 African-American newborns. Polygenetic factors are causative in some cases, but fetal viral infection, maternal corticosteroid therapy, radiation, dietary influence, and hypoxia have been associated factors. The combination of cleft lip and palate affects more male than female infants.

Treatment requires special feeding techniques, for example, the use of uniquely designed nipples. The cleft lip is repaired before palate repair and may be performed soon after birth if the newborn is free from infection, in good condition, and weighs at least 2500 g (5 lb 9 oz). Some clinicians suggest that lip repair (Fig. 27-20, *A*) is best undertaken when the infant weighs 4500 g (10 lb) or more because more tissue is available. Advantages of earlier labial (lip) repair include facilitating a positive parent-child relationship and permitting the infant to learn to use and strengthen musculature around the mouth. Infants with palatolabial fissures often look grotesque and repulsive to the parents. After initial labial repair and with collaborative health team support, the mother commonly is able to assume responsibility for the newborn's care until palatal repair is feasible (Fig. 27-20,

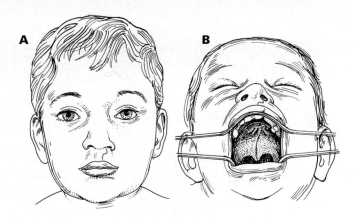

FIG. 27-20 Surgical repair of unilateral complete cleft lip **(A)** and of unilateral complete cleft palate **(B).** (Courtesy Ross Laboratories, Columbus, OH.)

B). Repair usually occurs between 16 and 24 months of age (9 kg [20 lb] body weight or more). The plastic surgeon, pediatrician, orthodontist, hospital and community nurses, speech therapist, and social worker comprise the collaborative health team that has made possible the effective treatment available today. Until repair of the palate is performed, a prosthesis is fitted to aid the infant's feeding and speech development and to reduce respiratory tract infections.

Musculoskeletal Disorders

The two most common musculoskeletal deviations seen in the neonatal period are congenital dysplasia of the hip and congenital clubfoot. Both conditions are easily recognized. Early detection and definitive treatment are mandatory for successful correction. Delay makes repair more difficult and prognosis less favorable.

Congenital Hip Dysplasia

Also known as *congenital dislocation of the hip,* hip dysplasia is an often hereditary disorder occurring more commonly in girls because of the structure of the pelvis. In this condition the acetabulum is abnormally shallow. The head of the femur becomes dislocated upward and backward to lie on the dorsal aspect of the ilium. The pressure of the displaced femoral head may form a false acetabulum on the ilium. A stretched joint capsule results, and ossification of the femoral head is delayed.

Before dislocation occurs, reduced movement, splinting of the affected hip, limited abduction, and asymmetry of the hip may be noted. After dislocation, all these signs are present, together with the external rotation and shortening of the leg. A clicking sound may be noted on gentle forced abduction of the leg (Ortolani's sign), and a bulge of the femoral head is felt or seen. X-ray films reveal a deformity in congenital dysplasia of the hip.

Treatment involves pressing the femoral head into the acetabulum to form an adequate socket before ossifica-

tion is complete. Several abduction devices such as the following are available:

- Thick diapers abduct and externally rotate the leg and flex the hip (pin anterior flaps of diapers under posterior flaps). Double or triple disposable diapers also can be used.
- The Pavlik harness is worn continuously for 3 to 6 months (see Fig. 14-12).
- A spica cast is used to maintain abduction, extension, and internal rotation when a stable reduction cannot be maintained with other devices (Schaming et al, 1990).

Polydactyly

Extra digits on the hands or feet occur occasionally. In some instances polydactyly is hereditary. If there is little or no bone involvement, the extra digit is tied with silk suture soon after birth. The finger falls off within a few days, leaving a small scar. When there is bone involvement, surgical repair is indicated.

Genitourinary Tract Anomalies

Abnormally low-set or misshapen ears may indicate other, often genitourinary, anomalies (such as renal agenesis).

Exstrophy of the Bladder

Exstrophy of the bladder (Fig. 27-21) is a rare congenital anomaly of unknown cause. With this anomaly a separation of the symphysis pubis and anterior abdominal wall structures results in exteriorization of the bladder trigone and surrounding mucosa. The exposed mucosa is deep red, has numerous folds, and is sensitive to touch. A direct passage of urine to the outside occurs. The infant should be examined for associated anomalies, such as undescended testes, inguinal hernia, absence of the vagina, and bowel defects. Surgical correction, often elimination of the bladder and construction of an ileal conduit, rarely is justified in the neonatal period. A prosthesis for collection of the urine and protection of the bladder may be employed.

Nursing management in the presence of exstrophy of the bladder focuses on the prevention of urinary tract infection and ulceration of adjacent skin from the constant seepage of urine. The child's touching and cuddling needs are met. Parents require considerable support and teaching to care for the defect if surgery is scheduled when the infant is several weeks or months of age.

Hypospadias and Epispadias

Hypospadias is a developmental anomaly in which the urethral meatus is placed lower than normal. In a male infant the meatus opens in the midline of the undersurface of the penis or on the perineum. In a female infant the meatus opens into the vagina. This condition tends to be hereditary.

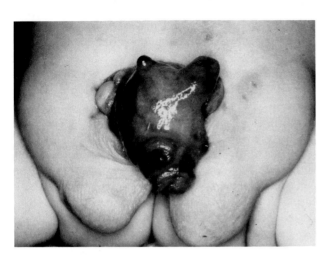

FIG. 27-21 Exstrophy of bladder. (Courtesy Edward S Tank, MD, Division of Urology, University of Oregon Health Sciences Center, Portland.)

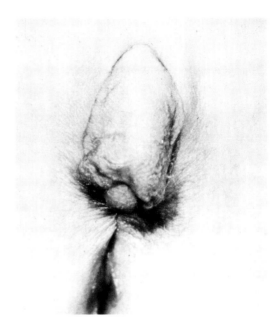

FIG. 27-22 Ambiguous external genitals (e.g., structure can be enlarged clitoral hood and clitoris or malformed penis). (Courtesy Edward S Tank, MD, Division of Urology, University of Oregon Health Sciences Center, Portland.)

Epispadias, also occurring in both sexes but predominating in boys, is a congenital absence of the upper urethral wall. In girls it often is associated with exstrophy of the bladder. In boys the meatal opening is located anywhere along the dorsum (upper side) of the penis.

Most instances of hypospadias are minor and require no corrective surgery. Pronounced defects require extensive urethroplasty. If needed, surgery is completed before the boy enters school so that he can urinate from a standing position like other boys. The more serious defects often coexist with other, multiple anomalies.

Nursing management of the physical care of the infant with hypospadias is the same as that for the normal infant. Should urethroplasty be required, circumcision is not performed because the foreskin is used in the surgical procedure. The parents are taught how to care for the urethral meatus and foreskin to prevent infection and to promote cleanliness.

Sexual Ambiguity

Sexual ambiguity in the newborn (Fig. 27-22) often is discovered by the nurse, who usually is the first one to perform a physical assessment.

Erroneous or abnormal sexual differentiation may be a genetic aberration (e.g., congenital adrenal hypoplasia), or it may be caused by maternal problems (such as steroid sex hormone therapy for threatened abortion). It is imperative to establish the genetic sex and the sex of child rearing as soon as possible. Early determination of genetic sex is important to permit the surgical correction of anomalies before an individual or social pattern is set. Prompt consultation with a surgeon who is experienced in the area of intersexuality should be arranged without delay. Meanwhile, parents need supportive care as they await the decision.

Teratoma

Teratoma, a solid or semisolid neoplasm, is composed of the three embryonal tissue types (ectoderm, mesoderm, endoderm). A teratoma in the newborn may occur in the skull, mediastinum, or abdomen. A solid or semisolid tumor in the sacral area also may prove to be a teratoma. It is protected by sterile dressings before surgical removal. Many teratomas diagnosed in the newborn are malignant. If the lesion cannot be removed entirely by surgery, x-ray therapy and chemotherapy are used. Long-term survival rate for infants with sacrococcygeal teratoma is 85% after surgical removal in the neonatal period. The survival rate is only 50% if surgery is delayed until the infant is more than 1 month old. Rectal and anal function can always be preserved.

Parental Support

Clarifying information is an important nursing function. A newly diagnosed disorder often implies the implementation of a therapeutic regimen. For example, the disorder in question may be an inborn error of metabolism such as PKU or galactosemia that requires consistent and rigid adherence to a diet. The family may need help to secure the necessary formula and counseling from dietetic services. The importance of maintaining the diet, especially keeping an adequate supply of special preparations and avoiding unauthorized substitutions, must be impressed on the family.

Referral to appropriate agencies is another essential part of the follow-up management. Many organizations and foundations help provide services and equipment for affected children, for example, the Cystic Fibrosis Foundation and the Muscular Dystrophy Association. Early Infant Stimulation Foundation programs are available for a child with Down syndrome. There also are numerous parent groups with whom the family can share experiences and derive mutual support in coping with similar problems. Nurses need to become familiar with services available in their community that provide assistance and education to families with these special problems (see Appendix H).

Probably the most important of all nursing functions is providing *emotional support* to the family during all aspects of the care of the child born with a defect or disorder. Feelings that are generated under the real or imagined threat posed by a genetic disorder are as varied as the persons being counseled. Responses may include all stress reactions, such as apathy, denial, anger, hostility, fear, embarrassment, grief, and loss of self-esteem.

Parents benefit from seeing before and after pictures of other babies born with the same defect. Coupled with other verbal and nonverbal supportive care, this visual reassurance is effective. Parents can be referred to other parents (or organizations of parents such as the Cleft Palate Club) for continuing mutual support.

Guilt and self-blame are universal reactions. Many look on the disorder as a stigma—especially if the disorder is visible to others. Knowledgeable persons involved with the family often are able to dispel fears and even absolve the family from guilt simply by explaining the random nature of cell division and segregation. Parents may derive comfort from knowing that everyone carries defective genes, which, when combined with the same genes in a partner, can produce undesirable consequences. Old wives' tales, superstitions, and long-held misconceptions are all factors that may influence a parents' reaction to a disorder. Religious beliefs, intellectual level, and prior attitudes toward the disease affect the way in which families respond.

The attitude of other family members and relatives can have a significant impact on some persons—especially situations in which the cause can be pinpointed (such as a dominant or an X-linked disorder). Recessive disorders are less likely to cause blaming because both partners carry the defective gene. Unfortunately most families tend to view a congenital disorder as shameful. Its presence in a family may cause altered plans for marriage or childbearing even when the probability of recurrence is no more than a random risk. The way a family views the probability of recurrence varies tremendously. For example, one family will consider a 10% risk as reassuring, whereas another may consider it too great a risk to contemplate marriage or childbearing.

The nature of a newborn's condition also influences the way families respond to a disorder. Factors such as the severity or chronicity of a disease, the age of onset,

the threat of early death, a lengthy period of deterioration, presence or absence of pain, mental retardation, or cosmetic disfiguration all determine the impact a condition has on a family. One family may risk having a child with a disorder that produces a minor defect or even an early death but will not risk having a child with a lifelong physical or mental disability.

Sometimes counselors and other health personnel create barriers through their own attitudes toward a specific disease. It is often difficult to be nonjudgmental and objective in all instances. Nurses may intentionally or unintentionally influence families in making decisions. This is especially true when the client's intellectual level makes it difficult or impossible for that person to comprehend the ramifications of a situation. Even persons who can repeat information accurately often fail to grasp its significance in their case. Families may pressure the nurse to make decisions for them with questions such as, "What would you do if you were me?"

Families and individuals need ongoing education, guidance, and support (Sammons, Lewis, 1985). They should be given the facts and possible consequences and all the assistance they need in problem solving, but the final decision regarding a course of action must be their own.

INFANT OF THE SUBSTANCE ABUSING MOTHER

Certain maternal behaviors result in perinatal risk. Maternal habits hazardous to the fetus and newborn are drug addiction, smoking, and alcohol abuse. Occasional withdrawal reactions have been reported in newborns of mothers who use to excess drugs such as barbiturates, alcohol, and amphetamines. Serious reactions are seen in newborns whose mothers abuse psychoactive drugs (see Chapter 23) or are treated with methadone. Almost 50% of pregnancies of women addicted to opioids result in LBW infants who are not necessarily preterm. Alcohol is a teratogen. Maternal ethanol abuse during gestation can cause a readily identifiable fetal alcohol syndrome (FAS).

The adverse effects of exposure of the fetus to drugs are varied. They include transient behavioral changes such as fetal breathing movements or irreversible effects such as fetal death, IUGR, structural malformations, and mental retardation. Some maternal drug use is for the pharmacologic control of disease processes (e.g., insulin) or for symptomatic relief of benign problems (e.g., aspirin). It has been shown that 92% to 100% of all pregnant women take at least one physician-prescribed drug, and 65% to 80% also take self-prescribed drugs. In addition to the therapeutic use of drugs, the nontherapeutic use of drugs—such as alcohol, nicotine, and narcotics—poses threats to fetal well-being. Critical determinants of

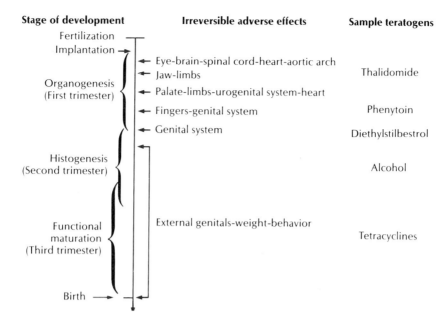

FIG. 27-23   Critical periods in human embryogenesis. (From Fanaroff AA, Martin RJ, editors: *Neonatal-perinatal medicine: diseases of the fetus and infant,* ed 5, St Louis, 1992, Mosby.)

the effect of the drug on the fetus include the specific drug, the dosage, the route of administration, the genotype of the mother or fetus, and the timing of the drug exposure. Fig. 27-23 shows critical periods in human embryogenesis and the teratogenic effects of drugs.

Care Management

✤ ASSESSMENT

Assessment of the newborn requires a review of the mother's prenatal record. A medical and social history of drug abuse and detoxification is noted. Some obstetric problems are seen in pregnancies complicated by substance abuse. The obstetric events include PROM, amnionitis, preterm labor, precipitous labor, abruptio placentae, placenta previa, and spontaneous abortion. Perinatal and neonatal mortality and morbidity also occur. There is an increase in stillbirths and in the births of newborns who have IUGR or are LBW and preterm.

The woman who is addicted to narcotics may have infections that compound the risk to the infant. These infections include hepatitis, septicemia, and STDs, including AIDS (Niebyl, 1988).

The nurse often is the first to observe the signs of drug dependence in the newborn. The nurse's observations help other health care providers differentiate between drug dependence and other conditions, such as tracheoesophageal fistula, CNS disorder, sepsis, hypoglycemia, and electrolyte imbalance.

The newborn is assessed and the gestational age and maturity are noted. In utero exposure to some drugs results in observable malformations or dysmorphism (ab-

normality of shape). Neonatal behavior may arouse suspicion. Lethargy, decreased visual alertness and auditory response to the Brazelton neonatal behavioral assessment scale, or withdrawal symptoms are noted. Urine screening may be used to identify substances abused by the mother. Because many women are multidrug users, the newborn infant initially may exhibit a confusing complex of signs.

✤ NURSING DIAGNOSES

The following nursing diagnoses, which depend on the assessment findings, are tailored to the individual needs of the newborn and the family.

Newborn

High risk for infection related to
- Maternal risk behaviors
- PROM

Altered growth and development related to
- Effects of maternal substance abuse

Sleep pattern disturbance related to
- Drug withdrawal

Parents

Actual or potential altered parenting related to
- Continuation of substance abuse or detoxification program
- Guilt about infant's condition
- Inability to cope with care needs of a special infant

Anxiety related to knowledge deficit related to
- Care needs of an affected infant

High risk for violence, self-directed or directed toward infant, related to
- Drug-dependent lifestyle

✤ EXPECTED OUTCOMES

Planning for care of the newborn presents a challenge to the health care team. Parents are included in the planning for the newborn's care and also are encouraged to plan for their own care. A multidisciplinary approach is needed that includes home health or community resource personnel (e.g., regulatory agencies such as child protective services).

Expected outcomes are stated in patient-centered terms and include the following:

1. The newborn will suffer no adverse sequelae to drug withdrawal.
2. The infant's malformations and dysfunction will be identified, and appropriate curative and rehabilitative measures will be instituted.
3. Parents will accept the newborn's condition and participate in the newborn's management.

✤ COLLABORATIVE CARE

Education and social support to prevent the abuse of drugs provide the ideal approach. However, given the scope of the drug abuse problem, total prevention is unrealistic.

Nursing care of the drug-dependent newborn involves supportive therapy for fluid and electrolyte balance, nutrition, infection control, and respiratory care. Medications are given as ordered. The newborn's narcotic withdrawal signs may require a schedule of weaning from the drug. Phenobarbital—6 mg per kilogram of body weight every 24 hours administered intramuscularly—or 2 mg given orally four times a day for 3 or 4 days may be ordered. The dosage is reduced by one third every 2 days for about 2 weeks, at which time treatment is discontinued. Paregoric may be ordered: 2 to 4 drops per kilogram orally every 4 to 6 hours initially to as much as 20 to 30 drops per kilogram orally every 4 to 6 hours, depending on the symptoms.

Swaddling, holding, reducing stimuli, and feeding as necessary may be helpful in easing withdrawal.

Drug dependence in the newborn is physiologic, not psychologic. Thus a predisposition to dependence later in life is not thought to be a factor. However, the psychosocial environment in which the infant is raised may create a tendency to addiction.

The mother requires considerable support. Her need for and her abuse of drugs result in a decreased capacity to cope. The newborn's withdrawal signs and decreased consolability stress her coping abilities even further. Home health care, treatment for addiction, and education are important considerations. Sensitive exploration of the woman's options for the care of her infant and herself and for future fertility management may help her see that she has choices. This approach helps communicate respect for the new mother as a person who can make responsible decisions.

✤ EVALUATION

Final evaluation may not be possible. Short-term expected outcomes include the following examples:
- The newborn suffers no adverse sequelae to drug withdrawal.
- The infant's malformations and dysfunction are identified, and appropriate curative and rehabilitative measures are instituted.
- The parents come to terms with the newborn's condition and management.

However, both the infant and the parent have long-term needs. The extent to which expected outcomes have been achieved may not be known for years.

Alcohol

The incidence of **fetal alcohol syndrome (FAS)** in the United States is about 2.2 in 1000 live births, and worldwide it is 1.9 in 1000 births. Milder effects may be seen in as high as 23 to 29 in 1000 births (Barbour, 1990; Eliason, Williams, 1990).

According to Barbour (1990) FAS is a set of symptoms that includes prenatal and postnatal growth retardation and CNS malfunctions, including mental retardation. Infants born to social or modest drinkers may exhibit *fetal alcohol effects (FAE)*. These effects run the gamut from learning disabilities and behavioral problems to speech and language problems and hyperactivity. Often these problems are not detected until the child goes to school and learning problems become evident.

Predictable abnormal patterns of fetal and neonatal morphogenesis are attributed to severe, chronic alcoholism in women who continue to drink heavily during pregnancy. The pattern of growth deficiency begun in prenatal life persists after birth, especially in the linear growth rate, rate of weight gain, and growth of head circumferences.

Ocular structural anomalies are common findings (Fig. 27-24). Limb anomalies and a variety of cardiocirculatory anomalies, especially ventricular septal defects, pose problems for the child. Mental retardation (IQ of 79 or below at 7 years of age) and fine motor dysfunction (poor hand-to-mouth coordination, weak grasp) add to the handicapping problems that maternal alcoholism can impose. Genital abnormalities are seen in daughters of alcohol-addicted mothers. Two thirds of newborns with FAS are girls; the cause of this altered sex birth ratio is unknown. Severe and chronic alcoholism (ethanol toxicity), not maternal malnutrition, is responsible for the severity and consistency of postnatal perfor-

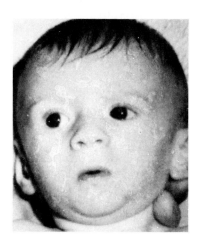

FIG. 27-24 Fetal alcohol anomaly. (Courtesy Dr. Charles Linder, Medical College of Georgia. From Goodman RM, Gorlin RJ: *Atlas of the face in genetic disorders,* ed 2, St Louis, 1977, Mosby.)

mance problems (Fanaroff, Martin, 1992). High alcohol levels are lethal to the developing embryo. Lower levels cause brain and other malformations. Long-term prognosis (no studies are available as yet) is discouraging even in an optimum psychosocial environment, when one considers the combination of growth failure and mental retardation.

Alcohol effects, however, depend not only on the amount of alcohol consumed but on the interaction of quantity, frequency, type of alcohol, and other drug abuse. Other drugs such as cigarettes, caffeine, and marijuana may potentiate the fetal effects of alcohol consumption during gestation (Fanaroff, Martin, 1992).

The newborn of a mother who abuses alcohol is faced with a number of clinical problems. Identification of the problems leads to the medical diagnosis of FAS. The newborn may suffer respiratory distress related to preterm birth, neurologic damage, and a floppy epiglottis and small trachea. Tracheoepiglottal anomalies may cause cardiopulmonary arrest. Other disorders include recurrent otitis media and hearing loss. Craniofacial features may be important in diagnosing craniofacial and oral anomalies, dental development abnormalities, and long-term body growth patterns (Jackson, Hussain, 1990). Feeding difficulties are related to preterm birth, poor sucking ability, and possible cleft palate. The newborn may exhibit brain dysfunction, microcephaly, and grand mal seizures.

Long-term effects into childhood may include impaired visual-motor perception and performance, lowered IQ scores, and delayed receptive and expressive language (Hill, Hegemier, Tennyson, 1990), as well as reduced capacity to process and store factual data (Becker, Warr-Leeper, Leeper, 1990). FAS follows the infant into childhood and adulthood with continuing negative results. It is now recognized as one of the leading causes

of mental retardation in the United States. Although the distinctive facial features of the infant tend to become less evident, the mental capacities never become normal. Long-term effects of the disorder persist, manifested in low IQ scores, poor ability in mathematics, distractibility, and poor judgment (Streissguth et al, 1991).

Nursing care involves many of the same strategies used for the care of preterm infants. Special efforts are made to involve the parents in their child's care and to encourage opportunities for parent-child attachment. The application of the nursing process to the care of a newborn with FAS is presented in the Plan of Care (p. 810).

Children placed in a warm, caring environment with an understanding caregiver who can deal with the infant's hyperirritability can be helped to lead a more normal existence than their condition might warrant (Barbour, 1989). These caregivers provide extensive cuddling and human contact and can deal with the eating problems that commonly lead to a diagnosis of *failure to thrive.*

Tobacco

Pregnant women need to be aware of the harmful effects of smoking on their unborn baby's health. Cigarette smoking in pregnancy is associated with birth weight deficits of up to 250 g for a full-term neonate (Fanaroff, Martin, 1992). Maternal cigarette smoking is implicated in 21% to 39% of LBW infants. The rate of preterm birth is increased. Nicotine and cotinine, the two pharmacologically active substances in tobacco, are found in higher concentrations in infants whose mothers smoke. These substances can be secreted in breast milk for up to 2 hours after the mother has smoked. Cigarette smoke contains more than 2000 compounds, including carbon monoxide, dioxin, cyanide, and cadmium. Long-term studies show residual effects beyond the neonatal period (Niebyl, 1988). Deficits in growth, in intellectual and emotional development, and in behavior have been documented.

The fetal tobacco syndrome is a diagnostic term applicable to infants who fit the following criteria (Nieberg et al, 1985):

1. The mother smoked five or more cigarettes a day throughout pregnancy.
2. The mother had no evidence of hypertension during pregnancy, specifically (a) no preeclampsia and (b) documentation of normal blood pressure at least once after the first trimester.
3. The newborn has symmetric growth retardation at term (up to or greater than 37 weeks), defined as (a) a birth weight less than 2500 g and (b) a ponderal index ([weight in g]/[length in m]) greater than 2.32.
4. There is no other obvious cause of IUGR (e.g., congenital infection or anomaly).

Mothers (and all others) need to refrain from smok-

PLAN OF CARE

Fetal Alcohol Syndrome

Case History
Albert was born 3 hours ago. His birth weight was 5½ lb (2464 g). His mother, age 24, drank heavily during the pregnancy. Albert exhibits clinical problems of FAS: microcephaly, hypotonia, irritability, poor suck, and increased respiratory effort. Both his mother and father are anxious to care for their baby.

EXPECTED OUTCOMES	IMPLEMENTATION	RATIONALE	EVALUATION
Nursing Diagnosis: Ineffective breathing pattern related to FAS			
Albert will maintain a patent airway. Albert will be able to maintain adequate ventilation by his own respiratory effort.	Place Albert in position where he exhibits least distress (prone or side). Suction mouth and nose as necessary. Implement seizure precautions. Have resuscitation equipment available. Place Albert on cardiopulmonary monitor (set close alarm limits).	Hypotonia and poor suck predispose Albert to distress from diminished ability to handle secretions and fluids; seizures may occur as Albert withdraws from alcohol.	Albert maintains a patent airway. Albert maintains adequate ventilation through his own respiratory effort. Albert has no seizures.
Nursing Diagnosis: Altered nutrition, less than body requirements, related to irritability and poor suck			
Albert will ingest and retain nutrients sufficient for growth.	Elevate Albert's head during and after feeding. Feed in small frequent amounts. Evaluate different nipples for feeding. Burp well after feedings. Feed by oral gavage as necessary. Obtain daily weight; maintain strict intake and output. Keep suction ready to use; aspirate nares as circumstances require.	Engages gravity to help fluids move downward to gastrointestinal tract. Prevents overfilling of stomach to diminish chance of aspiration. Compensates for infant's poor suck. Diminishes chance of aspiration. Provides nourishment as needed. Evaluates feeding method. Diminishes chance of aspiration.	Albert takes and retains enough nutrients for growth.

PLAN OF CARE—cont'd

Fetal Alcohol Syndrome

EXPECTED OUTCOMES	IMPLEMENTATION	RATIONALE	EVALUATION

Nursing Diagnosis: Altered family processes related to need to care for and love a child with a handicap, as well as lack of knowledge of infant's special needs and expected sequelae

EXPECTED OUTCOMES	IMPLEMENTATION	RATIONALE	EVALUATION
Albert will be successfully cared for by his parents. Parents will learn about infant's special needs. Parents will begin process of bonding and attachment to Albert.	Encourage frequent parental visits to the special care nursery, and promote physical contact with Albert. Teach parents about Albert's anomalies and their possible sequelae. Help parents state concerns. Be realistic when discussing Albert's potential for future development. Involve the parents in Albert's care (diapering, holding, bathing).	Parent-child bonding and attachment are essential for well-being of parent and child. Knowledge and practice increase parents' self-confidence and perhaps self-esteem and sense of some control over the situation.	Parents learn about Albert's anomalies and their possible effects on the child's future. Parents recognize and eventually accept Albert's handicaps. Parents verbalize their concerns. Parents learn and demonstrate child-care activities.
	Refer to outside resources (e.g., infant developmental/stimulation programs). Introduce parents to CPR skills; observe return demonstration.	Mobilization of community resources provides reassurance.	Parents utilize community resources as needed.

ing near the newborn infant. There is an increasing concern over second-hand smoke and its potential effects on infants. Several studies have reported a positive association between maternal smoking and SIDS (Niebyl, 1988). It is not clear whether this association reflects in utero exposure or passive exposure postnatally, or both.

Marijuana

Marijuana is believed to be the most abused drug in the United States, with an estimated 20 million users. It crosses the placenta. Its use during pregnancy may result in a shortened gestation and a higher incidence of precipitous labor (less than 3 hours) (Niebyl, 1988). Some investigators have found a higher incidence of meconium staining (Fanaroff, Martin, 1992; Niebyl, 1988). No increased incidence of congenital complications or effects on the infant's growth and physical parameters specific to marijuana use alone have been identified. However, the use of marijuana with alcohol results in decreased birth weight and a fivefold increase in risk for FAS. Compounding this issue is multidrug use, especially among adolescents, thus combining the harmful effects of marijuana, tobacco, alcohol, and cocaine. Long-term follow-up studies on exposed infants are needed.

Cocaine

Cocaine is another commonly abused drug among all social classes. It is the most powerfully addictive drug available. It is often used with other drugs such as marijuana and alcohol. Its use is blamed for a higher incidence of spontaneous abortion and abruptio placentae secondary to frequent episodes of vasospastic hypertension. It crosses the placenta and is found in breast milk.

Infants born to cocaine-abusing mothers show a high rate of perinatal morbidity, IUGR, microcephaly, preterm birth, cerebral hemorrhage or infarction, and congenital anomalies (Chasnoff, 1989). Cocaine-dependent newborns often experience significant and agonizing symptoms that can last 2 to 3 weeks or longer. Irritability, marked nervousness, rapid changes in mood, and hypersensitivity to noise and external stimuli characterize the infant's behavior. These neonates exhibit poor feeding, irregular sleep patterns, tachypnea, tachycardia, and often diarrhea. Chasnoff et al (1989) identified significant depression in interactive behavior and a poor organization response to environmental stimuli.

The infants exposed to cocaine typically have visual attention problems in that they are unable to focus on their parent's face. These children often have been subjected to numerous small strokes because of abrupt changes in their mothers' blood pressure during pregnancy. Renal problems, lack of coordination, developmental retardation, and perhaps visual problems may be related. There may be an increased risk for SIDS (Bauchner et al, 1988; Chasnoff et al, 1989).

Heroin

Heroin crosses the placenta. Of the infants born to heroin-addicted mothers, 50% are LBW and 50% are SGA. Heroin may have a direct growth-inhibiting effect on the fetus. There is an increased rate of stillbirths but not of congenital anomalies. Maternal detoxification during gestation is not advised because of the risk of fetal demise.

Heroin withdrawal occurs in 50% to 75% of infants born to addicted mothers, usually within the first 24 to 48 hours of life. The signs depend on the length of maternal addiction, the amount of drug taken, and the time of injection before birth. The infant whose mother is taking methadone may not demonstrate signs of withdrawal until a week or so after birth. The symptoms of newborns whose mothers used heroin or methadone are similar. Initially the infant may be depressed. The withdrawal syndrome may consist of a combination of any of the following signs. The newborn may be jittery and hyperactive. Commonly the newborn's cry is shrill and persistent. The infant may yawn or sneeze frequently. The deep tendon reflexes are increased, but the Moro reflex is decreased. The neonate may exhibit poor feeding and sucking, tachypnea, vomiting, diarrhea, hypothermia or hyperthermia, and sweating. In addition, an abnormal sleep cycle, with absence of quiet sleep and disturbance of active sleep, has been described in these infants (Fanaroff, Martin, 1992).

If withdrawal is not treated, vomiting, diarrhea, dehydration, apnea, and convulsions may develop. Death may follow. Therapy is individualized. Dehydration and electrolyte imbalance are prevented or treated. Usually the following drugs are ordered: phenobarbital, paregoric (compound tincture of opium), or diazepam, singly or in combination.

The long-term effect on these newborns is being studied. Researchers have found that "many serious" mental and physical problems are evident in the child's first few months of life, as well as "numerous indications . . . [of] serious abnormalities in the brain structure that will not be revealed until later years" (Howard, 1986).

Methadone

Methadone, a synthetic opiate, has been the therapy of choice for heroin addiction since 1965. By blocking the euphoric effects, it reduces the craving for heroin. It does cross the placenta. An increasing number of infants have been born to methadone-maintained mothers, who seem to have better prenatal care and a somewhat better lifestyle than those taking heroin (Fanaroff, Martin, 1992).

There is some question as to the benefits of methadone therapy during pregnancy because of its effect on the fetus. In one study (Davis, Templer, 1988) children exposed to methadone in utero demonstrated more pathologic problems and scored significantly lower on IQ testing than did those who had been exposed to heroin. These findings question the benefits of methadone treatment for pregnant heroin abusers and the related ethical issues. Multiple drug abuse, however, is a problem for many. The drugs include alcohol, barbiturates, tranquilizers, and other psychoactive drugs. Many of these women are heavy smokers as well. Methadone withdrawal occurs in about 70% to 90% of newborns born to these women.

Methadone withdrawal resembles heroin withdrawal syndrome but tends to be more severe and prolonged. In addition, the incidence of seizures is higher. Seizures usually occur between days 7 and 10. The infants exhibit a disturbed sleep pattern similar to that seen in heroin withdrawal. The newborns have higher birth weight, usually appropriate for gestational age. No increased incidence of congenital anomalies is seen.

Late-onset withdrawal occurs at 2 to 4 weeks and may continue for weeks or months. A higher incidence of SIDS also has been reported in these infants. This factor is important for perinatal nurses who coordinate follow-up care for the infant and education for the mother or other caregiver. That is, community health nurses need to know about the potential for withdrawal symptoms to occur.

Therapy for methadone withdrawal is similar to that for heroin withdrawal. The few available follow-up studies of these infants reveal a higher incidence of hyperactivity, learning and behavior disorders, and poor social adjustment (Fanaroff, Martin, 1992).

Phencyclidine (Angel Dust)

Phencyclidine (PCP) is one of the most dangerous of the available abused drugs. It may have extremely unpredictable, bizarre, and violent effects, especially when combined with crack (cocaine free base) (a combination known as "space base"). PCP increases the risk of injury to the user and therefore also to her passively dependent fetus. The user may be unaware that she is ingesting PCP because it commonly is misrepresented as another drug of abuse or mixed with other drugs.

PCP crosses the placenta and is found in breast milk. Literature about newborns is limited. The infants exposed to PCP appear to be alert, active babies. "Their mothers often think they are smarter. They hold their heads up faster. . . . But, in fact, it is abnormal behavior. Although we aren't sure why, the tone of the muscles in the head is of the kind that we see in [children with] cerebral palsy," a disorder of the CNS characterized by spastic paralysis or other forms of defective motor ability (Bean, 1986).

Miscellaneous Substances

Methamphetamine ("ice") is one of the most potent stimulants available. It is used commonly by adolescents and young adults. The fetal and neonatal effects of maternal use of methamphetamine in pregnancy are not well known, but they appear to mimic the effects of cocaine and seem to be dose related. LBW, preterm birth, and perinatal mortality may be consequences of higher doses used throughout pregnancy. Newborns may be drowsy and jittery and may also experience respiratory distress soon after birth. Lethargy may continue for several months, along with frequent infections and poor weight gain. Emotional disturbances and delays in gross and fine motor coordination may be seen during early childhood.

Phenobarbital is another commonly abused drug in all social classes. It crosses the placenta readily and is subsequently found in high levels in the fetal liver and brain. Because of its slow metabolic rate, when withdrawal does occur, onset is generally at 2 to 14 days after birth and duration is about 2 to 4 months. Irritability, crying, hiccoughs, and sleepiness mark the initial response. During the second stage the infant is extremely hungry, regurgitates and gags frequently, and demonstrates episodic irritability, sweating, and a disturbed sleep pattern.

Treatment consists of swaddling, frequent feedings, and protection from noxious external stimuli. If there is no improvement with the use of these methods, the newborn should be given phenobarbital and then slowly withdrawn from this drug after control of symptoms (Fanaroff, Martin, 1992).

Caffeine has not been implicated as a teratogen in humans, but it may be a factor in the incidence of preterm labor and birth (McDonald, Armstrong, Sloan, 1992). The FDA (1980) suggests that "prudence dictates that pregnant women and those who may become pregnant avoid caffeine-containing products or use them sparingly."

DISCHARGE TO HOME FOR THE COMPROMISED NEWBORN

Discharge planning for the compromised newborn begins on admission. The admission history should include important information regarding the family of the infant that can affect discharge. Who makes up the immediate family? Does the mother have others who depend on her for support? How are they being taken care of during this period?

Questions about the home environment should be asked as soon as possible. Is there gas or electric heating in the home, or is the family dependent on a fireplace or wood-burning stove? Is there access to a telephone for emergencies? Is there a home at all, or is the family living in a shelter? Problems posed by these questions require the intervention of social services and can take a long time to resolve.

Successful discharge of the compromised infants to their home or community hospital requires a multidisciplinary approach. Medical, nursing, and social services are crucial to the smooth transition of these infants and their families to the community and home. If the infant is transported back to the community hospital that referred either the mother before birth or the infant after birth, interfacility communication is essential to continuity of care.

Discharge to home, whether from the regional center or community hospital setting, requires parental competence. Discharge teaching begins as soon as the infant is stable and the parents wish to become involved in the care. Discharge teaching must include normal newborn care as well as specific information pertinent to the medical condition of the infant. Discharge teaching for the compromised newborn is extensive, requires time, and cannot be adequately accomplished on the day of discharge. Important considerations in the discharge teaching of the parents of compromised newborns are listed in the Teaching Approaches box below.

Discharge to home for compromised infants does not mean they can be treated like normal newborns. Follow-up by a pediatrician or nurse practitioner familiar with the complications common to the compromised newborn is essential. Further follow-up of specific complications by qualified specialists and referral to high-risk centers for developmental interventions can help ensure the best outcome possible for these fragile infants.

TEACHING APPROACHES

DISCHARGE TEACHING FOR PARENTS OF COMPROMISED NEWBORNS

Discharge teaching includes (but is not limited to) the following:
- Helping parents understand their baby's condition
- Infant/child car safety
- Safety measures in the home
- Feeding
- Elimination
- Bathing
- Cord care
- Taking the baby's temperature
- Medication administration
- CPR for infants
- Impact of environmental factors (maintaining thermoregulation at home)
- Teaching related to the infant's specific condition (signs and symptoms of deterioration, etc.)
- Developmental concerns related to their infant
- Follow-up appointments/consultations

KEY POINTS

- Infection in the newborn may be acquired in utero, during birth, during resuscitation, and from within the nursery.
- Preterm infants are at risk for problems related to the immaturity of organ systems.
- Nurses who work with preterm infants have an important role: to observe for respiratory distress and other early symptoms of physiologic functioning problems.
- Parental adaptation to preterm infants is different from that of parents who have given birth to full-term infants.
- The high incidence of fetal distress among postmature infants is related to progressive placental insufficiency.
- Prepregnancy planning and good diabetic control, coupled with strict diabetic control during pregnancy, may prevent the embryonic/fetal/neonatal conditions associated with pregnancies complicated by diabetes mellitus.

- Hyperbilirubinemia has a variety of etiologic factors, including maternal-fetal Rh and ABO incompatibility.
- Major congenital defects are now the leading cause of death in term neonates born to mothers who had good perinatal care.
- The curative and rehabilitative problems of a child with a congenital disorder are often complex, requiring a multidisciplinary approach to care.
- Providing high-quality perinatal care to a varied population with multiple conditions is complicated by the special needs of high-risk drug-dependent pregnant women.
- Rehabilitative measures must be included in the plan for care for the newborn and the parent to offer the infant an opportunity for optimum growth and development after discharge.

CRITICAL THINKING EXERCISES

1. Review and discuss the medical and nursing records of infants whose mothers experienced a diabetic pregnancy. Identify the findings that identified the particular risk(s) to the infants. Discuss the nursing and medical management of the infants. Compare the finding with the text.

2. You have been assigned to care for Emilie Gibson, an 18-year-old, unwed mother who has just given birth to a son, John who has a cleft lip and palate. You are bringing the baby to the mother for the first time.
   a. Identify your feelings about the infant and his physical defect.
   b. Anticipate how the mother is likely to react to this encounter.

References

Als H, Brazelton TB: A new model of assessing the behavioral organization in preterm and full term infants, *J Am Acad Child Psychiatry* 20:239, 1981.

Anderson GC: Current knowledge about skin-to-skin (kangaroo) care for preterm infants, *J Perinat* 11:216, 1991.

Angelini DJ, Whelan Knapp CM, Gibes RM: *Perinatal/neonatal nursing: a clinical handbook,* Boston, 1986, Blackwell Scientific Publications.

Bancalari E, Gerhardt T: Bronchopulmonary dysplasia, *Pediatr Clin North Am* 33:1, 1986.

Barbour BG: Alcohol and pregnancy, *J Nurse Midwife* 35:78, 1990.

Barbour BG: Is fetal alcohol syndrome completely irreversible? *MCN* 14:44, 1989.

Bauchner H et al: Risk of sudden infant death syndrome among infants with in utero exposure to cocaine, *J Pediatr* 113:831, 1988.

Bean Y: Report of ongoing research on the infants of mothers using cocaine and PCP, *Los Angeles Times,* Jan 1986.

Becker M, Warr-Leeper GA, Leeper HA: Fetal alcohol syndrome: a description of oral motor, articulatory, short-term memory, grammatical, and semantic abilities, *J Commun Disord* 23:97, 1990.

Bennett EC: Sexually transmitted diseases: current approaches, *NAACOG Newsletter* 14:1, 1987.

Brambati B et al: Genetic diagnosis before the eighth gestational week, *Obstet Gynecol* 77:318, 1991.

Brown AA et al: Effects on infants of a first episode of genital herpes during pregnancy, *N Engl J Med* 317(2):1249, 1987.

Chasnoff IJ: Cocaine, pregnancy, and the neonate, *Women Health* 15:23, 1989.

Chasnoff IJ et al: Prenatal cocaine exposure is associated with respiratory pattern abnormalities, *Am J Dis Child* 143:583, 1989.

Cherry SH, Merkatz IR: *Complications of pregnancy: medical, surgical, gynecologic, psychosocial, and perinatal,* ed 4, Baltimore, 1991, Williams & Wilkins.

Creasy R, Resnik R: *Maternal-fetal medicine: principles and practice,* ed 2, Philadelphia, 1989, WB Saunders.

Davis DD, Templer DI: Neurobehavioral functioning in children exposed to narcotics in utero, *Addict Behav* 13:275, 1988.

Eliason MJ, Williams JK: Fetal alcohol syndrome and the neonate, *J Perinat Neonat Nurs* 3:64, 1990.

Fanaroff AA, Martin RJ: *Neonatal-perinatal medicine: diseases of the fetus and infant*, ed 5, St Louis, 1992, Mosby.

Field TM: Interaction patterns of preterm and term infants. In Field TM, editor: *Infants born at risk*, Jamaica, NY, 1979, Spectrum Publications.

Food and Drug Administration: Caffeine and pregnancy, *FDA Drug Bull* 10:19, 1980.

Frigoletto FD, Little GA: *Guidelines for perinatal care*, ed 2, 1988, American Academy of Pediatrics and American College of Obstetricians and Gynecologists.

Greene MF, Benacerraf BR: Prenatal diagnosis in diabetic gravidas: utility of ultrasound and maternal serum alpha-fetoprotein screening, *Obstet Gynecol* 77:520, 1991.

Harnish DG et al: Early detection of HIV infection in a newborn, *N Engl J Med* 316:272, 1987.

Hill RM, Hegemier S, Tennyson LM: The fetal alcohol syndrome: a multihandicapped child, *Neurotoxicology* 10:585, 1990.

Hodson WA, Truog WE: *Critical care of the newborn*, ed 2, Philadelphia, 1989, WB Saunders.

Hoffman JI: Congenital heart disease: incidence and inheritance, *Pediatr Clin North Am* 37:31, 1990.

Howard J: Report of ongoing research on the infants of mothers using cocaine and PCP, *Los Angeles Times,* Jan 1986.

Jackson IT, Hussain K: Craniofacial and oral manifestations of fetal alcohol syndrome, *Plast Reconstr Surg* 85:505, 1990.

Johnson JP, Nair P, Alexander S: Early diagnosis of HIV infection in the neonate, *N Engl J Med* 316:273, 1987.

Korones S: *High-risk newborn infants: the basis for intensive nursing care*, ed 4, St Louis, 1986, Mosby.

Lemna WK et al: Mutation analysis for heterozygote detection and the prenatal diagnoses of cystic fibrosis, *N Engl J Med* 322:291, 1990.

McDonald A, Armstrong E, Sloan M: Cigarette, alcohol, and caffeine consumption and prematurity: public health brief, *Am J Public Health* 82(1)87, 1992.

Merenstein GB, Gardner SL: *Handbook of neonatal intensive care*, ed 3, St Louis, 1993, Mosby.

Nieberg P. et al: The fetal tobacco syndrome, *JAMA* 253:2998, 1985.

Niebyl JR: *Drug use in pregnancy*, ed 2, Philadelphia, 1988, Lea & Febiger.

Newman L: Parents' perceptions of their low birth weight infants, *Paediatrician* 9:182, 1980.

Philip A: *Neonatology: a practical guide*, ed 3, Philadelphia, 1987, WB Saunders.

Polin RA, Fox WW: *Fetal and neonatal physiology*, Philadelphia, 1992, WB Saunders.

Prenatal care and HIV screening, *JAMA* 258:2693, 1987 (letter to editor).

Prober CG: Low risk of herpes simplex virus infections in neonates exposed to the virus at the time of vaginal delivery to mothers with recurrent genital herpes simplex virus infections, *N Engl J Med* 316:240, 1987.

Pyun KH et al: Perinatal infection with human immunodeficiency virus: specific antibody responses by the neonate, *N Engl J Med* 317:611, 1987.

Sammons W, Lewis J: *Premature babies: a different beginning*, St Louis, 1985, Mosby.

Schaming D et al: When babies are born with orthopedic problems, *RN* 53(4):62, 1990.

Schraeder BD: Attachment and parenting despite lengthy intensive care, *MCN* 5:37, 1980.

Sosa R, Grua P: Perinatal responses to normal and premature birth experiences, *J Calif Perinat Assoc* 2:36, 1982.

Streissguth AP et al: Fetal alcohol syndrome in adolescents and adults, *JAMA* 265:1961, 1991.

Wenstrom K et al: Magnetic resonance imaging of fetuses with intracranial defects, *Obstet Gynecol* 77:529, 1991.

Whaley LF, Wong DL: *Nursing care of infants and children*, ed 5, St Louis 1995, Mosby.

Wolfe HM et al: Maternal obesity: a potential source of error in sonographic prenatal diagnosis, *Obstet Gynecol* 76:339, 1990.

Zacharias JF: The new genetics, *JOGNN* 19:122, 1990.

Bibliography

Becker PT et al: Outcomes of developmentally supportive nursing care for very low birth weight infants, *Nurs Res* 40:150, 1991.

Beckman CA: Postterm pregnancy: effects on temperature and glucose regulation, *Nurs Res* 39:21, 1990.

Boeckling AC: Exogenous surfactant therapy for premature infants, *J Perinat Neonat Nurs* 6(2)59, 1992.

Damato EG: Discharge planning from the neonatal intensive care unit, *J Perinat Neonat Nurs* 5:43, 1991.

Gennaro S et al: Concerns of mothers of low birthweight infants, *Pediatr Nurs* 16:459, 1990.

Harrison MJ: A comparison of parental interactions with term and preterm infants, *Res Nurs Health* 13:173, 1990.

Hoffman JI: Congenital heart disease: incidence and inheritance, *Pediatr Clin North Am* 37:31, 1990.

Kandall S et al: Relationship of maternal substance abuse to subsequent sudden infant death syndrome in offspring, *J Pediatr* 123(1):120, 1993.

Ladden M: The impact of preterm birth on the family and society: psychologic sequelae of preterm birth, *Pediatr Nurs* 16:515, 1990.

Ludington-Hoe SM, Hadeed AJ, Anderson GC: Physiologic responses to skin-to-skin contact in hospitalized premature infants, *J Perinat* 11:19, 1991.

Phibbs RH et al: Initial clinical trial of Exosurf, a protein-free synthetic surfactant, for the prophylaxis and early treatment of hyaline membrane disease, *Pediatrics* 88:1, 1991.

Pletsch PK: Birth defect prevention: nursing interventions, *JOGNN* 19:482, 1990.

Robbins JC: Diagnosis and management of neural-tube defects today, *N Engl J Med* 324:690, 1991.

Roberts PM: NEC: etiology, treatment, prevention, and nursing care, *Crit Care Nurse* 10(4):38, 1990.

Symanski ME: Action stat! Neonatal sepsis, *Nursing 91* 21:33, 1991.

Urrutia NL: Sorting the complexities of respiratory distress syndrome, *MCN* 16:308, 1991.

Walden M, Sala D: Controversies in the resuscitation of infants of borderline variability, *AWHONN's Clin Issu Perinat Womens Health Nurs* 4(1):570, 1993.

28

Loss and Grief

S A R A   R I C H   W H E E L E R

LEARNING OBJECTIVES

Define the key terms listed.

Describe the bereavement process, including physiologic, psychosocial, behavioral, and cultural grief responses to loss.

Formulate an example of an appropriate nursing diagnosis related to grief.

Describe how the nurse helps meet the special needs of the woman and her family experiencing loss and grief.

Develop expected outcome criteria to evaluate nursing care for grieving families.

Develop possible responses the nurse might use in caring for patients experiencing loss and grief.

KEY TERMS

anticipatory grief
bereavement
bittersweet grief
complicated bereavement
disorganization
ectopic pregnancy
grief responses
miscarriage
mourning
newborn death
reorganization
searching and yearning
shock and numbness
stillbirth

RELATED TOPICS

Cesarean birth *(Chap. 24)* • Ectopic pregnancy *(Chap. 21)* • Family dynamics *(Chap. 2)* • Infertility *(Chap. 30)* • Preterm birth *(Chap. 24)* • Newborn complications *(Chap. 27)*

During pregnancy new roles and relationships begin to develop between the mother, father, siblings, extended family and friends, and the baby. The childbearing process is one of giving up and letting go of previous lifestyles, body image and relationships, as well as taking on new roles and responsibilities and learning how to love someone before meeting him or her. Before and during pregnancy parents imagine who the baby will look like, how their lives will be changed, and what the birth experience will be like. However, the reality of the experience of childbirth is rarely what the parents have dreamed of or hoped for.

Situational life crises can be superimposed on the experience of childbearing when a family experiences infertility, preterm labor or preterm birth, a cesarean birth, any perception of loss of control during their birthing experience, having a boy when they wanted a girl, the birth of a handicapped child, a maternal death, or the death of their baby during pregnancy or shortly after (Limbo and

Wheeler, 1986b). All of these situations have a common denominator—they are losses of what was hoped for, dreamed about, or planned.

Certainly from the perspective of health care providers, these crises vary in degrees. But from the perspectives of the parents their perceived loss may be the most terrible thing that has ever happened to them. They never thought this experience could happen to them. Instead of celebrating life, they are mourning at a birth. They are among those who have experienced a loss and are bereaved. The feelings and emotions associated with bereavement are called grief responses to loss.

The statistics on losses in the childbearing years are grim. Out of 1000 births, 180 babies are stillborn or die shortly after birth (Cunningham et al, 1993). Approximately 750,000 babies die from **miscarriage,** a pregnancy that ends before 20 weeks' gestation; there are approximately 30,000 **stillbirths,** babies who die in utero or are born after 20 weeks' gestation or at a weight of

350 g, depending on the state laws regarding stillbirth. **Newborn death,** babies born showing signs of life such as respiratory effort, heart rate, pulsating cord, or muscle irritability at birth, regardless of the week of gestation, accounts for 30,000 deaths a year in the United States (Borg, Lasker, 1981). Over 1.4% of all pregnancies are an **ectopic pregnancy,** a pregnancy that takes place outside of the uterus, usually in a fallopian tube (Cunningham et al, 1993).

When an individual or family perceives they have experienced a loss, the role of the nurse is critical. Nurses must be prepared to put aside their own values and beliefs and meet each family member at the point of his/her need. Their needs are based on the perception each individual family member has regarding their personal loss. In many instances the nurse is also grieving.

GRIEF RESPONSES

When an individual experiences the loss of a relationship, hopes and dreams for the future end. The reestablishment of life without that particular relationship involves a process called **bereavement** or **mourning.** The subsequent feelings and emotions are called **grief responses.** This process may be brief and nonconscious—perhaps a sigh when looking at a daughter when a son was hoped for. For others, their mourning may last days, months, or years. The intensity and length of grief responses depends on the perception of the loss, age, religious beliefs, the changes the loss brought to their lives, their personal ability to cope with the loss, and their support systems (Sanders, 1998). Bowlby and Parks (1970) and Davidson (1984) described the characteristics of grief and the bereavement process in their research on separation and loss. The four dimensions of mourning were identified as follows:

1. **Shock and numbness** are experienced by parents as they express feelings of stunned disbelief, panic, distress, or anger. This experience can be interrupted by outbursts of emotion. It is difficult to make decisions during this time, and normal functioning is impeded. This phase predominates during the first 2 weeks after a loss. Parents have said they feel like they are in a bad dream and that they will wake up and everything will be all right.
2. **Searching and yearning** can be identified by feelings of restlessness, anger, guilt, and ambiguity. It is yearning for what could have been and searching for the answer for why the loss occurred. This phase is present at the time of the loss and peaks from 2 weeks to 4 months after the loss. Parents have stated that their arms ache to hold a baby, they wake to the sound of a baby crying, and they have disturbing dreams. They are preoccupied with thoughts about what happened, what they

did or did not do to have caused this terrible thing to happen, and the event of the death itself.
3. **Disorganization** is identified when the mourner turns from testing what is real to an awareness of the reality of the loss. Feelings of depression, difficulty in concentrating on work and solving problems, and a general sense of not feeling well about oneself physically and emotionally exist. This phase peaks around 5 to 9 months and slowly subsides. Many parents feel that they will never get over the loss, that they are losing their mind, and feel physically ill.
4. **Reorganization** occurs when the mourner is better able to function at home and work with an increase in self-esteem and confidence. The mourner has the ability to cope with new challenges and has placed the loss in perspective. This phase is present when parents laugh and when they begin to enjoy the simple pleasures of life without feeling guilty. Reorganization begins to peak sometimes after the first year as parents begin to move on with their lives. Families have said that they will never forget their baby who has died, but they have resumed life, which for them has a "new normal."

Both men and women express feeling loss of control and loss of self-esteem when unexpected outcomes have been perceived as more than a disappointment. The physical, emotional, and social grief responses to loss encompass many feelings and emotions (Box 28-1).

BOX 28-1

Signs and Symptoms of Grief

PHYSICAL EFFECTS

- Exhaustion
- Loss of appetite
- Sleeping problems
- Lack of strength
- Weight loss
- Headaches
- Blurred vision
- Breathlessness
- Palpitations
- Weight gain
- Aching arms
- Restlessness

EMOTIONAL AND/OR PSYCHOLOGIC EFFECTS

- Denial
- Guilt
- Anger
- Resentment
- Bitterness
- Depression
- Time confusion
- Irritability
- Sadness
- Sense of failure
- Concentration on problems
- Failure to accept reality
- Preoccupation with deceased

SOCIAL EFFECTS

- Withdrawal from normal activity
- Isolation (emotional and physical) from spouse, family, or friends

Mourning is not a neat and orderly process that moves smoothly from one dimension to another. All the dimensions of bereavement exist at the same time with one or more predominating at any given moment. There is much movement back and forth between the dimensions. The bereaved reveal their mourning through their language, intensity and duration of grief responses, and in their ability to regain their life without that which was lost.

Anticipatory grief occurs when families have knowledge of an impending loss, such as when the baby is admitted to an NICU with problems or when a diagnosis of an anencephalic baby is made by ultrasound. The baby is still alive, but the prognosis is poor. Being able to anticipate the loss gives families an opportunity to plan, feel more in control of their situation, and be able to say goodbye in a special way. However, some individuals or family members may distance or detach themselves from the experience or their loved one as a way of protecting or avoiding the pain of loss and grief.

TASKS OF MOURNERS

Worden (1991) identified four tasks of mourners. For the woman and her family to adapt to the loss of their baby or loved one, these tasks must be accomplished:

1. Accepting the reality of the loss
2. Working through the pain of grief
3. Adjusting to the environment
4. Moving on with life (reorganization)

Accepting the reality of the loss occurs when the woman and family come to grips with the reality of the loss. Their baby has died and their lives have changed. Seeing, holding, touching, and memorialization are all ways the bereaved can perceptually confirm the baby's death. It is important for the woman and family to tell their story about the events and the experiences and feelings surrounding the loss to cognitively and emotionally come to terms that their baby has died. Caregivers need to use the words *dead* and *died* rather than *lost* or *gone* to assist the bereaved in accepting the reality. This task interfaces with the first two initial phases of grief.

Working through the pain of grief means the mourner must feel and express the intense emotions of grief. Not all parents or families experience the same intensity of pain, but it is unlikely to experience the death of a baby and not feel some grief. Society in general tends to minimize the death of a baby because no real social relationship with or attachment to the baby existed. However, mothers, fathers/partners, and siblings many times have developed images and feel a relationship to the unborn baby no matter what stage of the pregnancy. Often society equates the number of years of life and visibility of a relationship to how much mourning is appropriate.

Families who experience a perinatal loss may suppress or deny their feelings because it seems, on the surface, to be more socially acceptable. The nurse can be instrumental in preparing the woman and family for reactions they may receive from others once they leave the hospital or clinic setting. If a supportive social network is not available, and even if it is, a perinatal bereavement support group can help the parents work through their pain by nonjudgmental sharing of feelings (see Appendix H). To deny the pain of grief will lead sooner or later to physical and emotional illness. Unfortunately, it is more acceptable in our society to be treated for physical problems than emotional ones. When no physical reasons for illness can be found, complicated bereavement (p. 833) may be the source.

Adjusting to the environment after the loss means learning how to accommodate to the changes the loss has wrought. The loss of a baby means not being able to fulfill the role of a mother, father/partner, older sibling, or grandparent. Issues such as deciding what to do about the nursery and baby clothes, going back to work, parenting other children, getting pregnant again, and learning how to cope with insensitive family members and friends are problems the bereaved must face.

Detachment needs to occur for the parents to adapt to their loss. Over time the bereaved have the opportunity to change their view on how the event of the loss has affected their lives. This does not mean they have forgotten about their baby. It means that as the weeks and months go by, they have an opportunity to develop a new

---

BOX 28-2

To Jessica

The candles are lit,
  but no song will be sung.
No laughter, no glee, of my little one
  who would have been three.
If you only knew the plans that would be
  made by your dad and me.
The cake to be baked . . .
The presents wrapped . . .
  and all the funny party hats.
The pictures taken by your dad,
  of course,
As loving friends fill the house.
All of this is not meant to be,
  since you were taken away from me.
  No birthday cake . . .
  No presents unwrapped . . .
  No pictures of you in your party hat.
But the candles are lit,
  Never to go out.
For they burn forever in my heart.

perspective, different feelings, and various ways of coping.

Moving on with life, or reorganization, means to love and live again. Once more being able to enjoy things that gave previous pleasure, being able to nurture oneself and others, developing new interests, and reestablishing relationships are all signs of moving on. For some people the birth of a subsequent child is necessary for them to be able to move on with their lives. Bereaved parents never forget their precious child, but their memories become bittersweet.

Bittersweet grief, a term coined by Kowalski (1984), refers to the memories that linger after the loss has occurred (Boxes 28-2 and 28-3). This grief occurs when someone is reminded about the loss. This can typically happen at birthdays, death days, anniversaries, school events, changes in the seasons, and months of the year when the loss occurred. The bereaved have conscious and unconscious psychologic triggers that enable them to remember their loved one according to what was significant to them about their relationship with the loved one and the events surrounding the loss.

BOX 28-3

Bittersweet Grief

To Jessica Mayo—on her 11th Birthday
    Sunday, November 18, 1990
"The child born on the Sabbath day,
is bonny and blithe and good and gay."
    Sundays are special days.
  . . . a day of rest, a day to play.
  A day to reflect on days past.
  . . . a day to thank God for all that we bless.
    I bless your memory.
    I wish you were here.
On your eleventh birthday I still want to share.
    . . . Your dreams of the future.
    . . . Our memories past.
     My baby's first cry.
    My daughter's first laugh.
I was told you were an angel in heaven above.
    Eleven years later, I'm an expert . . .
    At long-distance love.
    On your third birthday I wrote my first poem
to you.
    Eight years later, it's still true
    ". . . no birthday cake,
    no presents unwrapped . . .
no pictures of you in your party hat.
    But the candles are lit,
     Never to go out
For they burn forever in my heart.
     Love, Mom"
Kathie Rataj Mayo
1990

CARING

Swanson-Kauffman's research (1986, 1988, 1990) on women and their families who have experienced perinatal loss has identified a theoretical framework on caring for the bereaved. The framework identifies five components in a caring concept:

- Knowing
- Being with
- Doing for
- Enabling
- Maintaining belief

Knowing implies that the nurse has taken the time to ask questions of the bereaved to help understand what the perception of the loss is and the meaning of the loss to the woman and her family.

Being with is how the nurse conveys acceptance to the woman and her family and how the nurse is able to understand the various feelings and perceptions each family member may have.

Doing for refers to the activities performed by the nurse that provide for the physical care, comfort, and safety of the woman and her family. This may include offering pain medication, sitz baths, maintaining the patency of the IV, postpartum checks, and back rubs.

Enabling requires the nurse to offer the woman and her family options for their care. The nurse must first understand how each family member perceives the loss and what the loss means to that family member. Offering information, anticipatory guidance, choices for decision making and support during hospitalization and after discharge helps the family feel more in control in a situation where they feel very much out of control. Enabling raises their self-esteem, allows them to feel more comfortable in asking for options based on *their* needs for memories and closure, rather than what the nurse thinks their needs are.

Maintaining belief refers to the nurse encouraging the woman and her family to believe in their own ability to pick up the pieces and begin to heal. The nurse avoids cliché treatment of the bereaved but rather spends time with the family, learns their inner strengths and coping abilities, and points them out to the family.

Care Management

The critical intervention time is in the immediate crisis period after the loss. The goal of the nurse is to provide care, support, information, and anticipatory guidance as a help to decision making. Families usually do not expect a loss to happen to them. The suddenness and unexpected nature of their loss leaves them unprepared both in life experiences and knowledge about grief responses and the mourning process but, more importantly, what they might need for positive memories of this tragic time in their lives. It is the nurse's responsibility to do the following:

- Be knowledgeable about grief
- Anticipate what families might need or appreciate for future memories
- Create a nonjudgmental environment where families can express their feelings and emotions, make decisions based on needs, and feel support for those decisions.

✤ ASSESSMENT

Families who experience a loss may have many and varied feelings and responses. Assessment of the feelings, the perception of the loss, and the events surrounding the loss is important. It is immaterial in supporting bereaved families how the nurse or others view the event. Feelings of loss and grief are real. No one should be made to feel guilty or hurt for feelings they may not have, nor should anyone feel their needs for support, information, and decision making went unmet because their loss was perceived by others as not important.

Some people view an early pregnancy as the union of cells; others have visions of a baby; and still others are wrapped up in thinking about the thrill of being pregnant. There appears to be a time when cognition and emotion join, and acceptance of the pregnancy means "pregnant with baby" (Limbo, Wheeler, 1986a,b). The point when this occurs varies for each individual man, woman, and child. Assessment of family members' perception of the loss and the events surrounding the loss is crucial before intervention, especially in the instance of miscarriage, ectopic pregnancy, stillbirth, newborn death and loss of the perfect child.

Helpful information to gather in making assessments of the perception of loss might be:

- When did you find out you were pregnant?
- Who have you told about your pregnancy?
- What plans had you made for this pregnancy?
- When was your due date?

What the nurse should listen for is the word *baby*. The language people choose to express the perception of the event reveals what the person believes has been lost, or what is being grieved.

Attention should be paid to their verbal and nonverbal responses when they are questioned about the event, such as:

- Did they cry?
- Were there verbalizations of anger, guilt, or disbelief?
- What did their face look like when they were telling you their story?
- Did they look at you when you asked them questions?
- Was it hard to get their attention?
- How did they answer your questions?

- Did they have a hard time answering even the simplest of questions?
- Did their answer make sense?

Answers to these are indications of a grief response. Ability or inability to respond to open-ended questions is a clue to help the nurse decide which interventions and how much intervention are needed at any given time.

Pregnancy and birth bring about many changes in role expectations, relationships, and how one views oneself. The perceptions of loss that may be associated with pregnancy and birth may be any or all of the following:

- Feelings of being out of control
- Decrease in self-esteem
- Concerns about their fertility or their ability to bear children
- Changes in their relationships with others, most specifically the father of the baby and their mother
- Changes in body image
- Changes in role expectations
- Loss of their precious baby or perfect child

Listening for the words that are used to describe their experiences can help the nurse formulate appropriate nursing diagnoses and plan of care.

✤ NURSING DIAGNOSES

Nursing diagnoses may include physiologic and psychosocial problems related to grieving or problems occurring in the grieving process. Examples of nursing diagnoses include the following:

Powerlessness related to
- Hospitalization
- Inability to care for self
- Inability to communicate
- Lack of knowledge

Sleep pattern disturbance related to
- Grieving process
- Anticipatory grief

Spiritual distress related to
- Loss of baby, mother, or perfect child
- Loss of self-esteem

Alteration in family processes related to
- Loss of family member (i.e., mother, baby, or birth of child with a disorder)
- Dissatisfaction over loss of control
- Inability to make decisions
- Anxiety for not achieving a pregnancy (infertility)
- Acting out behaviors, depression, apathy, or anxiety
- Social isolation

✤ EXPECTED OUTCOMES

During this important step in the nursing process, expected outcomes are set in patient-centered terms, based on the mutual goals chosen by the woman/family and the case manager. The expected outcomes are prioritized. Nursing actions are then selected to meet the expected outcomes.

Expected outcomes may include the following:

1. Family members will be able to share their experiences and verbalize the feelings that have contributed to their sensation of powerlessness, loss of self-esteem, and changes in their relationships.
2. The mother and her family will show increasing independence in participating in and making decisions regarding their plan of care.
3. The family will be able to make decisions that reflect their religious and cultural beliefs.
4. The woman and her family will be able to use family and community resources for support.
5. The woman and her family will verbalize satisfaction with their health care professionals.

When these individual expected outcomes are achieved, the ultimate expected outcome of positive integration of the perceived loss experience within the individual and family can, over time, be met. What families experience during hospitalization can either be positive memories or memories that have the capacity to haunt them for a lifetime. The overall goal of the nurse

---

CULTURAL CONSIDERATIONS

CULTURAL AND RELIGIOUS ASPECTS OF DEATH

BURIAL

Cremation is forbidden, discouraged, or allowed only under unusual circumstances for Baha'is, Roman Catholics, Jews, and members of the Christian and Missionary Alliance, Church of Jesus Christ of Latter-Day Saints, and Greek Orthodox Church. Cremation is customary for Hindus and Unitarian Universalists.

EMBALMING

The body is not to be embalmed, unless required by state law, for Jews and Baha'is.

SACRAMENTS

Baptism is performed only if the baby is living, for most Protestant and Roman Catholic Churches. Rituals in preparing the body for burial are performed in Judaism, Hinduism, and Islam.

SPECIAL MEMENTOS

Picture taking may be in conflict with beliefs of some cultures, such as Native Americans, Indian, Eskimo, Amish, Hindu, and Moslem. It would be important to offer a choice for these families. Within the culture as a whole, this may not be acceptable, but within a family it may be a desired memento.

---

is to create a nonjudgmental atmosphere, which provides a listening ear, anticipatory guidance, support and information to help with decision making at the time of the loss and during any follow-up contact.

✤ COLLABORATIVE CARE

Mothers, father/partners, and extended families look to the medical and nursing staff for support and understanding during the time of loss. They take cues from their health care providers to determine what to do and what their behavior or responses should be to their loss. Many families do not know what they need at the time of loss. Their hopes, dreams, self-esteem, and role expectations have been shattered. However, all families can make a choice once it has been offered and they have some time to consider what their needs might be. It is the rare mother or family who knows exactly what they need and are willing to verbalize or demand their needs. When a mother or family is able to verbalize their needs, it is extremely important for the nurse to respond positively to that need. The nurse should do everything possible to see that the need is met. Unmet needs may be the base of "if only's" that can plague the mother for a lifetime and can be the foundation for the development of complicated bereavement (p. 833).

Regardless of the type of loss experienced, all families need the listening ear of the nurse. Therapeutic communication and counseling techniques help the mother, father/partner, and other family members express their feelings and emotions, understand their responses to the loss, and empower them to make decisions.

Communicating and Caring Techniques

Listening is the single most important communication technique nurses have in providing support, care, and understanding. To be a good listener, the nurse should be seated comfortably in a chair positioned at a 45-degree angle about 2 to 4 feet from the person talking. The nurse's facial expression and demeanor should be one of concern and caring.

Ask only one question at a time for the bereaved person to respond to. Leaning forward, nodding your head, saying "Uh-huh" or "Tell me more" are encouragement enough for the bereaved mother to tell her story. The use of silence many times gives the mother the opportunity to collect her thoughts and to respond to your question. Grief responses in the initial days of crisis makes it difficult for individuals to concentrate on what is being asked, to think what the question means, and to respond to the question.

Listen patiently while people tell you their story of loss or grief. When needed, ask questions that help people talk specifically about their grief and the experiences surrounding the loss. Encourage the bereaved to talk about their loved one and what their loss means to them. Resist the temptation to give advice or to use clichés in offering support to the bereaved (Box 28-4).

Nurses need to become more comfortable with their own feelings of grief and loss to effectively support and care for the bereaved. It is all right to cry with bereaved families and to share the moment with them; it is not all right to be more emotional than the bereaved so that they have to comfort the nurse.

Worden (1991) identified several counseling techniques the nurse might want to use in helping the family share and express their grief. These include the following.

Actualize the Loss

Ask the bereaved family questions that help them in expressing the experience of the loss. Make sure you use the name of their baby and, in the case of a death, that you have seen the baby first, before you speak with family members. Questions might include:

"Tell me about your labor and birth with Lucas."

"When did you know you were miscarrying?"

"What was the most significant thing you remember about Jessica's funeral?"

"Who does Angela resemble in your family?

Help the Survivors Identify and Express Feelings

The feelings and emotions of expressed grief can feel overwhelming to the health care professionals. The feelings of anger, guilt, and sadness are paramount in the early days and months following a loss. When the be-

reaved family members are expressing feelings of anger, it can be helpful to identify the feeling by simply saying, "You sound angry," or "You look angry. Where is this anger coming from?" Being willing to sit down and talk with them about their feelings of anger can help them move past those feelings into the underlying feelings of powerlessness and helplessness in not being able to control many aspects of the situation they are experiencing.

Bereaved individuals have many questions surrounding the event of their loss. "What did I do?" "What caused this to happen?" "Do you think I should have, could have done something?" These are all issues of searching and yearning. Part of grief process is to figure out what happened, what their role was in the loss, why them, why their baby. The nurse needs to recognize that the answers to these questions need to be answered by the bereaved. It is part of their healing. When a bereaved mother asks, "Do you think that I shouldn't have painted the baby's room? Did that cause my baby to die?" An appropriate response to her might be, "I understand you need to find an answer for why your baby died. What are some of the other things you've been thinking about?"

Giving the bereaved advice or answering their questions does not help them process their grief. And in reality many times there are no definite answers for why this terrible thing has happened to them. Nurses can speculate, but for the most part they don't know why. The "why" is unknown.

Being with someone who is terribly sad, crying, or sobbing can be extremely difficult. The initial impulse is to touch the person or to hand her a tissue. Although this may seem supportive at the time, what may happen is that the expression of emotion is stopped or stifled. The bereaved person will let you know when she is ready for a tissue by wiping her eyes or nose, raising her head and looking around, or reaching for a tissue.

Careful assessment before using touch as a therapeutic technique is important. If touch is used inappropriately, the bereaved person will stiffen, pull away, look at where she was touched, or stop the expression of feelings and emotions.

The nurse should have the presence of mind and the willingness to be alongside, quietly supporting the bereaved person in whatever expression of feelings or emotions is appropriate for her. It is the presence that leaves mourners with the feeling that they were cared for.

Provide Time to Grieve

Families become unaware of time frames when they first learn and come to grips with their loss. They do not care about the change of shifts or the needs the hospital system might have in "moving things along." When families are pushed or rushed into making decisions, in most cases they will make a decision based on the health care system's need, not theirs. Nurses need to be sensitive to

---

BOX 28-4

What to Say and What Not to Say

WHAT YOU CAN SAY

"I'm sad for you."

"How are you doing with all of this?"

"This must be hard for you.'

"What can I do for you?"

"I'm sorry."

"I'm here, and I want to listen."

WHAT NOT TO SAY

"You're young, you can have others."

"You have an angel in heaven."

"This happened for the best."

"Better for this to happen now, before you knew the baby."

"There was something wrong with the baby anyway."

Calling the baby a "fetus" or "it."

From La Crosse Lutheran Hospital, La Crosse, WI, 1984.

the needs families might have in spending time with their baby. Providing time to see and hold their baby in private, making arrangements for their baby to be returned to them for further viewing, and not processing consent forms for autopsy or removal from the hospital offer the family the opportunity to further accept the reality of the loss and say goodbye.

Interpret Normal Feelings

Many bereaved parents have feelings of losing control or going crazy with the thoughts that plague them about their loved one. It is essential for the nurse to verbally reassure and educate bereaved parents about the grief process, including the physical, social, and emotional responses of individuals and families. Offering reading material on the grief process, miscarriage and ectopic pregnancy, responses of family and friends, talking with children, planning a special goodbye, and the differences between men and women who are grieving can satisfy some of the educational needs of bereaved families.

Offering health teaching on the bereavement process alone is not enough. In the initial days following a loss, it is difficult for parents to cognitively understand what they have been told, as well as remember what has been said. During hospitalization or contact with the nurse, the combination of written material and the verbal sharing of information can help provide the bereaved with an understanding of their own as well as others' grief. After discharge, other strategies for providing information and education on the grief process can be done by making follow-up phone calls to bereaved families, offering them the opportunity to talk with other bereaved parents in one-on-one support over the phone, referring them to a mutual self-help perinatal bereavement support group, or providing a reading list that identifies books and articles on loss, grief, and perinatal bereavement.

Allow for Individual Differences

Grief is very personal and private. How a person responds to loss and grief depends on age, sex, culture, religion, socioeconomic status, how others around respond to the loss, and how the person coped with prior losses. Within a family the nurses may observe many different types of responses. Typically men want to protect their partner from further pain, and parents and grandparents want to protect their children from more hurt. The underlying feelings of powerlessness and helplessness can be hidden behind expressions of anger, resistance to ideas, overcontrol of situations, or blame. These feelings can leave the partner or grandparent feeling isolated and alone, when in fact it is the care and concern for their loved one that perpetuates the expression of their feelings. The nurse can respond to these underlying feelings by doing the following:

1. Recognizing what a difficult time this is for the mother, father/partner, parent, grandparent, or child.
2. Acknowledging how hard it must be for them to feel responsible for making sure everything and everyone is taken care of.
3. Eventually asking them about their own hopes, dreams, and subsequent feelings of loss.

These communication techniques can help the nurse move the person who is resistive to a position of support where personal needs can also be met.

Families should be asked at least three times during their hospitalization when important decisions need to be made. This gives them the opportunity to change their mind, to express their needs to each other, and to make a decision based on their needs as individuals and as family members.

Physical Comfort

Coping with loss and grief after childbirth can be an overwhelming experience for the woman and her family. Many times these families request the mother to be moved off the maternity unit. Their baby has died, and for them the thought of being on the same unit with other mothers and babies is more than they want to handle. Other mothers, however, may want to remain on the maternity unit, where the staff nurses are better prepared to meet their physical and emotional needs. It should be the mother's choice in terms of where she wants to spend her postpartum stay.

When a mother does choose to move to another floor, it is the nurse's responsibility to ensure that her needs for physical assessment of breasts, fundus, lochia flow, perineum, and pain medication needs are continued. This may be done through inservice education of nursing staff on units where the bereaved mother and her family are transferred by maternity nurses or through consultation with the perinatal clinical nurse specialist. Also, the nurse caring for the family at the time of the loss should visit the family after transfer so the family will not feel forgotten.

The physical needs of a bereaved mother are the same as any mother who has given birth. The cruel reality for many bereaved mothers is their milk may come in and there is no baby to breastfeed, their afterpains remind them of their emptiness, and gas pains feel like there is still a baby moving inside them. Many struggle with the frustration of having to go through all the pain of childbearing only to be discharged home with empty arms. "What was this for?" they wonder. "All they did is cut me up and take my baby from me. I got nothing for all of this pain and suffering when they wheeled me out." For a bereaved mother to not even have her physical needs met after childbirth in terms of postpartum checks, sitz baths, perineal care, pain medication, information about inhibiting lactation, afterpains, lochia flow, perineal care, and sexuality after a loss sends her a strong message that she is not worthy, that she "did not do it right."

Hands-on interventions such as help with getting out of bed the first few times, bathing, answering call lights as soon as possible, and back massages convey caring in a tangible way. Being sensitive to the needs of the father, such as offering another meal tray, juice, and a place to sleep or perhaps shower in the mother's room, shows that the nurse understands their needs to be together in this time of crisis.

The grieving process makes it difficult for the bereaved to sleep. Their appetite may be nonexistent or voracious. Adequate rest, diet, and fluids must be offered to replenish the woman's physical strength. Discharge instructions should be both in verbal and written forms. They should include the need for eating foods from each of the basic food groups, decreasing food or fluids that contain caffeine, limiting alcohol consumption and nicotine, increasing fluids to at least a quart a day, exercising regularly, and strategies for rest when unable to sleep. Suggestions for helping the bereaved rest or sleep at night might be a warm bath or milk before bedtime, limit alcohol and nicotine after 12 PM, relaxation exercises or a nightly walk before bedtime, restful music, massage, or when necessary, sleeping medication. It is recommended that sleeping medication be used only every third night to allow the bereaved to do their needed grief work, but not become sleep deprived. Sleep deprivation, poor nutrition, and inadequate fluids can be the forerunner to the development of a clinical depression, which can complicate the mourning process.

Options for Memories

Families need to be involved in the decision-making process. The decisions made during the time of their loss will be their memories for a lifetime. Offering a choice to parents implies they have the freedom to choose. Choices or options need to be offered in a gentle manner. Parents should not be rushed, pushed, or feel forced to make a decision their health care provider feels would be best for them. In the initial phases of grief, families need to be asked at least three times about the important options of seeing and holding their baby. Shock and numbness make it difficult for them to fully understand the ramifications of what the option means, let alone making the decision. Time and an environment that understands the needs of grieving families offer family members the opportunity to change their minds and not feel bad or inconvenient to someone for doing so.

Nurses walk a fine line between offering the bereaved what they have a right to have and making them feel guilty for not wanting to choose those options. Communicating with parents that options are their right, not their obligation, is vital.

Seeing and Holding

One of the first options to be discussed is whether the family wants to see their baby or, in the case of miscarriage or ectopic pregnancy, the products of conception. A statement such as "Some parents have found it helpful to see their baby" or "the products of conception" gives the parents permission to do what might seem odd or distasteful. Responses can vary greatly between someone who experiences a miscarriage or ectopic pregnancy and someone who has experienced stillbirth or newborn death, as well as between family members.

Parents appreciate preparation for how their baby looks (e.g., red, peeling skin like a bad sunburn, dark discoloration similar to bruises, molding of the head that makes the head look soft and swollen, or any defects). This helps them know what to expect. The nurse should make the baby look as sweet as possible. Always remember, parents see their baby with very different eyes than health care professionals. Bathing the baby, applying lotion to the baby's skin, combing hair, placing identification bracelets on the arm and leg, dressing the baby in a diaper and special outfit, sprinkling powder in the baby's blanket, and wrapping the baby in a pretty blanket conveys to the parents that their baby is cared for the same as any baby in the nursery. The olfactory sense is greatly heightened in the bereaved. The use of powder and lotion stimulates the parent's senses and provides pleasant memories of their baby for in the future.

Caring for a baby who has died can be a difficult task for the nurse. It can be made more difficult if the baby has been dead for several days or weeks. It may be helpful to have a colleague help in making the baby look presentable and in taking pictures. In some cases decapitation or dismemberment has occurred. Consultation with a local funeral director can help the nurse prepare the baby to meet the parents. If the baby has been in the morgue, he or she can be placed underneath a warmer for 20 to 30 minutes and wrapped in a warm blanket before being brought to the parents. Cold cream rubbed over stiffened joints can help in repositioning the baby.

When bringing the baby to the parents, it is important to treat the baby as one would a live baby. Holding the baby close, touching a hand or cheek, using the baby's name, and talking with the parents about the special features of their child conveys that it is all right for them to do likewise. If a baby has a congenital anomaly, the nurse can desensitize the family by having a perfect hand or foot showing as they approach the parents. Help them explore the baby's body as they desire, pointing out family resemblances or characteristics you find especially attractive.

Be sure to offer the parents time alone. Parents will need to know when the nurse will return and how to call should they need anything. It is difficult to predict how long or how many times parents will need to spend with their baby. These moments are the only ones they will have to parent their child while their child's physical presence is still with them. Some parents need only a few minutes, others hours and still others days.

A rocking chair can be a soothing place for parents to

sit when holding their baby. When parents are ready to return their baby to the nursery or morgue or discharged to the funeral director, they will tell the nurse. It is extremely painful for some parents to say goodbye to their baby. They will tell the nurse they are ready verbally and nonverbally. Being sensitive to their needs of actualizing the loss and coping with the reality of the death is essential for their healing.

Knowing the Baby's Sex/Naming the Baby

This is an option that can be offered whether the sex can be determined or not. Genetic studies are an option to determine the cause of death, as well as the sex of the baby. Naming the baby is an important decision parents can make. In choosing a name, the baby is made a member of their family, the loss is more real, and it makes it easier for the baby to be remembered in a special way. If the sex of the baby is unable to be determined and the parents would like to name their baby, they could choose a special name for their baby, use a name already chosen for the sex of child they hoped for, or a unisex name could be chosen.

Autopsy/Organ Donation

An autopsy can be instrumental in determining the cause of death. For some families this information is helpful in understanding why their loss occurred, processing their grief, and perhaps preventing another loss. Other parents may feel their baby has been through enough. They prefer not to have further information about the cause of death. Also, some religions prohibit autopsy.

Options for the type of autopsy are available to parents, such as excluding the head. Parents may need plenty of time to make this decision. There is no need to rush them unless there was evidence of contagious disease or maternal infection at the time of death.

Organ donation can be an aid to grieving, an opportunity for the family to see something good come from this experience. The health care provider is usually the first one to offer this opportunity to the family. The parents may be offered the opportunity to donate the baby's eyes. Organ donation of eyes from a baby can occur if the baby was born alive and is at least 36 weeks' gestation or more.

Bathing and Dressing

When possible, families should be given the opportunity to bathe, dress, and annoint their baby. This can be a very symbolic ritual for many families. Some babies' skin is fragile and may crack or ooze when touched. Parents can still apply lotion with cotton balls, sprinkle the powder, tie ribbons, fasten the diaper, and place amulets, medallions, rosaries, or special toys or mementos in their baby's hands or alongside their baby. They may want to do other parenting responsibilities such as combing hair, wrapping the baby in a blanket, placing the baby in a bassinet, or carrying their baby to the nursery. They may have special clothes at home or they may want to purchase a special outfit in which to dress their baby.

Privacy

If at all possible, the mother should be admitted to a private room. This enables her and her partner to have special time together, with their baby and with other family members. Marking the door to the room with a special card indicating that this family has experienced a loss can prevent any embarrassment on behalf of the staff and uncomfortable feelings for the family (Fig. 28-1).

Visitation with other Family Members or Friends

Families need to be offered the opportunity to have their children, grandparents, extended family members, and friends visit with them during hospitalization and to see and hold their baby. This affords others the opportunity to become acquainted with the baby, to understand the parents' loss, to offer their support, and to say goodbye.

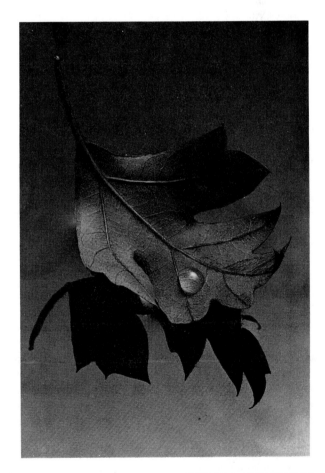

Resolve Through Sharing®

FIG. 28-1 Door card for room of mother who has experienced perinatal loss. (From Resolve Through Sharing, La Crosse, WI.)

This experience helps parents explain to their surviving children who their brother or sister was and what death means, offers the children concrete answers to their questions, and helps the children express their grief. Involving extended family and friends enables the parents to mobilize their circle of friends who will support them not only at the time of loss but also in the future.

Lock of Hair

A lock of hair may be an important keepsake for the parents' memories. Parents need to be asked first, for permission, before cutting a lock of hair. Hair can be removed from the nape of the baby's neck where it is not noticeable.

Rituals of Remembrance

The spiritual needs at the time of a loss can be an important aspect of care. Support from the clergy is an option that should be offered to all parents. Parents may wish to have their own pastor, priest, rabbi, or spiritual leader contacted. Or, they may wish to see the hospital's chaplain.

Members from the clergy may offer the parents the opportunity for baptism, when appropriate. Other rituals that might be offered are a blessing, naming ceremony, last rites, ritual of the sick, memorial service, a prayer, or just their physical presence as a representative of a higher being.

Funeral Arrangements

Parents should be given information about the choices for the final disposition of their baby, regardless of the stage of gestation. In the instance of a baby under 20 weeks' gestation, many hospitals offer to make the final disposition arrangements. Babies under 20 weeks' gestation are considered to be products of conception. Embryos, fallopian tubes removed because of an ectopic pregnancy, tissue from a pregnancy obtained during a dilatation and curettage, and babies under 20 weeks are all considered tissue. Should parents want to know what arrangements the hospital makes for those babies, the nurse should know the hospital's process and answer the parents' questions as honestly as possible. Many hospitals are currently reviewing and changing their policy on the cremation and burial of babies under 20 weeks' gestation to reflect more respect and dignity for these babies. In most states, if a baby is over 20 weeks and 1 day of gestation or is born alive, it is the parents' responsibility to make the final arrangements for their baby (see the Legal Tip).

Final disposition of all identifiable babies, regardless of weeks of gestation, includes burial or cremation. Nurses need to be knowledgeable about arrangement for transportation of the deceased and the role of the funeral director in working with bereaved families. Depending on the cemetery's policies, casketed babies or the ashes

Legal Tip: Definition of Live Birth

In all states there are laws that govern what constitutes a live birth. In most states a "live birth" is considered to be any products of conception expelled from a woman that show any signs of life. Signs of life are considered to be any muscle irritability, respiratory effort, or heart rate regardless of weeks of gestation. All nurses should know what their state considers a live birth and what forms need to be completed in the case of fetal death, stillbirth, or neonatal death.

from cremated babies can be buried in a special place designated for babies, at the foot of an already deceased relative, in a plot by themselves, in a mausoleum, or scattered in a designated area. Many states have regulations where cremated bodies can be scattered. A local funeral director or a state's Vital Statistics Bureau should have information about their state's rules, codes, and regulations regarding live births, burial requirements, transportation of the deceased by parents, and cremation.

In making final arrangements for their baby, parents may want a special service. They may choose to have a service in the hospital chapel, visitation at a funeral home or their home, a funeral service, and/or a graveside service. Parents can make any of these services as special, personal, and memorable as they like. They can choose special music, poetry, or prose written by others or themselves.

At the funeral home parents may want to hold their infant again, take pictures, dress their baby, and position their baby in the casket. All of these things are possible with a supportive funeral director who understands the needs of bereaved parents.

Special Memories

Parents need tangible mementos of their baby. This again allows for actualizing the loss. Parents may want to bring in a baby book already purchased. Special memory books, cards, and information on grief and mourning are available through national perinatal bereavement organizations for purchase by parents or hospitals and clinics.

The nurse records the baby's weight, length, and head circumference. Footprints and handprints are taken and placed with the other information on a special card, memory, or baby book. Sometimes it is difficult to obtain good handprints and footprints. Using alcohol or acetone on the palms or soles first can help the ink adhere to make the prints clearer, especially for small babies. When making prints, have a hard surface underneath the paper to be printed. Place the baby's heel or palm down first, roll the foot or hand forward, and keep the toes and fingers extended. It may be helpful to have a partner when doing this procedure. If the print does not turn

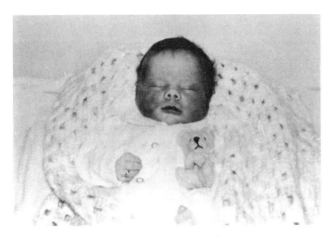

FIG. 28-2   Miranda. Full-term newborn death. (Used with permission, La Crosse Lutheran Hospital, La Crosse, WI.)

out, trace around the baby's hand and feet. This distorts the actual size. A form of plaster of Paris can also be used to make an imprint of the baby's hand or foot.

Any article that comes in contact or is used in caring for the baby is saved, placed in a sealable bag, and given to the parents. Articles should not be washed or cleaned beforehand so the parents can keep the smell of their baby. Some articles parents have appreciated receiving are the tape measure used to measure the baby, lotions, combs, clothing, hats, blankets, pacifier, crib cards, and identibands. Identibands should be placed on the baby before being given to the parents. The identibands help the parents to remember the size of the baby and enable them to directly touch something their baby touched.

Pictures

Pictures are the most important memento a parent can have. Photographs should be taken in any instance where there is an identifiable baby (Fig. 28-2). It does not matter how tiny, what the baby looks like, or how long the baby has been deceased, nor does it matter if other nursing staff members think pictures should not be taken because of how the baby looks.

Pictures should be taken by an instant print camera as well as a 35-mm camera. Every effort should be made to make the baby special, as if a portrait has been taken. Pictures should include closeups of the baby's face, hands, and feet. In some of the pictures the baby should be wrapped in a blanket with a hat or gown. They should also be taken of the baby unclothed. If there are any congenital anomalies, closeups of the anomalies should also be taken. Flowers, blocks, stuffed animals, or toys can also be placed in the background to make the picture more special, like a portrait. The parents or siblings may also want to have their picture taken holding the baby. Keeping a camera nearby and taking pictures when parents are spending special time with their baby can provide wonderful memories later.

Some parents may have their own camera or video camera with them and would like for the nurse to record them holding or parenting their baby during the bath, dressing or diapering their baby. Asking families what special times they had wanted to record prior to the knowledge of their baby's death usually makes the most special memories for the family at the time and in the future.

Taking the Baby to the Morgue

The baby's skin should be prepared by gently putting cold cream on the eyelids, hands, and face to keep the skin from dehydrating during refrigeration, before being placed in the morgue. The baby should be undressed, placed on a large smooth blanket, hands and arms positioned at the baby's sides, and wrapped carefully to avoid making impressions on the face.

When taking the baby to the morgue, the nurse should hold the baby close to her chest, with the face covered or transported per hospital protocol. Walking in a purposeful manner and not making eye contact with anyone along the way should keep interested individuals from asking questions. Should the nurse be asked, a response such as, "Baby's not seeing any visitors today," will keep people from being further interested. The nurse may want the accompaniment of a colleague, mainly for support.

The baby should be placed face up in the refrigeration unit of the morgue, making sure the blanket is loose over the face. If the baby is to be placed in a casket, the baby should be positioned comfortably. Should the baby be too large for the casket, the arms can be positioned on the chest or the baby can be placed on the stomach with the head turned and knees tucked under the chest.

Documentation

Many hospitals have a checklist that is used in providing care, mobilizing members of the multidisciplinary health care team, communicating options the family has chosen, and keeping track of all the details in meeting the needs of bereaved parents (Limbo, Wheeler, and Gensch, 1988) (Boxes 28-5 and 28-6). This checklist may or may not be a permanent part of the chart. Documentation in the nursing notes on primary concerns, grief responses, health teaching, health care advice, and referrals of the mother or any other family members is essential for continuity and consistency of care.

Follow-Up after Discharge

Follow-up phone calls after a loss occurs are important. The grief of the mother and her family does not end with discharge, but rather really begins once they return home, attend the funeral, and start to live their life without their baby. The calls are made to let the parents know they are still thought of and cared about. The calls are made at predictable, difficult times, such as the first week

BOX 28-5

Resolve Through Sharing
Checklist for Assisting Parent(s) Experiencing Miscarriage/Ectopic Pregnancy

RTS counselor _____   Date _____

Mother's name _____   Age _____ Due date _____

Date of beginning of miscarriage _____   Date of surgery _____

# of miscarriages _____ # of children _____   Religion _____

Address _____   Occupation _____

Phone number( ) _____   Marital status _____

Father's name _____   Age _____ Occupation _____

Address _____   Phone number ( ) _____

Baby's name _____   Sex _____

Support people available _____   Children's names: _____

Problem areas _____   Physician _____

O.K. to send written material to home address ☐ Yes ☐ No

Date	Time	See Miscarriage Protocol RTS Manual Sec. II p. 21-22	Comments	Initials
		Notify/Assign RTS counselor ☐ Yes ☐ No		
		Pastoral care ☐ Yes ☐ No		
		Offered: ☐ Blessing ☐ Memorial Service ☐ Naming Ceremony		
		Asked: "Would you like someone with you now?" ☐ Yes ☐ No		
		D&C/Surgical procedure discussed ☐ Yes ☐ No		
		Saw baby or tissue ☐ Mother ☐ Father		
		Touched and/or held baby ☐ Mother ☐ Father		
		If RH negative, RhoGAM given within 72 hrs ☐ Yes ☐ No		
		Patient's room flagged with door card ☐ Yes ☐ No		
		Photos taken: ☐ 35 mm ☐ Polaroid ☐ Given to Parents ☐ On file		
		Footprints & handprints/weight & length: ☐ Given to Parents ☐ On file		
		Grief process discussed ☐ Yes ☐ No		
		Incongruent grief discussed ☐ Yes ☐ No		
		Grief packet given ☐ Yes ☐ No		
		Info Brochure given to parents re: RTS PSG ☐ Yes ☐ No		
		Name/business card given ☐ Yes ☐ No		
		Regular OB/Midwife notified_____ ☐ Memo ☐ Vervally		
		Childbirth Educator notified_____ ☐ Yes ☐ No		
		Telephone number verified ☐ Yes ☐ No Optimal call time_____		
		Preg & Inf Loss Card sent to RTS Secretary ☐ Yes ☐ No		
		Given option to transfer from Maternity Unit ☐ Yes ☐ No		
		Genetic Studies ordered/Kevin Josephson, Genetic Associate notified 2771 or 783-6321 ☐ Yes ☐ No		
		Sex determination desired (tissue in NS only) ☐ Yes ☐ No		
		Would like another parent to call: ☐ Yes ☐ No ☐ Ask Later Parent contact:_____		
		Follow-up calls: eg. ☐ 1 wk, ☐ 3 wk, ☐ 4 mo, ☐ due date/anniv date		

Forms for burial or cremation of:

a) Products of Conception–2 copies of "Request for Return of Products of Conception to Patients" (1 copy-chart, 1 copy-lab). Obtain forms from Histology.

b) Identifiable Baby less than 20 wk or less than 350 gm–2 copies of "Request for Return of Products of Conception to Patients" (1-chart, 1-lab). "Notice of Removal" #DOH 5043–Responsible party for burial signs this form (either parent or a funeral director). Pink copy goes to responsible party. "Final Disposition of a Human Corpse" #DOH 5045 is required for any age identifiable baby that goes across state lines.

Note: Some cemeteries may require a "Final Disposition of Human Corpse" report for their own record keeping.

BOX 28-6

Resolve Through Sharing
Checklist for Assisting Parent(s) Experiencing Stillbirth or Newborn Death

Mother's discharge date: _____ Religion: _____
Mother's name: _____ Age ____ Gr ____ Para ____ L.C. ____ Due date _____
Address: _____ Previous loss: _____
Phone number: (   ) _____ Date/time of birth: _____
Father's name: _____ Date/time death: _____
Address: _____ Baby's name: _____ Sex: _____
Phone number: (   ) _____ Children's Name(s): _____ Age: _____
Optimal call time   _____ Age: _____
RTS counselor: _____   _____ Age: _____
Unit: _____ Ext _____ Support people: _____
Regular OB MD/midwife: _____ Attending MD &/or pediatrician _____

Date	Time	Follow Protocol in RTS manual Sec. II, P. 3-8		Comments	Initials
		Notify/Assign RTS counselor	☐ Yes ☐ No		
		Pastoral Care notified:	☐ Yes ☐ No		
		Communications notified:	☐ Yes ☐ No		
		Saw baby when born and/or after birth	☐ Mother ☐ Father		
		Touched and/or held baby	☐ Mother ☐ Father		
			☐ Siblings ☐ Grandparents ☐ Friends		
		Offered private time with their baby:	☐ Yes ☐ No		
		Baptism offered: (use seashell as vessel, give to parents)	☐ Yes ☐ No		
		Remembrance of Blessing offered:	☐ Yes ☐ No		
			☐ given to parents		
		Given option to transfer off Maternity Unit:	☐ Yes ☐ No		
		Patient's room flagged with door card:	☐ Yes ☐ No		
		Autopsy: ☐ Yes ☐ No Genetic Studies:	☐ Yes ☐ No		
		Genetic Associate notified: (see note)	☐ Yes ☐ No		
		Regular Physician/Midwife notified of death:	☐ Yes ☐ No		
		Memo sent to Physician/Midwife:	☐ Yes ☐ No		
		Section of Fetal Monitor Strip:	☐ Given to Parents ☐ On file		
		ID Bands/Crib Cards/Tape Measure:	☐ Given to Parents ☐ On file		
		Footprints/Handprints/Weight/Length recorded on "In Memory Of" sheet:	☐ Given to Parents ☐ On file		
		Lock of hair offered:	☐ Yes ☐ No		
			☐ Given to Parents ☐ On file		
		Mementos (clothing, hat, blanket, pacifier, crib cards, basin, thermometer, silk flower)	☐ Given to Parents ☐ On file		
		Complimentary birth certificate:	☐ Given to Parents ☐ On file		
		Resolve Through Sharing Photos taken: (clothed, unclothed, w. props, family photo)			
		1) Polaroid–3 or more	☐ Given to Parents ☐ On file		
		2) 35 mm (6-12 pictures)	☐ Given to Parents ☐ On file		
		3) Medical photos:	☐ Yes ☐ No		
		Informed about postponing funeral until mother is able to attend:	☐ Yes ☐ No		
		Services/Funeral arrangements, options discussed: ☐ Self-transport ☐ Gravesite services ☐ Visitation ☐ Hospital chapel ☐ Cremation ☐ Funeral home ☐ Burial at foot or head of relative's grave ☐ Specific area for babies in cemetery			
		Funeral arrangements made by: ☐ Mother ☐ Father Discussed: ☐ Seeing baby at funeral home ☐ Taking pictures there ☐ Providing outfit/toy for baby ☐ Dressing baby at funeral home			

Continued.

BOX 28-6

Resolve Through Sharing
Checklist for Assisting Parent(s) Experiencing Stillbirth or Newborn Death—cont'd

Date	Time	Follow Protocol in RTS manual Sec. II, P. 3-8	☐Mother ☐ Father	Comments	Initials
		Grief information packet given to:	☐ Mother ☐ Father		
		Discussed grief process/incongruent grief with:	☐ Mother ☐ Father		
		Discussed grief conference:	☐ Yes ☐ No		
		RTS Parents Support Group brochure given to:	☐ Mother ☐ Father		
		RTS business card given to:	☐ Mother ☐ Father		
		Pregnancy & Infant Loss Card sent to RTS secretary:	☐ Yes ☐No		
		Follow-up calls: 1 week: . . . . 3 weeks: . . . . Due date: . . . . 6-10 months: . . . . Anniversary date:			
		Grief conference planned with parents: Date _____ Time _____ Place _____ Letter of confirmation sent:	☐ Yes ☐ No		
		Parent Support Group, first meeting attended: Date: _____ Follow-up meetings attended: Dates _____			
		Would like another parent to call: Parent contact: _____	☐ Yes ☐ No ☐ ask later		

Note: Genetic Associate, Kevin Josephson, ext. 2771 or home 783-6321. Medical Media is available 8-4:30 weekdays for photos (or "on call" nights and weekends if needed for medical photos).
Forms: Report of Fetal Death #5402 Rev. 12-86 for ≥20 week or 350 gm wt. or more (Photocopy and save for parents)
Autopsy if ordered LLH 40-04P
Record of Death LLH 40-459 if SB or NB death
Genetics Protocol (folder) if ordered–follow checklist front of folder
Notice of Removal of a Human Corpse from an Institution #5043 Rev. 11/86-SB or NB death
Final Disposition from #5045 Rev. 11/86 for SB or NB transported across state lines by parents or for family burial (see note)
If funeral home involved–final Disposition will be completed by them.
Original Certificate of Death (for NB death only) #5040 Rev. 6-84
Note: If a live birth (NB) death occurs, parent should go to courthouse with Original Certificate of Death and R.D. will assist with forms for Family Burial. A copy of death certificate can be obtained from courthouse for $5.

at home, 1 month to 6 weeks later (parents should be invited to attend a support group at this time), 4 to 6 months after the loss, the due date, and at the anniversary of the death. Families who experienced a miscarriage, ectopic pregnancy, or preterm birth appreciate a phone call on their due dates. The calls are an opportunity for parents to ask questions, share their feelings, seek advice, and receive information to help them process their grief.

A grief conference is an opportunity for families to sit down with their health care providers and receive information about the baby's autopsy report, genetic studies, or just to ask questions they have been wondering about since their baby's death. Parents appreciate the opportunity to review the events of hospitalization, to go over the baby's and/or mother's chart with their primary health care provider, and to talk with those who cared for them during hospitalization. The grief conference gives health care professionals the opportunity to assess how the family is coping with their loss, to provide additional information on grief, and to share their own feelings and experiences with the family.

✦ EVALUATION

The evaluation of nursing care is made more difficult because of the shock and numbness of the bereavement process and the varied grief responses of the parents and other family members during hospitalization. Families need time to make decisions, the opportunity to change their minds, information on grief responses and the bereavement process, and the caring support of the nursing staff to ensure their needs are anticipated and met. Gathering mementos and saving them until the parents are ready to have them, ensuring an opportunity for parents to spend as much time with their baby as desired, and creating precious memories are all important to families healing after a loss. However, it is just as impor-

Case History

Ann, age 27, is primigravida at 20 weeks' gestation who was admitted to the labor and birth unit after complaining of severe abdominal cramping and leaking small amounts of pink vaginal discharge. Ann and her husband, John, are placed in a private labor room. As the nurse enters the room she hears Ann state, "I don't want to lose this baby—I feel so close to it now that I have felt it move—I'm scared." After several unsuccessful trials of drug therapy to stop labor, this situation is assessed as persistent preterm labor. There is no longer a fetal heart rate, and the couple has been informed of their baby's death. Ann is being prepared for the imminent birth. She is scared and upset. She is crying. John has been holding her hand and supporting her. He has said nothing about his feelings. The couple would like Ann's mother to be called and want someone from pastoral care to support them at this time. They have no understanding of the labor and birth process and are unsure if they want to see or hold the baby after birth. Neither Ann nor John has experienced any prior losses.

EXPECTED OUTCOMES	IMPLEMENTATION	RATIONALE	EVALUATION
Nursing Diagnosis: Anxiety and fear related to lack of knowledge of the labor and birth process			
Ann and John will be able to cope with the labor and birth process.	Explain labor and birth phases, including pushing and what to expect physically and emotionally. Explain comfort measures for support person to use in caring for the mother, such as ice chips, back massage, and encouragement. Discuss options at the time of birth.	Prenatal fear of loss of control during labor can be avoided by preparing a mother and her significant other for the process.	Ann and John worked well together during labor and birth. He held her hand and helped her to breathe.
Nursing Diagnosis: Powerlessness related to loss and grief			
Parents will be able to express their needs and make decisions regarding the loss of their baby.	Offer family options for decision making. Provide information when needed and time to make decisions. Use therapeutic communication and counseling skills to support the family's grief responses and help with decision making.	Acceptance of the loss is the first task of mourners. Shock and numbness make it difficult to make decisions. Offering information and time to make decisions can help to raise self-esteem and promote feelings of some control over the situation.	They spent 2 hours with their baby in recovery and asked to have her brought to them in the postpartum unit.
Nursing Diagnosis: High risk for ineffective individual (family) coping related to death of baby			
Ann and family will be able to cope with the loss and experience uncomplicated bereavement.	Mobilize family's identified support systems, such as grandmother and chaplain. Secure tangible mementos such as footprints, handprints, and pictures. Follow-up after discharge can include phone calls, grief conference, and referral to support group.	Involving family, friends, and clergy mobilizes support for the bereaved parent at the time of the loss and after. Mementos are a tangible memory of their baby and their loss. Follow-up is crucial for the bereaved family not to feel alone and isolated after a loss.	Ann's mother came in to support Ann and John. She saw her granddaughter. Pastoral care offered a blessing. The baby is named Emily Ann. Ann and John verbalize appreciation for their mementos. One month later the couple joins a support group.

tant to respect family systems, culture, and religious practices and to support families when they choose to do things their way.

The evaluation of nursing care should rest on building an environment in which families can express their grief as well as their needs. The achievement of the expected outcomes is assured when the positive integration of the perceived loss is experienced by the family (see Plan of Care on p. 831).

OTHER LOSSES
Perinatal Diagnosis with a Negative Outcome

Early prenatal diagnostic tests such as ultrasonography, chorionic villus sampling, and amniocentesis can determine the well-being of the embryo or fetus. Reasons for doing prenatal testing include a history of chromosomal abnormality in the family, three or more miscarriages, maternal age, lack of fetal growth, movement, or heartbeat, diabetes mellitus or other chronic illnesses.

If the diagnosis of the health care provider is 99% sure that the baby has a serious genetic defect that would lead to death in utero or after birth (e.g., congenital anomalies incompatible with life or genetic disorders with severe mental retardation), the choice of *medical interruption of a pregnancy (abortion)* may be offered. The subject of abortion is controversial and may prevent parents from sharing this decision with other family members or friends. This of course limits their support systems after their loss.

The decision to terminate the pregnancy paves the way for feelings such as guilt, despair, sadness, and anger. The nurse's role is to be a good listener. It is important to assess how these families feel about the experience and to offer options for their memories as appropriate. The healing can take place when words can be given to feelings and when needs can be met. The parent who decides to continue the pregnancy will require emotional support as well. Remember, parents may be grieving not only the loss of the perfect child but the loss of expectations for their child's future (see Clinical Application of Research below).

✣ LOSS OF ONE IN A MULTIPLE PREGNANCY

The death of a twin or babies in a multifetal pregnancy during pregnancy, labor, and birth or after birth requires parents to parent and grieve at the same time. It imposes a very confusing and ambivalent induction into parenthood (Swanson-Kauffman, 1988). Parents feel they cannot do anything right. They cannot parent their surviv-

---

 CLINICAL APPLICATION OF RESEARCH

GRIEVING AFTER TERMINATION OF PREGNANCY FOR FETAL ANOMALY

With the increased availability of prenatal diagnosis, early identification of fetal anomalies is possible. Termination of planned pregnancies may be chosen by some couples. The purpose of this study was to compare the grief responses of women whose pregnancies were terminated to the grief responses of women who had a spontaneous loss of pregnancy. The index group included 23 women who had terminations of pregnancy and agreed to a psychiatric evaluation 2 months after termination. The comparison group compared 23 women in a longitudinal study of perinatal loss. At the end of the psychiatric interview each patient was assigned a Global Assessment of Functioning score. Participants completed the Beck Depression Inventory, the Perinatal Grief Scale, the Nethelp (to measure social support), and the Life Experiences Survey (to measure stressful life events). The groups were different in ages of the women (those electing termination were older) and gestational age when the loss occurred (terminations were earlier than the other perinatal losses). Gestational age was not related to depression, grief, despair, or difficulty in coping, but maternal age was related to these variables, with younger women experiencing more symptoms. In subsequent analyses maternal age was adjusted statistically. The re-

searchers found no differences between the two groups in grief responses. Four (17%) women in the index group met criteria for major depression, and 13 others had symptoms of depression. There were no differences in feelings of guilt between the two groups. Women reported preoccupation with the loss of a wanted baby rather than with the termination. Women who elected to terminate pregnancies usually had good outcomes.

The researchers suggested that the psychologic adaptation of women who terminate pregnancies following prenatal diagnosis is more like that of women who have spontaneous perinatal losses than that of women who have elective termination of a pregnancy. Nurses who work with women who have a perinatal loss, either spontaneously or by elective termination, must assess them for adaptation to the loss. Significant grief responses that require psychiatric intervention may occur; nurses should be alert to the need for referral. Follow-up of these women to assess adaptation over time is necessary.

Reference: Zeanah CH et al: Do women grieve after terminating pregnancies because of fetal anomalies? A controlled investigation, *Obstet Gynecol* 82:270, 1993.

ing child with all the joy and enthusiasm of new parents because the baby reminds them of what they have lost. They cannot give over completely to grieve in the manner they would want to because the surviving child demands their attention. These parents are at high risk for dysfunctional parenting, as well as developing complicated bereavement. They might repress their grief to parent their surviving child or they may be overwhelmed in their grief and unable to parent the surviving children.

It is important to help the parent's acknowledge the birth of all their babies. They should be treated as bereaved families, and all the options discussed previously should be offered. Pictures should be taken of the babies together and separately. Parents should be offered the opportunity to hold all their babies in their arms, as well as to have private time to say goodbye to the baby who has died.

Bereaved parents should be warned that well-meaning family members or friends may say, "Well at least you have the other baby." implying that there should be no grief because they are lucky to have one. Parents need to be able to anticipate insensitivity to their loss and empowered to say to those people, "That is not how I feel." By simply setting a boundary on what their feelings are, they are able to acknowledge their baby who died, and then have an opportunity to share more about their feelings if they so choose.

Bereaved parents of twins have special problems in coping with their life without their anticipated "extra special" family, telling their surviving child about his or her twin, dealing with the possibility of that child's feelings of survivor guilt, plus deciding on how to celebrate birthdays, death days, and special holidays.

Adolescent Grief

Adolescent pregnancy accounts for approximately 20% of all births in the United States (ACOG, 1989). Adolescent participants have been included in the samples of research done in all areas of perinatal bereavement. This indicates that adolescents do grieve the loss of their babies during pregnancy or shortly after (Bright, 1987; Shodt, 1982).

The relationship of the pregnant woman to her mother has been highlighted as significant by Lederman (1984). Many mothers and health care professionals may feel the adolescent's loss of her baby was for the best. Adolescents may not feel the same way and may be grieving the loss of a much wanted, needed baby.

The first step for the nurse in caring for a bereaved adolescent is to acknowledge the significance of giving birth no matter what age the mother might be. Second, the nurse should make additional efforts in developing a trusting relationship in working with an adolescent. Third, the nurse offers all of the options, anticipatory guidance, support, and information to meet the adolescent at the point of her need. It may take longer for an adolescent to process her grief due to her level of cognitive and psychoemotional maturation. Being patient, saving mementos, and giving the adolescent information on how to contact the nurse, can help the adolescent accept the reality of the loss and process their grief.

Maternal Death

It is extremely rare for a woman to die in childbirth, but it can happen. Families may be faced with not only mourning the death of a wife and mother, but also the death of the baby. Or they may be faced with parenting a baby without a surviving mother. "Death of the mother completely disrupts the family structure and often leaves the father with the care of a baby at a time when his emotional reserves are lowest" (Johnson, 1986). The same bereavement process and tasks need to be accomplished for the surviving partner, children, grandparents, other family members, and friends for them to heal after such a devastating loss.

The nursing care of families at this time is similar to what has already been described. Options need to be offered, memories made, and mementos obtained and held for the family until they are ready for them. These families are at high risk for developing complicated bereavement and dysfunctional parenting of the surviving baby and other children in the family. Referral to social services to help the family mobilize support systems, as well as for counseling, can combat potential problems before they develop and can be beneficial not only at the time of the loss, but also in the future.

Complicated Bereavement

Working with the bereaved in the weeks and months after a loss occurs requires knowledge of how to identify **complicated bereavement.** The difficulties an individual or a family experience may be in the grieving of the loss itself or an exacerbation of prior problems that were simply intensified during mourning. Referral to a competent therapist is part of one's professional responsibility to the family experiencing complicated bereavement.

Who needs referral? The list includes, but is not limited to, those who:
- Have symptoms of anxiety or depression that interfere with functioning in any of the three major areas of life: social/family, work, and physical health
- Have persistent thoughts of suicide that become almost constant, or express serious suicide intents or the development of a plan
- Are stuck in the searching and yearning phase, which is evident by persistent anger, guilt, or obsessive thinking about the loss
- Abuse mood-altering chemicals;
- Have relationship difficulties (partner, children, family, friends, co-workers)

It is the responsibility of a qualified mental health professional to distinguish between uncomplicated bereavement or an adjustment disorder with depressed mood and a major depression. However, there are certain symptoms that signal the likelihood of major depression, something for which a person should be immediately referred:

- Loss or gain of 15% of one's body weight
- Inability to maintain or initiate basic living activities, including care of surviving children
- Persistent suicidal thoughts with or without intent or plan
- Reclusiveness

These are all red flags for depression. An individual experiencing uncomplicated bereavement who does not have a major depression feels better over time; is sad but functional; and can perform the usual activities of daily living though not with as much enthusiasm and energy as before the loss.

Finding a mental health professional with whom one can consult is imperative for the nurse doing bereavement follow-up. That person could be anyone who does therapy and is knowledgeable about bereavement and the referral process. Bereavement complications seem to be best handled by a strong individual therapist with knowledge of family systems or a marriage and family therapist who also does individual work.

Families should be told about the therapy process and what to expect.

1. Change in their symptoms should occur within four sessions or there is something wrong with the therapist or therapy, or the mix of patient and therapist is not right.
2. All therapists should be willing to discuss with a patient their professional degrees, experience, particular strengths, and how they usually work with similar patients.
3. The patient should have input into the treatment plan; know what the goals of therapy are; and approximately how long it will take to accomplish them (e.g., is the therapist thinking about 4 to 6 weeks or 6 to 12 months?)

Going for therapy is a big step for people to make. The highest number of cancellations and "no shows" in a therapist's practice are intakes or first visits; therefore anything the nurse can do for a family or individual to help with that major hurdle would accomplish a great deal. However, it is also important to remember that for whatever reason, people with symptoms might not be ready to work on those issues.

KEY POINTS

- Parental and infant attachment can begin prior to pregnancy with many hopes and dreams for the future.
- The gestational age of the baby does not influence the severity of the grief response or bereavement process.
- When a baby dies, all members of a family are affected, but no two family members will grieve in the same way.
- When birth represents death, the role of the nurse is critical in caring for the woman and her family regardless of the age of the woman.
- An understanding of grief responses and the bereavement process is fundamental in the implementation of the nursing process.

- Careful assessment of each family member's perception of the loss is important prior to intervention.
- Therapeutic communication and counseling techniques can help families in identifying their feelings, to feel comfortable in expressing their grief, and in understanding their bereavement process.
- Follow-up after discharge is an essential component in providing care to families who have experienced a loss.
- Nurses need to be aware of their own feelings of grief and loss to provide a nonjudgmental environment of care and support for bereaved families.

CRITICAL THINKING EXERCISES

1. Discover what community resources and support groups exist to assist parents who have experienced:
   a. A preterm birth
   b. Birth of a less than perfect child
   c. A cesarean birth
   d. The death of a baby through miscarriage, stillbirth, or newborn death
2. Ask permission of the group leader to attend a support group meeting.
   a. Discuss your reactions to the meeting.

   b. Describe what information you identified as useful in providing care to grieving families.
3. After viewing a film on death and grieving, discuss the kinds of grief responses observed.
4. Role play a situation where a family has experienced a newborn death and the nurse is bringing their baby to them.
5. Practice taking pictures of different size baby dolls.

References

American College of Obstetricians and Gynecologists: *Fact sheet,* Washington, DC, 1989, ACOG.

Borg S, Lasker J: *When pregnancy fails,* Boston, 1981, Beacon Press.

Bowlby J, Parkes CM: Separation and loss within the family. In Anthony EJ, Koupernik C, editors: *The child and his family,* New York, 1970, Wiley.

Bright P: Adolescent pregnancy and loss, *MCN* 16:1, 1987.

Cunningham FG et al: *Williams obstetrics,* ed 19, Norwalk, CT, 1993, Appleton & Lange.

Davidson GW: *Understanding mourning,* Minneapolis, 1984, Ausburg Pub. House.

Johnson SH: *Nursing assessment and strategies for the family at risk: high risk parenting,* ed 2, Philadelphia, 1986, JB Lippincott.

Kowalski K: *Perinatal death: an ethnomethological study of factors influencing perinatal bereavement,* Unpublished doctoral dissertation, Denver, 1984, University of Colorado.

Lederman R: *Psychosocial adaptation to pregnancy,* Englewood Cliffs, NJ, 1984, Prentice Hall.

Limbo RK, Wheeler SR: Coping with unexpected outcomes, *NAACOG Update Series,* 5(3):1, 1986a.

Limbo RK, Wheeler SR: *When a baby dies: a handbook for healing and helping,* La Crosse, WI, 1986b, Lutheran Hospital.

Limbo RK, Wheeler SR, Gensch BK: *Resolve through sharing counselor's certification manual,* La Crosse, WI, 1988, Lutheran Hospital.

Sanders CM: *Grief, the mourning after: dealing with adult bereavement,* New York, 1989, Wiley Interscience.

Schodt C: Grief in adolescent mothers after an infant death, *Image J Nurs Sch* 14:20, 1982.

Swanson-Kauffman KM: Caring in the instance of unexpected early pregnancy loss, *Topics Clin Nurs* 8(2):37, 1986.

Swanson-Kauffman KM: Providing care in the NICU: sometimes an act of love, *Adv Nurs Science* 13(1):60, 1990.

Swanson-Kauffman KM: There should have been two: nursing care of parents experiencing perinatal death of a twin, *J Perinat Neonat Nurs* 2(2):78, 1988.

Worden WJ: *Grief counseling and grief therapy: a handbook for the mental health practitioner,* New York, 1991, Springer.

Bibliography

Gifford BJ, Cleary BB: Supporting the bereaved, *Am J Nurs* 2:49, 1990.

Gilbert E, Harmon J: Pregnancy loss and perinatal grief. In Gilbert E, Harmon J, editors: *Manual of high risk pregnancy and delivery,* ed 2, St Louis, 1993, Mosby.

Kimble DL: Neonatal death: a descriptive study of fathers' experiences, *Neonatal Network* 9(8):45, 1991.

Lawson L: Culturally sensitive support for grieving parents, *MCN* 16(2):76, 1991.

Page-Lieberman J, Hughes CB: How fathers perceive perinatal death, *MCN* 15:320, 1990.

Parkman S: Helping families say goodbye, *MCN* 17(1):14, 1992.

Peppers L, Knapp R: *Motherhood and mourning,* New York, 1990, Praeger.

Reed K: Influence of age and parity on the emotional care given to women experiencing miscarriages, *Image J Nurse Sch* 22(2):89, 1990.

Sexton P, Stephen S: Postpartum mothers' perceptions of nursing interventions for perinatal grief, *Neonatal Network* 9(5):47, 1991.

Eight

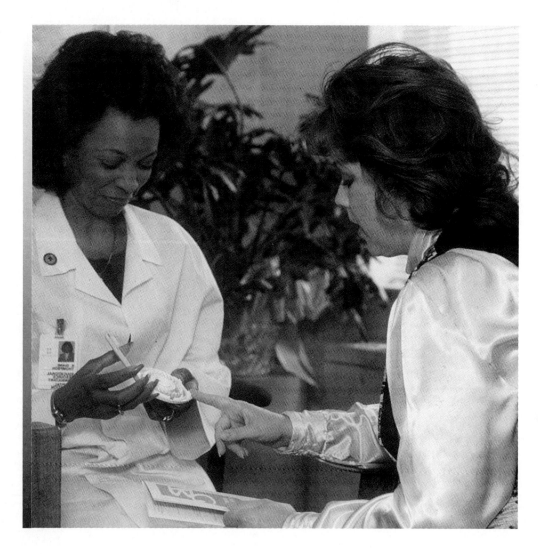

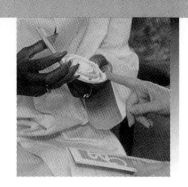

Women's Health

29 Health Promotion and Screening

30 Common Reproductive Concerns

CHAPTER

29 Health Promotion and Screening

E D N A   B.   Q U I N N

LEARNING OBJECTIVES

Define the key terms listed.
List factors influencing a woman's contact with the health care system.
Outline the schedule for women's health promotion and screening.
Identify reasons women enter the health care delivery system.
Explain how well-woman health assessment varies with culture, age, physical handicaps, and family abuse.
Review important assessments in screening for cervical and breast cancer.
Review patient teaching of breast self-examination.
Suggest community resources for well-woman health care.

KEY TERMS

breast self-examination (BSE)
cervical intraepithelial neoplasm (CIN)
Kegel exercises
mammography
Papanicolaou (Pap) smear
vulvar self-examination (VSE)

RELATED TOPICS

Battered women (Chap. 23) • Contraception (Chap. 18) • Nutrition history (Chap. 8) • Osteoporosis (Chap. 30) • Pelvic examination (Chap. 7) • Sexually transmitted diseases (Chap. 21) • Substance abuse assessment (Chap. 23)

This chapter deals with those aspects of women's health promotion and screening not covered elsewhere in this text. It highlights assessment of older women, abused women, and women with disabilities. Cultural considerations in gynecologic care are included, and concerns related to screening for breast and cervical cancer are discussed. Also included is anticipatory guidance for health promotion and preventive care.

In the reproductive years, health promotion takes place for most women in prenatal and family planning care settings. Their care is discussed elsewhere in this text. Newborn through adolescent assessment can be found in child nursing texts.

WELL-WOMAN HEALTH CARE

The rising expectations of women, as well as profound changes in the family, society, and sexual behavior, make women's health promotion a challenging field. For years the traditional medical system, either consciously or unconsciously, oppressed and exploited women "for their own good" (Ehrenreich, English, 1978). In the 1970s many women sought alternatives to what they perceived as insensitive and sexist treatment, and the women's self-help movement was born. Groups of women established and ran their own clinics, providing services and educational programs. Women in the movement were determined to learn more about their own bodies, and they demanded the right to make decisions regarding their health care in active participation with care providers.

Today "a host of alternative health care systems have emerged in response to the perceived inattention of the traditional medical community to wellness issues" (Stotland, 1990). Women are continuing to question and change the traditional system. The American Nurses Association made women's health issues a priority for 1992, focusing on two major concerns: the lack of women in scientific studies and the lack of research on diseases that disproportionately affect women, such as breast cancer and osteoporosis. Space does not permit a detailed discussion of the women's health movement and the issues that gave rise to it, but nurses should understand this historical background for women's health care.

A major thrust of care is educating women about the impact that lifestyle has on health status and the risks involved if they abuse their health. The fact that most women are interested in participating in decision making and self-care gives the nurse a unique opportunity. As a change agent and patient advocate, the nurse can increase women's knowledge and self-esteem so that they will become active and satisfied participants in their own health care. It is important for the nurse to ascertain what a woman is interested in learning and her baseline knowledge of a topic before teaching. The woman's interests may be significantly different from what the care provider believes she wants to know. However, many women believe a topic is important only if the care provider initiates the discussion, giving the nurse the opportunity to motivate learning and facilitate informed decision making (Freda et al, 1993).

Reasons for Entering the Health Care System

Many women first enter the health care delivery system for a Papanicolaou test or contraception. Visits to the gynecologist, nurse-practitioner, or nurse-midwife may be their only contact with the system unless they become ill. Some women postpone examination until a specific need arises, such as pregnancy, pain, abnormal vaginal bleeding, or incapacitating vaginal discharge. Other women report a minor symptom as a "ticket" for entering the health care system when other motives for seeking care, either conscious or unconscious, underlie their primary complaint. It is not uncommon for serious concerns (fear of pregnancy, sexually transmitted disease, cancer, sexual functioning, or perimenopausal events) to surface during the interview. Embarrassing signs and symptoms, such as urinary incontinence, dyspareunia (painful intercourse), and annoying vaginal discharge, are often only elicited by sensitive interviewing and careful examination.

Health care needs vary with culture, religion, age, and personal differences. The changing status and roles of women, socioeconomic status, education, and personal circumstances contribute to differences in the health behavior of women. Employment outside the home, physical disability, a change in residence, separation or divorce, single parenthood, and widowhood affect women's ability to seek care.

The Interview and History

The interview should be conducted in an unhurried manner, with questions phrased in a sensitive, nonjudg-

mental manner. Body language should match verbal communication. The nurse must recognize the women's *vulnerability* and assure the woman of *strict confidentiality*. For many women, modesty and fear of the unknown make the assessment—the interview, the physical examination, and particularly the pelvic examination—an ordeal. Many women are uninformed, misguided by myths, or afraid to appear stupid by asking questions about sexual and reproductive functioning. The nurse must be sensitive to these issues.

Biographic Information (Admission Form)

At a woman's first visit she fills out a form with biographic and historical data before meeting with the examiner. The examiner scans the admission form and welcomes her to the office. When the woman and examiner are comfortable, the examiner begins with the interview, clarifying, expanding, or completing the admission form. The nurse ensures that the woman's name, identification number, age, marital status, racial origin, ethnic background, address, phone numbers, occupation, and date of visit are recorded. Names of next of kin are noted for dependent adults. Identifying data should appear on all pages of the document.

Source and Reliability of Information

Old records are considered reliable sources. The nurse records a subjective judgment about the reliability of the person giving the history—the woman, the parent, or other historian.

Chief Concern

The chief concern is the *verbatim response* to the question, "What problem or symptom(s) brought you here today?" The onset and duration of the problem are also noted. If no specific problem is identified, the nurse can proceed to the medical history.

Present Problem or Illness

No single outline is applicable to all cases. The interviewer may feel most comfortable asking questions related to the chief concern. Other interviewers prefer to complete the history before returning to the present. It may be useful to ask the woman to sketch out the problem first. Using this method, the interviewer can see the relative importance of the features surrounding the problem from the woman's perception.

The woman's state of health before the onset of the present problem is determined. In addition, the earliest symptoms noted before the initial episode may reveal its cause. If the problem is of long standing, the reason for seeking attention at this time is elicited. Identification of associated symptoms and factors that precipitate, exacerbate, or relieve the condition provide important data. The woman is requested to describe how the problem has affected her usual lifestyle. The course of the problem is plotted from the onset to the present. The findings are summarized and reviewed with the woman/historian to confirm or correct the information obtained. When more than one significant problem is present, each one is treated in the same manner.

Medical History*

1. *General health and strength*
2. *Childhood illnesses:* measles, mumps, whooping cough, chickenpox, scarlet fever, acute rheumatic fever, diphtheria, poliomyelitis
3. *Major adult illnesses:* tuberculosis, hepatitis, hypertension, diabetes, myocardial infarction, tropical or parasitic diseases, sexually transmitted diseases, other infections; any nonsurgical hospital admissions (dates and reasons)
4. *Immunizations:* polio, diphtheria, pertussis, and tetanus toxoid, influenza, cholera, typhus, typhoid, last PPD or other skin tests, hepatitis B, unusual reactions to immunizations: tetanus or other antitoxin made with horse serum
5. *Surgery:* dates, hospital, diagnosis, complications
6. *Serious injuries:* resulting in disability; if the present problem has potential medicolegal relation to an injury, give full documentation
7. *Medications:* current and recent medications, including dosage; both prescription, over-the-counter, herbal, and home remedy
8. *Allergies:* especially to medications, but also to environmental allergens and foods
9. *Transfusions:* reactions, date and number of units transfused

Family History*

1. Do any members of the woman's family have illnesses with features that are similar to the woman's illness?
2. What is the health status or cause of death of parents and siblings, with ages at death?
3. Is there a history of heart disease, high blood pressure, cancer, tuberculosis, stroke, diabetes, gout, kidney disease, thyroid disease, asthma and other allergic states, blood diseases, sexually transmitted diseases, any familial disease?
4. What are the ages and health status of spouse and children?
5. If there is a hereditary disease in the family, such as hemophilia, Tay-Sachs disease, or sickle cell anemia, what is the condition of the grandparents, aunts, uncles, and cousins? A pedigree diagram is often helpful in recording this type of family information.

Social and Experiential History*

1. *Personal status:* birthplace, where raised, home environment as youth (e.g., parental divorce or separation, socioeconomic class, cultural background), education, position in family, marital status, general life satisfaction, hobbies, interests, perception of "being healthy"
2. *Nutrition:* diet; regularity of eating; quantity of coffee, tea, and alcohol consumed; use of vitamin and mineral supplementation
3. *Activity-exercise:* quantity and type
4. *Sleep-rest:* regularity of sleeping, hours, usual times for sleep-rest
5. *Coping–stress tolerance:* typical stressors, estimate of level of stress on a typical day at home or work, usual ways of coping, relaxing, use of illicit drugs (frequency, type, and amount)
6. *Sexuality:*
   a. Has she had a pelvic examination before?
   b. Times and frequency of coitus if sexually active
   c. Contraceptive history: type, when used, any problems, time and reasons for discontinuation
   d. Attitudes concerning range of acceptable sexual behavior as defined by such factors as culture, religion, family, and peer group (1) Is it all right for married people to masturbate? (2) How do your ideas and feelings about sex differ from those of your partner?
   e. Sexual self-concept (how one sees oneself sexually influences how one relates to others)
   f. Level of knowledge, including understanding of how the body functions, sexual anatomy and physiology, and myths and misinformation about sex
   g. Sexual behavior: marital or alternative relationship
   h. Any difficulties or fears?
7. *Home conditions:* housing, economic condition, type of health insurance if any, pets and their health
8. *Occupation:* description of usual work and present work if different; conditions and hours, physical or mental strain; duration of employment, present and past exposure to heat and cold, industrial toxins (especially lead, arsenic, chromium, asbestos, beryllium, poisonous gases, benzene, and polyvinyl chloride or other carcinogens); any protective devices required; exposure to cigarette smoke
9. *Environment:* travel and other exposure to contagious diseases, residence in tropics, water and milk supply, other sources of infection if applicable
10. *Military record:* dates and geographic area of assignments

---

*Modified from Seidel HM et al: *Mosby's guide to physical examination,* ed 3, St Louis, 1995, Mosby.

11. *Religious preference:* determine any religious proscriptions concerning health care
12. *Culture and ethnicity:* determine any proscriptions or prescriptions affecting health care

Review of Systems*

It is probable that all of the questions in each system will not be included every time you take a history. Nevertheless, some questions regarding each system should be included in every history. The essential areas to be explored are listed in the following outline. If the woman gives a positive response to a question about an essential area, then more detailed questions should be asked. Keep in mind that these lists do not represent an exhaustive list of questions that might be appropriate within an organ system. Even more detailed questions may be required depending on the woman's problem.

1. *General constitutional symptoms:* energy level, feelings of well-being, fever, chills, malaise, fatigability, night sweats; weight (average, preferred, present, change, appetite)
2. *Skin:* rash or eruption, itching, pigmentation or texture change; excessive sweating; abnormal nail or hair growth
3. *Musculoskeletal:* joint stiffness, pain, restriction of motion, swelling, redness, heat, bony deformity, muscle tone and cramping, vascularity, bone fragility, flat feet, curvature of spine
4. *Head*
   a. General: frequent or unusual headaches, dizziness, syncope, severe head injuries
   b. Eyes: visual acuity or problems, pain, discharge; use of eye drops or other eye medications; history of trauma or familial eye disease; prescription glasses or contact lenses; last eye examination
   c. Ears: hearing loss, pain, discharge, tinnitus, vertigo
   d. Nose: sense of smell, frequency of colds, obstruction, epistaxis, postnasal discharge, sinus pain
   e. Throat and mouth: hoarseness or change in voice, frequent sore throats, bleeding or swelling of gums, recent tooth abscesses or extractions, soreness of tongue or buccal mucosa, ulcers, disturbance of taste, dentures, last visit to a dentist, frequency of dental care, problems with chewing or swallowing
   f. Neck: pain, restriction of movement, swelling
5. *Endocrine:* thyroid enlargement or tenderness, heat or cold intolerance, unexplained weight change, diabetes, polydipsia, polyuria, changes in facial or body hair, increased hat and glove size, skin striae
   a. Menses: regularity, duration and amount of flow, dysmenorrhea, last menstrual period (LMP), previous menstrual period (PMP), last normal menstrual period (LNMP), intermenstrual discharge or bleeding, itching, date of last Papanicolaou smear, age at menopause, libido, frequency of intercourse, sexual difficulties
   b. Pregnancies: number, miscarriages/abortions, duration of pregnancy in each and any complication during any pregnancy or postpartum period; use of oral or other contraceptives
   c. Breasts: pain, tenderness, discharge, lumps, mammograms
6. *Respiratory:* pain relating to respiration, dyspnea, cyanosis, wheezing, cough, sputum (character and quantity), hemoptysis, night sweats, exposure to TB; date and result of last chest x-ray study; frequency and types of infection; number of cigarettes smoked per day and for how many years
7. *Cardiovascular:* history of congenital heart disease, rheumatic fever, hypertension, hypotension, pain, dyspnea, palpitations, number of pillows (to evaluate head) needed to sleep comfortably, estimate of exercise tolerance, past ECG or other cardiac tests
8. *Hematologic:* blood type, Rh factor, anemia, tendency to bruise or bleed easily, thromboses, thrombophlebitis, any known abnormality of blood cells, transfusions
9. *Immune:* lymph node enlargement, tenderness, or suppuration, infections (type, response to therapy, complications), autoimmune disorders
10. *Gastrointestinal:* appetite, digestion, intolerance for any class of foods, dysphagia, heartburn, nausea, vomiting, regularity of bowels, constipation, diarrhea, change in stool color or contents (clay colored, tarry, fresh blood, mucus, undigested food), flatulence, hemorrhoids, hepatitis, jaundice, dark urine, history of ulcers, gallstones, polyps, or tumor, previous x-ray studies (where, when, findings)
11. *Genitourinary:* dysuria, flank or suprapubic pain, urgency, frequency, nocturia, hematuria, polyuria, hesitancy, dribbling, loss of force of stream, passage of stone, edema of face, stress incontinence, hernias, sexually transmitted disease (inquire what kind and symptoms)
12. *Neurologic:* syncope, seizures, weakness or paralysis, abnormalities of sensation or coordination, tremors, loss of memory, unusual frequency, distribution, or severity of headaches, serious head injury in past

---

*Modified from Seidel HM et al: *Mosby's guide to physical examination,* ed 3, St Louis, 1995, Mosby.

13. *Psychiatric:* depression, mood changes, difficulty concentrating, nervousness, tension, suicidal thoughts, irritability, sleep disturbances, drug or alcohol abuse

Concluding Questions

At the conclusion of the history, the woman is asked, "Is there anything else that you think would be important for me to know?" If several complaints are mentioned and discussed in the history, it is often useful to ask, "What problem concerns you most?" With vague, complicated, or contradictory histories, it may be helpful to ask, "What do you think is the matter with you?"

Cultural Considerations

Recognition of signs and symptoms of disease, as well as deciding when to seek treatment, are influenced by *cultural perceptions.* Every society has culture-specific beliefs and extensive prescriptions regarding sexuality and reproduction.

In the United States premarital sexual activity, often with multiple partners or a partner of the same or opposite sex, has become increasingly acceptable, contributing to the increased incidence of unplanned pregnancy, sexually transmitted diseases, and cervical dysplasia and neoplasms. On the other hand, in many other cultures, knowledge of sexual matters is limited, and explicit graphic reproduction of the genitals is forbidden. The reputation and status of the entire family may rest on the woman's marital fidelity and premarital virginity (Laffin, 1975). Therefore, to ensure an intact hymen (or proof of virginity) tampons and douches are avoided, and medical examination of the vaginal vault is limited to a one-finger internal examination and the use of the small-

est available speculum (see Fig. 7-3). A female attendant should always be present when the examiner is male. Women examiners are often preferred.

The Older Woman

The older woman can present a challenge in taking a history. Multiple chronic and debilitating health problems often overlap with the process of aging, and signs and symptoms of disease may be less dramatic, producing only vague complaints. Confusion, for example, may be the only symptom of an infection or cerebrovascular accident. Older people are at greater risk of developing painful conditions or injuries, but pain may be an unreliable symptom. They seem to lose pain perception or experience pain differently.

Some women fail to report symptoms because they fear the complaint will be attributed to old age or that nothing can be done (see Clinical Application of Research box below). They may have lived with a chronic condition for so long that they have come to accept the symptoms as part of daily life.

The tendency for multiple problems to be treated with many drugs puts the older person at risk for iatrogenic disorders. A complete medication history is essential, with special attention to the interaction of drugs, diseases, and the aging process.

Functional assessment should be included as part of the older woman's history. In the review of systems, the nurse needs to ask about self-care activities such as walking, getting out of bed, getting to the bathroom, bathing, combing the hair, dressing, and eating. Questions about driving a car or using public transportation, dialing the telephone, hanging up clothes, getting groceries, and preparing meals should also be included. It is

CLINICAL APPLICATION OF RESEARCH

PHYSICAL HEALTH AND PSYCHOLOGIC WELL-BEING IN ELDERLY WOMEN

The majority of the aged are women. Elderly women have more acute illnesses and injuries, are more likely to be poor and live alone, and have more chronic illnesses than elderly men. However, most elderly women state that they are doing well. The purpose of the study was to examine relationships among age, health, and well-being in elderly women living in the community. Participants were 240 women, 65 years of age or older. Physical health was assessed by self-report measures of illness, activities of daily living, and bothersome symptoms. Psychologic well-being was measured by assessing autonomy, personal growth, purpose in life, and positive relations with others. Depression and anxiety were also measured. Questionnaires were completed and returned in postage-paid envelopes. The researcher found that, as women grow older, they report less purpose in life, less personal growth, and fewer positive relationships.

Women who report poor health, regardless of age, also report more depression and anxiety and fewer positive relationships and less autonomy. Physical symptoms, rather than number of health problems, affect the well-being of elderly women (21% reported being depressed). Since treating symptoms may relieve depression, nursing assessment and treatment of bothersome symptoms are important. Efforts need to be directed toward helping women in advanced old age maintain a purpose in life and a feeling of social connectedness. Viewing women within a life-span developmental perspective is important in assessing well-being in old age.

Reference: Heidrich SM: The relationship between physical health and psychological well-being in elderly women: a developmental perspective, *Res Nurs Health* 16:123, 1993.

important to assess whether the woman is able to take medications correctly.

The Woman with a Disability

Women with serious physical or emotional disorders— the deaf, the blind, the depressed, the physically disabled, the mentally retarded, and the brain-injured—must all be respected and fully involved in the assessment to the limit of their ability. The nurse should communicate directly with the woman with a disability, maintaining eye contact: it is best to learn about the disability from her. When the family is available, they can often advise on communication techniques used successfully at home. If there is a language barrier, a translator should be used. A translator who signs may be available for the deaf, but most deaf people read, write, and read lips, so an interviewer who speaks and enunciates each word slowly and in full view may be understood. The blind can usually hear, and the nurse should avoid two common pitfalls with these women—trying to communicate with gestures, and talking louder in hopes of being understood (Care providers also tend to speak louder when trying to communicate with non–English-speaking women).

Women with emotional problems may not be able to give a reliable history, but their points of view and attitudes should be obtained from *them* to the extent possible. The woman's record and, when necessary, the family and other health professionals involved in care, must be consulted.

Abused Women

When seeing any woman, the nurse must keep in mind the possibility that violence against the woman may have occurred. Abuse is a life-threatening health problem that affects millions of women and their children. Many care providers defer questions about family violence because they are unaware of the extent of the problem or they find it difficult to ask about violence. Just as they learn to ask other intimate questions, nurses can learn to inquire about this problem. Help depends on early detection and intervention. Fear, guilt, and embarrassment keep many women from giving information about family violence. Clues in the history (e.g., numerous injuries and stress-related symptoms) and evidence on physical examination of injuries, such as burns or lacerations, should alert the nurse to the problem. Assessment requires a detailed history of the woman's investment in her situation and active listening. The nurse helps the woman formulate a plan: What referral options (local agencies and shelters) can help her? If she plans to return home, how will she manage? The nurse's goal is to empower the woman: she needs to gain a feeling of control over her life, to set her own goals and make her own decisions. Misinformation and resorting to legal avenues can be dangerous. There is a national toll-free number

(1-800-333 SAFE) for information regarding abuse and local shelters (Parker, McFarlane, 1991).

Schedule for Screening

Protocols may recommend periodic visits every 1 to 3 years, depending on the age and risk status of the woman. Annual visits that include history, height, and weight, blood pressure, clinical breast examination, pelvic examination, Papanicolaou smear (Pap test), and digital rectal examination are the norm.

The optimum frequency for screening examinations is debatable in the absence of strong baseline data that relate the frequency of examinations and tests with outcomes. The American College of Obstetricians and Gynecologists (ACOG), (1989) recommends the first gynecologic examination by age 18 or earlier if the woman has menstrual problems, a vaginal discharge, is sexually active or about to become sexually active, or is planning a pregnancy. The frequency of visits after the initial examination depends on the plan of care or presence of risk factors.

Annual oral, skin, and digital rectal examinations are recommended, beginning at age 50 (*Healthy People 2000*, 1990). Malignant melanoma, a skin cancer, has a 90% 5-year survival rate if localized, but only a 12% survival rate if the disease has spread (*Healthy People 2000*, 1990). Box 29-1 illustrates a periodic screening program for women ages 40 to 65.

Physical Examination

Physical examination may not always include a pelvic examination. Regardless of whether a complete gynecologic examination is indicated, an atmosphere conducive to privacy, with respect for the woman's dignity and culture, should be provided. Basic content on the physical examination is found in Chapter 7. Since the most critical parts of the examination are the breast examination and the Papanicolaou (Pap) smear included in the pelvic examination, this chapter focuses on them.

Breast Self-Examination (BSE)

Breast cancer is the leading cause of cancer deaths in women. An estimated 175,000 (or one in nine) American women develop breast cancer annually, and about 44,500 die. Despite years of research and improvements in diagnosis, death rates have remained the same since the 1970s. The nurse has a critical role to play in breast cancer screening and teaching. When the tumor is detected early while it is still localized, the survival rate approaches 100% (Nemcek, 1990). Most tumors are discovered by the woman herself.

Breast examination by a health care provider is recommended every 3 years for women between 20 and 40 years of age and every year after age 40. The breast examination provides an ideal opportunity to teach or re-

Sample Screening Program for Women Ages 40 to 65

RECOMMENDED FOR ALL MIDLIFE WOMEN EVERY 1 TO 3 YEARS

Physical examination
  Height and weight
  Breast exam
  Pelvic exam
  Vulvar exam
  Rectal exam
Blood pressure check
Laboratory tests/diagnostic tests
  Pap smear
  Mammogram
  Nonfasting total blood cholesterol
  Urinalysis
  Stool guiac
  Hgb/Hct

RECOMMENDED AS NEEDED FOR MIDLIFE WOMEN AT RISK

Physical examination
  Skin exam
  Oral cavity exam
Laboratory tests/diagnostic tests
  Tuberculin testing
  VDRL
  Chlamydial testing
  Gonorrhea culture
  HIV testing
  Electrocardiogram
  Endometrial biopsy
  Bone density screening
  Proctoscopic exam
  Fasting plasma glucose

Modified from United States Preventive Services Task Force, National Health Information Center, USDHS: *Guide to clinical preventive services,* Baltimore, 1989, Williams & Wilkins.

view **breast self-examination (BSE)**. Monthly BSE is recommended, but most women practice it far less often, and some women do not perform it at all. Nursing research indicates that positive attitudes toward the BSE, social influences, and the stated intention to perform BSE correlate well with the behavior (Lierman et al, 1990). The nurse should explore these influences and encourage the woman to verbalize (and thereby reinforce) her intention to perform BSE monthly. Return demonstration is essential; this allows for correction where there is error, and reinforcement of the woman's confidence in self-care ability (see the Teaching Approaches box on p. 846).

Nemeck (1990) found that difficulty in remembering when to perform BSE, fear of finding a lump, perceived

inability to recognize lumps, and embarrassment were barriers to BSE in a study of 95 African-American women. For each woman, barriers must be assessed and strategies to overcome them must be individualized. The extra time these efforts take may save a life.

Pelvic Examination

The gynecologic examination (see Chapter 7) does not differ markedly from the rest of the physical examination except that it is a more intimate and invasive procedure and requires specialized skills and greater sensitivity on the part of the examiner. A positive attitude can do much to make it less threatening. Women need procedure-specific, concrete, objective information along with self-care instructions during stressful medical procedures (Barsevick, Lauver, 1990).

Vulvar Self-Examination (VSE)

The pelvic examination provides a good opportunity for the practitioner to emphasize the need for regular **vulvar self-examination (VSE)** and to teach this procedure. Because there has been a dramatic increase in cancerous and precancerous conditions of the vulva in recent years, VSE should be performed as an integral part of preventive health care by all women who are sexually active or 18 years of age or older, monthly between menses or more frequently if there are symptoms or a history of serious vulvar disease (Lawhead, 1990). Most lesions, including malignancy, condyloma acuminata, and Bartholin's cysts, can be seen and/or palpated and are easily treatable if diagnosed early.

The examination can be performed by the practitioner and woman together, using a mirror. A simple diagram of the anatomy of the vulva can be given to the woman, with instructions to perform the examination herself that evening to reinforce what she has learned. She does the examination in a sitting position with adequate lighting, holding a mirror in one hand and using the other hand to expose the tissues surround the vaginal introitus. She then systematically examines the mons pubis, clitoris, urethra, labia majora, perineum, and perianal area, and palpates the vulva, noting any changes in appearance or abnormalities, such as ulcers, lumps, warts, and changes in pigmentation. The number of women who seek early treatment for vulvar symptoms, resulting in timely diagnosis and treatment, should increase as a result of this simple screening procedure.

Laboratory and Diagnostic Procedures

The following laboratory and diagnostic procedures are ordered at the discretion of the clinician: hemoglobin, nonfasting total blood cholesterol, fasting plasma glucose, urinalysis for bacteria, VDRL and other screening

TEACHING APPROACHES

BREAST SELF-EXAMINATION

1. The best time to do breast self-examination is after your period, when breasts are not tender or swollen. If you do not have regular periods or sometimes skip a month, do it on the same day every month.
2. Lie down and put a pillow under your right shoulder. Place your right arm behind your head (Fig. 1).

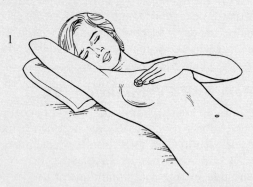

3. Use the finger pads of your three middle fingers on your left hand to feel for lumps or thickening. Your finger pads are the top third of each finger.
4. Press firmly enough to know how your breast feels. If you're not sure how hard to press, ask your health care provider. Or try to copy the way your health care provider uses the finger pads during a breast examination. Learn what your breast feels like most of the time. A firm ridge in the lower curve of each breast is normal.
5. Move around the breast in a set way. You can choose either the circle (**Fig. 2,A**), the up and down line (**Fig. 2,B**), or the wedge (**Fig. 2,C**). Do it the same way every time. It will help you to make sure that you've gone over the entire breast area and to remember how your breast feels.

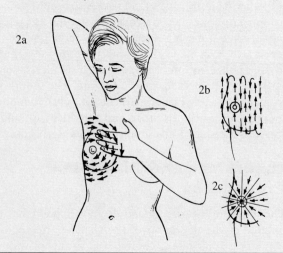

6. Now examine your left breast using right hand finger pads.
7. If you find any changes, see your health care provider right away.
8. You might want to check your breasts while standing in front of a mirror right after you do your breast self-examination each month. See if there are any changes in the way your breasts look: dimpling of the skin, changes in the nipple, or redness or swelling.
9. You might also want to do an extra breast self-examination while you're in the shower (Fig. 3). Your soapy hands will glide over the wet skin, making it easy to check how your breasts feel.

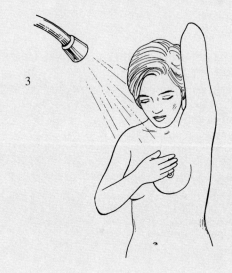

tests for sexually transmitted diseases, tuberculin skin test, hearing, electrocardiogram, fecal occult blood, and bone mineral content.

Fecal occult blood testing is recommended every 1 to 2 years in women age 50 years or older. Colon cancer is the second leading cause of cancer death for both sexes. Since many colorectal cancers are undetected through fecal occult blood testing or rectal digital examination, *proctosigmoidoscopy* (examination of the rectum and sigmoid colon with a sigmoidoscope) is indicated every 3 to 5 years after age 50 (*Healthy People 2000*, 1990).

HIV and drug screening may be offered or encouraged with informed consent, especially in high-risk populations.

Papanicolaou Smear

All women who are 18 or older or who have been or are currently sexually active should have a yearly **Papanicolaou (Pap) smear** and pelvic examination (Procedure 29-1). After three or more consecutive negative tests a year apart, the Pap smear may be performed less frequently if the woman and her health care provider wish. There does not seem to be any benefit from more frequent screening, especially in women over the age of 65 who have had many normal Pap smears. It is more im-

portant to obtain Pap smears on unscreened women, who account for over 50% of cervical cancers, than to rescreen women who have had numerous previous normal smears (Table 29-1) (Harlan, Bernstein, Kessler, 1991; U.S. Dept. of Health and Human Services, 1989).

Elderly women who have not been screened, African-Americans, lower socioeconomic groups, and more sexually active women are at higher risk for cervical carcinoma. A woman exposed to diethylstilbestrol (DES) in utero should have a Pap smear twice a year (Clay, 1990).

Learning about an abnormal Pap smear over the telephone can be terrifying. Fear can immobilize a woman so that she does not return for treatment. Before the examination the nurse should explain the purpose of the smear and that early cellular changes that could become cancerous can be treated with a 100% cure rate.

A woman with a Pap smear indicating infection should be treated and the smear repeated in 3 months. Results showing kilocytosis (indicating human papillomavirus [HPV]) or squamous and endocervical atypia must be referred to a gynecologist. Follow-up may include endocervical curettage, colposcopy, and biopsy. **Cervical intraepithelial neoplasia (CIN)** requires colposcopy. CIN risk factors include sexual intercourse before age 18, multiple sexual partners, smoking one or more packs of

---

PROCEDURES 29-1

Papanicolaou Smear

In preparation, make sure the woman has not douched, used vaginal medications, or had sexual intercourse for at least 24 hours prior to the procedure. Reschedule the test if the woman is menstruating.

The woman is assisted into a lithotomy position. A speculum is inserted in the vagina.

Explain to the woman the purpose of the test and what sensations she will feel as the specimen is obtained (i.e., pressure but not pain).

The cytologic specimen is obtained before any digital examination of the vagina is made, or endocervical bacteriologic specimens are taken with cotton swabbing of the cervix.

The specimen is taken by placing the S-shaped end of the cervical spatula just *within the cervical canal at the external os* (Fig. 29-1, *A*). The blade is rotated 360 degrees so that the surface at the squamocolumnar junction is firmly scraped. If the junction is inside the cervical canal, a swab may be used to obtain cells (Fig. 29-1, *B*). If gross exudate or mucus is present, the excess is gently pushed away from the os with the end of the spatula.

The mucus is spread on a slide without drying or rubbing, sprayed lightly with fixative, and allowed to dry.

Some mucus is obtained from the *posterior fornix* (vaginal pool) with the rounded end of the spatula, spread on another slide, sprayed, and dried.

Label the slides with woman's name and site. Include on the form to accompany the slides the woman's name, age, parity, and chief complaint or reason for taking the cytologic specimens.

Send specimens to the pathology laboratory promptly for staining, evaluation, and a written report, with special reference to abnormal elements, including cancer cells.

Advise the woman that repeat smears may be necessary if specimen is not adequate.

Instruct the woman concerning routine check-ups for cervical and vaginal cancer. The American Cancer Society advises that women over the age of 18 and those under 18 who are sexually active have the test at least every 3 years, *but only after they have had three negative Papanicolaou tests a year apart*. A pelvic examination is recommended every 3 years from age 20 to 40 and every 1 to 3 years there after.

Record the examination date and untoward reactions on the woman's record.

A

B

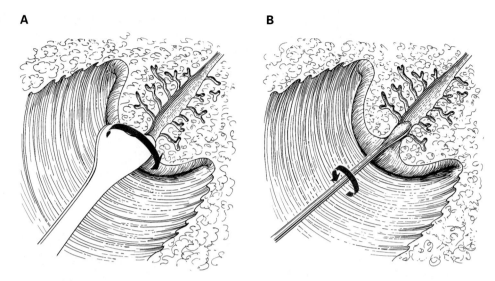

FIG. 29-1 **A,** Cervical smear. **B,** Endocervical smear. (From Malasanos L et al: *Health assessment,* ed 4, St. Louis, 1990, Mosby.)

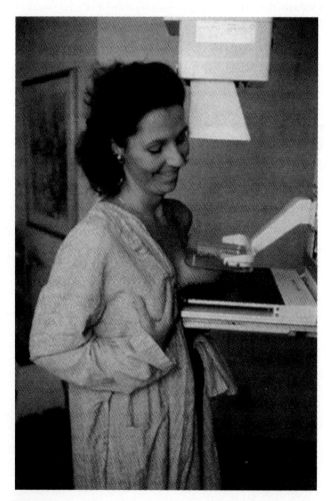

FIG. 29-2 Mammography. (From Edge V, Miller M: *Women's health care,* Clinical Nursing Series, St Louis, 1994, Mosby.)

cigarettes per day, and history of HPV. CIN is classified into categories I, II, and III according to severity. Dysplasia (disordered growth) is the term given to all disorders that are considered precancerous (Clay, 1990).

Mammography

Breast masses too small to be detected by BSE or by the health care provider may be detected by **mammography,** a low-dose x-ray of the breast (Fig. 29-2) Concerns about mammography include possible carcinogenic effects of regular x-rays (less than 1%), the cost, discomfort, and a relatively high frequency of false positive results, causing unnecessary biopsy. It is generally believed, however, that the advantages of mammography in older women outweigh the disadvantages. Studies that compare cancer deaths in women who have regular mammograms with cancer deaths in women who are unscreened indicate that regular mammography reduces death rates from breast cancer by about 25% to 30%; that would correspond to saving the lives of over 10,000 American women annually (Cooper, 1992).

After a recent Canadian National Breast Screening Study suggested that mammography provided no long-term survival benefit to women under age 50 (Elwood, Cox, Richardson, 1993), it was anticipated that the recommended starting age for mammography would be changed. However, experts continue to believe that mammography is useful for women 40 to 50 years of age. Currently the American Cancer Society recommends a screening mammogram by age 40, mammography for women ages 40 to 49 every 1 to 2 years if they are asymptomatic, and annual mammography of women 50 or over (American Cancer Society, 1994). The National Cancer Institute (NCI) advocates routine screening every 1 to 2 years with mammography for women over the age of 50 (NCI, 1993).

TABLE 29-1   Pap Smear Classification

OLD TERMINOLOGY	CURRENT TERMINOLOGY	CHARACTERISTICS
Class I	Within normal limits	Minimal or no inflammation; no malignant cells
Class II	Inflammatory atypia	Inflammation; mild atypia
Class III	Cervical intraepithelial neoplasia	
Mild dysplasia	CIN Grade I	Abnormal nucleus; normal cytoplasm
Moderate dysplasia	CIN Grade II	Abnormal nucleus; minimal cytoplasm abnormalities
Severe dysplasia	CIN Grade III	Abnormal chromosome and cytoplasm; abnormal cells
Carcinoma *in situ*		predominate; many undifferentiated cells

From Beal MW: Cervical cytology, *NAACOG's Clin Issu Perinat Womens Health Nurs* 1(4):475, 1990.

Mammography involves taking two x-rays of each breast, one with the breast compressed from top to bottom, and one compressed side to side, to get a clear picture of the breast tissue. The procedure takes about 15 minutes and involves minimal, discomfort. The nurse should discuss the advantages of mammography with the woman (peace of mind or early detection), explain the procedure to her, and review the preparation for the test: she should wear an easily removable top; she should bathe but not use any deodorant or creams, ointments, or body powder on the breast area or underarms the day of the test; and she should avoid any medications or beverages, such as coffee, containing caffeine during the week before the test, since caffeine dilates the blood vessels and may confound the results. She should be reassured that her health care provider will share the results of the test with her in a follow-up visit or telephone call.

Health promotion and screening include being sure the woman knows the American Cancer Society's seven warning signs (see the Teaching Approaches box at right).

ANTICIPATORY GUIDANCE FOR PREVENTION AND HEALTH PROMOTION

The fact that women are living longer today is shifting the focus of women's health care from childbearing to a more comprehensive approach to women's health. *Healthy People 2000* (1990) emphasizes the responsibility that all Americans must take for their individual health. Nurses have a major opportunity and responsibility to help women understand risk factors and to motivate them to adopt healthy lifestyles that prevent disease. Lifestyle factors that affect health over which the woman has some control include diet, tobacco, alcohol, and substance use, exercise, sunlight exposure, stress management, and sexual practices. Other influences, such as genetic and environmental factors, may be beyond the woman's control, although some opportunities

TEACHING APPROACHES

CANCER'S SEVEN WARNING SIGNALS

1. Change in bowel or bladder habits
2. A sore that does not heal
3. Unusual bleeding or discharge
4. Thickening or lump in breast or elsewhere
5. Indigestion or difficulty in swallowing
6. Obvious change in wart or mole
7. Nagging cough or hoarseness
   If you have a warning signal, see your health care provider.

for prevention exist (e.g., through environmental legislation activism or genetic counseling services).

Knowledge is not enough to bring about healthy behaviors. The woman must be convinced that she has some control over her life and that healthy life habits, including periodic health examinations, are a sound investment. She must believe in the efficacy of prevention, early detection, and therapy and in her ability to perform self-care practices, such as BSE. Many people believe that they have little control over their health, or they become immobilized by fear and anxiety in the face of life-threatening illnesses, such as cancer, so that they delay seeking treatment. The nurse must explore the reality of each woman's perceptions about health behaviors and individualize teaching if it is to be effective. The model illustrated in Fig. 29-3 incorporates the major aspects to be included when counseling women.

Nutrition

According to *Healthy People 2000* (1990), poor diet is associated with five of the 10 leading causes of death in the United States: coronary heart disease, certain types of cancer, stroke, non–insulin-dependent diabetes mellitus, and suicide associated with excessive alcohol intake. The intake of foods high in fats and low in dietary fiber and inadequate calcium intake are of particular concern for women, as are eating disorders, such as anorexia ner-

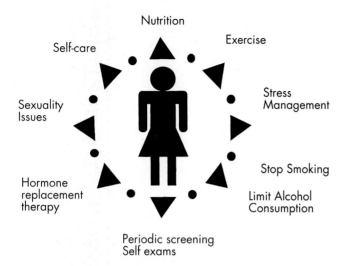

Nutrition

Self-care

Exercise

Sexuality
Issues

Stress
Management

Hormone
replacement
therapy

Stop Smoking

Limit Alcohol
Consumption

Periodic screening
Self exams

FIG. 29-3 Nursing care model. (Courtesy Design Center, University of North Carolina at Chapel Hill School of Nursing, Chapel Hill, NC.)

vosa and bulimia. Finally, hunger and the marginal nutritional status of many elderly women, Native Americans on reservations, poor women, and the homeless are other significant nutritional problems.

Overweight affects a large proportion of Americans. Diets high in fat are associated with an increased risk of obesity, cancers of the breast, colon, and possibly gallbladder disease. A greater risk of coronary heart disease is associated with high blood cholesterol and the high saturated fat intake of the typical American diet. Fewer calories are required as exercise and metabolic rate decrease with age, so women typically put on weight as they leave the childbearing years. Therefore a comprehensive approach that includes diet and exercise should be recommended. Extremely low-calorie diets and fad weight-loss programs may be unsafe and do not lead to long-term ideal weight maintenance. Extreme behaviors, such as those which occur in bulimia and anorexia, require medical treatment.

Healthy People 2000 (1990) recommends that dietary fat intake be reduced to an average of 30% or less of total caloric intake, with average saturated fat intake reduced to less than 20% of calories. Complex carbohydrate and fiber-containing foods should be increased to include five or more servings of vegetable and fruits per day, and six or more servings of grain products per day. These foods are generally low in fat, and there is evidence that fiber and fruits and vegetables rich in vitamins A and C protect against certain types of cancer. Foods high in fiber and at least six to eight glasses of fluid per day also help to promote good bowel and bladder hygiene. Preventing constipation and cystitis is especially important in older women. Cranberry juice and juices or foods high in vitamin C are recommended to help to keep urine acidic; drinking coffee, tea, and alcohol should be dis-

couraged in women prone to cystitis, since these appear to irritate the bladder. Most Americans need to reduce sugar and salt intake; 1 to 3 g of sodium per day are sufficient for healthy adults.

The technique of basic nutrition counseling does not differ markedly from that used with pregnant women. The diet can be assessed using a standard assessment form—a 24-hour recall is adequate and quick—and then food likes and dislikes, including cultural variations and typical food portions and dietary habits, should be discussed and incorporated into counseling. The woman should be actively involved in evaluating her intake with the nurse, using a standard food group guide, and should suggest modifications in the diet, where needed. Many women have a fair knowledge of food groups and their importance for various nutrients; with guidance they can critique their own intake and suggest changes to improve nutrition. A nonjudgmental approach is important, since many women, especially if they are obese or know they are not eating as they should are sensitive about diet. Unless the motivation to change food habits is intrinsic, efforts to change the diet will fail. If the nurse is supportive, this approach can increase the woman's self-esteem and reinforce good practices while motivating change where needed.

The nurse can provide information about the risks associated with high fat intake and ways to reduce dietary fat intake and increase fiber intake. Although many people are aware of the association between high fat and cholesterol and disease, they may be ignorant of the major sources of saturated fat and need help in changing eating patterns established during childhood. Since there are more than twice as many calories in fat as they are in protein and carbohydrate, gram for gram, weight control can be facilitated by encouraging women to choose foods relatively low in fat and calories. Fiber-rich foods can be substituted for foods high in fat; they delay digestion and absorption and increase the feeling of satiety.

Most women do not recognize the importance of calcium to health, and their diets are insufficient in calcium. If an adequate bone mass is not achieved at skeletal maturity (usually by about age 20) the woman is at increased risk of developing osteoporosis in later life. Osteoporosis is a disabling, life-threatening disease of epidemic proportions in the United States. Although canned fish, certain greens (kale, broccoli), legumes, calcium-enriched products, and seeds and nuts contain some calcium, the major source of calcium in the diet is the mild group (milk, cheese, yogurt). Calcium intake is probably insufficient if intake from this group is insufficient. The ideal daily calcium intake is unknown, but it is agreed that most women, especially adolescents, should increase their intake. Women under age 50 need 800 mg of calcium per day and postmenopausal women over age 50 need 1000 mg. Pregnant and lactating women have special needs. The nurse should explore every woman's knowledge of the importance of calcium to health and personalize the risk factors for osteoporosis. If diet assessment indicates her intake compared with the recommended number of dairy group servings is low, good food sources of calcium from lower fat dairy products can be suggested. Poor women and racial and ethnic minority women present a special challenge in recommending inexpensive or culturally appropriate calcium food sources. Women who are unlikely to get enough calcium in the diet may need calcium supplements in the form of calcium carbonate, which contains more elemental calcium than other preparations.

Long-standing dietary habits are difficult to modify but, given the potential health benefits and positive influence a woman can have on the nutrition of other family members, she may respond to the nurse's encouragement and reinforcement of her good intentions. Chances of success may be enhanced if she becomes involved in a support group or enlists significant others in goal setting.

Exercise

One of the goals of *Healthy People 2000* (1990) is to increase the number of primary care providers who routinely assess and counsel patients about physical activity practices. Nurses are respected care providers who can influence patients to become more active and help them to develop an exercise program geared to their age and personal fitness and goals. Regular physical activity is associated with the prevention and management of coronary heart disease, hypertension, non–insulin-dependent diabetes mellitus, osteoporosis, obesity, and mental health problems. Aerobic exercise or vigorous exercise 3 or more days per week for 20 or more minutes each time improves cardiovascular fitness and may decrease other risk factors associated with heart disease, such as obesity and hypertension (Fig. 29-4). The rate of coronary heart disease is twice as high in physically inactive people.

Unfortunately, few Americans exercise daily for 30 minutes or longer, as recommended; and physical inactivity increases with age, especially during adolescence and early adulthood. Even small increases in activity can be beneficial. Resistance training or weight lifting increases muscular strength and endurance. Other benefits of exercise include decreased carbohydrate intolerance, increased serum lipid profiles, weight control, decreased fatigue, increased relaxation and mental function, and, with other factors, the prevention of osteoporosis.

The nurse should stress the importance of daily exercise throughout life for weight management and health promotion, suggesting exercises that are enjoyable to the individual. Weight-bearing exercises, such as jogging, racquet sports, cycling, and dancing are excellent. Walking, as a part of the daily routine is more vigorous activities cannot be performed, is feasible for most women. Swimming is good for cardiorespiratory fitness but will

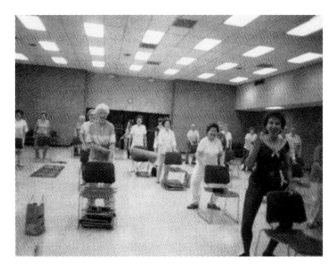

FIG. 29-4 Aerobic exercise improves cardiovascular fitness. (From Edge V, Miller M: *Women's health care,* Clinical Nursing Series, St Louis, 1994, Mosby.)

not prevent osteoporosis, since it is not a weight-bearing exercise. Many women who are sedentary during leisure time can profit from gradually increasing their physical activity. They may be encouraged to exercise with their children or in groups. Worksite fitness programs or community-based programs are increasing. Young women can be involved in physical education activities, games and group sports, and more active pursuits. Home maintenance, yard work, and gardening are other activities that promote health and a sense of well-being, especially for older adults. Attention to safety factors and clothing and shoes appropriate to each activity are advised.

Kegel Exercises

Advice about exercise to women in the childbearing years and in later life is incomplete without a discussion of pelvic floor (**Kegel**) exercises. First developed by Dr. Kegel to strengthen the pelvic-vaginal muscles to control stress incontinence, the exercises are also beneficial during pregnancy and childbirth and postpartum. They strengthen the muscles of the pelvic floor, providing support for the pelvic organs and control of the muscles surrounding the vagina and urethra. Strengthening of the pubococcygeus muscle, which surrounds the vagina, has also been reported to improve sexual response. Kegal exercises are described on p. 137.

Stress Management

Women today contrast sharply with the woman of past generations who devoted their lives entirely to their families. Today a woman is more likely to spend much of her life as a single, independent adult and to participate in the work force throughout her life, whether she is married or has children. The effects of heightened expectations, new lifestyles, changing gender roles and norms, and resources for women may have detrimental effects on women's mental health and health-related behaviors (see Clinical Application of Research below).

The study by Woods, Lentz, Mitchell (1993) suggests that stress in women is linked with depression, which may be specifically linked with health-damaging behaviors, such as smoking or too little sleep. They conclude:

> Women who have more stressors in their lives, less education, low self-esteem, no partner, no employment, contemporary gender role norms, and more depressed mood are at increased risk of practicing the health-damaging behaviors of smoking and alcohol use. In contrast, having a lifestyle of social advantage, including having access to education, being partnered and employed, and being exposed to fewer stressors, promotes women's involvement in health-related behaviors such as exercise and healthy eating and sleeping patterns.

Healthy People 2000 (1990) confirms that stress-related problems are of epidemic proportions, citing evidence from physicians and employers (worker compensation data). Adverse health effects of stress include common symptoms such as nervousness, tension, anger, irritation, depression, anxiety, and an inability to cope as well as headache, muscle ache or tension, stomach ache or tension, and fatigue. Clinical illnesses associated with stress include anxiety, eating disorders, depression, gastrointestinal and cardiovascular illnesses, immune disorders, suicide and other forms of aggression, substance abuse, and intentional and unintentional injuries.

Most women experience a great deal of stress. Living conditions are a major contributing factor. Role strain is another. Since it is neither possible nor desirable to avoid all stress, women need to learn how to manage stress. The nurse should assess each woman for signs of stress, using therapeutic communication skills to determine risk factors and the woman's ability to function.

Some women must be referred for counseling or other mental health therapy. Women are two to three times more likely to suffer from major depressive disorder than men, and the problem is commonly underdiagnosed and undertreated by primary care providers (Depression Guideline Panel, 1993). Nurses need to be alert to the symptoms of serious mental disorders, such as depression and anxiety, and make referrals to mental health practitioners when necessary. Many women who are treated for physical symptoms—sleep, appetite problems, headaches, and other unexplained complaints—are experiencing undiagnosed depression or other serious problems. If there has been a previous episode of depression, a family history of depression, or prior suicide attempts, and the woman is sad or depressed, further mental status evaluation is indicated. Women experiencing major life changes, such as divorce and separation, bereavement, serious illness, and unemployment, also need special attention.

For many women the nurse is able to provide comfort, reassurance, and advice concerning helping resources, such as support groups. Many centers offer support groups to help women prevent or manage stress. The nurse can help her become more aware of the relationship between good nutrition, rest, relaxation and exercise/diversion, and her ability to deal with stress. In

---

 CLINICAL APPLICATION OF RESEARCH

HEALTH-PROMOTING AND HEALTH-DAMAGING BEHAVIORS OF WOMEN

Women today are better educated, live alone longer, and work throughout their lives irrespective of their marital status and ages of their children. These changes in lifestyle affect patterns of health-promoting and health-damaging behavior and may change morbidity and mortality figures. Interest in health-promoting and health-damaging behaviors increased following publication of a study that linked health behaviors to health status and mortality. The purpose of this study was to develop models to relate "women's roles, gender role norms, social demands and social resources, well-being, and distress to health-promoting and health-damaging behavior." Participants in the study, women ($N = 656$) who lived in ethnically mixed and middle-income neighborhoods, were interviewed in their homes. The average age of the women was 32 years, their average education level was 14 years, and average income ranged from $29,000 to $30,999. The majority were married or partnered (57%)

and worked outside the home (76%). Health-promoting behaviors included regular exercise, three meals a day, and 7 to 8 hours of sleep per night. Health-damaging behaviors included drinking alcohol and smoking. More health-promoting behaviors were performed by women who had fewer life stresses and were better educated. Health-damaging behaviors were engaged in by women who were stressed, had less education, had a contemporary attitude about women, had no partner, or were depressed. Nurses working with women need to consider social factors and role stressors in their efforts to promote healthy behaviors. Health promotion activities can be directed toward encouraging women to exercise, eat regularly, and obtain adequate sleep at night and to reduce alcohol intake and smoking.

Reference: Woods NF, Lentz M, Mitchell E: The new woman: health-promoting and health-damaging behaviors, *Health Care Women Internat* 14:389, 1993.

the case of role overload, learning to set realistic expectations and determining what needs immediate attention and what can wait are important. Practical advice includes regular breaks, taking time for friends, developing interests outside of work or the home, and learning self-acceptance. Discussing how the woman can maintain meaningful relationships is very important. Social support and good coping skills can improve a woman's self-esteem and give her a sense of mastery. Anticipatory guidance for developmental or expected situational crises can help her plan strategies for dealing with potentially stressful events.

There is a great deal of literature on an array of stress management interventions. Role-playing, relaxation techniques, biofeedback, meditation, desensitization, imagery, assertiveness training, yoga, diet, exercise and weight control are techniques the nurses can include in their repertoire of helping skills. Insufficient time prevents one-on-one assistance in many situations, but the more nurses know about these resources, the better able they are to intervene, counsel, and direct women to appropriate resources. Careful follow-up of all women experiencing difficulty in dealing with stress is important.

Substance Use

Tobacco use causes more preventable disease and death in the United States than any other known factor. It is responsible for one in every six deaths and is considered a major risk factor for diseases of the heart and blood vessels, chronic respiratory diseases, stomach ulcers, and cancers of the lung, larynx, pharynx, oral cavity, esophagus, pancreas, and bladder. People who smoke more than two packs per day are 15 to 25 times more likely to die of lung cancer than people who have never smoked. Smoking accounts for about 10% of all infant mortality, 20% to 30% of low-birth-weight babies, and up to 14% of preterm births. Passive, or involuntary, smoking causes lung cancer and other diseases in healthy non-smoking family members, and severe respiratory problems and ear infections are more frequent in children of parents who smoke (*Healthy People 2000*, 1990).

Cigarette smoking has declined dramatically over the past 25 years, despite its addictive power and strong efforts by advertisers and lobbyists on the part of cigarette manufacturers and tobacco farmers. However, nearly one third of all adults in the United States are smokers, and the decline is slower in women than in men. Nearly 18% to 19% of all high school seniors smoke; high school dropouts have an even higher smoking rate. Young African-Americans, Hispanics, and blue-collar workers are more likely to be smokers, and smoking may actually be increasing among young women while it is decreasing among most other groups (*Healthy People 2000*, 1990).

Women who smoke and use oral contraceptives are at increased risk for heart attack and stroke (*Healthy People 2000*, 1990). Lung cancer death rates for women are still increasing and have surpassed breast cancer death rates. Death rates for chronic obstructive pulmonary disease due to smoking have paralleled rates for lung cancer and have been on the increase over the past 25 years.

Since there is no effective cure for lung cancer, prevention is the key. Ten to 20 years after quitting, former smokers have lung cancer rates approaching the rates of those who have never smoked. Lost ventilatory function in cigarette smokers with chronic lung disease cannot be regained, but the development of more serious symptoms and disability can be prevented.

New approaches to increase cessation among smokers and to discourage smoking among young women—especially in adolescence and during pregnancy—are needed. Health care providers can have an impact on smoking behavior and should attempt to motivate smokers to stop. Raising questions about social consequences—stained teeth, foul-smelling breath and clothes—is sometimes effective with young people. It is very difficult for regular smokers to quit, and most people require multiple attempts. The March of Dimes and the American Lung Association provide self-help smoking cessation materials with which nurses working in primary health care should be familiar.

Alcohol and other drugs exact a staggering toll on society, not only in terms of personal health, but in their association with poverty and homelessness, family disorganization, violence, crime, motor vehicle injuries, reduced productivity, and economic costs. Cirrhosis of the liver related to alcohol abuse is the ninth leading cause of death among adults (*Healthy People 2000*, 1990). The abuse of alcohol and other drugs increases the risk of victimization and date rape and of acquiring the human immunodeficiency virus (HIV) through shared needles or sexual contact. Alcohol use and drug use are the leading preventable causes of birth defects.

Drug abuse, especially the use of crack cocaine, is becoming worse in the inner cities, with an increase in violent crime. Lower income, inner city youth, especially school dropouts and pregnant teenagers, are high-risk populations. Alcohol use among high school seniors appears to be declining, but binge drinking is still a serious problem.

A national awareness of the seriousness of problems associated with substance abuse has led to raising the legal drinking age to 21 in all states and tighter controls on advertising. Stronger regulation of advertising and tougher laws and law enforcement for alcohol- and drug-related offenses are needed. There is still much that must be done to increase the accessibility to care for low-income people, minorities, and young people. Women have special needs that must be addressed, especially mothers of young children and pregnant women.

All primary care providers should screen for alcohol and other drug use problems, with an understanding of the obvious problems in relying on self-reporting of these behaviors. The use of over-the-counter drugs by women should also be explored. Counseling women who appear to be drinking excessively or using drugs may include strategies to increase self-esteem and teaching new coping skills to resist and maintain resistance to alcohol abuse and drug use. Appropriate referrals should be made, with the health care provider arranging the contact and then following up to be sure that appointments are kept. Anticipatory guidance includes teaching about the health and safety risks of alcohol and mind-altering substances, and discouraging drug experimentation among preteen and high school students, since the use of drugs at an early age tends to predict greater involvement later.

Sexuality Issues

Sexuality is central to a person's identity, and assessing sexual function and discussing sexual issues should be an integral part of holistic health care. Many women need knowledge about sexual matters, and a sensitive nurse can supply information and correct myths and misconceptions in a manner that communicates to the woman an appreciation of the importance and appropriateness of these concerns. Social mores have a great deal to do with sexual attitudes and practices, and advice should be individualized and appropriate to the woman's age and life situation.

Sexual sharing and open communication with one's partner are healthy parts of a mature sexual relationship. If the woman indicates that there is sexual dysfunction—such as a lack of sexual desire or orgasm, vaginismus, or dyspareunia—further assessment, treatment, or, if necessary, referral are indicated.

Health objectives outlined in *Healthy People 2000* (1990) include reducing sexual intercourse and pregnancies among adolescents, reducing unintended pregnancies among all women, and increasing the number of people who use contraception. Dealing with issues such as decision making about sexual activity and childbearing must be a part of general practice. Preconception counseling before sexual activity starts can be initiated by asking about plans the woman may have for starting a family.

The nurse should encourage mothers to discuss appropriate sexual behavior with their children by simply stating what they believe or feel without making the child feel defensive. It has been shown that family support and guidance have a significant effect on sexual activity in young people, whereas school-based sex education has little effect (*Healthy People 2000*, 1990). Nurses can provide parents with practical advice about communicating with children and their need for time and positive feedback, and they can recommend parenting skills programs and specific educational programs in the community.

Women in the childbearing years need an accurate knowledge of the various contraceptive methods, and all women need to know how to prevent sexually transmitted diseases, which are almost entirely preventable.

Health promotion and disease prevention provide the best opportunities for addressing the major health problems of women. Nurses have a vital role to play in these activities, providing hands-on care, teaching and counseling, or directing and participating in clinical research. They must also become more conscientious role models and become more active in the public arena, establishing networks with others interested in promoting women's health and supporting legislation sensitive to the unique needs of women.

KEY POINTS

- Culture, religion, socioeconomic status, personal circumstances, the uniqueness of the individual and stage of development are among the factors that influence a person's recognition of need for care and responses to the health care system and therapy.
- The changing status and roles for women affect their health, needs, and ability to cope with problems.
- Assessment is more comprehensive and learning is best in a safe environment in which the atmosphere is nonjudgmental and sensitive, and the interaction is strictly confidential.
- Every woman is entitled to be respected and fully involved in the assessment process to the fullness of her capacity.

- A health assessment includes a comprehensive interview and physical examination and diagnostic testing.
- The Papanicolaou smear will detect approximately 90% of early cervical dysplasias.
- The risk of American women developing cancer of the breast is 1 in 9.
- An estimated 90% of all breast lumps are detected by the woman during breast self-examination.
- Monthly breast self-examination, routine screening mammography, and yearly breast examinations by practitioners are recommended for early detection of breast cancer.

CRITICAL THINKING EXERCISES

1. Interview at least two women of different cultures.
   a. Ask them about their beliefs in relation to seeking health care.
   b. Identify reasons for differences and how these would influence planning to teach about preventive health care and health promotion.

2. You are assigned to a woman's clinic to do breast self-examination (BSE) teaching in a small group setting. In the group are a 17-year-old high school student, a 25-year-old unemployed mother of 2, a 40-year-old single professional woman who has never had children, and a 60-year-old postmenopausal grandmother.
   a. What factors unique to these women will influence your teaching strategy?

   b. What information about BSE is essential to all the women?
   c. What information about BSE needs to be different based on the ages of the women?
   d. Develop a teaching plan, including outcome criteria.

3. Interview nursing students and other students regarding the knowledge and use of screening methods for cancer detection.
   a. Analyze your findings to determine the degree of awareness among nonnursing students and nursing students.
   b. Examine reasons for the differences and similarities.
   c. Propose an educational strategy to increase awareness of resources for cancer detection and prevention.

References

ACOG: *Your health and the Ob/Gyn exam,* Washington, DC, 1989, The American College of Obstetricians and Gynecologists.

American Cancer Society: *1994 cancer facts and figures,* New York, 1994, ACS.

Barsevick AM, Lauver D: Women's informational needs about colposcopy, *Image J Nurs Sch* 22(1):23, 1990.

Beal MW: Cervical cytology, *NAACOG Clin Issu Perinat Womens Health Nurs* 1(4):470, 1990.

Breast cancer screening guidelines remain unchanged, *Cancer News* p. 19 Summer 1993.

Clay LS: Midwifery assessment of the well woman: the Pap smear, *J Nurs Midwife* 35(6):341, 1990.

Cooper GM: *Elements of human cancer,* Boston, 1992, Jones & Bartlett.

Depression Guideline Panel: *Depression in primary care: vol 1, Detection and diagnosis, Clinical Practice Guideline, no 5,* Rockville, MD. U.S. Department of Health and Human Services, Public Health Service, Agency for Health Care Policy and Research, AHCPR Pub No 93-0550, April 1993.

Ehrenreich B, English D: *For her own good: 150 years of the experts' advice to women,* New York, 1978, Anchor Press.

Elwood JM, Cox B, Richardson AK. The effectiveness of breast cancer screening by mammography in younger women, *Online J Curr Clin Trials (serial online)* 2:25, Feb 1993.

Freda MC et al: What pregnant women want to know: a comparison of client and provider perceptions, *JOGNN* 22(3):237, 1993.

Harlan LC, Bernstein AB, Kessler LG: Cervical cancer screening: who is not screened and why? *Am J Public Health* 81(7):885, 1991.

Healthy People 2000: national health promotion and disease prevention objectives, Washington, DC, US Department of Health and Human Services, DHHS Pub No (PHS) 91-50212, 1990.

Laffin J: *The Arab mind considered: a need for understanding,* New York, 1975, Paplinger Publishing.

Lawhead RA: Vulvar examination: what your patients should know, *Female Patient* 15(1):33, 1990.

Lierman LM et al: Predicting breast self-examination using the theory of reasoned action, *Nurs Res* 39(2):97, 1990.

National Cancer Institute (NCI): *International workshop on screening of breast cancer* (press release), Bethesda, MD, March 4, 1993.

Nemcek MA: Health beliefs and breast self-examination among black women, *Health Values* 14(5):41, 1990.

Parker B, McFarlane J: Identifying and helping battered pregnant women, *MCN* 16(3):161, 1991.

Seidel H et al: *Mosby's guide to physical examination,* ed 3, St Louis, 1995, Mosby.

Stotland NL: Social change and women's reproductive health care, *Women's Health Issues* 1(1):4, 1990.

US Department of Health & Human Services (Public Health Service, Office of Population Affairs/Family Planning): *Improving the quality of clinician Pap smear education, and the evaluation of Pap smear laboratory testing,* Sept 1989.

Woods NF, Lentz M, Mitchell E: The new woman: health-promoting and health-damaging behaviors, *Health Care Women Internat* 14:389, 1993.

Bibliography

Brucker MC, Scharbo-HeHaan M: Breast disease: the role of the nurse-midwife, *J Nurs Midwife* 36(1):63, 1991.

Cook M: Perimenopause: an opportunity for health promotion, *JOGNN* 22(3):223, 1993.

Dignan M et al: The role of focus groups in health education for cervical cancer among minority women, *J Community Health* 15(6):369, 1990.

Ebersole P, Hess P: *Toward healthy aging: human needs and nursing response*, ed 4, St Louis, 1994, Mosby.

Freda MC: Childbearing reproductive control, aging women and health care: the projected ethical debates, *JOGNN* 23(2): 144, 1994.

Giger JN, Davidhizar RE: *Transcultural nursing: assessment and intervention*, St Louis, 1991, Mosby.

Rubin MM, Lauver D: Assessment and management of cervical intraepithelial neoplasia, *Nurs Pract* 15(9):23, 1990.

Sevel F: Designing effective health promotion and disease prevention programs: a course model, *Health Values* 14(1):32, 1990.

Speake DL, Cowart ME, Stephens R: Healthy lifestyle practices of rural and urban elderly, *Health Values* 15(1):45, 1991.

Walker S et al: A Spanish language version of the health-promoting lifestyle profile, *Nurs Res* 39(5):268, 1990.

30 Common Reproductive Concerns

E D N A   B.   Q U I N N

D E I T R A   L E O N A R D   L O W D E R M I L K

LEARNING OBJECTIVES

Define key terms
Describe sequelae associated with injuries of the birth canal.
Develop a nursing plan of care for the woman with primary dysmenorrhea.
Outline patient teaching about premenstrual syndrome.
Relate the pathophysiology of endometriosis to associated symptoms.
List common causes of impaired fertility.
Discuss the psychologic impact of impaired fertility.
List the common diagnoses and treatments for impaired fertility.
Describe the techniques used for surgical interruption of pregnancy.
Recognize the various ethical and legal considerations of impaired infertility and termination of fertility.
List teaching strategies utilized by the nurse in assisting women and couples regarding reproductive concerns.
Develop an assessment guide for women experiencing the climacterium.
Develop a nursing plan of care for the woman experiencing the postclimacterium.
Suggest community resources for women with common reproductive concerns.
Describe the various alternative treatments for breast cancer.

KEY TERMS

assisted reproductive therapies (ART)
climacterium
culdocentesis
cystocele
dilatation and curettage (D & C)
elective abortion (EAB)
endometriosis
enterocele
estrogen replacement therapy (ERT)
fistula
hormone replacement therapy (HRT)
hot flushes
hypogonadotropic amenorrhea
impaired fertility
isoimmunization
laminaria
lumpectomy
menopause
modified radical mastectomy
osteoporosis
pelvic inflammatory disease (PID)
pelvic relaxation
pessary
premenstrual syndrome (PMS)
primary dysmenorrhea
rectocele
referred shoulder pain
secondary dysmenorrhea
semen analysis
simple mastectomy
stress urinary incontinence
therapeutic abortion (TAB)
therapeutic intrauterine insemination
vacuum or suction curettage
varicocele
urethrocele
uterine prolapse

RELATED TOPICS

Basal body temperature *(Chap. 18)* • Breast self-examination *(Chap. 29)* • Conception *(Chap. 4)* • Contraception *(Chap. 18)* • Ectopic pregnancy *(Chap. 21)* • Loss and grief *(Chap. 28)* • Mammography *(Chap. 29)* • Menstrual cycle *(Chap. 3)* • Sexually transmitted diseases *(Chap. 21)* • Spontaneous abortion *(Chap. 21)* • Toxic shock syndrome *(Chap. 21)* • Ultrasound examination *(Chap. 20)* • Vaginal infections *(Chap. 21)*

This chapter deals with the most common problems associated with the menstrual cycle—infertility, unwanted pregnancy, long-term sequelae of childbirth trauma, and difficulties during the climacteric and postclimacteric periods associated with normal changes in the reproductive and genitourinary systems. Breast cancer is also included as the most frequent reproductive cancer occurring in women.

COMMON MENSTRUAL DISORDERS

Common menstrual disorders that have a negative effect on the quality of the lives of women and their families are discussed in this chapter (refer to Chapter 3 for a review of the normal menstrual cycle and endocrine physiology).

Hypogonadotropic Amenorrhea

Hypogonadotropic amenorrhea reflects a problem in the central hypothalamic-pituitary axis. In rare instances a pituitary lesion or genetic inability to produce follicle-stimulating hormone (FSH) and luteinizing hormone (LH) is at fault. A diagnostic workup including thyroid-stimulating hormone (TSH) and prolactin levels, x-rays or computed tomography (CT) scan of the sella turcica, and a progestational challenge is done to determine the cause.

Hypogonadotropic amenorrhea most commonly results from hypothalamic suppression as a result of two principal influences: *stress* (in the home, school, or workplace) or a *critical body fat-to-lean ratio* (underweight for height, rapid weight loss, and eating disorders such as anorexia nervosa or bulimia, or strenuous exercise such as competitive athletics or dancing, especially ballet). Menstrual regularity requires the maintenance of weight and body fat above a critical level.

The history often reveals a weight-conscious woman engaging in significant physical exercise and concerned with control over her own body. She may weigh less than 115 lb and may have lost 10 lb or more through exercising. The serious female athlete may have an adequate weight but a reduced proportion of body fat. Peripheral levels of endorphins increase with strenuous exercise and are believed to have a suppressive effect on the hypothalamus. A loss of calcium from the bone, comparable to that seen in postmenopausal women, may occur with this disturbance of ovulation (Prior et al, 1990).

If counseling is ineffective in altering the woman's lifestyle of exercise and weight control, **hormone replacement therapy (HRT)** may be indicated. Yearly reevaluation for return of normal menstrual function is necessary. HRT does not protect against pregnancy if normal function returns; therefore caution is advised. Therapy usually includes conjugated estrogen for days 1 through 24 of each month (starting with the first calendar day of the month) and medroxyprogesterone acetate (Provera) for days 10 through 24. Withdrawal bleeding usually occurs on day 27.

Dysmenorrhea

Dysmenorrhea, or painful menstruation, is one of the most common gynecologic problems in women of all ages. It is estimated that American women lose 1.7 million working days each month because of dysmenorrhea.

Primary Dysmenorrhea

Primary dysmenorrhea occurs in the absence of organic disease, usually appearing from 6 months to 2 years after menarche. It often improves by age 25 or following pregnancy with vaginal birth. Psychogenic factors may influence symptoms, but symptoms are definitely related to ovulation and do not occur when ovulation is suppressed. During the luteal phase and subsequent menstrual flow, prostaglandin F_2 alpha ($PGF_2\alpha$) is secreted. Excessive release of $PGF_2\alpha$ increases the amplitude and frequency of uterine contractions and causes vasospasm of the uterine arterioles, resulting in ischemia and cyclic lower abdominal cramps. Systemic responses to $PGF_2\alpha$ include backache, weakness, sweats, gastrointestinal symptoms (anorexia, nausea, vomiting, and diarrhea), and central nervous system symptoms (dizziness, syncope, headache, and poor concentration) (Heitkemper et al, 1991). The cause of excessive prostaglandin release is unknown.

For some women heat (heating pad or hot bath), massage, distraction, exercise, and sleep are sufficient to relieve primary dysmenorrhea. Heat relieves ischemia by decreasing contractions and increasing circulation. Orgasm may bring relief by reducing tension and increasing a sense of well-being, increasing menstrual flow, and relieving pelvic vasocongestion. Diet changes to decrease salt and increase natural diuretics, such as asparagus or parsley, may help reduce edema and related discomforts.

Several over-the-counter (OTC) preparations—analgesics, nonsteroidal antiinflammatory drugs (NSAIDs), and diuretics—are available. Cope and Midol contain both aspirin and caffeine: Midol also contains cinnamedrine, a mild uterine relaxant. Many products contain pamabrom (similar to caffeine in its diuretic effect) and pyrilamine maleate, an antihistamine with sedative and analgesic properties. Aspirin, acetaminophen (recommended dosage, 650 mg every 4 hours not to exceed 4000 mg in a 24-hour period), and ibuprofen (Motrin, Advil, Nuprin), an NSAID, in doses of 200 to 400 mg every 4 to 6 hours, work by inhibiting prostaglandin synthesis. Other prostaglandin-synthesis inhibitors include naproxen (Naprosyn and Anaprox) and mefenamic acid (Ponstel). They are most effective if started several days before menses. Exposing an early unsuspected pregnancy to drugs must be avoided (Lubianezki, Fischer, 1987; Sohn, Korberly, Tannenbaum, 1986).

As a last resort for intractable dysmenorrhea, surgery

may be indicated. Approximately 70% of women who undergo presacral neurectomy or sympathectomy obtain relief.

Secondary Dysmenorrhea

Secondary dysmenorrhea is associated with organic pelvic disease, such as endometriosis, pelvic inflammatory disease, cervical stenosis, uterine or ovarian neoplasms, and uterine polyps. An IUD can also be a cause. Secondary dysmenorrhea may be misdiagnosed as primary dysmenorrhea or may be confused with complications of early pregnancy. Treatment must be directed toward the underlying cause.

Premenstrual Syndrome

Symptoms of **premenstrual syndrome (PMS)** begin in the luteal phase about 7 to 10 days before menses and end with the onset of menses. There may be a heightened sense of creativity and increased mental and physical energy. Negative symptoms are related to edema (abdominal bloating, pelvic fullness, edema of the lower extremities, breast tenderness, and weight gain) or emotional instability (depression, crying spells, irritability, panic attacks, and impaired ability to concentrate). Headache, fatigue, and backache are common complaints (Hsia, Long, 1990). A small percentage of women find PMS so incapacitating that normal activities are disrupted for several days during each cycle. A lack of understanding of PMS may result in poor self-esteem and stress relationships to the breaking point.

The cause of PMS is unknown. Theories include progesterone deficiency, prolactin and prostaglandin excesses, and dietary deficiencies. PMS has a significant psychosocial component.

There is little agreement on management. A careful, detailed history and daily log of symptoms and mood fluctuations spanning several cycles may give direction to a plan of management. Counseling, in the form of support groups or individual/couple counseling, may be helpful. Medications, such as prostaglandin inhibitors and diuretics for edema, bromocriptine (Parlodel) for breast tenderness, and a well-balanced diet, low in caffeine and sodium or with naturally diuretic foods, may ease symptoms. Exercise and vitamin supplements (B_6 and E) are often recommended.

Endometriosis

Endometriosis is characterized by the presence and growth of endometrial tissue outside of the uterus. It may be implanted on the ovaries, cul-de-sac, uterosacral ligaments, rectovaginal septum, sigmoid colon, round ligaments, pelvic peritoneum, or urinary bladder (Fig. 30-1). A chocolate cyst is a cystic area of endometriosis in the ovary. The dark coloring of the contents of the cyst is caused by old blood.

Ectopic endometrial tissue responds to hormonal stimulation in the same way that the uterine endome-

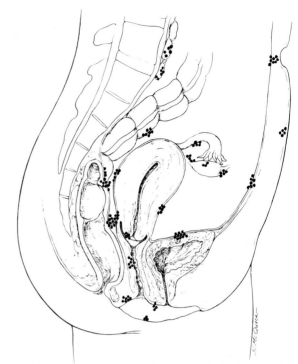

FIG. 30-1   Common sites of endometriosis. (From Herbst AL et al: Comprehensive Gynecology, ed 2, St Louis, 1992, Mosby.)

trium does. During the proliferative and secretory phases of the cycle, the endometrium grows. During or immediately after menstruation, the tissue bleeds, resulting in an inflammatory response with subsequent fibrosis and adhesions to adjacent organs. Scar tissue and distortion or blockage of surrounding organs may result.

The exact number of women with endometriosis is unknown, but 5% to 15% of women who undergo pelvic surgery are observed to have endometriosis. The condition usually develops in the third decade of life and worsens with repeated cycles, or it may remain asymptomatic and undiagnosed, eventually disappearing during the climacterium. However, women who have symptoms require medical management and nursing intervention.

Several theories to account for the cause of endometriosis have been suggested. The most accepted theory is *transtubal migration* or *retrograde menstruation*. According to this theory, endometrial tissue is regurgitated from the uterus during menstruation to the fallopian tubes and into the peritoneal cavity, where it implants on the ovaries and other organs.

Symptoms vary among women and change over time. The major symptom is secondary dysmenorrhea. Women also complain of pain on defecation around the time of the menstrual cycle, pelvic heaviness, and pain radiating into the thighs. Less common symptoms include pain with exercise or during intercourse as a result of adhesions, and abnormal bleeding—hypermenorrhea, menorrhagia, or premenstrual staining—possibly as a result of ovarian adhesions that have disrupted normal ovarian hormone production.

Impaired fertility may result from adhesions around the uterus that pull the uterus into a fixed, retroverted position. Adhesions around the fallopian tubes may prevent the spontaneous movement that carries the ovum to the uterus or blocks the fimbriated ends. Approximately 30% to 45% of women with endometriosis are infertile, compared with only 12% of women in the general population.

Treatment is based on the severity of symptoms and the goals of the woman or couple. Women without pain who do not want to become pregnant need no treatment. Women with mild pain who may desire a future pregnancy may require analgesics. Those who have severe pain and can postpone pregnancy may be treated with low estrogen-to-progestin–ratio oral contraceptives to shrink endometrial tissue. Another treatment method is danazol (Danocrine), a mildly androgenic synthetic steroid that suppresses FSH and LH secretion. Most women note relief from pain within 6 weeks. Danazol is continued for 9 months; when it is discontinued, menstruation returns.

Danazol can produce side effects that necessitate its discontinuation. These include masculinizing traits in the woman (which often disappear when treatment is discontinued), weight gain, edema, decreased breast size, oily skin, hirsutism, deepening of the voice, decreased libido, vasomotor symptoms (e.g., hot flushes), atrophic vaginitis, emotional lability, and seborrhea. Migraine headaches, dizziness, fatigue, and depression are also reported.

Danazol should never be prescribed when pregnancy is suspected, and contraception should be used with it since ovulation may not be suppressed. Danazol can produce pseudohermaphroditism in female fetuses. The drug is contraindicated in women with liver disease and should be used with caution in women with cardiac and renal disease. Because it is an expensive drug, danazol may not be available to all women. The recommended dosage is 400 to 800 mg a day for 6 to 9 months, and one 200-mg tablet costs about $2.

A gonadotropin-releasing hormone (GnRH) agonist (Nafarelin) has shown promise of being an effective alternative to danazol. Clinical trials indicate that Nafarelin is as effective as danazol, with fewer side effects, in the treatment of endometriosis when 200 to 400 μg are administered twice daily. Because it is destroyed by digestive enzymes, it must be used either intranasally or subcutaneously (Few, 1988).

Endometriosis may not be cured by hormonal treatments, and pain may return within 3 to 9 months when treatment is discontinued. Pregnancy may well be a "treatment" for endometriosis—both pregnancy and lactation are excellent prophylaxis in the presence of endometriosis because they suppress menstruation and cause ectopic endometrial tissue to shrink. Relief from pain may persist for years following pregnancy.

Surgical intervention, most commonly laparoscopy or laparotomy with bowel wedge resection, may be appropriate for some women. It is possible to lyse adhesions, resect implants, and cauterize or use a laser via the laparoscope. There is a 50% improved fertility rate following surgery.

During the climacterium, endometrial tissue atrophies, and endometriosis ceases to be a problem. However, women who use HRT for problems associated with menopause should be aware that endometriosis can be reactivated during this therapy.

Care Management

✦ ASSESSMENT

In addition to taking a careful menstrual, obstetric, sexual, and contraceptive history, the nurse should explore the woman's perceptions of her condition, cultural or ethnic influences, experiences with other caregivers, lifestyle, and patterns of coping (see Cultural Considerations). The amount of pain experienced and its effect on daily activities, home remedies, and prescriptions to relieve discomfort are noted. A symptom diary, in which the woman records emotions, behaviors, physical symptoms, diet, and exercise and rest patterns, is a useful diagnostic tool.

✦ NURSING DIAGNOSES

Examples of nursing diagnoses for women experiencing menstrual disorders include:

High risk for ineffective individual or family coping related to
- Insufficient knowledge of the cause of the disorder
- Emotional and physiologic effects of the disorder
Knowledge deficit related to
- Self-care
- Available therapy for the disorder
High risk for body image disturbance related to
- Menstrual disorder
High risk for low self-esteem related to
- Others' perception of her discomfort
- Inability to conceive
Pain related to
- Menstrual disorder

✦ EXPECTED OUTCOMES

After data collection and review, mutual expected patient outcomes are established and a plan of care is developed. Expected patient outcomes may include:
1. The woman will verbalize her understanding of reproductive anatomy, etiology of her disorder, medication regimen, and diary use.
2. The woman (couple) will understand and accept

CULTURAL CONSIDERATIONS

SOME CULTURAL ASPECTS OF WOMEN'S HEALTH PROBLEMS

In assessing for health problems experienced by women, nurses need to know who is at high risk for certain problems. The following list may be used to assist the nurse in assessment.

- African-American women are at greater risk for certain women's health problems than Caucasian women. These include leiomyomas or fibroids and cervical cancer.
- Caucasian women are more at risk for endometriosis, prolapse of the uterus, and edometrial cancer.
- Caucasian and Asian women are at higher risk for osteoporosis.

her emotional and physical responses to her menstrual cycle.

3. The woman (couple) will develop personal goals that benefit her (them) emotionally and physically.
4. The woman (couple) will choose appropriate therapeutic measures.
5. The woman (couple) will adapt successfully to the condition if cure is not possible.

✧ COLLABORATIVE CARE

During the history and diagnostic workup, the health care provider's concern and acceptance of the woman's symptoms are in themselves therapeutic. Data from the daily log of emotional status, subjective feelings, and physical state are correlated with physiologic changes. If the woman has a male partner, both the woman and her partner keep separate logs that include how each perceives the other's responses day by day. Through the log, feelings are vented, problems are identified and clarified, insights occur, and possible solutions begin to develop. The health care provider facilitates insights and suggests therapeutic options. The woman (couple) makes choices considered best for her (them).

Nurses need to discuss the options available to women with menstrual disorders. They must understand basic information about the anatomy and physiology, pathophysiology, psychologic impact, and treatment for the condition.

Support groups are an important resource. Nurses can use a local women's center or clinic to bring together women who want to learn more about their condition and support each other.

✧ EVALUATION

Disorders associated with menstruation disrupt the quality of life for affected women and their families. Reviewing the monthly diary provides a basis for evaluation and further revision of the nursing care plan. Care has been effective when the woman reports improvement in the quality of her life, skill in self-care, and a positive self-concept and body image (see p. 862 for a case study and plan of care for a patient with endometriosis.)

INFECTIONS

Common vaginal infections such as bacterial vaginitis, *Trichomonas vaginalis,* and vulvovaginal candidiasis can occur throughout a woman's life. Toxic shock syndrome, an uncommon but potentially life-threatening system disorder, can occur in women who use tampons during menstruation and vaginally inserted methods of contraception such as the diaphragm, cervical cap, and vaginal sponge. These infections are discussed in Chapter 21.

Pelvic Inflammatory Disease

Pelvic inflammatory disease (PID) may be a generalized infection of the female pelvic organs and supporting structures, or it may be confined to the fallopian tubes, in which case it is called salpingitis. Salpingitis is synonymous with acute PID in common usage. It is a significant cause of infertility, and 15% to 25% of women who have had the disease are affected. Ectopic pregnancy may also be a complication of PID. Chronic pain, dyspareunia, and dysmenorrhea may be sequelae.

The disease is most frequently caused by the sexually transmitted organisms *Neisseria gonorrhoeae, Chlamydia,* and *Mycoplasma,* and less frequently by *Escherichia coli, Streptococcus, Haemophilus,* and other organisms. These pathogens usually invade the cervix during sexual intercourse, during or after childbirth, or after an abortion (Swearingen, 1990). PID frequently occurs at the end of a menstrual period, since blood is a rich medium for the growth of bacteria. Occasionally PID is the result of the secondary spread of infection from adjacent structures, such as a perforated appendix or intraabdominal abscess, resulting in pelvic peritonitis.

Women with multiple sexual partners are at greater risk for PID, and there is an increased incidence in young women (Swearingen, 1990). Women with a history of PID are at greater risk. The disease is more common in women using IUDs than in women using other contraceptive methods; oral contraceptives and barrier methods of contraception, such as spermicidal foams and jellies, condoms, and diaphragms, may decrease risk. PID is also seen in HIV-infected women (see Clinical Application of Research box on p. 863). At least 13 women per 1000 between 14 and 34 years of age develop PID each year (Swearingen, 1990).

PLAN OF CARE

Endometriosis

Case History

Terry Smith is a 28-year-old married woman who is referred to the clinic nurse for instruction and counseling after seeing the physician. A tentative diagnosis of endometriosis has been made. Danazol, 400 mg bid, is prescribed, and a laparoscopy to confirm the diagnosis is scheduled.

Terry complains of heavy menstrual periods, accompanied by severe pelvic and abdominal pain that may radiate down her thighs or be accompanied by a sensation of pelvic fullness. Her pain has gradually worsened over time. Terry reports that she and her husband have a strong relationship, but there is a lot of tension: "We both are under a lot of stress." She confides that she has painful intercourse (dysparunia) and no longer enjoys sexual relations. "We just can't be spontaneous," she adds. She and her husband would like to have a child, but she has been unable to conceive, although she has been married 3 years. She states, "I feel like such a failure. I'm trying to get pregnant, and it's not working." Terry reports that she has been feeling tired and weak. "I come home from work and just collapse." Her hemoglobin is 10.5 g. Terry asks, "What will this prescription do for me?" She appears anxious and states, "I'm scared of what the doctor is going to do. I'm afraid of what he is going to find and that there is nothing he can do."

EXPECTED OUTCOMES	IMPLEMENTATION	RATIONALE	EVALUATION
Nursing Diagnosis: Pain related to endometriosis			
Terry's pain will be relieved or minimized.	Assess location, type, and duration of pain and history of discomfort. Give analgesics prn.	After pain is assessed and diagnosis is established, interventions to assist with pain relief are implemented.	Terry's pain is localized and minimized.
Nursing Diagnosis: Knowledge deficit related to condition and treatment			
Terry will demonstrate knowledge of endometriosis and its treatment.	Teach about endometriosis and comfort measures and use and side effects of medications.	Knowledge dispels the unknown and empowers the patient to become a partner in her care.	Terry understands condition and uses medication and comfort measures correctly.
Nursing Diagnosis: Body image disturbance and self-esteem disturbance related to symptoms of diagnosis			
Terry will maintain her self-esteem.	Provide time to discuss feelings. Refer to support group.	Interventions promote positive body image and self-esteem.	Terry joins a support group. Terry reports she feels positive about herself.
Nursing Diagnosis: Anxiety related to diagnosis			
Terry will report decreased anxiety.	Discuss feelings and concerns about diagnosis. Provide support and realistic hope. Teach about endometriosis and treatment.	Ventilation of feelings and knowledge about the cause and management can decrease anxiety.	Terry verbalizes understanding of information presented. Terry is less anxious about her diagnosis.

CLINICAL APPLICATION OF RESEARCH

PELVIC INFLAMMATORY DISEASE IN HIV-INFECTED WOMEN

Pelvic inflammatory disease is a major cause of morbidity in the reproductive tract of females. The Centers for Disease Control and Prevention recently revised the classification system for human immunodeficiency virus (HIV) infection to include pelvic inflammatory disease (PID) in category B-2. This study was conducted to determine whether women who are hospitalized for PID and are HIV-seropositive differ in presenting symptoms, complications, and failure of treatment from women who are HIV-seronegative. The medical records of all women admitted for PID during a 6-year period and who were tested for HIV serostatus were reviewed. Twenty-three patients with PID were identified as HIV-seropositive; 108 patients with PID who were tested and found to be HIV-seronegative served as a control group. The researchers found no significant differences between the groups in most demographic characteristics. More HIV-positive women had a history of IV drug use (78% vs. 20%). HIV-positive women had less abdominal tenderness then did the HIV-negative women. More HIV-

negative women than HIV-positive women had cervical smears positive for *N. gonorrhoeae* and *C. trachomatis*. The duration of treatment and length of hospitalization did not differ between groups. More HIV-positive women received surgical treatment than did HIV-negative women. The authors explained the lower incidence of abdominal tenderness by noting that pain associated with PID is due to the inflammatory process; immune-suppressed women will not have inflammation as a response to infection. Nurses caring for women should recognize that the incidence of PID and that of HIV infection are related. For women at risk for either PID or HIV infections, careful histories must be obtained and referrals for diagnosis and treatment of women with symptoms made. Anticipatory guidance related to risk factors and health promotion activities such as the use of condoms must be encouraged for sexually active women.

Reference: Korn AP et al: Pelvic inflammatory disease in human immunodeficiency virus–infected women, *Obstet Gynecol* 82:765, 1993.

Symptoms of acute PID include severe lower abdominal pain and tenderness. Purulent vaginal discharge, fever, and dysuria may also be present. On pelvic examination, any manipulation of the cervix causing motion of the edematous adnexae (tubes and ovaries) results in severe pain and abdominal guarding. Ectopic pregnancy must be ruled out through pregnancy testing or sonography. **Culdocentesis,** in which peritoneal fluid is aspirated form the cul-de-sac for culture of the offending organism, may aid in the diagnosis; laparoscopy, with direct inspection of the adnexae, is the definitive test. Laboratory studies include white blood cell count, sedimentation rate, and cultures of specimens from the cervix, urethra, and rectum.

Treatment consists of specific antibiotics and analgesia, depending on the severity of symptoms. If hospitalization is indicated, intravenous antibiotics may be administered for 4 to 5 days, followed by oral therapy for 7 to 10 days. Most women with uncomplicated PID can be treated as outpatients with oral antibiotics or a combined one-time dose of an intramuscular antibiotic followed by oral therapy over a period of 10 to 14 days. These women must be reevaluated 49 to 72 hours after antibiotic therapy is initiated to ensure the infection is responding to treatment. Nonpharmaceutical pain measures include sitz baths and heat applied to the lower abdomen or back. Bed rest in semi-Fowler's position to promote drainage and comfort is recommended. A few women who do not respond to treatment will require

laparotomy through a small subumbilical incision to remove an abscess or pelvic mass.

Care Management

A detailed history, including a history of sexual activity, contraceptive use, and previous episodes of PID or sexually transmitted diseases (STDs), is obtained. Presenting symptoms are elicited. A nonjudgmental approach by the nurse will help dispel the woman's embarrassment or any guilt feelings if the problem is associated with an STD. Physical examination and laboratory studies as previously discussed confirm the diagnosis. The woman will need emotional support and reassurance during the examination because it may be painful.

The nurse needs to assess the woman's knowledge of PID and risk factors for the disease. Health teaching should include information about PID and increased risk related to multiple sex partners and the IUD as a birth control measure; the need for frequent pad changes during menses and careful washing of the perineal area, wiping from front to back to prevent rectal contamination of the vagina; and the need to seek early medical care, should symptoms of PID occur. Women with a history of PID should not risk STDs and should avoid intercourse during menstruation. If children are desired, early childbearing may be recommended, since tubal scarring increases the risk of infertility.

Nursing care during hospitalization for acute PID includes providing information about hospital routines and procedures, comfort measures, and emotional support. If the woman is anxious, the nurse provides an atmosphere conducive to asking questions and expressing feelings. If future fertility is a concern, reassurance regarding the advantages of early treatment, advances in infertility surgery, and information about support groups can be shared. Significant others should be involved in the plan of care.

When the woman demonstrates a knowledge of PID—signs and symptoms, treatment, and possible outcomes—and expresses her intention to lower risks of infection through good health practices, the goals of health education have been accomplished. When PID is present, if the woman becomes asymptomatic, expresses less discomfort and anxiety regarding her condition, and confidence in her ability to cope with anxiety about future fertility and to seek help, the plan of care has been satisfactory.

IMPAIRED FERTILITY

The inability to conceive and bear a child comes as a surprise to 15% to 20% of otherwise healthy adults (Evans et al, 1989). It is difficult to be denied the experiences of pregnancy and birth, parenthood, and the expression of love through the care and nurturing of another human being. Disturbance in one's sexual self-concept is often experienced. Couples requesting assistance with impaired fertility have already decided that they want a child. They seek acceptance and assistance from the health care provider in coping with and possibly resolving this problem.

The traditional definition of **impaired fertility** is the inability to conceive after at least 1 year of unprotected intercourse. A contemporary definition does not consider a time limit. It is the inability to conceive or carry to live birth at a time the couple has chosen to do so.

Impaired fertility is *primary* if the woman has never been pregnant or the man has never impregnated a woman. It is *secondary* if the woman has been pregnant at least once but has not been able to conceive again or sustain a pregnancy.

The incidence of impaired fertility seems to be increasing. An estimated one out of every six couples in the United States is involuntarily childless (Willson, Carrington, 1991). Probable causes include the trend to delay pregnancy until later in life when fertility decreases naturally, the increase in pelvic inflammatory disease, and the increase in substance abuse. Environmental agents (e.g., pesticides and lead) negatively affect both male and female reproductive systems (Mattison et al, 1990). Diagnosis and treatment of impaired fertility require considerable physical, emotional, and financial investment over an extended period. Frank (1990b) found that per-

sonal beliefs, physician advice, and emotional stress are the critical factors influencing infertility treatment decisions. Men tend to make decisions based on potential side effects and women on the potential effectiveness of treatment (Frank, 1990a).

The attitude, sensitivity, and caring nature of health team members who are involved in the assessment of impaired fertility lay the foundation for the patient's ability to cope with the subsequent therapy and management. All members of the health team must respect the patient's rights to privacy and the confidentiality of the patient records.

Special Considerations
Religious Considerations

Civil laws and religious proscriptions about sex must always be kept in mind by the health care provider. For example, the Orthodox Jewish husband and wife may face infertility investigation and management problems because of religious laws that govern marital relations. According to Jewish law the couple may not engage in marital relations during menstruation and through the following 7 "preparatory days." The wife then is immersed in a ritual bath (Mikvah) before relations can resume. Fertility problems can arise when the woman has a short cycle (i.e., a cycle of 24 days or fewer; when ovulation would occur on day 10 or earlier).

The Roman Catholic Church regards the embryo as a human being from the first moment of existence and regards technical procedures such as in vitro fertilization, artificial insemination, and freezing embryos as unacceptable (White, 1992). Both Orthodox Jewish and Roman Catholic women may at times question proposed diagnostic and therapeutic procedures because of religious proscriptions. These women are encouraged to consult their rabbi or priest for a ruling.

Other religious groups may also have ethical concerns about infertility tests and treatments.

Psychosocial Considerations

Within the United States, feelings connected to impaired fertility are many and complex. The origin of some of these feelings are myths, superstitions, misinformation, or "magical" thinking about the cause of infertility. Other feelings arise from the need to undergo many tests and examinations and from being different from others.

Infertility is recognized as a major life stressor that can affect self-concept, relations with the spouse, family and friends, and careers. Couples often need assistance in separating their concepts of success and failure related to treatment for infertility from personal success and failure. Recognizing the significance of infertility as a loss and resolving these feelings are crucial to putting infertility into perspective, even if treatment is successful (Olshansky, 1992).

Cultural Considerations

Worldwide, cultures continue to employ symbols and rites that celebrate fertility. One fertility rite that persists today is the custom of throwing rice at the bride and groom. Other fertility symbols and rites include the passing out of congratulatory cigars, candy, or pencils by a new father as well as baby showers held in anticipation of a child's birth.

In many cultures the responsibility for infertility is usually attributed to the woman. A woman's inability to conceive may be due to her sins, to evil spirits, or to the fact that she is an inadequate person. The virility of a man in some cultures remains in question until he demonstrates his ability to reproduce by having at least one child (Geissler, 1994).

Factors Associated with Infertility

The couple is a biologic unit of reproduction. Many factors, both male and female, contribute to normal fertility. A normally developed reproductive tract is essential. Normal functioning of an intact hypothalamic-pituitary-gonadal axis supports gametogenesis—the formation of sperm and ova. The life span of the sperm and ovum is short. Although sperm remain viable in the female's reproductive tract for 48 hours or more, probably only a few retain fertilization potential for more than 24 hours. Ova remain viable for about 24 hours, but the optimum time for fertilization may be no more than 1 to 2 hours (Cunningham et al, 1993). It is likely that viable sperm may need to be present in the uterine tube at the time of ovulation for optimum fertilization (Cunningham et al, 1993). Thus timing of intercourse becomes critical.

The male must produce sperm that are normal, adequate in number, and motile. Accessory glands must provide supportive secretions to the sperm to form semen. The tube system to the urethra must be patent. Ejaculation must deposit semen around the cervix at the appropriate time of the female's menstrual cycle. After being deposited, sperm must be able to penetrate and be sustained by receptive and supportive cervical mucus. Sperm must undergo capacitation to prepare for fertilization. Then they migrate through the uterus to the ampulla of the uterine tube to fertilize a receptive normal ovum.

In the female, a graafian follicle must mature and release a healthy ovum able to be fertilized. The ovum must be drawn by the fimbria into a healthy, patent uterine tube and fertilized within a few hours. The conceptus must migrate down the tube into a well-developed normal uterus. Implantation of the blastocyst must occur within 7 to 10 days in a hormone-prepared endometrium. The conceptus must develop normally, reach viability, and be born in good condition for extrauterine life.

An alteration in one or more of these structures, functions, or processes results in some degree of impairment of fertility. Causes of impaired fertility are sometimes difficult to assign to either the male or the female (Willson, Carrington, 1991). A male factor may be solely responsible in 30% of infertile couples, but it may be contributory in another 10%. Tubal factors are identified in about 25% of infertile couples, an ovulatory disorder in about 20%,* or a cervical factor in approximately 15%. Miscellaneous (5%) or unexplained factors (5%) account for the remaining causes.

Unexplained infertility and recurrent (habitual) abortion may be the result of aberrations of the immune system (e.g., antisperm antibodies, failure of implantation and growth of a blastocyst) (Evans et al, 1989).

Investigation of Female Infertility

Since multiple factors involving both partners are common, the investigation of impaired fertility is conducted systematically. Both partners must be interested in the solution to the problem. The medical investigation requires time and considerable financial expense, as well as causes emotional distress and strain on the couple's interpersonal relationship. Nurses can be instrumental in providing information about the latest tests and treatment (Nero, 1988). A thorough investigation usually requires 3 to 4 months and sometimes more.

Investigation of impaired fertility begins with a complete history and physical examination. The history explores the duration of infertility and past obstetric events and contains a detailed sexual history. Medical and surgical conditions are evaluated. Exposure to reproductive hazards in the home (e.g., mutagens such as plastic-vinyl chlorides, teratogens such as alcohol, and emotional stresses) and workplace are explored.

A complete general physical examination is followed by a specific assessment of the reproductive tract. Evidence of endocrine system abnormalities is sought. Inadequate development of secondary sex characteristics (e.g., inappropriate distribution of body fat and hair) may point to problems with the hypothalamic-pituitary-ovarian axis or genetic aberrations (e.g., Turner's syndrome). Women with Turner's syndrome are typically short, have underdeveloped breasts, and abnormal gonads. These women are infertile. A woman may have an abnormal uterus and tubes as a result of exposure to diethylstilbestrol (DES) in utero. Evidence of past infection of the genitourinary system is sought. Bimanual examination of the internal organs may reveal lack of mobility of the uterus or abnormal contours of the uterus and adnexa.

Laboratory data are assembled. Data from routine

---

*Other authors (Evans et al, 1989) suggest that ovulation disorders are implicated in 40% to 50% of infertile couples.

urine and blood tests are obtained along with other tests (see following discussion).

Tests and Examinations

There are several examinations and tests for impaired fertility. The basic infertility survey involves evaluation of the cervix, uterus, tubes, and peritoneum; detection of ovulation; assessment of immunologic compatibility; and evaluation of psychogenic factors (Scott et al, 1990).

A discussion of the most common tests follows.

Detection of Ovulation

Documentation of time of ovulation is important in the investigation of impaired fertility. Direct proof of ovulation is pregnancy or the retrieval of an ovum from the uterine tube. There are several indirect or presumptive methods for detection of ovulation. These include assessment of BBT (for discussion of BBT, see p. 486) and cervical mucus characteristics (for discussion of cervical mucus, see p. 487), as well as endometrial biopsy. These clinical tests more or less determine whether progesterone is secreted in significant amounts (Table 30-1) to accommodate implantation and maintain pregnancy. Occurrence of mittelschmerz and midcycle spotting provides unreliable presumptive evidence of ovulation (Scott et al, 1990).

Hormone Analysis

Hormone analysis is performed to assess endocrine function of the *hypothalamic-pituitary-ovarian axis*. Blood

and urine specimens are obtained at varying times during a woman's menstrual cycle. Blood specimens are drawn to determine levels of progesterone, estrogen, FSH, and LH. Urine specimens provide information about the levels of 17-ketosteroids and 17-hydroxy-corticosteroids.

Blood is drawn late in the woman's menstrual cycle to assess the function of the *corpus luteum*. This test can be done in a serial manner to determine if the levels of plasma progesterone correlate well with the woman's BBT and cervical mucus characteristics.

Timed Endometrial Biopsy

Endometrial biopsy is scheduled after ovulation during the luteal phase of the menstrual cycle. Late in the menstrual cycle, 3 to 4 days before expected menses, a sample of the endometrium is removed for histologic study to assess the function of the corpus luteum and the receptivity of the endometrium for implantation. There are two methods of performing a timed endometrial biopsy; neither method requires hospitalization. The first method is implemented 3 to 4 days before expected menses. With the woman draped and in the lithotomy position, a vaginal speculum is inserted into the vagina. Using a small-lumen vabra aspirator, a sample of the endometrium is obtained.

The second method includes the following steps:

1. The couple is cautioned to abstain from intercourse during preceding "fertile" period to avoid dislodging a possible embryo during the procedure.

TABLE 30-1 Tests for Impaired Fertility

TEST/EXAMINATION	TIMING (MENSTRUAL CYCLE DAYS)	RATIONALE
Hysterosalpingogram	7 to 10	Late follicular, early proliferative phase will not disrupt a fertilized ovum; may open uterine tubes before time of ovulation
Postcoital (Huhner test)	Peak cervical mucus flow*	Ovulatory late proliferative phase—look for normal motile sperm in cervical mucus
Sperm immobilization antigen-antibody reaction		Immunologic test to determine sperm and cervical mucus interaction
Assessment of cervical mucus		Cervical mucus should have low viscosity, high spinnbarkheit
Ultrasound observation of follicular collapse	Ovulation	Collapsed follicle is seen after ovulation
Serum assay of plasma progesterone	20 to 25	Midluteal midsecretory phase—check adequacy of corpus luteal production of progesterone
Basal body temperature (BBT)		Elevation occurs in response to progesterone
Endometrial biopsy	26 to 27	Late luteal, late secretory phase—check endometrial response to progesterone and adequacy of luteal phase

*Exogenous estrogen may be given to induce mucus flow if spontaneous and reasonably regular ovulation does not occur.

2. The cervix is dilated with laminaria 4 to 24 hours before the procedure, which requires no analgesia (Fig. 30-2). **Laminaria** are small, thin inserts of packed seaweed or synthetic osmotic dilators that, when inserted into the cervix, absorb moisture, expand, and thus dilate the cervix.)

3. The woman assumes the lithotomy position and is draped, and the speculum is inserted.

4. The laminaria are removed.

5. If not previously dilated with laminaria, the cervix is dilated at this time with metal rod dilators. Analgesia or anesthesia is often necessary.

6. A small specimen of endometrium is removed from the side wall in the fundus to avoid dislodging an embryo should conception have occurred. (When implantation occurs, it is usually high in the fundus, either in the anterior or posterior portion).

Findings favorable to fertility include an endometrium that is negative for tuberculosis, polyps, or inflammatory conditions and that reflects secretory changes normally seen in the presence of adequate luteal (progesterone) phase.

Hysterosalpingography

Radiographic (x-ray) film allows visualization of the uterine cavity and tubes after the instillation of radiopaque contrast material through the cervix (Fig. 30-3). It is possible to see abnormalities of the uterus such as congenital defects or defects produced by submucous myomas and endometrial polyps. Distortions of the uterine cavity or uterine tubes as a result of current or past pelvic inflammatory disease (PID) are identified. Scar tissue and adhesions from inflammatory processes can immobilize the uterus and tubes, kink the tubes, and surround the ovaries. PID may follow infection from sexually transmitted diseases (STDs) or rupture of an inflamed appendix.

Hysterosalpingography is scheduled 2 to 5 days after menstruation to avoid flushing a potential fertilized ovum out through a fallopian tube into the peritoneal cavity. Also at this time there are no open vessels, and all menstrual debris has been discharged. This decreases the risk of embolism or of forcing menstrual debris out through the tubes into the peritoneal cavity. If the woman has PID, she is treated with antimicrobials and the test is rescheduled in 2 to 3 months.

Referred shoulder pain may occur during this procedure. The referred pain is indicative of subphrenic irritation from the contrast material if it is spilled out of the patent uterine tubes or if the tubes are occluded. The discomfort subsides with position change. It usually disappears within 12 to 14 hours and can be controlled with mild analgesics.

This procedure may be therapeutic as well as diagnostic. The passage of contrast medium may clear tubes of mucous plugs, straighten kinked tubes, or break up adhesions within the tubes (secondary to salpingitis). The procedure may stimulate cilia in the lining of the tubes to facilitate transport of the ovum. It also may aid healing as a result of the bacteriostatic effect of the iodine within the contrast medium.

Laparoscopy

Laparoscopy is usually scheduled early in the menstrual cycle. During the procedure a small telescope is inserted through a small incision in the anterior abdominal wall. Cold fiberoptic light sources allow for superior visualization of the internal pelvic structures (Fig. 30-4). The woman is usually admitted shortly before surgery, having taken nothing by mouth (NPO) for 8 hours. She voids before surgery. A general anesthetic is usually given and the woman is placed in the lithotomy position. Her pubic hair is shaved only if this examination is likely to be followed by laparotomy. A needle is inserted and carbon dioxide gas is pumped into the peritoneum to elevate the abdominal wall from the organs, thereby creating an empty space that permits visualization and exploration with the laparoscope. If tubal patency is being assessed, a cannula is used to instill a dye contrast medium through the cervix. Visualization of the peritoneal cavity in infertile women may reveal endometriosis, pelvic adhesions, tubal occlusion, or polycystic ovaries. Fulguration (destruction of tissue by means of electricity) of small endometrial implants, lysis of the adhesions, and taking ovarian biopsies are some of the procedures possible through the use of a laparoscope. After surgery, deflation of most of the gas is done by direct expression. Trocar (and needle) sites are closed with a single subcuticular absorbable suture or skin clip, and an adhesive bandage is applied. Postoperative recovery requires taking of vital signs, assessing level of consciousness, pre-

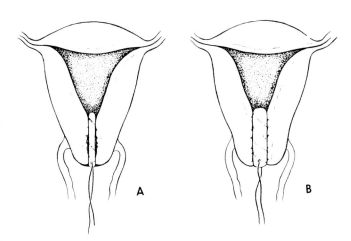

FIG. 30-2 Laminaria. **A,** Inserted through narrow cervical canal beyond the internal os. **B,** Cervix dilated 4 to 12 hours later. (From Sanberg EC: *Synopsis of obstetrics,* ed 10, St. Louis, 1978, Mosby.)

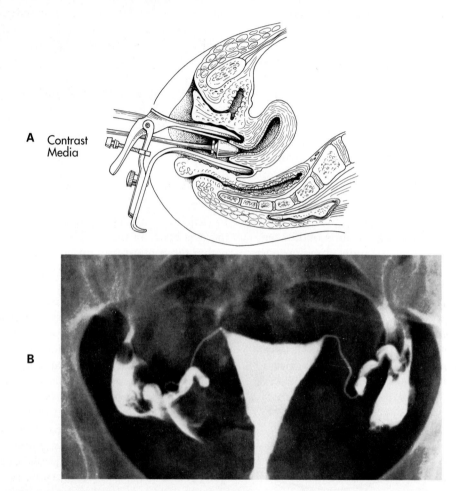

A Contrast
Media

B

FIG. 30-3 **A,** Hysterosalpingography. Sagittal section showing technique. Contrast medium blows through intrauterine cannula and out through tubes, the cervix being closed by a rubber stopper. **B,** Normal hysterosalpingogram showing passage of radiopaque material through fimbriated ends of tubes. (**B** from Willson JR, Carrington ER: *Obstetrics and gynecology,* ed 9, St. Louis, 1991, Mosby.)

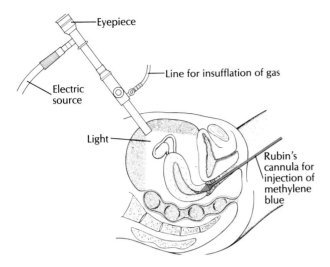

FIG. 30-4   Laparoscopy.

venting aspiration, monitoring intravenous fluids, and reassuring the patient regarding referred shoulder discomfort. Discharge from the hospital usually occurs in 4 to 6 hours. Referred shoulder pain or subcostal discomfort usually lasts only 24 hours and is relieved with a mild analgesic. The woman must be cautioned against heavy lifting or strenuous activity for 4 to 7 days, at which time she is usually asymptomatic.

Ultrasound Pelvic Examination

Abdominal or transvaginal ultrasound is also used to assess pelvic structures (Fig. 30-5). This procedure is used to visualize pelvic tissues for a variety of reasons (e.g., to identify abnormalities, to verify follicular development and maturity, or to confirm intrauterine [vs. ectopic] pregnancy).

Reproductive Structures and Factors Implicated in Infertility

Congenital or Developmental Factors

If the woman has abnormal external genitals, surgical reconstruction of abnormal tissue and construction of a functional vagina may permit normal intercourse. If internal reproductive tract structures are absent, there is no hope for fertility. Vaginal and uterine anomalies and their surgical repair vary from individual to individual. If a functional uterus can be reconstructed, pregnancy may be possible.

Ovarian Factors

Anovulation may be primary or secondary. *Primary anovulation* may be caused by a pituitary or hypothalamic hormone disorder or an adrenal gland disorder such as congenital adrenal hyperplasia. *Secondary anovulation* may be caused by ovarian disease. In amenorrheic states and instances of anovulatory cycles, hormone studies usually reveal the problem.

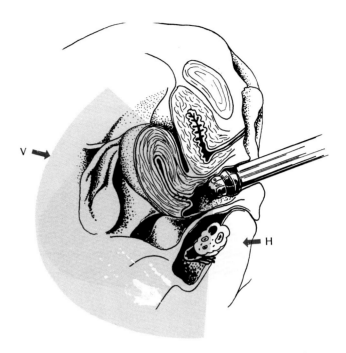

FIG. 30-5   Vaginal ultrasonography. Major scanning planes of transducer. *H,* Horizontal, *V,* vertical.

Care Management

Drug therapy is often an important but expensive component of patient care. *Ovulatory stimulants* may be warranted. *Clomiphene* (Clomid, Serophene), an oral preparation, is a follicular maturing agent. It is used to treat anovulation caused by hypothalamic suppression when the hypothalamic-pituitary-ovarian axis is intact. *Bromocriptine* (Parlodel), a synthetic ergot alkaloid that inhibits the release of prolactin, is used to treat anovulation caused by elevated levels of prolactin. *Thyroid-stimulating hormone* (TSH) is indicated if the woman has hypothyroidism; *human menopausal gonadotropin* (hMG) (Pergonal), if she has hypogonadotropic amenorrhea. When anovulation is caused by hypothalamic-pituitary dysfunction, hypothalamic failure, or failure to respond to clomiphene, *gonadotropin-releasing hormone* (GnRH) may be prescribed.

Hormone replacement therapy may be indicated. The woman who has low levels of estrogen is a candidate for *conjugated estrogens and medroxyprogesterone.* A hypoestrogenic condition may result from a high stress level or decreased percentage of body fat as a result of an eating disorder (e.g., anorexia nervosa) or excessive exercise. *Hydroxyprogesterone* supplementation with vaginal suppositories or intramuscular injection is used to treat luteal phase defects. The nurse may encounter other medications as well. In the presence of adrenal hyperplasia, *prednisone,* a glucocorticoid, is taken orally. *Danazol* is the drug of choice in the management of endometriosis. Infections are treated with appropriate antimicrobial formulations.

Ovarian tumors must be excised. Whenever possible, functional ovarian tissue is left intact. Scar tissue adhesions caused by chronic infection may cover much or all of the ovary. These adhesions usually necessitate surgery to free and expose the ovary so that ovulation can occur.

Thyroid gland dysfunction may be associated with menstrual abnormalities, impaired fertility, or recurrent fetal wastage. Therapy consists of management of the thyroid condition coupled with careful scrutiny of BBT charts (p. 486) to promote sperm deposition at the same time as ovulation. Continuous monitoring and management of thyroid function during pregnancy are also carried out.

Tubal (Peritoneal) Factors

The motility of the tube and its fimbriated end may be reduced or absent as a result of infections, adhesions, or tumors. Chlamydial infection negatively influences tubal function and impedes fertility (Eggert-Kruse et al, 1990). In rare instances there may be congenital absence of one tube. It is also possible to find one tube relatively shorter than the other. This condition is often associated with an abnormally developed uterus.

Inflammation within the tube or involving the exterior of the tube or the fimbriated ends represents a major cause of impaired fertility. Tubal adhesions resulting from pelvic infections (e.g., ruptured appendix) may impair fertility. When infection with purulent discharge eventually heals, scar tissue adhesions form. In the process the tube may be blocked anywhere along its length. It can be closed off at the fimbriated end, or it can be distorted and kinked by adhesions. Adhesions may permit the tiny sperm to pass through the tube but may prevent a fertilized egg from completing the journey into the intrauterine cavity. This results in an ectopic pregnancy that may completely destroy the tube. In other cases, adhesions of the tubes to the ovary or bowel may follow *endometriosis* (p. 859).

Care Management

Treatment must include prevention and early adequate management of infection with appropriate antibiotics. Surgery may be necessary when drainage of a serious focus of infection is required. Hysterosalpingography is useful for identification of tubal obstruction and also for the release of blockage. During laparoscopy, delicate adhesions may be divided and removed and endometrial implants may be destroyed by electrocoagulation or Nd:YAG laser. Women with severe endometriosis have an improved chance for pregnancy when treated with gamete intrafallopian transfer (GIFT) (Yovich, Matson, 1990) (see p. 876). Laparotomy and even microsurgery

may be required to do extensive repair of the damaged tube. Prognosis is dependent on the degree to which tube patency and function can be restored.

Uterine Factors

Congenital abnormalities of the uterus are far more common than might be expected. Minor developmental anomalies of the uterus are fairly common; major anomalies occur rarely. Hysterosalpingography may reveal double uteri or other anomalous congenital variations. Endometrial and myometrial *tumors* (e.g., polyps or myomas) may also be revealed by x-ray studies of infertile women.

Asherman's syndrome, uterine adhesions or scar tissue, is characterized by hypomenorrhea or amenorrhea. The adhesions, which may partially or totally obliterate the uterine cavity, are sequelae to surgical interventions such as too vigorous curettage (scraping) after an abortion (elective or spontaneous). The hysteroscope is useful in the verification of intrauterine anomalies.

Endometritis (inflammation of the endometrium) may result from any of the causes of infection of the cervix or uterine tubes (e.g., chlamydial). Women who have numerous sex partners are more susceptible to endometrial infection than are women in monogamous relationships.

Care Management

A woman with a relatively small uterus may become pregnant, but the uterus may be incapable of accommodating the enlarging fetus, and a spontaneous abortion may result. In such cases recurrent or habitual (three or more) spontaneous abortions often occur. No medical therapy has been effective for the enlargement of an abnormally small uterus. Observation suggests that women who do become pregnant but who miscarry often abort at a later time with each successive pregnancy. Finally, after two or three pregnancy losses, they may give birth to a viable infant. Apparently actual growth of the uterus occurs with each pregnancy. Plastic surgery—for example, the unification operation for bicornuate uterus—often improves a woman's ability to conceive and carry the fetus to term.

Surgical removal of tumors or fibroids involving the endometrium or uterus often improves the woman's chance of conceiving and maintaining the pregnancy to viability. Surgical treatment of uterine tumors or maldevelopment that results in successful pregnancy usually requires birth by cesarean surgery near term gestation. The uterus may rupture as a result of weakness of the area of surgical healing.

Vaginal-Cervical Factors

Vaginal-cervical infections (e.g., trichomoniasis vaginitis) increase the acidity of the vaginal fluid and reduce the alkalinity of the cervical mucus. Thus vaginal infection often destroys or drastically reduces the number of viable motile sperm before they enter the cervical canal. The amount of mucus and its physical changes are influenced by the presence of blood, pathogenic bacteria, and irritants such as an IUD or a tumor. Severe emotional stress, antibiotic therapy, and diseases such as diabetes mellitus alter the acidity of mucus.

About 20% of infertile women have sperm antibodies. The production of antibodies by one member of a species against something that is commonly found within that species is termed **isoimmunization.** Sperm may be immobilized within the cervical mucus, or they become incapable of migration into the uterus (see postcoital test, p. 872). A greater incidence of sperm agglutination occurs in women with otherwise unexplained impaired fertility. However, the true significance and reliability of tests for sperm immobilization or agglutination are uncertain.

Care Management

Therapy for lower genital factors requires the elimination of vaginitis or cervicitis. Appropriate antibiotic or chemotherapeutic drugs generally resolve this problem. In addition to antibiotics, radial chemocautery (destruction of tissue with chemicals) or thermocautery (destruction of tissue with heat, usually electrical) of the cervix, cryosurgery (destruction of tissue by application of extreme cold, usually liquid nitrogen), or conization (excision of cone-shaped piece of tissue from the endocervix) is effective in eliminating chronic inflammation and infection. When the cervix has been deeply cauterized or frozen or when extensive conization has been performed, extreme limitation of mucus production by the cervix may result. Therefore sperm migration may be difficult or impossible because of the absence of a mucous bridge from the vagina to the uterus. Therapeutic intrauterine insemination may be necessary to carry the sperm directly through the *internal os* of the cervix.

Treatment is available for women who have *immunologic reactions to sperm.* Exposure to semen via the orogenital and anal modes is avoided. The use of condoms during genital intercourse for 6 to 12 months will reduce female antibody production in the majority of women who have elevated antisperm antibody titers. After the serum reaction subsides, condoms are used at all times except at the expected time of ovulation. Approximately one third of couples with this problem conceive by following this course of action.

The prognosis for the infertile woman is generally good provided a serious genital or inflammatory disorder is not identified. Most women present numerous so-called minor problems that, although compounded, may be relatively easy to correct (e.g., chronic cervicitis, hypothyroidism). If successful treatment has not been achieved after a year, for example, other alternatives may be considered (e.g., adoption, childfree living, therapeutic insemination, or in vitro fertilization).

Investigation of Male Infertility

The systematic investigation of impaired fertility in the male, as it does for the female, begins with a thorough history and physical examination. Assessment of the man proceeds in a manner similar to that of the woman, starting with noninvasive tests. Male reproductive failure may be caused by many of the difficulties that also affect women, such as nutritional, endocrine, and psychologic disorders. Exposure to reproductive hazards in the workplace and home is evaluated.

Substance abuse can be a major factor in male infertility. *Alcohol* consumption causes erectile problems (impotence). Cigarette smoking has been associated with abnormal sperm, a decreased number of sperm, and chromosome damage. The degree of abnormality is related to the number of cigarettes smoked per day (Mattison et al, 1989). *Marijuana (Cannabis sativa)* adversely affects spermatogenesis (e.g., it depresses the number and motility of sperm and increases the percentage of abnormally formed sperm). *Monoamine oxidase* (MAO), an antidepressant, adversely affects spermatogenesis. *Amyl nitrate, butyl nitrate, ethyl chloride,* and *methaqualone* (used to prolong orgasm) causes changes in spermatogenesis. *Heroin, methadone,* and *barbiturates* decrease libido.

Tests and Examinations

The basic infertility survey of the male includes a semen analysis. The postcoital test evaluates characteristics of the sperm within the cervical mucus of the man's sexual partner.

Semen Analysis

Examination of semen is an important part of investigation of impaired fertility, since the male is often at least partially responsible (Willson, Carrington, 1991). A complete **semen analysis,** study of the effects of cervical mucus on sperm forward motility and survival, and evaluation of the sperm's ability to penetrate an ovum provide basic information. Sperm counts vary from day to day and are dependent on emotional and physical status and sexual activity. Therefore a single analysis may be inconclusive (Willson, Carrington, 1991). Usually three specimens taken at monthly intervals are evaluated.

Semen is collected by ejaculation into a clean, wide-mouthed plastic or glass jar with a screw top (Willson, Carrington, 1991). The specimen is usually collected by masturbation following 2 to 5 days of abstinence from ejaculation. A specimen can also be collected during genital intercourse if a special nonrubber, unpowdered condom is used.

The semen is taken to the laboratory in a sealed container within 1 hour of ejaculation. Exposure to excessive heat or cold is avoided. Normal values for semen characteristics are given in the Box 30-1.

The fertility potential of sperm is difficult to evaluate solely by semen analysis, which gives little insight into sperm survival, cervical penetration, migration to the uterine tubes, or capacity for ovum penetration and fertilization (Cunningham et al, 1993). In addition, there is insufficient knowledge of the method by which male and female antibodies can act to inhibit fertility potential of sperm. An immunologic disorder as yet not identified may be the basis for unexplained infertility (Cunningham et al, 1993).

Seminal deficiency may be attributable to one or more of a variety of factors. The male is assessed for these factors (Scott et al, 1990): hypopituitarism, nutritional deficiency, debilitating or chronic disease, trauma, exposure to environmental hazards such as radiation and toxic substances, gonadotropic inadequacy, and obstructive lesions of the epididymis and vas deferens. A genetic basis such as Klinefelter's syndrome is ruled out. Hormone analyses are done for testosterone, gonadotropin, FSH, and LH. Testicular biopsy may be warranted.

Postcoital Test

The postcoital test is one method used to test for adequacy of coital technique, cervical mucus, sperm, and degree of sperm penetration through cervical mucus. The test is performed within 2 hours after ejaculation of semen into the vagina. A specimen of cervical mucus is obtained. Intercourse is synchronized with the expected time of ovulation (as determined from evaluation of BBT, cervical mucus changes, and usual length of menstrual cycle). It is performed only in the absence of vaginal infection. Couples may experience some difficulty abstaining from intercourse for 2 to 4 days before expected ovulation and then having intercourse with ejaculation on schedule. Sex on demand may strain the couple's interpersonal relationship. A problem may arise if the expected day of ovulation occurs when facilities or the physician is unavailable (such as over a weekend or holiday). If no sperm is found, the coital technique used must be evaluated (e.g., extreme obesity may prevent adequate penile penetration).

General Therapies

The difficulty may be caused by timing and frequency of intercourse. The couple is taught about the menstrual cycle, the peak cervical mucus symptom, and the appropriate timing of intercourse.

Penile insertion into the vagina is often difficult because of chordee (painful downward curvature on erection) and obesity. The couple is advised to alter positions used for intercourse. Heavy use of alcohol makes penile erection difficult to achieve and maintain until ejaculation. The man is advised to avoid drinking alcohol during the time of the woman's ovulation.

Medical therapy for male infertility has been disappointing, especially when pituitary or testicular disease is discovered. Occasionally it is possible to suppress the production of sperm with injections of testosterone and in that way cause a reduction in the number of autoimmune antibodies present in the man. Following the reduction in sperm autoantibodies, sperm quality improves, and a pregnancy sometimes occurs.

Drug therapy may be indicated for male infertility. Infections are identified and treated promptly with antimicrobials. Problems with the thyroid or adrenal glands are corrected with appropriate medications. Testosterone enanthate (Delatestyl) and testosterone cypionate (Depo-Testosterone) by injection are used to stimulate virilization, especially in the adolescent. Human chorionic gonadotropin (hCG) (Pregnyl) given intramuscularly virilizes a hypogonadotropic male to restore Leydig cell function and spermatogenesis. FSH and hMG aid hCG for completion of spermatogenesis. Bromocriptine, an ergot derivative and dopamine agonist, is used to treat hypogonadotropic hypogonadism–associated prolactin-producing hypothalamic or pituitary tumors and may reduce the tumor. Clomiphene may be given for idiopathic subfertility.

Surgical repair of **varicocele** (enlargement of the veins of the spermatic cord) has been relatively successful. A

BOX 30-1

Semen Analysis

1. Liquefaction: usually complete within 10 to 20 minutes
2. Semen volume — 2 to 5 ml (range: 1 to 7 ml)
3. Semen pH — 7.2 to 7.8
4. Sperm density — 20 to 200 million/ml
5. Normal morphology (%) — ≥60% normal oval
6. Motility (important consideration in sperm evaluation), percentage of forward-moving sperm (swim-up test) estimated in relation to abnormally motile and nonmotile sperm. This requires evaluation by a technician with some degree of experience, but since the test provides a more accurate diagnosis, it is well worth the time involved: ≥50% is normal.
7. Cell count: average normal, 60 million or more per milliliter or a total of 150 to 200 or more million per ejaculate; minimum normal standards: 40 million/ml, with a total count of at least 125 million per ejaculate (average of counts on two or preferably three separate specimens).

Note: These values are not absolute, but only relative to the final evaluation of the couple as a single reproductive unit.

8. Ovum penetration test.

varicocele on the left side is found in a substantial number of subfertile men. Ligation of the varicocele does lead to improvement of the sperm quality and commonly to pregnancy.

Simple changes in lifestyle may be effective in the treatment of subfertile men. Poor nutritional state is corrected if it exists. High temperatures in the groin area reduce the number of sperm produced. High temperatures may be caused by wearing brief shorts and tight jeans that keep the scrotal sac pressed against the body regardless of environmental temperature changes. The testes are kept at temperatures too high for efficient spermatogenesis. Frequent and prolonged hot tubbing has also been implicated in relative infertility. It must be remembered that these conditions lead to relative infertility only and should not be employed as a means of contraception. Lubricants used during intercourse should not contain spermicides or have spermicidal properties.

Care Management

The nurse assists in the *assessment* by obtaining data relevant to fertility through interview and physical examination. The data base needs to include information to identify whether infertility is primary or secondary. Religious, cultural, and ethnic data are noted.

Some of the data needed to investigate impaired fertility are of a sensitive, personal nature. Obtaining these data may be viewed as an invasion of privacy. The tests and examinations are occasionally painful and intrusive and can take the romance out of lovemaking. A high level of motivation is needed to endure the investigation.

Many couples have already visited various physicians and have read extensively on the subject. Their previous experiences are recorded. The depth and breadth of their knowledge base are explored. *Nursing diagnoses* are derived from the data base. Examples of nursing diagnoses related to impaired fertility include:

Anxiety related to
- Unknown outcome of diagnostic workup

Body image or self-esteem disturbance related to
- Impaired fertility

High risk for impaired individual/family coping related to
- Methods used in the investigation of impaired fertility

Decisional conflict related to
- Therapies for impaired fertility
- Alternatives to therapy: childfree living or adoption

Altered family processes related to
- Unmet expectations for pregnancy

Anticipatory grieving related to
- Expected poor prognosis

Acute pain related to
- Effects of diagnostic tests (or surgery)

Powerlessness related to
- Lack of control over prognosis

Altered patterns of sexuality related to
- Loss of libido secondary to medically imposed restrictions

High risk for social isolation related to
- Impaired fertility, its investigation and management

Planning requires sensitivity to the couple's needs. Equipped with a knowledge of impaired fertility, the nurse can help develop a plan of care for the couple with impaired fertility. The *expected outcomes* are phrased in patient-centered terms and may include the following:

1. The couple will understand the anatomy and physiology of the reproductive system.
2. The couple will verbalize understanding of treatment for any abnormalities identified through various tests and examinations (e.g., infections, blocked uterine tubes, sperm allergy, and varicocele) and will be able to make an informal decision about treatment.
3. The couple will verbalize understanding of their potential to conceive.
4. The couple will resolve guilt feelings and will not need to focus blame.
5. The couple will conceive or, failing to conceive, decide on an alternative acceptable to both of them (e.g., childfree living or adoption).
6. The couple will demonstrate acceptable methods for handling pressure they may feel from peers and relatives regarding their childless state.

Nursing actions vary with the nurse's level of education, position held, and policies of the agency. The nurse acts on the woman's or man's readiness to learn and her or his level of understanding of impaired fertility. Although primary responsibility for teaching rests with the primary care provider, the nurse assists in the identification of the gaps in knowledge, clarifies information, and reinforces explanations and instructions. Occasionally the nurse acts as an advocate by helping the patient state a concern or question or request further explanation from other health care providers.

During the period of diagnostic testing, the nurse's nonverbal behavior before and during the procedure can reassure and support the woman. Often the woman feels inadequate because of the necessity for testing and the intimidating nature of the tests.

Written and verbal instructions for specific preparation for tests will increase the woman's feeling of adequacy. Supportive nursing actions include providing privacy while giving instructions for obtaining specimens and changing clothes, encouraging the woman to void before draping, creating a comfortable physical environment, padding the stirrups of the examination table, warming the speculum, and coaching for relaxation.

In addition to discussing the specifics of common tests for impaired fertility, nurses can provide sensory information about these future tests. Providing preparatory information can help patients form a mental image of what an experience will include and thus help make the testing experience more tolerable and less distressing.

Women often experience anxiety when undergoing a pelvic examination. After any procedure, when the woman or man is fully dressed and comfortably seated (at the same level as the health care provider), she or he benefits from an opportunity to talk about the experience in an unhurried manner. Not only do these behaviors help the patient relax, but also they indicate that the recipient of such care is worthy and thus helps build self-esteem. The goal of nursing-medical care is to encourage the patient to become an active partner in care as well as to establish rapport to ensure that therapy and counseling are facilitated.

The nurse needs to know the correct method for obtaining, labeling, and transporting specimens to the laboratory. A mishandled specimen may lead to misdiagnosis or the need to obtain another specimen. These errors create added expense and stress for the patient as well as significant time delays before therapy can be instituted.

The primary care provider is responsible for informing patients fully about the prescribed medications. However the nurse must be ready to answer patient's questions and to confirm their understanding of the drug, its administration, potential side effects, and expected outcomes. Since information varies with each drug, the nurse needs to consult the medication package inserts, pharmacology references, physician, and pharmacist as necessary.

Nurses can help patients express and discuss their feelings as honestly as possible. Ventilation may help couples unburden themselves of negative feelings (Davis, Dearman, 1991). Current research reveals an infertility strain profile including tension, worry, depressive symptoms, and interpersonal alienation (Berg, Wilson, 1990; Wright et al, 1989). Professional referral may be necessary.

The myriad of psychologic responses to a diagnosis of impaired fertility may tax a couple's giving and receiving of physical and sexual closeness. The prescriptions and proscriptions for achieving conception may add tension to a couple's sexual functioning. Couples are instructed about frequency and timing of intercourse as well as use of certain coital positions. It is no wonder that these couples complain of decreased desire for intercourse, orgasmic dysfunction, and midcycle erectile disorders. A once-spontaneous act of expressing love has become a mechanical act for creating a baby.

During evaluation of impaired fertility, the previously private act of intercourse becomes a topic of discussion. Even in the sexually liberated culture of the 1990s, few people eagerly share the frequency of coitus and positions used during intercourse.

To be able to deal comfortably with a couple's sexuality, nurses must be comfortable with their own sexual-

ity. Nurses need to have up-to-date factual knowledge about human sexual practices, be able to accept the preferences and activities of others without being judgmental, acquire skill in interviewing and in therapeutic use of self, develop sensitivity to the nonverbal cues of others, and be knowledgeable of the couple's sociocultural and religious tenets. Once nurses are comfortable with their own sexuality, they can better help couples understand why the private act of lovemaking needs to be shared with health care professionals.

Because of the interference with the spontaneity of coitus, many infertility specialists limit the period of investigation. These specialists have found that the shorter the diagnostic period, the less the disruption of a couple's sexual lifestyle.

The woman or couple facing impaired fertility exhibits behaviors that resemble the *grieving process* associated with loss. The loss of one's genetic continuity with the generations to come leads to loss of self-esteem, of a sense of adequacy as a woman (or man), of control over one's destiny, and of a sense of self. Infertile individuals experience impaired self-concept and greater dissatisfaction with their marriages (Hirsch, Hirsch, 1989). The investigative process leads to a loss of spontaneity and control over the couple's marital relationship and sometimes over progress toward career and life goals. All people do not experience every one of the reactions described, nor can it be predicted how long any one reaction will last for an individual.

The support systems of the couple with impaired fertility need to be explored. This exploration should include persons available to assist, their relationship to the couple, their ages, their availability, and the cultural or religious support that is available. This type of assessment is suitable for a health team conference in which representatives of several disciplines can share ideas and work cooperatively in developing a plan for management.

If the couple conceives, nurses need to be aware that the concerns and problems of the previously infertile couple may not be over. Many couples are overjoyed with the pregnancy. However, some are not. Some couples rearrange their lives, sense of self, and personal goals within their acceptance of their infertile state. The couple may feel that those who worked with them to identify and treat impaired fertility expect them to be happy with the pregnancy. The couple may be shocked to find that they themselves feel resentment because the pregnancy, once a cherished dream, now necessitates another change in goals, aspirations, and identities. Bernstein et al (1988) found interpersonal sensitivity, hostility, and depression among previously infertile women. The normal ambivalence toward pregnancy may be perceived as reneging on the original choice to become parents. The couple might choose to abort the pregnancy at this time. Other couples worry about spontaneous abortion. If the couple wishes to continue with the pregnancy, they will need the

ETHICAL CONSIDERATIONS

ASSISTED REPRODUCTIVE THERAPIES (ARTS)

ISSUES	QUESTIONS
The right to reproduce	Should IVF be available only to married couples?
Ownership of embryo	Should the embryo be frozen for later use? Who has ownership—the woman, the man, or both?
Parenthood and parent-child bonding	Who are the parents—the biologic or adoptive parents?
Rights of research subjects and research initiatives	Is compensation for egg donors acceptable?
Truth telling and confidentiality	Should donors be anonymous?
Intergenerational responsibilities	What are the long-term effects of the medications and treatments on women, children, and families?

care other expectant couples need. The couple may need extra preparation for the realities of pregnancy, labor, and parenthood, because they have developed fantasies about childbearing when they thought it was beyond their reach. *A history of impaired fertility is considered to be a risk factor for pregnancy.*

The couple too may desire information about contraception after the birth of this baby. If the previously infertile couple desires additional children, they are advised about contraceptive methods that are least likely to cause damage and impair fertility.

If the couple does not conceive, they are assessed regarding their desire to be referred for help with adoption, therapeutic intrauterine insemination, other reproductive alternatives, or choosing a childfree state. The couple would find a list of such agencies within their particular community helpful.

REPRODUCTIVE ALTERNATIVES
Assisted Reproductive Therapies

There have been remarkable developments in reproductive medicine (Evans et al, 1989). **Assisted reproductive therapies (ARTs)** are creating ethical and legal issues. The Ethical Considerations box above lists the ethical issues related to new reproductive technologies as identified by the Office of Technological Assessment (1988). The lack of information or misleading information about success rates and the risks and benefits of treatment alternatives prevents couples from making informed decisions. Nurses can provide information so that couples have an accurate understanding of their chances for a successful pregnancy and live birth. Nurses can also provide anticipatory guidance about the moral and ethical dilemmas regarding the use of ARTs (White, 1992).

Some of the ARTs for treatment of infertility include in vitro fertilization–embryo transfer, (IVF-ET), gamete intrafallopian transfer (GIFT), zygote intrafallopian transfer (ZIFT), ovum transfer (oocyte donation), em-

bryo adoption, embryo hosting, and surrogate parenting. Table 30-2 describes these procedures and the possible indications for the ARTs.

Therapeutic Insemination

When the husband's sperm has poor quality or motility, several semen samples are collected from him. The samples consist of split ejaculates, that is, the sperm-rich *first portion* only is collected for freezing and later pooling for **therapeutic intrauterine insemination.** Donor semen may also be used for therapeutic intrauterine insemination. Rapid freezing with liquid nitrogen and subsequent thawing do not cause genetic damage even after 10 years' storage using glycerol. Pooling should increase the sperm count and improve the placement of a portion of the total semen specimen at the cervical os.

Assuming normal female fertility, therapeutic intrauterine insemination at or about the time of ovulation has resulted in pregnancy in as many as 70% of cases. Numerous inseminations may be necessary to ensure proper timing of ovulation. Ovulation detection kits using urinary LH or serial ultrasound offer more reliable evidence of impending ovulation than do BBT charts (Ory, 1989).

Tubal Reconstruction

Microsurgery to reanastomose (restoration of tubal continuity) the sperm ducts can be accomplished successfully in 90% of cases (i.e., sperm in the ejaculate) (Jarow, 1987). However, the fertility (pregnancy) rate is much lower (40% to 60%). The rate of success decreases as the time since the procedure increases. The vasectomy may result in permanent changes in the testes that leave men unable to father children. The changes are those ordinarily seen only in the elderly (e.g., interstitial fibrosis [scar tissue between the seminiferous tubules]). Some men develop antibodies against their own sperm (autoimmunization). The role of antisperm antibodies in fertility after vasectomy reversal has not been completely determined. Fallopian tube reconstruction is discussed in Chapter 18 on p. 501.

TABLE 30-2 Defining the ARTs

PROCEDURE	DEFINITION	INDICATION
In vitro fertilization (IVF)	The process by which a woman's eggs are collected from her ovaries, fertilized in the laboratory with sperm, and transferred to her uterus after normal embryo development has occurred.	Tubal disease or blockage; severe male infertility; endometriosis; unexplained infertility; cervical factor; immunologic infertility
Gamete intrafallopian transfer (GIFT)	The process by which oocytes are retrieved from the ovary, placed in a catheter with washed motile sperm, and immediately transferred into the fimbriated end of the fallopian tube(s). Fertilization occurs in the fallopian tube (in vivo) rather than in the laboratory (in vitro).	Same as for IVF *except* there must be normal tubal anatomy, patency and absence of previous tubal disease
IVF and GIFT with donor sperm	The process as described above except in cases where the husband's fertility is severely compromised and donor sperm can be used, if donor sperm is used, the wife must have indications for IVF and GIFT.	Severe male infertility; azoospermia; indications for IVF or GIFT
Donor oocyte	The process by which eggs are donated by an IVF procedure and the donated eggs are inseminated. The embryos are transferred into the recipient's uterus, which is hormonally prepared with estrogen/progesterone therapy.	Premature ovarian failure; surgical removal of ovaries; congenitally absent ovaries; autosomal or sex-linked disorders; lack of fertilization in repeated IVF attempts because of subtle oocyte abnormalities or defects in oocyte/spermatozoa interaction
Donor embryo (embryo adoption)	Process by which a donated embryo is transferred to the uterus of an infertile woman at the appropriate time (normal or induced) of the menstrual cycle.	Infertility not resolved by less aggressive forms of therapy; absence of ovaries; male partner is azoospermic or is severely compromised
Gestational carrier (embryo host)	The process by which a couple undertakes an IVF cycle and the embryo(s) are transferred to another woman's uterus (the carrier) who has contracted with the couple to carry the child to term. The carrier has no genetic investment in the child, which distinguishes it from surrogate motherhood.	Congenital absence or surgical removal of uterus; a reproductively impaired uterus, myomas, uterine synechiae, or other congenital abnormalities; a medical condition that might be life-threatening during pregnancy, such as diabetes, immunologic problems, or severe heart, kidney, or liver disease

From Braverman A, English M: Creating brave new families with advanced reproductive technologies, *NAACOGs Clin Issu Perinat Womens Health Nurs* 3(2):354, 1992.

THERAPEUTIC AND ELECTIVE ABORTION

Therapeutic abortion (TAB) is the termination of a previable pregnancy to safeguard the life or health of the mother. Elective abortion (EAB) is the purposeful interruption of a previable pregnancy. Indications for therapeutic abortion are as follows:

1. Preservation of the life or health of the mother (e.g., class III or IV heart disease)
2. Avoidance of the birth of an offspring with a serious developmental or hereditary disorder (e.g., Tay-Sachs disease)
3. Rape or incest

The indication for an elective abortion is by request of the mother but not for reasons of maternal risk or fetal disease.

Many women report more than one factor contributing to the decision (Torres, Forrest, 1988).

The control of birth, dealing as it does with human sexuality and the question of life and death, is one of the most emotionalized components of health care. Abortion as one of the surgical alternatives to contraception and is regulated in most countries (Cohen, 1990; Henshaw, 1990). Regulations exist presumably to protect the mother from the complications of abortion or because of religious constraints. The U.S. Supreme Court set aside previous antiabortion laws in January 1973, holding that first-trimester abortion is permissible inasmuch as the mortality from interruption of early gestation is now less than the mortality after normal term birth. Second-trimester abortion was left to the discretion of the individual states (Annas, 1989; Chavkin, Rosenfield, 1990; Rhodes, 1988; Rhodes, 1990; Rogers et al, 1991). Roman Catholic hospitals and some of those maintained by strict fundamentalists forbid abortion (and often sterilization) despite legal challenge (see Legal Tip).

LEGAL TIP: **Abortion**

Before providing abortion counseling, nurses need to know the laws regarding such activity for the state in which they practice.

Before the legalization of abortion, many illegal abortions took place, with little-documented sequelae other than death from infection or hemorrhage or both. Although studies indicate that biologic sequelae do occur after abortion (e.g., ectopic pregnancy) rates of biologic complications tend to be low, especially if the woman aborts during the first trimester (Holt et al, 1989; Seidman et al, 1988). Studies related to psychologic sequelae (e.g., anxiety) suggest that they are short lived (Adler et al, 1990; Llewelyn, Putches, 1988; Rogers et al, 1989). Sequelae are related to circumstances surrounding the abortion, such as rape or the attitudes reflected by friends, family, and health care workers. It must be remembered that the woman facing an abortion is pregnant and will exhibit the emotional responses shared by all pregnant women, including postpartum depression.

The values and moral convictions involve nurses to the same extent as those of pregnant women. The conflicts and doubts of the nurse can be readily communicated to women who are already anxious and overly sensitive. Health professionals need assistance to identify and come to terms with their own feelings. It is not uncommon for confusion to arise as beliefs are challenged by the reality of care. A nursing student reacted to learning experiences associated with in-hospital abortions in the following manner:

■ I really feel I believe in the rightness of elective abortion, but when I watched the health care provider insert the needle

and then inject the dose of prostaglandin, I felt an unreasoning rage sweep over me. I could have attacked him. Funny, I felt no anger toward the woman at all. I really need to rethink my beliefs.

Responses can also change with life experiences. A nurse who before her marriage had worked as a counselor in a municipal clinic established a reputation as a supportive and concerned counselor of young persons with regard to birth control. Four years later she remarked:

■ I've been trying to get pregnant for the past 3 years. I didn't realize how important it would be to me. You know I can't counsel about abortion any more. I can't be objective. I keep feeling, "Have your baby and please give it to me." I am more concerned about myself now, not them [the pregnant women], and counseling won't work that way.

Care Management

A thorough *assessment* is conducted through history, physical examination, and laboratory tests. If the woman is Rh negative and the pregnancy is greater than 8 weeks' gestation, she is a candidate for prophylaxis against Rh isoimmunization. She receives $Rh_o(D)$ immune globulin within 72 hours after the abortion if she is D^u negative and if Coombs' test results are negative (if she is unsensitized or has not developed isoimmunization). Compelling medical, surgical, or psychiatric indications for therapeutic abortion, though not numerous, are possible factors. The following conditions probably would qualify; class IV coronary heart disease, fulminating (pelvic) Hodgkin's disease, stage 1B carcinoma of the cervix, and Marfan's syndrome with early aortic aneurysm. The length of pregnancy and the condition of the woman need to be determined to select the appropriate type of abortion procedure.

The woman's understanding of alternatives, the types of abortions, and expected recovery are assessed. Misinformation and gaps in knowledge are identified and corrected. The record is reviewed for the signed informed consent, and the patient's understanding is verified. General preoperative, operative, and postoperative assessments are performed.

Analysis of data leads to the identification of the appropriate *nursing diagnoses*. Following are examples of nursing diagnoses for the woman undergoing abortion:
Decisional conflict related to:
 ▪ Perceived threat to value system
Fear related to:
 ▪ The abortion procedure
 ▪ Potential complications
 ▪ Implications for future pregnancies
Anticipatory grieving related to:
 ▪ Distress at loss and/or feelings of guilt

High risk for infection related to:

- Effects of the procedure
- Lack of understanding of preoperative and postoperative self-care

Acute pain related to:

- Effects of the procedure and/or postoperative events

Planning is a collaborative effort among the woman, her sexual partner (as appropriate), and the health care providers. *Expected outcomes* are established collaboratively, should be stated in patient-centered terms, and may include the following:

1. The woman will state that she understands all information necessary to give informed consent.
2. The woman will experience a successful procedure, and recovery will be uneventful.
3. The woman will verbalize that she is satisfied with the decision for elective abortion, the procedure, and the experience with the health care team.

Counseling about abortion includes help for the woman in identifying how she perceives the pregnancy: information about the choices available (i.e., having an abortion or carrying the pregnancy to term and then either keeping the child or placing the child for adoption); and information about types of abortion procedures. *The goal is to assist the woman in making an informed decision.*

Preoperative preparation, postoperative care, and discharge planning parallel the methods used for sterilization (see p. 500).

First-Trimester Abortion

Methods for performing abortion include the following:

1. Menstrual extraction—early aspiration of the endometrium in women who have not yet missed a menstrual period
2. Surgical D&C when aspiration equipment is unavailable
3. Uterine aspiration after one or two missed periods

Surgical D&C refers to cervical **dilatation and curettage (D&C)** of the uterine endometrium. Curettage is the scraping of the uterine lining with a metal curette or a flexible aspiration tip to remove the products of conception implanted in the endometrium. The procedure is similar to that of uterine aspiration. Cervical trauma and uterine performation, infection, or hemorrhage are possible though rare complications.

Uterine aspiration (**vacuum or suction curettage**) abortion is the most common procedure. The insertion of a small laminaria tent retained by a vaginal tampon for 4 to 24 hours usually will facilitate the purposeful interruption of a first-trimester pregnancy greater than 10 weeks' gestation by dilating the cervix atraumatically (see Fig. 30-2). On removal of the moist, expanded laminaria, the cervix will have dilated two or three times its original (dry) diameter. Rarely will further mechanical dilata-

tion of the cervix be required. The insertion of an adequate-sized aspiration cannula (8.5 to 10.5 mm) is almost always possible. Cervical laceration and bleeding are reduced by the use of laminaria. A disadvantage is the delay necessary and the need for an additional visit to the office or clinic.

The woman comes to the clinic on the day before the abortion procedure. An antiseptic solution is used to prepare the pelvic area. A vaginal speculum is inserted, and the vaginal canal and cervix are cleansed. Injection of a local anesthetic agent into the cervix may follow (see paracervical block, Chapter 10). Again the area is cleansed, and the laminaria tent is inserted into the endocervical canal. Prophylactic use of an antibiotic is usually begun. Some women experience a mild cramping or have light spotting from the anesthetic injection. Discomfort can usually be controlled with mild analgesics (e.g., acetaminophen).

Aspiration abortion may be performed in the office, clinic, or in the hospital setting. If the woman chooses a hospital setting, she is admitted the day after insertion of the laminaria tent and is given preoperative sedation. The vaginal area is cleansed (shaving is not necessary). The suction procedure for accomplishing an early elective abortion (ideal time is 8 to 12 weeks since last menstrual period) usually requires less than 5 minutes and can easily be effected under paracervical block anesthesia and sedation. Independent nursing interventions have the potential to reduce pain during the procedure (Wells, 1989). During the procedure the woman is kept informed about what to expect next: for example, menstrual-like cramping and sounds of suction machine. The nurse assesses the woman's vital signs. The aspirated uterine contents must be carefully inspected to ascertain whether all fetal parts and adequate placental tissue have been evacuated. A single dose of oxytocin is used occasionally to control bleeding. The woman may remain in the health care facility for 1 to 3 hours for detection of unstable vital signs, excessive cramping, or excessive bleeding; then she is discharged. If the procedure is done in the clinic, preoperative sedation is usually not given, and the anesthetic of choice is usually paracervical block. After the abortion the woman rests on the table until she is ready to stand. Then she remains in the waiting room until she feels she can travel. She may be discharged alone or in the company of a relative or friend, depending on the anesthetic used.

Bleeding after the operation is normally about the equivalent of a heavy menstrual period, and cramps are rarely severe. Infection such as endometritis or salpingitis occurs in about 8% of women. Subsequently, a D&C procedure for bleeding or sepsis caused by retained placental tissue is necessary in about 2% of women. A recent study reported an overall complication rate of less than 1% (Hakim-Elahi et al, 1990). Serious depression or other psychiatric problems are rare.

Postabortal instructions differ among health care providers (e.g., use of tampons may be discouraged for only 3 days or for up to 3 weeks, and resumption of sexual intercourse may be permitted within 1 week or discouraged for 3 weeks). The woman may shower daily. Instruction is given to watch for excessive bleeding (i.e., more than one large pad per hour for 4 hours), cramps, or fever and to avoid douches of any type. The woman may expect her menstrual period to resume 4 to 6 weeks from the day of the procedure. The nurse offers information about the birth control method the woman prefers, if this has not been done previously during the counseling interview that usually precedes the decision to have an abortion. The woman must be strongly encouraged to return for her follow-up visit so that complications can be avoided and an acceptable contraceptive method prescribed.

Second-Trimester Abortions

There are several techniques used for second-trimester abortions.

Transabdominal Intrauterine Injection of Hypertonic Sodium Chloride

The woman is admitted to the hospital for this procedure. Amniocentesis is performed. The health care provider determines where the needle (an 18-gauge, 7.5 cm [3 in] spinal needle) will be inserted. The area is cleansed, and if desired, a local anesthetic agent is given. Approximately 200 ml of amniotic fluid is withdrawn, and a similar amount of sterile hypertonic sodium chloride solution is injected. The woman is instructed to report to the nurse when uterine contractions begin—generally, within 8 to 48 hours. In most cases augmentation with oxytocin is necessary to effect uterine evacuation in a reasonable time. Occasionally reinjection is required. Labor begins, in theory at least, because the hypertonic saline solution releases the placental uterine progesterone blockade that normally prevents the onset of labor. The same careful monitoring of uterine contractions is as necessary as for a term birth. Instruction in relaxation and breathing techniques is indicated, and an analgesic can be administered for discomfort. The assistance of a supportive person at the time of birth of the dead fetus is essential. If the woman wishes to see the fetus, emotional support should be provided before and after the procedure. Many women are relieved to find the fetus normal and commonly inquire as to its sex. After the abortion the standard observations and postpartum care are carried out (see Chapter 18). Contraceptive counseling is given before discharge. The woman is advised to return should excessive bleeding occur.

Complications of hypertonic saline injection for second-trimester abortion may occur. Complications with the approximate frequency of their occurrence include infection (10%), need for D&C to remove retained tissue (15%), failure to abort (10%), and excessive bleeding, necessitating transfusion (2%). Symptoms related to saline solution (hypernatremia) include tinnitus, tachycardia, and headache, those of water intoxication, edema, oliguria ($\leq$200 mg/8 hours), dyspnea, thirst, and restlessness. Rarely, disseminated intravascular coagulation (DIC) or expulsion of the fetus through the uterine isthmus occurs.

Dilatation and Evacuation (D&E)

This procedure extends the D&C and vacuum curettage up to 20 weeks of gestation (Hatcher et al, 1994). The cervix requires more dilatation because the products of conception are larger. Often laminaria are inserted on the 2 preceding days of the procedure (i.e., two to three may be inserted on the first day; on the second day these are removed, and four to six may be inserted). This allows slow dilatation of the cervix. The procedure is performed on the third day. Larger instruments are employed and additional anesthetic is required. Nursing care includes monitoring vital signs, providing emotional support, administering analgesics, and postoperative monitoring.

Injection of Urea Solution after Amniocentesis

After the removal of about 200 ml of amniotic fluid, 200 ml of 30% solution of urea in 5% dextrose in water is introduced into the uterus by gravity drip. After 1 hour a solution of 5 units of oxytocin in 500 ml of 5% dextrose in water is started intravenously. Fetal death occurs, and abortion ensues in most cases within 12 hours. Complications are less common and are less serious than with hypertonic saline solution.

Prostaglandins

Prostaglandins are now widely used for inducing second-trimester abortion (Hatcher et al, 1994). Prostaglandins can be administered in suppository form, as a gel, or by intrauterine injection. Unpleasant side effects (e.g., nausea, vomiting, and diarrhea) will occur. Repeated doses may be needed for expulsion of the products of conception.

Abdominal Hysterotomy

Hysterotomy may be chosen after more than 14 to 16 weeks of pregnancy, after failure of intrauterine injection of saline solution or $PGF_2\alpha$, and when sterilization is desired. The management is comparable to that of cesarean birth.

Complications after Abortion

The most common complications after abortion include infection, retained products of conception or intrauterine blood clots, continuing pregnancy, cervical or uterine trauma, and excessive bleeding (Hatcher et al, 1990). Women are advised to report fever, pelvic pain, and excessive bleeding. Prophylactic chlamydia and gonorrhea treatment and the use of an oral ergotrate postoperatively may reduce the incidence of infection and retained products of conception.

RU 486 (Mifepristone)

Progesterone is essential for maintaining pregnancy. RU 486 (mifepristone) is a progesterone antagonist that prevents implantation of a fertilized egg. It is most effective in early gestation, during the luteal phase, within 10 days of the expected onset of what would be the first missed period after conception. It can be taken up to 5 weeks after conception. The effectiveness of RU 486 is inversely related to gestational age as determined by β-hCG levels and duration of amenorrhea (Donaldson et al, 1994). However, it is considered to be an effective and safe method for termination of early pregnancy.

Uterine bleeding begins within 4 days of administration of the first dose. Usually a period of painless, heavy bleeding is reported. Termination of pregnancy occurs for most women. For the woman in whom abortion does not occur, evacuation of the uterus by aspiration is facilitated by the softening of the uterine cervix caused by RU 486. Some women experience slight nausea and fatigue during the period of bleeding.

Supporters of this method feel that even with known disadvantages, RU 486 offers a reasonable alternative to surgical abortion, which carries the risks of anesthesia, surgical complications, infertility, and psychologic sequelae (Couzinet et al, 1986; Debate, 1987a). Others have taken a strong stand against the use of RU 486 (Debate, 1987b). Its use in the United States remains in the investigational state (FDA, 1993).

The nurse can be reasonably assured that care was effective when the expected outcomes of care have been achieved: the woman understands all information necessary to give informed consent; the procedure is successful, recovery is uneventful, and the woman continues to be satisfied with the decision for elective abortion, the procedure, and the experience with the health care team.

NORMAL CLIMACTERIUM AND POSTCLIMACTERIUM

Climacterium refers to the period of a woman's life when she passes from the reproductive to the nonreproductive stage with regression of ovarian function.

Premenopause is the first phase of the climacterium when fertility decreases and menses become irregular. This phase lasts a few months or a few years. Troublesome symptoms, such as vasomotor instability, fatigue, headaches, and emotional disturbances, may appear during this phase.

Menopause is the point at which menstruation ceases. The average age for menopause is 51.4, but 10% of

women stop menstruation by age 40 and 5% do not stop until 60. Surgical menopause occurs with hysterectomy and bilateral oophorectomy.

Perimenopause, roughly the same period as the climacterium, includes premenopause, menopause, and at least 1 year after menopause.

Postmenopause is the phase following menopause, when symptoms associated with decreased ovarian hormones, such as vaginal atrophy and osteoporosis, can develop.

Symptoms of Climacterium

Approximately 20% of women never experience symptoms. Most women experience mild or moderate symptoms and rarely require medical attention, and a few women have severe symptoms.

Vasomotor Instability

Vasomotor instability is the most common disturbance of the climacterium. Women experience changeable vasodilation and vasoconstriction as **hot flushes** (flashes) and night sweats. A hot flush is a sudden sensation of warmth of varying duration and intensity, in the head, neck, and chest. *Mild* flushes do not interfere with daily activities. *Moderate* flushes cause discomfort, with noticeably elevated temperature, accompanied by perspiration. *Severe* flushes produce extreme discomfort that interfere with activities of daily living.

Hot flushes may continue for several months or years. Several factors can precipitate an episode, including crowded or warm rooms, alcohol, hot drinks, spicy foods, and proximity to a source of heat (Scharbo-DeHaan, Brucker, 1991).

Night sweats are another form of vasomotor instability experienced by many women. Sleep may be interrupted nightly, since bed clothes and linens may be soaked, and many women complain of not being able to go back to sleep. Estrogen replacement therapy (ERT) has been recommended to relieve symptoms.

Emotional Disturbances

Mood swings, irritability, anxiety, and depression are often associated with perimenopause. Women feel more emotionally labile, nervous, or agitated. Women often associate mood swings and irritability of the climacterium with feelings they experienced during and immediately after pregnancy. The biochemical process that underlies variations in emotional responses in the climacterium is unknown, however.

Midlife stress may aggravate menopause. Dealing with teenage children, helping aging parents, becoming widowed or divorced, and grieving for friends and family who are ill or dying are among the many stresses that increase the risk of serious emotional problems.

The ability to cope with any stress involves at least three factors: the person's perception or understanding of the event, her support system, and coping mechanisms. Nurses must therefore assess how much information about the climacterium the woman has, her perception of stressful experiences, whom she can depend on for help, and her repertoire of coping skills.

Cultural messages also influence emotional status during perimenopause. Many women perceive the inability to bear children as a significant loss. Others see menopause as the first step to old age and associate it with a loss of attractiveness. Western culture values youth and physical attractiveness and the elderly suffer a loss of status, function, and role. For women who perceive menopause as a time of loss, depression is likely to occur.

For other women, menopause is not a loss but a relief from the fear of pregnancy, the hassle of menstruation, and the inconveniences of contraception. In spite of a strong cultural message that youth is valued above age, women who value themselves adjust well to menopause.

Fatigue and headaches are other common problems during menopause. Their cause is unknown.

Symptoms of Postclimacteric Period

Symptoms that occur in the postmenopausal phase are related to genital atrophy and osteoporosis.

Genital Atrophy and Sexuality Changes

As estrogen levels decrease, the vaginal epithelium thins and there is an increase in the vaginal pH, resulting in dryness, burning, irritation, and dyspareunia. In some women the shrinking of the uterus, vulva, and distal portion of the urethra leads to disturbing symptoms, including urinary frequency, dysuria, uterine prolapse, stress incontinence, and constipation.

Itching around the vulva occurs as the vulva becomes thinner, less elastic, and more prone to inflammation.

Dyspareunia (painful intercourse) can occur because the vagina becomes smaller, vaginal walls become thinner and dryer, and lubrication during sexual stimulation takes longer. Intercourse may result in postcoital bleeding, and women may decide to forego intercourse altogether. Sexual activity does not end with menopause. However, women and their partners may change their expression of sexuality during and after menopause, depending on physical changes, changes in the partner, and cultural myths and messages. For people who see aging as loss, sexuality may become difficult to incorporate into what they perceive to be a less attractive identity. The fear of rejection is always present. As men age, they take longer to reach orgasm: erections take longer to occur and are less firm. Women may believe their partners are losing interest in them. Couples may need counseling to understand these changes.

The lack of available male partners has a devastating effect on sexual expression. Women outlive men, and older widowed and divorced women have fewer opportunities to develop relationships because they are less sought after. Older women who do engage in intercourse cannot assume that new or nonmonogamous partners are HIV-free and therefore need to use condoms.

As long as women are able to bear children, some accept intercourse as part of their responsibility as wives. When menopause frees them from this duty, they may choose to forgo intercourse. For other women, libido may increase without the fuss of contraception, fear of pregnancy, or interruption from menses.

Urinary frequency occurs sometimes because the distal portion of the urethra, which has the same embryologic origin as the reproductive organs, shrinks. Irritants have easier access to the urinary tract with its shorter urethra and cause frequency and cystitis. Urine culture results in postmenopausal women may be negative for pathogens.

Urinary incontinence and *uterine displacement* are two other common findings during this period. These conditions are discussed on pp. 888 and 890. *Constipation* or pain during bowel movements may indicate that a rectocele is present (see p. 884).

Not all women experience symptoms of genital atrophy. Endogenous estrogen has been found to provide stimulation a decade after menopause. ERT often brings relief.

Osteoporosis

Osteoporosis is an age-related reduction in bone mass associated with an increased susceptibility to fractures. The postmenopausal drop in estrogen levels causes old bone to deteriorate faster than new bone is formed, resulting in a slow thinning of the bones.

Estrogen is required for the conversion of vitamin D into calcitonin, which is essential in the absorption of calcium by the intestine. A reduced calcium absorption, as well as the thinning of bones, places postmenopausal women at risk for problems associated with osteoporosis.

Approximately one in four women is affected. During the first 5 to 6 years after menopause, women lose bone six times more rapidly than men. By the time women reach age 80, they have lost 47% of their trabecular bone, concentrated in the vertebrae, pelvis and other flat bones, and in the epiphyses. Women at risk are likely to be white or Asian, small boned, and thin. Up to 80% of the differences in peak bone mass are due to genetic factors.

Low calcium intake is a risk factor, particularly during adolescence (Johnston, Longcope, 1990). A high protein or caffeine intake increases calcium excretion. Smoking, excessive alcohol intake, and a greater phosphorus than calcium intake (which occurs with soft drink consumption) are other risk factors (Erickson, Jones, 1992).

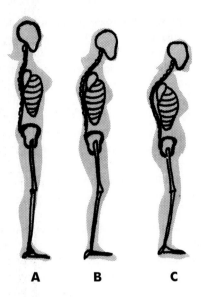

FIG. 30-6 Skeletal changes secondary to osteoporosis assessed by height and body shape at age 55 (**A**), age 65 (**B**), and age 75 (**C**).

Radiographic techniques to identify women at risk are imprecise and expensive. Osteoporosis cannot be detected by x-ray examination until 30% to 50% of the bone mass has been lost.

The first sign of osteoporosis is often loss of height resulting from vertebral fracture and collapse (Fig. 30-6). Back pain may or may not be present. Later signs include dowager's hump, in which the vertebrae can no longer support the upper body, and fractured hip. The fracture often precedes a fall.

Coronary Heart Disease

Although coronary heart disease is the leading cause of death in American women, no large well-designed studies have been done on women (Eaker et al, 1992). Postmenopausal women are at risk for coronary artery disease because there is a decline in serum levels of high-density lipoprotein (HDL) cholesterol and an increase in low-density lipoprotein (LDL) levels. ERT reverses this process (Barrett-Connor, Bush, 1991).

Care Management

A thorough health history, physical examination, and laboratory tests are essential for distinguishing pathologic states from the normal climacterium. Recent changes in menstrual history help to identity the phase of the climacterium the woman is experiencing and the woman's perception of her health, ethnic and cultural factors, and knowledge and concerns.

The plan of care may include ERT, weight-bearing exercise and calcium supplements, which involve consider-/able expense and possible side effects. Therefore, mutual negotiation of expected outcomes is of the utmost importance. Whenever possible, include the woman's spouse or partner and family members in planning.

Women need to know what to expect, why it happens, and what measures will help make them more comfortable. They need to know their symptoms have a normal physiologic basis and that other women experience similar complaints. There is a need for women's support groups and menopause clinics, where collaborative care by various specialties, such as endocrinology, radiology, psychosocial resources, exercise physiology, and nutrition, can be coordinated and research on various treatments can be implemented.

Hormone Replacement Therapy

Estrogen replacement therapy (ERT) increases serum levels of calcitonin, which prevents bone resorption, maintains bone density, and decreases the risk of fracture (Avioli, 1992). ERT should be started as soon as possible after menopause and continued for life if acceptable to the woman (McKeon, 1990; Youngkin, 1990). The dose needed to prevent osteoporosis is 0.625 mg of conjugated equine estrogen.

With any drug there is a benefit to risk ratio. ERT is controversial, but many authorities recommend treatment for all women without contraindications at the time of menopause (McKeon, 1990).

Intramuscular and once-a-week oral estrogen regimens are available, but daily medication appears safer. Transdermal estradiol, in the form of a patch applied twice a week to the skin, provides a relatively constant level of estrogen (Whitehead et al, 1990). Some women develop skin irritation in the area of the patch or injection.

The type of estrogen used for postmenopausal ERT is much less potent than ethinyl estradiol used in oral contraceptives and has fewer serious side effects. It is unlikely that ERT causes hypertension, gallbladder disease, or an increased incidence of thrombophlebitis or thromboembolism in postmenopausal women. Postmenopausal ERT is associated with reduced cardiovascular morbidity and mortality, even in women who smoke (Matthews et al, 1989).

Neoplastic Effects

The breast and endometrium are target tissues of estrogen, and estrogen is contraindicated in women with a history of breast or endometrial malignancies. Carcinoma of the breast may exist for as long as 8 years before it is palpable. Therefore a mammogram must be obtained for all women before ERT, and the importance of regular BSE and follow-up should be emphasized.

Studies to determine an association between estrogen use and breast cancer have been controversial as a result of methodologic problems. Although the risk appears to be minimal, caution is advised. In a prospective cohort study of 121,700 female nurses, a significant increase in breast cancer associated with current or recent use or postmenopausal hormones was found. This effect is reversible within 2 years of discontinuing therapy (Colditz et al, 1990).

Long-term unopposed estrogen therapy (estrogen without progestin) increases the risk of developing endometrial cancer five times. The risk of developing cancer decreases with hormone replacement therapy (HRT)—adding a progestin for 10 days beginning on day 16 of the estrogen cycle each month, or as prescribed. Several authorities recommend that women without a uterus not be given progestins because of the positive effects of unopposed estrogen on lipids (McKeon, 1990).

Decisions with regard to taking estrogen alone or in combination with progestin must be made after weighing the benefits and risks of each protocol. Cancer is a serious threat, but heart disease is a more common cause of mortality (Box 30-2).

Alternative Methods of Management

There are many women who cannot or will not take ERT. A progestogen is the next best therapy. It provides significant relief from hot flushes and may also decrease the excretion of calcium, but it will not prevent vaginal or urethral atrophy (Herbst et al., 1992). Some women can obtain relief from other products, if they do not have physical conditions that contraindicate their use.

Bellergal-S tablets, composed of phenobarbital, ergotamine tartrate, and belladonna, may significantly reduce symptoms related to autonomic nervous system activity. Bellergal-S is contraindicated for women with peripheral vascular disease, coronary heart disease, hypertension, impaired hepatic or renal function, sepsis, glaucoma, or hypersensitivity to any of the drug's components. *Vitamin E* can relieve hot flushes, leg cramps, and loss of energy. Dosage varies widely; between 50 and 400 IU can be taken daily during meals without any ill effects (Nachtigall, 1977).

Certain plants used in Chinese *herbal medicine,* European folk medicine, and Native American medicine may have properties that relieve hot flushes. Ginseng and dong quai are Oriental herbs that some women use to prevent hot flushes. Claims for herbal remedies have not been substantiated by scientific research.

BOX 30-2

Hormone Replacement Therapy

- Menopause, the permanent cessation of menses, occurs spontaneously about age 51.
- In most women, the loss of ovarian function and subsequent fall in estrogen production result in vasomotor flushes, genitourinary symptoms, mood changes, and osteoporosis.
- Estrogen replacement therapy (ERT) can relieve these symptoms and is recommended for symptomatic women who have no contraindications to estrogen.
- ERT decreases the risk of cardiovascular disease in older women, but increases the risk of endometrial cancer. Adding a progestin to hormone replacement therapy (HRT) greatly decreases this risk but also reverses the protective influence of estrogen

in cardiovascular disease. It is not known whether ERT increases the risk of breast cancer; ERT is contraindicated in women at high risk for breast cancer.
- HRT should be continued indefinitely (which may mean lifelong treatment) for women who are at high risk for osteoporosis. High-risk factors include advanced age; white or Asian race; thin, small-framed body; history of low calcium intake; early menopause; sedentary lifestyle; nulliparity; cigarette smoking; and diet high in protein, phosphate, alcohol, or caffeine.
- The benefits of HRT outweigh the risks for most women. HRT, combined with general health promotion strategies, enhances health and well-being.

Muscle tone around the reproductive organs decreases after menopause. *Kegel exercises* strengthen these muscles, and, if practiced regularly, help prevent prolapsed uterus and stress incontinence. This is a low-cost, effective, noninvasive intervention. However, symptoms return if exercises are discontinued (Ferguson et al, 1990).

K-Y Lubricating Jelly and coconut oil are two examples of *water-soluble lubricants* that provide relief from painful intercourse. They may be applied directly to the vulva and the penis. Oil-based lubricants such as petroleum jelly (Vaseline) should not be used because they clog vaginal glands, which can then be sites for bacterial infection.

Another consequence of genital atrophy is urinary frequency and dysuria, often associated with asymptomatic bacteriuria. Older women may not experience typical symptoms (cramping, pain, or burning on urination). A daily intake of at least eight glasses of water to decrease urine concentration and the growth of bacteria, may prevent serious infection. Most urinary tract infections are limited to the urethra and the bladder, but occasionally the kidneys are involved. Signs of serious infection include fever, chills, vomiting, and costovertebral angle (CVA) tenderness (pain in the back over the kidneys).

Prevention of Complaints Associated with Osteoporosis

ERT is the only well-documented prevention of osteoporosis. *Calcitonin* is effective in preventing and treating osteoporosis, but must be given subcutaneously (Avioli, 1992). *Etidronate disodium* has been shown to reduce fractures by half and significantly increase bone mass. It is poorly absorbed and must be given on an empty stomach, followed by 2 hours of fasting (Johnston, Longcope, 1990; Storm et al, 1990).

Calcium Supplementation

The role of calcium supplementation in treating osteoporosis is controversial, but it appears to retard bone loss from cortical bone and to reduce the incidence of fractures (Dawson-Hughes, Dallal, Krall, 1990). Although calcium cannot reverse loss of bone mass or prevent fractures, calcium supplementation may retard the development of osteoporosis after menopause. Oral calcium should be taken daily as early as premenopause. The recommended dose is 1 to 1.5 g daily, usually taken at bedtime. However, calcium supplements are best taken with meals because of the increase in acid secretions and extended time in the stomach. At least 8 oz of water to increase solubility is recommended. Calcium is most commonly available as calcium carbonate, calcium lactate, and calcium phosphate. Over half of the calcium preparations on the market are useless because they do not dissolve.

Foods high in calcium and low in phosphorus are rec-

ommended. Women should avoid excessive alcohol, soft drinks, and caffine.

Exercise and Safety

Exercise alone cannot prevent or reverse osteoporosis, but weight-bearing exercise, such as walking and stair-climbing 30 to 60 minutes a day, may be beneficial (Erickson, Jones 1992; Urrows, 1991). Examples of exercises are available from the National Osteoporosis Foundation (Fig. 30-7).

Osteoporosis-related fractures are often the result of falls. Accident prevention, including proper storage of articles and correction of poor lighting and loose carpeting, should be discussed with the older woman (Box 30-3). The nurse can be reasonably assured that care was effective if the woman can explain the changes associated with menopause and the measures that can make them more comfortable.

SEQUELAE OF CHILDBIRTH TRAUMA
Alterations in Pelvic Support

The term **pelvic relaxation** refers to the weakening and lengthening of fascial supports of the pelvic organs. In most cases it is the delayed but direct result of childbearing. Although extensive damage may be noted and repaired shortly after birth, symptoms related to pelvic relaxation most often appear during the perimenopausal period, when the effects of ovarian hormones on pelvic tissues are lost and atrophic changes begin. Pelvic trauma, stress and strain, and the aging process are contributing causes. Neither exercise nor rest will correct the problem or restore normal anatomic relations and physiologic function.

Generally, symptoms of pelvic relaxation relate to the structure involved: urethra, bladder, uterus, vagina, cul-de-sac, or rectum. The most common complaints are pulling and dragging sensations, pressure, protrusions, fatigue, and low backache. Symptoms may be worse after prolonged standing or deep penile penetration during intercourse. Urinary stress incontinence may be present.

During distention of the birth canal, levator ani bundles separate, and the fascia is stretched. Although external damage may be minimal or not visible, extensive damage may have occurred in the deep supporting structures. When lacerations occur in the levator muscles, the muscle fibers contract so that the muscle separates and retracts laterally, eliminating the perineal body and normal support of the rectum.

Permanent defects in support, such as rectocele and cystocele, may occur in childbirth and in women who have never been pregnant. **Rectocele** is the herniation of the anterior rectal wall through the relaxed or rup-

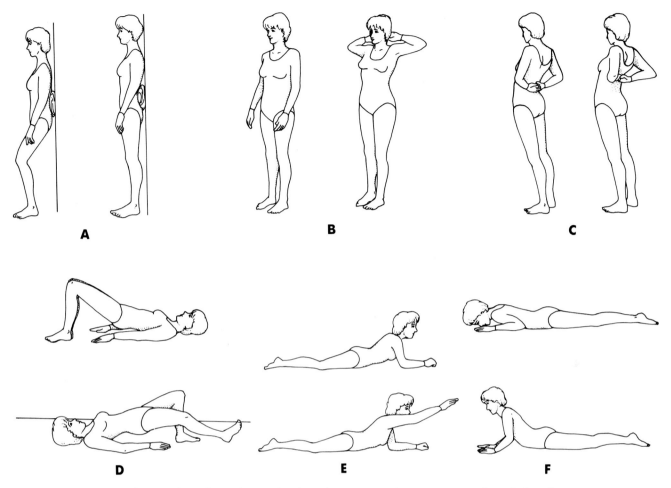

FIG. 30-7 **A,** Wall standing and pelvic tilt. **B,** Isometric posture correction. **C,** Standing back bend. **D,** Bridge. **E,** Elbow prop. **F,** Prone press-ups with deep breathing. (From *Boning Up on Osteoporosis,* with special permission from the National Osteoporosis Foundation.)

BOX 30-3

Prevention of Osteoporosis

- Osteoporosis is primarily a disease that affects postmenopausal women. It is characterized by lower back pain, a loss of height, and fractures of the back and hip. More women die each year from complications of osteoporosis than from cervical and breast cancer combined.
- Postmenopausal women naturally lose bone mass when the ovaries stop producing estrogen, which is necessary for calcium metabolism. Risk factors for osteoporosis include a family history of the disease, small build, early menopause, nulliparity, long-term low intake of dairy products, high intake of soft drinks and caffeine, smoking, alcoholism, inadequate exercise, and certain diseases and medications such as phenytoin (Dilantin), furosemide (Lasix), and corticosteroids.
- Estrogen replacement therapy (ERT) can be pre-

scribed to prevent fractures from osteoporosis. The risks and benefits of ERT must be weighed on an individual basis with the health care provider.
- Significant bone loss can be prevented by a well-balanced diet, including 200 to 400 IU of vitamin D and 1000 to 1500 mg of calcium a day, and regular weight-bearing exercise. Good sources of calcium are dairy products, fish, oysters, tofu, dark-green leafy vegetables, and whole-wheat bread.
- Supplements of vitamin D and calcium can be prescribed, but the body cannot use them without the right balance of other vitamins and minerals.
- Eliminating environmental hazards in the home can decrease the risk of falls.
- Weight-bearing exercise 30 to 60 minutes per day may delay bone loss and increase bone mass.

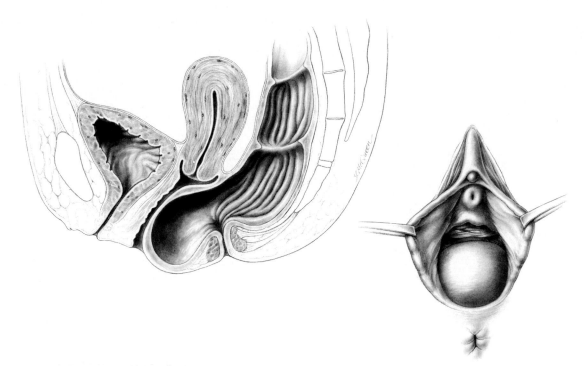

FIG. 30-8   Side and direct views of rectocele. (Redrawn from Symmonds RE: Relaxations of pelvic supports. In Benson RC, editor: *Current obstetric and gynecologic diagnosis and treatment,* ed 5, Los Altos, CA, 1984, Lange Medical Publications.)

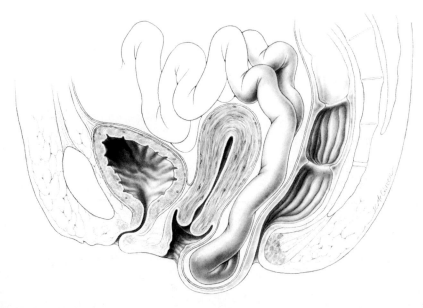

FIG. 30-9   Lateral view of enterocele and prolapsed uterus. (Redrawn from Symmonds RE: Relaxations of pelvic supports. In Benson RC, editor: *Current obstetric and gynecologic diagnosis and treatment,* ed 5, Los Altos, CA, 1984, Lange Medical Publications.)

tured vaginal fascia and rectovaginal septum: it appears as a large bulge that may be seen through the relaxed introitus (Fig. 30-8). Symptoms are absent when the woman is lying down. A rectocele causes a disturbance in bowel function, the sensation of bearing down or that the pelvic organs are falling out. With a very large rectocele, it may be difficult to have a bowel movement. Each time the woman strains during bowel evacuation, the feces are forced against the thinned rectovaginal wall, stretching it more. This is usually repaired surgically.

Enterocele (Fig. 30-9), or posterior vaginal hernia, is the herniation of the peritoneum of the posterior cul-de-sac between the uterosacral ligaments into the rectovaginal septum. The sacculation contains loops of small bowel but no rectum. The woman may be unaware of the problem or complain of pressure or a bearing-down or dragging sensation with low backache. The defect is closed surgically through the vagina by approximating the uterosacral ligaments and the levator muscles in the middle.

With fetopelvic disproportion, prolonged labor, or a preipitous birth, structures of the vesical and vaginal walls are stretched and may be injured. The bladder neck and urethra may be compressed between the presenting part and the pubic bones or forced downward ahead of the presenting part. Since soft-tissue damage usually occurs behind an intact vaginal epithelium, there is nothing visible to repair. Cystocele, urethrocele, and vaginal prolapse are possible sequelae.

Cystocele (Fig. 30-10) is the protrusion of the bladder downward into the vagina that develops when supporting structures in the vesicovaginal septum are injured. Anterior wall relaxation gradually develops over time—often after several babies. When the woman stands, the weakened anterior vaginal wall cannot support the weight of the urine in the bladder: the vesicovaginal septum is forced downward, the bladder is stretched, and its capacity is increased. With time the cystocele enlarges until it protrudes into the vagina. Complete emptying is difficult because the cystocele sags bellow the bladder neck.

Cystocele is recognized as a bulging of the anterior wall of the vagina. Unless the bladder neck and urethra are damaged, urinary continence is unaffected, but recurrent cystitis and ascending urinary tract infection may develope. Surgical support is accomplished through the vagina. Plication (taking a fold, tuck, or running stitch to gather material together) of the bladder wall reduces the cystocele.

Urethrocele is a herniation of the paravaginal fascia under the urethra that allows the urethra to protrude into the vagina. The condition may be asymptomatic, or the woman may complain of a vaginal protrusion or stress urinary incontinence if there is relaxation of fascial supports in the area of the posterior urethrovesical angle.

Vaginal prolapse is an uncommon but greatly distressing condition that may occur after vaginal or abdominal hysterectomy. It must be repaired surgically.

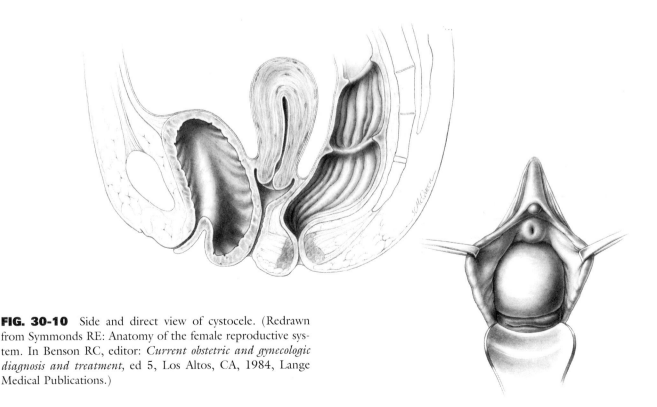

FIG. 30-10 Side and direct view of cystocele. (Redrawn from Symmonds RE: Anatomy of the female reproductive system. In Benson RC, editor: *Current obstetric and gynecologic diagnosis and treatment,* ed 5, Los Altos, CA, 1984, Lange Medical Publications.)

Urinary Incontinence

Many women experience uncontrollable leakage of urine as a result of childbirth injury. Conditions that disturb urinary control include **stress urinary incontinence,** due to sudden increases in intraabdominal pressure (such as that due to sneezing or coughing); *urge incontinence,* caused by disorders of the bladder and urethra, such as urethritis and urethral stricture, trigonitis, and cystitis; *neuropathies,* such as multiple sclerosis, diabetic neuritis, and pathologic conditions of the spinal cord; and *congenital and acquired urinary tract abnormalities.*

Stress urinary incontinence may follow injury to bladder neck structures. A sphincter mechanism at the bladder neck compresses the upper urethra, pulls it upward behind the symphysis, and forms an acute angle at the junction of the posterior urethral wall and the base of the bladder (Fig. 30-11). To empty the bladder, the sphincter complex relaxes and the trigone contracts to open the internal urethral orifice and pull the contracting bladder wall upward, forcing urine out. The angle between the urethra and the base of the bladder is lost or increased if the supporting pubococcygeus muscle is injured. This change, coupled with urethrocele, causes incontinence. Urine spurts out when the woman is asked to bear down or cough in the lithotomy position.

Performing Kegel exercises 80 to 100 times a day can relieve mild stress incontinence. HRT may improve urinary control for postmenopausal women, but surgical correction is often indicated to relieve symptoms.

Injuries to Pelvic Joints

Separation of the *symphysis pubis* occurs to some degree during birth. If forcible extraction or birth of a large baby occurs, serious injury is likely. The woman suffers severe pain on movement in the symphysis pubis and *sacroiliac joints.* Palpation reveals tenderness over the symphysis, wide separation of the ends of the pubic bones, and unusual mobility (several centimeters) of the bone ends when she shifts her weight from one foot to the other.

Uterine Displacement

Uterine prolapse occurs when the cardinal ligaments that support the uterus and vagina do not return to normal after childbirth and when the relationship of the axis of the uterus to that of the vagina is altered (Fig. 30-12). Cystocele and rectocele almost always accompany uterine prolapse, causing it to sag even further backward and downward into the vagina. There are varying degrees of prolapse—with procidentia (complete prolapse), the cervix and body of the uterus protrude through the vagina and the vagina is inverted. Transvaginal surgical correction of severe prolapse to correct the cystocele and rectocele return the uterus to its normal position, shorten the elongated cervix, and shorten the cardinal ligaments is indicated. When surgery is contraindicated (e.g., in aged and debilitated women) a **pessary** may be inserted to support the uterus (Fig. 30-13, *A*).

Retroversion, the most common simple displacement of the uterus, may be congenital or a sequel to child-

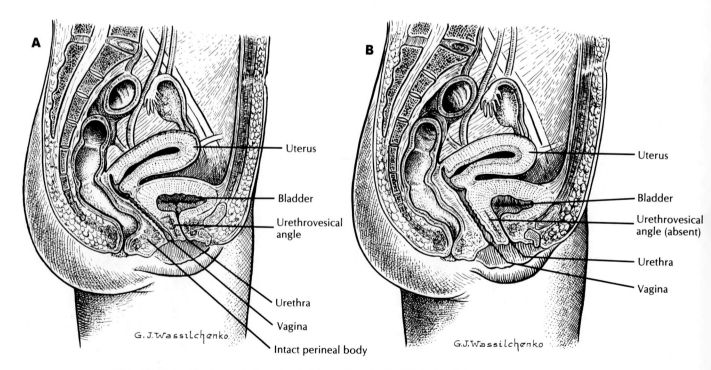

FIG. 30-11 Urethrovesical angle. **A,** Normal angle. **B,** Widening (absence) of angle.

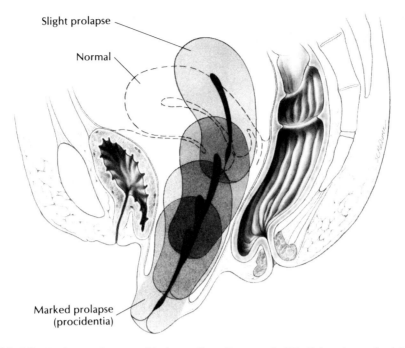

FIG. 30-12   Prolapse of uterus. (Redrawn from Symmonds RE: Relaxations of pelvic supports. In Benson RC, editor: *Current obstetric and gynecologic diagnosis and treatment,* ed 5, Los Altos, CA, 1984, Lange Medical Publications.)

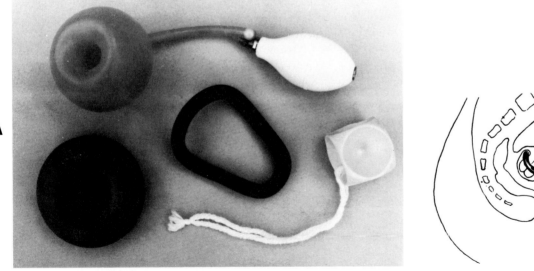

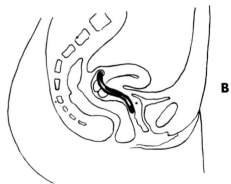

FIG. 30-13   **A,** Examples of pessaries (Smith-Hodge, donut, inflatable). **B,** Pessary in place to hold posterior vaginal fornix and, with it, attached cervix wall backward and upward in pelvis. (**B** from Beacham DW, Beacham WD: *Synopsis of gynecology,* ed 10, St. Louis, 1982, Mosby.)

birth. *Lateral displacement* may signal adnexal disease such as a large ovarian tumor, inflammation, or scar tissue.

Normally the round ligaments hold the uterus in anteversion, and the uterosacral ligaments pull the cervix backward and upward (see Figs. 3-4, 3-5, and 3-6). By 2 months postpartum these ligaments should return to normal length, but in approximately one third of women, the uterus remains retroverted. This condition is rarely symptomatic, but conception may be difficult because the cervix points toward the anterior vaginal wall and away from the posterior fornix, where seminal fluid pools after coitus. Symptoms may include deep pelvic and low back pain, difficulty with elimination, exaggeration of premenstrual tension, and dyspareunia.

Insertion of a pessary (Fig. 30-13, *B*) to replace the uterus in the anterior position may confirm that symptoms were related to malposition of the uterus. Usually a pessary is used only for a short time; it can lead to pressure necrosis and vaginitis. Good hygiene is important: some women can be taught to remove the pessary at night, cleanse it, and replace it in the morning. If the pessary is always left in place, regular douching to remove increased secretions and frequent checkups are indicated. After a period of treatment most women are free from symptoms and do not require the pessary. Surgical correction is rarely indicated.

Genital Fistulas

A **fistula** is an abnormal communication between one hollow viscus and another or from one hollow viscus to the outside. Genital fistulas may occur between the bladder and the genital tract (e.g., vesicovaginal); between the ureter and the vagina (ureterovaginal); and between the rectum or sigmoid colon and other structures (e.g., enterovesical) (Fig. 30-14). They may be a result of a congenital anomaly, gynecologic surgery, obstetric trauma, cancer, radiation therapy, gynecologic trauma, or infection.

Vesicovaginal fistula, the most common urinary tract fistula, forms in the anterior vaginal wall. It is usually a result of injury near the uterovesical junction during radical hysterectomy for cancer. Urine is lost through the vagina, resulting in partial or complete incontinence. A transvaginal surgical repair is possible in most cases.

Rectovaginal fistula is most often caused by an infection in the episiotomy, a suture placed through the rectal wall during repair, or an unrecognized rectal injury during childbirth. Fistulas may also be a result of extension of cervical cancer or radiation therapy. Surgical repair is possible but is often complicated by infection, which delays healing or causes the repair to break down.

Care Management

Assessment focuses primarily on the genitourinary tract, the reproductive organs, bowel elimination, and psychosocial and sexual factors. A complete health history, physical examination, and laboratory and diagnostic tests are done to support the appropriate medical diagnosis. The woman's knowledge of the disorder, its management, and possible prognosis is also assessed.

Possible nursing diagnoses include physical problems, such as *constipation or diarrhea* related to anatomic changes; *pain* related to relaxation of pelvic support and/or elimination difficulties; and *high risk for injury* related to lack of skill in self-care procedures or lack of understanding of the need to comply with therapy. Psychosocial diagnoses include *anxiety* related to possible surgical procedures; *ineffective coping* related to changes in body image; *altered family processes or interpersonal relationships* related to anatomic and functional changes; *social isolation, spiritual distress, body image disturbance,* and *low self-esteem* related to changes in anatomy and function.

Nursing interventions are directed toward educating the woman about childbirth sequelae and symptoms. This content is especially important in view of the current trend toward hospital discharge of both mother and baby within 24 hours following normal birth or within 3 days following a cesarean birth. Before hospital discharge, the mother must be alerted to signs of potential problems and advised to contact her caregiver without hesitation if she has questions or doubts regarding her well-being. New strategies for anticipatory guidance and teaching about potential problems and self-care postpar-

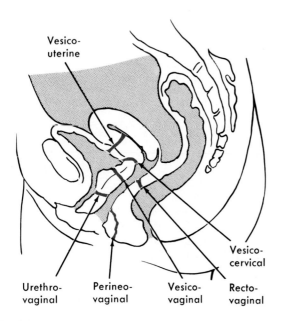

FIG. 30-14 Types of fistulas that may develop in vagina, uterus, and rectum. (From Phipps WJ et al: *Medical-surgical nursing: concepts and clinical practice,* ed 4, St. Louis, 1991, Mosby.)

tum may include greater emphasis in prenatal classes or home visits.

The nurse should encourage yearly physical examinations that promote early diagnosis and treatment, and facilitate self-care and cooperation with recommended medical and surgical regimens. Through support and acceptance, the nurse can promote self-esteem and a positive body image and self-concept, despite altered body functions.

The woman should be instructed in good hygiene and measures that prevent problems related to pelvic support alterations. This requires great sensitivity and tact because the client may be embarrassed about odors and soiling of her clothing beyond her control. She may withdraw or, conversely, become hostile. It is not uncommon for the woman to become so accustomed to the odors that she is no longer aware of them. Commercial deodorizing douches are available, or noncommercial solutions, such as chlorine solution (1 teaspoon of chlorine household bleach to 1 quart of water) may be used. Sitz baths and thorough washing of the genitals with unscented, uncolored, mild soap and warm water help. Sparse dusting with deodorizing powders such as sodium borate can be useful. Hygienic care is time consuming and must be repeated frequently throughout the day; protective pads or pants must be worn. All of these activities are demoralizing to the woman and her family.

If a rectovaginal fistula is present, high enemas, given before leaving the house, provide temporary relief from oozing of fecal material in the preoperative period.

Much of the nurse's efforts with these problems are directed toward participating in a team effort to prepare the woman for surgery. The nurse in the health promotion setting is usually most aware of the woman's living circumstances, physical limitations, and social problems and therefore may be best suited to coordinate continuity of care. If function cannot be fully restored through surgery, medication, or other therapy, goals related to compliance with the medical regimen, regaining or maintaining self-esteem, and satisfactory family and interpersonal processes are appropriate.

BREAST CANCER

When a woman finds a lump in her breast, she reacts with fear, anxiety, and apprehension about the possibility of breast cancer. The disease may or may not be malignant, but the woman's emotional responses will influence the effectiveness of her care.

Since there is no clear method for prevention of breast cancer, women must be educated about early detection, screening, and risk factors, as described in Chapter 29. Early detection can lead to treatment of localized cancer, which is associated with a 5-year survival rate of over 90% (American Cancer Society, 1994).

Care Management

Controversy continues regarding the best treatment of breast cancer. The women is faced with difficult decisions about the various surgical options (Fig. 30-15). Most health care providers recommend that the malignant mass be removed as well as the axillary nodes for staging purposes. The treatment can be conservative or more radical. *Breast conserving surgery,* such as a **lumpectomy** (Fig. 30-15, *A*) or quadrectomy (Fig. 30-15, *B*), involves the removal of the tumor and is often followed by radiation therapy. Many women who wish to avoid breast removal because of its psychologic effects may choose this option. A **simple mastectomy** is the removal of the breast containing the tumor. A **modified radical mastectomy** (Fig. 30-15, *D*) is the removal of the breast tissue, skin, and axillary nodes. These procedures have similar 5-year survival and recurrence rates (Harris et al, 1992a). After surgery, follow-up treatment may include radiation, chemotherapy, or hormonal therapy. The decision to include follow-up therapy is based on the stage

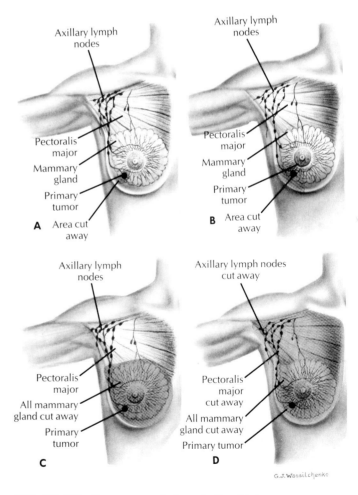

FIG. 30-15   Four ways to deal surgically with breast cancer. **A,** Lumpectomy (tylectomy). **B,** Quadrectomy (segmental resection). **C,** Total (simple) mastectomy. **D,** Radical mastectomy.

of disease, age and menopausal status of the woman, the woman's preference, and her hormonal receptor status. Follow-up treatment is usually used to decrease the risk of recurrence in women who have no evidence of metastasis.

Radiation is usually recommend for women who have stage I or II cancer. Hormone therapy with tamoxifen, an estrogen agonist, is given to women who have estrogen receptor–positive tumors. Therapy for more advanced tumors is still controversial, but usually includes surgery followed by chemotherapy and/or radiation (Harris et al, 1992b).

Preoperatively women need to be assessed for psychologic preparation as well as specific teaching needs. A visit from a woman who has had a similar experience may be beneficial preoperatively as well as postoperatively.

Postoperative nursing care focuses on recovery. Precautions should be taken to avoid taking the blood pressure, giving injections, or taking blood from the arm on the affected side. The woman may have drainage tubes from the incision site that will need to be assessed and drained. Incisional care may include dressing changes. If postoperative arm exercises are appropriate, these may be initiated during the early postoperative period. The woman is usually discharged to home after being given self-care instructions after 1 or 2 days (see the Teaching Approaches box.

Information about reconstruction surgery should be given before surgery, although not all women will be candidates for the procedure or are interested in it. Available options include grafts of muscle and skin from the woman's back, abdomen, or hip, and saline-filled prostheses. Silicone gel implants were restricted by the FDA in 1992 to women in safety studies (NAACOG, 1992).

Concerns about appearance after breast surgery may affect the woman's self-concept. Before surgery the woman and her partner need information about what the woman's postoperative appearance will be like. Both the

TEACHING APPROACHES

DISCHARGE TEACHING FOR THE WOMAN WITH A MASTECTOMY

1. Perform arm exercises as indicated.
2. Call physician if inflammation of incision or swelling of the incision or the arm occurs.
3. Wash hands well before touching incision area.
4. Avoid constriction of circulation in affected area.
5. Contact Reach for Recovery regarding external prosthesis, if desired.
6. Avoid depilatory creams, strong deodorants, and shaving of affected axilla.
7. Empty drainage tube every 8 hours, and record amounts.
8. Sponge bath until drains are removed; shower after drainage tube removed
9. Continue with monthly BSE on unaffected side.
10. Change dressing, if present, as instructed.
11. Note that sensation around the wound and the affected area may be diminished or absent.

woman and her partner need to be able to discuss feelings and concerns about accepting the changes. Nurses can assist the couple to communicate these feelings and concerns. Information about community resources and support groups such as Reach to Recovery may be beneficial.

Care of the woman with breast cancer is effective if the woman verbalizes satisfaction with the decision-making process about treatment options and if she gets appropriate support from significant others through all stages of treatment and recovery.

KEY POINTS

- Gynecologic disorders diminish the quality of life for affected women and their families.
- Premenstrual syndrome (PMS), no longer considered a purely psychologic problem, is a disorder that begins approximately 7 to 10 days before menses and ends with the onset of menses.
- Endometriosis is characterized by secondary amenorrhea, dyspareunia, abnormal uterine bleeding, and infertility.
- Impaired fertility is the inability to conceive and carry a child to term gestation at a time the couple has chosen to do so.

- Impaired fertility affects between 15% and 20% of otherwise healthy adults.
- Male and female factors each separately account for 40% of impaired fertility. Factors from both partners are responsible for the remaining 20%.
- Common etiologic factors of impaired fertility include decreased sperm production, interference with hypothalamic-pituitary-ovarian axis, tubal occlusion, and varicocele.
- It is estimated that 40% to 50% of couples with impaired fertility who seek assistance will be able to become pregnant and carry the child to viability.

- Reproductive alternatives to achieve parenthood include IVF-ET, GIFT, ZIFT, therapeutic insemination, surrogate motherhood, and adoption.
- Abortion accomplished in the first trimester is safer than one performed in the second trimester
- The climacterium is a normal developmental phase during which a woman passes from the reproductive to the nonreproductive stage.
- During the climacterium, women seek care for symptoms that arise from vasomotor instability, emotional disturbances, fatigue, genital atrophy, and changes related to sexuality. Estrogen and progestin therapy (HRT) is recommended for relief of menopause symptoms.
- Osteoporosis, a progressive loss of bone mass that results from decreasing levels of estrogen after menopause, can be prevented or minimized with estrogen replacement therapy.
- Sexuality and the ability for sexual expression continue after menopause.
- Pelvic relaxation and lengthening of fascial supports are most often the delayed sequelae of childbirth trauma, but they may be seen in young or childless women.
- Approximately 80% of breast lumps are found by the woman; only a fourth of these are cancerous.
- There is controversy regarding the best treatment for breast cancer, but most care providers agree that the mass should be removed and that the axillary nodes be removed for staging purposes.

CRITICAL THINKING EXERCISES

1. Interview a woman with PMS to determine her responses to the condition.
   a. What are her perceptions about how others view her condition?
   b. Examine how her responses compare to theoretic responses as well as your own perceptions.
   c. Analyze the woman's responses to identify positive and negative aspects of PMS.
   d. Formulate a plan of care using the data from the interview.
2. You are assigned to the infertility clinic. A couple has arrived to begin diagnostic workup for infertility.
   a. Interview the couple to determine how infertility has affected their lives.
   b. Examine what your feelings would be if you were told that you were infertile.
   c. Identify ways you can assist the couple in coping with the diagnosis of infertility. Justify your interventions.
   d. Discuss in your clinical group the ethical issues resulting from treatment of infertility (i.e., *in vitro* fertilization, surrogate motherhood, and artificial insemination by donor).
3. You are assigned to a clinic where women are assessed and treated for menopausal symptoms.
   a. What are some generalizations about women and menopause?
   b. What are your perceptions about women who have numerous complaints/symptoms that they attribute to menopause?
   c. What impact could these perceptions have on providing care to menopausal women?
   d. How can nurses effect a positive change in the care of midlife and older women?

References

Adler NE et al: Psychological responses after abortion, *Science* 248(4951):41, 1990.

American Cancer Society: *Facts and figures 1994,* New York, 1994, ACS.

Annas GJ: The supreme court, privacy, and abortion, *N Engl J Med* 321(17):1200, 1989.

Avioli LA: Osteoporosis syndromes: patient selection for calcitonin therapy, *Geriatrics* 47(4):58, 1993.

Barrett-Connor E, Bush TL: Estrogen and coronary heart disease in women, *JAMA* 265(14):1861, 1991.

Berg BJ, Wilson JF: Psychiatric morbidity in the infertile population: a reconceptualization, *Fertil Steril* 53(4):654, 1990.

Bernstein JL, et al: Psychosocial status of previously infertile couples after successful pregnancy, *JOGNN* 17(6):404, 1988.

Chavkin W, Rosenfield A: A chill wind blows. Webster, obstetrics, and the health of women, *Am J Obstet Gynecol* 163(2):450, 1990.

Cohen SS: Health care policy and abortion: a comparison, *Nurs Outlook* 38(1):20, 1990.

Colditz GA et al: Prospective study of estrogen replacement therapy and risk of breast cancer in postmenopausal women, *JAMA* 264(20):2648, 1990.

Couzinet B et al: Termination of early pregnancy by the progesterone antagonist RU 486 (mifepristone), *N Engl J Med* 315(25):1565, 1986.

Cunningham FG et al: *Williams obstetrics,* ed 19, Norwalk, 1993, Appleton & Lange.

Davis DC, Dearman CN: Coping strategies of infertile women, *JOGNN* 20(3):221, 1991.

Dawson-Hughes B, Dallal GE, Krall EA: A controlled trial of the effect of calcium supplementation on bone density in postmenopausal women, *N Engl J Med* 323(13):878, 1990.

The debate: abortion pill (RU 486): we should test this drug in the USA, *USA Today* p. 10A, Jan 15, 1987a.

The debate: abortion pill: keep this chemical killer out of the USA (an opposing view), *USA Today* p. 10A, Jan 15, 1987b.

Donaldson K et al: RU 486: an alternative to surgical abortion, *JOGNN* 23(7):555, 1994.

Eaker ED et al: Heart disease in women: how different? *Patient Care* 191:204, 1992.

Eggert-Kruse W et al: Chlamydial infection—a female and/or male infertility factor? *Fertil Steril* 53(6):1037, 1990.

Erickson GP, Jones JA: Osteoporosis risk assessment of mature working women: primary and secondary prevention strategies, *AAOHN Journal* 40(9):423, 1992.

Evans MI et al, editors: *Fetal diagnosis and therapy: science, ethics and the law,* Philadelphia, 1989, JB Lippincott.

Ferguson K et al: Stress urinary incontinence: effect of pelvic muscle exercise, *Obstet Gynecol* 75:671, 1990.

Few BJ: Treating endometriosis with nafarelin, *MCN* 13(5): 323, 1988.

Frank DT: Factors related to decisions about infertility treatment, *JOGNN* 19(2):162, 1990a.

Frank DT: Gender differences in decision making about infertility treatment, *Appl Nurs Res* 3(2):56, 1990b.

Geissler E: *Pocket guide to cultural assessment,* St Louis, 1994, Mosby.

Hakim-Elahi et al: Complications of first-trimester abortion: a report of 170,000 cases, *Obstet Gynecol* 76(1):129, 1990.

Harris JR et al: Breast cancer: first of three parts, *N Engl J Med* 327:319, 1992a.

Harris JR et al: Breast cancer: second of three parts, *N Engl J Med* 327:390, 1992b.

Hatcher RA et al: *Contraceptive technology: 1994-1996,* ed 16, New York, 1994, Irvington Publishers.

Heitkemper M et al: GI symptoms, function, and psychophysiological arousal in dysmenorrheic women, *Nurs Res* 40(1):20, 1991.

Henshaw SK: Induced abortion: a world review, *Family Planning Perspectives* 22(2):76, 1990.

Herbst AL et al: *Comprehensive gynecology,* ed 2, St Louis, 1992, Mosby.

Hirsch AM, Hirsch SM: The effects of infertility on marriage and self concept, *JOGNN* 18(1):13, 1989.

Holt VL et al: Induced abortion and the risk of subsequent ectopic pregnancy, *Am J Public Health* 79(9):1234, 1989.

Hsia LS, Long MH: Premenstrual syndrome: current concepts in diagnosis and management, *J Nurs Midwif* 35(6):351, 1990.

Jarow JP: Vasectomy: autoimmunity and reversal, *JAMA* 257(15):2087, 1987.

Johnston CC, Longcope C: New treatments for osteoporosis, *Lancet* 335(8697):1065, 1990.

Llewelyn SP, Putches R: An investigation of anxiety following termination of pregnancy, *J Adv Nurs* 13(4):468, 1988.

Lubianezki N, Fischer RG: OTC menstrual pain preparations, *Pediatr Nurs* 13(6):435, 1987.

Matthews KA et al: Menopause and risk factors for coronary heart disease, *N Engl J Med* 32(10):641, 1989.

Mattison DR et al: Effects of drugs and chemicals on the fetus, *Contemp OB/GYN* 33(3):164, 1989.

Mattison DR et al: Reproductive toxicity; male and female reproductive systems as targets for chemical injury, *Med Clin North Am* 74(2):391, 1990.

McKeon VA: Estrogen replacement therapy: current guidelines for education and counseling, *J Gerontol Nurs* 16(1):6, 1990.

NAACOG: FDA limits access to breast implants, *NAACOG Newsletter* 19(6):3, 1992.

Nachtigall L: *The Lila Nachtigall Report,* New York, 1977, G P Putnam's Sons.

Nero FA: When couples ask about infertility, *RN* 51(11):26, 1988.

Office of Technology Assessment: *Infertility: medical and surgical consequences (Congress of the United States),* Washington DC, U.S. Government Printing Office, 1988.

Olshansky EF: Redefining the concepts of success and failure in infertility treatment, *NAACOGs Clin Issu Perinat Womens Health Nurs* 3(2):343, 1992.

Ory SJ: Keeping up to date on donor insemination, *Contemp OB/GYN* 33(3):88, 1989.

Prior JC et al: Spinal bone loss and ovulatory disturbances, *N Engl J Med* 323:1221, 1990.

Rhodes AM: Options and issues for pregnant adolescents, *MCN* 13:427, 1988.

Rhodes AM: Issue update: abortion, *MCN* 15:289, 1990.

Rogers JL et al: Impact of the Minnesota parental notification law on abortion and birth, *Am J Public Health* 81(3):294, 1991.

Rogers JL et al: Psychological impact of abortion: methodological and outcomes summary of empirical research between 1968 and 1988, *Health Care Women Int* 10(4):347, 1989.

Scharbo-DeHaan M, Brucker MC: The perimenopausal period: implications for nurse-midwifery practice, *J Nurs Midwife* 36(1):9, 1991.

Scott JR et al: *Danforth's obstetrics and gynecology,* ed 6, Philadelphia, 1990, JB Lippincott.

Seidman DS: Childbearing after induced abortion: reassessment of risk. *J Epidemiol Comm Health* 42(3):294, 1988.

Sohn C, Korberly B, Tannenbaum R: Menstrual products, *Handbook of Nonprescription Drugs* 17:371, 1986.

Storm T et al: Effect of intermittent cyclical etidronate therapy on bone mass and fracture rate in women with postmenopausal osteoporosis, *N Engl J Med* 322(18):1265, 1990.

Swearingen P: *Manuel of nursing therapeutics,* ed 2, St Louis, 1990, Mosby.

Torres A, Forrest JD: Why do women have abortions? *Fam Plann Perspect* 20(4):169, 1988.

Urrows ST, Freston MS, Pryor DL: Profiles in osteoporosis, *Am J Nurs* 91:33, 1991.

Wells N: Management of pain during abortion, *J Adv Nurs* 14:56, 1989.

White GB: Understanding the ethical issues in infertility nursing practice, *NAACOGs Clin Issu Perinat Womens Health Nurs* 3(2):347, 1992.

Whitehead MI et al: Transdermal administration of oestrogen/progestagen hormone replacement therapy, *Lancet* 335(8685):310, 1990.

Willson JR, Carrington ER: *Obstetrics and gynecology,* ed 9, St Louis, 1991, Mosby.

Wright J et al: Psychological distress and infertility: a review of controlled research, *Int J Fertil* 34(2):126, 1989.

Youngkin EQ: Estrogen replacement therapy and the estraderm transdermal system, *Nurs Pract* 15(5):19, 1990.

Yovich JL, Matson PL: The influence of infertility etiology on the outcome of IVF-ET and GIFT treatments, *Int J Fertil* 35(1):26, 1990.

Bibliography

Bernhard L, Sheppard L: Health, symptoms, self-care, and dyadic adjustment in menopausal women, *JOGNN* 22(5):456, 1993.

Bernstein J et al: Coping with infertility: a new nursing perspective, *NAACOGs Clin Issu Perinat Womens Health Nurs* 3(2):335, 1992.

Blanchard DS: What women can do to protect against osteoporosis, *RN* 53(10):60, 1990.

Christian A: The relationship between women's symptoms of endometriosis and self esteem, *JOGNN* 22(4):370, 1993.

Devor M et al: Estrogen replacement therapy and venous thrombosis, *Am J Med* 92:275, 1992.

Goode CJ, Hahn SJ: Oocyte donation and in vitro fertilization: the nurse's role with ethical and legal issues, *JOGNN* 22(2):106, 1993.

Hunter M: The Southeast England longitudinal study of the climacteric and postmenopause, *Maturitas* 14:117, 1992.

Jossens M, Sweet R: Pelvic inflammatory disease: risk factors and microbial etiologies, *JOGNN* 22(2):169, 1993.

Lang N: *Quality of health care for older people in America: a review of nursing research,* Kansas City, 1991, ANA.

McElmurry BJ, Huddleston DS: Self-care and menopause: critical review of research, *Health Care for Women International* 12:15, 1991.

McKinlay SM et al: The normal menopause transition, *Maturitas* 14:102, 1992.

Nachtigall LE, Nachtigall LB: Protecting older women from their growing risk of cardiac disease, *Geriatrics* 45(5):24, 1990.

Quinn AA: A theoretical model of the perimenopausal process, *J Nurs Midwif* 36(1):25, 1991.

Reame N et al: Infertility, *NAACOGs Clin Issu Perinat Womens Health Nurs* 3(2):291, 1992.

Tilyard M et al: Treatment of postmenopausal osteoporosis with calcitriol of calcium, *N Engl J Med* 326(6):357, 1992.

Trice LB: Meaningful life experience to the elderly, *Image J Nurs Sch* 22(4):248, 1990.

Glossary

ABC Alternative Birthing Center. Birthing areas in hospitals located away from the traditional obstetric department.

abdominal Belonging or relating to the abdomen and its functions and disorders.

a. birth Birth of a child through a surgical incision made into the abdominal wall and uterus; cesarean birth.

a. gestation Implantation of a fertilized ovum outside the uterus but inside the peritoneal cavity.

ABO incompatibility Hemolytic disease that occurs when the mother's blood type is O and the newborn's is A, B, or AB.

abortion Termination of pregnancy before the fetus is viable and capable of extrauterine existence, usually less than 20 weeks' gestation (or when the fetus weighs less than 500 g).

complete a. Abortion in which fetus and all related tissue have been expelled from the uterus.

elective a. Termination of pregnancy chosen by the woman that is not required for her physical safety.

habitual (recurrent) a. Loss of three or more successive pregnancies for no known cause.

incomplete a. Loss of pregnancy in which some but not all the products of conception have been expelled from the uterus.

induced a. Intentionally produced loss of pregnancy by woman or others.

inevitable a. Threatened loss of pregnancy that cannot be prevented or stopped and is imminent.

missed a. Loss of pregnancy in which the products of conception remain in the uterus after the fetus dies.

septic a. Loss of pregnancy in which there is an infection of the products of conception and the uterine endometrial lining, usually resulting from attempted termination of early pregnancy.

spontaneous a. Loss of pregnancy that occurs naturally without interference or known cause.

therapeutic a. Pregnancy that has been intentionally terminated for medical reasons.

threatened a. Possible loss of a pregnancy; early symptoms are present (e.g., the cervix begins to dilate).

abruptio placentae Partial or complete premature separation of a normally implanted placenta.

abstinence Refraining from sexual intercourse periodically or permanently.

access to care Opportunity to receive health care services.

accreta, placenta See *placenta accreta*.

acidosis Increase in hydrogen ion concentration resulting in a lowering of blood pH below 7.35.

acini cells Milk-producing cells in the breast.

acme Highest point (e.g., of a contraction).

acrocyanosis Peripheral cyanosis; blue color of hands and feet in most infants at birth that may persist for 7 to 10 days.

acromion Projection of the spine of the scapula (forming the point of the shoulder); used to explain the presentation of the fetus.

adnexa Adjacent or accessory parts of a structure.

uterine a. Ovaries and fallopian tubes.

adolescence That period of an individual's transformation from a child to an adult.

adult respiratory distress syndrome (ARDS) Set of symptoms including decreased compliance of lung tissue, pulmonary edema, and acute hypoxemia. The condition is similar to respiratory distress syndrome of the newborn.

afibrinogenemia Absence or decrease of fibrinogen in the blood such that the blood will not coagulate. In obstetrics, this condition occurs from complications of abruptio placentae or retention of a dead fetus.

afterbirth Lay term for the placenta and membranes expelled after the birth of the child.

afterbirth pains Painful uterine cramps that occur intermittently for approximately 2 or 3 days after birth and that result from contractile efforts of the uterus to return to its normal involuted condition.

AGA Appropriate (weight) for gestational age.

agenesis Failure of an organ to develop.

agonist-antagonist compounds An agonist is an agent that actives something; an antagonist is an agent that blocks something.

albuminuria Presence of readily detectable amounts of albumin in the urine.

alkalosis Abnormal condition of body fluids characterized by a tendency toward an increased pH, as from an excess of alkaline bicarbonate or a deficiency of acid.

amenorrhea Absence or suppression of menstruation.

amniocentesis Procedure in which a needle is inserted through the abdominal and uterine walls into the amniotic fluid; used for assessment of fetal health and maturity and for therapeutic abortion.

amnioinfusion Infusion of normal saline warmed to body temperature, via an intrauterine catheter into the uterine cavity in an attempt to increase the fluid around the umbilical cord and prevent compression during uterine contractions.

amnion Inner membrane of two fetal membranes that form the sac and contain the fetus and the fluid that surrounds it in utero.

amnionitis Inflammation of the amnion, occurring most frequently after early rupture of membranes.

amniotic Pertaining or relating to the amnion.

a. fluid Fluid surrounding fetus derived primarily from maternal serum and fetal urine.

a. fluid embolism Embolism resulting from aniotic fluid entering the maternal blood stream during labor and birth after rupture of membranes; this is often fatal to the woman if it is a pulmonary embolism.

a. sac Membrane "bag" that contains the fetus before birth.

amniotomy Artificial rupture of the fetal membranes (AROM).

analgesia Lack of pain without loss of consciousness.

analgesic Any drug or agent that will relieve pain.

android pelvis Male type of pelvis.

anencephaly Congenital deformity characterized by the absence of cerebrum, cerebellum, and flat bones of skull.

anesthesia Partial or complete absence of sensation with or without loss of consciousness.

aneuploidy Having an abnormal number of chromosomes.

announcement phase The first developmental task experienced by expectant fathers as identified by May. During this phase the expectant father accepts the biological fact of pregnancy.

anomaly Organ or structure that is malformed or in some way abnormal with reference to form, structure, or position.

anovulatory Failure of the ovaries to produce, mature, or release eggs.

anoxia Absence of oxygen.

antenatal Occurring before or formed before birth.

antepartal Before labor.

anterior Pertaining to the front.

    a. fontanel See *fontanel, anterior.*

anthropoid pelvis Pelvis in which the anteroposterior diameter is equal to or greater than the transverse diameter.

antibody Specific protein substance made by the body that exerts restrictive or destructive action on specific antigens, such as bacteria, toxins, or Rh factor.

anticipatory grief Grief that predates the loss of a beloved object.

antigen Protein foreign to the body that causes the body to develop antibodies (e.g., bacteria, dust, Rh factor).

Apgar score Numeric expression of the condition of a newborn obtained by rapid assessment at 1, 5, and 15 minutes of age; developed by Dr. Virginia Apgar.

apnea Cessation of respirations for more than 10 seconds associated with generalized cyanosis.

Apt test Differentiation of maternal and fetal blood when there is vaginal bleeding. It is performed as follows: Add 0.5 ml blood to 4.5 ml distilled water. Shake. Add 1 ml 0.25N sodium hydroxide. Fetal and cord blood remains pink for 1 or 2 minutes. Maternal blood becomes brown in 30 seconds.

areola Pigmented ring of tissue surrounding the nipple.

    secondary a. During the fifth month of pregnancy, a second faint ring of pigmentation seen around the original areola.

artificial insemination Introduction of semen by instrument injection into the vagina or uterus for impregnation.

asphyxia Decreased oxygen and/or excess of carbon dioxide in the body.

fetal a. Condition occurring in utero, with the following biochemical changes: hypoxemia (lowering of Po_2), hypercapnia (increase in Pco_2), and respiratory and metabolic acidosis (reduction of blood pH).

aspiration pneumonia Inflammatory condition of the lungs and bronchi caused by the inhalation of vomitus containing acid gastric contents.

aspiration syndrome See *meconium aspiration syndrome.*

ataractic Drug capable of promoting tranquility; a tranquilizer.

atelectasis Pulmonary pathosis involving alveolar collapse.

atony Absence of muscle tone.

atresia Absence of a normally present passageway.

    biliary a. Absence of the bile duct.

    choanal a. Complete obstruction of the posterior nares, which open into the nasopharynx, with membranous or bony tissue.

    esophageal a. Congenital anomaly in which the esophagus ends in a blind pouch or narrows into a thin cord, thus failing to form a continuous passageway to the stomach.

attachment Relationship between two persons (e.g., a parent and a child).

attitude Body posture or position.

    fetal a. Relation of fetal parts to each other in the uterus (e.g., all parts flexed, all parts flexed except neck is extended, etc.).

augmentation of labor Artificial stimulation of uterine contractions after labor has started spontaneously but is not progressing satisfactorily.

autoimmune disease Body produces antibodies against itself, causing tissue damage.

autoimmunization Development of antibodies against constituents of one's own tissues (e.g., a man may develop antibodies against his own sperm).

autolysis "Self-digestive" process by which the uterus returns to a nonpregnant state following childbirth. The decrease in estrogen and progesterone levels following childbirth results in this destruction of excess hypertrophied uterine tissue.

autosomal inheritance Characteristics transmitted by genes on the autosomes, not the sex chromosomes.

autosomes Any of the paired chromosomes other than the sex (X and Y) chromosomes.

azoospermia Absence of sperm in the semen.

bacteremic shock Shock that occurs in septicemia when endotoxins are released from certain bacteria in the bloodstream.

bag of waters Lay term for the sac containing amniotic fluid and fetus.

ballottement (1) Movability of a floating object (e.g., fetus). (2) Diagnostic technique using palpation: a floating object, when tapped or pushed, moves away and then returns to touch the examiner's hand.

Bandl's ring Abnormally thickened ridge of uterine musculature between the upper and lower segments that follows a mechanically obstructed labor, with the lower segment thinning abnormally.

Bartholin's glands Two small glands situated on either side of the vaginal orifice that secrete small amounts of mucus during coitus and that are homologous to the bulbourethral glands in the male.

basal body temperature Lowest body temperature of a healthy person taken immediately after awakening and before getting out of bed.

basalis, decidua See *decidua basalis.*

behavioral assessment Assessment of activity, feeding and sleeping patterns, responsiveness.

Bell's palsy See *palsy, Bell's.*

bereavement The feelings of loss, pain, desolation, and sadness that occur after the death of a loved one.

bicornuate uterus Anomalous uterus that may be either a double or single organ with two horns.

biliary atresia See *atresia, biliary.*

bilirubin Yellow or orange pigment that is a breakdown product of hemoglobin. It is carried by the blood to the liver, where it is chemically changed and excreted in the bile or is conjugated and excreted by the kidneys.

Billings method See *ovulation method.*

bimanual Performed with both hands.

  b. palpation Examination of a woman's pelvic organs done by placing one hand on the abdomen and one or two fingers of the other hand in the vagina.

biophysical profile (BPP) Noninvasive assessment of the fetus and its environment using ultrasonography and uterine fetal monitoring; includes fetal breathing movements, gross body movements, fetal tone, reactive fetal heart rate, and qualitative amniotic fluid volume.

biopsy Removal of a small piece of tissue for microscopic examination and diagnosis.

biparietal diameter Largest transverse diameter of the fetal head; extends from one parietal bone to the other.

birth plan A tool by which parents can explore their childbirth options and choose those that are most important to them.

Bishop score Rating system to evaluate inducibility of the cervix; a higher score increases the rate of successful induction of labor.

bittersweet grief The resurgence of feelings and emotions that occur upon remembering a loved one after the bereavement process has lessened.

blastocyst Stage in the development of a mammalian embryo, following the morula, that consists of an outer layer, or trophoblast, and a hollow sphere of cells enclosing a cavity.

blended family Family form which includes step-parents and step-children.

bloody show Vaginal discharge that originates in the cervix and consists of blood and mucus; increases as cervix dilates during labor.

body boundaries Boundaries that serve to separate the self from the nonself and provide a feeling of safety.

body image Person's subjective concept of his or her physical appearance.

bonding See *attachment.*

born out of asepsis (BOA) Pertaining to birth without the use of sterile technique.

Bradley method Preparation for parenthood with active participation of father and mother.

Braxton Hicks sign Mild, intermittent, painless uterine contractions that occur during pregnancy. These contractions occur more frequently as pregnancy advances but do not represent true labor.

Brazelton assessment Criteria for assessing the interactional behavior of a newborn.

breakthrough bleeding Escape of blood occurring between menstrual periods; may be noted by women using chemical contraception (birth control pill).

breast milk jaundice See *jaundice, breast milk.*

breast self-examination (BSE) Self-examination of the breasts.

breech presentation Presentation in which buttocks and/or feet are nearest the cervical opening and are born first; occurs in approximately 3% of all births.

  complete b.p. Simultaneous presentation of buttocks, legs, and feet.

  footling (incomplete) b.p. Presentation of one or both feet.

  frank b.p. Presentation of buttocks, with hips flexed so that thighs are against abdomen.

bregma Point of junction of the coronal and sagittal sutures of the skull; the area of the anterior fontanel of the fetus.

brim Edge of the superior strait of the true pelvis; the inlet.

bronchopulmonary dysplasia Emphysematous changes caused by oxygen toxicity.

brown fat Source of heat unique to neonates that is capable of greater thermogenic activity than ordinary fat. Deposits are found around the adrenals, kidneys, and neck, between the scapulas, and behind the sternum for several weeks after birth.

bruit, uterine Sound of passage of blood through uterine blood vessels, synchronous with fetal heart rate.

calendar method See *rhythm method.*

Candida vaginitis Vaginal, fungal infection; moniliasis.

capsularis, decidua See *decidua capsularis.*

caput Occiput of fetal head appearing at the vaginal introitus preceding birth of the head.

  c. succedaneum Swelling of the tissue over the presenting part of the fetal head caused by pressure during labor.

cardiac decompensation   Inability of the heart to maintain a sufficient cardiac output.

cardinal movements of labor   The mechanism of labor in a vertex presentation includes engagement, descent, flexion, internal rotation, extension, external rotation (restitution), and expulsion.

carpal tunnel syndrome   Pressure on the median nerve at the point at which it goes through the carpal tunnel of the wrist. It causes soreness, tenderness, and weakness of the muscles of the thumb.

carrier   Individual who carries a gene that does not exhibit itself in physical or chemical characteristics but that can be transmitted to children (e.g., a female carrying the trait for hemophilia, which is expressed in male offspring).

caudal epidural block   Type of regional anesthesia used in childbirth in which the anesthetic agent is injected into the caudal area of the spinal canal through the sacral hiatus, affecting the caudal nerve roots and thereby anesthetizing the cervix, vagina, and perineum. Medication does not mix with cerebrospinal fluid (CSF).

caul   Hood of fetal membranes covering fetal head during birth.

cephalhematoma   Extravasation of blood from ruptured vessels between a skull bone and its external covering, the periosteum. Swelling is limited by the margins of the cranial bone affected (usually parietals).

cephalic   Pertaining to the head.

   c. presentation   Presentation of any part of the fetal head.

cephalocaudal development   Principle of maturation that development progresses from the head to the feet.

cephalopelvic disproportion (CPD)   Condition in which the infant's head is of such a shape, size, or position that it cannot pass through the mother's pelvis.

cerclage   Use of nonabsorbable suture to keep an incompetent cervix closed; released when pregnancy is at term to allow labor to begin.

cervical cap (custom)   Individually fitted contraceptive covering for the cervix.

cervical intraepithelial neoplasm (CIN)   Uncontrolled and progressive abnormal growth of cervical epithelial cells.

cervical mucus method   See *ovulation method.*

cervical os   "Mouth" or opening to the cervix.

cervicitis   Cervical infection.

cervix   Lowest and narrow end of the uterus; the "neck." The cervix is situated between the external os and the body or corpus of the uterus, and its lower end extends into the vagina.

cesarean birth   Birth of a fetus by an incision through the abdominal wall and uterus.

cesarean hysterectomy   Removal of the uterus immediately after the cesarean birth of an infant.

Chadwick's sign   Violet color of mucous membrane that is visible from about the fourth week of pregnancy; caused by increased vascularity of the vagina.

chloasma   Increased pigmentation over bridge of nose and cheeks of pregnant women and some women taking oral contraceptives; also known as *mask of pregnancy.*

choanal atresia   See *atresia, choanal.*

cholelithiasis   Presence of gallstones in the gallbladder.

chorioamnionitis   Inflammatory reaction in fetal membranes to bacteria and /or viruses in the amniotic fluid, which then become infiltrated with polymorphonuclear leukocytes.

chorion   Fetal membrane closest to the intrauterine wall that gives rise to the placenta and continues as the outer membrane surrounding the amnion.

chorionic villi   See *villi, chorionic.*

chorionic villi sampling (CVS)   Removal of fetal tissue from placenta for genetic diagnostic studies.

chromosome   Element within the cell nucleus carrying genes and composed of DNA and proteins.

circumcision   Excision of the male's prepuce (foreskin).

cleft lip   Incomplete closure of the lip; harelip.

cleft palate   Incomplete closure of the palate or roof of mouth; a congenital fissure.

climacterium   The period of a woman's life when she is passing from a reproductive to a nonreproductive state, with regression of ovarian function. The cycle of endocrine, physical, and psychosocial changes that occurs during the termination of the reproductive years.

clitoris   Female organ analogous to male penis; a small, ovoid body of erectile tissue situated at the anterior junction of the vulva.

   prepuce of the c.   See *prepuce of the clitoris.*

clonus (ankle)   Spasmodic alternation of muscular contraction and relaxation.

coitus   Penile-vaginal intercourse.

   c. interruptus   Intercourse during which penis is withdrawn from vagina before ejaculation.

cold stress   Excessive loss of heat which results in increased respirations and nonshivering thermogenesis to maintain core body temperature.

colostrum   Yellow secretion from the breast containing mainly serum and white blood corpuscles preceding the onset of true lactation 2 or 3 days after birth.

complement   Naturally occurring blood component that is a factor in the destruction of bacteria.

complete abortion   See *abortion, complete.*

complete breech presentation   See *breech presentation, complete.*

conception   Union of the sperm and ovum resulting in fertilization; formation of the one-celled zygote.

conceptional age   In fetal development, the number of completed weeks since the moment of conception. Because the moment of conception is almost impossible to determine, conceptional age is estimated at 2 weeks less than gestational age.

conceptus Embryo or fetus, fetal membranes, amniotic fluid, and the fetal portion of the placenta.

condom Mechanical barrier worn on the penis for contraception; "rubber."

confinement Period of childbirth and early puerperium.

congenital Present or existing before birth as a result of either hereditary or prenatal environmental factors.

congenital rubella syndrome Complex of problems including hearing defects, cardiovascular abnormalities, and cataracts caused by maternal rubella in the first trimester of pregnancy.

conjoined twins See *twins, conjoined.*

conjugate

diagonal c. Radiographic measurement of distance from *inferior border* of SP to sacral promontory; may be obtained by vaginal examination; 12.5 to 13 cm.

true c. (c. vera) Radiographic measurement of distance from *upper margin* of symphysis pubis (SP) to sacral promontory; 1.5 to 2 cm less than diagonal conjugate.

conjunctivitis Inflammation of the mucous membrane that lines the eyelids and that is reflected onto the eyeball.

conscious relaxation Technique used to release the mind and body from tension through conscious effort and practice.

contraception Prevention of impregnation or conception.

contractions

contraction stress test (CST) Test to stimulate uterine contractions for the purpose of assessing fetal response; a healthy fetus does not react to contractions while a compromised fetus demonstrates late decelerations in the FHR that are indicative of uteroplacental insufficiency.

duration The period of time from the beginning of the contraction to the end.

frequency How often the contractions occur—the period of time from the beginning of one contraction to the beginning of the next.

intensity The strength of the contraction at its peak.

interval The period of time between uterine contractions—timed from the end of one contraction to the beginning of the next.

resting tone The tension in the uterine muscle between contractions.

contraction ring See *Bandl's ring.*

Coombs' test Indirect: determination of Rh-positive antibodies in maternal blood; direct: determination of maternal Rh-positive antibodies in fetal cord blood. A positive test result indicates the presence of antibodies or titer.

coping mechanism Any effort directed at stress management. It can be task oriented and involve direct problem-solving efforts to cope with the threat itself or be intrapsychic or ego defense oriented with the goal of regulating one's emotional distress.

copulation Coitus; sexual intercourse.

corpus Discrete mass of material; body.

c. cavernosum Term referring to one of two cylinders of spongy tissue within the penis or tissue within the clitoris that engorges with blood during sexual excitement resulting in erection.

c. luteum Yellow body. After rupture of the graafian follicle at ovulation, the follicle develops into a yellow structure that secretes progesterone and some estrogen in the second half of the menstrual cycle, atrophying about 3 days before sloughing of the endometrium in menstrual flow. If impregnation occurs, it continues to produce the hormones until the placenta can take over this function.

c. spongiosum One of the spongy cylinders of tissue within the penis; has a protective function.

cotyledon One of the 15 to 28 visible segments of the placenta on the maternal surface, each made up of fetal vessels, chorionic villi, and an intervillous space.

couplet care One nurse, educated in both mother and infant care, functions as the primary nurse for both mother and infant (also known as mother-baby care or single room maternity care).

couvade Custom whereby the husband goes through mock labor while his wife is giving birth.

Couvelaire uterus See *uterus, Couvelaire.*

CPAP Continuous positive airway pressure.

cradle cap Common seborrheic dermatitis of infants consisting of thick, yellow, greasy scales on the scalp.

craniotabes Localized softening of cranial bones.

creatinine Substance found in blood and muscle; measurement of levels in maternal urine correlates with amount of fetal muscle mass and therefore fetal size.

crib death Unexpected and sudden death of an apparently normal and healthy infant that occurs during sleep and with no physical or autopsic evidence of disease. Also referred to as sudden infant death syndrome (SIDS).

cri-du-chat syndrome Rare congenital disorder recognized at birth by a kittenlike cry, which may prevail for weeks, then disappear. Other characteristics include low birth weight, microcephaly, "moon face," wide-set eyes, strabismus, and low-set misshaped ears. Infants are hypotonic; heart defects and mental and physical retardation are common. Also called cat-cry syndrome.

crowning Stage of birth when the top of the fetal head can be seen at the vaginal orifice.

cryptochidism Failure of one or both of the testicles to descend into the scrotum. Also called undescended testis.

cul-de-sac of Douglas Pouch formed by a fold of the peritoneum dipping down between the anterior wall of the rectum and the posterior wall of the uterus; also called *Douglas' cul-de-sac, pouch of Douglas,* and *rectouterine pouch.*

culdocentesis Puncture of Douglas's cul-de-sac through the vagina for aspiration of fluid.

Cullen's sign Faint, irregularly formed, hemorrhagic patches on the skin around the umbilicus. The discolored skin is blue-black and becomes greenish brown or yellow. Cullen's sign may appear 1 to 2 days after the onset of anorexia and the severe, poorly localized abdominal pains characteristic of acute pancreatitis. Cullen's sign is also present in massive upper gastrointestinal hemorrhage, ruptured ectopic pregnancy.

cultural context A situation which considers the individual and family's beliefs and practices (culture).

curettage Scraping of the endometrium lining of the uterus with a curet to remove the contents of the uterus (as is done after an inevitable or incomplete abortion) or to obtain specimens for diagnostic purposes.

cystocele Bladder hernia: injury to the vesicovaginal fascia during labor and birth may allow herniation of the bladder into the vagina.

cytology The study of cells, including their formation, origin, structure, function, biochemical activities, and pathology.

daily fetal movement counts (DFMC) Maternal assessment of fetal activity; the number of fetal movements within a specific time period are counted.

death Cessation of life.

fetal d. Intrauterine death. Death of a fetus weighing 500 g or more of 20 weeks' gestation or more.

infant d. Death during the first year of life.

maternal d. Death of a woman during the childbearing cycle.

neonatal d. Death of a newborn within the first 28 days after birth.

perinatal d. Death of a fetus of 20 weeks' gestation or older or death of a neonate 28 days old or younger.

decidua Mucous membrane, lining of uterus, or endometrium of pregnancy that is shed after giving birth.

d. basalis Maternal aspect of the placenta made up of uterine blood vessels, endometrial stroma, and glands. It is shed in lochial discharge after delivery.

d. capsularis That part of the decidual membranes surrounding the chorionic sac.

d. vera Nonplacental decidual lining of the uterus.

decrement Decrease or stage of decline, as of a contraction.

deep tendon reflexes (DTRs) Reflex caused by stimulation of tendons, such as elbow, wrist, knee, triceps, and ankle jerk reflexes.

ΔOD$_{450}$ (read delta OD$_{450}$) Delta optical density (or absorbance) at 450 nm, obtained by spectral analysis of amniotic fluid. This prenatal test is used to measure the degree of hemolytic activity in the fetus and to evaluate fetal status in women sensitized to Rh(D).

demand feeding Infant feeds when hungry, not by schedule.

deoxyribonucleic acid (DNA) Intracellular complex protein that carries genetic information, consisting of two purines (adenine and guanine) and two pyrimidines (thymine and cytosine).

depressive reactions Depression related to the postpartum period including postpartum blues, postpartum non-psychotic depression, and postpartum psychosis.

DES Diethylstilbestrol, used in treating menopausal symptoms. Exposure of female fetus predisposes her to reproductive tract malformations and (later) dysplasia.

desquamation Shedding of epithelial cells of the skin and mucous membranes.

developmental crisis Severe, usually transient, stress that occurs when a person is unable to complete the tasks of a psychosocial stage of development and is therefore unable to move on to the next stage.

developmental task Physical or cognitive skill that a child must accomplish during a particular age period in order to continue developing, as walking, which precedes the development of sense of autonomy in the toddler period.

developmental theory Theoretical approach for viewing the family. The developmental perspective sees family members pass through phases of growth from dependence through active independence to interdependence.

diabetes mellitus A systemic disorder of carbohydrate, protein, and fat metabolism; because of deficient insulin production or ineffective use of insulin at the cellular level.

diaphragmatic hernia Congenital malformation of diaphragm that allows displacement of the abdominal organs into the thoracic cavity.

diastasis recti abdominis Separation of the two rectus muscles along the median line of the abdominal wall. This is often seen in women with repeated childbirths or with a multiple gestation (triplets, etc.). In the newborn it is usually because of incomplete development.

Dick-Read method An approach to childbirth based on the premise that fear of pain produces muscular tension, producing pain and greater fear. The method includes teaching physiological processes of labor, exercise to improve muscle tone, and techniques to assist in relaxation and prevent the fear-tension-pain mechanism.

dilatation of cervix Stretching of the external os from an opening a few millimeters in size to an opening large enough to allow the passage of the infant.

dilatation and curettage (D and C) Vaginal operation in which the cervical canal is stretched enough to admit passage of an instrument called a *curet.* The endometrium of the uterus is scraped with the curet to empty the uterine contents or to obtain tissue for examination.

diploid number Having two sets of chromosomes; found normally in somatic (body) cells; 23 sets or 46 chromosomes.

discordance Discrepancy in size (or other indicator) between twins.

disparate twins See *twins, disparate.*

disseminated intravascular coagulation (DIC) A pathological form of coagulation in which clotting factors are consumed to such an extend that generalized bleeding can occur; associated with abruptio placentae, eclampsia, intrauterine fetal demise, amniotic fluid embolism, and hemorrhage.

dizygotic Related to or proceeding from two zygotes (fertilized ova).

dizygotic twins See *twins, dizogotic.*

Döderlein's bacillus Gram-positive bacterium occurring in normal vaginal secretions.

dominant trait Gene that is expressed whenever it is present in the heterozygous gene state (e.g., brown eyes are dominant over blue).

doppler blood flow analysis Device for measuring blood flow noninvasively in the fetus and placenta to detect intrauterine growth retardation.

Douglas' cul-de-sac See *cul-de-sac of Douglas.*

Down syndrome Abnormality involving the occurrence of a third chromosome, rather than the normal pair (trisomy 21), that characteristically results in a typical picture of mental retardation and altered physical appearance. This condition was formerly called *mongolism* or *mongoloid idiocy.*

drug dependence (addiction) Physical or psychological dependence or both on a substance.

dry labor Lay term referring to labor in which amniotic fluid has already escaped. A "dry birth" does not exist.

Dubowitz assessment Estimation of gestational age of a newborn, based on criteria developed for that purpose.

ductus arteriosus In fetal circulation, an anatomic shunt between the pulmonary artery and arch of the aorta. It is obliterated after birth by a rising Po_2 and change in intravascular pressures in the presence of normal pulmonary function. It normally becomes a ligament after birth but in some instances remains patent.

ductus venosus In fetal circulation, a blood vessel carrying oxygenated blood between the umbilical vein and the inferior vena cava, bypassing the liver. It is obliterated and becomes a ligament after birth.

Duncan's mechanism Delivery of placenta with the maternal surface presenting, rather than the shiny fetal surface.

dys- Prefix meaning abnormal, difficult, painful, faulty.

dysfunctional labor Abnormal uterine contractions that prevent normal progress of cervical dilatation and effacement.

dysmaturity See *intrauterine growth retardation (IUGR).*

dysmenorrhea

    primary dysmenorrhea Painful menstruation beginning 2 to 6 months after menarche, related to ovulation.

    secondary dysmenorrhea Painful menstruation related to organic disease such as endometriosis, pelvic inflammatory disease, uterine neoplasm.

dysmorphogenesis Development of ill-shaped or malformed structures.

dyspareunia Painful sexual intercourse.

dystocia Prolonged, painful, or otherwise difficult birth because of mechanical factors produced by the passenger (the fetus) or the passage (the pelvis and soft tissues of the birth canal of the mother), inadequate powers (uterine and other muscular activity), or maternal position.

ecchymosis Bruise; bleeding into tissue caused by direct trauma, serious infection, or bleeding diathesis.

eclampsia Severe complication of pregnancy of unknown cause and occurring more often in the primigravida; characterized by tonic and clonic convulsions, coma, high blood pressure, albuminuria, and oliguria occurring during pregnancy or shortly after birth.

ectoderm Outer layer of embryonic tissue giving rise to skin, nails, and hair.

ectopic Out of normal place.

    e. pregnancy Implantation of the fertilized ovum outside of its normal place in the uterine cavity. Locations include the abdomen, fallopian tubes, and ovaries.

EDB Expected date of birth; "due date."

effacement Thinning and shortening or obliteration of the cervix that occurs during late pregnancy or labor or both.

effleurage Gentle stroking used in massage.

ejaculation Sudden expulsion of semen from the male urethra.

elective abortion See *abortion, elective.*

electronic fetal monitoring (EFM) Electronic surveillance of fetal heart rate by external and internal methods.

embolus Any undissolved matter (solid, liquid, or gaseous) that is carried by the blood to another part of the body and obstructs a blood vessel.

embryo Conceptus from the second or third week of development until about the eighth week after conception, when mineralization (ossification) of the skeleton begins. This period is characterized by cellular differentiation and predominantly hyperplastic growth.

emotional lability Rapid mood changes.

endocervical Pertaining to the interior of the canal of the cervix of the uterus.

endocrine glands Ductless glands that secrete hormones into the blood or lymph.

endometriosis Tissue closely resembling endometrial tissue but aberrantly located outside the uterus in the pelvic cavity. Symptomatology may include pelvic pain or pressure, dysmenorrhea, dyspareunia, abnormal bleeding from the uterus or rectum, and sterility.

endometrium Inner lining of the uterus that undergoes changes caused by hormones during the menstrual cycle and pregnancy; decidua.

endorphins Endogenous opioids secreted by the pituitary gland that act on the central and peripheral nervous systems to reduce pain.

engagement In obstetrics, the entrance of the fetal presenting part into the superior pelvic strait and the beginning of the descent through the pelvic canal.

engorgement Distension or vascular congestion. In obstetrics, the process of swelling of the breast tissue brought about by an increase in blood and lymph supply to the breast, which precedes true lactation. It lasts about 48 hours and usually reaches a peak between the third and fifth postbirth days.

engrossment Sustained involvement of a parent with an infant.

enterocele Herniation of the peritoneum of the posterior cul-de-sac between the uterosacral ligaments into the rectovaginal septum.

entoderm Inner layer of embryonic tissue giving rise to internal organs such as the intestine.

entrainment Phenomenon observed in the microanalysis of sound films in which the speaker moves several parts of the body and the listener responds to the sounds by moving in ways that are coordinated with the rhythm of the sounds. Infants have been observed to move in time to the rhythms of adult speech but not to random noises or disconnected words or vowels. Entrainment is thought to be an essential factor in the process of maternal-infant bonding.

epicanthus Fold of skin covering the inner canthus and caruncle that extends from the root of the nose to the median end of the eyebrow; characteristically found in certain races but may occur as a congenital anomaly.

epidural anesthesia Injection of anesthetic outside the dura mater (anesthetic does not mix with spinal fluid).

epidural block Type of regional anesthesia produced by injection of a local anesthetic into the epidural (peridural) space.

epidural blood patch A patch formed by a few millimeters of the mother's blood repairing a tear or hole in the dura mater around the spinal cord.

episiotomy Surgical incision of the perineum at the end of the second stage of labor to facilitate birth and to avoid laceration of the perineum.

epispadias Defect in which the urethral canal terminates on dorsum of penis or above the clitoris (rare).

Epstein's pearls Small, white blebs found along the gum margins and at the junction of the soft and hard palates. They are a normal manifestation and are commonly seen in the newborn. Similar to Bohn's nodules.

epulis Tumorlike benign lesion of the gingiva seen in pregnant women.

equilibrium A state of balance or rest owing to the equal action of opposing forces, as calcium and phosphorus in the body. In psychiatry, a state of mental or emotional balance.

Erb-Duchenne paralysis Paralysis caused by traumatic injury to the upper brachial plexus, occurring most commonly in childbirth from forcible traction during birth. The signs of Erb's paralysis include loss of sensation in the arm and paralysis and atrophy of the deltoid, the biceps, and the branchialis muscles. Also called Erb's palsy.

ergot Drug obtained from *Claviceps purpurea*, a fungus, which stimulates the smooth muscles of blood vessels and the uterus, causing vasoconstriction and uterine contractions.

erythema toxicum Innocuous pink papular neonatal rash of unknown cause, with superimposed vesicles appearing within 24 to 48 hours after birth and resolving spontaneously within a few days.

erythroblastosis fetalis Hemolytic disease of the newborn usually caused by isoimmunization resulting from Rh incompatibility or ABO incompatibility.

esophageal atresia See *atresia, esophageal.*

estimated date of birth Approximate date of birth. Usually determined by calculation using Nagele's rule.

estradiol An estrogen.

estriol Major metabolite of estrogen that increases during the second half of pregnancy with an intact fetoplacental unit (normal placenta, normal fetal liver and adrenals) and normal maternal renal function.

estrogen Female sex hormone produced by the ovaries and placenta.

estrogen replacement therapy (ERT) Exogenous estrogen given to women during and after menopause to prevent hot flashes, mood changes, osteoporosis, and genitourinary symptoms.

eutocia Normal or natural labor or birth.

exchange transfusion Replacement of 75% to 85% of circulating blood by withdrawing the recipient's blood and injecting a donor's blood in equal amounts, the purposes of which are to prevent an accumulation of bilirubin in the blood above a dangerous level, to prevent the accumulation of other by-products of hemolysis in hemolytic disease, and to correct anemia and acidosis.

expressive style Expectant father's strong emotional response to partner's pregnancy.

expulsive Having the tendency to drive out or expel.

    e. contractions Labor contractions that are characteristic of the second stage of labor.

extended family Family form that includes the nuclear family and other blood-related persons.

extension Straightening of a body part; opposite of flexion.

external cephalic version (ECV) Turning the fetus to a vertex position by exerting pressure on the fetus externally through the maternal abdomen.

extrauterine Occurring outside the uterus.

  e. pregnancy Ectopic pregnancy in which the fertilized ovum implants itself outside the uterus.

extrusion reflex Infant automatically extends tongue when it is stimulated.

facies Pertaining to the appearance or expression of the face; certain congenital syndromes typically present with a specific facial appearance.

FAD Fetal activity determination.

failure to thrive Condition in which neonate's or infant's growth and development patterns are below the norms for age.

fallopian tubes Two canals or oviducts extending laterally from each side of the uterus through which the ovum travels, after ovulation, to the uterus.

false labor Uterine contractions that do not result in cervical dilatation, are irregular, are felt more in front, often do not last more than 20 seconds, and do not become longer or stronger.

false pelvis The part of the pelvis superior to a plane passing through the linea terminalis (brim or outlet).

family dynamics The process by which family members assume appropriate social roles.

family functions Activities carried out within families for the well-being of family members; including biologic, economic, educational, psychologic and sociocultural.

family violence Interpersonal violence including child, elder, sibling, and spouse.

fantasy child The imagined dream child; the "ideal" unborn child.

Ferguson's reflex Reflex contractions of the uterus after stimulation of the cervix.

ferning (arborization) test The appearance of a fernlike pattern found on slides of certain fluids.

  ovulation f. t. Test in which cervical mucus, placed on a slide, dries in a branching pattern in the presence of high estrogen levels at the time of ovulation.

fertile period The period before and after ovulation during which the human ovum can be fertilized; usually 3 days before and 4 days after ovulation.

fertility Quality of being able to reproduce.

fertility rate Number of births per 1000 women aged 15 through 44 years.

fertilization Union of an ovum and a sperm.

fetal Pertaining or relating to the fetus

  f. alcohol syndrome Congenital abnormality or anomaly resulting from maternal alcohol intake above 3 oz. of absolute alcohol per day. It is characterized by typical craniofacial and limb defects, cardiovascular defects, intrauterine growth retardation, and developmental delay.

  f. asphyxia See *asphyxia, fetal.*

  f. attitude See *attitude, fetal.*

  f. death See *death, fetal.*

  f. distress Evidence such as a change in the fetal heartbeat pattern or activity indicating that the fetus is in jeopardy.

  f. lie Relation of the fetal spine to the maternal spine; i.e., in vertical lie, maternal and fetal spines are parallel and the fetal head or breech presents; in transverse lie, fetal spine is perpendicular to the maternal spine and the fetal shoulder presents.

  f. presentation The part of the fetus that presents at the cervical os.

  f. heart rate (FHR) Beats per minute (bpm) of the fetal heart. Normal range is 110 to 160 bpm.

    acceleration Increase in fetal heart rate, usually seen as a reassuring sign.

    baseline The average fetal heart rate between uterine contractions.

    bradycardia Baseline fetal heart rate below 110 bpm.

    deceleration Slowing of fetal heart rate contributed to a parasympathetic response and described in relation to uterine contractions.

    early Onset corresponding to onset of uterine contraction, related to fetal head compression.

    late Onset after peak of contraction, continuing into interval after contraction; caused by uteroplacental insufficiency.

    variable Onset anytime unrelated to contraction; caused by cord compression.

    prolonged deceleration Slowing of fetal heart rate lasting longer than 2 minutes.

  f. scalp spiral electrode Internal signal source for electronically monitoring the fetal heart rate.

α-fetoprotein (AFP) Fetal antigen; elevated levels in amniotic fluid associated with neural tube defects.

fetotoxic Poisonous or destructive to the fetus.

fetus Child in utero from about the eighth week after conception, until birth.

fibroid Fibrous, encapsulated connective tissue tumor, especially of the uterus.

fimbria Structure resembling a fringe, particularly the fringelike end of the fallopian tube.

fissure Groove or open crack in tissue.

fistula Abnormal tubelike passage that forms between two normal cavities, possibly congenital or caused by trauma, abscesses, or inflammatory processes.

flaccid Having relaxed, flabby, or absent muscle tone.

flaring of nostrils Widening of nostrils (alae nasi) during inspiration in the presence of air hunger; sign of respiratory distress.

flexion In obstetrics, resistance to the descent of the baby down the birth canal causes the head to flex, or bend, so that the chin approaches the chest. Thus the smallest diameter (suboccipitobregmatic) of the vertex presents.

fluid, amniotic   See *amniotic fluid.*

focusing phase   The third developmental task experienced by expectant fathers as identified by May. This phase is characterized by the father's active involvement in both the pregnancy and his relationship with his child.

follicle   Small secretory cavity or sac.

   graafian f.   Mature, fully developed ovarian cyst containing the ripe ovum. The follicle secretes estrogens, and after ovulation, the corpus luteum develops within the ruptured graafian follicle and secretes estrogen and progesterone.

follicle-stimulating hormone (FSH)   Hormone produced by the anterior pituitary during the first half of the menstrual cycle. Stimulates development of the graafian follicle.

fomites   Nonliving material on which disease-producing organisms may be conveyed (e.g., bed linen).

fontanel   Broad area, or soft spot, consisting of a strong band of connective tissue contiguous with cranial bones and located at the junctions of the bones.

   anterior f.   Diamond-shaped area between the frontal and two parietal bones just above the baby's forehead at the junction of the coronal and sagittal sutures.

   mastoid f.   Posterolateral fontanel usually not palpable.

   posterior f.   Small, triangular area between the occipital and parietal bones at the junction of the lambdoidal and sagittal sutures.

   sagittal f.   Soft area located in the sagittal suture, halfway between the anterior and posterior fontanels; may be found in normal newborns and in some neonates with Down's syndrome.

   sphenoid f.   Anterolateral fontanel usually not palpable.

footling (incomplete) breech presentation   See *breech presentation, footling.*

foramen ovale   Septal opening between the atria of the fetal heart. The opening normally closes shortly after birth, but if it remains patent, surgical repair usually is necessary.

forceps-assisted birth   Birth in which two curved-bladed instruments are used to assist in delivery of the fetal head.

foreskin   Prepuce, or loose fold of skin covering the glans penis.

fornix   Any structure with an arched or vaultlike shape.

   f. of the vagina   Anterior and posterior spaces, formed by the protrusion of the cervix into the vagina, into which the upper vagina is divided.

fourth stage of labor   The initial period of recovery from childbirth. It is usually considered to last for the first 1 to 2 hours after the expulsion of the placenta.

fourth trimester of pregnancy   Another term for the puerperium, the six-week interval between the birth of the newborn and the return of the reproductive organs to their nonpregnant state.

Fowler's position   Posture assumed by patient when head of bed is raised 18 or 20 inches and individual's knees are elevated.

frank breech presentation   See *breech presentation, frank.*

fraternal twins   Nonidentical twins that come from two separate fertilized ova.

free standing birth center   A center that provides prenatal care, labor and birth, and postbirth care outside of a hospital setting.

frenulum   Thin ridge of tissue in midline of undersurface of tongue extending from its base to varying distances from the tip of the tongue.

friability   Easily broken. May refer to a fragile condition of the cervix especially during pregnancy that causes the cervix to bleed easily when touched.

Friedman's curve   Labor curve; pattern of descent of presenting part and of dilatation of cervix; partogram.

FSH   See *follicle-stimulating hormone.*

fulguration   Destruction of tissue by means of electricity.

fundus   Dome-shaped upper portion of the uterus between the points of insertion of the fallopian tubes.

funic souffle   See *souffle, funic.*

funis   Cordlike structure, especially the umbilical cord.

galactosemia   Inherited, autosomal recessive disorder of galactose metabolism, characterized by a deficiency of the enzyme galactose-1-phosphate uridyl transferase.

gamete   Mature male or female germ cell; the mature sperm or ovum.

gastroschisis   Abdominal wall defect at base of umbilical stalk.

gastrostomy   Surgical creation of an artificial opening into the stomach through the abdominal wall, performed to feed a client when oral feeding is not possible.

gate control theory   Proposed in 1965 by Melzack and Wall, this theory explains the neurophysical mechanism underlying the perception of pain.

gavage   Feeding by means of a tube passed to the stomach.

gender identity   The sense or awareness of knowing to which sex one belongs. The process begins in infancy, continues throughout childhood, and is reinforced during adolescence.

gene   Factor on a chromosome responsible for hereditary characteristics of offspring.

genetic   Dependent on the genes. A genetic disorder may or may not be apparent at birth.

genetic counseling   Process of determining the occurrence or risk of occurrence of a genetic disorder within a family and of providing appropriate information and advice about the courses of action that are available, whether care of a child already affected, prenatal diagnosis, termination of a pregnancy, sterilization, or artificial insemination is involved.

genitalia Organs of reproduction.

genotype Hereditary combinations in an individual determining physical and chemical characteristics. Some genotypes are not expressed until later in life (e.g., Huntington's chorea); some hide recessive genes, which can be expressed in offspring; and others are expressed only under the proper environmental conditions (e.g., diabetes mellitus appearing under the stress of obesity or pregnancy).

gestation Period of intrauterine fetal development from conception through birth; the period of pregnancy.

gestational age In fetal development, the number of completed weeks counting from the first day of the last normal menstrual cycle.

gestational diabetes Glucose intolerance first recognized during pregnancy.

gingivitis Inflammation of the gums characterized by redness, swelling, and tendency to bleed.

glabella Bony prominence above the nose and between the eyebrows.

glans penis Smooth, round head of the penis, analogous to the female glans clitoris.

glomerulonephritis Noninfectious disease of the glomerulus of the kidney, characterized by proteinuria, hematuria, decreased urine production, and edema.

glucose tolerance test A test of the body's ability to utilize carbohydrates; used as a screening measure for gestational diabetes.

glycosuria Presence of glucose (a sugar) in the urine.

glycosylated hemoglobin A measurement of glycemic control over time (usually 4 to 6 weeks).

gonad Gamete-producing, or sex, gland; the ovary or testis.

gonadotropic hormone Hormone that stimulates the gonads.

Goodell's sign Softening of the cervix, a probable sign of pregnancy, occurring during the second month.

graafian follicle (vesicle) See *follicle, graafian.*

gravid Pregnant.

grieving process A complex of somatic and psychological symptoms associated with some extreme sorrow or loss, specifically the death of a loved one.

grunt, expiratory Sign of respiratory distress (hyaline membrane disease [respiratory distress syndrome, or RDS] or advanced pneumonia) indicative of the body's attempt to hold air in the alveoli for better gaseous exchange.

gynecoid pelvis Pelvis in which the inlet is round instead of oval or blunt; heart shaped. Typical female pelvis.

gynecology Study of the diseases of the female, especially of the genital, urinary, and rectal organs.

habitual (recurrent) abortion See *abortion, habitual.*

habituation An acquired tolerance from repeated exposure to a particular stimulus. Also called negative adaptation; a decline and eventual elimination of a conditioned response by repetition of the conditioned stimulus.

haploid number Having half the normal number of chromosomes found in somatic (body) cells; 23 chromosomes.

harlequin sign Rare color change of no pathologic significance occurring between the longitudinal halves of the neonate's body. When infant is placed on one side, the dependent half is noticeably pinker than the superior half.

Hawthorne effect A general beneficial effect on a person or group of people as a result of a therapeutic encounter with a health care provider or as a result of a change in the environment (lighting, temperature, type of room [family-centered versus four-bed unit]).

Hegar's sign Softening of the lower uterine segment that is classified as a probable sign of pregnancy and that may be present during the second and third months of pregnancy and is palpated during bimanual examination.

HELLP syndrome Condition characterized by hemolysis, elevated liver enzymes, and low platelet count; is a form of severe preeclampsia.

hematocrit Volume of red blood cells per deciliter (dl) of circulating blood; packed cell volume (PCV).

hematoma Collection of blood in a tissue; a bruise or blood tumor.

hemoconcentration Increase in the number of red blood cells resulting from either a decrease in plasma volume or increased erythropoiesis.

hemodilution An increase in fluid content of blood, resulting in diminution of the proportion of formed elements.

hemoglobin Component of red blood cells consisting of globin, a protein, and hematin, an organic iron compound.

h. electrophoresis Test to diagnose sickle cell disease in newborns. Cord blood is used.

hemolytic disease of the newborn Breakdown of fetal red blood cells by maternal antibodies, usually from an Rh-negative mother.

hemorrhagic disease of newborn Bleeding disorder during first few days of life based on a deficiency of vitamin K.

hemorrhagic shock A clinical condition in which the peripheral blood flow is inadequate to return sufficient blood to the heart for normal function, particularly oxygen transport to the organs/tissue.

hereditary Pertaining to a trait or characteristic transmitted from parent to offspring by way of the genes; used synonymously with *genetic.*

hermaphrodite Person having genital and sexual characteristics of both sexes.

heterozygous Having two dissimilar genes at the same site, or locus, on paired chromosomes (e.g., at the sites for eye color, one chromosome carrying the gene for brown, the other for blue).

high risk An increased possibility of suffering harm, damage, loss, or death. See also *risk factor.*

hirsutism Condition characterized by the excessive growth of hair.

Homans' sign Early sign of phlebothrombosis of the deep veins of the calf in which there are complaints of pain when the leg is in extension and the foot is dorsiflexed.

home birth Planned birth of the child at home. Usually under the supervision of a midwife.

homoiothermic Referring to the ability of warm-blooded animals to maintain internal temperature at a specified level regardless of the environmental temperature. This ability is not fully developed in the human neonate.

homologous Similar in structure or origin but not necessarily in function.

homologous insemination Insemination in which the semen specimen is provided by the husband. The procedure is used primarily in cases of impotence or when the husband is incapable of sexual intercourse because of some physical disability.

homosexual family Family form where parents form a homosexual union. Children may be the offspring of a previous heterosexual union or may be conceived by one member of a lesbian couple through artificial insemination.

homozygous Having two similar genes at the same locus, or site, on paired chromosomes.

hormone Chemical substance produced in an organ or gland that is conveyed through the blood to another organ or part of the body, stimulating it to increased functional activity or secretion. See also *specific hormones.*

hormone replacement therapy (HRT) Progestin is added to estrogen replacement therapy to prevent endometrial cancer. See *estrogen replacement therapy.*

hour-glass uterus Uterus in which a segment of circular muscle fibers contracts during labor. The resultant "constriction ring" dystocia is characterized by lack of progress in spite of adequate contractions; by pain experienced prior to palpation of a uterine contraction and persisting after the observer feels the contraction end; and by recession of the presenting part during a contraction, instead of descent of the presenting part.

human chorionic gonadotropin (hCG) Hormone which is produced by chorionic villi; the biologic marker in pregnancy tests.

hyaline membrane disease (HMD) Disease characterized by interference with ventilation at the alveolar level, theoretically caused by the presence of fibrinoid deposits lining alveolar ducts. Membrane formation is related to prematurity (especially with fetal asphyxia) and insufficient surfactant production (L/S ratio less than 2:1). Otherwise known as *respiratory distress syndrome (RDS).*

hydramnios (polyhydramnios) Amniotic fluid in excess of 1.5L; often indicative of fetal anomaly and fre-

quently seen in poorly controlled, insulin-dependent, diabetic pregnant women even if there is no coexisting fetal anomaly.

hydrocele Collection of fluid in a saclike cavity, especially in the sac that surrounds the testis, causing the scrotum to swell.

hydrocephalus Accumulation of fluid in the subdural or subarachnoid spaces.

hydrops fetalis Most severe expression of fetal hemolytic disorder, a possible sequela to maternal Rh isoimmunization; infants exhibit gross edema (anasarca), cardiac decompensation, and profound pallor from anemia and seldom survive.

hymen Membranous fold that normally partially covers the entrance to the vagina in the virgin.

hymenal caruncles Small, irregular bits of tissue that are remnants of the hymen.

hymenal tag Normally occurring redundant hymenal tissue protruding from the floor of the vagina that disappears spontaneously in a few weeks after birth.

hymenotomy Surgical incision of the hymen.

hyperbilirubinemia Elevation of unconjugated serum bilirubin concentrations.

hyperemesis gravidarum Abnormal condition of pregnancy characterized by protracted vomiting, weight loss, and fluid and electrolyte imbalance.

hyperesthesia Unusual sensibility to sensory stimuli, such as pain or touch.

hyperglycemia Excess glucose in the blood.

hyperplasia Increase in number of cells; formation of new tissue.

hyperreflexia Increased action of the reflexes.

hyperthyroidism Excessive functional activity of the thyroid gland.

hypertonic uterine dysfunction Uncoordinated, painful, frequent uterine contractions that do not cause dilatation and effacement; primary dysfunction labor.

hypertrophic cardiomyopathy (HCM) Enlargement of heart walls and septum impacting on the size of the heart chambers.

hypertrophy Enlargement, or increase in size, of existing cells.

hyperventilation Rapid, shallow (or prolonged, deep) respirations resulting in respiratory alkalosis: a decrease in H^+ concentration and P_{CO_2} and an increase in the blood pH and the ratio of $NaHCO_3$ to H_2CO_3. Symptoms may include faintness, palpitations, and carpopedal (hands and feet) muscular spasms. Relief may result from rebreathing in a paper bag or into one's cupped hands to replace the CO_2 "blown off" during hyperventilation.

hypofibrinogenemia Deficient level of a blood clotting factor, fibrinogen, in the blood; in obstetrics, it occurs following complications of abruptio placentae or retention of a dead fetus.

hypogastric arteries Branches of the right and left iliac arteries carrying deoxygenated blood from the fetus through the umbilical cord, where they are known as *umbilical arteries,* to the placenta.

hypoglycemia Less-than-normal amount of glucose in the blood, usually caused by administration of too much insulin, excessive secretion of insulin by the islet cells of the pancreas, or by dietary deficiency.

hypoglycemia Low glucose level in the blood.

hypospadias Anomalous positioning of urinary meatus on undersurface of penis or close to or just inside the vagina.

hypotensive drugs Drugs that lower the blood pressure.

hypothalamus Portion of the diencephalon of the brain forming the floor and part of the lateral wall of the third ventricle. It activates, controls, and integrates the peripheral autonomic nervous system, endocrine processes, and many somatic functions, as body temperature, sleep, and appetite.

hypothyroidism Deficiency of thyroid gland activity with underproduction of thyroxine.

hypotonic uterine dysfunction Weak, ineffective uterine contractions usually occurring in the active phase of labor; often related to cephalopelvic disproportion (CDC) or malposition of the fetus.

hypoxemia Reduction in arterial Po_2 resulting in metabolic acidosis by forcing anaerobic glycolysis, pulmonary vasoconstriction, and direct cellular damage.

hypoxia Insufficient availability of oxygen to meet the metabolic needs of body tissue.

hysterectomy Surgical removal of the uterus.

panhysterectomy Removal of entire uterus, but ovaries and tubes remain.

subtotal h. Removal of fundus and body of the uterus, but the cervical stump remains.

total h. Removal of entire uterus, including the cervix, but the ovaries and tubes remain.

hysterosalpingography Recording by x-ray of the uterus and uterine tubes after injecting them with radiopaque material.

hysterotomy Surgical incision into the uterus.

iatrogenic Caused by a health care provider's words, actions, or treatment.

icterus neonatorum Jaundice in the newborn.

idiopathic peripartum cardiomyopathy A primary disease of the heart muscle with no apparent cause, occurring during the peripartum period.

idiopathic respiratory distress syndrome (hyaline membrane disease) Severe respiratory condition found almost exclusively in preterm infants and in some infants of diabetic mothers regardless of gestational age. See also *hyaline membrane disease (HMD).*

IDM Infant of a diabetic mother.

IgA Primary immunoglobulin in colostrum.

IgG Transplacentally acquired immunoglobulin that confers passive immunity against the infections to which the mother is immune.

IgM Immunoglobulin neonate can manufacture soon after birth. Fetus produces it in the presence of amnionitis.

immunity

acquired immunity Protection against microorganisms that develops in response to actual infection or transfer of antibody from an immune donor.

active immunity Protection against specific microorganisms that develops in response to actual infection or vaccination.

natural immunity Nonspecific protection against microorganisms. Natural immunity is the first line of defense and includes skin and phagocytic cells.

passive immunity Protection against specific microorganisms that develops in response to the transfer of antibody or lymphocytes from an immune donor.

immunocompetent The ability of the immune system to respond appropriately to foreign antigens and to develop antigen-specific antibodies.

immunology The study of the components essential to the recognition and disposal of foreign (nonself or antigenic) material and maintenance of body defenses.

impaired fertility Inability to conceive or carry to live birth at a time a couple chooses to do so.

implantation Embedding of the fertilized ovum in the uterine mucosa; nidation.

impotence Archaic term designating a man's inability, partial or complete, to perform sexual intercourse or to achieve orgasm; erectile dysfunction.

inborn error of metabolism Hereditary deficiency of a specific enzyme needed for normal metabolism of specific chemicals (e.g., deficiency of phenylalanine hydroxylase results in phenylketonuria [PKU]; a deficiency of hexosaminidase results in Tay-Sachs disease).

incompetent cervix Cervix that is unable to remain closed until a pregnancy reaches term, because of a mechanical defect in the cervix resulting in dilatation and effacement usually during the second or early third trimester of pregnancy.

incomplete abortion See *abortion, incomplete.*

increment An increase, or buildup, as of a contraction.

induced abortion See *abortion, induced.*

induction Artificial stimulation or augmentation of labor.

inertia Sluggishness or inactivity; in obstetrics, refers to the absence or weakness of uterine contractions during labor.

inevitable abortion See *abortion, inevitable.*

infant A child who is under 1 year of age.

infective endocarditis Inflammation of the lining membrane of the heart due to invasion of microorganisms.

infertility Decreased capacity to conceive.

inhalation analgesia Reduction of pain by administration of anesthetic gas. Occasionally given during the second stage of labor. Consciousness is retained to allow the woman to follow instructions and to avoid the adverse effects of general anesthesia.

inlet Passage leading into a cavity.

    pelvic i. Upper brim of the pelvic cavity.

instrumental style Characteristic style displayed by expectant fathers which emphasizes tasks to be accomplished.

insulin A hormone produced by the beta cells of the pancreatic islets of Langerhans; promotes glucose transport into the cells; aids in protein and lipid synthesis.

internal os Inside mouth or opening.

interstitial cell-stimulating hormone (ICSH) Hormone that stimulates production of testosterone; analogous to LH in the female.

intertuberous diameter Distance between ischial tuberosities. Measured to determine dimension of pelvic outlet.

intervillous space Irregular space in the maternal portion of the placenta, filled with maternal blood and serving as the site of maternal-fetal gas, nutrient, and waste exchange.

intimate partner abuse Violence between intimate adults.

intrapartum During labor and birth.

intrathecal Within the subarachnoid space.

intrauterine device (IUD) Small plastic or metal form placed in the uterus to prevent implantation of a fertilized ovum.

intrauterine growth retardation (IUGR) Fetal undergrowth of any etiology, such as deficient nutrient supply or intrauterine infection, or associated with congenital malformation.

intrauterine pressure catheter (IUPC) Catheter inserted into uterine cavity to assess uterine activity and pressure by electronic means.

introitus Entrance into a canal or cavity such as the vagina.

intromission Insertion of one part or object into another (e.g., introduction of penis into vagina).

intussusception Prolapse of one segment of bowel into the lumen of the adjacent segment.

in utero Within or inside the uterus.

in vitro fertilization Fertilization in a culture dish or test tube.

inversion Turning end for end, upside down, or inside out.

    i. of the uterus Condition in which the uterus is turned inside out so that the fundus intrudes into the cervix or vagina, caused by a too vigorous removal of the placenta before it is detached by the natural process of labor.

involution (1) Rolling or turning inward. (2) Reduction in size of the uterus after birth and its return to its nonpregnant condition.

isoimmune hemolytic disease Breakdown (hemolysis) of fetal/neonatal Rh-positive RBCs because of Rh antibodies formed by an Rh-negative mother who had been previously exposed to Rh-positive RBCs.

isoimmunization Development of antibodies in a species of animal with antigens from the same species (e.g., development of anti-Rh antibodies in an Rh-negative person).

ITP Abbreviation for idiopathic thrombocytopenic purpura.

jaundice Yellow discoloration of the body tissues caused by the deposit of bile pigments (unconjugated bilirubin); icterus.

    breast milk j. Yellowing of infant's skin from pregnanediol (in mother's milk) inhibition of enzyme (glucuronyl transferase) necessary for conjugation of bilirubin.

    pathologic j. Jaundice usually first noticeable within 24 hours after birth; caused by some abnormal condition such as an Rh or ABO incompatibility and resulting in bilirubin toxicity (e.g., kernicterus).

    physiologic j. Jaundice usually occurring 48 hours or later after birth, reaching a peak at 5 to 7 days, gradually disappearing by the seventh to tenth day, and caused by the normal reduction in the number of red blood cells. The infant is otherwise well.

karyotype Schematic arrangement of the chromosomes within a cell to demonstrate their numbers and morphology.

Kegel exercises Exercises to strengthen the pubococcygeal muscles.

kernicterus Bilirubin encephalopathy involving the deposit of unconjugated bilirubin in brain cells, resulting in death or impaired intellectual, perceptive, or motor function, and adaptive behavior.

ketoacidosis The accumulation of ketone bodies in the blood as a consequence of hyperglycemia; leads to metabolic acidosis.

Kleihauer-Betke test Laboratory test which detects the presence of fetal blood cells in the maternal circulation.

labia Lips or liplike structures.

    l. majora Two folds of skin containing fat and covered with hair that lie on either side of the vaginal opening and from each side of the vulva.

    l. minora Two thin folds of delicate, hairless skin inside the labia majora.

labor Series of processes by which the fetus is expelled from the uterus; parturition; childbirth.

laceration Irregular tear of wound tissue; in obstetrics, it usually refers to a tear in the perineum, vagina, or cervix caused by childbirth.

lactase Enzyme necessary for the digestion of lactose.

lactation Function of secreting milk or period during which milk is secreted.

lactation suppression Stopping the production of breast

milk through the use of medication and/or nonpharmacologic interventions.

lactogen Drug or other substance that enhances the production and secretion of milk.

lactogenic Stimulating the production of milk.

l. hormone Gonadotropin produced by anterior pituitary and responsible for promoting growth of breast tissue and lactation; prolactin; lutcotropin.

lactose intolerance Inherited absence of the enzyme lactose.

lactosuria Presence of lactose in the urine during late pregnancy and during lactation. Must be differentiated from glycosuria.

Lamaze method Method of psychophysical preparation for childbirth developed in the 1950s by a French obstetrician, Fernand Lamaze. It requires classes, practice at home, and coaching during labor and birth.

lambdoid Having the shape of the Greek letter lambda.

l. suture Suture line extending across the posterior third of the skull, separating the occipital bone from the two parietal bones, and forming the base of the triangular posterior fontanel.

laminaria tent Cone of dried seaweed that swells as it absorbs moisture. Used to dilate the cervix nontraumatically in preparation for an induced abortion or in preparation for induction of labor.

lanugo Downy, fine hair characteristic of the fetus between 20 weeks' gestation and birth that is most noticeable over the shoulder, forehead, and cheeks but is found on nearly all parts of the body except the palms of the hands, soles of the feet, and the scalp.

laparoscopy Examination of the interior of the abdomen by inserting a small telescope through the anterior abdominal wall.

large for dates (large for gestational age [LGA]) Exhibiting excessive growth for gestational age.

last menstrual period The date of the first day of the last normal menstrual bleeding.

labor, delivery, recovery (LDR) A single room where all steps of the birth process occur. Avoids having to move the woman to different rooms for each phase of the birth process. The woman is moved to a postpartum room after recovery.

labor, delivery, recovery, postpartum (LDRP) A single room where all steps of the birth process and hospitalization occur. The woman stays in the same room throughout her hospitalization.

lecithin A phospholipid that decreases surface tension; surfactant.

lecithin/sphingomyelin ratio Ratio of lecithin to sphingomyelin in the amniotic fluid. This is used to assess maturity of the fetal lung.

Leopold's maneuver Four maneuvers for diagnosing the fetal position by external palpation of the mother's abdomen.

let-down reflex Oxytocin-induced flow of milk from the alveoli of the breasts into the milk ducts.

letting go phase Interdependent phase after birth in which the mother and family move forward as a system with interacting members.

leukorrhea White or yellowish mucous discharge from the cervical canal or the vagina that may be normal physiologically or caused by pathologic states of the vagina and endocervix (e.g., *Trichomonas vaginalis* infections).

LH See *luteinizing hormone (LH)*.

libido Sexual drive.

lie Relationship existing between the long axis of the fetus and the long axis of the mother. In a longitudinal lie, the fetus is lying lengthwise or vertically, whereas in a transverse lie the fetus is lying crosswise or horizontally in the mother's uterus.

ligation Act of suturing, sewing, or otherwise tying shut.

tubal l. Abdominal operation in which the fallopian tubes are tied off and a section is removed to interrupt tubal continuity and thus sterilize the woman.

lightening Sensation of decreased abdominal distention produced by uterine descent into the pelvic cavity as the fetal presenting part settles into the pelvis. It usually occurs 2 weeks before the onset of labor in nulliparas.

linea nigra Line of darker pigmentation seen in some women during the latter part of pregnancy that appears on the middle of the abdomen and extends from the symphysis pubis toward the umbilicus.

linea terminalis Line dividing the upper (false) pelvis from the lower (true) pelvis.

lithotomy position Position in which the woman lies on her back with her knees flexed and abducted thighs drawn up toward her chest.

live birth Birth in which the neonate, regardless of gestational age, manifests any heartbeat, breathes, or displays voluntary movement.

local infiltration anesthesia Process by which a substance such as a local anesthetic drug is deposited within the tissue to anesthetize a limited region.

lochia Vaginal discharge during the puerperium consisting of blood, tissue, and mucus.

l. alba Thin, yellowish to white, vaginal discharge that follows lochia serosa on about the tenth day after birth and that may last from 2 to 6 weeks postpartum.

l. rubra Red, distinctly blood-tinged vaginal flow that follows birth and lasts 2 to 4 days.

l. serosa Serous, pinkish brown, watery vaginal discharge that follows lochia rubra until about the tenth day after birth.

low-birth-weight (LBW) Infant weighing 2500 g or less at birth.

lunar month Four weeks (28 days).

lutein Yellow pigment derived from the corpus luteum, egg yolk, and fat cells.

l. cells Ovarian cells involved in the formation of the corpus luteum and that contain a yellow pigment.

luteinizing hormone (LH) Hormone produced by the anterior pituitary that stimulates ovulation and the development of the corpus luteum.

luteotropin (LTH) Lactogenic hormone; prolactin; an adenohypophyseal hormone.

lysozyme Enzyme with antiseptic qualities that destroys foreign organisms and that is found in blood cells of the granulocytic and monocytic series and is also normally present in saliva, sweat, tears, and breast milk.

maceration (1) Process of softening a solid by soaking it in a fluid. (2) Softening and breaking down of fetal skin from prolonged exposure to amniotic fluid as seen in a postterm infant. Also seen in a dead fetus.

macroglossia Hypertrophy of tongue or tongue large for oral cavity; seen in some preterm neonates and in neonates with Down's syndrome.

macrophage Any phagocytic cell of the reticuloendothelial system including Kupffer cell in the liver, splenocyte in the spleen, and histocyte in the loose connective tissue.

macrosomia Large body size as seen in neonates of diabetic or prediabetic mothers; macrosomatia.

magnetic resonance imaging (MRI) Noninvasive nuclear procedure for imaging tissues with high fat and water content; in obstetrics, uses include evaluation of fetal structures, placenta, amniotic fluid volume.

malpractice Professional negligence that is the proximate cause of injury or harm to a patient, resulting from a lack of professional knowledge, experience, or skill that can be expected in others in the profession or from a failure to exercise reasonable care or judgment in the application of professional knowledge, experience, or skill.

mammary gland Compound gland of the female breast that is made up of lobes and lobules that secrete milk for nourishment of the young. Rudimentary mammary glands exist in the male.

mask of pregnancy See *chloasma*.

mastectomy Excision, or removal, of the mammary gland.

   modified radical Removal of breast tissue, skin, and axillary nodes.

mastitis Inflammation of mammary tissue of the breasts.

maternal mortality Death of a woman related to childbearing.

maturation (1) Process of attaining maximum development. (2) In biology, a process of cell division during which the number of chromosomes in the germ cells (sperm or ova) is reduced to one half the number (haploid) characteristic of the species.

maturational crisis Crisis that arises during normal growth and development, e.g., puberty.

McDonald's sign Easy flexion of the fundus on the cervix.

mean arterial pressure (MAP) Average of systolic and diastolic blood pressures. A MAP of 90 in the second trimester is associated with an increase in the incidence of PIH in the third trimester.

meatus Opening from an internal structure to the outside (e.g., urethral meatus).

meconium First stools of infant: viscid, sticky; dark greenish brown, almost black; sterile; odorless.

   m. aspiration syndrome Function of fetal hypoxia: with hypoxia, the anal sphincter relaxes and meconium is released; reflex gasping movements draw meconium and other particulate matter in the amniotic fluid into the infant's bronchial tree, obstructing the air flow after birth.

   m. ileus Lower intestinal obstruction by thick, puttylike, inspissated (dried) meconium that may be the result of deficiency of trypsin production in the newborn with cystic fibrosis.

   m.-stained fluid In response to hypoxia, fetal intestinal activity increases and anal sphincter relaxes, resulting in the passage of meconium, which imparts a greenish coloration.

meiosis Process by which germ cells divide and decrease their chromosomal number by one half.

membrane Thin, pliable layer of tissue that lines a cavity or tube, separates structures, or covers an organ or structure; in obstetrics, the amnion and chorion surrounding the fetus.

membrane rupture Tearing of the fetal membranes (amnion and chorion) with the release of amniotic fluid.

menarche Onset, or beginning, of menstrual function.

meningomyelocele Saclike protrusion of the spinal cord through a congenital defect in the vertebral column.

menopause From the Latin word *mensis* (month) and Greek word *pausis* (to cease), the actual permanent cessation of menstrual cycles.

menorrhagia Abnormally profuse or excessive menstrual flow.

menses (menstruation) Periodic vaginal discharge of bloody fluid from the nonpregnant uterus that occurs from the age of puberty to menopause.

mentum Chin, a fetal reference point in designating position (e.g., "Left mentum anterior" [LMA], meaning that the fetal chin is presenting in the left anterior quadrant of the maternal pelvis).

mesoderm Embryonic middle layer of germ cells giving rise to all types of muscles, connective tissue, bone marrow, blood, lymphoid tissue, and urogenital system.

metritis Inflammation of the endometrium and myometrium.

metrorrhagia Abnormal bleeding from the uterus, particularly when it occurs at any time other than the menstrual period.

microcephaly Congenital anomaly characterized by abnormal smallness of the head in relation to the rest of the body and by underdevelopment of the brain, resulting in some degree of mental retardation.

midwife One who practices the art of helping and aiding a woman to give birth.

milia Unopened sebaceous glands appearing as tiny, white, pinpoint papules on forehead, nose, cheeks, and chin of a neonate that disappear spontaneously in a few days or weeks.

milk ejection Milk leaking from the breasts, often before a feeding.

milk-leg See *phlegmasia alba dolens.*

miscarriage Spontaneous abortion; lay term usually referring specifically to the loss of the fetus between the fourth month and viability.

missed abortion See *abortion, missed.*

mitosis Process of somatic cell division in which a single cell divides, but both of the new cells have the same number of chromosomes as the first.

mitral valve prolapse (MVP) A disorder in which the cusp(s) of the mitral valve drop into the left atrium during systole characterized by midsystolic click and late systolic murmur.

mitral valve stenosis Narrowing of the opening of the mitral valve due to stiffening of value leaflets obstructing free flow from atrium to ventricle.

mittelschmerz Abdominal pain in the region of an ovary during ovulation, which usually occurs midway through the menstrual cycle. Present in many women, mittelschmerz is useful for identifying ovulation, thus pinpointing the fertile period of the cycle.

molding Overlapping of cranial bones or shaping of the fetal head to accommodate and conform to the bony and soft parts of the mother's birth canal during labor.

mongolian spot Bluish gray or dark nonelevated pigmented area usually found over the lower back and buttocks present at birth in some infants, primarily nonwhite. The spot fades by school age in black or Oriental infants and within the first year or two of life in other infants.

mongolism See *Down syndrome.*

moniliasis Infection of the skin or mucous membrane by a yeast-like fungus, *Candida albicans;* see *thrush.*

monitrice One trained in psychoprophylactic methods and who supports women during labor.

monosomy Chromosomal aberration characterized by the absence of one chromosome from the normal diploid complement.

monozygotic Originating or coming from a single fertilized ovum, such as identical twins.

monozygotic twins See *twins, monozygotic.*

mons veneris Pad of fatty tissue and coarse skin that overlies the symphysis pubis in the woman and that, after puberty, is covered with short curly hair.

Montgomery's glands tubercles Small, nodular prominences (sebaceous glands) on the areolas around the nipples of the breasts that enlarge during pregnancy and lactation.

mood disorders Depression or depression with manic episodes (bipolar disorders).

moratorium phase The second developmental task experienced by expectant fathers as identified by May. During this phase the expectant father adjusts to the reality of pregnancy.

morbidity (1) Condition of being diseased. (2) Number of cases of disease or sick persons in relationship to a specific population; incidence.

morning sickness Nausea and vomiting that affect some women during the first few months of their pregnancy; may occur at any time of day.

Moro's reflex Normal, generalized reflex in a young infant elicited by a sudden loud noise or by striking the table next to the child, resulting in flexion of the legs, an embracing posture of the arms, and usually a brief cry. Also called startle reflex.

mortality (1) Quality or state of being subject to death. (2) Number of deaths in relation to a specific population; incidence.

  fetal m. Number of fetal deaths per 1000 births (or per live births). See also *death, fetal.*

  infant m. Number of deaths per 1000 children 1 year of age or younger.

  maternal m. Number of maternal deaths per 100,000 births.

  neonatal m. Number of neonatal deaths per 1000 births (or per live births). See also *death, neonatal.*

  perinatal m. Combined fetal and neonatal mortality. See also *death, perinatal.*

morula Developmental stage of the fertilized ovum in which there is a solid mass of cells resembling a mulberry.

mosaicism Condition in which some somatic cells are normal, whereas others show chromosomal aberrations.

mourning The process of finding the answers to the questions surrounding the loss, coping with grief responses and determining how to live again.

mucous membrane Specialized thin layer of tissue lining certain cavities and passages that is kept moist by the secretion of mucus.

multigravida Woman who has been pregnant two or more times.

multipara Woman who has carried two or more pregnancies to viability, whether they ended in live infants or stillbirths.

multifetal pregnancy Pregnancy in which there is more than one fetus in the uterus at the same time; multiple pregnancy.

mutation Change in a gene or chromosome in gametes that may be transmitted to offspring.

Naegele's rule Method for calculating the estimated date of birth (EDB) or "due date."

narcotic antagonist A compound such as naloxone (Narcan) which promptly reverses the effects of narcotics such as meperidine (Demerol).

natal Relating or pertaining to birth.

navel Depression in the center of the abdomen, where the umbilical cord was attached to the fetus; umbilicus.

necrotizing enterocolitis (NEC) Acute inflammatory bowel disorder that occurs primarily in preterm or low-birth-weight neonates. It is characterized by ischemic necrosis (death) of the gastrointestinal mucosa that may lead to perforation and peritonitis.

negligence Commission of an act that a prudent person would not have done or the omission of a duty that prudent person would have fulfilled, resulting in injury or harm to another person. In particular, in a malpractice suit a professional person is negligent if harm to a patient results from such an act or such a failure to act, but it must be proved that other prudent persons of the same profession would ordinarily have acted differently under the same circumstances.

neonatal mortality Statistical rate of infant death during the first 28 days after live birth, expressed as the number of such deaths per 1000 live births in a specific geographic area or institution in a given period of time.

neonatology Study of the neonate.

neural tube Tube formed from fusion of the neural folds from which develops the brain and spinal cord.

  n. t. defect improper development of tube resulting in malformation of brain and/or spinal cord; see α-*fetoprotein*.

nevus Natural blemish or mark; a congenital circumscribed deposit of pigmentation in the skin; mole.

  n. flammeus Port-wine stain; reddish, usually flat, discoloration of the face or neck. Because of its large size and color, it is considered a serious deformity.

  n. vasculosus (strawberry hemangioma) Elevated lesion of immature capillaries and endothelial cells that regresses over a period of years.

nidation Implantation of the fertilized ovum in the endometrium, or lining, of the uterus.

Nipple cup A device used to make inverted nipples erectile.

Nonreassuring fetal heart rate pattern Fetal heart rate pattern that indicates the fetus is not well oxygenated and requires intervention.

nonshivering thermogenesis Infant's method of producing heat from brown fat by increasing metabolic rate.

nonstress test (NST) Evaluation of fetal response (fetal heart rate) to natural contractile uterine activity or to an increase in fetal activity.

normoglycemia Blood glucose level within normal limits; glycemic control.

nosocomial Pertaining to a hospital.

nuchal cord Encircling of fetal neck by one or more loops of umbilical cord.

nuclear family Family form consisting of parents and their dependent children.

nulligravida Woman who has never been pregnant.

nullipara Woman who has not yet carried a pregnancy to viability.

nursing practitioner Registered nurse who has additional education to practice nursing in an expanded role.

observer style Characteristic style displayed by expectant fathers who show a detached approach to involvement in his partner's pregnancy.

occipitobregmatic Pertaining to the occiput (the back part of the skull) and the bregma (junction of the coronal and sagittal sutures) or anterior fontanel.

occiput Back part of the head or skull.

oligohydramnios Abnormally small amount or absence of amniotic fluid; often indicative of fetal urinary tract defect.

oliguria Diminished secretion of urine by the kidneys.

omphalic Concerning or pertaining to the umbilicus.

omphalitis Inflammation of the umbilical stump characterized by redness, edema, and purulent exudate in severe infections.

omphalocele Congenital defect resulting from failure of closure of the abdominal wall or muscles and leading to hernia of abdominal contents through the navel.

oocyte Primordial or incompletely developed ovum.

oogenesis Formation and development of the ovum.

operculum Plug of mucus that fills the cervical canal during pregnancy.

ophthalmia neonatorum Infection in the neonate's eyes usually resulting from gonorrheal or other infection contracted when the fetus passes through the birth canal (vagina).

opisthotonos Tetanic spasm resulting in an arched, hyperextended position of the body.

oral GTT Test for blood sugar following oral ingestion of a concentrated sugar solution.

orchitis Inflammation of one or both of the testes, characterized by swelling and pain, often caused by mumps, syphilis, or tuberculosis.

orifice Normal mouth, entrance, or opening, to any aperture.

os Mouth, or opening.

  external o. (o. externum) External opening of the cervical canal.

  internal o. (o. internum) Internal opening of the cervical canal.

  o. uteri Mouth, or opening, of the uterus.

ossification Mineralization of fetal bones.

-otomy Combining form meaning cutting, incision, section.

outlet Opening by which something can exit.

  pelvic o. Inferior aperture, or opening, of the true pelvis.

ovary One of two glands in the female situated on either side of the pelvic cavity that produces the female reproductive cell, the ovum, and two known hormones, estrogen and progesterone.

ovulation Periodic ripening and discharge of the unimpregnated ovum from the ovary, usually 14 days prior to the onset of menstrual flow.

  o. method Evaluation of cervical mucus throughout the menstrual cycle; ovulation occurs just after the appearance of the peak mucus sign; Billings method.

ovum Female germ, or reproductive cell, produced by the ovary; egg.

oxygen toxicity Oxygen overdosage that results in pathologic tissue changes (e.g., retinopathy of prematurity, bronchopulmonary dysplasia).

oxytocics Drugs that stimulate uterine contractions, thus accelerating childbirth and preventing postdelivery hemorrhage. They may be used to increase the let-down reflex during lactation.

oxytocin Hormone produced by the posterior pituitary that stimulates uterine contractions and the release of milk in the mammary gland (let-down reflex).

  o. challenge test (OCT) Evaluation of fetal response (fetal heart rate) to contractile activity of the uterus stimulated by exogenous oxytocin (Pitocin).

Paco$_2$ Partial pressure of carbon dioxide in arterial blood.

Palmer erythema Rash on the surface of the palms sometimes seen in pregnancy.

palsy Permanent or temporary loss of sensation or ability to move and control movement; paralysis.

  Bell's p. Peripheral facial paralysis of the facial nerve (cranial nerve VII), causing the muscles of the unaffected side of the face to pull the face into a distorted position.

  Erb's p. See *Erb-Duchenne paralysis.*

Pao$_2$ Partial pressure of oxygen in arterial blood.

Papanicolaou (Pap) smear Microscopic examination using scrapings from the cervix, endocervix, or other mucous membranes that will reveal, with a high degree of accuracy, the presence of premalignant or malignant cells.

para Term used to refer to past pregnancies that reached viability regardless of whether the infant(s) was dead or alive at birth.

paracervical block Type of regional anesthesia produced by injection of a local anesthetic into the lower uterine segment just beneath the mucosa adjacent to the outer rim of the cervix (9 and 3 o'clock positions) after the cervix is more than 5 cm dilated.

parity Number of pregnancies that reached viability.

parturient Woman giving birth.

parturition Process or act of giving birth.

patent Open.

pathogen Substance or organism capable of producing disease.

pathologic jaundice See *jaundice, pathologic.*

pedigree Shorthand method of depicting family lines of individuals who manifest a physical or chemical disorder.

pelvic Pertaining or relating to the pelvis.

  p. inflammatory disease (PID) Infection of internal reproductive structures and adjacent tissues usually secondary to STD infections.

  p. inlet See *inlet, pelvic.*

  p. outlet See *outlet, pelvic.*

  p. relaxation Refers to the lengthening and weakening of the fascial supports of pelvic structures.

  p. tilt (rock) An exercise used to help relieve low back discomfort during pregnancy.

pelvimetry Measurement of dimensions and proportions of the pelvis to determine its capacity and ability to allow the passage of the fetus through the birth canal.

pelvis Bony structure formed by the sacrum, coccyx, innominate bones, and symphysis pubis, and the ligaments that unite them.

  android p. See *android pelvis.*

  anthropoid p. See *anthropoid pelvis.*

  gynecoid p. See *gynecoid pelvis.*

  platypelloid p. See *platypelloid pelvis.*

  true p. Pelvis below the linea terminalis.

penis Male organ used for urination and copulation.

percutaneous umbilical blood sampling (PUBS) Procedure during which the fetal umbilical vessel is accessed for blood sampling or for transfusions.

perinatal Of or pertaining to the time and process of giving birth or being born.

perinatal period Period extending from the twentieth or twenty-eighth week of gestation through the end of the twenty-eighth day after birth.

perinatologist Physician who specializes in fetal and neonatal care.

perineum Area between the vagina and rectum in the female and between the scrotum and rectum in the male.

periodic breathing Sporadic episodes of cessation of respirations for periods of 10 seconds or less not associated with cyanosis commonly noted in preterm infants.

periods of reactivity (newborn infant) *First period* (within 30 minutes after birth): brief cyanosis, flushing with crying; rales, nasal flaring, grunting, retractions; heart sounds loud, forceful, irregular; alert; mucus; no bowel sounds; followed by period of sleep. *Second period* (4 to 8 hours after birth): swift color changes; irregular respiratory and heart rates; mucus with gagging; meconium passage; temperature stabilizing.

petechiae Pinpoint hemorrhagic areas caused by numerous disease states involving infection and thrombocytopenia and occasionally found over the face and trunk of the newborn because of increased intravascular pressure in the capillaries during birth.

pH Hydrogen ion concentration.

phenotype Expression of certain physical or chemical characteristics in an individual resulting from interaction between genotype and environmental factors.

phenylketonuria (PKU) Recessive hereditary disease that results in a defect in the metabolism of the amino acid phenylalanine caused by the lack of an enzyme, phenylalanine hydroxylase, that is necessary for the conversion of the amino acid phenylalanine into tyrosine. If PKU is not treated, brain damage may occur, causing severe mental retardation.

phimosis Tightness of the prepuce, or foreskin, of the penis.

phlebitis Inflammation of a vein with symptoms of pain and tenderness along the course of the vein, inflammatory swelling and acute edema below the obstruction, and discoloration of the skin because of injury or bruise to the vein, possibly occurring in acute or chronic infections or after operations or childbirth.

phlebothrombosis Formation of a clot or thrombus in the vein; inflammation of the vein with secondary clotting.

phlegmasia alba dolens Thrombophebetis of femoral vein resulting in edema of leg and pain; may occur after difficult vaginal birth.

phocomelia Developmental anomaly characterized by the absence of the upper portion of one or more limbs so that the feet or hands or both are attached to the trunk of the body by short, irregularly shaped stumps, resembling the fins of a seal.

phototherapy Utilization of lights to reduce serum bilirubin levels by oxidation of bilirubin into water-soluble compounds that are then processed in the liver and excreted in bile and urine.

physiologic hyperbilirubinemia Hemolysis of excessive fetal red blood cells in the early neonatal period; jaundice not apparent during first 24 hours. Levels are nontoxic to the individual.

physiologic jaundice See *jaundice, physiologic.*

pica Unusual craving during pregnancy (e.g., of laundry starch, dirt, red clay).

pinch test Determines if nipples are erectile or retractile.

placenta Latin, flat cake; afterbirth, specialized vascular disc-shaped organ for maternal-fetal gas and nutrient exchange. Normally it implants in the thick muscular wall of the upper uterine segment.

    abruptio p. See *abruptio placentae.*

    battledore p. Umbilical cord insertion into the margin of the placenta.

    circumvallate p. Placenta having a raised white ring at its edge.

    p. accreta Invasion of the uterine muscle by the placenta, thus making separation from the muscle difficult if not impossible.

    p. previa Placenta that is abnormally implanted in the thin, lower uterine segment and that is typed according to proximity to cervical os: total—completely occludes os; partial—does not occlude os completely; and marginal—placenta encroaches on margin of internal cervical os.

    p. succenturiata Accessory placenta.

placental Pertaining or relating to the placenta.

    p. infarct Localized, ischemic, hard area on the fetal or maternal side of the placenta.

    p. souffle See *souffle, placental.*

platypelloid pelvis Broad pelvis with a shortened anteroposterior diameter and a flattened, oval, transverse shape.

plethora Deep, beefy-red coloration ("boiled lobster" hue) of a newborn caused by an increased number of blood cells (polycythemia) per volume of blood.

podalic Concerning or pertaining to the feet.

    p. version Shifting of the position of the fetus so as to bring the feet to the outlet during labor.

polycythemia Increased number of erythrocytes per volume of blood, which may be caused by large placental transfusion, fetofetal transfusion, or maternal-fetal transfusion, or it may be due to hypovolemia resulting from movement of fluid out of vascular into interstitial compartment.

polydactyly Excessive number of digits (fingers or toes).

polyhydramnios See *hydramnios.*

polyuria Excessive secretion and discharge of urine by the kidneys.

position Relationship of an arbitrarily chosen fetal reference point, such as the occiput, sacrum, chin, or scapula on the presenting part of the fetus to its location in the front, back, or sides of the maternal pelvis.

positive sign of pregnancy Definite indication of pregnancy (e.g., hearing the fetal heartbeat, visualization and palpation of fetal movement by the examiner, sonographic examination).

posterior Pertaining to the back.

    p. fontanel See *fontanel, posterior.*

postmature infant Infant born at or after the beginning of week 43 of gestation or later and exhibiting signs of dysmaturity.

postnatal Happening or occurring after birth (newborn).

postpartum Happening or occurring after birth (mother).

postpartum blues A letdown feeling, accompanied by irritability and anxiety, which usually begins 2 to 3 days after giving birth and disappears within a week or two. Sometimes called the "baby blues."

postpartum depression Depression occurring within 6 months of childbirth, lasts longer than postpartum blues, and is characterized by a variety of symptoms.

postpartum psychosis Symptoms begin as postpartum blues or depression but are characterized by a break with reality. Delusions, hallucinations, confusion, delirium, and panic can occur.

postterm birth Birth of an infant after 42 weeks of gestation.

precipitous labor Rapid or sudden labor of less than 3 hours' duration beginning from onset of cervical changes to completed birth of neonate.

preconception care Care designed for health maintenance before pregnancy.

preeclampsia Disease encountered after 20 weeks' gestation or early in the puerperium; a vasopastic disease process characterized by increaseing hypertension, proteinuria, and hemoconcentration.

pregnancy Period between conception through complete birth of the products of conception. The usual duration of pregnancy in the human is 280 days, 9 calendar months, or 10 lunar months.

    abdominal p. See *abdominal gestation*.

    ectopic p. See *ectopic pregnancy*.

    extrauterine p. See *extrauterine pregnancy*.

pregnancy-induced hypertension (PIH) Hypertensive disorders of pregnancy including preeclampsia, eclampsia, and transient hypertension.

premature infant Infant born before completing week 37 of gestation, irrespective of birth weight; preterm infant.

premenstrual syndrome Syndrome of nervous tension, irritability, weight gain, edema, headache, mastalgia, dysphoria, and lack of coordination occurring during the last few days of the menstrual cycle preceding the onset of menstruation.

premonitory Serving as an early symptom or warning.

prenatal Occurring or happening before birth.

prepartum Before birth; before giving birth.

prepuce Fold of skin, or foreskin, covering the glans penis of the male.

    p. of the clitoris Fold of the labia minora that covers the glans clitoris.

presentation That part of the fetus which first enters the pelvis and lies over the inlet: may be head, face, breech, or shoulder.

    breech p. See *breech presentation*.

    cephalic p. See *cephalic presentation*.

presenting part That part of the fetus which lies closest to the internal os of the cervix.

pressure edema Edema of the lower extremities caused by pressure of the heavy pregnant uterus against the large veins; edema of fetal scalp after cephalic presentation (caput succedaneum).

presumptive signs Manifestations that suggest pregnancy but that are not absolutely positive. These include the cessation of menses, Chadwick's sign, morning sickness, and quickening.

preterm birth See *premature birth*.

previa, placenta See *placenta previa*.

primigravida Woman who is pregnant for the first time.

primipara Woman who has carried a pregnancy to viability without regard to the child's being dead or alive at the time of birth.

primordial Existing first or existing in the simplest or most primitive form.

probable signs Manifestations or evidence which indicates that there is a definite likelihood of pregnancy. Among the probable signs are enlargement of abdomen, Goodell's sign, Hegar's sign, Braxton Hicks' sign, and positive hormonal tests for pregnancy.

prodromal Serving as an early symptom or warning of the approach of a disease or condition (e.g., prodromal labor).

progesterone Hormone produced by the corpus luteum and placenta whose function is to prepare the endometrium of the uterus for implantation of the fertilized ovum, develop the mammary glands, and maintain the pregnancy.

prolactin See *lactogenic hormone*.

prolapsed cord Protrusion of the umbilical cord in advance of the presenting part.

proliferative phase of menstrual cycle Preovulatory, follicular, or estrogen phase of the menstrual cycle.

PROM Premature (before 38 weeks' gestation) rupture of membranes.

promontory of the sacrum Superior projecting portion of the sacrum at the junction of the sacrum and the L-5.

prophylactic Pertaining to prevention or warding off of disease or certain conditions; condom, or "rubber."

proscription Establish taboos.

prostaglandin (PG) Substance present in many body tissues; has a role in many reproductive tract functions.

proteinuria Excretion of protein into urine.

pruritus Itching.

pseudocyesis Condition in which the woman has all the usual signs of pregnancy, such as enlargement of the abdomen, cessation of menses, weight gain, and morning sickness, but is not pregnant; phantom or false pregnancy.

pseudopregnancy See *pseudocyesis*.

psychoprophylaxis Mental and physical education of the parents in preparation for childbirth, with the goal of minimizing the fear and pain and promoting positive family relationships.

ptyalism Excessive salivation.

puberty Period in life in which the reproductive organs mature and one becomes functionally capable of reproduction.

pubic Pertaining to the pubis.

pubis Pubic bone forming the front of the pelvis.

pudendal block Injection of a local anesthetizing drug at the pudendal nerve root in order to produce numbness of the genital and perianal region.

puerperal infection Infection of the pelvic organs during the postbirth period; childbed fever.

puerperium Period of time following the third stage of labor and lasting until involution of the uterus takes place, usually about 3 to 6 weeks.

pulse oximetry Noninvasive method of monitoring oxygen levels by detecting the amount of light absorbed by oxygen-carrying hemoglobin.

Pyrosis A burning sensation in the epigastric and sternal region from stomach acid (heartburn).

quickening Maternal perception of fetal movement; usually occurs between weeks 16 and 20 of gestation.

radioimmunoassay Pregnancy test that tests for the beta subunit of HCG using radioactively labeled markers.

RDS See *respiratory distress syndrome (RDS)*.

recessive trait Genetically determined characteristic that is expressed only when present in the homozygotic state.

referred pain Discomfort originating in a local area such as cervix, vagina, or perineal tissues and the discomfort is felt in the back, flanks, or thighs.

reflex Automatic response built into the nervous system that does not need the intervention of conscious thought (e.g., in the newborn, rooting, gagging, grasp).

regional anesthesia Anesthesia of an area of the body by injecting a local anesthetic to block a group of sensory nerve fibers.

regurgitate Vomiting or spitting up of solids or fluids.

residual urine Urine that remains in the bladder after urination.

respiratory distress syndrome (RDS) Condition resulting from decreased pulmonary gas exchange, leading to retention of carbon dioxide (increase in arterial Pco_2). Most common neonatal causes are prematurity, perinatal asphyxia, and maternal diabetes mellitus; hyaline membrane disease (HMD).

restitution In obstetrics, the turning of the fetal head to the left or right after it has completely emerged from the introitus as it assumes a normal alignment with the infant's shoulders.

resuscitation Restoration of consciousness or life in one who is apparently dead or whose respirations or cardiac function or both have ceased.

retained placenta Retention of all or part of the placenta in the uterus after birth.

retinopathy of prematurity Associated with hyperoxemia, resulting in eye injury and blindness.

retraction (1) Drawing in or sucking in of soft tissues of chest, indicative of an obstruction at any level of the respiratory tract from the oropharynx to the alveoli. (2) Retraction of uterine muscle fiber. After contracting, the muscle fiber does not return to its original length but remains slightly shortened, a unique attribute of uterine muscle that aids in preventing postdelivery hemorrhage and results in involution.

retroflexion Bending backward

   r. of the uterus Condition in which the body of the womb is bent backward at an angle with the cervix, whose position usually remains unchanged.

retrolental fibroplasia (RLF) See *Retinopathy of prematurity*.

retroversion Turning or a state of being turned back.

   r. of the uterus Displacement of the uterus; the body of the uterus is tipped backward with the cervix pointing forward toward the symphysis pubis.

retrovirus A single piece of RNA surrounded by a protein coat, or envelope. A unique enzyme, reverse transcriptase, allows this RNA retrovirus to go backward, against the "flow of life." The RNA becomes a piece of DNA, which infects the cell's DNA nucleus and remains in the cell until its death (e. g., HIV). (The normal flow of genetic information in life is from DNA to RNA to proteins.)

Rh factor Inherited antigen present on erythrocytes. The individual with the factor is known as *positive* for the factor.

Rh immune globulin Solution of gamma globulin that contains Rh antibodies. Intramuscular (IM) administration of Rh immune globulin (trade name RhoGam) prevents sensitization in Rh negative women who have been exposed to Rh positive red blood cells.

rheumatic heart disease Permanent damage of heart valves secondary to an autoimmune reaction in the heart tissue precipitated by rheumatic heart disease.

rhythm method Contraceptive method in which a woman abstains from sexual intercourse during the ovulatory phase of her menstrual cycle and at least 3 days before and 1 day after the ovulation date.

ribonucleic acid (RNA) Element responsible for transferring genetic information within a cell; a template, or pattern.

ring of fire Burning sensation as vagina stretches and fetal head crowns.

risk factors Factors that cause a person or a group of people to be particularly vulnerable to an unwanted, unpleasant, or unhealthful event.

risk-taking Intentional behaviors with uncertain outcomes.

rite of passage Significant life event indicating movement from one maturational level to another.

Ritgen maneuver Procedure used to control the birth of the head.

roll-over test Sometimes used in the second trimester as a predictor of a potential hypertensive problem in the third trimester.

rooming-in unit Maternity unit designed so that the newborn's crib is at the mother's bedside or in a nursery adjacent to the mother's room.

rooting reflex Normal response in newborns when the cheek is touched or stroked along the side of the mouth to turn the head toward the stimulated side, to open the mouth, and to begin to suck. The reflex disappears by 3 to 4 months of age but in some infants may persist until 12 months.

rotation In obstetrics, the turning of the fetal head as it follows the curves of the birth canal downward.

rubella vaccine Live attenuated rubella virus given to patients who have not had rubella or who are serologically negative. Exposure to the rubella virus through vaccination causes the patient to form antibodies, producing active immunity.

Rubin's test Transuterine insufflation of the fallopian tubes with carbon dioxide to test their patency.

rugae Folds of vaginal mucosa.

sac, amniotic See *amniotic sac.*

sacroiliac Of or pertaining to the sacrum and ilium.

sacrum Triangular bone composed of five united vertebras and situated between L-5 and the coccyx; forms the posterior boundary of the true pelvis.

safe passage Normal uneventful birth process for mother and child.

safe period The days in the menstrual cycle that are not designated as fertile days, i.e., before and after ovulation.

sagittal suture Band of connective tissue separating the parietal bones, extending from the anterior to the posterior fontanel.

salpingo-oophorectomy Removal of a fallopian tube and an ovary.

Schultze's mechanism Delivery of the placenta with the fetal surfaces (shiny in appearance) presenting.

scrotum Pouch of skin containing the testes and parts of the spermatic cords.

secondary areola See *areola, secondary.*

secretory phase of menstrual cycle Postovulatory, luteal, progestational, premenstrual phase of menstrual cycle; 14 days in length.

secundines Fetal membranes and placenta expelled after childbirth; afterbirth.

self-care Patient provides care for self as part of plan of care.

semen Thick, white, viscid secretion discharged from the urethra of the male at orgasm; the transporting medium of the sperm.

semen analysis Examination of semen specimen to determine liquefaction, volume, pH, sperm density, and normal morphology.

sensitization Development of antibodies to a specific antigen.

sensory behavior Responses of the five senses; indicate a readiness for social interaction.

septic abortion See *abortion, septic.*

sepsis Bacterial infections of the bloodstream in infants during the first 4 weeks of life.

sex chromosome Chromosome associated with determination of gender: the X (female) and Y (male) chromosomes. The normal female has two X chromosomes and the normal male has one X and one Y chromosome.

sexual decision-making Selection of choices concerned with intimate and sexual behavior.

sexual history Past and present health conditions, lifestyle behaviors, knowledge, and attitudes related to sex and sexuality.

sexual response cycle The phases of physical changes that occur in response to sexual stimulation and sexual tension release.

sexuality The part of life that has to do with being male or female.

sexually transmitted diseases (STDs) Disease acquired as a result of sexual activity with an infected individual.

shake test "Foam" test for lung maturity of fetus; more rapid than determination of L/S ratio.

sibling rivalry Competition that occurs between brothers and sisters.

sickle cell hemoglobinopathy Abnormal crescent shape red blood corpuscles in the blood.

Sims' position Position in which the patient lies on the left side with the right knee and thigh drawn upward toward the chest.

single-parent family Family form characterized by one parent in the household. This may result from loss of spouse by death, divorce, separation, desertion, or out of wedlock birth of a child.

singleton Pregnancy with a single fetus.

situational crisis Crisis that arises suddenly in response to an external event or a conflict concerning a specific circumstance. The symptoms are transient, and the episode is usually brief.

sitz bath Application of moist heat to the perineum by sitting in a tub or basin filled with warm water.

sleep-wake cycles Variations in states of newborn consciousness.

small for dates (small for gestational age [SGA]) Refers to inadequate growth for gestational age.

smegma Whitish secretion around labia minora.

somatic pain Perineal discomfort resulting from stretching of perineal tissues.

souffle Soft, blowing sound or murmur heard by auscultation.

funic s. Soft, muffled, blowing sound produced by blood rushing through the umbilical vessels and synchronous with the fetal heart sounds.

placental s. Soft, blowing murmur caused by the blood current in the placenta and synchronous with the maternal pulse.

uterine s. Soft, blowing sound made by the blood in the arteries of the pregnant uterus and synchronous with the maternal pulse.

sperm Male sex cell. Also called spermatozoon.

spermatogenesis Process by which mature spermatozoa are formed, during which the diploid chromosome number (46) is reduced by half (haploid, 23).

spermicide Chemical substance that kills sperm by reducing their surface tension, causing the cell wall to break down by a bactericidal effect or by creating a highly acidic environment. Also called spermatocide.

spina bifida occulta Congenital malformation of the spine in which the posterior portion of laminas of the vertebras fails to close but there is no herniation or protrusion of the spinal cord or meninges through the defect. The newborn may have a dimple in the skin or growth of hair over the malformed vertebras.

spinal (saddle) block anesthesia Type of regional anesthesia produced by injection of a local anesthetic solution into the cerebrospinal fluid intrathecal (subarachnoid) space in the spinal canal.

spinnbarkheit Formation of a stretchable thread of cervical mucus under estrogen influence at time of ovulation.

splanchnic engorgement Excessive filling or pooling of blood within the visceral vasculature that occurs after the removal of pressure from the abdomen, e.g., birth of a child, removal of an excess of urine from bladder (1000 ml), removal of large tumor.

spontaneous abortion See *abortion, spontaneous.*

square window Angle of wrist between hypothenar prominence and forearm; one criterion for estimating gestational age of neonate.

standard body weight An appropriate weight for height, a body mass index (BMI) within the normal range.

state-related behavior Behavioral responses dependent on current state of infant.

station Relationship of the presenting fetal part to an imaginary line drawn between the ischial spines of the pelvis.

sterility (1) State of being free from living microorganisms. (2) Complete inability to reproduce offspring.

sterilization Process or act that renders a person unable to produce children.

stillbirth The birth of a baby after 20 weeks' gestation and 1 day and/or 350 gm (depending on the state code) that does not show any signs of life.

striae gravidarum ("stretch marks") Shining reddish lines caused by stretching of the skin, often found on the abdomen, thighs, and breasts during pregnancy. These streaks turn to a fine pinkish white or silver tone in time in fair-skinned women and brownish in darker-skinned women.

subinvolution Failure of a part (e.g., the uterus) to reduce to its normal size and condition after enlargement from functional activity (e.g., pregnancy).

suboccipitobregmatic diameter Smallest diameter of the fetal head—follows a line drawn from the middle of the anterior fontanel to the under surface of the occipital bone.

subtotal hysterectomy See *hysterectomy, subtotal.*

succedaneum See *caput succedaneum.*

supine hypotension Shock; fall in blood pressure caused by impaired venous return when gravid uterus presses on ascending vena cava, when woman is lying flat on her back; vena caval syndrome.

support systems Network from which people receive help in times of crisis.

surfactant Phosphoprotein necessary for normal respiratory function that prevents the alveolar collapse (atelectasis). See also *lecithin* and *L/S ratio.*

suture (1) Junction of the adjoining bones of the skull. (2) Operation uniting parts by sewing them together.

symphysis pubis Fibrocartilaginous union of the bodies of the pubic bones in the midline.

syndactyly Malformation of digits, commonly seen as a fusion of two or more toes to form one structure.

systemic analgesia Analgesics administered either intramuscular (IM) or intravenous (IV) that cross the blood-brain barrier and provide central analgesic effects.

systemic lupus erythematosus A connective tissue disease affecting the mucous membranes, skin, kidneys, and nervous system. It is inflammatory and chronic in nature.

taboo Proscribed (forbidden) by society as improper and unacceptable.

tachypnea Excessively rapid respiratory rate (e.g., in neonates, respiratory rate of 60 breaths/min or more).

taking-in phase Period after birth characterized by the woman's dependency; maternal needs are dominant, talking about the birth is an important task.

taking-hold phase Period after birth characterized by the woman becoming more independent and more interested in learning infant care skills.

talipes equinovarus Deformity in which the foot is extended and the person walks on the toes.

telangiectasia Permanent dilatation of groups of superficial capillaries and venules.

telangiectatic nevi ("stork bites") Clusters of small, red, localized areas of capillary dilatation commonly seen in neonates at the nape of the neck or lower occiput, upper eyelids, and nasal bridge that can be blanched with pressure of a finger.

teratogenic agent Any drug, virus, or irradiation, the exposure to which can cause malformation of the fetus.

teratogens Nongenetic factors that cause malformations and disease syndromes in utero.

teratoma Tumor composed of different kinds of tissue, none of which normally occur together or at the site of the tumor.

term infant Live infant born between weeks 38 and 42 of completed gestation.

testis One of the glands contained in the male scrotum that produces the male reproductive cell, or sperm, and the male hormone testosterone; testicle.

tetany, uterine Extremely prolonged uterine contractions.

thalassemia anemia Affecting Mediterranean and Southeast Asian populations in which there is an insufficient amount of globin produced to fill the red blood cells.

therapeutic abortion See *abortion, therapeutic.*

therapeutic intrauterine insemination See *artificial insemination.*

therapeutic rest Administration of analgesics to decrease pain and induce rest for management of hypertonic uterine dysfunction.

thermogenesis Creation or production of heat, especially in the body.

thermoneutral environment Environment that enables the neonate to maintain a body temperature of 36.5° C (97.7° F) with minimum use of oxygen and energy.

thermoregulation Control of temperature.

threatened abortion See *abortion, threatened.*

thrombocytopenia Abnormal hematologic condition in which the number of platelets is reduced, usually by destruction of erythroid tissue in bone marrow owing to certain neoplastic diseases or to an immune response to a drug.

thrombocytopenic purpura Hematologic disorder characterized by prolonged bleeding time, decreased number of platelets, increased cell fragility, and purpura, which result in hemorrhages into the skin, mucous membranes, organs, and other tissue.

thromboembolism Obstruction of a blood vessel by a clot that has become detached from its site of formation.

thrombophlebitis Inflammation of a vein with secondary clot formation.

thrombus Blood clot obstructing a blood vessel that remains at the place it was formed.

thrush Fungal infection of the mouth or throat characterized by the formation of white patches on a red, moist, inflamed mucous membrane and is caused by *Candida albicans.*

toco- (toko-) Combining form that means childbirth or labor.

tocolytic drug Drug used to suppress preterm labor.

tocotransducer Electronic device for measuring uterine contractions.

TORCH organisms Organisms that damage the embryo or fetus; acronym for *t*oxoplasmosis, *o*ther (e.g., syphilis), *r*ubella, *c*ytomegalovirus, and *h*erpes simplex.

toxemia Term previously used for hypertensive states of pregnancy.

tracheoesophageal fistula Congenital malformation in which there is an abnormal tubelike passage between the trachea and esophagus.

transition—labor Last phase of first stage of labor; 8 to 10 cm cervical dilatation.

transition period—newborn Period from birth to 4 to 6 hours later; infant passes through period of reactivity, sleep, and second period of reactivity.

translocation Condition in which a chromosome breaks and all or part of that chromosome is transferred to a different part of the same chromosome or to another chromosome.

trial of labor (TOL) Period of observation to determine if a laboring woman is likely to be successful in progressing to a vaginal birth.

Trichomonas vaginitis Inflammation of the vagina caused by *Trichomonas vaginalis,* a parasitic protozoon and characterized by persistent burning and itching of the vulvar tissue and a profuse, frothy, white discharge.

trimester Time period of 3 months.

trisomy Condition whereby any given chromosome exists in triplicate instead of the normal duplicate pattern.

trophoblast Outer layer of cells of the developing blastodermic vesicle that develops the trophoderm or feeding layer which will establish the nutrient relationships with the uterine endometrium.

trophoblastic disease A condition in which trophoblastic cells covering the chorionic villi proliferate and undergo cystic changes which may be malignant.

tubal ligation See *ligation, tubal.*

tubercles of Montgomery Small papillae on surface of nipples and areolae that secrete a fatty substance that lubricates the nipples.

twins Two neonates from the same impregnation developed within the same uterus at the same time.

   conjoined t. Twins who are physically united; Siamese twins.

   disparate t. Twins who are different (e.g., in weight) and distinct from one another.

   dizygotic t. Twins developed from two separate ova fertilized by two separate sperm at the same time; fraternal twins.

   monozygotic t. Twins developed from a single fertilized ovum; identical twins.

ultrasonography High frequency sound waves to discern fetal heart rate or placental location or body parts.

ultrasound transducer External signal source for monitoring fetal heart rate electronically.

umbilical cord (funis) Structure connecting the placenta and fetus and containing two arteries and one vein encased in a tissue called *Wharton's jelly.* The cord is ligated at birth and severed; the stump falls off in 4 to 10 days.

umbilicus Navel, or depressed point in the middle of the abdomen that marks the attachment of the umbilical cord during fetal life.

urethra Small tubular structure that drains urine from the bladder.

urinary frequency Need to void often or at close intervals.

urinary meatus Opening, or mouth, of the urethra.

uterine Referring or pertaining to the uterus.

   u. adnexa See *adnexa, uterine.*

   u. bruit Abnormal sound or murmur heard while auscultating the uterus.

   u. ischemia Decreased blood supply to the uterus.

   u. prolapse Falling, sinking, or sliding of the uterus from its normal location in the body.

   u. souffle See *souffle, uterine.*

uteroplacental insufficiency Decline in placental function—exchange of gasses, nutrients, and wastes—leading to fetal hypoxia and acidosis; evidenced by late fetal heart rate decelerations in response to uterine contractions.

uterus Hollow muscular organ in the female designed for the implantation, containment, nourishment of the fetus during its development, and expulsion of fetus during labor and birth.

Couvelaire u. Interstitial myometrial hemorrhage following premature separation (abruptio) of placenta. A purplish-bluish discoloration of the uterus and boardlike rigidity of the uterus are noted.

inversion of the u. See *inversion of the uterus.*

retroflexion of the u. See *retroflexion of the uterus.*

retroversion of the u. See *retroversion of the uterus.*

vaccination Intentional injection of antigenic material given to stimulate antibody production in the recipient.

vacuum curettage Uterine aspiration method of early abortion.

vacuum extraction Birth involving attachment of vacuum cup to fetal head and using negative pressure to assist in birth of the fetus.

vagina Normally collapsed musculomembranous tube that forms the passageway between the uterus and the entrance to the vagina.

vaginal birth after cesarean (VBAC) Giving birth vaginally after having had a previous cesarean birth.

vaginismus Intense, painful spasm of the muscles surrounding the vagina.

valsalva maneuver The process of making a forceful attempt at expulsion while holding one's breath and tightening the abdominal muscles (as in pushing during the second stage of labor).

variability Normal irregularity of fetal cardiac rhythm; short term—beat to beat changes; long term—rhythmic changes (waves) from the baseline, usually 3 to 5 bpm.

varicocele Enlargement of veins of the spermatic cord.

varicosity (varicose veins) Swollen, distended, and twisted veins that may develop in almost any part of the body but are most commonly seen in the legs, caused by pregnancy, obesity, congenital defective venous valves, and occupations requiring much standing.

vasectomy Ligation or removal of a segment of the vas deferens, usually done bilaterally to produce sterility in the male.

VDRL test Abbreviation for Venereal Disease Research Laboratory test, a serological flocculation test for syphilis.

vernix caseosa Protective gray-white fatty substance of cheesy consistency covering the fetal skin.

version Act of turning the fetus in the uterus to change the presenting part and facilitate birth.

podalic v. shifting of the fetus' position so as to bring the feet to the outlet during birth.

vertex Crown or top of the head.

v. presentation Presentation in which the fetal skull is nearest the cervical opening and is born first.

very low-birth-weight (VLBW) Infant weighing 1500 g or less at birth.

viable Capable of living, such as a fetus that has reached a stage of development, usually 22 menstrual (20 weeks of gestation), which will permit it to live outside the uterus.

villi Short, vascular processes or protrusions growing on certain membranous surfaces.

chorionic v. Tiny vascular protrusions on the chorionic surface that project into the maternal blood sinuses of the uterus and that help to form the placenta and secrete hCG.

visceral pain Discomfort from cervical changes and uterine ischemia located over the lower portion of the abdomen and radiates to the lumbar area of the back and down the thighs.

voluntary abortion See *abortion, elective.*

vulva External genitalia of the female that consist of the labia majora, labia minora, clitoris, urinary meatus, and vaginal introitus.

vulvar self-examination (VSE) Systematic examination of the vulva by the patient.

weaning Process of changing from breast-feeding or bottle feeding to drinking from a cup.

Wharton's jelly White, gelatinous material surrounding the umbilical vessels within the cord.

witch's milk Secretion of a whitish fluid for about a week after birth from enlarged mammary tissue in the neonate, presumably resulting from maternal hormonal influences.

womb See *uterus.*

X chromosome Sex chromosome in humans existing in duplicate in the normal female and singly in the normal male.

X linkage Genes located on the X chromosome.

Y chromosome Sex chromosome in the human male necessary for the development of the male gonads.

zona pellucida Inner, thick, membranous envelope of the ovum.

zygote Cell formed by the union of two reproductive cells or gametes; the fertilized ovum resulting from the union of a sperm and an ovum.

Appendices

A Standards for the Nursing Care of Women and Newborns

B NANDA-Approved Nursing Diagnoses (Through the 10th Conference, 1992)

C Nursing Responsibilities in Implementing Intrapartum Fetal Heart Rate Monitoring

D Standard Laboratory Values: Pregnant and Nonpregnant Women

E Human Fetotoxic Chemical Agents

F Standard Laboratory Values in the Neonatal Period

G Relationship of Drugs to Breast Milk and Effect on Infant

H Resources

APPENDIX

A Standards for the Nursing Care of Women and Newborns

I: NURSING PRACTICE

Comprehensive nursing care for women and newborns focuses on helping individuals, families, and communities achieve their optimum health potential. This is best achieved within the framework of the nursing process.

The nurse is responsible for decisions and actions within the domain of nursing practice, which may include:

- integration of the nursing process components of assessment, planning, implementation, and evaluation in all areas of nursing practice;
- individualization and prioritization of nursing care to meet the physical, psychologic, spiritual, and social needs of patients;
- collaboration with the individual, family, and other members of the health care team;
- promotion of a safe and therapeutic environment for both the recipients and providers of nursing care;
- demonstration and validation of competence in nursing practice;
- acquisition of specialized knowledge and skills and additional formal education to provide specialized care; and
- provision for complete and accurate documentation of care.

The written or computerized patient record is the documented means of communication among all members of the health care team. It also promotes continuity of care and provides a mechanism for evaluating care. The record should contain accurate and complete recordings

From NAACOG: *Standards for the nursing care of women and newborns,* ed 4, Washington, DC, 1991, NAACOG.

of the patient's history and physical examination, as well as the nursing plan of care, including goals, interventions, health education, and evaluation of patient and family responses. Additional documentation may include planned follow-up and appropriate referrals. All information contained in the patient record and related to the care of the patient and family is confidential and should be released only according to institutional policy.

Note: To apply this universal standard to a specific area of gynecologic, obstetric, or neonatal nursing practice, refer directly to the specialty-specific nursing practice standards section.

II: HEALTH EDUCATION AND COUNSELING

Health education for the individual, family, and community is an integral part of comprehensive nursing care. Such education encourages participation in, and shared responsibility for, health promotion, maintenance, and restoration.

Comprehensive health education includes:

- identification of the needs and abilities of the learner;
- collaboration with the patient and other health care providers in design, content, and follow-up of the educational plan;
- provision of accurate and current information;
- provision of information based on educationally sound principles of teaching and learning;

- recognition of patient rights, responsibilities, and alternative choices;
- utilization of available educational resources in the practice environment;
- utilization of available educational resources to provide health education information to individuals/families in the community; and
- documentation and evaluation of health education including patient response.

The nurse participates in and/or coordinates the health education and counseling process. It begins with the initial patient contact or admission to the unit or service and is an ongoing, continuous process.

Note: To apply this universal standard to a specific area of gynecologic, obstetric, or neonatal nursing practice, refer directly to the specialty-specific nursing practice standards section.

III: POLICIES, PROCEDURES, AND PROTOCOLS

Written policies, procedures, and protocols clarify the scope of nursing practice and delineate the qualifications of personnel authorized to provide care to women and newborns within the health care setting.

The components of policies, procedures, and protocols are based on:
- recognition of the organization's philosophy;
- recognition of the unit's philosophy;
- coordination with the overall mission of the organization;
- assessment of the practice setting and determination of types of services to be provided;
- incorporation of a multidisciplinary approach in their development;
- identification of specific areas of practice to be addressed;
- reflection of current practice, standards, and local regulations; and
- anticipated use as references for health care providers, orientation of new personnel and students, quality assurance activities, and/or guiding nursing actions in emergency situations.

The development of policies, procedures, and protocols should include consideration of staff availability, skill, and licensure; the physical plant and equipment; effects on other departments; and fiscal impact. Policies, procedures, and protocols should be reviewed and revised at least on an annual basis or more frequently as science/technology changes.

Note: To apply this universal standard to a specific area of gynecologic, obstetric, or neonatal nursing practice, refer directly to the specialty-specific nursing practice standards section.

IV: PROFESSIONAL RESPONSIBILITY AND ACCOUNTABILITY

Comprehensive nursing care for women and newborns is provided by nurses who are clinically competent and accountable for professional actions and legal responsibilities inherent in the nursing role.

Responsibility and accountability for newborns include:
- awareness of changing practices and professional and ethical issues;
- knowledge and clinical skills gained through inservice education, professional continuing education, research data, and professional literature;
- implementation of newly acquired knowledge and skills;
- collaboration through networking and sharing with other professionals;
- participation in the development of standards and policies, procedures, and protocols;
- participation in periodic peer and self-evaluations; and
- recognition of certification as one mechanism for the demonstration of special knowledge within a specialty area of practice.

Legal accountability extends to the:
- nurse practice acts;
- parameters of professional practice established by professional organizations;
- institutional standards;
- legislative changes that affect practice; and
- policies, procedures, and protocols within the practice environment.

V: UTILIZATION OF NURSING PERSONNEL

Nursing care for women and newborns is conducted in practice settings that have qualified nursing staff in sufficient numbers to meet patient-care needs.

Each practice setting should have sufficient nursing personnel to meet patient-care requirements. Nursing staff who provide direct care to women and newborns should be supervised by registered nurses who are clinically proficient in the specialty area of practice. The patient-care unit or service is managed by a professional nurse who is prepared educationally and clinically to assume a leadership position. In all practice settings, the nurse may practice independently or collaboratively with other health care team members. It is essential that nurses know both the responsibilities and the limitations of professional nursing practice specific to the practice setting.

Many variables are considered in determining both the number and type of nursing staff needed for a practice setting. Among these variables are those related to the patient, practice, organization, and personnel. Patient-related variables may include:

- patient demographics and acuity of patients served;
- length of stay;
- educational needs;
- cultural factors and level of comprehension;
- communication barriers; and
- discharge or home care needs.

Practice-related variables may include:

- difference in educational and experiential level of nursing staff;
- nursing philosophy;
- type of nursing care delivery system;
- use of assistive personnel;
- use of nurses in expanded roles; and
- participation in teaching programs.

Organizational variables may include:

- scope of services provided;
- availability of support services;
- patient volume;
- mission or philosophy of the organization;
- risk-management concerns;
- quality assurance programs;
- policies, procedures, and protocols;
- physical plant;
- marketing strategies; and
- fiscal considerations.

Personnel variables relate to the type and number of professional and nonprofessional staff and may include:

- education, skill, and experience of the nursing leadership;
- educational preparation, skill, and experience of staff;
- types and mix of nursing staff;
- availability of qualified alternative staff to deal with emergencies or unanticipated volumes;
- distribution of staff, e.g., temporary reassignment, floating, on-call, cross-training, and supplemental staffing;
- responsibilities for orientation, precepting, or students;
- turnover rates; and
- clinical and technical support.

Competency-based job descriptions should be available for each level of nursing staff. Orientation for all personnel should include a general overview of the organization and specific information about the individual practice setting. Performance evaluations for all personnel should be conducted, documented, and discussed on a regular basis with input from the individual, colleagues, and supervisory staff.

VI: ETHICS

Ethical principles guide the process of decision making for nurses caring for women and newborns at all times and especially when personal or professional values conflict with those of the patient, family, colleagues, or practice setting.

The nurse should have the opportunity to participate in the ethical decision-making process. To participate actively, nurses should:

- clarify their own personal and professional values;
- recognize the difficulty in selecting a course of action that is morally and ethically acceptable to all parties;
- communicate openly and assertively;
- identify options; and
- seek consultations.

Nurses must carefully examine their own value systems, since values influence the decision-making process. Opportunities should be provided in the practice setting for discussion of potential ethical issues. Each practice setting should have a framework for decision making regarding bioethical dilemmas. Ethical dilemmas generally arise when there is a conflict between loyalties, rights, duties, or values.

For nurses, most ethical dilemmas occur when there is a real or perceived requirement to act in a manner contrary to personal values or when care ordered or provided does not seem compatible with the best interest of the patient. Common areas of concern may include:

- nursing autonomy and decision making;
- maternal interests versus fetal interests;
- issues of duty, obligation, and loyalty (for example, employer to employee, professional to public, professional to professional);
- patients' rights to resources, privacy, confidentiality, information, participation in decision making, and refusal of therapy;
- the right to live or die;
- life cycle concerns, including contraception, sterilization, pregnancy termination, genetic manipulation, infanticide, sexuality and choices of lifestyle, and euthanasia;
- fetal or neonatal conditions incompatible with life;
- fetal tissue use; and
- biomedical intervention.

The bioethics literature can provide nurses with strategies to cope with or resolve decisions in situations when conflicts of values occur. For ethical decision-making frameworks to be applied to practice situations, working relationships must be established in which individuals may express their own points of view. All persons potentially affected by an ethical decision have the right to participate in the decision-making process.

VII: RESEARCH

Nurses caring for women and newborns utilize research findings, conduct nursing research, and evaluate nursing practice to improve the outcomes of care.

Knowledge of the research process and participation in scientific inquiry are necessary to

- conduct or participate in the conduct of research according to ethical guidelines;
- use research findings to provide appropriate and safe nursing care;
- use research findings as a basis for validating standards of nursing care;
- evaluate the relevance and application of research findings from nursing and related disciplines; and
- validate the effect of nursing practice on patient outcomes.

VIII: QUALITY ASSURANCE

Quality and appropriateness of patient care are evaluated through a planned assessment program using specific, identified clinical indicators.

Each unit or service should have a written quality assurance plan that reflects a philosophy that is coordinated with the organization's mission and overall quality assurance program. Objectives of the unit-based or service-based quality assurance plan should include:

- assurance of consistent quality patient outcomes;
- identification and correction of potential nursing practice deficiencies;

- promotion of professional nursing practice based on appropriate nursing standards; and
- education and participation of staff in quality assurance activities.

The unit nurse manager is responsible for developing and implementing the unit-based quality assurance plan. The plan should include:

- responsibilities of all personnel in the quality assurance process;
- the scope of service provided;
- important aspects of care or service involving high-risk, high-volume, and problem-prone patients or activities;
- clinical indicators or measurable standards that affect the aspects of care and service that have been identified as important;
- specific criteria and thresholds for use in monitoring clinical indicators;
- methods for the collection and analysis of data, including reference to collection tools, sample size, time frame, and staff responsibility;
- determination of appropriate corrective action, when indicated, that will fall into one of three categories; educational, organizational, or behavioral change;
- follow-up assessment of identified problems;
- documentation of all aspects of the quality assurance program, including results; and
- a process for communication related to quality assurance activities within the total organization.

B NANDA-Approved Nursing Diagnoses

Activity intolerance
Activity intolerance, high risk for
Adjustment, impaired
Airway clearance, ineffective
Anxiety
Aspiration, high risk for
Body image disturbance
Body temperature, altered, high risk for
Bowel incontinence
Breastfeeding, effective
Breastfeeding, ineffective
Breastfeeding, interrupted
Breathing pattern, ineffective
Cardiac output, decreased
Caregiver role strain
Caregiver role strain, high risk for
Communication, impaired verbal
Constipation
Constipation, colonic
Constipation, perceived
Coping, defensive
Coping, family, potential for growth
Coping, ineffective family, compromised
Coping, ineffective family, disabling
Coping, ineffective individual
Decisional conflict (specify)
Denial, ineffective
Diarrhea
Disuse syndrome, high risk for
Diversional activity deficit
Dysfunctional ventilatory weaning response (DVWR)
Dysreflexia

Family processes, altered
Fatigue
Fear
Fluid volume deficit (1)
Fluid volume deficit (2)
Fluid volume deficit, high risk for
Fluid volume excess
Gas exchange, impaired
Grieving, anticipatory
Grieving, dysfunctional
Growth and development, altered
Health maintenance, altered
Health-seeking behaviors (specify)
Home maintenance management, impaired
Hopelessness
Hyperthermia
Hypothermia
Incontinence, functional
Incontinence, reflex
Incontinence, stress
Incontinence, total
Incontinence, urge
Infant feeding pattern, ineffective
Infection, high risk for
Injury, high risk for
Knowledge deficit (specify)
Mobility, impaired physical
Noncompliance (specify)
Nutrition, altered, less than body requirements
Nutrition, altered, more than body requirements
Nutrition, altered, high risk for more than body requirements
Oral mucous membrane, altered
Pain
Pain, chronic

Parental role conflict
Parenting, altered
Parenting, altered, high risk for
Peripheral neurovascular dysfunction, high risk for
Personal identity disturbance
Poisoning, high risk for
Posttrauma response
Powerlessness
Protection, altered
Rape-trauma syndrome
Rape-trauma syndrome, compound reaction
Rape-trauma syndrome, silent reaction
Role performance, altered
Self-care deficit, bathing/hygiene
Self-care deficit, dressing/grooming
Self-care deficit, feeding
Self-care deficit, toileting
Self-esteem disturbance
Self-esteem, chronic low
Self-esteem, situational low
Self-mutilation, high risk for
Sensory/perceptual alterations (specify) (visual, auditory, kinesthetic, gustatory, tactile, olfactory)
Sexual dysfunction
Sexuality patterns, altered
Skin integrity, impaired
Skin integrity, impaired, high risk for
Sleep pattern disturbance
Social interaction, impaired
Social isolation
Spiritual distress (distress of the human spirit)

(Through the 10th Conference, 1992)

Stress syndrome, relocation

Suffocation, high risk for

Swallowing, impaired

Therapeutic regimen (individual), ineffective management of

Thermoregulation, ineffective

Thought processes, altered

Tissue integrity, impaired

Tissue perfusion, altered (specific type) (renal, cerebral, cardiopulmonary, gastrointestinal, peripheral)

Trauma, high risk for

Unilateral neglect

Urinary elimination, altered patterns

Urinary retention

Ventilation, inability to sustain spontaneous

Violence, high risk for, self-directed or directed at others

C Nursing Responsibilities in Implementing Intrapartum Fetal Heart Rate Monitoring

The primary goal of perinatal care is to ensure optimal maternal and neonatal outcomes. The intrapartum period represents a time of risk for the mother and the fetus. Assessment of fetal heart rate (FHR) has been recognized as a vital aspect in the evaluation of fetal well-being in response to the stresses of labor and birth.

Auscultation and electronic fetal monitoring (EFM) are the basic techniques used to assess FHR. Each method has its advantages and limitations, necessitating individualized decision making for appropriate use. The method of FHR monitoring selected and the frequency of FHR evaluation should be based on consideration of maternal-fetal risk factors and the availability of nursing personnel who are skilled in the monitoring techniques. The patient's preference regarding the method of FHR monitoring should be taken into consideration.

Nurses who perform FHR monitoring are responsible for their actions and will be held to the established standards of care as defined by their professional organizations, the standards of practice in their institutions, and the scope of practice as defined by their nurse practice act.

METHODOLOGY

Auscultation of the FHR is an auditory assessment procedure that, when properly performed, allows evaluation of FHR both during and immediately following the stress of a uterine contraction. Auscultation between contractions establishes the baseline FHR. Auscultation as a primary technique of FHR surveillance requires a thorough knowledge of the basic principles of the fetal heart and uterine physiology and pathophysiology. Clini-

cal experience in the recognition of and the response to significant FHR changes is required. Validation of competency in the use of this technique must be in accordance with established institutional policy.

Intermittent auscultation of the fetal heart with a 1:1 nurse patient ratio at 15-minute intervals during the active phase of the first stage of labor and at 5-minute intervals during the second stage has been shown to be equivalent to EFM (American Academy of Pediatrics and The American College of Obstetricians and Gynecologists [ACOG], 1992). For low-risk patients, the suggested auscultation frequency is 30-minute intervals in active first-stage labor and 15-minute intervals in second-stage labor (NAACOG,* 1990). For high-risk patients, the suggested auscultation frequency is 15-minute intervals in active first-stage labor and 5-minute intervals in second-stage labor (NAACOG, 1990). Therefore, if auscultation is prescribed as the primary technique of FHR surveillance in the second stage of labor, a minimum of a 1:1 nurse-fetus ratio is required.

EFM is an auditory and visual assessment procedure that provides data for the evaluation of uterine activity and fetal heart responses, including baseline heart rate, variability, and FHR change over time. Further, EFM produces a printed record. The use of EFM requires knowledge of its equipment and thorough knowledge of the basic principles of the fetal heart and uterine physiology and pathophysiology. Nurses who use EFM must be able to recognize FHR patterns, variability, and uterine activity.

---

*Approved by the Executive Board, October 1988. Revised February 1992. Reaffirmed 1994. NAACOG became the Association for Women's Health, Obstetric, and Neonatal Nurses in January 1993.

Fetal monitoring patterns have been given descriptive names, for example, accelerations and early, late, and variable decelerations. Nurses should use these terms in written chart documentation and verbal communication. Deviations from a normal heart rate pattern should be documented. When such changes in a FHR pattern occur, the nurse also should document a subsequent return to a normal pattern.

The patient's medical record should include observations and assessments of FHR and characteristics of uterine activity, as well as specific actions taken when changes in FHR patterns are observed. The monitor tracing is a legal part of the medical record and should include identifying information about the patient, as well as times and events related to the patient's ongoing care.

After identification of a nonreassuring pattern, the nurse is responsible for initiating and documenting appropriate nursing interventions as indicated by the pattern identified and for notifying a physician or certified nurse-midwife. Documentation of such notification should be entered in the patient's medical record. The nurse can expect the physician or certified nurse-midwife to respond after being notified of a nonreassuring pattern. An institutional policy should be established for the nurse to follow in the event that the physician or certified nurse-midwife is unable to respond in a timely fashion.

Core competencies in FHR monitoring have been published by NAACOG (1991). Competency validation of this expertise must be in accordance with established institutional policy (NAACOG, 1988).

EVALUATION AND DOCUMENTATION

The institution should establish policies, procedures, and protocols that define evaluation and documentation of FHR monitoring. In developing policies, procedures, and protocols, the institution should address the following:

- method(s) for assessment (EFM, auscultation, or a combination of both)
- maternal-fetal risk factors
- stage of labor
- frequency of assessment
- qualifications of health care providers performing assessments
- nurse-fetus ratios
- methods of documentation

Documentation of the evaluation of FHR monitoring information during labor is applicable regardless of the method of monitoring selected and may be accomplished in narrative nurses' notes and/or by the use of comprehensive flow sheets at the time of assessment. Documentation also may be achieved by the use of abbreviated nurses' notes with follow-up summary nurses' notes at intervals specified by institutional policy. The format for abbreviated notes may include initialing the EFM tracing, annotating the EFM tracing, or annotating basic flow sheets.

Suggested frequencies for interval evaluation of FHR information using auscultation have been addressed. For high-risk patients being monitored with auscultation during the active phase of the first stage and during the second stage of labor, intervals for both the evaluation and recording of FHR information are suggested at 15 and 5 minutes, respectively (NAACOG, 1990). For the same group of patients being monitored electronically, evaluation of the tracing is suggested at the same intervals (ACOG, 1989). For low-risk patients being monitored with auscultation, the suggested intervals for evaluation and recording are at 30 and 15 minutes in the active phase of the first and the second stage of labor, respectively. The standard practice for low-risk patients being monitored electronically is to evaluate and record the FHR at least every 30 minutes following a contraction in the active phase of the first stage of labor and at least every 15 minutes in the second stage of labor (ACOG, 1989).

Evaluation of FHR information may take place at the intervals suggested above or more frequently as necessitated by the individual patient-care situation. Written documentation of these FHR evaluations, however, may occur at longer intervals in narrative, abbreviated, and/or summary formats, in accordance with institutional policy and procedure.

CONFLICT RESOLUTION

The potential for conflict exists in terms of professional judgment and decision making regarding which method of monitoring is best for a particular patient in a given situation. Institutional policies, procedures, and protocols must provide a mechanism that will allow nurses the flexibility to decline to implement the prescribed method of FHR monitoring if any question exists regarding the ability to meet the required staffing ratios or if the methodology is beyond the individual nurse's expertise. Ultimately, the responsibility for implementing the prescribed method of FHR monitoring remains with the prescriber. In the event of differences of opinion among professionals regarding the ability to implement the prescribed method, the established institutional policy for resolution of conflict should be followed.

References

American Academy of Pediatrics and American College of Obstetricians and Gynecologists: *Guidelines for Perinatal Care,* ed 3, Washington, DC, 1992, American Academy of Pediatrics and ACOG.

Nurses Association of the American College of Obstetricians and Gynecologists: *OGN nursing practice resource: fetal heart rate auscultation,* Washington, DC, 1990, NAACOG.

Nurses Association of the American College of Obstetricians and Gynecologists: *Nursing practice competencies and educational guidelines: antepartum fetal surveillance and intrapartum fetal heart monitoring,* Washington, DC, 1991, NAACOG.

Nurses Association of the American College of Obstetricians and Gynecologists: *Essentials of electronic fetal monitoring competency validation,* Washington, DC, 1991, NAACOG.

American College of Obstetricians and Gynecologists: *ACOG technical bulletin: intrapartum fetal heart rate monitoring,* Number 132, Washington, DC, 1989, ACOG.

D

Standard Laboratory Values: Pregnant and Nonpregnant Women

	NONPREGNANT	PREGNANT
HEMATOLOGIC VALUES		
Complete Blood Count (CBC)		
Hemoglobin, g/dl	12 to 16*	>11*
Hematocrit, PCV, %	37 to 47	>33
Red cell volume, ml	1600	1500 to 1900
Plasma volume, ml	2400	3700
Red blood cell count, million/mm³	4.2 to 5.4	4.2 to 5.4
White blood cells, total per mm³	5000 to 10,000	5000 to 15,000
Polymorphonuclear cells, %	55 to 70	60 to 85
Lymphocytes, %	20 to 40	15 to 40
Erythrocyte sedimentation rate, mm/h	20/hr	Elevated second and third trimesters
MCHC, g/dl packed RBCs (mean corpuscular hemoglobin concentration)	32 to 36	No change
MCH/(mean corpuscular hemoglobin per picogram [less than a nanogram])	27 to 31	No change
MCV/μm³ (mean corpuscular volume per cubic micrometer)	80 to 95	No change
Blood coagulation and fibrinolytic activity†		
Factors VII, VIII, IX, X		Increase in pregnancy, return to normal in early puerperium; factor VIII increases during and immediately after birth
Factors XI, XIII		Decrease in pregnancy
Prothrombin time (PT)	12 to 14 sec	Slight decrease in pregnancy
Partial thromboplastin time (PTT)	60 to 70 sec	Slight decrease in pregnancy and again decrease during second and third stage of labor (indicates clotting at placental site)
Bleeding time	1 to 3 min (Duke) 2 to 4 min (Ivy)	No appreciable change
Coagulation time	6 to 10 min (Lee/White)	No appreciable change
Platelets	150,000 to 400,000/mm³	No significant change until 3 to 5 days after birth, then marked increase (may predispose woman to thrombosis) and gradual return to normal
Fibrinolytic activity		Decreases in pregnancy then abrupt return to normal (protection against thromboembolism)

*At sea level. Permanent residents of higher levels (e.g., Denver) require higher levels of hemoglobin.
†Pregnancy represents a hypercoagulable state.

	NONPREGNANT	PREGNANT
Fibrinogen	300 mg/dl	600 mg/dl
Mineral/Vitamin Concentrations		
Vitamin B$_{12}$, folic acid, ascorbic acid	Normal	Moderate decrease
Serum proteins		
Total, g/dl	6.0 to 8.0	5.5 to 7.5
Albumin, g/dl	3.2 to 4.5	3 to 5
Globulin, total, g/dl	2.3 to 3.4	3 to 4
Blood sugar		
Fasting, mg/dl	115	65
2-hour postprandial, mg/dl	70 to 140	Under 140 after a 100 g carbohydrate meal is considered normal
CARDIOVASCULAR DETERMINATIONS		
Blood pressure, mm Hg	90 to 140/60 to 90	114/65 during midtrimester, then return to usual value by end of third trimester
Pulse, rate/min	70	80
Stroke volume, ml	45±12	75
Cardiac output, L/min	3.6	6
Circulation time (arm-tongue), sec	15 to 16	12 to 14
Blood volume, ml		
Whole blood	4000	5600
Plasma	2400	3700
Red blood cells	1600	1900
Chest x-ray studies		
Transverse diameter of heart	—	1 to 2 cm increase
Left border of heart	—	Straightened
Cardiac volume	—	70 ml increase
HEPATIC VALUES		
Bilirubin total	Not more than 1 mg/dl	Unchanged
Serum cholesterol	150 to 200 mg/dl	↑ 60% from 16 to 32 weeks of pregnancy; remains at this level until after birth
Serum alkaline phosphatase	2 to 4.5 units (Bodansky)	↑ from week 12 of pregnancy to 6 weeks after birth
Serum globulin albumin	2.3 to 3.4 g/dl	↑ slight
	3.2 to 4.5 g/dl	↓ 3.0 g by late pregnancy
RENAL VALUES		
Bladder capacity	1300 ml	1500 ml
Renal plasma flow (RPF), ml/min	490 to 700	Increase by 25%
Glomerular filtration rate (GFR), ml/min	88 to 128	Increase by 50%
Nonprotein nitrogen (NPN), mg/dl	25 to 40	Decreases
Blood urea nitrogen (BUN), mg/dl	10 to 20	Decreases
Serum creatinine, mg/kg/24 hr	20 to 22	Decreases
Serum uric acid, mg/kg/24 hr	250 to 750	Decreases
Urine glucose	Negative	Present in 20% of pregnant women
Intravenous pyelogram (IVP)	Normal	Slight-to-moderate hydroureter and hydronephrosis; right kidney larger than left kidney

APPENDIX

E Human Fetotoxic Chemical Agents

MATERNAL MEDICATION	REPORTED EFFECTS ON FETUS OR NEONATE
ANALGESICS	
Indomethacin (Indocin)	Prolongs gestation (monkey); in neonates, used to close patent ductus arteriosus
Narcotics	70% of maternal level; death, apnea, depression, bradycardia, hypothermia
Salicylates	Death in utero; hemorrhage, methomoglobinemia, ↓ albumin-binding capacity, salicylate intoxication, difficult birth, (?) prolonged gestation
ANESTHESIAS	
Conduction	Indirect effect of maternal hypotension; direct effect—convulsions, death, acidosis, bradycardia, myocardial depression, fetal hypotension, methemoglobinemia
Paracervical	Methemoglobinemia, fetal acidosis, bradycardia, neurologic depression, myocardial depression
ANTICOAGULANTS	
Coumarins	Fetal death, hemorrhage, calcifications
ANTICONVULSANT AGENTS	
Barbiturates	Irritability and tremulousness 4 to 5 months after birth, hemorrhage, enzyme inducer
Phenytoin and barbiturate	Congenital malformations, cleft lip and palate, congenital heart disease (CHD), CNS and skeletal anomalies, failure to thrive, enzyme inducer, hemorrhage
ANTIMICROBIALS	All antimicrobials cross placenta
Ampicillin	↓ Maternal urinary and plasma estriol levels
Chloramphenicol	Crosses placenta with no reported effect; interferes with biotransformation of tolbutamide, phenytoin, biohydroxycoumarin (i.e., hypoglycemia may occur if used in combination)
Chloroquine	Death, deafness, retinal hemorrhage
Erythromycin	Possible hepatic injury
Nitrofurantoin	Megaloblastic anemia, G6PD deficiency
Novobiocin	Hyperbilirubinemia
Streptomycin	Therapeutic levels reached, nerve deafness
Sulfonamides	Icterus, hemolytic anemia, kernicterus, growth retardation (?), thrombocytopenia
Tetracycline	Placental transfer after 4 months' gestation; enamel hypoplasia, delay in bone growth, congenital cataract (?)
ANTITUBERCULOSIS	
Isoniazid	Toxic blood level in fetus; no reported effect; mother should be on pyridoxine supplement
Pyridoxine	*See* vitamins

MATERNAL MEDICATION	REPORTED EFFECTS ON FETUS OR NEONATE
CANCER CHEMOTHERAPEUTIC AGENTS	
Aminopterin 6-Mercaptopurine Methotrexate	Abortion, congenital anomalies (first trimester); combination of drugs detrimental to fetus; skeletal and cranial malformations, hydrocephalus; questionable long-term effects such as slow somatic growth; ovarian agenesis; ↓ immune mechanisms
CARDIOVASCULAR AGENTS	
Digitoxin	Placental transfer, no reported effect
Propranolol	Indirect effect of delay in cervical dilatation
CHOLINESTERASE INHIBITORS	Myasthenia-like symptoms for 1 week; muscle weakness in 10% to 20% of infants
Cigarette smoking	Effect equal to number of cigarettes smoked; ↑ incidence of stillbirth; low-birth-weight; effect on later somatic growth and mental development (?); reduction in O_2 transport to fetus
DIURETICS	
Ammonium chloride Thiazide	Maternal and fetal acidosis; thrombocytopenia, hemorrhage, hypoelectrolytemia, convulsions, respiratory distress, death, hemolysis
DRUGS OF ABUSE (USUALLY MULTIPLE DRUGS CONSUMED)	
Alcohol	Blood level equal to mother's; convulsions, withdrawal syndrome, hyperactivity, crying, irritability, poor sucking reflex, low-birth-weight; cleft palate, ophthalmic malformation, malformation of extremities and heart; poor mental performance, microencephaly, small for dates, growth deficiency
Barbiturates	Withdrawal symptoms, convulsions, onset immediately after birth or at 2 weeks of age
Cocaine	Abruptio placentae, preterm labor
"Ice"—methamphetamine	Preterm labor, IUGR, abnormal sleep patterns, poor feeding, tremors, hypertonia
LSD (lysergic acid diethylamide)	Chromosome breakage, limb and skeletal anomalies

Narcotics
  Heroin
  Methadone
	Small for dates, 4% to 10% mortality, habituation, withdrawal symptoms, convulsions, sudden infant death syndrome (SIDS), indirect effect of maternal complications (i.e., infection, hepatitis, STD), permanent effect on somatic growth (?)

HORMONES	
Androgens Estrogens Progestins	Labioscrotal fusion before week 12; after 12 weeks, phallic enlargement; other anomalies (?); ↑ bilirubin (?), vaginal cancer; cleft lip and palate, CHD; tracheo-esophageal fistula and atresia; cancer of prostate, testes, and bladder
Corticosteroids	Adrenal insufficiency, cleft palate, small-for-dates infant
Ovulatory agents	Anencephaly (?), chromosomal abnormalities in abortus (?), multiple pregnancy
PSYCHOTROPIC DRUGS	
Diazepam (Valium)	High fetal levels; hypotonia, poor sucking reflex, hypothermia; ↑ low Apgar score; ↑ resuscitation, ↑ assisted births; dose related
Lithium carbonate	Neonatal serum levels reach adult toxic range; lethargy, cyanosis for 10 days; teratogenic—dose related
RADIATION	Microencephaly, mental retardation, many unknown effects; nondisjunction of chromosomes
SEDATIVES	
Barbiturate	Apnea, depression, depressed EEG, poor sucking reflex, slow weight gain; concentration of drug in brain; enzyme inducer, lower bilirubin level
Bromides	Growth failure, lethargy, dilated pupils, dermatitis, hypotonia, ? effect on mental development
Magnesium sulfate	Neonatal blood level does not correlate with clinical condition; respiratory depression, hypotonia, convulsions, death; exchange transfusion may be required
Paraldehyde	Apnea, depression
Thalidomide	Administered between days 34 and 50 of gestation causes phocomelia, malformation of cord, angiomas of face, CHD, intestinal stenosis, eye defects, absence of appendix

MATERNAL MEDICATION	REPORTED EFFECTS ON FETUS OR NEONATE
TOXINS	
Carbon monoxide	Stillbirth, brain damage equal to anoxia
Heavy metals	
Arsenic	Concentrated in brain
Lead	Abortion, growth retardation, congenital anomalies, sterility
Mercury	Cerebral palsy, mental retardation, convulsions, involuntary movements, defective vision; mother asymptomatic
Naphthalene	Hemolysis
VITAMINS	
A and D	Congenital anomalies
K (water-soluble analogs)	Icterus, anemia, kernicterus
Pyridoxine	Withdrawal seizures

Modified from Babson SG et al: *Diagnosis and management of the fetus and neonate at risk: a guide for team care,* ed 4, St Louis, 1980, Mosby.

F Standard Laboratory Values in the Neonatal Period

	NEONATAL	

1. HEMATOLOGIC VALUES

Clotting factors

Activated clotting time (ACT)	2 min	
Bleeding time (Ivy)	2 to 7 min	
Clot retraction	Complete 1 to 4 hr	
Fibrinogen	125-300 mg/dl*	

	TERM	PRETERM
Hemoglobin (g/dl)	14.5 to 22.5	15 to 17
Hematocrit (%)	44 to 72	45 to 55
Reticulocytes (%)	0.4 to 6	Up to 10
Fetal hemoglobin (% of total)	40 to 70	80 to 90
Nucleated RBC/mm^3 (per 100 RBC)	200(0.05)	(0.2)
Platelet count/mm^3	84,000 to 478,000	120,000 to 180,000
WBC/mm^3	9000 to 30,000	10,000 to 20,000
Neutrophils (%)	54 to 62	47
Eosinophils and basophils (%)	1 to 3	
Lymphocytes (%)	25 to 33	33
Monocytes (%)	3 to 7	4
Immature WBC (%)	10	16

	NEONATAL	

2. BIOCHEMICAL VALUES

Bilirubin, direct			0 to 1 mg/dl
Bilirubin, total	Cord:		<2 mg/dl
	Peripheral blood:	0 to 1 day	6 mg/dl
		1 to 2 day	8 mg/dl
		3 to 5 day	12 mg/dl
Blood gases		Arterial:	pH 7.31 to 7.45
			P$_{CO_2}$ 33 to 48 mm Hg
			P$_{O_2}$ 50 to 70 mm Hg
		Venous:	pH 7.28 to 7.42
			P$_{CO_2}$ 38 to 52 mm Hg
			P$_{O_2}$ 20 to 49 mm Hg
α_1-fetoprotein			0
Fibrinogen			150 to 300 mg/dl
Serum glucose mg/dl			40 to 60 mg/dl

*dl refers to decilter (1dl=100ml); this conforms to the SI system (standardized international measurements)

	NORMAL RANGES NEWBORN

3. URINALYSIS

Color	Clear, straw
Specific gravity	1.001 = 1.018
pH	5 to 7
Protein	Negative
Glucose	Negative
Ketones	Negative
RBC	Rare
WBC	0 to 4
Casts	Rare
17-Ketosteroids	Under 1
17-Hydroxycorticosteroids	Same
Urinary calcium	5 mg/kg body weight
Urinary sodium	20% of adult values
Urinary vanillymandelic acid (VMA)	1.40 to 15.0

Volume: 20 to 40 ml executed daily in the first few days; by week 1, 24-hour wrine volume close to 200 ml.
Protein: may be present in first 2 to 4 days.
Casts and WBCs: may be present in first 2 to 4 days.
Osmolarity: (m Osm/L): 100 to 600.Protein

4. URINE SCREENING TESTS FOR INBORN ERRORS OF METABOLISM

Benedict's test: for reducing substances in the urine—glucose, galactose, fructose, lactose; phenylketonuria, alkapto-nuria, tyrosyluria, and tryosinosis may give a positive Benedict's test result.

Ferric chloride test: an immediate, green color for phenylketonuria, histidinemia, and tyrosinuria, a gray to green color for presence of phenothiazines, isoniazid, red to purple color for presence of salicylates or ketone bodies.

Dinitrophenylhydrazine test: for phenylketonuria, maple syrup urine disease, Lowe's syndrome.

Cetyltrimethyl ammonium bromide test: for mucopolysaccharides: immediate positive reaction in gargoylism (Hurler's syndrome); delayed, moderately positive reaction for Marfan's, Morquio-Ullrich, and Murdoch syndromes.

Metachromatic stain (or *urine sediment*): Granules (free or as inclusion bodies in cells) are seen in metachromatic leukodystrophy; may also be seen rarely in Tay-Sachs and other lipid diseases of the central nervous system.

Amino acid chromatography: Aminoaciduria may be normal in newborns; chromatography may be helpful to detect hypophosphatasia and argininosuccinicaciduria.

Diaper test, Phenistix test, and *Dinitrophenyl-hydrazine (DNPH) test:* simple, inexpensive tests for PKU (phenylketon-uria): used for screening; most useful when infant is at least 6 weeks of age.

5. BLOOD SERUM PHENYLALANINE TESTS

Guthrie inhibition assay methods: drops of blood placed on filter paper; laboratory uses bacterial growth inhibition test; phenylalanine level above 8 mg/dl blood: diagnostic of PKU. Effective in newborn period; used also to monitor PKU diet; blood easily obtained by heel or finger puncture; inexpensive; used for wide-scale screening

G Relationship of Drugs to Breast Milk and Effect on Infant

The drugs listed in this appendix have been categorized by their major use. The ratings given are those published by the American Academy of Pediatrics Committee on Drugs (AAP). These ratings label drugs that transfer into human milk. Drugs without a rating were not included in the AAP list. The ratings are described as:

1 Drugs that are contraindicated during breastfeeding
2 Drugs of abuse that are contraindicated during breastfeeding
3 Radioactive compounds that require temporary cessation of breastfeeding
4 Drugs with unknown effects on breastfeeding, but may be of concern
5 Drugs that have been associated with significant effects on some nursing infants and should be given to breastfeeding mothers with caution
6 Maternal medication usually compatible with breastfeeding
7 Food and environmental agents: effect on breastfeeding

DRUG	EXCRETED IN MILK	% ADULT DOSE IN MILK	AAP RATING	COMMENTS
ANALGESICS AND ANTIINFLAMMATORY DRUGS (NONNARCOTIC)				
Acetaminophen (Datril, Tylenol)	Yes	0.04 to 1.85	6	Detoxified in liver. Avoid in immediate postbirth period; otherwise no problems with therapeutic dose.
Aspirin (Bayer, Anacin, Bufferin, Excedrin, etc.)	Yes	10.55 ± 10.45	6	Long history of experience shows complications rare. Can cause interference with platelet aggregation and diminished factor XII (Hageman factor) at birth. When mother requires high, continuing level of medication for arthritis, aspirin is drug of choice. Observe infant for bruisability. Platelet aggregation can be evaluated. Salicylism only seen in maternal overdosing. Mother should increase vitamin C and vitamin K intake.
Ibuprofen (Advil, Nuprin, Motrin, etc.)	Yes	<0.8	6	No apparent effects in therapeutic doses.
Indomethacin (Indocin)	Yes	0.11 to 0.98	6	Convulsions in breastfed neonate (case report). Used to close patent ductus arteriosus. Insufficient data as to effect on other vessels. May be nephrotoxic.

DRUG	EXCRETED IN MILK	% ADULT DOSE IN MILK	AAP RATING	COMMENTS
Mefenamic acid (Ponstel)	Yes	0.036 to 0.8	6	No apparent effect on infant at therapeutic doses; infant able to excrete via urine.
Naproxen (Naproxyn, Anaprox, Naprosyn, Aleve)	Yes	1.1		Less toxic in adults than some other organic derivatives.
Propoxyphene (Darvon)	Yes	Trace amounts	6	Only symptoms detectable would be failure to feed and drowsiness. On daily, around-the-clock dosage, infant could consume 1 mg/day.

ANTIINFECTIVES (MAY CHANGE INTESTINAL FLORA OF INFANT AND SENSITIZE FOR LATER ALLERGIC REACTION.)

DRUG	EXCRETED IN MILK	% ADULT DOSE IN MILK	AAP RATING	COMMENTS
Acyclvir (Zovirax)	Yes	5.6 + 4.4	6	Minimal absorption through maternal skin.
Ampicillin (Polycillin, Amcill, Omnipen, Penbritin)	Yes	0.05 to 0.04		Sensitivity resulting from repeated exposure; diarrhea or secondary candidiasis.
Carbenicillin (Pyopen, Geopen)	Yes	0.001		Levels not significant. Drug is given to neonate. Not well absorbed from GI tract.
Cefazolin (Ancef, Kefzol)	Yes	0.075	6	Probably not significant. Detected in milk if given IV.
Cephalexin (Keflex)	Yes	0.86 ± 0.35		Completely gone by 8 hours; absorption less in first few months.
Cephalothin (Keflin)	Yes	0.4		Negligible.
Chloramphenicol (Chloromycetin)	Yes	1.6	4	Gray syndrome. Infant does not excrete drug well, and small amounts may accumulate. Contraindicated. May be tolerated in older infant with mature glycuronide system.
Colistin (Colymycin)	Yes	0.07		Not absorbed orally.
Demeclocycline (Declomycin)	Yes	Trace		Not significant in therapeutic doses. Can be given to infants. Drug remains in milk 3 days after dose.
Erythromycin (Ilosone, E-Mycin, Erythrocin)	Yes	0.1 to 2.1	6	Higher concentrations have been reported in milk than in plasma. Should not be given under 1 month of age because of risk of jaundice. Dose in milk higher when given IV to mother.
Gentamicin	Yes	Trace		Not absorbed from gastrointestinal tract, may change gut flora. Drug is given to newborns directly.
Isoniazid (Nydrazid)	Yes	2.3		Infant at risk for toxicity, but need for breast milk may outweigh risk.
Kanamycin (Kantrex)	Yes	0.95	6	Infant absorbs little from gastrointestinal tract. Infants can be given drug.
Metronidazole (Flagyl)	Yes	0.13 to 36	4	Caution should be exercised because of its high milk concentrations. Contraindicated when infant under 6 months; may cause neurologic disorders and blood dyscrasia. AAP says to discard milk for 12 hours if mother takes 2 g dose.
Nitrofurantoin (Furadantin, Macrodantin)	Yes	0.6	6	Not significant in therapeutic doses to affect child except in G6PD deficiency.
Novobiocin (Albamycin, Cathomycin)	Yes	0.15		Infant can be given drug directly.

DRUG	EXCRETED IN MILK	% ADULT DOSE IN MILK	AAP RATING	COMMENTS
Nystatin (Mycostatin)	No	Not absorbed orally		Can be given to infant directly.
Oxacillin (Prostaphlin)	No	Trace		
Penicillin G, benzathine (Bicillin)	Yes	0.8		Clinical need should supersede possible allergic responses.
Penicillin G, potassium	Yes	0.8		Infant can be given penicillin directly. Parents should be told to inform physician that infant has been exposed to penicillin because of potential sensitivity.
Streptomycin	Yes	0.5	6	Not to be given more than 2 weeks. Ototoxic and nephrotoxic with long use. Is given to infants directly.
Sulfisoxazole (Gantrisin)	Yes	0.45	6	To be avoided during first month after birth; may cause kernicterus.
Tetracycline HC1 (Achromycin, Panmycin, Sumycin)	Yes	0.3 to 4.8	6	Not enough to treat an infection in an infant. May cause discoloration of the teeth in the infant; the antibiotic, however, may be largely bound to the milk calcium. Do not give longer than 10 days or repeatedly.

ANTICOAGULANTS

DRUG	EXCRETED IN MILK	% ADULT DOSE IN MILK	AAP RATING	COMMENTS
Coumarin derivatives Dicumarol (bishydroxycoumarin) Warfarin (Panwarfin)	Yes	0.5	6	Monitor prothrombin time. Give vitamin K to infant. Discontinue if surgery or trauma occurs. Drug of choice if mother to continue breastfeeding. May cause bleeding.
Heparin	No			Heparin ineffective orally.

Anticonvulsants and Sedatives (barbiturates may pass into milk but do not sedate infant)

DRUG	EXCRETED IN MILK	% ADULT DOSE IN MILK	AAP RATING	COMMENTS
Magnesium sulfate	Yes	0.5	6	May produce sedation in infant.
Pentobarbital (Nembutal)	Yes	Traces		Depends on liver for detoxification so may accumulate in first week of life until infant is able to detoxify. No problem for older infant in usual doses.
Phenytoin (Dilantin)	Yes	1.4 to 7.2	6	No problem if mother's dose is in therapeutic range.
Phenobarbital (Luminal)	Yes	1.5	5	Sleepiness and decreased sucking possible. On usual analeptic doses infants alert and feed well. On hypnotic doses infants depressed and difficult to rouse.
Sodium bromide (Bromo-Seltzer and across-the-counter sleeping aids)	Yes		6,7	Drowsy, decreased crying, rash, decreased feeding. No longer available in the United States.

Antihistamines (may suppress lactation; administer after nursing; all pass into breast milk.)

DRUG	EXCRETED IN MILK	% ADULT DOSE IN MILK	AAP RATING	COMMENTS
Brompheniramine (Dimetane)	Yes	Unknown		Drugs used in neonates. May cause sedation, decreased feeding, or may produce stimulation and tachycardia. Should avoid long-acting preparations, which may accumulate in infant.
Diphenhydramine (Benadryl)	Yes	Unknown		When combined with decongestants, may cause decrease in milk.
Promethazine (Phenergan)	Yes	Unknown	6	Passage into breast is expected; increases serum prolactin levels.

AUTONOMIC DRUGS

DRUG	EXCRETED IN MILK	% ADULT DOSE IN MILK	AAP RATING	COMMENTS
Atropine sulfate*	Yes	Traces	6	Hyperthermia, atropine toxicity, infants especially sensitive; also inhibits lactation. Infant dose 0.01 mg/kg.

*An ingredient in many prescription and nonprescription drugs.

DRUG	EXCRETED IN MILK	% ADULT DOSE IN MILK	AAP RATING	COMMENTS
Ergotamine	Yes	Unknown	1	May inhibit lactation.
Neostigmine	No			No known harm to infant.
Propranatheline bromide (Pro-Banthine)	No	Uncontrolled data indicate no measurable levels.		Drug rapidly metabolized in maternal system to inactive metabolite. Mother should avoid long-acting preparations, however.
Scopolamine (Hyoscine)	Yes	Traces	6	Usually given as single dose and of no problem to neonate. No data on repeated doses.

CARDIOVASCULAR DRUGS

DRUG	EXCRETED IN MILK	% ADULT DOSE IN MILK	AAP RATING	COMMENTS
Diazoxide (Hyperstat)				Arteriolar dilators and antihypertensive, only given IV, not active orally.
Digoxin	Yes	0.07 to 14	6	Not detected in infant's plasma.
Hydralazine (Apresoline)	Yes	0.8	6	Jaundice, thrombocytopenia, electrolyte disturbances possible.
Methyldopa (Aldomet)	Yes	0.02 to 0.09		Galactorrhea. No specific data except as affects mother's milk production.
Propranolol (Inderal)	Yes	Traces		Insignificant amount. Infants reported had no symptoms noted. Should watch for hypoglycemia and/or "β-blocking" effects.
Quinidine	Yes	4.1	6	Arrhythmia may occur.

CATHARTICS

DRUG	EXCRETED IN MILK	% ADULT DOSE IN MILK	AAP RATING	COMMENTS
Cascara	Yes	Low	6	Caused colic and diarrhea in infant.
Milk of magnesia	No	None	6	No effect.
Mineral oil	No	None	6	No effect.
Phenolphthalein	Unknown	Unknown	6	Reported to cause symptoms in some.
Rhubarb	Unknown	None	6	None in syrup form. Fresh rhubarb may give symptoms of colic and diarrhea.
Saline cathartics	No	None	6	No effect.
Senna	No	None	6	None.
Stool softeners and bulk-forming laxatives	No	None	6	No effect.
Suppositories (for constipation)	No	None	6	Not absorbed.

DIURETICS

DRUG	EXCRETED IN MILK	% ADULT DOSE IN MILK	AAP RATING	COMMENTS
Furosemide (sulfamoylanthranilic acid) (Lasix)	Possible	Not found in all samples		Drug is given to children under medical management.
Spironolactone (Aldactone)	Yes	Canrenone, a metabolite, appears	6	Acts as antagonist of aldosterone; causes sodium excretion and potassium retention. The metabolite apparently has some activity.

DRUG	EXCRETED IN MILK	% ADULT DOSE IN MILK	AAP RATING	COMMENTS
Thiazides (Diuril, Enduron, Esidrix, Hydrodiuril, Oretic, Thiuretic tablets)	Yes	0.25 to 0.43	6	Risk of dehydration and electrolyte imbalance, especially sodium loss, which would require monitoring. Watching weight and wet diapers and taking an occasional specific gravity reading of urine and serum sodium would indicate status of infant. Risk, however, is extremely low. May suppress lactation because of dehydration in mother.
ENVIRONMENTAL AGENTS				
Benzene hexachloride (BHC)	Yes	Varies by location	7	Not a reason to wean from breast. No need to test milk unless inordinate exposure.
Dichlorodiphenyltrichlorethane (DDT or DDE)	Yes	Varies by location	7	Not a reason to wean from breast. No need to test milk unless inordinate exposure.
Methyl mercury	Yes	Varies by location	7	Infant blood level 600 ng/ml in heavy exposure. Only in excessive exposure is testing and/or weaning necessary.
Polybrominated biphenyl (PBB)	Yes	Varies by location	7	If mother at high risk from the environment or the diet, milk sample should be measured. If level in milk is high, then breastfeeding should be discontinued. Those at risk are workers who handle PBB/PCB and individuals who eat game fish from contaminated waters. Crash diets mobilize fats and should be avoided especially if PBB or PCB is present.
Polychlorinated biphenyl (PCB)	Yes	Varies by location	7	
HEAVY METALS				
Arsenic	Yes	Can be measured for given woman.		Can accumulate. Check infant's blood level if there is reason to suspect exposure.
Fluorine	Yes	0.19		Monitor for excessive dose. Depends on level in water supply.
Iron	Yes			
Lead	Unknown			Nursing contraindicated if maternal serum 40 μg; conflicting reports, breast milk not always cause of lead poisoning in breastfed infant.
Mercury	Yes		7	Hazardous to infant.
HORMONES AND CONTRACEPTIVES				
Chlorotrianisene (Tace)	Yes			Has estrogenic effect although does not change consistency of milk. May have feminizing effect on infant. May suppress lactation.
Contraceptives (oral) Ethinyl estradiol, Mestranol, 19-Nortestosterone, Norethindrone (Norlutin)	Yes	0.16 ± 0.14	6	May diminish milk supply. May decrease vitamins, protein, and fat in milk. Most significant concern is long-range impact of hormone on young infant, which is not certain. Reports of feminization of infant.
Corticotropin	Yes	1.1	6	May decrease quantity and quality of milk.

DRUG	EXCRETED IN MILK	% ADULT DOSE IN MILK	AAP RATING	COMMENTS
Cortisone	Yes	Significant amounts.		May affect infant in therapeutic doses.
Epinephrine (Adrenalin)	Yes			Destroyed in gastrointestinal tract of infant.
Estrogen	Yes	0.1	6	Risks as with oral contraceptives. May alter quality and quantity of milk
Insulin	No			Destroyed in intestinal tract.
Medroxyproges-terone acetate (Provera)	Yes	0.86 to 5	6	6-month injection may affect milk supply; 3-month injection should not decrease supply.
Prednisone	Yes	0.06 to 3.6	6	Minimum amount not likely to cause effect on infant in short course.
Tolbutamide (Ori-nase)	Yes	18	6	Watch for jaundice.
NARCOTICS				
Cocaine	Yes	Significant levels in milk.	1,2	No metabolites or drug found in milk after 36 hours or in infant's urine after 60 hours.
Codeine		5 ± 2	6	No effect in therapeutic level and transient usage. Can accumulate. Individual variation. Watch for neonatal depression.
Heroin	Yes		2	Chinese metabolize drug less than Caucasians.
Marijuana (Cannabis)	Yes		2	Shown in laboratory animals to produce structural changes in nursling's brain cells; impairs DNA and RNA formation. Infant at risk of inhaling smoke during feeding or when held by person who is smoking.
Meperidine (Demerol)	Yes	Trace		Trace amounts may accumulate if drug taken around the clock when infant is neonate. Watch for drowsiness and poor feeding.
Methadone	Yes	2.2	6	When dosage not excessive, infant can be breastfed if monitored for evidence of depression and failure to thrive. Suggest mother get daily dose after evening feeding and supplement formula at next feeding.
Morphine	Yes	0.8 to 1.2	6	Single doses have minimum effect. Potential for accumulation. May be addicting to neonate. Breastfeeding no longer considered appropriate means of weaning infant of an addict.
Percodan [oxyco-done (derived from opiate thebaine) aspirin, phenacetin, caffeine]	Yes	Unknown		Consider for its component parts. In neonatal period sleepiness and failure to feed, which increase maternal engorgement and neonatal weight loss, have been observed, probably caused by oxycodone.

DRUG	EXCRETED IN MILK	% ADULT DOSE IN MILK	AAP RATING	COMMENTS
PSYCHOTROPIC AND MOOD-CHANGING DRUGS				
Alcohol (ethanol)	Yes	1 to 19.5	6	Milk may smell like alcohol. Ethanol in doses of 1 to 2 g/kg to mother causes depression of milk-ejection reflex (dose dependent). No acetaldehyde found as infant cannot metabolize ethanol.
Amphetamine	Yes	6.1 ± 0.1	2	Has caused stimulation in infants with jitteriness, irritability, sleeplessness. Long-acting preparations cumulative.
Benzodiazepines* Chlordiazepoxide (Librium)	Yes			Not sufficient to affect infant first week when glucuronyl system needed for detoxification. May accumulate. May cause jaundice. Older infant, no apparent problem.
Diazepam (Valium)	Yes	2 to 4.7	4	Detoxified in glucuronyl system. In first weeks of life may contribute to jaundice. Metabolite active. Effect on infant: hypoventilation, drowsiness, lethargy, and weight loss. Single doses over 10 mg contraindicated during breastfeeding. Accumulation in infant possible.
Haloperidol (Haldol)	Yes	0.15 to 2	4	A butyrophenone antidepressant: animal studies in nursings show behavior abnormalities.
Lithium carbonate (Eskalith, Lithane, Lithonate)	Yes	1.8		Measurable lithium in infant's serum. Infant kidney can clear lithium; however, lithium inhibits adenosine 3′:5′-cyclic monophosphate, significant for brain growth. Also affects amine metabolism. Report of cyanosis and poor muscle tone and ECG changes in nursing infant.
Meprobamate (Miltown, Equanil)	Yes	2 to 4 times maternal plasma level		If therapy continued, infant should be followed closely.
Phencyclidine (PCP)	Yes		1	Animal studies show PCP in milk even after drug has been discontinued for 40 days.
Phenothiazines Chlorpromazine (Thorazine)	Yes	0.07 to 0.2		Drowsiness and lethargy in infants.
Thioridazine (Mellaril)	Yes	No information		Thioridazine is less potent in general than other phenothiazines. Probably safe.
Trifluoperazine (Stelazine)	Yes	Minimum		
Tricyclic antidepressants				Apparently no accumulation. No infants that have been observed showed symptoms.
Amitriptyline (Elavil)	Yes	0.8 ± 0.2	4	Watch for depression or failure to feed. Increase maternal prolactin secretion.
Desipramine (Norpramin, Pertofrane)		1	4	
Imipramine (Tofranil)	Yes	0.1	4	
STIMULANTS				
Caffeine	Yes	0.66 to 10	6	Accumulates when intake moderate and continual. Causes jitteriness, wakefulness, and irritability. Caffeine present in many hot and cold drinks. Consider if infant very wakeful.

*Alcohol enhances the effects of these drugs.

DRUG	EXCRETED IN MILK	% ADULT DOSE IN MILK	AAP RATING	COMMENTS
Theobromine	Yes	20	7	No adverse symptoms observed in the infants. Chocolate the most common cause of exposure.
Theophylline	Yes	<1 to 15	6	Irritability, fretfulness.
THYROID AND ANTITHYROID MEDICATIONS				
Thiouracil	Yes	0.3 to 2.6	6	Get baseline levels of T3, T4, and TSH before and 6 weeks after mother starts medication.
Thyroid and thyroxine	Yes	0.3 to 2.6	6	Does not produce adverse symptoms on long-range follow-up. Noted to improve milk supply of hypothyroid mothers. No contraindication.
MISCELLANEOUS				
DPT	Yes	Minimum		Does not interfere with immunization schedule.
Methotrexate	Yes	0.93	1	Antimetabolite. Infant would receive 0.26 µg/dl, which researchers consider nontoxic for infant.
Nicotine	Yes		2	Decreases milk production. Smoking may interfere with let-down reflex if smoking started before onset of a feeding. Smoke exposure may be a concern.
Poliovirus vaccine	No			Live vaccine taken orally. Not necessary to withhold nursing 30 min before and after dose. Provide booster after infant no longer nursing.
Rh antibodies	Yes			Destroyed in gastrointestinal tract; not effective orally.
Rubella virus vaccine	Yes	Minimum		Will not confer passive immunity. Mother should not be given vaccine when at risk for pregnancy.
Tuberculin test	No			Tuberculin-sensitive mothers can adaptively immunize their infants through breast milk, and that immunity may last several years.
Chest x-ray				No effect.

Compiled from Lawrence RA: *Breastfeeding: a guide for the medical profession,* ed 4, St. Louis, 1994, Mosby and the Committee on Drugs, American Academy of Pediatrics: The transfer of drugs and other chemicals into human breast milk, *Pediatrics,* 93:137, 1994.

H Resources

This Appendix includes community and national resources, national clearinghouses, journals, and nursing organizations of interest to the maternity nurse.

COMMUNITY AND NATIONAL RESOURCES

AASK (Aid to the Adoption of Special Kids)
3530 Grand Avenue
Oakland, CA 94610
(415) 451-1748

AIDS Medical Foundation
10 East 13th Street, Suite LD
New York, NY 10003
(212) 206-0670

AMEND
Aiding a Mother Experiencing Neo-Natal Death
4324 Berrywick Terrace
St. Louis, MO 63141
(314) 487-7582

American Academy of Husband-Coached Childbirth
P.O. Box 5224
Sherman Oaks, CA 91413
(818) 788-6662

American Cancer Society, Inc.
1599 Clifton Road, NE
Atlanta, Georgia 30329
1-800-ACS-2345

American Cleft Palate Association
331 Salk Hall
Pittsburgh, PA 15261
(412) 681-9620

American Diabetes Association
Diabetes Information Service Center
1660 Duke Street
Alexandria, VA 22314
1-800-ADA-DISC

American Fertility Foundation
2131 Magnolia Avenue, Suite 201
Birmingham, AL 35256
(205) 251-9764

American Foundation for Maternal and Child Health, Inc.
(research on the perinatal period)
30 Beekman Place
New York, NY 10022
(212) 759-5510

American Red Cross
17th and E Streets
Washington, DC 20006
(202) 737-8300

American Society for Psychoprophylaxis in Obstetrics (ASPO)
1840 Wilson Boulevard
Suite 204
Arlington, VA 22201
(703) 524-7802

Association for the Aid of Crippled Children
345 East 46th Street
New York, NY 10017

Association of Birth Defects in Children
3201 E. Crystal Lake Avenue
Orlando, FL 32806

Association for the Care of Children's Health
7910 Woodmont Avenue, Suite 300
Bethesda, MD 20814
(301) 654-6549

Association for Childbirth at Home, International
P.O. Box 39498
Los Angeles, CA 90039
(213) 667-0839

Association of Voluntary Sterilization, Inc. (AVS)
122 E. 42nd Street
New York, NY 10168
(212) 351-2500

The Association of Women's Health, Obstetric, and Neonatal Nurses (AWHONN)
700 14th Street, NW, Suite 600
Washington, DC 20005-2019
(202) 662-1600

Black Male Youth Health Enhancement Project
Family Life Center
Shiloh Baptist Church
Washington, DC

Boston Women's Health Book Collective
47 Nichols Avenue
Watertown, MA 02172
(617) 921-0271

Centers for Disease Control and Prevention
1600 Clifton Road, NE
Atlanta, GA 30333
(404) 329-1819; (404) 329-3286

Center for Sickle Cell Disease
2121 Georgia Ave, NW
Washington, DC 20059
(202) 636-7930

Childbirth Graphics
P.O. Box 21207
Waco, TX 76702
1-800-229-3366

Child Study Association of America
9 East 89th St.
New York, NY 10028
    Provides parent education materials.

Cleft Palate Foundation
1218 Grandview Avenue
Pittsburgh, PA 15211
1-800-24-CLEFT

Compassionate Friends
(following death of an infant)
P.O. Box 1347
Oak Brook, IL 60521
(312) 990-0010

COPE (Coping with the Overall Pregnancy/Parenting Experience)
37 Clarendon Street
Boston, MA 02116
(617) 357-5588

C/SEC, Inc. (Cesarean/Support Education and Concern)
22 Forest Road
Framingham, MA 01701
(617) 877-8266

DES Action USA
Long Island Jewish Medical Center
New Hyde Park, NY 11040

ECMO Moms and Dads
c/o Blair and Gayle Willson
HCR1, Box 108
Plainview, TX 79072
(806) 889-3877

Ed-U-Press
760 Ostrum Ave.
Syracuse, NY 13210
    Offers series of excellent cartoon books for
    adolescents and parenting classes.

Educational and Scientific Plastics, Ltd.
76 Holmethorpe Avenue
Holmethorpe, Red Hill Surrey, RH1, 2PF, England
    Offers numerous plastic models.

Endometriosis Association
238 West Wisconsin Avenue
P.O. Box 92187
Milwaukee, WI 53202
(414) 962-8972

Environmental Protection Agency (EPA)
Public Information Center
Room PM 211-B
401 M Street, SW
Washington, DC 20460
(202) 382-7550

Equal Rights for Fathers
P.O. Box 90042
San Jose, CA 95109-3042
(408) 848-2323

Florence Crittenton Association of America
608 South Dearborn Street
Chicago, IL 60605
    Assists in bringing about a greater understanding of
    factors relating to unmarried mothers and adolescent
    girls with other problems in adjustment.

International Childbirth Education Association (ICEA)
P.O. Box 20048
Minneapolis, MN 55420

Lact-Aid
P.O. Box 1066
Athens, TN 37303
(614) 744-9090
    Provides information and services to promote
    breastfeeding.

La Leche League
P.O. Box 1209
Franklin Park, IL 60131-8209
(312) 455-7730 (24-hour line)

March of Dimes See *National Foundation/March of Dimes*

Maternal Health Society
Box 46563, Station G
Vancouver, BC V6R 4G8

Maternity Center Association, Inc.
48 East 92nd Street
New York, NY 10028
(212) 269-7300

National Abortion Rights Action League
1101 14th Street, NW
Washington, DC 20005
(202) 371-9779

National Association of Childbirth Education, Inc. (NACE)
3940 Eleventh Street
Riverside, CA 92501

National Association for Sickle Cell Disease
3345 Wilshire Blvd., Suite 1106
Los Angeles, CA 90010-1880
(213) 736-5455; 1-800-421-8453

National Association of Parents and Professionals for Safe Alternatives in Childbirth (NAPSAC)
P.O. Box 267
Marble Hill, MO 63764
(314) 238-2010

National Coalition Against Domestic Violence
2401 Virginia Avenue, NW, Suite 305
Washington, DC 20037
1-800-333-SAFE (24-hour line)

National Coalition Against Sexual Assault
c/o Fern Ferguson, President
Volunteers of America of Illinois
8787 State Street, Suite 202
East St. Louis, IL 62203

The National Coalition of Hispanic Health and Human Services Organizations (COSSMHO)
1030 15th Street, NW, Suite 1053
Washington, DC 20005
(202) 371-2100

National Conference of Catholic Charities
1346 Connecticut
Washington, DC 20036
Service for children and youth; i.e., foster care, counseling, adoption services, short-term counseling to families and youth, emergency material assistance.

National Down Syndrome Congress
1800 Dempster Street
Park Ridge, IL 60068-1146
1-800-232-6372

National Down Syndrome Society Hotline
141 Fifth Avenue
New York, NY 10010
1-800-221-4602

National Foundation/March of Dimes
1275 Mamaroneck Avenue
White Plains, NY 10605
(914) 428-7100

National Foundation for Jewish Genetic Diseases, Inc.
250 Park Avenue, Suite 1000
New York, NY 10177

National Institute of Child Health and Human Development (NICHD)
National Institutes of Health
9000 Rockville Pike
Bldg 31, Room 2A32
Bethesda, MD 20892
(301) 496-4000

National Organization of Mothers of Twins Clubs, Inc.
12404 Princess Jeanne, NE
Albuquerque, NM 87112-4640
(505) 275-0955

National Perinatal Association
101½ South Union Street
Alexandria, VA 22314-3323
(703) 549-5523

National Right to Life Committee
419 7th Street, NW, Suite 500
Washington, DC 20004
(202) 626-8800

National Sudden Infant Death Syndrome Foundation
10500 Little Patuxent Parkway, Suite 420
Columbia, MD 21044
1-800-221-7437; (301) 964-8000

Office of Minority Health Resource Center
P.O. Box 37337
Washington, DC 20013-7337
(301) 587-1938

Parent Care, Inc.
(neonatal intensive care unit family support)
101-½ South Union
Alexandria, VA 22314
(703) 836-4678

Parenthood After Thirty
451 Vermont
Berkeley, CA 94707
(415) 524-6635

Parents of Prematures
13613 NE 26th Place
Bellevue, WA 98005
(206) 883-6040

Parents Without Partners
8807 Colesville Road
Silver Spring, MD 20910
(301) 588-9354

Patient Counseling Library
Budlong Press Co.
5428 N. Virginia Avenue
Chicago, IL, 60625
(312) 541-7800
  Provides videotapes covering topics such as pregnancy, infant care, sexuality, breastfeeding, and weight control.

Planned Parenthood Federation of America, Inc.
810 Seventh Avenue
New York, NY 10019
1-800-829-7732

Pregnancy and Infant Loss
1421 East Wayzata Boulevard, Suite 40
Wayzata, MN 55391
(612) 473-9372

Premenstrual Syndrome Action
P.O. 16292
Irving, CA 92713
(714) 854-4407

Reach to Recovery
(breast cancer)
(see American Cancer Society)

Read Natural Childbirth Foundation
P.O. Box 956
San Rafael, CA 94915
(415) 456-8462

Resolve, Inc.
(impaired fertility)
5 Water Street
Arlington, MA 02174
(617) 643-2424

Resolve Through Sharing (RTS)
(perinatal bereavement)
Lutheran Hospital—La Crosse
1910 South Ave.
La Crosse, WI 54601
(608) 791-4747

Save the Children Federation, Inc.
345 East 46th Street
New York, NY 10017

SHARE (Source of Help in Airing and Resolving Experiences)
(for parents who have suffered loss of newborn baby)
St. Elizabeth's Hospital
211 South 3rd Street
Belleville, IL
(618) 234-2415

SIECUS
Human Science Press
72 Fifth Avenue
New York, NY 10011
  Provides publications (e.g., "Sexual relations in pregnancy and postpartum") and teaching aids.

Spina Bifida Association of America
1700 Rockville Pike, Suite 250
Rockville, MD 20852
1-800-621-3141; (301) 770-7222

Teen Obstetrical Perinatal Parenting Services Clinic (TOPPS)
University of Arkansas College of Medicine
Little Rock, AR

Twins Magazine,
P.O. Box 12045
Overland Park, KS 66212
1-800-821-5533

Victims Anonymous
9514-9 Reseda Blvd. #607
Northridge, CA 91324
(818) 993-1139

VBAC (Vaginal Birth After Cesarean)
10 Great Plain Terrace
Needham, MA 01292

Women Against Rape
P.O. Box 02084
Columbus, OH 43202
(614) 291-9751

Women Against Violence Against Women (WAVAW)
543 North Fairfax Avenue
Los Angeles, CA 90036

NATIONAL CLEARINGHOUSES

American Foundation for Maternal and Child Health
(research on the perinatal period)
300 Beekman Place
New York, NY 10022
(212) 759-5510

Food and Drug Administration (FDA)
Office of Consumer Affairs
Public Inquiries
5600 Fishers Lane (HFE-88)
Rockville, MD 20857
(301) 443-3170

National AIDS Information Clearinghouse
1-800-458-5231 (English and Spanish)

National Clearinghouse for Drug Abuse Information
P.O. Box 426
Dept DQ
Kensington, MD 20795
1-800-637-2045; 1-800-492-6605 (in Maryland only)

National Clearinghouse for Family Planning Information
P.O. Box 10716
Rockville, MD 20850
(703) 558-4990

National Clearinghouse for Human Genetic Disease
National Center for Education in Maternal and Child
  Health
38th and R Streets, NW
Washington, DC 20057
   Provides information about inherited diseases.

National Maternal and Child Health Clearinghouse
3520 Prospect St., NW, Ground Floor
Washington, DC 20057

Sudden Infant Death Syndrome Clearinghouse
8201 Greensboro Dr, Suite 600
McLean, VA 22102

NURSING JOURNALS

Birth: Issues in Prenatal Care and Education
(formerly Birth and Family Journal)
110 El Camino Real
Berkeley, CA 94705
(415) 658-5099

Bookmarks
ICEA Supplies Center
P.O. Box 20048
Minneapolis, MN 55420
   Complimentary annotated catalogue of book
   reviews.

Canadian Nurse
The Canadian Nurses Association
50 The Driveway
Ottawa, Canada K2P1E2

The Female Patient
Division Excerpta Medica
301 Gibraltar Drive

P.O. Box 528
Morris Plains, NJ 07950

Journal of Nurse-Midwifery
Editor
82 Willow Ln.
Tenafly, NJ 07670

Journal of Obstetric, Gynecologic and Neonatal Nursing (JOGNN)
J.B. Lippincott Co.
12107 Insurance Way
  Hagerstown, MD 21740

Journal of Perinatal and Neonatal Nursing
Aspen Publishers, Inc.
7201 McKinney Circle
Frederick, MD 21701

Maternal/Newborn Advocate
The National Foundation/March of Dimes
P.O. Box 2000
White Plains, NY 10602

MCN The American Journal of Maternal Child Nursing
555 W. 57th Street
New York, NY 10019

Nursing Network on Violence Against Women Newsletter
Trauma Program, UHN-66
Oregon Health Sciences University
3181 SW Sam Jackson Pk Rd
Portland, OR 97201-3098
Fax: (503) 494-4357

Nurse Practitioner: A Journal of Primary Nursing Care
3845 42nd Ave., N.E.
Seattle, WA 98105

Nursing Research
555 W. 57th Street
New York, NY 10019

Perinatal Press
Perinatal Press Subscriptions
The Perinatal Center
Sutter Memorial Hospital
52nd and F Sts.
Sacramento, CA 95819

Women's Health Nursing Scan
J.B. Lippincott Co.
Downsville Pike, Rte 3, Box 20-B
Hagerstown, MD 21740

Loss and Grief
"Bereavement" Magazine
305 Gradle Dr.
Carmel, IN 46032
(317) 846-9429

Newsletter
(a multiple birth loss support network)
P.O. 1064
Palmer, AK 99645
(907) 745-2706

NURSING ORGANIZATIONS

American College of Nurse Midwives
1522 K Street, NW, Suite 1120
Washington, DC 20005
(202) 347-5445

American Nurses Association
1101 14th Street, NW, Suite 200
Washington, DC 20005
(202) 789-1800;
Head office
600 Maryland Ave, SW
Washington, DC

The Association of Women's Health, Obstetric, and Neonatal Nurses (AWHONN).
700 14th Street, NW, Suite 600
Washington, DC 20005-2019
(202) 662-1600

Canadian Nurses Association
50 The Driveway
Ottawa, Ont. K2P 1E2

Midwives Alliance of North America
United States and Canada
c/o Concord Midwifery Service
30 South Main Street
Concord, NH 03301
(603) 225-9586

National League for Nursing (NLN)
Ten Columbus Circle
New York, NY 10019
(212) 582-1022

ORGANIZATIONS INVOLVED IN PARENT EDUCATION

American Academy of Husband-Coached Childbirth (AAHCC)
P.O. Box 5224
Sherman Oaks, CA 91413

American Society for Psychoprophylaxis in Obstetrics (ASPO)
1411 K Street NW, Suite 200
Washington, DC 20005

Council of Childbirth Education Specialists, Inc. (CCES)
168 West 86th Street
New York, NY 10024

International Childbirth Education Association (ICEA)
P.O. Box 20048
Minneapolis, MN 55420

Maternity Center Association
48 East 92nd St
New York, NY 10028

National Association of Childbirth Education, Inc. (NACE)
3940 11th Street
Riverside, CA 92501

Read Natural Childbirth Foundation
PO Box 956
San Rafael, CA 94915

Index

A

Abdomen
  in first stage of labor, 271, 272
  of newborn, 342, 349-350
    assessment of, 363, 366
    distention of, 761
  in postpartum period, 443
  prenatal examination of, 130
Abdominal discomfort, in pregnancy, 106
Abdominal pregnancy, 577
Abdominal surgery during pregnancy, 656-657
Abortion
  adolescent pregnancy and, 726
  assessment of, 574
  elective, 877-880
  grief response to, 832
  of hydatidiform mole, 579
  spontaneous, 572, 574-576
    diabetes and, 621
    nursing care for, 580
  types of, 572
Abortus, definition of, 4
Abrasion, as birth trauma, 373
Abruptio placentae, 582-583, 585
Abuse
  spousal, 677-683
    well-woman care and, 844
  substance, 668-677; *see also* Substance abuse
Accelerations of fetal heart rate, 249-254
  definition of, 249-250
Access to health care, 7
Accessory reproductive system gland, 48
Acculturation, 17
Acid, amino
  dietary deficiency of, 196
  essential, 182
  newborn requirements for, 409
Acid-base balance, 102
Acinus, of breast, 39
Acne vulgaris, 104
Acoustic stimulation, fetal, 549
Acquaintance, parental, 450-453
Acquired immunity, 51
Acquired immunodeficiency syndrome,
      595-597; *see also* Human immunodeficiency
      virus
Acrocyanosis, 753
Acroesthesia, 105
Active immunity, 51
Active transport, 76

Adaptation
  to extrauterine life
    dysfunctional, 752-753
    normal, 370, 387, 755
  to infant, 455-456
    preterm, 779-780
  to labor, 218-219
  to parenthood, 459-460, 475-482
    criteria for, 516
  to pregnancy
    by grandparent, 118-119
    maternal, 110-115
    paternal, 115-118
    by sibling, 118-119
Adaptive immunity, 51
Adjustment, to infant, 455-456
Admission to hospital
  diabetes and, 629
  form for, 264
  in labor, 266, 269
  of newborn, 364
  for preeclampsia, 566-567
Adnexa, anatomy of, 29
Adolescent
  adaptation to pregnancy by, 119
  death of infant of, 833
  development of, 722-724
  as parent, 729
    assessment of, 740-741
    collaborative care for, 741
    expected outcomes for, 741
    nursing diagnosis for, 741
  pregnancy in, 727-729
    assessment of, 732-733
    care plan for, 742-744
    evaluation of, 740
    expected outcomes for, 733-734
    nursing care for, 734-740
    nursing diagnosis for, 733
    risks and consequences of, 729-730
  sexuality of, 724-727, 730-731
  social networks for, 5
Adoption
  breastfeeding and, 415
  embryo, 876
  grief and, 739
Adrenal gland, fetal, 82
Adrenal hyperplasia, 389
Adult respiratory distress syndrome,
      652-653
Affecting skills, 450

African-American culture
  beliefs of, 19
  food patterns of, 193
Afterpains, 310-311, 441
  breastfeeding and, 414
Age
  birthrate according to, 4
  gestational; see Gestational age
  maternal adjustment and, 458-459
  pregnancy after age 35 and, 119-120
  as risk factor, 536
Agonist-antagonist compound, 229
AIDS; see Human immunodeficiency virus
Airway
  maternal, 641
  of newborn, 371-373
    resuscitation and, 374-375
Albumin, pregnancy and, 103
Alcohol abuse
  fetal effects of, 808-811
  male infertility and, 871
  prevention of illness and, 853-854
  psychological factors and, 669
  risk from, 142-143
Aldomet, 569
Alert state, 367
Allergic drug reaction, 239
  to local anesthetic, 230
Alpha-fetoprotein, 545
Alternative birth center, 165-166
Alveolus
  of breast, 39
  of newborn, 324
Ambiguity, sexual, 805
Ambivalence, to pregnancy, 111
Ambulation, 280
Ambulatory tokodynamometer, 714, 715
Amenorrhea, 858
Amino acid
  dietary deficiency of, 196
  essential, 182
  newborn requirements for, 409
Amniocentesis
  abortion and, 879
  in high-risk pregnancy, 544-546
  ultrasonography with, 541
Amnion
  development of, 78
  formation of, 68
Amniotic fluid
  assessment of, 278
  congenital anomaly and, 794
  function of, 78
  oligohydramnios and, 80
  swallowing of, 82
  volume of, 541
Amniotic fluid embolus, 301
Amniotic fluid index, 541
Amniotic membranes
  birth of head and, 298
  formation of, 68
  rupture of, 277-278, 698
Amniotitis, 278
Amniotomy, 698
Ampulla, of fallopian tube, 30
Amyl nitrate, male infertility and, 871
Amylase, newborn and, 326

Analgesia
  for dilatation and curettage, 580
  for labor pain, 221-245; see also Labor, pain
    management in
  for postpartum pain, 311
Android pelvis, 213
Anemia, 649-650, 651
  in newborn, 753
  physiologic, 178
  pregnancy and, 100
  as risk factor, 536
Anencephaly, 803
Anesthesia
  for cesarean birth, 703
  for dilatation and curettage, 580
  for labor, 228-238; see also Labor, pain management in
Aneurysm, cerebral, 301
Angioma, pregnancy and, 103
Angle, subpubic, 211
Announcement phase of pregnancy, 115
Anomalous venous return, 795
Anomaly; see Congenital disorder
Anovulation, 869
Anovulatory drug, 492-493
Antacid, general anesthesia and, 237
Antagonist, narcotic, 230
Antepartal period; see Fetal entries; Fetus;
    Pregnancy entries; Prenatal period
Anthropoid pelvis, 213
Anthropometry, 188
Antibiotic, for pelvic inflammatory disease, 863
Antibody-mediated immunity, 51-52
Anticipatory grief, preterm infant and, 779
Anticipatory guidance for health promotion, 849-854
Anticoagulant therapy
  epidural block and, 236
  heart disease and, 643
Anticonvulsant, eclampsia and, 569-570
Antihypertensive drug, 569
Anus
  examination of, 132
  imperforate, 801
  of newborn, 353
Anxiety
  about postpartum bleeding, 525-526
  care plan for, 169
  in second trimester, 148
Aorta, Marfan's syndrome and, 648-649
Apgar score, 362, 753
Appendicitis, 656-657
Appetite, in postpartum period, 444
Apresoline, 569
Apt test, 546
Areola, anatomy of, 39
Arm, of newborn, 352
Arrhythmia, of newborn, 761
Arterial blood gases, neonatal, 760
Arterial blood pressure, 99
Arterial pressure, mean, 760
Arthritis, rheumatoid, 655
Artificial rupture of membranes, 277-278, 698
Asian culture
  food patterns of, 195
  support during labor and, 288
Aspartame, 182
Asphyxia
  macrosomia and, 789

Asphyxia—cont'd
    neonatal, 752
    in small for gestational age infant, 787
Aspiration
    meconium, 786-787
    respiratory distress syndrome and, 652-653
Aspiration abortion, 878-879
Aspiration pneumonia, powder causing, 400
Aspirin, preeclampsia and, 557
Assessment
    of abortion, 574
    abuse, 678
    of adolescent, 732-734
    of amniotic fluid, 278
    of cardiac output, 583
    of cervical dilatation, 274, 275
    for elective abortion, 877
    fetal heart rate; see Fetal heart rate
    of grief response, 820
    for heart disease, 640-641
    of hemorrhage, 580
    home visit, 518-519
    of hypertension, 559-564
    of infant feeding, 413
    of infection, 606-608
    of labor, 238
        fourth stage of, 305, 307
    of newborn, 362-369
        compromised, 753, 755-758
    nutritional, 185-188
    postpartum, 464
    psychosocial
        during labor, 267
        postpartum, 464, 478-482
    risk assessment, preconception, 87, 88
    in second trimester, 146-151
    in third trimester, 159-160
Assimilation, 17
Assisted reproductive therapy, 875-876
    Catholic view of, 864
    Orthodox Jewish view of, 864
Asthma, 650, 652
Ataractic, labor and, 229-230
Atony, uterine, 308, 586-587
Atresia
    choanal, 795
    esophageal, 799-800
Atrial fibrillation, 648
Atrial septal defect, 795
Atrium, of newborn, 321
Attachment, parental, 450-453
Attitude, fetal, definition of, 207-208
Auditory response, of newborn, 367
Augmentation of labor, 698
Auscultation
    fetal, 254-255
        in first stage of labor, 271-272
    of newborn, 363
Autoimmune disorder, 654-656
    thrombocytopenic purpura as, 591
Autopsy, 825
Autosomal abnormalities, 62-63
Autosomal inheritance, 64
Aversion, food, 192, 196
Awake state, of newborn, 337
Azidothymidine, for HIV infection, 596

B
Babinski's reflex, 357, 358
Baby blues, 456, 480, 655, 665
Baby powder, aspiration of, 400
Back, of newborn, 353
Back blows, for airway obstruction, 372-373
Backache, in second trimester, 154
Bacteremic shock, 604
Bacteria, intestinal, in newborn, 326
Bacterial infection; see Infection
Ballottement, 96-97
Barrier, to infection, 50
Barrier contraceptive, 489-490
    diabetes and, 630
Basal body temperature, 42, 43
    contraception and, 486-487
    diagnosis of pregnancy and, 124
Basal metabolic rate
    of fetus, 82
    of newborn, 334
    nutrition and, 178
    pregnancy-related changes in, 101-102
Baseline fetal heart rate, 247-249
Bathing
    of infant, 381-383, 384-385
        after death, 825
    in second trimester, 152
Bearing-down efforts, 214-215, 295-296
Beating of spouse, 677-683
Bed, birthing, 295
Bed rest
    heart disease and, 647
    for hypertonic uterine dysfunction, 687
    preeclampsia and, 565
Behavior
    adaptive; see Adaptation
    bonding and, 450-453
    breastfeeding and, 412-422
    fetal, 218
    formula feeding and, 428
    mothering, 477
    of newborn, 331, 334-339
        assessment of, 366-369
        feeding and, 326, 408
        interpretation of, 476
    parenting, 453-459
    sexual, 725; see also Sexuality
Beliefs
    childbearing, 16
    food, 192, 196
Bellergal-S tablets, 883
Bell's palsy, 654
Bereavement, 816-835; see also Grief
Beta-adrenergic agonist, heart disease and, 644
Bilirubin
    excess of, 327-328, 377
        causes of, 793
        diabetes and, 790
        treatment of, 394-397
    in high-risk pregnancy, 545
Billings method of contraception, 486, 487
Bimanual palpation, 133-134
Biochemical assessment in high-risk pregnancy, 544-548
Biophysical profile of fetus, 542-543
Biorhythmicity, 452-453
Biotinidase deficiency, 389

Biparietal diameter, 208
Bipolar disorder, 667
Birth; *see* Labor
Birth canal, 209
Birth control; *see* Contraception
Birth plan, 129, 143
Birth setting, 165-167, 288-289
Birth trauma; *see* Trauma
Birthing bed or chair, 295
Birthing room, 294, 296-297
Birthmark, 344
Birthrate
    definition of, 4
    trends in, 3-4
Birthweight, 775-777
Bishop score, 697
Bite, stork, 329-330
Bittersweet grief, 819
Bladder
    extrophy of, 804
    in postpartum period, 444
    pregnancy-related changes in, 102
Blastocyst, 68
Blastomere, 68
Bleeding; *see also* Hemorrhage
    lochia and, 441-442
    withdrawal, 42
Bleeding disorder
    epidural block and, 236
    HELLP syndrome and, 559
Blended family, 13
Blood
    ABO incompatibility of, 793
    fetal circulation and, 79-80
    in first stage of labor, 277
    lochia and, 441-442
    placenta and, 75
    postpartal testing of
        maternal, 445
        of newborn, 390-391
    pregnancy-related changes in, 556
    prenatal testing of
        fetal, 257, 546-547
        maternal, 134, 548
    of preterm infant, 778
    Rh incompatibility of, 77, 793
        dilatation and curettage and, 581
    transfusion of, 590-591
    well-woman care and, 842
Blood cells
    folate and, 184
    HELLP syndrome and, 557, 559, 566-568
    labor and, 219
    pregnancy and, 100
Blood flow, placental, 247
Blood gases, neonatal, 760
Blood glucose testing, 627-628
    gestational diabetes and, 635
Blood pressure; *see also* Hypertension
    hemorrhagic shock and, 589
    hypovolemic shock and, 309
    labor and, 218-219
    maternal, 77-78
    measurement of, 561
    of newborn, 323, 341
    pregnancy-related changes in, 99, 100
    renal function and, 102
    in second trimester, 146, 148

Blood vessels
    of newborn, 321
    uterine, 33-34
Blood volume
    of newborn, 323
    nutrition and, 178
    pregnancy-related changes in, 99
Bloody show, 215, 265
Blues, baby, 456, 480, 655
Body
    birth of, 299
    ketone, 622
    perineal, 37
Body defense, 50
Body image, in pregnancy, 111
Body language, assessment of, 267
Body mass index, 175, 176
Body mechanics, in second trimester, 152, 155
Body temperature; *see* Temperature
Bonding, 311-312, 450-453
Bone; *see* Skeletal system
Bony pelvis, 37-38, 209-210
Borderline prematurity, 777
Borrelia burgdorferi, 605
Bottle feeding, 426-429
    prenatal preparation for, 157
Bowel disease, inflammatory, 653
Bowel elimination
    labor and, 281
    parent education about, 401
    in postpartum period, 444
Bowel sounds, of newborn, 326
Brachial pulse, in newborn, 375
Bradley childbirth method, 224
Bradycardia, fetal, 247
Brain
    anencephaly and, 803
    aneurysm of, 301
    fetal, 81
    hydrocephalus and, 802-803
    ischemia of, 649
    microcephaly and, 803
    of newborn, 331
Brassiere, maternity, 152
Braxton Hicks contractions, 162
Braxton Hicks sign, 96
Brazelton neonatal behavior assessment scale, 335
Breast
    anatomy of, 38-39
    cancer of, 891-892
    care of, 417, 427-428
    engorgement of, 414
    estrogen replacement therapy and, 883
    in first trimester, 139, 144
    infection in, 604-605
    mammography of, 848-849
    of newborn, 330
    in postpartum period, 444-445
    pregnancy-related changes in, 98-99
    prenatal examination of, 130
    self-examination of, 844-845, 846
Breast pump, 414
Breastfeeding, 416-433
    by adolescent mother, 738
    assessment of, 413
    birth control and, 426
    breast care and, 417
    breast development and, 410

Breastfeeding—cont'd
  breast tenderness and, 445
  care plan for, 431-432
  by diabetic mother, 630
  expected outcomes for, 416
  HIV transmission and, 595
  home care and, 418
  immediate, 302
  immune system and, 417
  infant response to, 421-422
  jaundice and, 328, 417
  knowledge deficit about, 526
  lactation process and, 410-413
  maternal nutrition and, 420
  nursing diagnosis for, 413
  planning for, 413
  positions for, 420-421
  postnatal period and, 417
  prenatal period and, 416-417
  prenatal preparation for, 157-158
  of preterm infant, 422
  problems with, 414-415, 425-426
  reflexes of, 411, 412
  stool and, 326
  storing and breast milk and, 422-425
  substance abuse and, 675
  supplemental feedings and, 430
  of twins, 422, 423
  vitamin and mineral supplements and, 430
Breathing, by newborn, 323-324
  abnormal, 372
  parent education about, 400-401
Breathing techniques for labor, 225-226
Breech presentation, 208, 689-692
  external cephalic version for, 696-697
Bromocriptine, infertility and, 872
Bronchial asthma, 650, 652
Bronchopulmonary dysplasia, 783
Brow presentation, 209
Bulbocavernous muscle, 36
Bulging of perineum, 297
Butorphanol, labor and, 229
Butyl nitrate, male infertility and, 871

C
Caffeine, risk from, 143
Calcium
  diabetes and, 790
  neonatal hypocalcemia and, 378
  newborn requirement for, 409
  osteoporosis and, 882
  pregnancy requirement for, 179
  requirement for, 183-184, 850-851
    for adolescent, 738
  teeth and, 105
Calcium gluconate, preeclampsia and, 568
Calendar method of contraception, 486
Calorie requirement, 179, 181-182
Cambodian food patterns, 195
Canal
  birth, 209-211
  cervical, 33
  testicular, 47-48
  uterine, 33
Cancer; see Malignancy
Candidiasis, neonatal, 774-775
Cap, cervical, 495, 498
Capacitation, 66

Capillary blood, for neonatal screening, 390-391
Capillary hemangioma, 330
Caput succedaneum, 329
Car seat, infant, 514
Carbohydrate, newborn requirement for, 409
Carbon dioxide, neonatal monitoring for, 760
Carcinoma; see Malignancy
Card, admission labor, 266
Cardiac output
  assessment of, 583
  labor and, 218
  maternal, 77
  in postpartum period, 445-446
  pregnancy and, 100
Cardiomyopathy, 647
  diabetes and, 790
Cardiopulmonary resuscitation; see Resuscitation
Cardiovascular system
  cocaine and, 671
  labor and, 218-219
  maternal heart disease and, 639-649
    antepartum care in, 643
    assessment of, 640-641
    cardiopulmonary resuscitation and, 641-642
    care plan for, 645-646
    cerebrovascular accident and, 649
    endocarditis as, 648
    evaluation of, 644, 647
    expected outcomes for, 642
    heart failure and, 647
    intrapartum care in, 643-644
    Marfan syndrome and, 648-649
    mitral valve prolapse as, 648
    nursing diagnosis for, 642
    postpartum care in, 644
    rheumatic, 647-648
  of newborn, 321-322
    compromised, 760-761, 797
    patent ductus arteriosus of, 784
    persistent pulmonary hypertension and, 786
    preterm, 777
  in postpartum period, 445-446
  pregnancy-related changes in, 99-100, 556
  well-woman care and, 842
Care clustering, for preterm infant, 782
Care path case management, postpartum, 509, 510-511
Care standards
  in first stage of labor, 279, 280
  prenatal, 136
Carpal tunnel syndrome, 105, 154
Carryover, 452
Catheter
  for airway suctioning, 371-372
  intrauterine pressure, 255, 256
Catheterization, labor and, 281
Catholic view of assisted fertility therapy, 864
Caudal regression syndrome, diabetes and, 790
Caul, 298
Cavity, pelvic, 210
Cell
  desquamation of, 97
  squamous, fetal, 277
Cell division, 60-61
Cell-mediated immunity, 50, 51
Central cyanosis, 753
Central nervous system; see Nervous system
Central venous pressure, 589
Cephalhematoma, 329

Cephalic presentation, 208
Cephalic version, external, 689, 695-696
Cephalocaudal development, 80
Cephalopelvic disproportion, 689
    adolescent pregnancy and, 729-730
Cerclage, McDonald, 576
Cerebral aneurysm, 301
Cerebral ischemia, 649
Cervical canal, 33
Cervical cap, 495, 498
Cervical intraepithelial neoplasia, 847-848
Cervical mucus method of contraception, 487
Cervix
    anatomy of, 32, 33
    dilation of, 214
    effacement of, 211, 214
    false vs. true labor and, 264
    incompetent, 575-576
        nursing care for, 579-580
    infertility and, 870-871
    laceration of, 304
    Papanicolaou smear and, 847-848
    in postpartum period, 442
    ripening of, 697-698
Cesarean birth, 702-713
    anesthesia for, 237, 702-703
    care plan for, 712-713
    complications of, 702-703
    emergency, 703
    indications for, 702
    nursing care during, 704, 708-709
    postpartum care for, 707
    prenatal preparation for, 703-704
    scheduled, 703
    surgical techniques for, 702
    vaginal birth after, 165, 707, 710
Chadwick's sign, 95, 97
Chair, birthing, 295
Chart, body mass index, 175
Chemical contraceptive barrier, 489-490
Chest, of newborn, 349
    assessment of, 366
    auscultation of, 363
    circumference of, 324, 342
Chest compression, of newborn, 375
Chest wall retractions, 757, 760
Chickenpox, 605
Childbearing, complications of, 533-553; see also Pregnancy,
        high-risk
Childbed fever, 603-605
Childbirth; see Labor
Childbirth preparation
    adaptation pregnancy and, 114, 129
    adolescent pregnancy and, 736-737
    education programs for, 164-167
    methods of, 223-225
Childbirth trauma, 884-890; see also Trauma, childbirth
Chilling, in postpartum period, 310
Chinese culture
    father prohibited from birth room, 288
    food patterns of, 193
    neonatal behavior and, 336
Chlamydia trachomatis, 133, 593-594, 773-774
    infertility and, 870
Chloasma, 103
Choanal atresia, 795
Choking, 372-373

Cholecystitis, 653
Cholelithiasis, 653
Chorioamnionitis, 603
Chorion, 78
Chorionic gonadotropin
    nausea and vomiting and, 107
    placenta and, 75
    pregnancy testing and, 92-93
Chorionic villus, function of, 68
Chorionic villus sampling, 547-548
Chromosome, 60
    abnormalities of, 62-63, 798
        infertility and, 865
    of hydatidiform mole, 579
    sex of fetus and, 82
Cigarette smoking
    male infertility and, 871
    in pregnancy, 143, 673, 809, 810
    prevention of illness and, 853
Circulatory system; see also Cardiovascular system
    fetal, 69-73, 79-80, 218
    maternal-placental-embryonic, 75
    pregnancy and, 100
Circumcision, 396, 397-400
Circumference
    of chest, 324, 342, 343
    of head, 342, 343, 366
Cleanliness, in postpartum period, 311
Cleavage, 68
Cleft lip and palate, 803-804
Climacterium, 44, 880-881
Clitoris, 27
Clomiphene
    hydatidiform mole and, 578
    for infertility, 869
Clonus, 562
Clothing
    for newborn, 383, 763
        after death, 825
    for pregnancy, 145
Clotting, normal, 591
Clotting factor
    in postpartum period, 445
    replacement of, 591
    vitamin K and, 82
    von Willebrand's disease and, 592
Coach, labor
    cesarean birth and, 704
    in first stage, 287-288
    in second stage, 296
Coagulation
    disseminated intravascular, 591-592
        preeclampsia and, 557
    HELLP syndrome and, 559
    normal, 591
    pregnancy and, 100
Coagulation factor
    in postpartum period, 445
    replacement of, 591
    vitamin K and, 82
    von Willebrand's disease and, 592
Cocaine abuse, 669, 671
    care plan for, 676
    effects of, 811-812
Coccygeus muscle, 35
Coccyx, 37
Cognitive development, 724

Cognitive skills, parenting and, 450
Coital position, 144
Cold stress, 334
    bilirubin and, 327-328
    of newborn, 370-371
Colitis, 653
Collection of specimens for neonatal screening, 390-393
Colloid oncotic pressure, 589
Color, of newborn, 366, 753, 755, 756
Colostrum, 99, 411
Columnar epithelium, uterine, 33
Comfort; *see also* Discomfort
    in grief, 823-824
    in postpartum period, 310-311
Commercial formula, 428-429
Communication
    assessment of, 267
    in family, 15
    in grief, 821-823
    infant-parent, 451-453
Complete abortion, 574
Complete breech presentation, 691
Complicated bereavement, 833-834
Complications
    of childbearing, 531-746; *see also* Pregnancy, high- risk
    neonatal; *see* Newborn, compromised
    postpartal, warning signs of, 514
Compression
    chest, of newborn, 375
    on umbilical cord, 282-284, 285
Conception, 65-66
Condom
    female, 490
    male, 490, 491
Conductive heat loss, 333
Condyloma, neonatal syphilis and, 770
Condyloma acuminata, 601-602
Congenital disorder, 793-806
    amniotic fluid volume and, 794
    anencephaly and microcephaly as, 803
    cleft lip and palate as, 803-804
    death caused by, 535
    diabetes and, 623, 624, 789
    diagnosis of
        genetic, 797-798
        perinatal, 794
        prenatal, 794
    diaphragmatic hernia as, 799
    dislocation of hip as, 376-377
    of gastrointestinal system, 797
    genitourinary, 804-805
    grief response and, 832
    of heart, 795-797
    hydrocephalus of, 802-803
    imperforate anus as, 801
    infectious; *see* Infection
    intestinal, 801
    musculoskeletal, 804
    myelomeningocele as, 801-802
    of neurologic system, 794-795
    noninherited, 85-86
    omphalocele as, 800-801
    of reproductive system, 869
    of respiratory system, 794
    syphilis and, 770-771
    transesophageal, 799-800
    of urogenital system, 797

Conjunctivitis, chlamydial, 773-774
Conscious relaxation, 157
Consciousness, level of
    in postpartum period, 310
    in third stage of labor, 301
Consent
    for anesthesia, 240
    for sterilization, 499-500
Consolability of newborn, 339, 368
Constipation
    care plan for, 197
    nutrition and, 192
    in second trimester, 154
Contaminant, in breast milk, 425
Contraception, 483-502
    adolescent and, 725-726
    barrier, 489-490
    breastfeeding and, 426
    diabetes and, 630
    hormonal, 490-494
    natural family planning and, 485-489
    oral, 490-494
    pelvic inflammatory disease and, 861
    periodic abstinence as, 485-489
    tuberculosis and, 605-606
Contraction, uterine
    Braxton Hicks, 96
        in third trimester, 162
    false labor and, 264
    fetal heart rate and, 247
    in first stage of labor, 273-274
    nerve impulses and, 216
    postpartum, -441
    suppression of, 715-718
    true labor and, 264
Contraction stress test, 550-551
Convective heat loss, 333
Cooper's ligament, 39
Coping mechanism, 20
    cultural factors in, 268
    in grief, 823-824; *see also* Grief
    mandatory bedrest and, 565
    for new parents, 480-482
    preterm infant and, 780
    social history and, 128
Cord
    spinal, fetal development of, 81
    umbilical; *see* Umbilical cord
Cordocentesis, 546-547
Coronary heart disease, postmenopausal, 882
Corpus luteum, 42
Cost of care, 7
Coumadin, 643
Counseling
    diabetic patient and, 621
    genetic, 84-85
    in hospital birth, 167
    nutrition
        for adolescent, 737-738
        in health promotion, 850-851
Cow milk, 428
    nutrients in, 409-410
Coxsackievirus, 605
Crack cocaine, 671
Cramp
    leg, 192
    menstrual, 858-859

Cravings, food, 153
Crawling reflex, 355
Creatinine, 545-546
Cri-du-chat syndrome, 63
Crisis
    in family, 18, 20-21
    maturational, pregnancy as, 110
Crossed extension reflex, 355, 356
Crown-to-rump measurement, fetal, 69-73
Cry, assessment of, 758
Crying
    hunger and, 422
    of newborn, 339
Cuddliness of newborn, 339, 368
Cul-de-sac of Douglas, 31
Culdocentesis, 863
Cultural factors, 16-18
    adolescent pregnancy and, 728
    birth practices and, 267
    of breastfeeding, 412-413
    father's participation and, 287-288
    fertility and, 865
    labor and, 268-269
    menopause and, 881
    newborn and, 378
    nutritional, 193-196
    pain and, 223
    parenting behavior and, 459
    in postpartum period, 311
    in prenatal care, 145-146
    psychosocial assessment and, 478-479
    well-woman assessment and, 843
Curettage
    dilatation and, 580
        for hydatidiform mole, 579
    vacuum, 878-879
Cyanosis
    neonatal, 366
    in newborn, 753
Cycle
    menstrual, 39-44
        breast changes and, 39
    sexual response, 48-50
    sleep-wake, 335, 366
Cyst, retention, 325
Cystic fibrosis, 653
    genetics of, 65
Cystocele, 887
Cytologic examination, 132-133, 798
Cytomegalovirus, 599, 772

D
Daily fetal movement count, 551
Danazol
    for endometriosis, 860
    for infertility, 869-870
Danish food patterns, 195
Data collection process, 21
Death
    fetal, 534
        abnormal labor and, 695
        chlamydial infection and, 594
        maternal hypertension and, 555
    grief response to, 816-835; see also Grief
    HELLP syndrome and, 557, 559
    maternal
        eclampsia and, 555

Death—cont'd
    maternal—cont'd
        grief response to, 833
        respiratory distress syndrome causing, 653
    mortality rate and, definition of, 4
    neonatal, 534
        documentation of, 827, 828-830
        of postterm infant, 785
        preterm, 777
        taking baby to morgue, 827
Decelerations of fetal heart rate, 250-254
    nonreassuring patterns of, 259, 261
Decidua basilis, 68
Decompensation, cardiac, 641, 643
Deep tendon reflex, 355
    hypertension and, 560-562
Delayed hypersensitivity reaction, 52
DeLee suction, 371-372
Deletion, chromosomal, 63
Delivery room, 296-297
Dental health, 142
    nutrition and, 188
Deodorizing agents, 891
Deoxygenated blood, 79-80
Dependent edema, hypertension and, 560
Dependent phase of maternal adjustment, 455-456
Depression
    baby blues and, 456, 480, 665
    grief and, 833-834
    postpartum, 665-666
Dermatitis, diaper, 383, 775
Dermatoglyphics, 798
Dermatologic disorder, 653-654; see also Skin
Descent of fetus, 216-217
Desquamation, 329
    of vaginal cells, 97
Development
    of embryo, 69-79
    fetal, 79-83
    of preterm infant, 779
Developmental factors in infertility, 869
Developmental tasks
    of adolescence, 723-724
    of parenthood, 729
    of pregnancy, 727-728
Developmental theory of family, 15-16
Diabetes mellitus, 618-636
    breastfeeding and, 425
    care plan for, 791-792
    classification of, 619, 620
    fetus and, 82
    gestational, 630, 633-636
    infant of diabetic mother and, 788-792
    metabolic changes in pregnancy and, 620
    pathogenesis of, 618
    pregestational, 621-630
        assessment of, 623-624
        care plan for, 631-633
        counseling about, 621
        evaluation of, 630
        expected outcomes for, 625
        intrapartum period, 629
        nursing diagnosis for, 624-625
        postpartum care and, 629-630
        prenatal care for, 625-629
        risks and complications with, 621-623

Diameter
  biparietal, 208
  suboccipitobregmatic, 208
Diaper rash, 383
  candidal, 775
Diaphoresis, postpartal, 444
Diaphragm
  contraceptive, 494-497
  pelvic, 35-36
Diaphragmatic hernia, 799
Diastasis recti abdominis muscle, 443
Dick-Read childbirth method, 223-224
Diet; see Feeding of infant; Nutrition
Difficult child, 339
Digestion, by newborn, 326
Digits, extra, 804
Dilatation and curettage, 580
  for abortion, 878, 879
  for hydatidiform mole, 579
Dilation, cervical, 214
  expected responses to, 286
Direct bilirubin, 327
Disabled patient, 129
  well-woman care for, 844
Discharge
  ferning of, 98
  in third trimester, 161-162
Discharge from hospital
  of compromised newborn, 813
  criteria for, 386
  early
    advantages and disadvantages of, 506-509
    preparation for, 512-515
  for general surgery, 657
  mastectomy and, 892
  planning for, 482-483
  of preterm infant, 779
  substance abuse and, 675
Discomfort
  of circumcision, 398
  during labor, 267; see also Labor, pain management in
  during pregnancy
    in first trimester, 138, 139
    nutrition-related, 191-192
    in second trimester, 153-154
    in third trimester, 159, 162
Dislocation of hip, congenital, 376-377
Disseminated intravascular coagulation
  preeclampsia and, 557
  respiratory distress syndrome and, 652
Diuresis
  postpartal, 444
  preeclampsia and, 568
Diverticulum, Meckel's, 79
Dizygotic twins, 83-84
DNA, cell division and, 61
Documentation
  birth/recovery, 306
  of death, 827
  of home visit, 517
  of infant care teaching, 379
  prenatal, review of, 264-265
  of recovery period, 313
Domestic violence, 677-683
Dominant gene, 60
Dominant inheritance, 64, 65

Donor
  of oocyte or sperm, 876
  organ, 825
Doppler blood flow measurement, 541
Dorsolumbar lordosis, 105
Down syndrome, 62
Dressing of infant, 385
  after death, 825
Drug
  for abortion, 880
  abuse of, 806-813; see also Substance abuse
  for amenorrhea, 858
  antihypertensive, 569
  in breast milk, 425
  for chlamydial infection, 594
  for dysmenorrhea, 858
  for eclampsia, 570
  for endometriosis, 860
  in first trimester, 142
  for gonorrhea, 595
  history of use of, 128
  for HIV infection, 596
  for human papillomavirus, 601-602
  for infertility
    female, 869-870
    male, 872
  labor and, 228-238
    consent for, 240
    for general anesthesia, 237
    for inhalation anesthesia, 237-238
    for nerve block, 230-236
    routes of administration of, 240-241
    sedatives and, 228
    systemic analgesics and, 228-230
  maternal, neonatal behavior and, 336
  for neonatal resuscitation, 752
  oral contraceptives and, 490-494
  for pelvic inflammatory disease, 863
  placental transfer of, 77
  for preeclampsia, 567-568
  psychotropic, 667
  for toxoplasmosis, 598
Drug abuse; see Substance abuse
Duct
  milk, 39
    plugging of, 414
  seminal, 46
  testicular, 47-48
Ductus arteriosus, 321
  fetal development and, 80
Ductus venosus, 321
Duncan's mechanism, 301
Dysfunctional labor, 687
Dysmaturity, 787-788
Dysmenorrhea, 858-859
Dysplasia of hip, 376-377, 804
Dyspnea, in third trimester, 162
Dystocia, 687-711
  abnormal labor and, 693-695
  assessment of, 695
  augmentation of labor and, 699
  cesarean birth and, 702-710
    vaginal birth after, 707, 710
  dysfunctional labor and, 687
  evaluation of, 711
  expected outcomes for, 696
  external cephalic version in, 696-697

Dystocia—cont'd
  fetal causes of, 689-692
  forceps-assisted birth and, 699-701
  induction of labor and, 697-699
  nursing diagnosis for, 695-696
  pelvic structure and, 687-689
  position of mother and, 692-693
  psychological response to, 693
  trauma secondary to, 367, 373
  trial of labor in, 697
  vacuum extraction and, 701-702

E

Ear
  congenital disorder of, 794
  of newborn, 338, 347
Early adolescence, pregnancy in, 730
Early decelerations of fetal heart rate, 250-254
Early discharge from hospital
  advantages and disadvantages of, 506-509
  preparation for, 512-515
Early pregnancy class, 164-165
Easy child, 339
Eclampsia
  definition of, 556
  as emergency, 568-570
  epilepsy vs., 654
  magnesium sulfate for, 568
Economic functions of family, 13
Economic security, pregnancy and, 116
Ectoderm, 79
Ectopic pregnancy, 576-578
  checklist for assisting parents, 828
  nursing care for, 580
Edema
  ankle, 162
  care plan for, 168
  hypertension and, 560
  neonatal, 758
  preeclampsia and, 556
  pregnancy and, 99
  vulvar, 98
Education
  for adolescent parent, 741
  in first trimester, 136-143
  as function of family, 13
  infant care teaching and, 379
  for parents of compromised newborn, 813
  in second trimester, 152, 155-158
  sex, 726-727
  in third trimester, 160-167
Effacement, 211, 214
Effleurage, 163, 226
Ejaculate, 48
Ejaculation, conception and, 66
Ejection, of milk, 411
Elderly patient, well-woman care for, 843-844
Elective abortion, 572, 877-880
Electrical nerve stimulation, transcutaneous, 228
Electrolytes, newborn and, 325
Electronic fetal monitoring, 255-257, 548-551
Elimination
  labor and, 281
  parent education about, 401
  in postpartum period, 444
Embolus, amniotic fluid, 301

Embryo
  development of, 66-68, 68-79
  donor, 876
Emergency
  cardiac, 641
  cesarean birth as, 703
  eclampsia as, 568-570
  in first stage of labor, 282-284
  metabolic, 641
  surgical, 799-801
Emergency childbirth, 299, 300
Emesis; see Vomiting
Emotional response; see Psychological response
Employment, in first trimester, 138-139
En face position, 311, 457-458
Endocarditis, 648
Endocrine disorder
  diabetes as
    gestational, 630, 633-636
    pregestational, 621-630, 631
  hyperemesis gravidarum and, 636-639
  hypothyroidism as, 639
  of thyroid; see Thyroid gland
Endocrine system
  of fetus, 82
  labor and, 219
  in postpartum period, 442-443
  pregnancy-related changes in, 106-107, 556
  in well-woman care, 842
Endoderm, 79
Endometrial cycle, 40-42
Endometriosis, 859-860
  care plan for, 862
Endometritis, postpartal, 603
Endometrium, 31
  estrogen replacement therapy and, 883
  timed biopsy of, 866-867
Endothelium, preeclampsia and, 557
Energy requirement
  of newborn, 408
  in pregnancy, 181-182
Engagement, 208, 216
Engorgement
  of breast, 414
  splanchnic, 310
    heart disease and, 644
Enlargement, uterine and abdominal, 94-95
Enteritis, regional, 653
Enterocele, 886, 887
Enterocolitis, necrotizing, 784
Entrainment, 452
Environment
  of home, 386, 390
  immune system and, 53
  neutral thermal, 762-763, 764
Environmental stimulus, newborn's response to, 338-339
Enzyme
  capacitation of sperm and, 66
  HELLP syndrome and, 557, 559, 566-568
Enzyme immunoassay for pregnancy, 93
Enzyme-linked immunosorbent assay, 93
Epidermis, fetal, 83
Epididymis, 46, 47-48
Epidural anesthesia
  for cesarean birth, 703
  plan of care for, 242
Epidural block, 234-236

Epilepsy, 654
Epinephrine, for drug reaction, 239
Episiotomy, 297, 302-304, 442
    pain of, 310
    vacuum extraction birth and, 701
Epispadias, 804-805
Epstein's pearls, 325
Epulis
    pregnancy and, 103-104
    in third trimester, 162
Equipment
    for childbirth, 293-295
    for newborn resuscitation, 752
Erection
    of nipple, 412
    of penis, 49
Ergonovine, 581
Erythema, birth trauma causing, 373
Erythema infectiosum, 605
Erythema neonatorum, 330
Erythema toxicum, 330
Erythropoiesis, folate and, 184
Esophageal atresia, 799-800
Esophagus, 105-106
Essential amino acid, 182
Estimated date of birth, 124-125
Estrogen
    breast and, 38
    malignancy and, 883
    in oral contraceptive, 490-494
    osteoporosis and, 881-883
    placenta and, 75
    in postpartum period, 440-441
    respiratory system and, 100, 101
Ethical issues, 8
    in assisted reproductive therapy, 875
    diabetes and, 629
    forced cesarean birth as, 702
Ethnocentrism, 17
Ethyl chloride, male infertility and, 871
Evaporated milk formula, 428
Evaporation, heat loss and, 333
Examination; see Physical examination
Excitement phase of sexual response, 49
Exercise
    diabetes and, 628
    in first trimester, 140-141, 142
    health promotion and, 851
    Kegel; see Kegel exercise
    nutrition and, 190
    osteoporosis prevention and, 884, 885
Exotoxin, pyrogenic, 606
Experiential history, 841-842
Expressing breast milk, 422-424
Expulsion of fetus, 218
Extended family, 12
    adolescent pregnancy and, 729
Extension of fetus, 218
External cephalic version, 689, 695-696
External electronic fetal monitoring, 255
External os, 32
External physical assessment, 362-363
External rotation of fetus, 218
Extra digits, 804
Extracellular fluid, sodium in, 185
Extraction, vacuum, 701-702

Extrauterine life, adaptation to
    dysfunctional, 752-753
    normal, 370, 387, 755
Extravasation, intravenous, in newborn, 758
Extremity
    birth of, 299
    of newborn, 351-352
Extremity restraint, 399
Extrophy of bladder, 804
Extrusion reflex, 354
Eye
    chlamydial infection of, 773-774
    fetal, 81
    of newborn, 336, 338, 346-347
    phototherapy and, 395
    prophylaxis for, 394
Eye-to-eye contact, 452

F
Face, rash on, 383
Face presentation, 689, 692
Facial melasma, 103
Facial paralysis, 654
Facies, of newborn, 347
Facilitated transport, 76
Factor VIII, von Willebrand's disease and, 592
Failure to thrive, flow chart for, 416
Faintness
    in pregnancy, 105
    in second trimester, 153
Fallopian tube, 28-30
    ectopic pregnancy in, 576-577
    infertility and, 870
    reconstruction of, 875
    sterilization procedures and, 500-501
Family
    adaptation of, 109-122; see also Adaptation
    adolescent pregnancy and, 728
    after childbirth
        adaptation to infant and, 459-460, 475-482
        bonding and, 450-453
        grandparent adaptation and, 460
        parental roles and, 453-459
        parenting process and, 450
        sibling adaptation and, 459-460
    of compromised newborn, 765
    crisis and, 18, 20-21
    cultural factors in, 16-18
    development of, 15-16
    dynamics of, 15
    functions of, 13, 15
    grief and, 825-826
    health of, 16
    life cycle of, 14
    migrant, 681
    social history and, 128
    structure and function of, 476, 478
    in third stage of labor, 302
    types of, 11-13
Family history, 128
    in well-woman care, 841
Family unit, 13
Family-centered care, 7-8
Fat
    body, amenorrhea and, 858
    dietary, 850
    newborn requirement for, 409

Fat metabolism, ketone bodies and, 622
Father
    adaptation to pregnancy by, 115-118
    adjustment of, 456-457
    adolescent, 728, 740
    during labor
        first stage, 287-288
        second stage, 296
Father-child relationship, 117-118
Fatigue
    in first trimester, care plan for, 147
    maternal, 456
Fat-soluble vitamins, requirement for, 180, 182-183
Feedback
    bonding and, 451
    relaxation and, 225
Feeding of infant, 380, 407-435
    by adolescent mother, 738
    assessment of, 413
    behavior during, 326
    breastfeeding and; see Breastfeeding
    care plan for, 431-432
    expected outcomes in, 416
    formula, 426-429
    frequency of, 429-430
    general considerations in, 416-417
    hyperbilirubinemia and, 327-328
    lactation and, 410-413
    necrotizing enterocolitis and, 784
    nursing diagnosis for, 413
    nutritional needs and, 407-410
    planning for, 413, 416
    prenatal preparation for, 157
    problems with, 425-426
    readiness of, 408
    rhythm of, 457-458
Female genitalia, of newborn, 350-351
    cleansing of, 385
Female infertility, 864-876; see also Infertility
Female reproductive system
    adult, 25-44; see also Reproductive system, female
    of newborn, 330
Female sterilization, 500-501
Femoral thrombophlebitis, 604
Fencing reflex, 355
Fentanyl, labor and, 229
Ferguson's reflex, 215
Ferning, 98, 277
Fertility
    cervical mucus and, 42
    contraception and; see Contraception
    impaired, 864-876; see also Infertility
    trends in, 3-4
Fertility awareness, 485-486
Fertility rate, 4
Fertilization, 66-68
Fertilized ovum, implantation of, 42
Fetal alcohol syndrome, 808-811
Fetal blood sampling, 257
Fetal circulation, 322
Fetal heart rate, 96, 254-261
    baseline, 247-249
    contraction stress test and, 550-551
    diabetic mother and, 629
    electronic monitoring of, 255-257
    fetal blood sampling and, 257
    fetal stimulation and, 257

Fetal heart rate—cont'd
    in first stage of labor, 271-272
    in high-risk pregnancy, 548-551
    history of, 246-247
    maternal hypertension and, 562
    nonreassuring patterns of, 259, 261, 285
    nonstress test and, 549
    normal, 80, 218
        in first trimester, 135
        periodic changes in, 249-254
        in second trimester, 150
    periodic auscultation for, 254-255
    protocol for monitoring of, 260
    reassuring patterns of, 259
    in second stage of labor, 296
Fetal hemoglobin, in newborn, 323
Fetopelvic disproportion, 689
Fetus; see also Fetal entries
    acoustic stimulation of, 549
    adaptation to labor by, 218
    biophysical profile of, 542-543
    birth of, 297-299
    blood sampling from, 257
    breech presentation of, 689-692
    cardiopulmonary resuscitation and, 641
    circulation of, 322
    death of, 534
        chlamydial infection and, 594
    of diabetic mother, 623, 624, 625
    dystocia and, 689-692
    engagement of head of, 208, 216
    false vs. true labor and, 264
    glucose and, 620
    heart rate assessment of, 246-262; see also Fetal heart rate
    high-risk
        biochemical assessment of, 544-548
        electronic monitoring of, 548-551
        ultrasonography of, 537-543
    labor and, 206-209
    lipid-containing exfoliated cells of, 546
    maternal concern about, 113
    maternal weight gain and, 176
    maturation of, 79-83
    movement of
        in high-risk pregnancy, 551
        in labor, 218
        in second trimester, 150
    rights of, 537
    risk factors for, 536
    in second trimester, 148-151
    squamous cells of, test for, 277
    in third trimester, 160
    at thirteen weeks, 135
    trauma to mother and, 659
    viability of, ultrasonography and, 539
Fever, childbed, 603-605
Fibrillation, atrial, 648
Fibrosis, cystic, 653
Fifth disease, 605
Filipino food patterns, 194
Fingernail, of fetus, 83
Finnish food patterns, 195
First stage of labor, 263-290; see also Labor, first stage of
First trimester abortion, 878-879
First trimester of pregnancy, 124-146; see also Pregnancy, normal, first trimester of

Fistula
  genital, 890
  tracheoesophageal, 799-800
Flaring, 756
Flatulence, in second trimester, 154
Flea-bite dermatitis, 330
Flexion
  fetal, 217
  as fetal attitude, 207
Fluid
  abruptio placentae and, 583
  amniotic; *see* Amniotic fluid
  as body defense, 50
  extracellular, sodium in, 185
  labor and, 281
  lung, 80
  newborn requirements for, 409
  overload of, 591
  patent ductus arteriosus and, 784
  in postpartum period, 311
  preeclampsia and, 566
  requirement for, 182
  respiratory distress and, 782
  vaginal, 34
Fluid and electrolytes
  newborn and, 325
  pregnancy-related changes in, 102-103
Fluorescent treponema antibody absorption test, 595
Fluoride
  breastfeeding and, 430
  newborn requirements for, 409-410
  pregnancy requirement for, 185
5-Fluorouracil, for human papillomavirus, 601
Flush, in menopause, 880
Focusing, relaxation and, 225
Focusing phase of pregnancy, 115
Folic acid
  deficiency of, 649-650
  requirement for, 181, 184
Follicle, infertility and, 865
Follicle-stimulating hormone, 42
  infertility and, 872
  in postpartum period, 443
Follicular phase of ovarian cycle, 42
Follow-up care, 509
  after death in infant, 827, 830
  by telephone, 521, 523-527
Food beliefs, 192, 196
Food cravings, 153
Food guide pyramid, 174, 190
Foramen ovale, 79-80, 321
Forceps assisted birth, 699-701
  trauma from, 373, 376
Forebrain, fetal, 81
Foregut, 81
Foreskin, 330
  circumcision and, 397-400
Formula feeding, 426-429
  iron and, 409
Fourchette, 28
Fourth stage of labor, 305-313; *see also* Labor, fourth
    stage of
Fourth trimester; *see* Postpartum period
Fracture, osteoporosis and, 884
Fragile X syndrome, inheritance of, 65
Frank breech presentation, 691
Freestanding birth center, 166

Frequency, urinary, 102
  in first trimester, 139
  genital atrophy and, 884
  in third trimester, 162
Friability, cervical, 97
Fruitarian diet, 197
FTA-ABS test for syphilis, 595
Fundal height
  maternal position affecting, 149
  in second trimester, 148-149
Fundal pressure, 299
Fundus, uterine
  anatomy of, 31
  massage of, 311
  palpation of, 308
  in postpartum period, 440
Funeral arrangements, 826
Funic souffle, 96

G

Gait, in pregnancy, 104
Galactosemia, 798
  screening for, 388
Gallbladder, 106
Gamete, 61
Gamete intrafallopian transfer, 876
Gametogenesis, 61, 62
Gastric emptying, fetal, 82
Gastric motility, in postpartum period, 444
Gastrointestinal system
  of fetus, 69-73, 81-82
  high-risk pregnancy and, 653
  labor and, 219
  of newborn, 325-326
    compromised, 761-762
    congenital disorders of, 801
    necrotizing enterocolitis and, 784
  in postpartum period, 444
  pregnancy-related changes in, 105-106
  well-woman care and, 842
Gate-control theory of pain, 223
Gene, 60
General anesthesia
  for cesarean birth, 703
  for labor, 237
Genetic counseling, 84-85
Genetic disorder
  amniocentesis for, 544
  diabetes as, 618
  postnatal diagnosis of, 797-798
  preeclampsia and, 557
Genetics, 60-65
Genital fistula, 890
Genital herpes, 599-601
Genital system; *see* Reproductive system
Genitalia
  circumcision and, 397-400
  of fetus, 82
  of newborn, 330, 331, 350-351
    assessment of, 366-367
    cleansing of, 385
  postmenopausal atrophy of, 881
Genitourinary system
  congenital anomalies of, 804
  well-woman care and, 842
German measles, 598, 599, 771-772

Gestational age, 775-777
  assessment of, 364
  behavior and, 335
  growth retardation and, 787-788
  postterm, 718-719
  in second trimester, 150
  ultrasonography and, 539
Gestational carrier, 876
Gestational diabetes; *see* Diabetes mellitus
Gestational trophoblastic neoplasm, 578
Gingival granuloma gravidarum, 103-104
Gingivitis, in third trimester, 162
Glabellar reflex, 354
Gland
  adrenal, of fetus, 82
  of male reproductive system, 48
  mammary, 38-39
  oil, of newborn, 329
  parathyroid, 107
  pituitary, prolactin and, 107
  Skene's, 131
  sweat, of newborn, 329
  thyroid
    of fetus, 82
    pregnancy-related changes in, 106-107
    prenatal examination of, 130
  vestibular, 27-28
Globulin
  pregnancy and, 103
  Rh$_o$ immune, 581
Glomerular filtration rate
  fetal, 81
  pregnancy and, 102
Glucocorticoid, for infertility, 869
Glucose
  diabetes and, 618, 790
    gestational, 635
    monitoring levels of, 627-628
  neonatal hypoglycemia and, 333, 378, 623, 765
  oral contraceptives and, 493
  placental transfer of, 620
  small for gestational age infant and, 787
Glucose intolerance of pregnancy, 619
Glucosuria, pregnancy and, 103
Gonadotropin, chorionic
  nausea and vomiting and, 107
  placenta and, 75
  pregnancy testing and, 92-93
Gonadotropin-releasing hormone, 42
  for endometriosis, 860
Gonorrhea, 594-595
  candidiasis and, 775
Goodell's sign, 95, 97
Graafian follicle, infertility and, 865
Grand mal seizure, 654
Grandparent
  adaptation of
    to newborn, 460
    to pregnancy, 118-119
  psychosocial assessment and, 481-482
Granuloma gravidarum, gingival, 103-104
Grasping reflex, 354
Gravidity, 92
Great vessels, transposition of, 795
Greater vestibular gland, 27-28

Grief, 816-835
  adolescent pregnancy and, 739, 833
  assessment of, 820
  care plan for, 832, 831830
  caring for persons in, 819
  communication techniques for, 821-823
  complicated bereavement and, 833-834
  discharge from hospital and, 827, 830
  evaluation of, 830, 832
  expected outcomes in, 820-821
  infertility investigation and, 874
  maternal death and, 833
  memories and, 824-827
  morgue and, 827
  multiple pregnancy and, 832-833
  nursing diagnosis for, 820
  physical comfort in, 823-824
  preterm infant and, 779
  signs and symptoms of, 817
  tasks of mourners and, 818-819
  therapeutic abortion and, 832
  types of responses to, 817-818
Group B streptococcal infection, 603
Growth, of preterm infant, 779
Growth retardation, intrauterine, 787-788
  cordocentesis for, 546-547
  definition of, 775
  diabetes and, 623
  ultrasonography and, 539-541
  weight gain and, 176
Grunting, 756
G-spot, 35
Gynecoid pelvis, 211, 213
Gynecologic disorder, surgery for, 657

H
Habituation, 339, 368, 458
Hair
  fetal, 83
  pubic
    in female, 26
    in male, 44
Halothane, -238
Hard measles, 605
Head
  fetal
    birth of, 298
    engagement of, 208, 216
    size of, 206
  hydrocephalus, 802-803
  of newborn
    assessment of, 345-346
    circumference of, 342, 343, 366
    molding of, 332
Headache
  in second trimester, 154
  tension, 105
Health promotion, 839-856
  preventive care and, 849-854
  well-woman health care and, 839-849
Healthy People 2000, 849-854
Hearing, of newborn, 338
Heart
  cocaine and, 671
  fetal, 79-80
  in postpartum period, 445

Heart disease
  congenital, 795-797
    patent ductus arteriosus as, 784
    persistent pulmonary hypertension and, 786
  maternal, 639-649
    antepartum care in, 643
    care plan for, 645-646
    endocarditis as, 648
    evaluation of, 644, 647
    expected outcomes for, 642
    intrapartum care in, 643-644
    Marfan syndrome and, 648-649
    mitral valve prolapse as, 648
    nursing diagnosis for, 642
    perinatal heart failure and, 647
    postpartum care in, 644
    rheumatic, 647-648
  postmenopausal, 882
Heart rate
  fetal; *see* Fetal heart rate
  of newborn, 322-323, 340, 366, 761-762
Heart sounds, of newborn, 322-323
Heartburn, 106
  care plan for, 197
  nutrition and, 191-192
  in second trimester, 153
Heat
  for dysmenorrhea, 858
  newborn and, 332-333
  small for gestational age infant and, 787-788
Heel stick, 390
Hegar's sign, 95
Height, fundal
  maternal position affecting, 149
  in second trimester, 148-149
HELLP syndrome, 557, 559, 566-568
Helpline services, 524, 527
Hemagglutination inhibition test, 93
Hemangioma, capillary, 330
Hematocrit, of newborn, 323, 762
Hematologic system; *see also* Blood
  of preterm infant, 778
  well-woman care and, 842
Hematoma, 308
  cephalhematoma and, 329
Hematopoietic system
  fetal, 80
  of newborn, 323
Hemodilution, 178
Hemoglobin
  fetal, 80
  of newborn, 323, 753
  pregnancy and, 100
Hemolytic disease
  HELLP syndrome and, 557, 559, 566-568
  prenatal diagnosis of, 546
Hemorrhage, 572-593
  anxiety about, 525-526
  clotting disorders causing, 591-593
  as contraindication for epidural block, 236
  in early pregnancy
    ectopic pregnancy causing, 576-578
    hydatidiform mole causing, 578
    incompetent cervix causing, 575-576
    nursing care for, 579-581
    spontaneous abortion and, 572, 574-576

Hemorrhage—cont'd
  elective abortion and, 879
  emergency interventions for, 285
  in late pregnancy, 581-585
  postpartum, 305, 308-309, 311
  as risk factor, 536
  shock caused by, 588-591
  standard of care for, 591
  subconjunctival, 373
  in third trimester, 161
Hemorrhoid, 106
  constipation and, 192
  examination for, 132
  pain of, 310
  in postpartum period, 442, 446
Heparin, heart disease and, 643
Hepatic system
  of fetus, 82
  HELLP syndrome and, 557, 559, 566-568
  of newborn, 326-328
  preeclampsia and, 557
  pregnancy and, 106
Hepatitis, 597, 599, 770
Hepatitis B vaccine, 393, 770
Herbal medicine, for postmenopausal patient, 883
Hereditary disorder; *see* Genetic disorder
Heredity, 60-65
Hernia
  diaphragmatic, 799
  hiatal, 105-106
  omphalocele and, 800-801
Heroin abuse, 672, 812
Herpes simplex virus, 772-773
  genital, 598, 599-601
Hiatal hernia, 105-106
Hierarchy, in family, 15
High altitude, 140
High-risk pregnancy, 533-746; *see also* Pregnancy, high-risk
Hindbrain, 81
Hindgut, 81
Hip, congenital dislocation of, 376-377, 804
Hirsutism, 104
Hispanic culture
  food patterns of, 194
  support during labor and, 288
History, patient
  diabetes and, 623-624
  in first trimester, 125-128
  of newborn, 365
  review of, 264-265
  in well-woman care, 840, 841-842
Holding of infant, 381
Home birth, 166-167
Home care, 506-529
  after hemorrhage, 585
  of newborn, 383, 386
  postpartal, 506-529
    breastfeeding and, 418
    early discharge and, 506-509
    evaluation of, 512
    expected outcomes in, 512
    home visits and, 515-521
    nursing diagnosis for, 512
    predischarge assessment and, 509
    preparatory instruction for, 512-515
    protocol for, 522

Home care—cont'd
  postpartal—cont'd
    support groups and, 527
    telephone follow-up and, 521, 523-527
  preeclampsia and, 565-566, 571-572
  trend to, 8
Home environment, 386, 390
Homocystinuria, screening for, 389
Homosexual family, 13
Hormone
  for breast cancer, 892
  endometriosis and, 860
  follicle-stimulating, 42
  gonadotropin-releasing, 42
  infertility investigation and, 866
  luteinizing, 42
  oral contraceptives and, 490-494
  placental, 75
  in postpartum period, 442-443
  pregnancy and, 93
  sex, 48
Hormone replacement therapy
  amenorrhea and, 858
  for infertility, 869-870
  postmenopausal, 882-883
Hosiery, support, 152
Hospital birth, 167
Hot flash, 880
Human chorionic gonadotropin, 107
  infertility and, 872
  placenta and, 75
  pregnancy testing and, 92-93
Human immunodeficiency virus, 595-597
  breastfeeding and, 425
  neonatal, 774
  pelvic inflammatory disease and, 863
  screening for, 135
Human papillomavirus, 601-602
Human placental lactogen, 75, 107
Humoral immunity, 50
Hydatidiform mole, 578-579
Hydralazine, 569
Hydramnios, 278
  diabetes and, 621
Hydrocephalus, 802-803
Hydrotherapy, labor and, 226-227
Hygiene
  labor and, 281
  in postpartum period, 311
Hymen, 27
Hyperbilirubinemia, 327-328, 377
  causes of, 793
  diabetes and, 790
  treatment of, 394-397
Hypercarbia, neonatal, 765
Hyperglycemia
  diabetes and, 618
  fetus and, 82
  ketoacidosis versus, 622
Hyperinsulinemia, fetus and, 82
Hyperplasia
  adrenal, screening for, 389
  cervical, 97
Hypersensitivity reaction, 52
Hypertension, 555-572
  assessment of, 559-564
  care plan for, 571-572

Hypertension—cont'd
  classification of, 555-556
  diabetes and, 621
  eclampsia and, 569-570
  etiology of, 556
  evaluation of, 570, 572
  expected outcomes in, 564
  HELLP syndrome and, 557, 559, 566-568
  morbidity and mortality from, 555
  nursing diagnosis for, 564
  pathophysiology of, 556-559
  persistent pulmonary, 786
  postpartum care and, 570
  preeclampsia and, 555-556, 564-568
  significance of, 555
Hypertonic sodium chloride, abortion with, 879
Hypertonic uterine dysfunctional, 687
Hypertrophic cardiomyopathy, 647
Hypertrophy, uterine, 440-441
Hyperventilation
  labor and, 225
  pregnancy and, 100-101
Hypocalcemia
  diabetes and, 790
  neonatal, 378
Hypoglycemia
  diabetes and, 790
  neonatal, 333, 378, 765
  in small for gestational age infant, 787
Hypogonadotropic amenorrhea, 858
Hyponatremia
  neonatal, 185
  water intoxication and, 409
Hypospadias, 804-805
Hypotension
  epidural block and, 236
  labor and, 219
  neonatal, 765
  placental perfusion and, 233
  in postpartum period, 310
  supine, 131, 153, 276
Hypothalamic-pituitary cycle, 41, 42
Hypothalamic-pituitary-gonadal axis, 48
  pregnancy and, 94
Hypothermia, neonatal, 371, 762-763
Hypothyroidism, 798
  maternal, 639
  screening for, 388
Hypotonia, uterine, 586-587
Hypotonic uterine dysfunction, 687
Hypovolemic shock, postpartum, 309
Hypoxemia, 763, 765
Hypoxia, 546
Hysterosalpingography, 867, 868
Hysterotomy, for abortion, 880

I

Ice pack, for postpartum pain, 310
Identity
  as developmental task of adolescent, 723-724
  fatherhood role and, 116
  pregnancy and, 112
Ileus, meconium, cystic fibrosis and, 65
Ilium, 37
Immune globulin, Rh_o, 581
Immune system
  breastfeeding and, 417

Immune system—cont'd
  infertility and, 871
  of newborn, 328
  in postpartum period, 447-448
  preeclampsia and, 557
  pregnancy-related changes in, 593
  well-woman care and, 842
Immunization, 51
  adolescent and, 732
  in first trimester, 142
  for hepatitis B, 393, 770
  HIV infection and, 596
Immunoglobulin
  breastfeeding and, 417
  fetal, 82-83
Immunologic system
  fetal, 82-83
  immunity and, 50-53
Impaired fertility, 864-876; see also Infertility
Imperforate anus, 801
Implantable contraceptive, 494, 495
Implantation of embryo, 42, 68
  low-lying, 581-582
In vitro fertilization, 876
Inborn errors of metabolism, 64-65, 797-798
Incompetent cervix, 575-576
  nursing care for, 579-580
Incomplete abortion, 574
Incomplete breech presentation, 691
Incontinence, 133
  odor of, 891
  postmenopausal, 881
Independent phase of maternal adjustment, 455-456
Index
  amniotic fluid, 541
  body mass, 175, 176
  of respiratory distress, 757
Indirect bilirubin, 327
Induction of labor, 697-699
Industrial nurse, 88
Inevitable abortion, 574
Infant; see Newborn
Infant car seat, 514
Infant care teaching record, 379
Infant mortality; see Death
Infant of diabetic mother; see Diabetes mellitus
Infection, 593-611
  amniotitis and, 278
  assessment of, 606-608
  breastfeeding and, 414
  care plan for, 609-610
  chlamydial, 593-594
  as contraindication for epidural block, 236
  control of, 608, 610
  diabetes and, 621-622
  endocarditis as, 648
  evaluation of, 608
  expected outcomes for, 608
  general, 605-606
  genital tract, 602-603
  heart disease and, 643
  hemorrhage and, 591
  immune system and, 83
  infertility and, 870-871
  nosocomial, 608, 610
  nursing diagnosis for, 608
  nutritional status and, 53

Infection—cont'd
  pelvic, 132-133, 861-864
  postpartal, 603-605
  preterm infant and, 778
  puerperal, heart disease and, 644
  as risk factor, 536
  sexually transmitted, 593-602; see also Sexually transmitted disease
  streptococcal, 603
  TORCH, 597-601, 769
  trichomoniasis and, 603
  vaginal, 97, 602-603
  viral
    cytomegalovirus, 599
    hepatitis, 597, 599
    herpes, 598, 599-601
    human immunodeficiency, 135, 425, 595-597
    human papillomavirus, 601-602
    mumps and, 605
    parvovirus B-19 and, 605
    placenta and, 77
    rubella and, 598, 599
    rubeola and, 605
Infertility, 864-876
  assisted reproductive therapies for, 875-876
  congenital or developmental factors in, 869-871
  cultural considerations in, 865
  incidence of, 864
  investigations of, 865-869
  male factors in, 865, 871-875
  religious considerations in, 864
Infiltration anesthesia, local, 230
Inflammatory bowel disease, 653
Inflammatory disease
  endometrial, 603, 859-860
  infertility and, 870
  pelvic, 861-864
Informed consent
  for anesthesia, 240
  sterilization and, 499-500
Infundibulum, of uterine tube, 30
Infusion
  of magnesium sulfate, 567
  postpartum hemorrhage and, 587
Inhalation anesthesia, 237-238
Inheritance, 60-65; see also Genetic disorder
Injectable contraceptive, 494
Injection
  insulin, 628
  intramuscular
    of magnesium sulfate, 567
    in newborn, 393-394
Injury; see Trauma
Inlet, pelvic, 209
Innominate bone, 37
Insemination, therapeutic, 875
Insomnia, 162
  care plan for, 168
Inspiratory time, 760
Instruments, for childbirth, 293-295
Insulin
  diabetes and, 618
    gestational, 635
    intrapartum period and, 629
    as therapy, 628
  fetus and, 82
  pregnancy and, 620, 621
Insulin shock, 622

Integumentary system
    disorders of, 653-654
    fetal, 83
    labor and, 219
    of newborn, 328-330, 344-345
    in postpartum period, 447
    pregnancy-related changes in, 103-104
Intercourse
    infertility testing and, 872
    in postmenopausal period, 881
    in postpartum period, 483
    during pregnancy, 143-145
Interdependent phase of maternal adjustment, 456
Internal electronic fetal monitoring, 256-257
Internal os, 32
Internal rotation of fetus, 217
Interstitium, of fallopian tube, 30
Interview
    in first trimester, 125
    at hospital admission, 265
    hypertension and, 559-560
    during labor, 238
    in nutritional assessment, 185-186
    in second trimester, 146
    in well-woman care, 840
Intestinal bacteria, in newborn, 326
Intestinal obstruction, congenital, 801
Intestine; see Gastrointestinal system
Intoxication, water, 409
Intraepithelial neoplasia, cervical, 847-848
Intramuscular injection
    during labor, 241
    of magnesium sulfate, 567
    in newborn, 393-394
Intrapartum care; see Labor
Intrauterine development
    of embryo, 69-79
    fetal, 79-83
Intrauterine device, 498-499
    diabetes and, 630
Intrauterine growth retardation, 787-788
    cordocentesis for, 546-547
    definition of, 775
    diabetes and, 623
    ultrasonography and, 539-541
    weight gain and, 176
Intrauterine insemination, 875
Intrauterine pressure catheter, 255, 256
Intravascular coagulation, disseminated, 591-592
    preeclampsia and, 557
Intravenous extravasation, in newborn, 758
Intravenous route, during labor, 240-241
Introitus, vaginal, 27
Inversion of uterus, 587-588
Involution of uterus, 440-441, 516
Iodine, 180
Iron, 179, 183
    adolescent pregnancy and, 738
    for newborn, 326, 409
Iron deficiency anemia, 649
Irritability, of newborn, 339, 367
Ischemia, cerebral, 649
Ischemic phase of endometrial cycle, 42
Ischial tuberosity, 37
Ischiocavernosus muscle, 36
Ischium, 37
Islet cell, fetus and, 82

Isoimmunization, 871
Isthmus, of fallopian tube, 30
Italian food patterns, 194

J
Japanese culture
    food patterns and, 194
    infant behavior and, 336
Jaundice, 793
    kernicterus and, 793
    neonatal, 327-328, 377, 756
        breastfeeding and, 417
        cause of, 396
Jelly, Wharton's, 79
Jet hydrotherapy, 226-227
Jewish culture
    assisted fertility therapy and, 864
    food patterns of, 195
Jitteriness, 378
Joint
    pain in, 154
    pelvic, 209
        injury to, 888
    rheumatoid arthritis and, 655
Junction, squamous columnar, 33

K
Kangaroo care, 785
Karyotype, 60, 798
Kegel exercise, 851
    for incontinence, 888
    for postmenopausal patient, 884
    in pregnancy, 130, 137
Kenyan culture, 412-413
Kernicterus, 793
Ketoacidosis, 618, 622
Ketone body, 622
Kick count, in high-risk pregnancy, 551
Kidney; see Renal system
Klinefelter's syndrome, 63, 798
Korean culture, breastfeeding and, 412
K-Y Lubricating Jelly, 884

L
Labetalol hydrochloride, 569
Labia majora, 26-27
Labia minora, 27
Labor, 205-317, 263-317
    abnormal patterns of, 693, 695
    adaptation to, 218-219
    adolescent and, 739
    anticipation of, 118
    assessment of, 238
    augmentation of, 699
    care plan for, 242-243
    collaborative care during, 239-241
    delivery, recovery, postpartum room, 166, 288-289
        transfer from, 312
    diabetic mother and, 624, 629
        gestational diabetes and, 635-636
    dystocia and, 686-711; see also Dystocia
    essential factors in, 206-215
    expected outcomes in, 239
    false, 264
    first stage of, 263-290
        abnormal patterns of, 693, 695
        breathing techniques in, 225

Labor—cont'd
  first stage of—cont'd
    care plan for, 290
    definition of, 216
    emergency during, 282-284, 285
    evaluation of, 289, 291
    expected outcomes for, 279
    father's participation during, 287-288
    grandparents' participation during, 288
    hospital admission and, 264, 269
    laboratory testing during, 277-278
    nursing diagnosis for, 278-279
    pain in, 222
    patient interview and, 265, 267
    physical care during, 280-282
    physical examination during, 269-277
    prenatal record and, 264-265
    preparation for giving birth and, 288-289
    psychological factors in, 267-269
    siblings and, 288
    standards of care during, 279, 280
    support measures during, 284, 286-287
  fourth stage of, 304-313
    assessment of, 305, 307
    bladder distention and, 309
    cleanliness and, 311
    comfort during, 310-311
    evaluation of, 312-313
    expected outcomes in, 305
    hemorrhage and, 305, 308-309
    nursing diagnosis for, 305
    psychosocial needs during, 311-312
    safety during, 309-310
    transfer from recovery area and, 312
  heart disease and, 643-644
  heart failure during, 647
  herpes infection and, 773
  HIV-positive mother and, 596-597
  induction of, 697-699
  normal patterns of, 694
  nursing diagnosis for, 239
  pain management in, 221-245, 290
    general anesthesia for, 236
    inhalation analgesia for, 237-238
    nerve blocks for, 230-236
    nonpharmacologic, 223-228
    sedatives for, 228
    systemic analgesia for, 228-230
  planning about, 143
  postterm, 718-719
  precipitous, 695
  preeclampsia and, 657
  process of, 215-218
  recognizing, 163-164
  second stage of, 291-299
    bearing-down efforts in, 295-296
    birth process and, 296-299
    birthing bed or chair and, 295
    coach during, 296
    definition of, 216
    duration of, 291-292
    emergency in, 299
    evaluation of, 299
    expected outcomes for, 293
    fetal heart rate in, 296
    nursing diagnosis for, 292-293
    pain in, 222

Labor—cont'd
  second stage of—cont'd
    positioning for, 295
    progress in, 292
    siblings during, 299
    supplies, instruments, and equipment for, 293-295
  substance abuse and, 675
  third stage of, 299-304, 301-304
  trial of, 697
  true vs. false, 264
Laboratory testing
  adolescent and, 734
  diabetes and, 624
  in dystocia, 695
  in first trimester, 134
  for heart disease, 641
  for HIV infection, 595
  hypertension and, 562, 564
  for infection, 607-608
  during labor, 239
  of newborn, 386
  in nutritional assessment, 186, 188
  in postpartum period, 464
  preeclampsia and, 559
  in second trimester, 148
  for septic shock, 604
  for syphilis, 595
  in third trimester, 160
  trauma and, 659
  in well-woman care, 845, 847
Labor-delivery-recovery room, 7-8
Laceration
  maternal
    of birth canal, 587
    perineal, 304
  of newborn, 373
Lact-Aid Nursing Trainer, 416
Lactation, 410-413; *see also* Breastfeeding
Lactiferous sinus, 39, 410
Lactoferrin, 417
Lactogen, human placental, 75
Lactogenesis, 411
Lactoovovegetarian, 196
Lactose intolerance, 184
Lactovegetarian, 196
Lamaze childbirth method, 224
  analgesia and, 228
Language, in data collection process, 21
Lanugo, 345
Lanugo hair, test for, 277
Laparoscopy, 867, 869
Large for gestational age infant, 775
  diabetes and, 623
Last menstrual period, 124
Late decelerations of fetal heart rate, 250, 252-253, 252-254, 259, 261
Late pregnancy class, 165
Latex agglutination inhibition test, 93
Learning needs assessment, for adolescent, 734
Lecithin/sphingomyelin ratio, 80, 324
  diabetes and, 790
  in high-risk pregnancy, 545
Leg, of newborn, 352
Leg cramps, 192
Leg pain, 168
Legal issues, 8
  of adolescent pregnancy, 728-729

Legal issues—cont'd
  cardiac emergency as, 641
  definition of live birth as, 826
  hemorrhage and, 591
  meconium aspiration and, 787
  psychological disorder and, 667
  seizures and, 591
  standard of prenatal care and, 136
  sterilization and, 499-500
Length, of newborn, 342
Leopold's maneuvers, 271, 272
Lesser vestibular gland, 27
Let-down reflex, 412
Lethargic infant, 759
Leukocytosis, neonatal, 323
Leukorrhea
  pregnancy and, 98
  in second trimester, 154
Level of consciousness
  in postpartum period, 310
  in third stage of labor, 301
Levothyroxine, 639
Lie, definition of, 207
Life cycle, of family, 14
Lifestyle
  immune system and, 53
  infertility and, 873
Ligament
  Cooper's, 39
  round, pain of, 154
Ligation, tubal, 501
Lightening, 96
  labor and, 215-216
Lightheadedness, 105
Linea nigra, 103
Lip, cleft, 803-804
Lipid-containing exfoliated cells, fetal, 546
Listeriosis, 605
Lithium, 665, 667
Lithotomy position, 130, 131, 296
Liver
  of fetus, 82
  HELLP syndrome and, 557, 559, 566-568
  of newborn, 326-328
  preeclampsia and, 557
  pregnancy and, 106
Local anesthesia, 230-236
Lochia, 441-442
Long-term variability of fetal heart rate, 248
Lordosis, dorsolumbar, 105
Loss; see Grief
Low-birth-weight infant, 775
  maternal age and, 178
  morbidity of, 777
  number of, 4-5
Lower extremity
  edema of, 162
  pain in, 168
Lower pelvic diaphragm, 35-36
Lumbar epidural anesthesia, 242
Lung
  bronchopulmonary dysplasia and, 783
  fetal, 80
    maturity of, 545-546, 718
  of newborn, 324, 753
    preterm, 781-782
  shock, 591

Lung cancer, 853
Lupus erythematosus, 655
Luteal phase, 42
Luteinizing hormone, 42
Lyme disease, 605
Lymphokine, 52
Lysozyme, 50

M

Maceration of skin, of newborn, 758
Macrosomia, 623
  maternal diabetes and, 789
Magnesium, 180
Magnesium sulfate
  eclampsia and, 569-570
  preeclampsia and, 567-568
  preterm labor and, 717-718
Magnet reflex, 357, 358
Magnetic resonance imaging, 543-544
Maladaptive behavior of parent, 476
Male genitalia
  adult, 44, 46-48
  of newborn, 330, 351
    cleansing of, 385
Male infertility, 865, 871-872
Male sterilization, 501-502
Malignancy
  breast, 891-892
  estrogen replacement and, 883
  hydatidiform mole and, 578-579
  screening for, 847-849
  smoking and, 853
  warning signals of, 849
Malposition of fetus, 689
Malpresentation of fetus, 689
Mammary gland
  anatomy of, 38-39
  pregnancy-related changes in, 98-99
Mammography, 848-849
Managed care, 7
Manic reaction, 665
Maple syrup urine disease, screening for, 389
Marfan syndrome, 648-649
Marginal placenta previa, 581
Marijuana, 672, 811
  male infertility and, 871
Mask of pregnancy, 103
Massage
  during labor, 226
  for postpartum pain, 311
Mastectomy, 892
Mastitis, 604-605
Masturbation, 144
Maternal adaptation; see Adaptation
Maternal mortality rate; see also Death
  definition of, 4
  trends in, 6
Maternal physiology in postpartum period, 439-448; see also
        Postpartum period, maternal physiology of
Maternal position; see Position
Maternal-fetal attachment, 113
Maternal-placental-embryonic circulation, 75
Maturational crisis, 18, 20
  pregnancy as, 110
Maturity
  of fetal lung, 545-546, 718
  of newborn, 363

McDonald cerclage, 576
McDonald's rule, 149
McDonald's sign, 95
McRoberts maneuver, 690
Mean arterial pressure, 760
    pregnancy and, 99
    in second trimester, 148
Measles, 605
    German, 598, 599, 771-772
Measurements, obstetric, 212
Meatus, urinary, 27
Mechanical contraceptive barrier, 489-490
Meckel's diverticulum, 79
Meconium
    in amniotic fluid, 278, 546
    aspiration of, 786-787
    cystic fibrosis and, 65
    definition of, 82
    passage of, 326
    staining of, 758
    suctioning of, 298
Median nerve, 105
Medical history; see History, patient
Mediolateral episiotomy, 303-304
Medroxyprogesterone, for infertility, 869
Meiosis, 61
    fertilization and, 66, 68
Melasma, facial, 103
Membrane
    amniotic
        birth of head and, 298
        formation of, 68
    fetal, 78
Memories of dead infant, 824-827
Menarche, 26, 40
Menopause, 44, 880-884
Menstrual cycle, 39-44
    assessment of, 860
    breast changes and, 39
    breastfeeding and, 425
    dysmenorrhea and, 858-859
    endometriosis and, 859-860
    evaluation of, 861
    hypogonadotropic amenorrhea and, 858
    nursing diagnosis for, 860
    oral contraceptives and, 492
    in postpartum period, 443
    premenstrual syndrome and, 859
    well-woman care and, 842
Mental illness, 667-668; see also Psychological
        response
Mental retardation
    Down syndrome and, 62
    fetal alcohol syndrome causing, 809
    fragile X syndrome and, inheritance of, 65
    screening for, 388-389
Meperidine, labor and, 229
Mesoderm, 79
Metabolic disorder, diabetes and, 623
Metabolic emergency, 641
Metabolism
    diabetes and, 620
    fetal, 82
    inborn errors of, 797-798
    of newborn, 334
Methadone, 675, 812
Methamphetamine abuse, 672, 813

Methaqualone, male infertility and, 871
Methyldopa, 569
Mexican culture
    beliefs of, 18
    breastfeeding and, 412
    food patterns of, 194
    infant behavior and, 336
Microcephaly, 803
Midbrain, fetal, 81
Middle Eastern food patterns, 193
Midforceps birth, 700
Midgut, 81
Midline episiotomy, 303
Midpregnancy class, 165
Mifepristone, 880
Migrant family, 681
Milestones, prenatal, 69-74
Milk
    breast
        inadequate, 414
        jaundice and, 328
        lactation process and, 410-412
    cow, 408-410, 428
    minerals and vitamins in, 409-410
Milk duct, plugging of, 414
Minerals
    newborn requirements for, 409-410
    pregnancy requirement for, 179
Miscarriage, 572, 574-576
    checklist for assisting parents, 828
Missed abortion, 574, 575
Mitleiden, 116
Mitosis, 60-61
    fertilization and, 68
Mitral valve prolapse, 648
Mittleschmerz, 42
Molding of head, 332
Mole, hydatidiform, 578-579
Mongolian spot, 329
Moniliasis, 774-775
Monitoring, fetal; see Fetal heart rate
Monosomy X, 63
Monozygotic twins, 84
Mons pubis, 26, 46
Montgomery's tubercle, 98
Mood disorder, 665-666
Moratorium phase of pregnancy, 115
Morgue, 827
Morning sickness; see Vomiting
Moro reflex, 355, 356
Mortality; see Death
Morula, 68
Mother; see also Maternal entries
    adaptation to pregnancy by, 110-115
    surrogate, 876
Mother-child interaction, 476
    heart disease and, 644
Mother-child relationship, 113-114
Mother-daughter relationship, 112
Mothering behavior, 477
Motility, gastric, 444
Motor function
    of newborn, 331, 368
    parenting and, 450
Mottling, 758
Mourning; see Grief

Mouth
  of newborn, 348
  pregnancy-related changes in, 105
Movement, fetal
  daily counts of, 551
  labor and, 218
  in second trimester, 150
Mucosa, vaginal, 34-35
Mucus
  as body defense, 50
  cervical, 42
    contraception and, 487
  ferning of, 98
Mucus-trap catheter, 371-372
Multifactorial inheritance, 65
Multigravida, 92
Multipara, 92
  over age 35, 119-120
Multiple pregnancy, 83-85
  loss of one in, 832-833
Multiple sclerosis, 654
Mummy restraint, 392, 393, 399
Mumps, 605
Muscle
  abdominal, 443
  myasthenia gravis and, 655-656
  pelvic, 35, 442
  pubococcygeal, 137
  spasm of, 163
Musculoskeletal system
  congenital disorders of, 804
  of fetus, 69-73
  labor and, 219
  in postpartum period, 446-447
  pregnancy-related changes in, 104-105
  in well-woman care, 842
Myasthenia gravis, 655-656
Mycotic stomatitis, 774-775
Myelomeningocele, 801-802
Myerson's reflex, 354
Myometrium, 31-32
Myotonia, in sexual response, 49
Myth
  about hymen, 27
  menstrual, 39-40

N

Nägele's rule, 124-125
Nail, of fetus, 83
Nalbuphine, labor and, 229
Narcotic, epidural or spinal, 235-236
Narcotic analgesic, systemic, 229
Narcotic antagonist, labor and, 230
Nasopharyngeal catheter, for suctioning, 372
Native American culture
  food patterns of, 193
  neonatal behavior and, 336
Natural family planning, 485-486
Natural immunity, 50
Nausea and vomiting; *see* Vomiting
Neck, of newborn, 348
Necrosis, intravenous extravasation and, 758
Necrotizing enterocolitis, 784
Neisseria gonorrhoeae, 594-595
Neonatal mortality; *see* Death
Neonatal reflex, 353-358
Neonate; *see* Newborn

Neoplasia, cervical intraepithelial, 847-848
Neoplasm; *see* Malignancy
Neopresol, 569
Nerve
  carpal tunnel syndrome and, 105
  labor contractions and, 216
Nerve block, 230-236
  technique for, 241
Nerve stimulation, transcutaneous electrical, 228
Nervous system
  behavior and, 335-336
  cocaine and, 671
  congenital disorders of, 794-795
  fetal, 69-73, 81
  fetal alcohol syndrome and, 809
  high-risk pregnancy and, 654
  hydrocephalus and, 802-803
  labor and, 219, 222
  of newborn, 331
    assessment of, 363-364
    compromised, 759
    preterm, 777
  in postpartum period, 446
  pregnancy-related changes in, 104-105
  vaginal, 34
  well-woman care and, 842
Network, social, 459
Neural tube, development of, 81
Neural tube defect, 65, 795
  myelomeningocele and, 801-802
Neurologic system; *see* Nervous system
Neuromuscular system, of newborn, 331
Neutral thermal environment, 762-763, 764
Nevus, 329-330
Newborn, 319-406
  adaptation to extrauterine life by, 370
  of adolescent mother, 730, 738
  assessment of, 362-367
  behavioral characteristics of, 334-339
  cardiovascular system of, 319-323
  care plan for, 402-403
  chlamydial infection and, 594
  compromised, 751-778
    cardiovascular system of, 760-761
    congenital anomalies and, 793-806; *see also* Congenital disorder
    of diabetic mother, 623, 788-792
    dysfunctional transition and, 752-753
    evaluation of, 765
    expected outcomes for, 762
    family of, 765
    gastrointestinal system of, 761-762
    gestational age and birthweight of, 775-778
    hyperbilirubinemia and, 793
    infection and, 768-775
    nervous system of, 759
    nursing diagnosis for, 762
    postterm, 785-787
    preterm, 775-785; *see also* Preterm infant
    quick assessment of, 753, 755-758
    respiratory system of, 760-761
    small for gestational age, 787-788
    stabilization of, 762-765
    substance abuse and, 806-813
    transient tachypnea and, 768
  environment of, 369-370
  epidural anesthesia and, 236
  expected outcomes for, 369

Newborn—cont'd
feeding of, 407-437; *see also* Feeding of infant
gastrointestinal system of, 325-326
hematopoietic system of, 323
hepatic system of, 326-328
of HIV-positive mother, 597
hyponatremia in, 185
immune system of, 328
immunity in, 52
integumentary system of, 328-330
mother's immediate reaction to, 302
myasthenia gravis in, 656
neuromuscular system of, 331
nursing diagnosis for, 367, 369
persistent pulmonary hypertension of, 786
physical assessment of, 339-358
renal system of, 324-325
reproductive system of, 330
respiratory distress syndrome in, 718
respiratory system of, 323-324
resuscitation of, 752-753
skeletal system of, 331
thermogenic system of, 332-334
Niacin, requirement for, 181
Night sweats, in menopause, 880
Nipple
anatomy of, 39
Montgomery's tubercles and, 98
pinch test of, 157, 158
soreness of, 414
Nipple erection reflex, 412
Nipple-stimulated contraction stress test, 550-551
Nitrazine test, 277
Nitroglycerin, for hypertension, 569
Nitrous oxide
for cesarean birth, 237
for labor, 238
Nodule, of breast, 39
Nondisjunction, 62
Non–English-speaking patient, in labor, 268-269
Nonsteroidal anti-inflammatory drug for dysmenorrhea, 858
Nonstress test, 549
Normodyne, 569
Norplant, 494, 495
Norwegian food patterns, 195
Nose, of newborn, 347
Nosocomial infection, 608, 610
Nuchal cord, 79, 298
Nuclear family, 12
Nullipara, 92
Nulliparous women, over 35, 120
Numbness, in second trimester, 154
Nursing process, 21-22
Nursing trainer, Lact-Aid, 416
Nurturing, in family, 15
Nutrasweet, 182
Nutrition
for adolescent, 733, 737-738
care plan for, 197-198
diabetes and, 626-627
gestational, 635
endocrine system and, 107
feeding of infant and, 407-435; *see also* Breastfeeding; Feeding of infant
food cravings and, 153
health promotion and, 849-851
heart disease and, 643

Nutrition—cont'd
immune system and, 53
for infant; *see* Breastfeeding; Feeding of infant
patient history of, 128
in postpartum period, 311
breastfeeding and, 420, 428
preeclampsia and, 566
pregnancy and, 105, 172-201
assessment of, 185-188
care plan for, 197-198
cultural differences in, 145-146, 192-196
discomforts and, 191-192
evaluation of, 199
exercise and, 190
expected outcomes in, 189
in first trimester, 137, 147
nursing diagnosis for, 189
nutrient needs in, 178-185
postpartum period and, 198-199
resources for, 189-190
urinary tract infection and, 137
weight gain and, 172, 175-178
for preterm infant, 777-778
Nystatin, candidiasis and, 775

O
Obesity, health promotion and, 850
Obstetric measurements, 212
Obstruction
airway, 372-373
of milk duct, 414
Occupational nurse, 88
Odor, 452
incontinence and, 891
Oil gland, of newborn, 329
Older age group, pregnancy in, 119
Older woman, health care for, 843-844
Oligohydramnios, 80, 794
Omphalitis, 761
Omphalocele, 800-801
Oncotic pressure, colloid, 589
Oocyte, 61
Oogenesis, 61
Opiate, labor and, 229
Oral contraceptive, 490-494
adolescent and, 726
diabetes and, 630
Oral-genital intercourse, 144
Organ donation, 825
Orgasmic phase of sexual response, 49
Oriental food patterns, 193
Orthodox Jewish view of assisted fertility therapy, 864
Orthostatic hypotension, 310
Os, cervical, 32, 33
Osteoporosis, 881-882
exercise for, 885
prevention of, 884
Outlet, pelvic, 209-210
Outlet forceps, 700
Ovarian cycle, 42
Ovarian cyst, 657
Ovary
anatomy of, 28
of fetus, 82
infertility and, 869
in postpartum period, 443
tumor of, 870

Ovulation, 28, 42
  infertility and, 866
  menarche and, 40
  in postpartum period, 443
  predictor test for, 488-489
Ovulatory stimulant, 869-870
Ovum
  fertilization of, 65-66
  gametogenesis and, 61
  implantation of, 42
Oximetry, neonatal, 765
Oxygen
  fetal well-being and, 247
  hypoxemia and, 763, 765
  newborn and, 371
    asphyxia of, 752-753
  placenta and, 75-76
  toxicity of, 591
Oxygen pressure, neonatal, 324
Oxygen-associated complications, 783-784
Oxytocin
  contraction stress test with, 551
  for induction of labor, 697, 698-699, 700
  postpartum hemorrhage and, 587
  preeclampsia and, 568

P

Pacifier, 401, 404
Pain
  cultural factors in, 268
  of grief, 818
  hysterosalpingography causing, 867
  labor, 221-245; *see also* Labor, pain management in
  postpartum, 310-311
  in premature infant, 758
  in second trimester, 154
Palate, cleft, 803-804
Pallor, 756, 758
Palmar erythema, 103, 153
Palmar grasp, 354
Palpation
  fundal, 308
  in prenatal examination, 131-134
Palpitation, in second trimester, 153
Palsy, Bell's, 654
Pancreas
  of fetus, 82
  pregnancy-related changes in, 107
Papanicolaou smear, 34-35, 133, 847-848
Papillomavirus, 601-602
Paracervical block, 236, 237
Paralysis, facial, 654
Parathyroid gland, 107
Parathyroid hormone, fat and, 107
Parenchyma, of breast, 38
Parent; *see also* Family
  adolescent as, 729, 740-741
    adapation and, 727-728, 729
    assessment of, 740-741
    collaborative care for, 741
    expected outcomes for, 741
    nursing diagnosis for, 741
  cesarean birth and, 704, 706
  congenital anomaly and, 805-806
  education programs for, 164-167
  feeding of infant by, 413
  impact of childbirth on, 475-476

Parent—cont'd
  of preterm infant, 779-780
  role of, 453-459
Parenthood, adjustment to, 516
Parent-infant interaction, 476
Parenting process, 450, 475-482
Parent-newborn relationship, immediate, 302
Parietal peritoneum, 32
Parity, 92
  as risk factor, 536
Parotitis, 605
Partial placenta previa, 581
Partial thromboplastin time, 652
Partogram for assessment of cervical dilatation, 274, 275
Parvovirus B-19, 605
Passageway, 209
Passive immunity, 51-52
Patent ductus arteriosus, 784
Pearls, Epstein's, 325
Pelvic examination
  of adolescent, 731
  in first trimester, 130-134
  in well-woman care, 845
Pelvic inflammatory disease, 861-864
Pelvic joint injury, 888
Pelvic muscle, in postpartum period, 442
Pelvis
  anatomy of, 35-38
  childbirth trauma and, 884-887
  dystocia and, 687-689
  types of, 213
Penis
  anatomy of, 46
  circumcision and, 397-400
  condom and, 490, 491
  erection of, 49
Perception of pain, 223
Perfusion
  in newborn, 756
  placental, 233
Perimenopause, 44, 880
Perinatal death; *see* Death
Perinatal period; *see* Labor
Perineal body, 37
Perineum
  anatomy of, 28, 35-37
  bulging of, 297
  episiotomy and, 302-304
  examination of, 132
  laceration of, 304
  in postpartum period, 442
  pregnancy-related changes in, 98
  in third trimester, 162
Periodic changes in fetal heart rate, 249-254
Peripheral cyanosis, 753
Peristalsis, of fetus, 82
Peritoneum, parietal, 32
Persistent pulmonary hypertension of newborn, 786
Pessary, 889, 890
Petechiae
  birth trauma causing, 373
  disseminated intravascular coagulation and, 591
pH, vaginal, 97-98
Phasic oral contraceptive, 492-493
Phencyclidine, 672-673, 812
Phenobarbital abuse, 813
Phenothiazine, labor and, 229-230

Phenylketonuria, 64, 798
  screening for, 388
Philippine culture, breastfeeding and, 412
Phosphorus, pregnancy requirement for, 179
Phosphotidiglycerol, 545
Photographing of dead infant, 827
Phototherapy for hyperbilirubinemia, 394-397
Physical activity
  in first trimester, 140-141
  of newborn, 334-336
  in second trimester, 152
Physical examination
  of adolescent, 733
  diabetes and, 624
  in dystocia, 695
  in first trimester, 129-134
  hypertension and, 560-562
  infection and, 607
  during labor, 238-239
  in labor, first stage, 269-277
  of newborn, 339-358, 364, 366-367
  nutritional assessment and, 188
  in third trimester, 160
Physiologic anemia, 178
  pregnancy and, 100
Physiologic jaundice, 327-328, 377
Pigmentation
  of pregnancy, 103
  in second trimester, 153
Pinch test of nipple, 157, 158
Pinocytosis, 76
Piper forceps, 701
Pitting edema, 560
Pituitary gland
  in postpartum period, 443
  prolactin and, 107
Placenta
  birth of, 299, 301-304
  blood flow and, fetal well-being and, 247
  herpes infection and, 772
  maternal hypotension and, 233
  postpartum period and, 441
  retained, 587
  structure and function of, 75-76
  variations of, 585-586
Placenta previa, 581-585
Placental hormone, 442-443
Plant protein, 196
Plantar grasp, 354
Plateau phase of sexual response, 49
Platelets
  HELLP syndrome and, 557, 559, 566 568
  of newborn, 323
  thrombocytopenia and, 592
Platypelloid pelvis, 213
Plethora, 756, 758
Pneumonia
  aspiration, powder causing, 400
  chlamydial, 774
Podophyllin, 601-602
Points of maximum intensity of fetal heart rate, 269, 271-272
Polish culture, food patterns of, 195
Polydactyly, 804
Port-wine stain, 330
Position
  coital, 144
  en face, 311, 457-458

Position—cont'd
  fetal, 208
  of infant, 381
    for breastfeeding, 419, 420
    respiratory distress and, 782
    when held, 457
  maternal
    dystocia and, 692-693
    in labor, 215
      in first stage of, 280
      lithotomy, 296
      in second stage, 295
Positive end-expiratory pressure, 760
Positive feedback, bonding and, 451
Positive signs of pregnancy, 124
Postcoital test, 872
Postmature infant, 785-787
  definition of, 775
Postmenopause, 880
Postpartum period, 304-313
  for adolescent, 739-740
  breastfeeding and, 417
  cesarean birth and, 707
  depression in, 480, 665
  diabetic mother and, 624, 629-630
    gestational diabetes and, 636
  heart disease and, 641, 644
  hemorrhage in, 305, 308-309, 585-588
  HIV infection and, 597
  infection in, 603-605
  maternal physiology in, 439-448
    abdomen and, 443
    breasts and, 444-445
    cardiovascular system and, 445
    cervix and, 442
    endocrine system and, 442-443
    gastrointestinal system and, 444
    immune system and, 447-448
    integumentary system and, 447
    musculoskeletal system and, 445-447
    neurologic system and, 446
    pelvic muscles and, 442
    perineum and, 442
    urinary system and, 443-444
    uterus and, 440-442
    vagina and, 442
  mental illness in, 667-668
  nutrition in, 198-199
  physical needs in
    assessment of, 464
    bladder distention and, 309
    bleeding and, 468-470
    breastfeeding promotion and, 471
    care plan for, 474-475
    cleanliness and, 311
    comfort and, 310-311, 470-471
    elimination patterns and, 471
    episiotomy care and, 467
    evaluation of, 312-313, 475
    expected outcomes in, 466
    infection prevention and, 466-468
    lactation suppression in, 473
    nursing diagnosis for, 464, 466
    rest and exercise and, 471, 472
    Rh isoimmunization and, 473, 475
    rubella vaccination in, 473
    safety and, 309-310

Postpartum period—cont'd
preeclampsia and, 570
psychosocial needs in, 311-312, 475-482
expected outcomes in, 478-479
nursing diagnosis for, 478
parenting skills and, 479-482
transfer from recovery area and, 312
Postterm infant, 785-787
definition of, 775
Postterm labor and birth, 718-719
Posture
of newborn, 340
in second trimester, 152, 155
Potentiator, analgesic, 229-230
Potter's syndrome, 794
Poverty, abuse and, 679-680
Powder, aspiration pneumonia from, 400
Power, in family, 15
Powers, contractions as, 211-215
Prebirth education, 164-167
Precautions, universal, 611
Precipitous labor, 695
Preconception care, 86-88
Preconceptional counseling, for diabetic patient, 621
Precordium, of newborn, 761-762
Predictor test for ovulation, 488-489
Prednisone, for infertility, 869
Preeclampsia, 555-559, 564-568
hospital care of, 573
mild vs. severe, 563
Pregestational diabetes; see Diabetes mellitus
Pregnancy, high-risk, 533-746
abdominal surgery and, 656-657
adolescent, 722-746; see also Adolescent
anemia and, 649-650, 651
autoimmune disorder and, 654-656
cardiovascular disorder and, 639-649
categories of, 536
dystocia and, 687-711; see also Dystocia
endocrine disorders and, 618-639
diabetes mellitus as, 618-636
hyperemesis gravidarum and, 636-639
hypothyroidism as, 639
gastrointestinal disorder and, 653
hemorrhage and, 572, 574-593; see also Hemorrhage
hypertension and, 555-572; see also Hypertension
infection and, 593-611; see also Infection
infertility and, 874-875
integumentary disorder and, 653-654
neurologic disorder and, 654
numbers of, 6
postterm, 718-719
prenatal diagnosis of, 794
preterm, 711-718, 715-718
psychological disorders and, 665-685; see also Psychological entries
respiratory disorders and, 650, 652-653
risk factor assessment for, 533-553
amniocentesis for, 544-546
chorionic villus sampling for, 547-548
daily fetal movement counts and, 551
electronic monitoring and, 548-551
magnetic resonance imaging for, 543-544
maternal blood testing and, 548
percutaneous umbilical blood sampling for, 546-547
scope of problem and, 533-535
ultrasonography for, 537-543

Pregnancy, high-risk—cont'd
spousal abuse and, 677-683
trauma causing, 658-659
Pregnancy, normal, 123-171
adaptation to, 93-94
by grandparent, 118-119
maternal, 110-115
paternal, 115-118
after age 35, 119-120
cardiovascular changes in, 99-100
embryonic stage of, 68, 75-79
endocrine system in, 106-107
fetal development and, 79-83
milestones of, 69-73
first trimester of, 123-146
abortion in, 878-880
care plan for, 147
cultural variation in care during, 145-146
diagnosis of pregnancy in, 123
education about, 136-143
estimated date of birth and, 123-124
expected outcomes in, 135
nursing diagnosis for, 135
patient history and, 124-129
physical examination and, 129-135
sexual counseling and, 143-145
gastrointestinal system in, 105-106
gravidity and parity in, 92
integumentary system in, 103-104
multiple, 83-85
musculoskeletal system in, 104-105
nutrition in, 172-201; see also Nutrition
renal function in, 102-103
reproductive system changes in, 94-99
respiratory system changes in, 100-102
second trimester of, 146-158
abortion in, 878-880
assessment of, 146-151
care plan for, 158
education about, 152-158
expected outcomes in, 151-152
nursing diagnosis for, 151
testing for, 92-93
third trimester of, 158-169
assessment of, 159-160
care plan for, 168-169
education about, 161-167
evaluation and, 167
expected outcomes in, 161
nursing diagnosis for, 160
Premature infant; see Preterm infant
Premenopause, 880-881
Premenstrual syndrome, 859
Prenatal period; see also Fetal entries; Fetus; Pregnancy entries
adolescent pregnancy and, 736
breastfeeding preparation and, 416-417
cesarean birth and, 703-704
diabetic mother and, 624, 626-629
diagnosis of abnormality in, 85, 533-553; see also Pregnancy, high-risk
gestational diabetes and, 635
heart disease and, 643
HIV infection and, 595-596
milestones of, 69-74
preeclampsia and, 567
psychologic disorder in, 667

Prenatal period—cont'd
  record of
    in first trimester, 125-128
    review of, during labor, 264-265
Preparation for childbirth
  adaptation to pregnancy and, 114, 129
  education programs for, 164-167
  methods of, 223-225
Prepuce
  of clitoris, 27
  of penis, circumcision and, 397
Presentation
  breech, 689-692
    external cephalic version and, 696-697
  definition of, 206-207
  dystocia and, 689-692
  face, 689, 692
  vertex, 209
    emergency birth in, 300
    normal birth in, 297-299
Pressure
  central venous, 589
  colloid oncotic, 589
  mean arterial, 760
  positive end-expiratory, 760
  pulmonary artery wedge, hemorrhagic shock and, 589-590
  sacral, 226
Pressure catheter, intrauterine, 255, 256
Presumptive signs of pregnancy, 124
Preterm infant, 777-785
  assessment of, 778-780
  borderline, 777
  breastfeeding of, 422
  definition of, 92, 775
  development of, 784-785
  evaluation of, 785
  expected outcomes for, 781
  immunity in, 52
  necrotizing enterocolitis and, 784
  nursing diagnosis for, 780-781
  oxygen-associated complications and, 782-784
  pain assessment in, 758
  patent ductus arteriosus and, 794
  respiratory distress syndrome and, 781-782
Preterm labor and birth, 711, 715-718
Preventive care, preconception, 87-88
Primary dysmenorrhea, 858
Primary germ layer, 79
Primary powers, 211, 214
Primigravida, 92
Primipara, 92
Probable signs of pregnancy, 124
Problem solving, in family, 15
Prodromal labor events, 215
Progestasert, 499
Progesterone
  acid-base balance and, 102
  fat and, 107
  gastrointestinal system and, 106
  placenta and, 75-76
  respiratory system and, 101
Progestin, 490-494
Progestogen, 883
Prolactin, 412, 443
  pregnancy and, 107

Prolapse
  of umbilical cord, 282-284, 285
  uterine, 886, 888-890
  of vagina, 887
Proliferative phase of endometrial cycle, 42
Prolonged decelerations of fetal heart rate, 254
Promethazine, labor and, 230
Prophylaxis, eye, 394
Prostaglandin inhibitor, for dysmenorrhea, 858
Prostaglandins
  abortion and, 879-880
  menstrual cycle and, 44
  postpartum hemorrhage and, 587
Protein
  newborn requirement for, 409
  plant, 196
  pregnancy requirement for, 179
Proteinuria
  preeclampsia and, 555-556, 562
  pregnancy and, 103
Protocol, 280
Protozoan infection, 597, 598
Pruritus, 153
Psychological disorder, 664-685
  antepartum hospitalization for, 667
  assessment of, 666
  complicated bereavement and, 833-834
  expected outcomes for, 666-667
  mood disorders and, 665-666
  nursing diagnosis for, 666
  in postpartum period, 311-312, 667-668
  substance abuse and, 668-677; *see also* Substance abuse
  violence and, 677-683
Psychological response
  by adolescent father, 740
  to cesarean birth, 702, 707
  to coagulation disorder, 591
  to congenital anomaly, 806
  to dystocia, 693
  grief, 816-835; *see also* Grief
  to hemorrhage and, 585
  to infertility, 864
  menopause and, 881
  to newborn, 378
  to pregnancy, 111
    by adolescent, 733
    by family, 13
    by father, 116
    in first trimester, 139
    by mother, 111
    in third trimester, 162
  to preterm infant, 780
  well-woman assessment and, 843
Psychosis, postpartum, 666
Psychosocial factors, assessment of, 267
Psychosomatic symptoms, 116
Psychotropic medication, 667
Ptyalism, 139
Pubarche, 26
Pubic hair
  in female, 26
  in male, 44
Pubis, 37
Pubococcygeal muscle, Kegel's exercises for, 137
Pudendal block, 230-231
Puerperal sepsis, 603-605

Puerperium; *see* Postpartum period
Puerto Rican food patterns, 195
Pulmonary artery wedge pressure, 570
    hemorrhagic shock and, 589-590
Pulmonary hypertension of newborn, 786
Pulmonary surfactant, 80
Pulmonary system; *see* Respiratory system
Pulse
    hemorrhagic shock and, 589
    of newborn, 340, 761
    resuscitation of newborn and, 375
Pulse oximetry, neonatal, 765
Pump, breast, 414
Purpura, thrombocytopenic, 591
    of newborn, 373
Pushing, before dilatation, 226
Pyramid, food guide, 174, 190
Pyridoxine, 181
Pyrogenic exotoxin, 606
Pyrosis, 197

Q

Questionnaire, nutritional, 187
Quick assessment of newborn, 753, 755-757
Quickening, 97, 150

R

Radiation, heat loss and, 333
Radiation therapy
    for breast cancer, 892
    occupational protection and, 88
Radioimmunoassay for pregnancy, 93
Rapid eye movement sleep, of fetus, 81
Rash, diaper, 383
Ratio, lecithin/sphingomyelin, 80
Reabsorption, renal tubular, 102-103
Reactivity, periods of, 335
Recessive gene, 60
Recessive inheritance, 64, 65
Recommended Dietary Allowance, 173, 178-181
    for newborn, 409
Record; *see* Documentation
Recovery area, transfer from, 312
Rectocele, 886
Rectovaginal fistula, 890
Rectovaginal palpation, 133, 134
Rectus abdominis muscle, 105
Red blood cells
    folate and, 184
    in newborn, 323
    in postpartum period, 445
    pregnancy and, 100
Referral, for congenital anomaly, 805-806
Reflex
    breastfeeding, 411, 412
    deep tendon, hypertension and, 560-562
    Ferguson's, 215
    neonatal, 331, 353-358
    vasocongestion, 49
Regional anesthesia, 230-236
    for cesarean birth, 703
Regional enteritis, 653
Relactation, 415
Relationship
    father-child, 117-118
    maternal-fetal attachment and, 113
    mother-child, 112-114

Relationship—cont'd
    partner
        father and, 117-118
        mother and, 112-113
Relativism, cultural, 17
Relaxation
    conscious, 157
    preeclampsia and, 565
Relaxation techniques, labor and, 225
Renal system
    agenesis of, 794
    creatinine and, 545-546
    disseminated intravascular coagulation and, 591
    fetal, 69-73, 80-81
    labor and, 219
    of newborn, 324-325
    in postpartum period, 443-444
    pregnancy-related changes in, 102-103
    of preterm infant, 778
Renal tubular reabsorption, 102-103
Repertoire, 458
Report; *see* Documentation
Reproductive system, 25-55
    female, 25-44
        bony pelvis and, 37-38
        breasts and, 38-39
        external structures of, 25-28
        fallopian tubes and, 28-30
        infection of, 602-603, 861-864
        labor and, 215-216
        menstrual cycle and, 39-44, 45; *see* Menstrual cycle
        ovaries and, 28
        pelvic floor and perineum and, 35-37
        pregnancy-related changes in, 94-99
        uterus and, 30-34
        vagina and, 34-35
    fertility problems and, 864-876; *see also* Infertility
    fetal, 69-73, 82
    immunology and, 50-53
    male, 44, 46-48
    of newborn, 330
    sexual ambiguity and, 805
    sexual response and, 48-50
Research, 8
    adolescent parent and, 742
Resolution phase of sexual response, 49
Resources, nutritional, 189-190
Respirations
    fetal, 218
    neonatal, 324, 341, 366, 760
    parent education about, 400-401
Respiratory distress syndrome
    adult, 652-653
    diabetes and, 790
    in newborn, 718
        preterm, 781-782
Respiratory effort, of newborn, 756, 768
Respiratory system
    admission assessment of, 265, 267
    bronchopulmonary dysplasia and, 783
    congenital disorders of, 794
    cystic fibrosis and, 653
        genetics of, 65
    fetal, 69-73, 80
    high-risk pregnancy and, 650, 652-653
    labor and, 219

Respiratory system—cont'd
  of newborn, 323-324
    compromised, 760-761
    preterm, 777
    transient tachypnea and, 768768
  pregnancy-related changes in, 100-102
  well-woman care and, 842
Responsivity, 458
Rest
  for hypertonic uterine dysfunction, 687
  in second trimester, 152, 157
Restitution, 218
Restraint, infant
  methods of, 399-400
  for venipuncture, 392, 393
Resuscitation
  neonatal, 374-375
    cesarean birth and, 704
    equipment for, 752
    overview of, 754
  in pregnancy, 641-642
Retained placenta, 587
Retardation
  intrauterine growth
    definition of, 775
    weight gain and, 176
  mental
    Down syndrome and, 62
    fetal alcohol syndrome causing, 809
    fragile X syndrome and, 65
    screening for, 388-389
Retention cyst, 325
Retinal hemorrhage, 373
Retinopathy of prematurity, 783-784
Retraction of chest wall, 757
Retroversion of uterus, 30, 888, 890
Rh incompatibility, 77, 793
  dilatation and curettage and, 581
Rhagades, 770
Rheumatic heart disease, 647-648
Rheumatoid arthritis, 655
Rh$_o$ immune globulin, 581
Rhythm, infant-parent, 457-458
Rib cage, pregnancy and, 100
Riboflavin, 181
Rights of fetus, 537
Ripening of cervix, 697-698
Risk assessment, preconception, 87, 88
Risk-taking behavior, 725
Rite of passage, pregnancy as, 111
Ritgen maneuver, 298
Ritodrine, 715-716
Ritual, in grief, 826
Rivalry, sibling, 459-460
Role
  in family, 15
  motherhood as, 112
  parental, 115
Roll-over test, 148
Rooting reflex, 353
Rotation of fetus
  external, 218
  internal, 217
Round ligament pain, 154
RU 486, 880
Rubella, 598, 599, 771-772
Rubeola, 605

Rule
  McDonald's, 149
  Nägele's, 124-125
Rupture of amniotic membranes, 277-278
  artificial, 698
  tests for, 277
Ruptured ectopic pregnancy, 577

S
Sacral pressure, 226
Sacroiliac joint injury, 889
Sacrum, 37
Safety
  of anesthesia, 241
  in bottle feeding, 427
  of newborn, 370
    parent education about, 401
  osteoporosis prevention and, 884
  in postpartum period, 309-310
    at home, 521
  during pregnancy, 140
Saline abortion, 879
Saliva, excessive, 139
Scalp injury, of newborn, 376
Scandinavian food patterns, 195
Schizophrenia, postpartum, 666
Schultze's mechanism, 301
Sclerosis, multiple, 654
Screening
  neonatal, 388-389
  in well-woman care, 844-849
Scrotum, 46
  of newborn, 330
Seat belt, during pregnancy, 140
Second stage of labor, 291-299; *see also* Labor, second stage of
Second trimester abortion, 879-880
Second trimester of pregnancy, 146-158; *see also* Pregnancy, normal, second trimester of
Secondary dysmenorrhea, 859
Secondary powers, 214-215
Second-time mother, 114-115
Secretory phase of endometrial cycle, 42
Seesaw respirations, 324
Seizure
  eclampsia and, 556, 568-570
  epilepsy vs. eclampsia and, 654
  neonatal, 759
  standard of care for, 591
Selenium, requirement for, 180
Self-care
  in first trimester, 136-143
  in second trimester, 152, 155-158
  in third trimester, 160-165
  trend in, 7
Self-effleurage, 163
Self-examination
  of breast, 844-845, 846
  vulvar, 845
Self-image, maternal, 476
Semen, 48
Semen analysis, 871-872
Seminal duct, 46
Seminiferous tubule, 48
Semivegetarian, 196
Sensory function, of newborn, 336, 338
Sensory organs, fetal, 69-73, 81

Sepsis
  neonatal, 768-769
  puerperal, 603-605
Septic abortion, 574-575, 580
Septic shock, 604
Sex chromosome, abnormalities of, 63
Sex education, 726-727
Sexual ambiguity, 805
Sexual identity, 723-724
Sexual response, 48-50
Sexuality
  adolescent, 724-727, 730-732
  contraception and, 483-502; see also Contraception
  in first trimester, 128-129
    care plan for, 148
  health promotion and, 854
  postmenopausal, 881
  in postpartum period, 483
  pregnancy and, 112-113, 143-145
Sexually transmitted disease
  in adolescent, 731, 732
  adolescent and, 727
  assessment of, 606-608
  care plan for, 609-610
  Chlamydia trachomatis as, 773-774
  chlamydial, 593-594
  gonorrhea as, 594-595, 775
  herpes as, 599-601, 772-773
  human immunodeficiency virus as, 595-597
  human papillomavirus as, 601-602
  pelvic inflammatory, 861, 863-864
  syphilis as, 595, 770-771
Sheath, vaginal, 490
Shirodkar, 576
Shock
  bacteremic, 604
  as drug reaction, 239
  as grief response, 817
  hemorrhagic, 309, 588-591
  insulin, 622
Short-stay maternity care
  advantages and disadvantages of, 506-509
  preparation for, 512-515
Shoulder
  birth of, 298-299
  pain in, 867
Shoulder presentation, 691
Show, bloody, 265
Sibling
  adaptation of
    to newborn, 302, 459-460
    to pregnancy, 118-119
  during labor, 288
    second stage, 299
  psychosocial assessment and, 482
Sickle cell anemia, 650, 651
Sign
  Chadwick's, 95, 97
  Goodell's, 95, 97
  Hegar's, 95
  McDonald's, 95
  of pregnancy, 93-94, 124
Signaling behavior, 451
Silverman-Anderson index of respiratory distress, 757
Sinciput presentation, 209
Single-parent family, 12-13
Sinus, lactiferous, 39, 410

Situational crisis, 20
Skeletal system; see also Musculoskeletal system
  birth trauma to, 376-377
  bony pelvis and, 37-38, 209-210
  congenital disorders of, 804
  of newborn, 331
  osteoporosis and, 881-882, 884
Skene's gland, 131
Skill, parenting, 450, 479-480
Skin
  of breast, 39
  childbirth and, 302-305
  disorders of, 653-654
  fetal, 83
  labor and, 219
  of newborn, 328-330, 366
  in postpartum period, 447
  pregnancy-related changes in, 103-104
  in well-woman care, 842
Skin-to-skin care, 785
Skull
  birth trauma to, 376
  of newborn, 331
Sleep
  of fetus, 81
  insomnia and, 168
  maternal, disturbance of, 520
  of newborn, 335, 337, 366
Slow-to-warm-up child, 339
Small for gestational age infant, 775, 787-788
Smear, Papanicolaou, 847-848
Smell, newborn and, 338
Smile, of newborn, 368
Smoking
  male infertility and, 871
  in pregnancy, 143, 673, 809, 810
  prevention of illness and, 853
Snuffles, 770
Soap for bathing of infant, 383
Social history, 128-129
  in well-woman care, 841-842
Social network, 459
Socialization, in family, 15
Sociocultural function, of family, 13, 15
Socioeconomic status
  of adolescent mother, 728, 730
  parenting behavior and, 459
  spousal abuse and, 679-681
Sodium
  hyponatremia and, 409
  newborn and, 325
  pregnancy requirement for, 185
Sodium chloride, abortion with, 879
Soft tissue
  of birth canal, 211
  of newborn, injury to, 373, 376
Solid food, introduction of, 430
Somatic pain, 222
Souffle, uterine, 96
Sounds
  bowel, 326
  heart, 322-323
Southeast Asian food patterns, 195
Spasm, muscle, 163
Specimen collection, for neonatal screening, 390-393
Speculum, vaginal, 132

Sperm
  conception and, 65-66
  immune reaction to, 871
  infertility and, 865
Spermatogenesis, 47, 62
Spermatogonia, 47
Spermicide, 489
  diaphragm with, 494-495
Sphincter, anal, 132
Spider, vascular, 103
  in second trimester, 153
Spina bifida, 801-802
Spinal anesthesia, 231-234
  for cesarean birth, 703
Spinal cord, fetal development of, 81
Spine, of newborn, 331
Spinnbarkheit, 42
Splanchnic engorgement, 310
  heart disease and, 644
Sponge bathing of infant, 384-385
Spontaneous abortion, 572, 574-576
  diabetes and, 621
  nursing care for, 580
Spot, G-, 35
Spousal abuse, 677-683
  well-woman care and, 844
Squamous cell, fetal, 277
Squamous columnar junction, 33
Squamous epithelium, uterine, 33
Stabilization of compromised newborn, 762-765
Stages of labor; see Labor
Standard of care
  in first stage of labor, 279, 280
  prenatal, 136
Staphylococcus infection, 606
Startle reflex, 355
Stasis, urinary, 102
State-related behaviors
  assessment of, 366-369
  definition of, 335
Station, 208-209
Status, in family, 15
Stenosis, mitral valve, 648
Stepping reflex, 355
Sterilization, 499-502
Steroidal contraceptive, 492-493
Stick, heel, 390
Stillbirth, 534; see also Death
  checklist for assisting parents, 828
  definition of, 4
Stimulation
  fetal, 257
  of newborn, 759
  transcutaneous electrical nerve, labor and, 228
Stimulus, behavior and, 335-336
Stomach
  of newborn, 326
  pregnancy-related changes in, 105-106
Stomatitis, mycotic, 774-775
Stool, of newborn, 326
  breastfed, 422
  Clinitest positive, 761
  formula-fed, 428
  parent education about, 401
Storing of breast milk, 422-424
Stork bites, 329-330
Straie gravidarum, 103

Strawberry mark, 330
Streptococcal infection, 603
  rheumatic heart disease and, 647-648
Stress
  cold, 334, 370-371
    bilirubin and, 327-328
  management of, 851-853
  menopause and, 881
Stress incontinence, 888
Stress test, contraction, 550-551
Stretch marks, 103
Stroke, 649
Subarachnoid block, 231-234
Subconjunctival hemorrhage, 373
Subculture, 16-17
Subcutaneous injection, insulin, 628
Suboccipitobregmatic diameter, 208
Subpubic angle, 211
Substance abuse, 668-677
  alcohol, 669
  approaches to, 853-854
  assessment of, 673
  breastfeeding and, 425
  care plan for, 675
  cocaine, 669, 671
  complications of, 671-672
  evaluation of, 675
  expected outcomes for, 673-674
  heroin, 672
  interventions for, 674-675
  marijuana, 672
  methamphetamine, 672
  newborn care and, 806-813
    alcohol and, 808-811
    assessment in, 807
    cocaine and, 811-812
    expected outcomes for, 808
    heroin and, 812
    marijuana and, 811
    methadone and, 812
    methamphetamine and, 813
    nursing diagnosis for, 807-808
    phencyclidine and, 812
    phenobarbital and, 813
  nursing diagnosis for, 673
  phencyclidine, 672-673
  smoking and, 673
Succenturiate placenta, 585
Succinylcholine, for cesarean birth, 237
Sucking, 325-326, 419
Sucking reflex, 353
Suction curettage, for hydatidiform mole, 579
Suctioning of airway, 371-373, 752
  of meconium, 298
Supine hypotension, 131, 153, 276
  labor and, 219
Supplement, nutrient, 185
Supplementation, iron, 183
Supplies, for childbirth, 293-295
Support hose, 152
Support system
  for adolescent, 733
  after childbirth, 527
  breastfeeding and, 426
  cesarean birth and, 704
  of family, 20-21

Support system—cont'd
in grief, 825-826
during labor, 284
Suppression of uterine activity, 715-718
Surfactant
preterm infant and, 781
pulmonary, 80
Surgery
for breast cancer, 892
during pregnancy, 656-657
Surgical emergency, 799-801
Surrogate mother, 876
Surveillance, fetal; *see* Fetal heart rate
Suture, cranial, 346
Swallowing reflex, 354
Swan-Ganz catheter, 589, 590
Sweat glands, of newborn, 329
Swedish food patterns, 195
Swelling of breast, of newborn, 330
Swimming, in second trimester, 152
Symphysis pubis, separation of, 889
Symptothermal method of contraception, 487-488
Synactive theory of infant development, 784
Syncope
in pregnancy, 105
in second trimester, 153
Synthroid, 639
Syntocinon, 644
Syphilis, 595, 770-771
Systemic analgesia, 228-229
Systemic lupus erythematosus, 655

T

Taboo, 145
Tachycardia
cocaine and, 671
fetal, 247
Tachypnea, transient, 768
Taking-hold phase of maternal adjustment, 456
Taste
fetal response to, 81
newborn and, 338
Tay-Sachs disease, 64-65
Teaching, of infant care, 379
Technology, trend to, 6-7
Teenage mother, social networks for, 5
Teeth, 105
Telangiectasia
pregnancy and, 103
in second trimester, 153
Telangiectatic nevus, 329-330
Telephone follow-up in postpartum period, 521, 523-527
Temperament of newborn, 338-339
Temperature
of air, 760
anticipatory guidance about, 400
jet hydrotherapy and, 227
of newborn, 340-341, 366, 370-371
hypothermia and, 762-763
phototherapy and, 395
preterm, 777
regulation of, 332-334
small for gestational age, 787-788
ovulation and, 486-487
puerperal infection and, 603-604
Tension headache, 105
Teratogen, types of, 87

Teratoma, 805
Terbutaline, 716-717
Term, definition of, 92
Test, pregnancy, 92-93
Testis
anatomy of, 46, 47
of newborn, 330
Testosterone, infertility and, 872
Thalassemia, 650
Theory, developmental, 15-16
Therapeutic abortion, 572
grief response to, 832
Therapeutic insemination, 875
Therapeutic rest
heart disease and, 647
for hypertonic uterine dysfunction, 687
preeclampsia and, 565
Thermal environment, neutral, 762-763, 764
Thermal regulation of newborn; *see also* Temperature
preterm, 777
small for gestational age, 787-788
Thermistor probe, 370
Thermogenic system, 332-334, 370
Thermometry, tympanic, 42
Thiamin, requirement for, 181
Thiopental sodium, 237
Third stage of labor, 299-304
definition of, 216
Third trimester of pregnancy, 159-169; *see also* Pregnancy, normal, third trimester of
Threatened abortion, assessment of, 574
Thrombocytopenic purpura, 591
of newborn, 373
Thrombophlebitis, 652
femoral, 604
Thrush, 774
Thumbsucking, 401
Thyroid gland
of fetus, 82
hypothyroidism and, 639, 798
infertility and, 870
pregnancy-related changes in, 106-107
prenatal examination of, 130
Tick-borne disease, 605
Tidal volume, pregnancy and, 100
Tingling, in second trimester, 154
Tobacco use
in pregnancy, 673, 809, 810
prevention of illness and, 853
Tocotransducer, 255
Toddler, 119
Toenail, of fetus, 83
Tokodynamometer, ambulatory, 714, 715
Tonic neck reflex, 355
TORCH infection, 597-601
Touch
infant-parent, 451-452
newborn and, 338
Towel support restraint, 399-400
Toxic shock syndrome, 606, 607
Toxicity
oxygen, 591
of podophyllin, 602
Toxin, pyrogenic, 606
Toxoplasmosis, 597-598, 769-770
Tracheoesophageal anomaly, 799-800
Tranquilizer, labor and, 229-230

Transabdominal intrauterine injection of sodium chloride, 879
Transcutaneous electrical nerve stimulation, 228
Transfer from recovery area, 312
Transferase deficiency, 388
Transfusion, hemorrhage and, 590-591
Transient hypertension, 556
Transient tachypnea of newborn, 768
Transition period of labor, 225
Transition to extrauterine life
    dysfunctional, 752-753
    normal, 370, 387, 755
Transplantation, of fetal tissue, 85
Transport, placental, 76-77
Transposition of great vessels, 795
Trauma
    childbirth, 884-890
        macrosomia and, 789
        to mother, 304
        to newborn, 373, 376
        pelvic relaxation and, 884-887
    during pregnancy, 658-659
Travel, in first trimester, 139-140
Tremor
    neonatal, 331
    postpartum, 310
Treponema pallidum, 595, 770-771
Trial of labor, 697
Trichomonas vaginalis, 133, 603, 861
Trichomoniasis, infertility and, 870
Tricuspid atresia, 795
Triphasic oral contraceptive, 492
Triplets, 538
Trisomy 21, 62
Trophoblast, 68
Trophoblastic neoplasm, 578
Trunk incurvation reflex, 357, 358
Tub bathing of infant, 385
Tube
    fallopian, 28-30
        ectopic pregnancy and, 576-577
        infertility and, 870
        reconstruction of, 501, 875
        sterility and, 500-501
    neural
        defect of, 65, 795, 801-802
        development of, 81
Tubercle, Montgomery's, 98
Tuberculosis, 605-606
    adolescent and, 732
Tuberosity, ischial, 37
Tubular reabsorption, renal, 102-103
Tubule, seminiferous, 48
Tumor, ovarian, 870; *see also* Malignancy
Turner's syndrome, 63, 798
    infertility and, 865
Twin pregnancy, 83-85
    loss of one in, 832-833
Twins, breastfeeding of, 422, 423
Two-week measles, 605
Tympanic thermometry, 42

U
Ulcerative colitis, 653
Ultrasonography
    for fetal monitoring, 255
    in high-risk pregnancy, 537-543
    in infertility examination, 869

Umbilical cord
    around neck, 298
    care of, 381
    compression of, 247
    cordocentesis and, 546-547
    development of, 79
    insertion abnormalities of, 585-586
    omphalitis and, 761
    prolapsed, 282-284, 285
Undescended testes, 330
Unifactorial inheritance, 63-65
Unit, family, 13
Universal precautions, 611
Upright position, in labor, 215
Urea, for abortion, 879
Ureter, 102
Urethra
    examination of, 131
    in postpartum period, 444
    stenosis of, 794
Urethrocele, 887
Urge incontinence, 888
Urgency, urinary, 102
    in third trimester, 162
Urgency of urination, in first trimester, 139
Urinalysis
    in first stage of labor, 277
    preeclampsia and, 562
Urinary frequency, 102
    genital atrophy and, 884
    in third trimester, 162
Urinary incontinence, 133
    childbirth trauma causing, 888
    postmenopausal, 881
Urinary meatus, 27
Urinary stasis, 102
Urinary system, in postpartum period, 443-444
Urinary tract infection
    pregnancy and, 603
    prevention of, 136-137
Urine
    diabetes and, 628
    hemorrhagic shock and, 589
    of newborn, 324-325, 762
    in postpartum period, 444
    pregnancy testing and, 92-93
    protein in
        preeclampsia and, 555-556, 562
        pregnancy and, 103
    specimen collection of, 391
Uterine aspiration, 878
Uterine canal, 33
Uterine contraction; *see* Contraction, uterine
Uterine souffle, 96
Uterine tube, 28-30
Uterosacral block, 236, 237
Uterus
    anatomy of, 29, 30-34
    atony of, 586-587
    displacement of, 888-890
    fourth stage of labor and, 305, 308
    hypertonic, 687
    hypotonic, 687
    inversion of, 587-588
    involution of, 516
    in postpartum period, 440-442
    pregnancy-related changes in, 94-95

Uterus—cont'd
prolapsed, 886
retroversion of, 889, 890

V

Vaccination, 51
in first trimester, 142
for hepatitis B, 393, 770
HIV infection and, 596
Vacuum curettage, 878-879
Vacuum extraction birth, 701-702
Vagina
anatomy of, 34-35
hematoma in, 308
infertility and, 870-871
laceration of, 304
in postpartum period, 442
pregnancy-related changes in, 97-98
prenatal examination of, 131
prolapse of, 887
Vaginal bleeding
emergency interventions for, 285
in third trimester, 161
Vaginal birth; *see also* Labor
after cesarean, 165, 707, 710
heart disease and, 644
nerve blocks for, 231-236
Vaginal discharge
ferning of, 98
in third trimester, 161-162
Vaginal examination, 269, 274
Vaginal infection, 602-603
Vaginal introitus, 27
Vaginal sheath, 490
Vaginal speculum, 132
Valsalva maneuver, 219, 296
Valve prolapse, mitral, 648
Variability of fetal heart rate, normal, 247-249
Variable decelerations of fetal heart rate
causes of, 250, 254
late deceleration versus, 252-253
nonreassuring patterns of, 259, 261
Varicella, 605
Varicella zoster virus, 605
Varicocele, infertility and, 872-873
Varicosity
hemorrhoids as, 106
of lower extremity, 154, 156
in postpartum period, 445-446
vulvar, 98
Vas deferens, 46
Vascular spider, 103
in second trimester, 153
Vascular system; *see also* Cardiovascular system
of breast, 39
fetal, 79-80
of fetus, 69-73
placenta and, 77-78
transposition of great vessels and, 795
uterine, 33-34
Vasectomy, 501-502
Vasocongestion reflex, in sexual response, 49
Vasomotor instability in menopause, 880
Vasospasm, preeclampsia and, 557
VDRL test for syphilis, 595
Vegetarian diet, 196
breastfeeding and, 430

Vein, varicose, 154, 156
Velamentous insertion of umbilical cord, 585
Veneral Disease Research Laboratory test, 595
Venipuncture, 392
Venous pressure
central, hemorrhagic shock and, 589
pregnancy and, 99
Venous return, anomalous, 795
Verbal communication, assessment of, 267
Vernix caseosa, 345
Version, external cephalic, 689, 695-696
Vertex presentation, 209
birth in
emergency, 300
normal, 297-299
external cephalic version and, 696-697
Very low-birth-weight infant, 777
Vesicovaginal fistula, 890
Vestibular glands, 27-28
Vestibule, 27
Viability of fetus, 79
definition of, 92
Vietnamese food patterns, 195
Villus, chorionic, 547-548
function of, 68
Violence, 677-683
Viral infection; *see* Infection, viral
Virginity, hymen and, 27
Visceral pain, 222
Visible poverty, 680
Vision
of fetus, 81
of newborn, 336, 338
Visitors, dealing with, 515
Visual response, of newborn, 367
Vital signs
of newborn, 340-341
in postpartum period, 445
Vitamin
newborn requirements for, 409-410
for postmenopausal patient, 883
requirement for, 180
requirements for, 182-183
Vitamin B_{12}, requirement for, 181
Vitamin K
bleeding and, 82
breastfeeding and, 430
in milk, 410
for newborn, 393
Voice, parent-infant child communication and, 452
Volume, blood, of newborn, 323
Vomiting
care plan for, 147
in first trimester, 105, 139
hyperemesis gravidarum and, 636-639
by newborn, 761
nutrition and, 191
von Willebrand's disease, 591-592
Vulva
hematoma of, 308
in pregnancy, 97-98
self-examination of, 845
Vulvovaginal infection, 602-603

W

Walking reflex, 355
Wall
chest, retractions of, 757

Wall—cont'd
   uterine, 31-32
   vaginal, examination of, 131
Warfarin, heart disease and, 643
Warm line services, 524, 527
Warm water gloves, 763
Warming of newborn, 371, 763
Warning signs
   in first trimester, 138
   in second trimester, 151, 158
   in third trimester, 161-162
Water excretion, pregnancy and, 103
Water intoxication, 409
Water-soluble vitamins, requirements for, 183
Weakness, myasthenia gravis and, 655-656
Weaning, 430
Wedge pressure, pulmonary artery, 589-590
Weight
   amenorrhea and, 858
   health promotion and, 850
   of newborn, 342, 343, 408
   preeclampsia and, 566
Weight gain, 173, 175-178
   care plan for, 197
   in second trimester, 146
Well-woman health care, 839-856; *see also* Health promotion
Wharton's jelly, 79

Whirlpool bath, labor and, 226-227
White blood cells
   labor and, 219
   of newborn, 323
   in postpartum period, 445
   pregnancy and, 100
Wife beating, 677-683
Withdrawal bleeding, 42
Women's health, 839-856; *see also* Health promotion

X

X chromosome, 60, 61
X-linked inheritance, 65
XXY phenotype, 63

Y

Y chromosome, 60, 61
   sex of fetus and, 82
Yolk sac, 78-79
Yutopar, 715-716

Z

Zidovudine, for HIV infection, 596
Zinc, requirement for, 179, 184-185
Zona pellicida, 66
Zygote, 68

TEMPERATURE EQUIVALENTS

CELSIUS	FAHRENHEIT	CELSIUS	FAHRENHEIT
34.0	93.2	38.6	101.4
34.2	93.6	38.8	101.8
34.4	93.9	39.0	102.2
34.6	94.3	39.2	102.5
34.8	94.6	39.4	102.9
35.0	95.0	39.6	103.2
35.2	95.4	39.8	103.6
35.4	95.7	40.0	104.0
35.6	96.1	40.2	104.3
35.8	96.4	40.4	104.7
36.0	96.8	40.6	105.1
36.2	97.1	40.8	105.4
36.4	97.5	41.0	105.8
36.6	97.8	41.2	106.1
36.8	98.2	41.4	106.5
37.0	98.6	41.6	106.8
37.2	98.9	41.8	107.2
37.4	99.3	42.0	107.6
37.6	99.6	42.2	108.0
37.8	100.0	42.4	108.3
38.0	100.4	42.6	108.7
38.2	100.7	42.8	109.0
38.4	101.1	43.0	109.4

To convert Fahrenheit to Celsius:
(Temperature minus 32) $\times$ 5/9
Example: To convert 98.6 degrees
Fahrenheit to Celsius:
98.6 − 32 = 66.6 $\times$ 5/9
= 37 degrees

To convert Celsius to Fahrenheit:
5/9 $\times$ temperature + 32
Example: To convert 40 degrees
Celsius to Fahrenheit:
5/9 $\times$ 40 = 72 + 32
= 104 degrees

CONVERSION OF POUNDS AND OUNCES TO GRAMS FOR NEWBORN WEIGHTS*

POUNDS	OUNCES																POUNDS
	0	1	2	3	4	5	6	7	8	9	10	11	12	13	14	15	
0	—	28	57	85	113	142	170	198	227	255	283	312	430	369	397	425	0
1	454	482	510	539	567	595	624	652	680	709	737	765	794	822	850	879	1
2	907	936	964	992	1021	1049	1077	1106	1134	1162	1191	1219	1247	1276	1304	1332	2
3	1361	1389	1417	1446	1474	1503	1531	1559	1588	1616	1644	1673	1701	1729	1758	1786	3
4	1814	1843	1871	1899	1928	1956	1984	2013	2041	2070	2093	2126	2155	2183	2211	2240	4
5	2268	2296	2325	2353	2381	2410	2438	2466	2495	2523	2551	2580	2608	2637	2665	2693	5
6	2722	2750	2778	2807	2835	2863	2892	2920	2948	2977	3005	3033	3062	3090	3118	3147	6
7	3175	3203	3232	3260	3289	3317	3345	3374	3402	3430	3459	3487	3515	3544	3572	3600	7
8	3629	3657	3685	3714	3742	3770	3799	3827	3856	3884	3912	3941	3969	3997	4026	4054	8
9	4082	4111	4139	4167	4196	4224	4252	4281	4309	4337	4366	4394	4423	4451	4479	4508	9
10	4536	4564	4593	4621	4649	4678	4706	4734	4763	4791	4819	4848	4876	4904	4933	4961	10
11	4990	5018	5046	5075	5103	5131	5160	5188	5216	5245	5273	5301	5330	5358	5386	5415	11
12	5443	5471	5500	5528	5557	5585	5613	5642	5670	5698	5727	5755	5783	5812	5840	5868	12
13	5897	5925	5953	5982	6010	6038	6067	6095	6123	6152	6180	6209	6237	6265	6294	6322	13
14	6350	6379	6407	6435	6464	6492	6520	6549	6577	6605	6634	6662	6690	6719	6747	6776	14
15	6804	6832	6860	6889	6917	6945	6973	7002	7030	7059	7087	7115	7144	7172	7201	7228	15
	0	1	2	3	4	5	6	7	8	9	10	11	12	13	14	15	
	OUNCES																

*To convert pounds and ounces to grams, multiply the pounds by 453.6 and the ounces by 28.35; add the totals.
To convert grams into pounds and decimals of a pound, multiply the grams by 0.0022.
To convert grams into ounces, divide the grams by 28.35 (16 oz = 1 lb).